BASIC MEDICAL MICROBIOLOGY

BASIC MEDICAL MICROBIOLOGY

FOURTH EDITION

Robert F. Boyd, Ph.D.
Wirtz, Virginia

Bryan G. Hoerl, Ph.D.
Associate Professor of Microbiology
Marquette University School of Dentistry
Milwaukee, Wisconsin

Little, Brown and Company
Boston/Toronto/London

1-800- 343-9204

To TJ, who taught me the meaning of friendship

R.F.B.

To my wife Pat, and to my children Bryan, Janet,
Michael, and Daniel, and their spouses

B.G.H.

CONTENTS

PREFACE

When we wrote the first edition of *Basic Medical Microbiology*, one of our primary aims was to present a concise and uncluttered view of medical microbiology. In this fourth edition, we have kept in mind these original aims but have made several changes, which we hope will make the text even more useful to students. These changes include the following:

1. We have added many more tables. These not only compare infectious agents but list specific laboratory features and other microbial characteristics.

2. Questions for study at the end of the chapters consist of multiple choice, matching, and/or completion. More than one answer may be appropriate for some questions.

3. Appendices are included. Appendix A provides tables of infectious agents based on the site of infection. Each table includes mode of transmission and method of treatment and/or prevention. In addition, the page number where the infectious disease or agent is discussed is also included. The tables should be helpful for reviewing the text material. Appendix B includes tables of the microbial agents that make up the flora of various body sites and the diseases with which they are associated.

4. The index for the fourth edition was prepared by R.F.B. Specific discussions and terminology that were not included in the third edition are now available for easy location by the student.

In addition, we have made changes in several sections of the book.

Section V, Bacteria That Cause Infectious Disease, is more concise and includes more tables. Diagnostic laboratory techniques have been updated to include more recent diagnostic methods. These chapters also contain updated material on mechanisms of pathogenesis. In addition, we have included discussions of more recently recognized pathogens such as *Helicobacter pylori*, *Ehrlichia* species, and *Chlamydia pneumoniae*.

In Section VI, Virology, Chapter 30, Viruses, was rewritten and condensed, with a discussion of animal viruses appearing first. In addition, there is a section called Diagnostic Virology that discusses the rapid methods now employed in the field. A brief discussion of the rationale for treatment and prevention of viral infections is also discussed. The last section of this chapter is devoted to bacterial viruses. Chapter 31, Viral Diseases, has also undergone revision. The discussion of smallpox has been shortened significantly since this disease has been declared eradicated. Included is a more encompassing discussion of enteroviral diseases. New headings include Hemorrhagic Fever Viruses; The Arboviruses, which now includes a discussion of dengue fever and dengue hemorrhagic fever; and Rotaviruses and Other Agents of Gastrointestinal Disease, which includes a discussion of caliciviruses and astroviruses. Perhaps the most significant change in the chapter is the inclusion of AIDS. Discussion of AIDS appeared originally in the chapter on immunological disorders in the third edition.

Section VII, Medical Mycology, is largely un-changed. However, we have added the pathogen *Pneumocystis carinii* to this section since RNA analysis suggests that it is a fungus and not a protozoan.

In Section VIII, Medical Parasitology, we have added comprehensive tables of all the major animal parasites. This inclusion should be of great help to students.

We would like to thank the reviewers of the third and fourth editions for their invaluable comments. A special thanks goes to the scientists and book and journal publishers who provided photomicrographs and allowed us to use various tables. We would like to thank Ruth Steinberger for the line drawings. We would also like to thank Jon Sarner, without whose efforts this book would have never been published.

R.F.B.
B.G.H.

I. GENERAL BACTERIOLOGY

1. SCOPE AND HISTORY OF MICROBIOLOGY

OBJECTIVES

To understand the importance of microbiology to medicine as well as to applied areas of science

To describe the contributions of the following scientists to microbiology: Leeuwenhoek, Pasteur, Koch, Lister, Jenner, and Ehrlich

To explain what is meant by the theory of spontaneous generation and the experiments that were performed to refute it

To list the steps that are required to identify the causative agent of an infectious disease

SCOPE

Microbiology is a science that is primarily concerned with the study of microorganisms and viruses. A distinction between microorganisms and viruses is made because viruses do not exhibit cellular characteristics. Viruses are entities that are totally dependent on the presence of a living cell for replication. Microorganisms are for the most part single-celled, but they also include certain multicellular types. When we speak of microorganisms, we must include bacteria, fungi (molds and yeasts), certain algae, and protozoa. Protozoa belong to the group called *animal parasites*, which also includes certain multicellular worms called *helminths*. Algae are not associated with disease in humans and will not be discussed in this text.

The explosion of microbiological information in recent years has been so great that it has resulted in the creation of specialties concerned with each of the representative groups of microorganisms being studied. For example, the bacteriologist may develop skills in various aspects of bacteriology such as bacterial physiology, bacterial genetics, or bacterial cytology. The microbiologist may specialize in the study of microorganisms as they relate to applied and environmental fields. There are now divisions of microbiology such as space microbiology, soil microbiology, aquatic microbiology, food microbiology, and industrial microbiology.

Medical microbiology, which deals primarily with microorganisms that cause infectious disease, is the branch of microbiology with which the student reading this book is primarily concerned. Since various representative types of microorganisms can cause disease in humans, the medical microbiologist must have a basic knowledge of the chemical and physical properties of the potentially harmful microbial agents—bacteria, viruses, yeasts, molds, and protozoa. The primary responsibility of the medical microbiologist is to understand the etiology (causation), disease manifestations, laboratory diagnosis, and treatment of infectious disease. The microbiologist's obligations may also include determining the epidemiology of disease (e.g., how diseases are transmitted) and developing measures for the control and prevention of diseases in the community. The fact that many major pestilences such as smallpox, diphtheria, and plague no longer decimate populations as they once did is testimony to the advances made in epidemiology, control, and prevention of infectious disease. Resistance or immunity to disease has been recognized for years. This area of study is referred to as *immunology* and deals specifically with the relationship of antigens or foreign substances to antibody production in the host. Because of its relationship to disease, immunology is also considered an important part of the medical microbiologist's background. The development of new concepts in molecular biology and cellular immunity has not only expanded our knowledge of the immune process but has also provided the microbiologist with new laboratory diagnostic tools. The medical microbiologist can now identify and classify microorganisms using immunological techniques.

In its early history, microbiology as a science was concerned with the identification and control of microorganisms. Major advances in microscopy and biochemical techniques from 1940 to the present have enabled scientists to use microorganisms as a model for the study of biological properties, particularly in the areas of genetics and metabolism. These studies are aided by the fact that microorganisms divide very rapidly and are easily cultivated and maintained in the laboratory—properties not common to higher forms of life.

During the development of microbiology, it was soon realized that many of the metabolic processes occurring in microbial systems were similar if not identical to those of cells in higher systems, including the human. In 1944 Avery, MacLeod, and McCarty discovered that isolated (cell-free) DNA was capable of transforming (producing a genetic change in) certain intact bacterial cells. This was one of several experiments proving that DNA was the hereditary material of the cell. The discovery of the structure of DNA by Watson and Crick in 1953 and the results obtained from experiments in microbial genetics provided the basic clues to genetic mechanisms not only in bacteria but in higher forms of life as well. Scientists are now able to manipulate genes and to transfer genes from one species of organisms into the DNA of totally unrelated microbial species. Such techniques referred to as *genetic engineering* are revolutionizing microbiology and related sciences. This technique, along with our greater understanding of molecular biology and biochemistry, is advancing us near the brink of conquering, or at the very least tempering, many of the major diseases, both infectious and noninfectious, that now afflict humankind. In addition, many biological properties unavailable to some organisms, such as plants' ability to fix nitrogen from the air or the capacity to produce large quantities of a single protein to be used as food, may become realities in the very near future. The future for microbiology, both medical and nonmedical, is so bright and promising that we can hardly wait for each day's new discoveries to be revealed. We hope that the importance of these discoveries will be imparted to you as you read each chapter. But keep in mind that you can fully appreciate these discoveries only if you understand the basic biological properties of microorganisms.

HISTORY

EARLY CONCEPTS OF DISEASE

Microbiology had its origins in the concepts that were first formulated to explain disease. In some ancient civilizations disease was believed to be a punishment sent from the gods for human wrong-doings. Many of the philosophers during these early periods in history, however, were of the belief that disease was transmitted by invisible "animals." Since the animals could not be seen, the theory remained just that, a theory. The Italian physician Fracastorius (1485–1553) later postulated that disease was transmitted by invisible particles or seeds from one person to another or from contact with the clothing or utensils of the infected. Two hundred years elapsed before a detailed description of microorganisms was made.

FIRST OBSERVATIONS OF MICROORGANISMS

Anton van Leeuwenhoek (c. 1685), who took up microbiology as a hobby, was an amateur microscope builder. Using a very primitive microscope, he described in some detail the structure of the red blood cells of humans and other animals. Leeuwenhoek was the first to describe microscopic organisms found in pond water and later made observations of bacteria he found in the debris surrounding teeth (Fig. 1-1). Leeu-

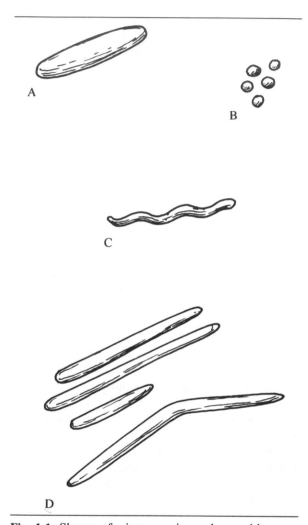

Fig. 1-1. Shapes of microorganisms observed by Leeuwenhoek in samples taken from the human mouth. A. Rod-shaped (bacillus). B. Spherical (cocci). C. Spiral-shaped (spirochete). D. Cigar-shaped rods.

wenhoek's microscope was a little over 2 inches in length and capable of magnifications approaching 160 to 200 times (Fig. 1-2).

SPONTANEOUS GENERATION

Even though his was the first description of microorganisms, most of Leeuwenhoek's peers

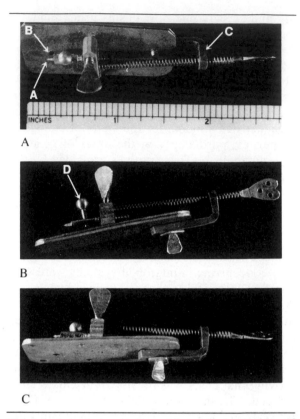

Fig. 1-2. Actual-size replica of Leeuwenhoek microscope from Leyden, Holland, showing various views of instrument. *A*, pin on which object is placed for viewing; *B*, lens; *C*, screw for coarse adjustment; *D*, screw for fine adjustment. (From D. A. Anderson and R. J. Sobieski, *Introduction to Microbiology* [2nd ed.]. St. Louis: Mosby, 1980.)

either ignored or denied the existence of these newly discovered organisms. Instead, most scientists accepted the theory of *spontaneous generation*, that is, that life can arise from dead organic matter—a theory first proposed by Aristotle in 384 B.C. For example, the scientific community was convinced that blowflies could arise spontaneously from rotted meat. Scientists such as Francisco Redi (1668) and Spallanzani (1776) performed experiments that showed that organic matter, if protected from contamination by boiling and preventing exposure to the air, did not give rise to new life. The spontaneous generation proponents refuted these experiments by suggesting that a *vital force,* such as air, had been destroyed by boiling.

Franz Schulze and Theodore Schwann in 1836 independently demonstrated that air was not the vital force. Schulze passed heated air into flasks of nutrient broth and showed that heating sterilized the air and prevented growth in the flasks. Schwann passed air through chemical solutions before it entered the flasks containing nutrient media and obtained the same results. The proponents of spontaneous generation were unswayed by these experiments. They countered that the treated air had been stripped of any life-generating forces. Despite these and other experiments that disproved spontaneous generation, the proponents of this theory were still unconvinced.

Only the experiments of Pasteur (Fig. 1-3) would finally put an end to the theory of spontaneous generation. Using swan-necked flasks

Fig. 1-3. Louis Pasteur (1822–1895). (From *Microbiology*, Fourth Edition by Philip L. Carpenter. Copyright © 1977 by W. B. Saunders Company. Reprinted by permission of CBS College Publishing.)

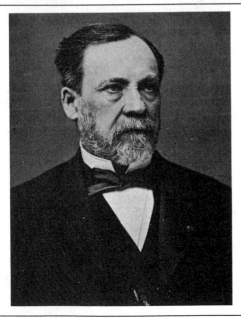

Table 1-1. Contributions of Louis Pasteur to Microbiology and Related Sciences

Development of attenuated vaccines for anthrax and chicken cholera

Immunization against rabies

Relationship of crystal structure to optical rotation

Study of diseases of swine and silkworms

Discovery of technique for selective destruction of microorganisms by heat (pasteurization)

Refutation of theory of spontaneous generation

Discovery of microorganisms that live in the absence of air (anaerobes)

Contributions to understanding the causes of fermentation

(Fig. 1-4), Pasteur boiled organic solutions to destroy any ''seeds'' (microorganisms) that might be present. There was no barrier to the passage of air in these flasks, and they could sit for several days with no visible turbidity, which would indicate the presence of life (seeds or microorganisms). In other words, air outside the flask could diffuse into the organic broth, but any microorganism carried in the air could go no farther than the walls of the flask's neck, where it would settle out. If the liquid in the flask was allowed to come in contact with the organisms in the neck, by tilting the flask and then returning the contaminated fluid by tilting the flask back again, the broth became turbid after 24 hours. Pasteur made many other important contributions to microbiology and related sciences (Table 1-1) and for this reason has been called the Father of Microbiology.

GERM THEORY OF DISEASE

The theoretical explanations of infectious disease as proposed by Fracastorius in 1546 were not supported by experimental proof until 200 years later. Physicians such as Semmelweis in Austria and Oliver Wendell Holmes in the United States implored their physician colleagues to wash their hands before examining pregnant women. Both of these physicians had demonstrated that the

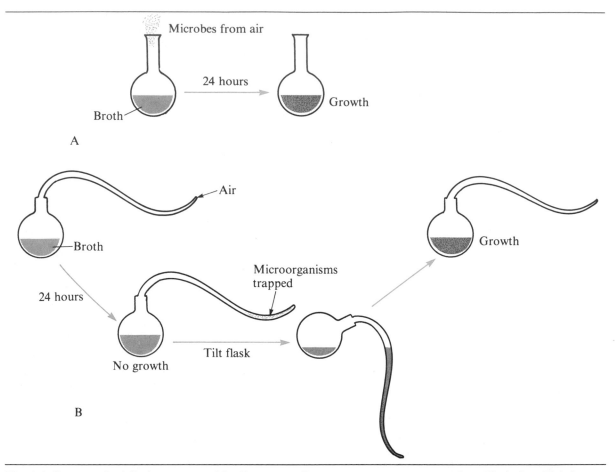

Fig. 1-4. Swan-necked flasks were used by Pasteur to disprove spontaneous generation. Flask A, which is not swan-necked, contains sterile broth that is directly exposed to the air and becomes turbid after 16 to 24 hours. Microorganisms in the air settle into the broth, where they reproduce and make the broth turbid. Flask B, which is swan-necked, also contains sterile broth. Because of its shape air, but not microorganisms, may enter the space above the broth. Microorganisms that are present in the air settle out by gravity in the curved neck of the flask. The broth in the swan-necked flask shows no turbidity even several days after exposure to air unless the flask is tilted and the broth makes contact with microorganisms.

agent of puerperal (childbed) fever was transmitted from an infected patient to an uninfected one by physicians who did not wash their hands. Their pleas were ignored by the majority of physicians who refused to believe they were unclean.

In 1857 Louis Pasteur formulated the theory of fermentation by microorganisms by demonstrating how microorganisms can convert sugar to lactic acid. From these experiments Pasteur theo-

rized that microorganisms could cause disease through similar chemical processes. In England at this time Joseph Lister, a surgeon, recognized the importance of Pasteur's experiments and proposed that infections of open wounds were due to microbes found in the air around the patient. It soon became Lister's policy to spray the air around the patient with phenol before surgical operations. The procedure of destroying or removing viable microorganisms from an environment is called *aseptic technique.* Although Lister's procedures dramatically decreased fatalities from surgical wound infections, his results were not totally accepted in the scientific community.

In the late 1800s a German physician named Robert Koch (Fig. 1-5) demonstrated the relationship between microorganisms and infectious disease. Koch studied anthrax, a disease of cattle that can secondarily affect humans. He isolated the organisms from infected cattle in *pure culture* (the cultivation of a single species of microorganism) and then injected an aliquot of the pure culture into healthy animals, which subsequently became infected. The infectious agent was later isolated from these infected animals. This sequence of isolation, reinfection, and recovery of the infective agent is called *Koch's postulates.* By following Koch's postulates it was now possible to establish the causative agent of many infectious diseases. Although numerous scientists at that time were busily engaged in isolating and characterizing microorganisms, men like Koch and Pasteur were also interested in developing techniques that would be effective in destroying bacteria and thus reduce human misery.

THE GOLDEN AGE OF MICROBIOLOGY (1870–1890)

Isolation Techniques

It was in the Koch-Pasteur era (1870–1890) that tremendous strides were made in microbiology. It was during this era, called the *Golden Age of Microbiology,* that the microbial agents responsible for so many of the fatal diseases of that time were isolated (Table 1-2). As you can see from Table 1-2, all of these diseases are caused by bacterial agents. During this period viruses had not been discovered and little was known about fungi or animal parasites as infectious agents. Perhaps one of the most important technical advances during this period was the discovery that *agar-agar* could be used with microbiological media for isolating microorganisms in pure culture. Agar-agar is a carbohydrate isolated from seaweed that is stable to heat, enzyme-stable, solid, transparent, and easily sterilized. Frau Hesse, the wife of a physician interested in the bacteriology of air, had been using agar-agar in her kitchen to prepare fruits and jellies. She suggested that agar-agar might be used in culture media. Dr. Hesse mentioned his wife's suggestion to Robert Koch, who adapted the new medium in his laboratory. The use of agar-agar in media made possible the isolation of single colonies on a solid medium, a technique that could not be accomplished with liquid media. This discovery, coupled with the design of the *Petri dish* (Fig. 1-6) in 1887 by J. R. Petri as a container for media, provided bacteriologists with a new tool for isolating bacteria in pure culture. Soon other microbiologists, using Koch's postulates and aided by these new isolation techniques, would

Fig. 1-5. Robert Koch (1843–1910). (From K. L. Burdon and R. P. Williams, *Microbiology* [6th ed.]. New York: Macmillan, 1968. Copyright © 1968 by Macmillan Publishing Company.)

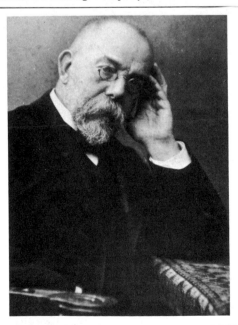

Table 1-2. Disease-producing Bacteria Discovered During the Golden Age of Microbiology (1870–1890)

Year	Disease	Causative agent	Researcher(s)
1872	Anthrax	*Bacillus anthracis*	Rayer and Devaine, Pasteur and Koch
1873	Relapsing fever	*Borrelia recurrentis*	Obermeier
1874	Leprosy	*Mycobacterium leprae*	Hansen
1879	Gonorrhea	*Neisseria gonorrhoeae*	Neisser
1880	Pneumonia	*Diplococcus pneumoniae*	Pasteur, Sternberg
1880	Abscesses	*Staphylococcus aureus*	Pasteur, Ogston, Rosenbach
1882	Tuberculosis	*Mycobacterium tuberculosis*	Koch
1883	Cholera	*Vibrio cholerae*	Koch
1884	Diphtheria	*Corynebacterium diphtheriae*	Klebs, Loeffler
1884	Tetanus	*Clostridium tetani*	Nicolaier, Kitasato
1885	Food-borne illness, paratyphoid	*Salmonella choleraesuis* and related species	Salmon and Smith, Gärtner, Schottmüller
1887	Epidemic meningitis	*Neisseria meningitidis*	Weichselbaum
1887	Brucellosis	*Brucella melitensis* and other species	Bruce, Bang

make major contributions to an understanding of the microbial agents causing disease.

Staining

Visualization of microorganisms was enhanced by the discovery of various staining agents. Weigert in 1878 was the first to stain bacteria using various aniline dyes. Further refinement in staining led to Gram's stain (1884), which can be used for most bacterial species, and the Ziehl-Neelsen stain, which is used for staining the organism causing tuberculosis. Loeffler utilized methylene blue stain to identify the organism causing diphtheria.

Immunology

It had been recognized for more than 2000 years that individuals who recovered from some diseases could not "catch" the disease a second time. In 1796 Edward Jenner discovered that milkmaids infected with the mild variety of pox called *cowpox* were immune to the more severe form of the disease, *smallpox*. Jenner inoculated fluid from a cowpox pustule into a healthy boy and later infected the same boy with smallpox fluid. The boy did not contract smallpox.

In 1879 Pasteur, while studying cholera in chickens, noted that if chicken cholera bacteria were left on laboratory media for extended periods of time, they lost their virulence (they became *attenuated*). The attenuated bacteria, when injected into healthy chickens, not only failed to cause cholera but protected them from infection by fresh virulent strains. These experiments eventually led to our present-day vaccination techniques and methods of immunization. Pasteur later developed immunization procedures in the treatment of anthrax in animals and rabies in humans. Today all of us are aware of vaccination procedures used against such diseases as tetanus, diphtheria, polio, and whooping cough.

Elie Metchnikoff, working in Pasteur's laboratory, observed that certain white blood cells could ingest microorganisms or other small foreign matter. Metchnikoff firmly believed that immunity to infection was totally dependent on the special white blood cells (phagocytic cells) that digested other cells. Paul Ehrlich, an associate of Robert Koch, was also interested in resistance to infection. He believed that immunity to infection was due to certain soluble substances in the

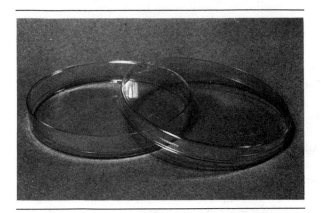

Fig. 1-6. Petri dish. The bottom portion of the dish (*left*) can be partially filled with a solid medium. The covering plate fits over the bottom portion. Petri dishes can be obtained presterilized and filled with sterilized media, or they may be unsterilized and filled with unsterilized media and then sterilized by autoclaving (steam under pressure).

blood called *antibodies*. Both mechanisms have since been shown to be important in immunity and are referred to as the *cellular* and *humoral* mechanisms of defense, respectively.

VIROLOGY

Viral diseases such as smallpox, rabies, polio, and others had been known for centuries. The nature of the infectious agent involved, however, did not become apparent until the late 1890s. Iwanowsky took the fluids pressed from tobacco plants afflicted with tobacco mosaic disease and filtered them through porcelain filters to remove bacteria. The fluid still caused disease in new plants, and thus the infectious agent was recognized as a filterable material that did not contain bacteria. Loeffler and Frosch (1898) were the first to demonstrate a filterable agent as the cause of an animal disease called *foot-and-mouth disease*. They concluded that the filterable agent was an organism smaller than a bacterium and capable of replication. Twort (1915) discovered bacterial viruses from the observation of bacte-

rial colonies growing on agar. Some of the colonies exhibited a glassy appearance. The material from the glassy colonies could be transferred to normal colonies and also cause the glassy appearance. d'Herelle in 1922 named the infectious material in these glassy colonies *bacteriophages* (bacteria eaters). d'Herelle also demonstrated that bacteriophages were capable of replication in their bacterial hosts.

Virology has seen many advances in the past 30 years, and most of the viral agents associated with infectious disease have been isolated and identified. In addition many vaccines have been successfully developed to prevent disease in mammalian hosts. Our current understanding of the molecular biology and genetics of viruses has led to important discoveries in mammalian genetics and the malignant processes caused by certain viruses.

CHEMOTHERAPY

In the late 1800s Paul Ehrlich, the German chemist, noted that dyes were selectively absorbed in some cell types and not in others. His observations led him to believe that certain chemicals taken into the body could selectively destroy bacteria and not affect normal body cells, a process he called "chemotherapy." Ehrlich began a systematic search for a chemical that could be used against the microorganism that caused syphilis. An arsenical compound, which Ehrlich called *606*, was found to be effective in the treatment of syphilis. (See Boxed Essay.) Until the discovery of penicillin, 606 (salvarsan) remained the major chemotherapeutic agent in the treatment of syphilis. Following Ehrlich's success many scientists began to test thousands of chemicals for antibacterial activity. In 1932, after years of research, Gerhard Domagk, a German chemist, prepared and tested a large number of dyes and discovered that the red dye Prontosil was highly effective in the treatment of numerous bacterial diseases. It was later discovered that in the body Prontosil is converted to a colorless derivative,

DR. EHRLICH'S "MAGIC BULLETS"

One of the most important contributions to the healing art of medicine was made by Paul Ehrlich, the father of modern chemotherapy. Ehrlich was born in Silesia, Germany, in 1854. He was primarily a chemist and his earliest work was in the field of histology and specifically in the staining of tissues. He proposed that certain dyes stain specific areas of the cell because of the chemical affinity between molecules in the tissue and molecules in the dye. He suggested that by changing the constitution of the chemical compound you could also change its effects.

Ehrlich proposed a theory that would be the guiding light in his later quest for chemotherapeutic agents. He stated that if a dye can stain just one type of tissue there must be one that does not stain tissue but only stains and kills the microorganism attacking the tissue. Ehrlich called these compounds, with affinity for microbes but not for tissue, "*magic bullets.*"

One of the compounds used by Ehrlich was called atoxyl, an organic molecule containing arsenic. Atoxyl had been used to treat human sleeping sickness, based on results with laboratory mice. The drug was so toxic to humans that it caused blindness before the patient had time to die of the disease. Chemists of the day said that atoxyl could not be chemically altered to decrease its toxicity and should not be used to treat human infections. Ehrlich, however, believed that atoxyl could be changed. For two years Ehrlich and his colleagues developed different derivatives of atoxyl. After six hundred and six trials a derivative was found that killed only parasites and did not adversely affect laboratory mice. Later, the drug, now called *606* or *salvarsan,* was used to treat syphilis, and the results were miraculous. Yet, despite saving thousands of lives, salvarsan adversely affected some patients. Ehrlich could not foresee that "magic bullets" can be two-edged swords.

called *sulfanilamide*, which was the active antibacterial component.

It had been known for several years before the turn of the century that certain bacteria and molds were capable of producing substances that killed or inhibited the growth of various types of microorganisms. In 1928 Sir Alexander Fleming discovered that a particular culture of *Staphylococcus* on an agar plate had become contaminated with mold from the air. Some of the bacterial colonies around one mold had stopped growing. The mold, later found to be *Penicillium notatum*, produced an antibacterial substance that Fleming called *penicillin*. In 1940 Chain and other scientists in Florey's laboratory in Oxford purified penicillin from culture fluids and demonstrated its potency. In 1942 penicillin was ready for injection into human subjects.

Selman Waksman, a Russian immigrant to the United States, during his undergraduate studies was interested in the types of microorganisms found in the soil. His work with a group of soil fungi called *actinomycetes* led to the discovery of the antibiotic actinomycin in 1940 and streptomycin in 1943. Streptomycin was soon shown to destroy bacteria not affected by penicillin, especially the tuberculosis bacillus. The experimentation and discoveries of Fleming and Waksman prompted a more extensive search for other antibiotics. After World War II a wider range of antibiotics, including tetracycline, chloramphenicol, and erythromycin, was discovered.

MODERN MICROBIOLOGY

Microbiology is now in the forefront of biological science. Many of the discoveries in microbiology have led to important discoveries in higher organisms and renewed interest and research in their biology. Much of this new interest has resulted from the development of gene-splicing techniques and the ability to produce large

amounts of specific antibody (monoclonal antibodies). Gene splicing (recombinant DNA or genetic engineering) is based on the ability of scientists to use DNA or genes from different sources and insert them into microbial DNA. The inserted DNA can then be expressed in the microbial cell. Gene splicing has already been used to produce various mammalian products in bacterial cells. Insulin, mammalian growth hormone, and interferon are just some of the mammalian proteins produced by bacterial cells. "Superbugs," or microorganisms containing foreign genes that code for highly degradative enzymes, have also been developed. They are being used to break down products such as petroleum compounds, herbicides, and pesticides that are environmental pollutants and are resistant to microbial attack in soil or water.

Monoclonal antibodies have enabled scientists to pinpoint specific components that are part of the structure of all cells. For example, monoclonal antibodies can be used to find the viral or microbial component that is responsible for the infectious disease process. This property will aid in the identification of microorganisms and will probably help us to develop better vaccines for the prevention of infectious diseases.

Despite our ability to isolate, identify, and control most of the microorganisms that cause disease in humans, we are still being confronted with new infectious agents. Diseases such as Legionnaires' disease, Lyme disease, and acquired immune deficiency syndrome (AIDS) make us realize that nature has found new ways to plague humankind. In addition, many of the drugs used to treat "old" infectious diseases are no longer effective, thus challenging the medical community to develop new solutions to old problems. Infectious disease is still a major problem in developing countries and a nagging problem in developed countries such as the United States, especially in the hospital community. The solution to these problems will require the combined efforts of both medical and allied health personnel.

SUMMARY

1. Microbiology is a science that involves the study of microorganisms such as bacteria, fungi, algae, and protozoa as well as noncellular viruses. Medical microbiology is but one branch of a field that also includes such divisions as environmental, industrial, and food microbiology. Immunology is also considered a major component of medical microbiology, even though it is a separate branch of biology.

2. Disease for many centuries was believed to be a divine punishment, but in the sixteenth century Fracastorius theorized that invisible seeds were transmitted from human to human to cause disease. Leeuwenhoek in the seventeenth century was the first to observe microorganisms, but up until the late nineteenth century many believed that microorganisms arose spontaneously from organic matter.

3. Many scientists, including Redi, Spallanzani, Schulze, and Schwann, designed experiments to disprove spontaneous generation but it was Pasteur in the late 1800s who finally laid the theory to rest. He demonstrated that microorganisms are carried in the air and can contaminate objects and solutions. Pasteur was responsible for many important discoveries in microbiology and he is considered the Father of Microbiology.

4. Robert Koch was one of the first to show the relationship of microorganisms to infectious disease. To show this relationship was valid, he demonstrated the pure culture technique and formulated what are now known as Koch's postulates. In the period between 1870 and 1890, the Golden Age of Microbiology, the bacterial agents causing many different infectious diseases were isolated and identified. These isolations and identifications were greatly enhanced by other developments including techniques for staining bacteria and the discovery of agar-agar, a component that provided a semi-solid medium in which a single species of bacteria could be isolated.

5. Edward Jenner in 1796 recognized the importance of immunity in resistance to infection, but it was Pasteur who first developed immunization practices in the form of vaccines. In the late 1800s Metchnikoff and Ehrlich postulated that immunity in humans relies on cellular and humoral mechanisms.

6. The nature of viruses was first recognized by Iwanowsky, who showed that they were filterable agents, that is, that they were smaller than bacteria. The relationship of the virus to animal disease was demonstrated in 1898 by Loeffler and Frosch, who showed that foot-and-mouth disease was caused by a filterable agent. Later, in 1915, Twort demonstrated that even bacteria can be infected by viruses.

7. The use of natural compounds to cure disease has been known for centuries, but it was Ehrlich who proposed that drugs can selectively destroy infectious microorganisms without causing undue harm to the tissue of the host. Domagk in 1932 synthesized dyes that were shown to be effective against certain infectious agents. Fleming in 1928 was the first to recognize that microorganisms can produce and release chemicals (antibiotics) that inhibit the activity of other microorganisms. From this discovery penicillin was isolated and purified by Florey, Chain, et al. in 1940.

8. Medical microbiology in the modern era still relies on the basic practices of isolation, identification, and treatment of infectious agents. These practices have been aided by the development of monoclonal antibodies and the new field of genetic engineering. The discovery of new diseases, such as acquired immune deficiency syndrome, and efforts to prevent new and old diseases offer many challenges to the medical community.

QUESTIONS FOR STUDY

Fill in the blank:

1. The "vital force" referred to by the proponents of spontaneous generation was _____.

2. The scientist who first used the term "chemotherapy" was _____.

3. The cultivation of a single species of microorganism in the laboratory is called _____.

4. Antibodies that have an affinity for one specific component are referred to as _____.

5. The process in which microorganisms can be altered in such a way as to lose their virulence but not their potential for immunization is called _____.

Select the best response or responses for each of the following:

6. What was (were) the major reason(s) that nearly all the infectious agents isolated before 1900 were bacteria and not viruses?
   A. Viruses had not evolved as infectious agents until after 1900.
   B. Only bacteria produced visible lesions from which the microbial agent could be isolated.
   C. Viruses pass through filters.
   D. Methods for culturing viruses were not yet available.

7. The reason that Pasteur used swan-necked flasks to disprove spontaneous generation was that
   A. Even if he tilted the medium into the neck of the flask, there would be no microbe contamination.
   B. Media could be easily introduced into the flask.
   C. If microbially contaminated air entered the flask, microorganisms would contaminate the neck of the flask and not the medium in the flask.
   D. He believed that bacterial spores were the only microbial agents in air and that they were too large to enter through the neck of the flask.

8. Which of the following discoveries or developments do you feel contributed most to the isolation of bacteria?
   A. Formulation of Koch's postulates
   B. Ehrlich's development of bacterial stains
   C. Frau Hesse's suggestion about a carbohydrate isolated from seaweed
   D. Development of filters that retained bacteria

9. Phenol was used by Joseph Lister in surgery to prove which of the following:
   A. That viruses could be killed by chemicals
   B. That many wound infections were caused by microorganisms present in the air
   C. That human blood contained microorganisms that contaminate the wound
   D. That microorganisms on the human skin are primarily anaerobes (that is, they live in the absence of air)

10. Which of the following types of microbial agents are most frequently associated with production of antibiotics?
   A. Soil microorganisms
   B. Microorganisms found on the surface of the body
   C. Soil viruses
   D. Aquatic fungi

ADDITIONAL READINGS

Bibel, D. J. William Bullock's pioneer women of microbiology. *ASM News* 51(7):328,1985.

Brock, T. D. (ed.). *Pasteur and Modern Science. Rene Dubos. New Illustrated Edition,* Madison, WI: Science Tech Publishers, 1988.

Brock, T. D. *Milestones in Microbiology.* Washington, DC: American Society for Microbiology, 1975.

Dixon, C. (ed.). *Magnificent Microbes.* New York: Atheneum, 1976.

Gest, H. *The World of Microbes.* Menlo Park, CA: Benjamin/Cummings, 1987.

Groschel, D. H. M. The etiology of tuberculosis: A tribute to Robert Koch on the occasion of the centenary of his discovery of the tubercle bacillus. *ASM News* 48(6):248,1982.

2. OBSERVATION OF MICROORGANISMS: MICROSCOPY AND STAINING

OBJECTIVES

To list the advantages and disadvantages of the following microscopes: compound bright-field, dark-field, phase-contrast, fluorescent, transmission electron, and scanning electron microscopes

To describe what is meant by resolving power and the factors affecting it

To describe the three ways in which biological material is prepared for electron microscopy

To differentiate between a simple and a differential stain

To describe the steps in the Gram stain and the significance of what is meant by gram-positive and gram-negative

To define: acid-fast stain, hanging drop technique, immunofluorescence, fluorochrome, immersion oil, refractive index

Probably one of the more exciting aspects of microbiology for the beginning student is the realization that individual microorganisms, as small as they are, have shape and are composed of structures that can be identified. Visualization of microorganisms is impossible with the naked eye because they are so small (Fig. 2-1). Microbial images can be magnified with the aid of a microscope. Most of the time, because of their transparency, microorganisms must be stained to enhance their visualization.

The purpose of this chapter is to discuss the various types of microscopes that are used in the research and clinical laboratory to identify and characterize microorganisms and viruses. In addition, we will also discuss the primary staining techniques used in the clinical laboratory.

MICROSCOPY

RESOLVING POWER

One of the purposes of a microscope is to enlarge or magnify the image, but magnification is of no value if the image is blurred. It is therefore important that the microorganism is clearly defined when observed. The property of definition is called the *resolving power,* and it is this property that determines the quality of the microscope. The resolving power of a microscope refers to the smallest detectable separation of two points or objects. In other words, how close can two objects be brought together and still be seen as two clearly defined objects? The resolving power of a microscope is dependent on the *wavelength* of light used in the optical system as well as a characteristic of the objective lens, called the *numerical aperture.* The formula for resolving power (RP) is:

$$RP = \frac{wavelength}{2 \times numerical\ aperture}$$

Since both the wavelength and the numerical aperture have narrow limits, the resolving power of the microscope using conventional light sources is very limited. Only with the advent of the electron microscope has it been possible to increase greatly the magnification and, more important, the resolving power of optical instruments.

TYPES OF MICROSCOPES

Compound Bright-Field

The compound bright-field microscope (Fig. 2-2) is called *compound* because the total magnifi-

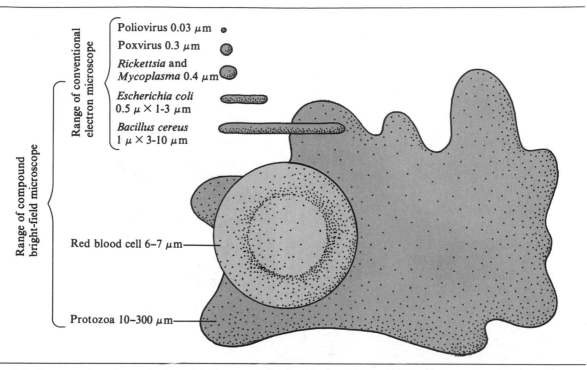

Fig. 2-1. Comparative sizes of microorganisms.

cation is due to the contribution of two magnifying lenses: an objective lens and an ocular lens. It is called *bright-field* because the light passing through it produces a brightly illuminated field around the object being viewed. The source of illumination is visible light, usually from an incandescent light bulb. The proper manipulation of the condenser and iris diaphragm is essential to achieve optimum contrast, depth of field, and resolution. The *condenser* contains lenses that bring the light rays into focus on the specimen, while the *iris diaphragm,* located between the condenser and the light source, controls the amount of light entering the condenser. The background surrounding the specimen will therefore appear very bright by using the conventional bright-field condenser.

Magnification in the compound bright-field microscope is equal to the product of the objective lens and ocular lens magnifications. The standard microscope has at least three objective lenses,

with magnifications of $10\times$, $44\times$, and $100\times$. The ocular lens has a magnification of $10\times$. Thus, the maximum magnification that can be obtained is $1000\times$. The $100\times$ objective lens is called the *oil immersion lens,* and when it is used oil is placed between the coverslip covering the specimen and the lens. By using the oil immersion lens with the $100\times$ objective the mathematical expression for the numerical aperture can be increased, thereby increasing the resolving power of the microscope. Immersion oil has the same refractive index* as the glass slide, and therefore light rays are not further refracted, as they would be in air. The resolving power of the compound bright-field microscope is approximately 0.2 μm; that is, if two bacterial cells 0.2 μm or more apart are examined, each can be clearly distinguished. If they

---

* Refractive index (RI) is a measure of the extent to which light is slowed down by a medium. Oil has the same RI as glass, but air has a smaller RI than glass.

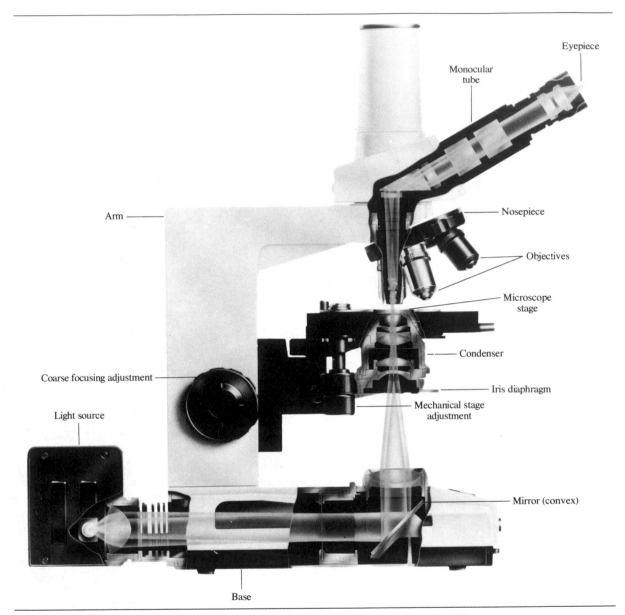

Fig. 2-2. Compound bright-field microscope. (Courtesy Nikon, Inc., Rochester, NY.)

are closer than 0.2 μm, they will appear as a blurred single cell.

Conventional bright-field illumination will not reveal brightness differences between the structural details of the specimen and its surroundings. In other words, the bacteria appear transparent. The transparency problem can be rectified by staining the cells or by using other microscopic techniques that take advantage of differences in optical density and refractive index produced in the specimen.

One of the advantages of bright-field microscopy is that living specimens can be examined. For example, it is relatively easy to determine the motility of bacteria.

Dark-Field

The dark-field microscope is frequently used to observe viable microorganisms that are very small or thin and whose morphology is best observed without staining. The condensers are the key to dark-field microscopy. A special light condenser is substituted for the customary bright-field condenser. Dark-field condensers channel the light rays at such an oblique angle that undiffracted rays are not collected by the objective lens. Only the rays diffracted by the specimen on the slide enter the objective. The background surrounding the specimen appears dark or black (Fig. 2-3). Organisms or structures whose diameter is less than the resolving power of the compound microscope can be observed by this technique. Bacterial flagella, which are only 0.02 μm in diameter, can be observed because they scatter enough light for their profile to be seen. Spirochetes, for example, are bacteria whose width is between 0.15 μm and 0.2 μm and they can be easily observed using dark-field microscopy (Plate I).

Phase Contrast

The phase contrast microscope has special condensers and objectives that are capable of altering light as it passes through and around the specimen. Light can be diffracted not only by the cell wall but also by any large structures in the cy-

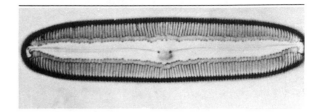

A

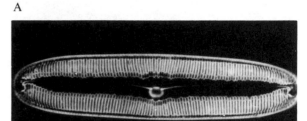

B

Fig. 2-3. Comparison of the images produced by (A) compound bright-field microscopy and (B) dark-field microscopy. (From R. F. Smith, *Microscopy and Photomicrography*. New York: Appleton-Century-Crofts, 1982.)

toplasm whose density is greater than the surrounding medium. Every object observed by this technique is surrounded by a halo of light (Fig. 2-4A), which does not represent a real structure. The internal structure of the cell can be revealed by this technique. For example, nuclear bodies and endospores (Fig. 2-5) are easily observed.

Nomarski Interference

Normarski interference microscopy is similar in many respects to phase-contrast microscopy. This technique requires specimens that are thicker than bacteria, for example, vegetative (growing) cells and spores of fungi. The presence of a polarizer and special prisms in the condenser result in the formation of a clearer image than that obtained with phase contrast. The object being examined, for example, has no halo and there is a three-dimensional appearance to the specimen (Fig. 2-4B). The resolving power in Nomarski interference microscopy is about twice that of the bright-field microscope, which is 0.1 μm.

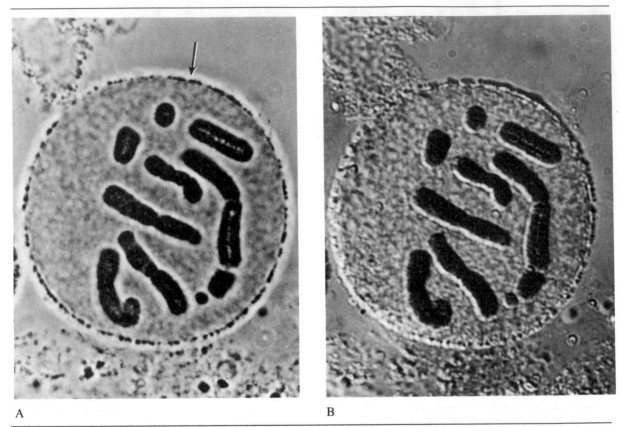

A

B

Fig. 2-4. A. Phase-contrast microscopy. Note the halo (*arrow*) around the spherical nucleus. B. Nomarski interference microscopy. Note that Nomarski interference microscopy appears to provide greater definition or clarity than does phase-contrast. (From R. F. Smith, *Microscopy and Photomicroscopy.* New York: Appleton-Century-Crofts, 1982.)

Fluorescent

Many materials are luminescent, that is, they absorb energy and release light. If the material absorbs a quantity of light and, after a delay of less than one-millionth of a second, re-emits a quantity of light of a larger wavelength, the material is called *fluorescent.* A few compounds fluoresce when illuminated with ultraviolet light or other short wavelengths of light and they are called *fluorochromes.* One of the most frequently used fluorochromes is called *fluorescein.* Microbiological material can be studied by coating it with fluorochromes. An important type of fluorescent microscopy is called *immunofluorescent micros-*

copy. In this technique fluorochromes may be conjugated (complexed) to specific antibodies to identify unknown specimens or structures, or, conversely, they may be conjugated to specific antigens to detect antibodies. *Antibodies* are proteins induced in mammalian systems in response to foreign molecules called *antigens.* For example, a bacterium could be the foreign agent and when injected into an animal will induce the animal to produce antibodies. These antibodies are specific for the bacterium (usually a protein or carbohydrate on the surface of the bacterium) and aid the host in destroying the infectious agent. Figure 2-6 illustrates how the technique is

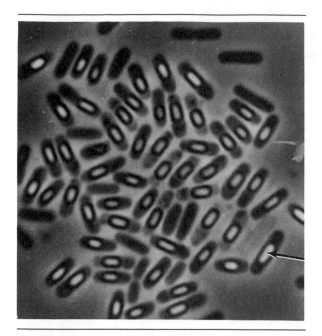

Fig. 2-5. Phase-contrast (× 3600) micrograph of bacterial cells in which endospores (*arrow*) have been produced. (Courtesy of P. C. Fitz-James.)

utilized in the clinical laboratory. Commercially prepared conjugated antibodies are readily available for detecting specific antigens of microbial species. If antibody is specific for the antigen in the clinical specimen, a complex of antigen, fluorochrome, and antibody is formed. The complex is then exposed to wavelengths of 350 nm produced by a high-pressure mercury vapor lamp or halogen lamp. The ultraviolet wavelengths (350 nm) strike the complex and visible wavelengths of light are released to produce an image seen by the observer (Fig. 2-7 and Plate 2).

Electron

One of the most important developments that advanced our knowledge concerning cell structure and function was the electron microscope (Fig. 2-8). By utilizing wavelengths of radiation from electrons instead of light, resolving power is increased several thousand times (0.0005 μm, compared to 0.2 μm in light microscopy). In transmission electron microscopy (TEM) the electrons penetrate the specimen, while in scanning electron microscopy (SEM), a more recent development, the electrons do not penetrate the specimen. We will discuss SEM later.

Fig. 2-6. Technique for producing fluorescent antibodies. Bacterial capsule (composed of a polysaccharide that appears here as a ring surrounding the cell wall) is removed and injected into rabbit. Antibodies to capsule are produced in the rabbit and then removed. A fluorochrome is conjugated to the antibodies, which will bind to organisms possessing specific capsule. Organism will be seen to glow when observed microscopically.

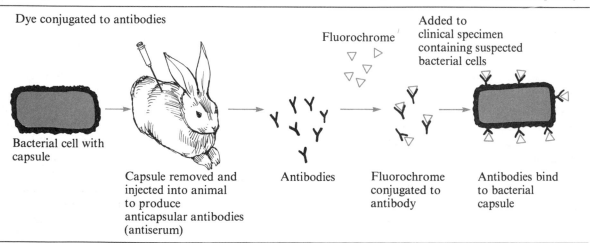

Dye conjugated to antibodies

Fluorochrome

Added to clinical specimen containing suspected bacterial cells

Bacterial cell with capsule

Capsule removed and injected into animal to produce anticapsular antibodies (antiserum)

Antibodies

Fluorochrome conjugated to antibody

Antibodies bind to bacterial capsule

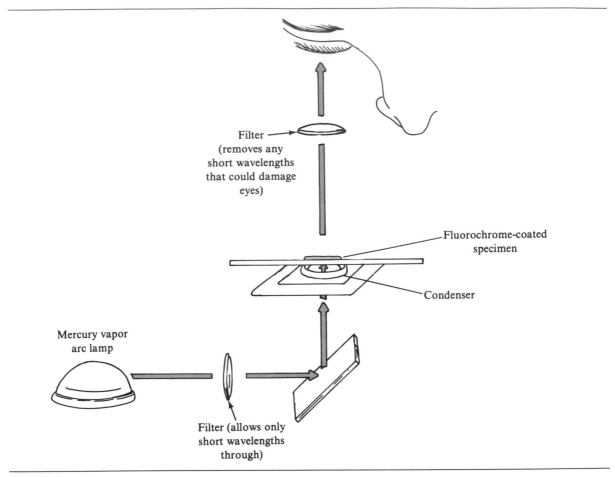

Filter ⟵
(removes any
short wavelengths
that could damage
eyes)

Fluorochrome-coated
specimen

Condenser

Mercury vapor
arc lamp

Filter (allows only
short wavelengths
through)

Fig. 2-7. Schematic of fluorescent microscopy.

An electrically heated tungsten filament is the source of radiation in both light and electron microscopy. In contrast to light microscopy, in which light is focused on the specimen, electron microscopy utilizes electrons to focus on the specimen (Fig. 2-9). Both light and electron microscopy use condensers to focus light and electrons, respectively, on the specimen. The condenser in the light microscope consists of glass lenses, but in the electron microscope large electromagnetic coils are used. In the light microscope the image is viewed through an ocular lens. The image in an electron microscope can be seen in two different ways: (1) the image can be viewed after projecting it on a movable zinc sulfide screen, so that when electrons hit the screen the zinc sulfide is excited and visible light is emitted, or (2) the image can be captured on photographic film in a camera mounted below the zinc sulfide screen. Magnifications in large electron microscopes are in the range of 500,000× and larger.

In transmission electron microscopy the electrons have to pass through the specimen; therefore, the specimen must be very thin. Electrons can reach the specimen only because the microscope is in a vacuum. The vacuum causes the

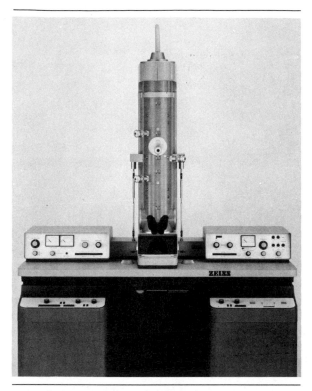

Fig. 2-8. Transmission electron microscope (Courtesy Carl Zeiss, Inc., New York, NY.)

specimen to dry out, and this prevents the investigator from observing cells in the living state as in light microscopy. There are basically three ways to prepare biological material for electron microscopy: *whole mount, ultrathin sectioning,* and *replication.*

Whole Mount. Whole mount preparations are usually objects that are thin enough for electrons to penetrate, for example, viruses. The specimen is placed on a copper grid and then stained with heavy metals such as lead or uranium salts. When electrons strike heavy metals they are deflected and this creates contrast. Specimen staining may involve three different techniques:

1. Positive staining. The object itself is stained with heavy metals such as osmium tetroxide.

2. Negative staining. The background around the object is stained with compounds of uranium or tungsten. The object appears bright against the dark background.

3. Evaporation of heavy metal. A thin layer of heavy metal atoms (platinum, for example) is deposited on a specimen at a precise angle so that the metal piles up on one side of the object in the specimen and leaves a clear area behind it. When photomicrographs are printed, shadows are cast, and this gives the observer an idea of the general size and shape of the object being viewed. This technique is referred to as *shadow casting.*

Ultrathin Sectioning. The biological material is fixed chemically (osmium tetroxide), stained with heavy metals, and embedded in epoxy resin. Ultrathin sections (less than 0.050 μm) are cut with an instrument called a microtome that uses diamond or glass knives.

Replication. Sometimes the object to be viewed cannot be brought into the electron microscope. Under these circumstances a thin replica is made by evaporating a layer of heavy metal on the specimen (see at 3 above). The replica is liberated from the object by digesting away any adhering organic material. The replication technique is used in a process called *freeze fracturing,* which utilizes three steps. First, the specimen is frozen to −150°C in liquid freon. Second, the frozen object is transferred to an evacuated chamber containing a microtome. The microtome produces a fracture plane that follows the topographic pecularities of the specimen. Freeze-fractured cells are three-dimensional because sometimes an entire organelle or object may be plucked out or left projecting while at other times the organelle may be cross-fractured, exposing its outer membrane and contents (Fig. 2-10). Third, a replica is made and depressions and protrusions receive a one-sided coating of the heavy metal that gives the image-shadowing effect. Freeze fracturing has been an important tech-

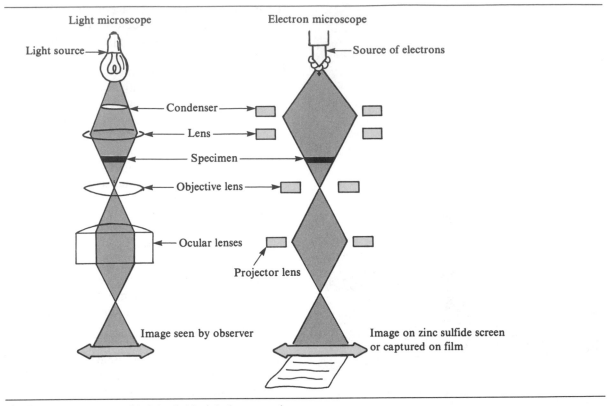

Light microscope

Electron microscope

Light source

Source of electrons

Condenser

Lens

Specimen

Objective lens

Ocular lenses

Projector lens

Image seen by observer

Image on zinc sulfide screen or captured on film

Fig. 2-9. Comparison of bright-field and electron microscopes.

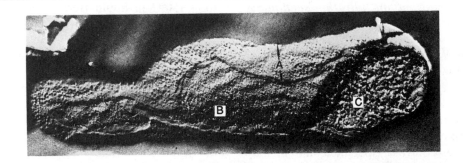

Fig. 2-10. Transmission electron micrograph of replica of freeze-fractured preparation of the bacterium *Escherichia coli*. The cell wall (A) is the outermost fraction, followed by the underlying cytoplasmic membrane (B), and, last, the cytoplasm (C) of the bacterial cell. (From J. W. Costerton, *Annu. Rev. Microbiol.* 33:459,1979.)

nique for observing organelles and membranes in both prokaryotic and eukaryotic cells.

In *scanning electron microscopy* (SEM) electrons do not penetrate the specimen but merely scan the surface topography. The resolution of the SEM is approximately 0.002 μm to 0.010 μm with direct magnifications up to 100,000 to 200,000×, but the most effective range of magnifications is between 15,000 and 50,000×. When the electrons hit the surface of the object, secondary electrons are released and directed to a scintillator. The scintillator converts the electrons into impulses that are relayed to a cathode ray tube. The result is an image similar to that produced in a television picture.

Samples examined by SEM are usually first coated with a metal such as gold-palladium alloy. The metal-coated sample is then affixed to a supporting disk that is placed in the path of the electron beam. The specimen can be rotated and thus different views of the object can be obtained from various angles. The image produced is three-di-

Fig. 2-11. Scanning electron micrograph of a freshwater diatom (Courtesy F. E. Round.)

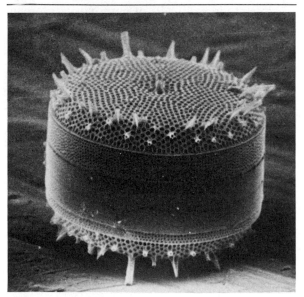

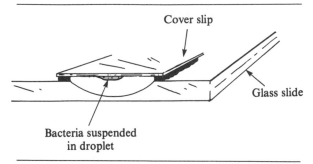

Fig. 2-12. The hanging drop preparation. The bacteria suspended in the concavity of the slide are free to move. Motility can be determined by observing bacterial movement with the high power of the compound microscope.

mensional and may be either observed directly or photographically recorded (Fig. 2-11).

PREPARATION OF LIVE SPECIMENS: THE HANGING DROP TECHNIQUE

Another technique, in addition to phase contrast and dark-field microscopy, for the microscopic examination of bacteria in the living state is called the *hanging drop preparation*. This technique is performed in the following way:

1. Petrolatum is placed on the periphery of a glass coverslip.
2. A drop of a bacterial suspension is transferred with an inoculating loop to the center of the coverslip.
3. A slide with a central depression is placed over the coverslip, and the preparation is inverted. The bacterial suspension will hang in the depression (Fig. 2-12) and can be observed under high power of the compound microscope.

The hanging drop technique is useful in determining the motility of bacteria and also gives an undistorted view of the morphology and arrangement of bacterial cells.

STAINING IN LIGHT MICROSCOPY

Bacteria are difficult to observe because of their transparency. Staining is therefore an important consideration in the observation and identification of microorganisms. The microbial surface is negatively charged because of the presence of phosphate and carboxyl groups; therefore, the types of dyes used to stain bacteria are limited. Basic dyes (those that ionize and become positively charged) are used to stain bacteria because they are attracted to the negatively charged bacterial surface. The basic dye will also stain internal components such as proteins and nucleic acids because they also contain many negative charges. Some of the preferred basic dyes used in the laboratory for staining bacteria are *crystal violet, safranin,* and *methylene blue*. In preparation for staining procedures, a bacterial suspension is first smeared with an inoculating loop onto the surface of a slide. The smear is air-dried and then heat-fixed to the slide. The slide is then ready for staining.

SIMPLE STAIN

In simple staining a suitable basic dye is applied to a heat-fixed smear for anywhere from a few seconds to a few minutes, depending on which dye is used. The excess dye is washed off and the stained preparation is observed microscopically.

DIFFERENTIAL STAINS

The chemical composition of many bacterial components is variable enough so that certain structural distinctions can be made between bacterial species or groups of bacteria. One way this objective can be accomplished is through the use of differential staining procedures, in which two stains and other reagents are applied sequentially to a heat-fixed bacterial smear. The two most widely used differential staining procedures are the *Gram-staining* procedure and the *acid-fast staining* procedure.

Gram Stain

Some years ago Dr. Christian Gram discovered that bacteria could be divided into two groups on the basis of the ability or inability of stained cells to resist decolorization by solvents such as alcohol and acetone. The sequence and function of each component in Gram's stain are as follows (Fig. 2-13):

1. Primary stain. The heat-fixed smear is stained with crystal violet, the primary stain. The excess stain is washed off the slide. The cells at this stage appear dark blue or purple.
2. Iodine. The crystal violet can be further fixed to the cell by the addition of a dilute solution of iodine. This produces a crystal violet-iodine complex.
3. Decolorization. A solution of 95 percent alcohol (or alcohol and acetone) is applied to the stained smear. The alcohol dehydrates carbohydrates, which are present in large amounts in cell walls of gram-positive organisms. Gram-positive organisms retain the stain (or stain-iodine complex). Walls of gram-negative bacteria contain a high concentration of lipids, for which alcohol is a solvent. Pore sizes are presumably enlarged and the dye complex escapes. Gram-negative organisms will therefore appear unstained after decolorization.
4. Counterstain. Safranin, a red dye, is the secondary stain applied to the fixed preparations. If the bacteria are decolorized with alcohol they will take up the safranin and appear red (gram-negative). If the cells are not decolorized, the safranin will have no effect on the already stained preparation, and the bacteria will remain blue or purple (gram-positive) (See Plates 3 and 4.)

Gram's stain is one of the first important iden-

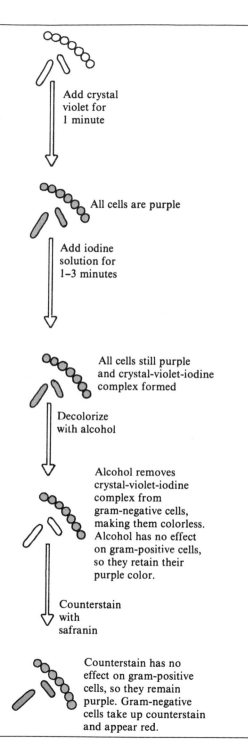

Add crystal
violet for
1 minute

All cells are purple

Add iodine
solution for
1–3 minutes

All cells still purple
and crystal-violet-iodine
complex formed

Decolorize
with alcohol

Alcohol removes
crystal-violet-iodine
complex from
gram-negative cells,
making them colorless.
Alcohol has no effect
on gram-positive cells,
so they retain their
purple color.

Counterstain
with
safranin

Counterstain has no
effect on gram-positive
cells, so they remain
purple. Gram-negative
cells take up counterstain
and appear red.

Fig. 2-13. Steps in the Gram-stain procedure.

tification procedures after the isolation of bacteria (see Boxed Essay, p. 30). This procedure allows one to divide the bacterial world into at least four categories: gram-positive cocci, gram-positive bacilli, gram-negative cocci, and gram-negative bacilli. When the Gram-staining characteristics of the cell have been determined, it is also possible to assign other general properties that apply to the group. They are outlined in Table 2-1.

The molecular basis of the Gram stain is not clear. Scientists originally suspected that the concentration of lipid in the cell wall determined the outcome of the Gram stain. Gram-negative cells possess more lipid in their cell walls than do gram-positive cells, and therefore alcohol produces pores in the gram-negative cell that result in loss of the primary stain. Other investigators propose that the shrinking, by alcohol, of the thicker peptidoglycan of the gram-positive cell wall retards the loss of the crystal-violet-iodine complex.

Acid-Fast Stain

The cell surface components of some bacteria, such as species of *Mycobacterium* and *Nocardia,* contain waxes and phospholipids that other bacteria do not possess. *Mycobacterium* and *Nocardia* are basically gram-positive if their waxes are removed, but in their natural state ordinary dyes cannot penetrate the waxy surface. These bacteria can be stained by the acid-fast technique. There are two major acid-fast staining techniques: *Kinyoun* and *Ziehl-Neelsen.*

In the Kinyoun method carbolfuchsin, a red dye, is applied to a smear of the bacteria for 3 minutes and then the smear is gently washed in water to remove excess stain. The smear is treated with acid alcohol until no more color appears in the washing and is then washed in water. The smear is counterstained with malachite green and then washed in water. Bacteria that are acid-fast retain the carbolfuchsin, while nonacid-fast bacteria do not retain carbolfuchsin and appear green.

THE GRAM STAIN: IMPORTANT TO THE MICROBIOLOGIST AND THE PHYSICIAN

One of the important aspects of the Gram stain is that it has helped microbiologists classify bacteria. The most widely accepted classification scheme for bacteria is called *Bergey's Manual of Determinative Bacteriology*. Upon examining this book one can immediately recognize the importance of the Gram stain, which is used to separate most of the major divisions of bacteria, for example, gram-negative rods, gram-positive rods, gram-negative cocci, gram-positive cocci, and gram-negative helical bacteria.

Identification of bacteria is greatly enhanced by first employing the Gram stain. The results of the Gram stain can also be a valuable piece of information to the physician. There are situations in which individuals with a bacterial infection are so in need of immediate treatment that the time for identification of the bacterium, based on biochemical tests as well as antibiotic sensitivity, is not realistic. The physician is faced with the decision as to which antibiotic to use in treatment. The microbiologist can help by providing the physician with the results of the Gram stain. The reason for this is that antibiotics, which are used to treat most bacterial infections, have different effects on the bacterial cell depending on cell wall composition. For example, many gram-negative bacteria are more resistant to certain antibiotics than are gram-positive bacteria. A knowledge of the Gram stain results could save a life.

Table 2-1. Some General Properties of Gram-Positive and Gram-Negative Bacteria Based on Cell Wall and Other Characteristics

Characteristic	Gram-positive	Gram-negative
Cell wall composition	Less complex; contains primarily peptidoglycan and very little lipid	More complex; little peptidoglycan but has outer membrane with considerable lipid, polysaccharide, and protein
Penicillin sensitivity	More sensitive	Less sensitive
Resistance to sonic disruption and other physical measures	More resistant	Less resistant
Resistance to cell wall lytic enzyme, i.e., lysozyme	Less resistant	More resistant
Dye inhibition	Inhibited by crystal violet	Not inhibited by crystal violet
Spore formation	Some bacilli are sporeformers	No bacilli are sporeformers
Toxin production	Toxins are not part of cell wall but are produced in the cytoplasm, i.e., *exotoxins*	One type of toxin is part of the cell wall and is called *endotoxin*

In the Ziehl-Neelsen method there are two major differences. First, the smear is flooded with carbolfuchsin and the slide is gently heated in a flame. Second, the counterstain, following the acid alcohol step, is methylene blue and non-acid-fast organisms will appear blue (see Plate 5).

NEGATIVE STAIN

Negative staining refers to the use of dyes that have no affinity for the microbial cell but will "stain" the background of a bacterial specimen. Two dyes that are used in negative staining are India ink and nigrosin. They can be added to the bacterial suspension, which is then spread on a microscopic slide and dried. A basic dye can be used to stain the bacterial cell proper if one so desires. Negative staining is valuable in determining the presence of sticky envelopes of carbohydrates, called *capsules,* that surround the cell wall of some bacteria (Fig. 2-14).

SPECIAL STAINS

Other staining techniques are available to the technician but are not so routinely used in the

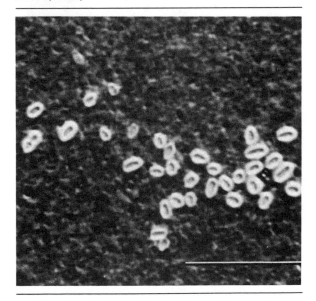

Fig. 2-14. Capsule-producing rod-shaped bacteria suspended in India ink and observed under oil immersion. Capsules appear as white halos around the rod-shaped bacterial cells. (From D. J. Politis and R. Goodman, *Appl. Environ. Microbiol.* 40:596,1980.)

Table 2-2. Characteristics of the Microscopes Used in Microbiology

Type	Resolving power	Useful magnification	Advantages	Disadvantages
Bright-field	0.2 μm	1000×	Microorganisms can be observed in living (unstained) state, for example, in hanging drop. Morphology of stained organisms can also be observed	Organisms less than 0.2 μm in diameter cannot be resolved
Dark-field	0.2 μm	1000×	Unstained organisms such as spirochetes whose diameter is at or just below resolving power of bright-field microscope can be observed	Manipulation of special condensers makes operation of instrument slightly more difficult than operation of bright-field microscope
Phase contrast	0.2 μm	1000×	Intensifies contrast between dense structures and transparent cytoplasm of live eukaryotic and prokaryotic microbes	Operation of instrument more difficult than bright-field microscope
Nomarski interference	0.1 μm	1000×	Produces clearer image than phase contrast and has resolving power twice that of phase contrast. Can be used on live specimens	Difficult to operate
Fluorescent	0.2 μm	1000×	Important diagnostic tool in clinical laboratory (immunofluorescence). Microorganisms can be detected in various types of specimens.	Personnel require training in its operation and evaluation of results
Transmission electron	0.0005 μm	200,000× and above	High resolving power. Molecular architecture of cells, microorganisms, and organelles can be identified. Objects can be viewed on screen or on film	Specimens in living state cannot be examined. Image produced is two-dimensional
Scanning electron	0.02 μm*	15,000– 50,000×	Three-dimensional appearance to specimen. Useful for evaluating surface of cells	Low resolving power. Specimen must be in nonliving state

* Some instruments may have a resolving power of 0.007 μm.

clinical laboratory as those previously discussed. They include the following:

1. Flagella stain. The flagella stain is used to stain the organ of motility in bacteria, called the *flagellum*. Flagella staining requires some skill and is sometimes used to classify some bacteria.
2. Spore stain. The spore is a specialized dormant form of the bacterium that is resistant to ordinary staining procedures. Spore location in the bacterial cell is of value in differentiating some species.
3. Metachromatic granule stain. Metachromatic granules are deposits of phosphates that accumulate in some bacteria. These phosphate deposits can be selectively stained to contrast with the cytoplasm.

SUMMARY

1. Microcopes are designed to magnify images while providing maximum resolution of them. There are a variety of microscopes, each having advantages and disadvantages. Table 2-2 outlines the characteristics of the various types of microscopes.

2. Staining is a very important technique in microscopic microbial identification. Staining is used in both light microscopy and electron microscopy to provide sufficient contrast. Positive staining techniques involve the use of dyes that are affixed to the organisms, while negative staining techniques involve dyes that stain the background.

3. In light microscopy positive stains are basic dyes that bind to the negatively charged surface of the microorganism or the negatively charged internal components. Simple staining techniques require but one stain, while differential stains involve more than one stain and enable the observer to differentiate certain groups of bacteria.

4. In light microscopy the Gram stain and acid-fast stain are the two most important differential staining techniques. The Gram stain enables the observer to differentiate the microbial world into groups (gram-positive and gram-negative) based on the complexity of the cell wall. The acid-fast stain is used to identify those microorganisms (mycobacteria) whose waxy surface is impenetrable by dyes from other staining procedures.

5. In transmission electron microscopy biological materials can be prepared in three ways: whole mount, ultrathin sectioning, and replication. In each process the material is stained with heavy metals to provide contrast. The replication technique is used in a process called freeze fracturing, which is especially useful in characterization of membranes.

QUESTIONS FOR STUDY

Fill in the blank:

1. A measure of the extent to which light is slowed down by a medium is called _____ .

2. The type of light microscopy that would enable one to view nuclear bodies is _____ .

3. The group of bacteria that are stained by the acid-fast stain are the _____ .

4. The chemical component whose concentration and time of application are critical in the Gram stain is _____ .

5. In _____ electron microscopy, electrons pass through the specimen, while in _____ electron microscopy, electrons scan the surface of the specimen.

Select the best response or responses for each of the following:

6. Under which of the following conditions would the resolving power of a microscope be the highest?
   A. Wavelength is 350 nm and numerical aperture is 1.0.
   B. Wavelength is 400 nm and numerical aperture is 1.05.
   C. Wavelength is 500 nm and numerical aperture is 1.4.
   D. Wavelength is 400 nm and numerical aperture is 1.4.

7. The primary advantage of the bright-field (BF) microscope and its principal disadvantage are that
   A. The BF microscope can be used to observe living material but the magnification is relatively low.
   B. The BF microscope enables one to observe both living and stained material but microbial motility cannot be detected.
   C. All types of microbial agents causing infectious disease can be observed but unstained bacterial capsules cannot be observed.
   D. Structures inside the bacterial cell can be differentiated from one another but the magnification is relatively low.

8. Which of the following statements concerning the fluorescent antibody technique is *not* true?
   A. The fluorescing material affixed to the object being observed or antibody is called a fluorochrome.
   B. The antibodies used in immunofluorescent microscopy to detect specific antigens in the host are usually derived from animals.
   C. Wavelengths of light used in fluorescent microscopy are between 400 nm and 500 nm
   D. The lamp used to generate the ultraviolet wavelengths for fluorescent microscopy is a pressure mercury vapor lamp or halogen lamp.

9. Which of the following statements about transmission electron microscopy is true?
   A. Heavy metals are used to stain specimens because when electrons strike them they are deflected and this produces contrast.
   B. The condenser in the electron microscope is an electromagnetic coil.
   C. The image from electron microscopy can be viewed on a screen or it can be captured on photographic film.
   D. The replication technique of electron microscopy is used when the specimen cannot be brought into the microscope.

10. The Gram stain is called *differential* because
   A. It differentiates bacteria from other microorganisms.
   B. It differentiates bacteria based on characteristics of the cytoplasmic membrane.
   C. It differentiates bacteria based on characteristics of their cell walls.
   D. None of the above, because the Gram stain is not a differential stain.

ADDITIONAL READINGS

Barer, R. Microscopes, microscopy and microbiology. *Annu. Rev. Microbiol.* 28:371,1974.

Kopp, F. *Electron Microscopy.* Burlington, NC: Scientific Publications Division, Carolina Biological Supply Co., 1981.

Slayter, E. M. *Optical Methods in Biology.* New York: Wiley-Interscience, 1970.

Smith, R. F. *Microscopy and Photomicrography.* New York: Appleton-Century-Crofts, 1982.

Spenser, M. *Fundamentals of Light Microscopy.* Cambridge, England: Cambridge University Press, 1982.

Wilson, M. B. *The Science and Art of Basic Microscopy.* Bellaire, TX: American Society for Medical Technology, 1976.

3. CHARACTERISTICS OF BACTERIA

OBJECTIVES

To describe the characteristics that differentiate
  prokaryotes from eukaryotes

To differentiate the terms genus, species, and strain

To explain the basis of bacterial taxonomy and what
  procedures are used to classify a bacterium

To list the components of a bacterial cell and their
  chemical composition

To describe the functions of the cytoplasmic
  membrane

To describe the ways in which solute can pass into
  and out of the cell

To describe the chemical similarities and differences
  in the cell wall of gram-positive and gram-negative
  bacteria

To describe the functions of the capsule and slime
  layer of bacteria

To illustrate the importance of flagella and pili to the
  bacterial cell

To describe the process of sporulation and its
  importance to bacteria

To define: taxonomy, coccus, bacillus,
  pleomorphism, mesosome, peptidoglycan,
  periplasm, porin, endotoxin, osmosis, protoplast,
  spheroplast, capsule, slime layer, flagellum,
  chemotactic, nucleoid, ribosome, endospore,
  vegetative cell

Each day new microbial properties are revealed by our advances in microscopy, biochemistry, and molecular biology. These advances have not only given us greater insight into microbial life and the factors that affect it, but they also give us insight into the properties of higher forms of life. The results obtained from the study of metabolic, physiological, and genetic characteristics in microbial models have provided us with a better understanding of many human functions.

In this chapter we will examine the chemistry and function of the various structures that make up the anatomy of the microbial cell. An understanding of microbial anatomy is important because the ability of chemical and physical agents to inhibit the growth of, or kill, infectious microorganisms is related to the presence or absence of specific microbial components. First, however, we will briefly discuss how microorganisms are classified.

CLASSIFICATION AND NOMENCLATURE

Classification is one branch of a science called *taxonomy*. The purpose of classification is to arrange organisms into specific groups, called *taxa,*
based on a similarity of characteristics. Until the discovery of microorganisms the biological world was divided into two major groups: plants and animals. Bacteria were originally classified as plants. Unicellular microorganisms possess characteristics that are neither plant nor animal, and for this reason some authorities preferred to place them in a separate group called the *Protista.* Even among the unicellular microorganisms, however, there was one important feature that showed that the term protista was not practical. This unique feature was the presence or absence of a nuclear membrane (the membrane surrounding the hereditary information of the cell). Organisms devoid of a nuclear membrane were called *prokaryotes* (from the Greek *protos,* primitive and *karyon,* nucleus) while organisms possessing a nuclear membrane were called *eukaryotes* (Greek *eu,* true, and *karyon,* nucleus). One of the most widely accepted classification schemes now divides the biological world into two superkingdoms, Prokaryotae and Eukaryotae. This classification scheme is arranged as follows:

Superkingdom: Prokaryotae
    Kingdom: Monera (Bacteria)

Table 3-1. Important Characteristics Distinguishing Prokaryotes from Eukaryotes*

Characteristic or structure	Eukaryote	Prokaryote	Virus
Size (average based on unicellular species)	5–10 μm	1–3 μm	0.025 μm–0.2 μm
Cell wall	Present in fungi and algae	Present except in *Mycoplasma*	Absent
Cytoplasmic membrane	Membrane possesses sterols	Membrane contains no sterols except in *Mycoplasma*	Absent, but a lipid membrane surrounds some viruses
Nuclear membrane	Present	Absent	Absent
Nucleolus	Present	Absent	Absent
Hereditary information	DNA; more than one chromosome in nucleus; proteins associated with chromosomes	DNA; single chromosome; no associated proteins	DNA or RNA and may be single- or double-stranded; some have enzymes associated with them
Ribosomes	Larger than prokaryotes (sedimentation constant of 80S**)	Smaller than eukaryotes (sedimentation constant of 70S**)	Absent
Respiration	Associated with mitochondrion	Associated with particles in cytoplasmic membrane	Absent
Reproduction	Sexual and asexual	Asexual (binary fission)	Asexual
Habitat	Found almost exclusively in environments containing oxygen; does not require an intracellular habitat in which to reproduce	Can be found equally in environments that may or may not contain oxygen; some (e.g., *Rickettsia*) require a living host in order to reproduce	Can reproduce only within the environment of a living host

* We have also included the acellular viruses to make the comparison of microorganisms more complete.
** S refers to Svedberg, which is a relative size unit derived from sedimentation studies.

Superkingdom: Eukaryotae
  Kingdom: Protista
    Branch: Protophyta (Plantlike; for example, primitive algae)
    Branch: Protomycota (funguslike; for example, slime molds)
    Branch: Protozoa (animallike; for example, protozoans)
  Kingdom: Fungi (unicellular yeasts and multicellular molds)
  Kingdom: Plantae (complex algae and plants such as mosses and ferns)
  Kingdom: Animalia (multicellular vertebrate and invertebrate animals)

In addition to the presence or absence of a nuclear membrane, other characteristics distinguish prokaryotes from eukaryotes (Table 3-1). Bacteria as a group possess the largest number of species that are infectious to humans and their classification will be discussed in more detail. Classification of infectious fungi, protozoa, and helminths will be discussed in Chapters 32 and 33, respectively.

Nomenclature is the assignment of names to a taxonomic group that has been defined by similarities in certain characteristics. The scientific naming is based on the taxonomic group, which incorporates two names (*binomial nomenclature*) called *genus* and *species*. The bacterial species, which is the basic taxonomic group, signifies a distinct member of a group of microorganisms that possess similar characteristics but differ in important ways from related groups of bacteria in other independent characteristics. The genus (plural, genera) name is capitalized, while the species name is not. Both words are italicized, for example, *Pseudomonas aeruginosa.* Much can be learned from the genus and species names. The genus name of bacteria often indicates the morphology of the species, for example, *Streptococcus* (chain of spherical cells), *Bacillus* (rod-shaped), Spirochaeta (spiral-shaped), but it can also indicate the organism's discoverer, for example *Escherichia* (Theodor Escherich), as well as various other characteristics. The species name frequently indicates a metabolic feature, biochemical characteristic, or disease association, for example, *Staphylococcus aureus,* in which *aureus* refers to a golden pigment produced by the species, or *Klebsiella pneumoniae,* in which *pneumoniae* refers to the type of disease caused by the species. The term *strain* will be seen in this book. A species may be composed of a group of related strains. For example, *Klebsiella pneumoniae* may consist of strains each of which is attacked by a different group of related bacterial viruses. *K. pneumoniae* could therefore be described as *K. pneumoniae* A1, A2, A3, A4. Letters or numbers or their combinations are used after the species name to indicate a strain that has properties distinct from other strains of the species.

The classification of bacteria is based on the wide variety of characteristics, or properties, associated with the organism. Related genera of bacteria are grouped into families, related families into orders, and so on up to kingdoms or superkingdoms. There is no official classification of bacteria and artificial classification schemes have appeared from time to time. The most widely accepted is *Bergey's Manual of Determinative Bacteriology,* which is in its ninth edition. The current edition has classified prokaryotes into the *Kingdom Procaryotae,* under which there are

various *sections.* Each section represents a specific group of bacteria that has been separated on the basis of one or more features, such as staining characteristics, morphology, oxygen requirements, physiological responses, spore formation, and other characteristics. Each section, which may be further subdivided into families and orders, contains a number of genera. A breakdown of the various sections and some of their characteristics appears in Table 3-2.

TAXONOMIC METHODS

The arrangement of organisms into various taxonomic groups is based on their degree of relatedness. Classification of bacteria based on natural relationships, that is, a fossil record, is called *phylogenetic classification.* Unlike higher forms of life, which have a fossil record in which certain characteristics can be compared, the fossil record of bacteria is virtually absent. Even the few fossil records of bacteria that have been discovered reveal only age and little else. Morphological, biochemical, and physiological characteristics as well as staining properties are used most frequently to differentiate bacteria. The use of such characteristics in taxonomy, however, represents an artificial scheme. Morphological traits are usually stable characteristics that are not influenced by environmental factors. Physiological traits, however, are subject to some variation. The temperature and pH requirements for growth or the fermentation products released by bacteria may be influenced by the environment. The kind of trait that can be used to separate or classify certain groups of bacteria may vary from one group to another. By evaluating various morphological or nonmorphological characteristics, bacteria can be arranged into certain taxonomic groups. Unfortunately, not all scientists agree on which microbial characteristics are most important. Some microbial properties are given more weight than others by one investigator, while another investigator may suggest that these properties should not be considered for classification.

Table 3-2. Outline of Those Taxonomic Divisions Found in *Bergey's Manual of Determinative Bacteriology* That Contain the Major Human Pathogens

Section	Section description	Important genera	Diseases
1	The Spirochetes	*Treponema, Borrelia, Leptospira*	Syphilis (*Treponema*), undulant fever (*Borrelia*)
2	Aerobic/Microaerophilic, Motile, Helical/Vibroid, Gram-Negative Bacteria	*Spirillum, Campylobacter*	Rat-bite fever (*Spirillum*), intestinal disease (*Campylobacter*)
4	Gram-Negative Aerobic Rods and Cocci	*Pseudomonas, Legionella, Neisseria, Brucella, Bordetella, Francisella,*	Opportunistic* (*Pseudomonas*), legionnaires disease (*Legionella*), meningitis and gonorrhea (*Neisseria*), brucellosis (*Brucella*), whooping cough (*Bordetella*), tularemia (*Francisella*)
5	Facultatively Anaerobic Gram-Negative Rods	*Escherichia, Shigella, Salmonella, Klebsiella, Yersinia, Proteus, Vibrio, Hemophilus*	Intestinal disease (*Escherichia*), opportunistic* (*Escherichia, Klebsiella,* and *Proteus*) plague (*Yersinia*), cholera (*Vibrio*), meningitis (*Hemophilus*)
6	Anaerobic Gram-Negative, Straight, Curved and Helical Rods	*Bacteroides, Fusobacterium, Leptotrichia*	Infections of oral cavity, opportunistic*
9	The Rickettsias and Chlamydias	*Rickettsia, Chlamydia, Coxiella*	Typhus and Rocky Mountain spotted fever (*Rickettsia*), psittacosis and genitourinary tract disease (*Chlamydia*), Q fever (*Coxiella*)
10	The Mycoplasma	*Mycoplasma, Ureaplasma*	Pneumonia (*Mycoplasma*), genitourinary tract disease (*Ureaplasma* and *Mycoplasma*)
12	Gram-Positive Cocci	*Staphylococcus, Streptococcus*	Skin infections (*Staphylococcus*), rheumatic fever (*Streptococcus*), opportunistic* (*Staphylococcus*)
13	Endospore-Forming Gram-Positive Rods and Cocci	*Bacillus, Clostridium*	Anthrax (*Bacillus*); tetanus, botulism, and gas gangrene (*Clostridium*)
15	Irregular, Nonsporing, Gram-Positive Rods	*Corynebacterium, Actinomyces*	Diphtheria (*Corynebacterium*), lesions of face and lungs (*Actinomyces*)
16	Mycobacteria	*Mycobacterium*	Tuberculosis and leprosy
17	Nocardioforms	*Nocardia*	Lesions of skin

* Opportunistic pathogens are organisms that cause disease in individuals compromised by some underlying illness or condition. Most opportunistic infections occur in the hospital.

Source: From J. G. Holt (Ed.), *Bergey's Manual of Determinative Bacteriology* (9th ed.). Baltimore: Williams & Wilkins, 1984.

A technique called *numerical taxonomy* gives equal weight to all the characteristics examined. All the characteristics of the organism are evaluated by a computer. A percentage of the total number of traits held in common between the organisms is expressed as a similarity profile. Those organisms showing similarity in 80 percent or more of specific characteristics are considered part of the same species.

There are techniques for determining phylogenetic relatedness between microorganisms, and this is based on analysis of large molecules such as DNA, RNA, and protein. These large molecules (called macromolecules) are made up of many smaller subunits and their sequence in the macromolecule is an evolutionary profile. Thus, these molecules represent a fossil record of the bacterium. Methods are now available for measuring relatedness between the DNA molecules of two organisms. The DNA can be cleaved into fragments and the amount of DNA sequences that are common between two organisms determines the degree of relatedness.

The proper classification of organisms should consist of:

1. Measuring and comparing specific biochemical reactions (and other significant characteristics) of the microorganisms.
2. Testing the DNA-relatedness of the organisms that have been grouped together based on tests described in #1.
3. Reexamination of the biochemical characteristics of each DNA-related group in order to define the biochemical boundaries of each species.

BACTERIAL STRUCTURE AND FUNCTION

SIZE AND MORPHOLOGY

Bacteria show considerable variation in size, from cells barely visible with the compound light microscope (0.2 μm) to spiral organisms that may reach lengths up to 60 μm. Most bacteria infectious for humans have average lengths of 1 to 3 μm and can be observed with the compound light microscope. Some of the basic structures that can be observed microscopically in a typical bacterial cell are illustrated in Figure 3-1.

Bacteria have four basic shapes: spherical, rod, spiral, and square (Fig. 3-2). Spherical cells are called *cocci* (singular, *coccus*) and may exist in different arrangements. When cocci divide they usually remain attached to one another, and the arrangement that follows is based on the plane of cell division (Fig. 3-3). Cocci that divide along the same axis may form chains of cocci varying in length from 2 to 20 cocci. A pair of cocci are called *diplococci,* while chains of 4 to 20 are called *streptococci.* Cocci that divide in two planes form a *tetrad.* Division in three planes results in the formation of a group of eight called *sarcina* or large clusters of cocci called *staphylococci.* Rod-shaped bacteria are called *bacilli* (singular, bacillus). They divide in one plane and are sometimes observed to be in short chains, but usually they appear singly (see Fig. 3-2). The term bacillus, which signifies a type of morphology, should not be confused with the taxonomic genus called *Bacillus.* Spiral-shaped microorganisms, which appear in a helical or corkscrew shape, divide in one plane and separate at cell division. The square-shaped bacteria are a recently discovered group found in areas of high salt content (Great Salt Lake, for example). Square bacteria are not known to be infectious and therefore will not be discussed further in this text.

PLEOMORPHISM

Pleomorphism is defined as the existence of different morphological forms of the same species or strain (Fig. 3-4). Pleomorphism usually refers to changes in microbial shape within the organism's natural environment. In the natural environment of some microorganisms there is a differentiation process in which a change of shape is normal. Some bacteria (usually not infectious for humans) under the influence of nutrient star-

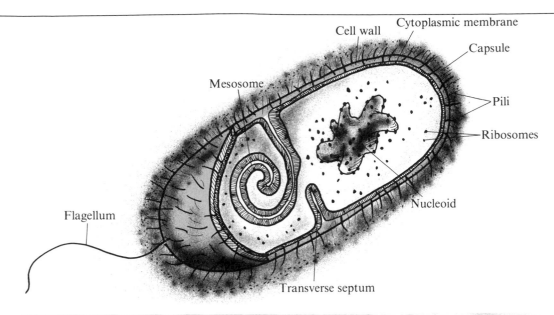

A

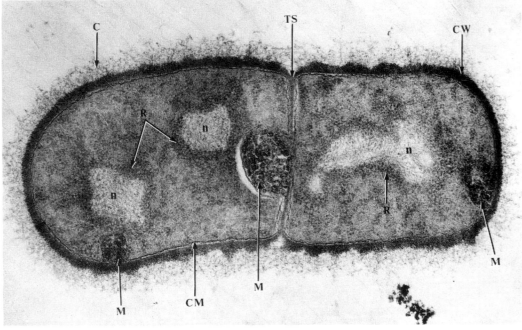

B

Fig. 3-1. A. Basic morphology of a bacterial cell. Some of the features, for example, flagella and extracellular polymeric substances (capsule) may not be present in all bacterial cells. B. Electron micrograph of a rod-shaped bacterium illustrating basic morphology. C = capsule; TS = transverse septum; CW = cell wall; M = mesosome; CM = cytoplasmic membrane; n = nuclear area or nucleoid; R = ribosome. The transverse septum is the site of cell division. (From D. J. Ellar, D. G. Lundgren, and R. A. Slepecky, *J. Bacteriol.* 94:1189,1967.)

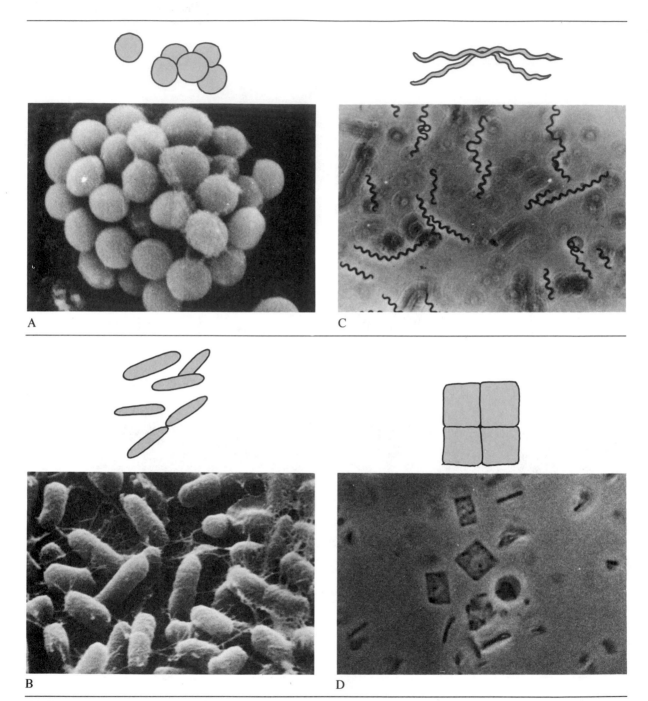

Fig. 3-2. Shapes of bacteria. A. Spherical (coccus). Scanning electron micrograph of staphylococci (×14,000). (Courtesy of Z. Yoshii.) B. Rod (bacillus). Scanning electron micrograph of bacilli. (From T. J. Kerr et al., *Appld. Environ. Microbiol.* 46:1201,1983.) C. Spiral. Micrograph of rumen treponemes. (From A. Ziolecki, *Appld. Environ. Microbiol.* 37:131,1979.) D. Square. Micrograph is phase contrast (×1,600 before 20 percent reduction). (From D. Stoeckenius, *J. Bacteriol.* 148:352,1981.)

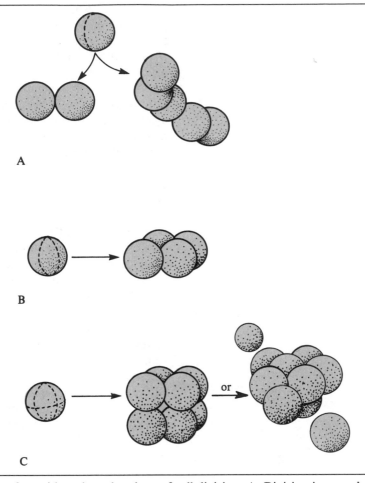

A

B

C

Fig. 3-3. Arrangements of cocci based on the plane of cell division. A. Division in one plane produces diplococci or streptococci. B. Division in two planes produces a tetrad. C. Division in three planes produces a group of eight (sarcina) or clusters (staphylococci).

vation, for example, change their morphology from ovoid to filamentous. Under adverse conditions in the laboratory (old cultures, for example) most bacteria show variations in shape (ballooning, bulging, branching, etc.), but this is not the normal state.

CYTOPLASMIC MEMBRANE

The cytoplasm of the cell is surrounded by a membrane referred to as the *cytoplasmic* or

plasma membrane. The cytoplasmic membrane is a dynamic, flexible structure that is actively and passively engaged in several cellular functions. Many of these functions are directly related to the structure of the cytoplasmic membrane.

The cytoplasmic membrane is made up of a phospholipid matrix into which are embedded various proteins. The phospholipid can be described as a molecule consisting of three units. One unit, called the head, contains a phosphate (PO_4) group, while the other two units are long-chain fatty acids that can be described as tails

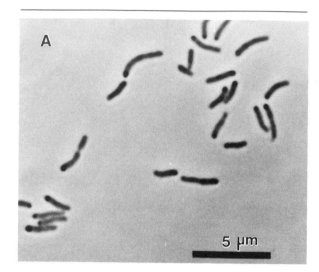

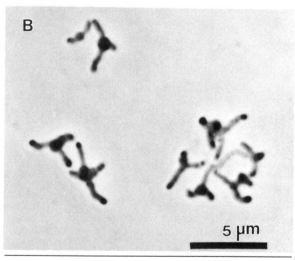

Fig. 3-4. Phase contrast (×4000) of soil microorganisms grown on different carbon sources. A. On one carbon source the organism is typically rod-shaped. B. On second carbon source organism shows branching. (From H. Reding and J. Lepo, *Appld. Environ. Microbiol.* 55:666,1988.)

(Fig. 3-5). When phospholipids are placed in water the phosphate heads are attracted to water (*hydrophilic*) but the fatty acid tails avoid water (*hydrophobic*) and huddle together. This results in a double layer (bilayer) of phospholipid (Fig. 3-6). The proteins that are superimposed onto the lipid bilayer are of two general types, those that span the membrane and those that do not. These proteins perform specific functions, which will now be discussed.

FUNCTIONS OF MEMBRANE PROTEINS

Nutrient Transport

The cytoplasmic membrane acts as a barrier to some molecules (for example, large ones such as proteins) but permits the entry of other molecules into the cytoplasm of the cell. Some molecules, such as oxygen and water, can move passively across the cytoplasmic membrane. The direction of this passive movement depends on the concentration of the dissolved molecules (solute) on either side of the cytoplasmic membrane. Solute will move from an area where its concentration is high to an area where its concentration is low (Fig. 3-7A) until the concentration of solute on either side of the membrane is the same. This type of solute transport mechanism is called *passive diffusion.*

Some solutes can be transported into the cytoplasm by exploiting carriers. The carriers are proteins located in the cytoplasmic membrane (Fig. 3-7B). They pick up solutes on one side of the cytoplasmic membrane and transport them, chemically unchanged, to the opposite side of the cytoplasmic membrane. This transport process is called *facilitated diffusion.**

The most important transport mechanism is called *active transport*. Microorganisms live primarily in environments where most nutrients are at a lower concentration outside the cell. Nutrients can, however, be transported into the cell

* Facilitated diffusion, like passive diffusion, is involved in the movement of solutes from an area of high concentration to an area of low solute concentration.

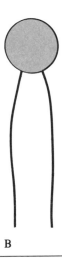

$$
\left.\begin{array}{l}
\text{H} \qquad\quad \text{O} \\
| \qquad\qquad || \\
\text{H}-\text{C}-\text{O}-\text{C}-\ (\text{CH}_2)_n \quad -\text{CH}_3 \\
| \qquad\qquad \text{O} \\
\qquad\qquad\quad || \\
\text{H}-\ \text{C}-\text{O}-\text{C}-\ (\text{CH}_2)_n \quad -\text{CH}_3
\end{array}\right\} \text{Fatty acid chains}
$$

$$
\left.\begin{array}{l}
| \qquad\qquad\ \text{O} \\
\qquad\qquad\quad || \\
\text{H}-\ \text{C}-\text{O}-\ \text{P}-\text{O}^- \\
| \qquad\qquad\ | \\
\text{H} \qquad\qquad \text{O}^-
\end{array}\right\} \text{Phosphate group}
$$

A

B

Fig. 3-5. Structure of phospholipid. A. Chemical structure B. Diagrammatic representation.

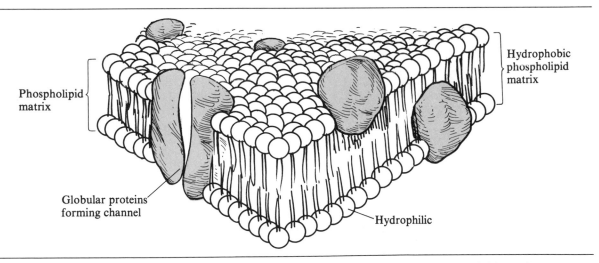

Phospholipid matrix

Hydrophobic phospholipid matrix

Globular proteins forming channel

Hydrophilic

Fig. 3-6. Model of cytoplasmic membrane. Globular proteins are embedded in a phospholipid matrix. (Adapted from S. J. Singer and G. I. Nicolson, *Science* 175:720,1972.)

45

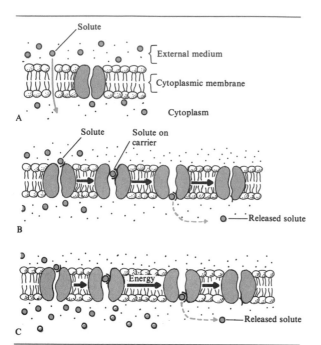

Fig. 3-7. Mechanisms for transport of nutrients across cytoplasmic membrane. A. Passive diffusion. B. Facilitated diffusion. C. Active transport.

against this concentration gradient through the use of carriers and by an expenditure of energy, i.e., active transport. Carrier proteins transport the solute through channels produced by other proteins that span the cytoplasmic membrane (Fig. 3-7C). The transported solute is not chemically changed during this transport process.

The final mechanism of nutrient transport is called *group translocation*. It is similar to active transport except that the solute is chemically altered during transfer.

Respiration
Several proteins associated with respiration, that is, electron transport and energy formation, are located in the cytoplasmic membrane. In eukaryotes these respiratory activities are associated with organelles called mitochondria. Respiration is discussed at more length in Chapter 4.

OTHER FUNCTIONS ASSOCIATED WITH THE CYTOPLASMIC MEMBRANE

Secretion
Many substances produced in the cytoplasm of the cell must be transferred to the surface of the cell or to those structures that are external to the cytoplasmic membrane. Proteins that are required for cell wall synthesis, for example, are produced in the cytoplasm. Various toxins that are produced by microorganisms, and may be involved in human disease or inhibit other bacteria, are also produced in the cytoplasm and must be transported to the exterior. In addition, many bacteria produce enzymes that are secreted outside the cell to break down macromolecules into smaller units that can be transported across the cytoplasmic membrane.

Cell Wall Biosynthesis
The enzymes involved in the assembly of cell wall components are located in the cytoplasmic membrane.

Site of DNA Synthesis
During the replication of the DNA molecule in the cell the cytoplasmic membrane is believed to be an anchoring site for the ends of the DNA molecule. These membrane attachment sites are believed to be invaginated areas of the cytoplasmic membrane called *mesosomes*. They are usually associated with the site of division of bacteria (*septum*) but can be found elsewhere in the cell (see Figure 3-1).

CELL WALL

The bacterial cell wall is a thick and relatively rigid layer that lies outside the cytoplasmic membrane. The wall protects the fragile cytoplasmic membrane and the contents it encloses. The wall is also responsible for maintaining the shape of the bacterium.

The bacterial world, with few exceptions, is divided into two basic cell wall types, *gram-positive* and *gram-negative,* on the basis of a staining procedure called the Gram's stain (see Chapter 2). Division into gram-positive and gram-negative is based on marked differences in the physical and chemical makeup of the cell wall. A cell is gram-positive if it resists decolorization by alcohol after the application of a primary stain and gram-negative if it is decolorized by alcohol after primary staining. The backbone material of both cell types is the *peptidoglycan* layer. The peptidoglycan is composed of layers of polysaccharide chains that are linked by short peptides (peptides are chains of amino acids of varying length). The peptidoglycan is composed of two alternating sugars, *N-acetylmuramic acid* (abbreviated NAM) and *N-acetylglucosamine* (abbreviated NAG). Let us compare the composition and structure of the two cell wall types.

GRAM-POSITIVE BACTERIA

The peptidoglycan layer of gram-positive bacteria is very thick compared to the gram-negative peptidoglycan layer and consists of layer upon layer of molecules. The peptidoglycan layer of gram-positive bacteria therefore accounts for 50 to 60 percent of the total dry weight of the cell wall. Much of the remaining cell wall material is a special polysaccharide called *teichoic acid* (Fig. 3-8A). The peptidoglycan of *Staphylococcus aureus,* a gram-positive bacterium, is illustrated in Figure 3-9. The degree of cross-linking of polysaccharide chains via peptides in the peptidolglycan of gram-positive bacteria is very high and this results in a very rigid cell wall. Teichoic acids not only permeate the peptidoglycan but also appear on the surface of the cell wall. Their function to the cell is not fully understood.

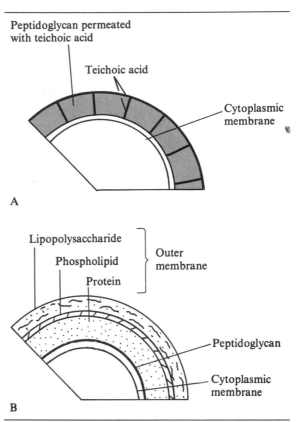

Fig. 3-8. Relative composition and structure of the bacterial cell wall. A. Gram-positive cell wall. Peptidoglycan is very thick and is permeated by teichoic acids that also cover the surface. B. Gram-negative cell wall. Wall is multilayered with peptidoglycan much thinner than in gram-positive cell. Figure shows only relative composition. More details of the precise location of cell wall components can be found in Figures 3-9 and 3-10.

GRAM-NEGATIVE BACTERIA

The gram-negative cell wall, unlike the gram-positive wall, is multilayered (Fig. 3-8B). The peptidoglycan layer of the gram-negative bacterium is only 1 to 2 molecules thick and accounts for only 5 to 10 percent of the total dry weight of the cell wall. External to the peptidoglycan is a complex cell wall layer called the *outer membrane.* The outer membrane is attached to the peptido-

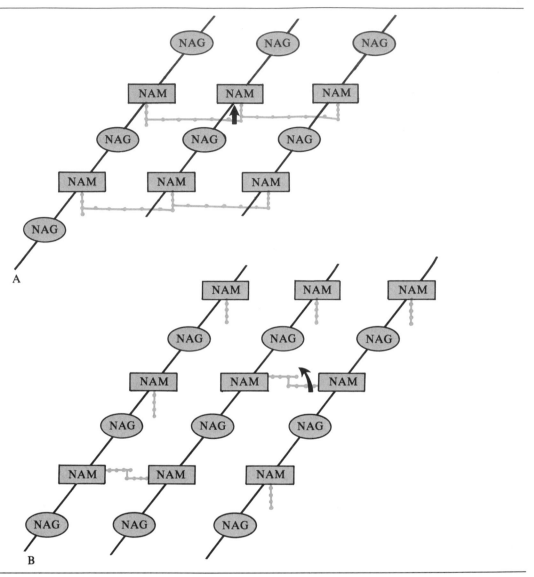

Fig. 3-9. Comparative peptidoglycan structure in gram-positive (A) and gram-negative bacteria (B). Arrows indicate sites where penicillin prevents linkage of adjacent strands.

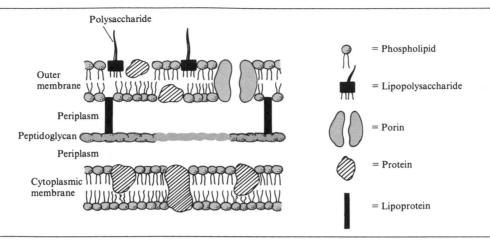

Fig. 3-10. More detailed illustration of the outer membrane of the gram-negative cell wall and its relationship to peptidoglycan. Note that this figure is not drawn to scale.

glycan by means of lipoprotein molecules (Fig. 3-10). The outer membrane is made up of phospholipid (20–30%), lipopolysaccharide (30%), and protein (40–50%). The phospholipid of the outer membrane resembles the bilayer arrangement seen in the cytoplasmic membrane. Located in the phospholipid are protein channels, called *porins*, that are involved in nutrient transport. Nutrients transported through porins must first enter the *periplasmic space,* an area between the cytoplasmic membrane and the outer membrane. The periplasmic space contains several types of molecules, including enzymes that process molecules before they enter the cytoplasm. The periplasmic space also contains protein molecules that act as carriers of nutrients and are similar to the carriers in the cytoplasmic membrane. Other molecules located in the periplasmic space that are of special interest are a group of enzymes that are capable of inactivating drugs such as antibiotics. These antibiotic-inactivating enzymes render the microorganism resistant to the affected antibiotic.

The lipid component of the lipopolysaccharide (LPS) is embedded in the phospholipid while the polysaccharide portion of the LPS projects from the surface of the cell (Fig. 3-10). Only the lipid component of the LPS, called Lipid A, is toxic,

but since the two molecules are released as a single unit the LPS is referred to as *endotoxin.* Endotoxin causes fever and can result in lysis of red blood cells. The polysaccharide portion of the LPS that projects from the surface of the cell is made of various sugars that vary from species to species. These sugars serve as markers that enable microbiologists to differentiate species in the laboratory.

OSMOSIS AND CELLS WITHOUT CELL WALLS

The cell wall is not a totally rigid structure but is capable of expanding and contracting. The solute concentration in the cell is usually greater than that outside the cell. In other words, the cytoplasm of the cell is *hypertonic,* while the environment or medium is *hypotonic.* In a hypotonic medium water moves from the solution outside the cell into the cell cytoplasm to establish an equilibrium—a process called *osmosis* (Fig. 3-11A,B). The cell contents swell but do not burst because of the rigidity of the cell wall. Without the cell wall the cytoplasmic membrane would expand and burst.

Sometimes in research it is necessary to remove the cell wall and produce a cellular unit that

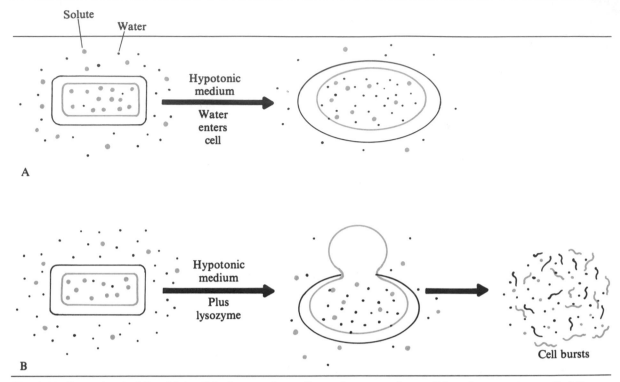

Fig. 3-11. Osmosis. A. Microbial cell in hypotonic medium takes water into cell but does not burst. B. Microbial cell in hypotonic medium containing lysozyme. As lysozyme degrades cell wall, water is taken into the cell, which causes cytoplasmic membrane to expand and eventually burst.

possesses an intact cytoplasmic membrane. This can be accomplished through the use of the enzyme *lysozyme,* which cleaves specific bonds in the peptidoglycan, and by placing the cells in a hypertonic medium. Once the wall has been digested, one of two types of intact cell membrane unit is produced: a *protoplast* or a *spheroplast.* Protoplasts possess no cell wall material and are produced from gram-positive cells but spheroplasts possess some cell wall remnants and are produced from gram-negative bacteria (Fig. 3-12). In a hypertonic medium the protoplast or spheroplast does not burst because a hypertonic medium contains a high concentration of solutes. These solutes exert enough pressure outside the cell to counterbalance the pressure from the solutes inside the cell that push against the cytoplasmic membrane.

One genus of bacteria called *Mycoplasma* lacks a cell wall. These bacteria can survive with-

out walls because their cytoplasmic membranes are fortified by the inclusion of large molecules called sterols. These organisms grow very slowly and require special media for laboratory cultivation.

EXTRACELLULAR POLYMERIC SUBSTANCES (CAPSULES AND SLIME LAYERS)

The bacterial cell may possess polymeric substances that are attached externally to the cell wall. These extracellular polymeric substances (EPS) are composed primarily of polysaccharides, but a few bacteria, such as *bacillus anthracis,* have polypeptide EPS. EPS are considered *capsules* if they exhibit some organization and adhere strongly to the cell wall. Loosely organized EPS that are not strongly attached to the cell wall are called *slime layers.* The EPS do not

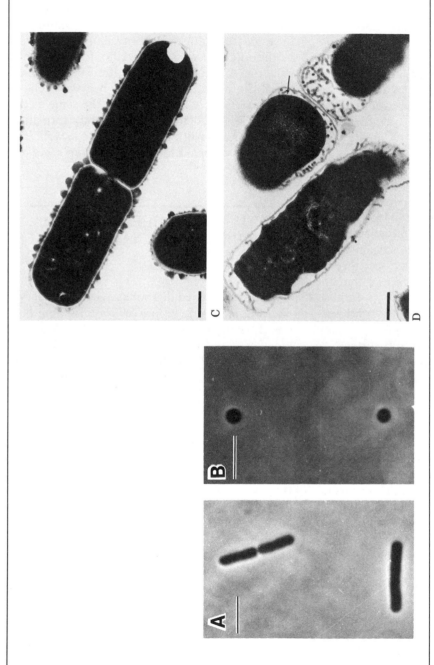

Fig. 3-12. Protoplast and spheroplast formation. Phase contrast micrographs of untreated bacillus (A) and spherical shape of protoplast (B). Bar = 2μm. Transmission electron micrograph of untreated bacillus (C) and spheroplast (D). Arrow points to cytoplasmic membrane, which is now widely separated from cell wall. Bar = 0.2μm. (From H. Connell, J. Lemmon, and G. W. Tannock, *Appld. Environ. Microbiol.* 54:1615,1988.)

take up ordinary stains; therefore they can be demonstrated by suspending the bacteria in a solution containing colloidal particles such as India ink or by using stains that "stain" the background (Plate 6). The particles cannot penetrate the EPS; therefore, the cell appears to have a halo. EPS are not necessary for the survival of the cell, and continued cultivation of an organism in the laboratory may result in the eventual loss of EPS. The capsule can perform some functions that may play a role in disease:

1. Adherence. Microorganisms can use the capsule for adherence to other members of their species to form colonies or to adhere to various surfaces. Adherence to human cells via EPS appears to be necessary for oral microorganisms such as *Streptococcus mutans,* the organism associated with the formation of cavities in teeth (caries). This organism synthesizes EPS that are polymers of glucose (glucans) as well as fructose (fructans). These polymers bind to the tooth surface and enable other bacteria to bind. Eventually a film called *plaque* covers the tooth surface.

2. Inhibition of phagocytosis. Phagocytosis is a process, carried out by certain blood or tissue cells, in which foreign objects, such as bacteria, are ingested. Ingested bacteria are usually destroyed by the phagocytic cells. Phagocytosis is, therefore, a defense measure on the part of the host's immune system. Some bacteria can resist phagocytosis because they possess extracellular molecules in the form of capsules or slime layers. *Streptococcus pneumoniae,* for example, can resist phagocytosis only if the strains of that species produce a capsule. The capsules and slime layers of some bacteria do not prevent phagocytosis. In addition, some of the encapsulated bacteria that are not ingested by phagocytes do not necessarily cause disease.

3. Antigenic activity. The term *antigen* refers to molecules, such as proteins and polysaccharides, that stimulate the formation of antibodies when injected into a mammalian host. Antibodies in effect can neutralize the activity of the antigen, which may be a molecule or a whole cell. The EPS of infectious microorganisms such as *Streptococcus pneumoniae* and *Hemophilus influenzae* are antigenic and have been purified and used as vaccines to prevent disease caused by these microorganisms. Antigenicity is also used in the identification of specific EPS-producing bacteria. Antibodies to a specific EPS can be applied to a culture of unknown bacterial cells. If the bacteria have an EPS that is the same as that of the EPS used to induce antibody formation, the antibodies will cause the EPS to swell. This swelling is referred to as the *quellung reaction.*

FLAGELLA AND OTHER STRUCTURES ASSOCIATED WITH MOVEMENT

Bacteria suspended in a solution can be observed microscopically to be moving in a random fashion. This random movement is called *brownian movement* and is due to bombardment by water molecules on the surface of the cell. Many bacteria, however, are capable of independent and directed movement that is directly related to the presence of protein appendages called *flagella.* A bacterial cell may have a single flagellum or more than one, depending on the species (Fig. 3-13). The flagellum, which consists of a filament, hook, and basal body, may be 20 μm in length (Fig. 3-14). The rings observed in the basal body differ between gram-positive and gram-negative bacteria, but their function remains the same—anchoring the flagellum to the cytoplasmic membrane and in some instances to the cell wall as well.

Flagella-like filaments called *axial filaments* are found in the group of bacteria called spirochetes. Axial filaments are chemically and structurally similar to flagella, but they do not emanate from the surface of the cell. Axial filaments are located beneath the outer surface of the bacterial cell. They appear to originate at the poles of the organism and then wrap themselves about the

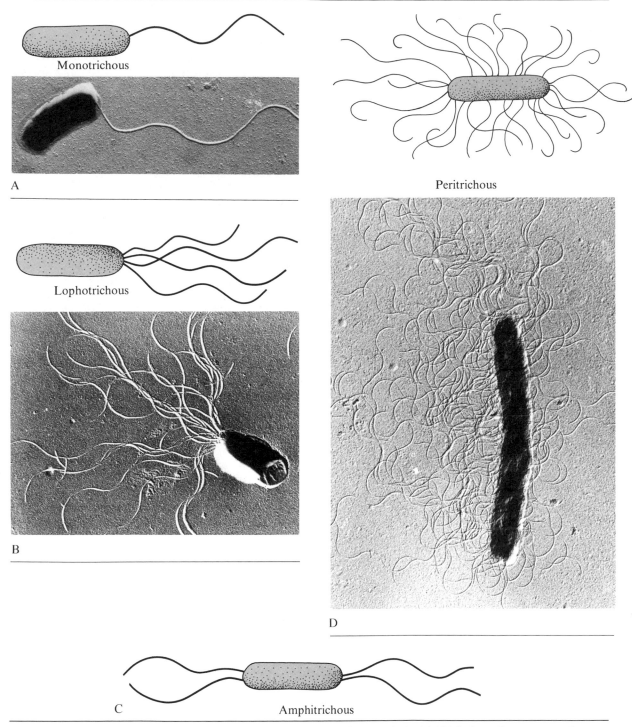

Fig. 3-13. Flagellar arrangement. A. Monotrichous. Electron micrograph ($\times$24,000 before 50 percent reduction). B. Lophotrichous. Electron micrograph ($\times$30,000 before 59 percent reduction). C. Amphitrichous. D. Peritrichous. Electron micrograph ($\times$24,000 before 44 percent reduction). (Electron micrographs courtesy of W. Hodgkiss.)

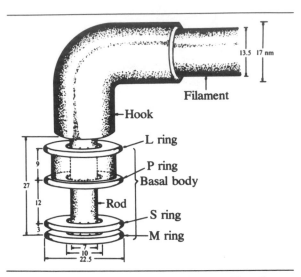

Fig. 3-14. Prokaryotic flagellar structure. Flagellum consists of filament, hook, and basal body. In gram-negative cells the L and P rings are anchored to the outer membrane of the cell wall, and the S and M rings are attached to the cytoplasmic membrane. In gram-positive cells the flagellum has only S and M rings. (From M. L. DePamphilus and J. Adler, *J. Bacteriol.* 105:384,1971.)

body of the spirochete (Fig. 3-15). Axial filaments are, therefore, not exposed to the external environment as are the flagella of other bacteria. Axial filaments are not hindered by the viscosity of the medium; thus, spirochetes can move more rapidly through viscous media than can flagellated bacteria.

Flagella are not an essential requirement for survival of the cell, but they do provide certain advantages. The involuntary movement of an organism in response to stimuli is called *taxis,* or a tactic response. Tactic responses are absolutely dependent on the possession of motility. Taxes result in the accumulation of bacteria in physiologically favorable environments; they may also prevent accumulation in unfavorable environments. Stimulants of taxes include nutrients (chemotaxis), air (*aerotaxis*), or light (*phototaxis*). Flagella may also help the bacterial cell to attach to surfaces including epithelial cells.

Rotation of flagella provides the cell with movement and is a consequence of the activity of the basal body. Flagellar rotation occurs in a direction opposite to that of the body of the cell (Fig. 3-16). When flagellar rotation is counter-

Fig. 3-15. Axial filaments. A. Electron micrograph of axial filaments (*arrow*) as they appear to wind around the body of the spirochete. B. A diagrammatic representation of the micrograph is also presented. (From M. A. Listgarten and S. S. Socransky, *J. Bacteriol.* 88:1087,1964.)

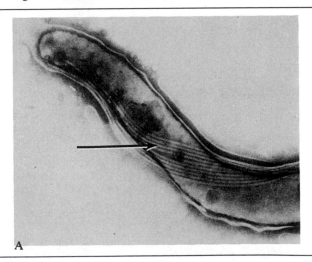

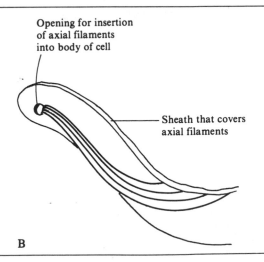

clockwise the bacterium swims smoothly toward an attractant. In the presence of a repellent the flagellar rotation is clockwise and the cell demonstrates a tumbling effect (Fig. 3-16B) in order to get away from the repellent.

PILI (FIMBRIAE)

Pili (singular, pilus) are protein appendages that project from the surface of the cell but are shorter than flagella (Fig. 3-17). Pili range in length from 0.03 μm to 0.2 μm. The term *fimbriae* frequently is used synonymously with pili by some in the scientific community. We will consider pili to be of two types, *sex pili* and *attachment* or *common pili*. Sex pili are found primarily on gram-negative bacteria. They are few in number (1–3) and are involved in transport of DNA between donor and recipient cell in the process called conjugation (see Chapter 6). Attachment or common pili, which are found in great numbers on the surface of the cell, are used for adhesion to various surfaces including plant and animal cells. Adherence to plant and animal cells is often an important factor in the infectious disease process (see Chapter 9). Attachment pili are found primarily in gram-negative bacteria, but some species of gram-positive bacteria, such as *Corynebacterium renale* and *Actinomyces naeslundii,* also possess them.

STRUCTURES WITHIN THE CYTOPLASM

NUCLEOIDS

Bacteria possess no nuclear membrane but do have areas of DNA concentration, called *nu-*

Fig. 3-16. Flagellar rotation. A. Rotation of a polar flagellum counterclockwise (*left*) results in smooth swimming with flagellum trailing cell. Clockwise rotation (*right*) causes cell to tumble with flagellum ahead of cell. B. In a peritrichously flagellated cell counterclockwise rotation causes flagella to form bundle and cell swims smoothly. When rotation of flagella is clockwise the flagella fly apart and cell tumbles.

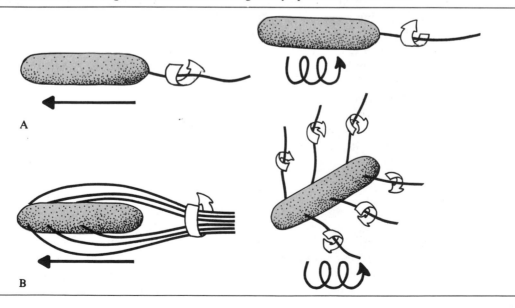

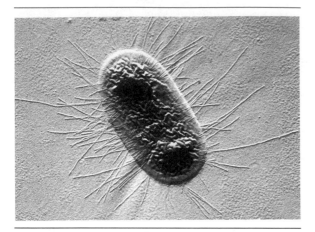

Fig. 3-17. Negatively stained electron micrograph of pili (fimbriae) covering the surface of *E. coli*. (From S. Knutton et al., *Infect. Immun.* 44:514,1984.)

cleoids (Fig. 3-18). The bacterial DNA molecule is circular and is not associated with proteins, as is eukaryotic DNA. The DNA in bacterial cells such as *Escherichia coli* can be carefully removed from the cell and when spread out is 1100 to 1400 μm long. DNA, therefore, is considerably condensed in the cell. Before bacterial cells divide, DNA is replicated while still attached to membranous areas called mesosomes (see Fig. 3-1). Since each cell will receive a copy of DNA, it is not surprising that the nuclear material can be observed at the center of the cell and site of cell division (septum). The number of nucleoids seen in the cell is usually dependent on the growth rate. When bacteria are dividing very rapidly, as many as four nucleoids can be observed in each bacterial cell, but only one nucleoid may be observed if the bacteria are dividing very slowly.

RIBOSOMES

Ribosomes are structures involved in protein synthesis in the cell. They are composed of approximately 60 percent RNA and 40 percent protein. When thin sections of bacteria are observed microscopically, ribosomes can be seen to fill the cytoplasm (Fig. 3-18). They may make up as much as 50 percent of the dry weight of the cell when it is growing very rapidly.

INCLUSION BODIES (INTRACELLULAR INCLUSIONS)

Bacterial growth under certain conditions can result in the accumulation of particles within the cytoplasm of the cell. These particles may or may not be covered with a membrane. Many of these inclusion bodies are observed in microorganisms found in the soil and water, where nutrient deprivation often occurs. These organisms are, however, not infectious for humans. *Gas vacuoles* in aquatic bacteria, *polyhedral bodies* in organisms that use CO_2 as a carbon source, and *sulfur granules* in bacteria that oxidize hydrogen sulfide are examples of inclusions in bacteria that do not cause disease in humans.

Inclusions found in bacteria that infect humans are *glycogen, lipid,* and *polyphosphate granules*. Glycogen is a polymer of glucose that can be used as a source of energy or carbon or both by the bacterial cell. Lipid storage in the cell often takes the form of polyhydroxybutyrate granules (Fig. 3-19). Inorganic phosphate is stored by the bacterial cell in the form of polyphosphate granules. These granules are also called volutin or *metachromatic granules*.

ENDOSPORES

Cells that are engaged in active growth and reproduction are referred to as *vegetative cells* or as being in the vegetative state of growth. There are several groups of microorganisms, including bacteria, that under environmental stress (nutrient depletion or oxygen depletion, for example) are capable of ceasing vegetative growth and producing intracellular bodies called *endospores*. Endospores are produced by gram-positive bacteria. The two most important genera of bacteria

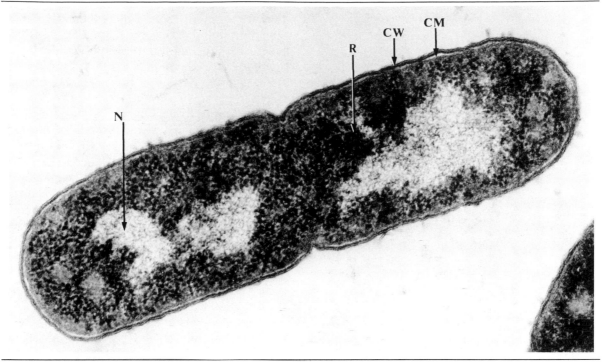

Fig. 3-18. Electron micrograph of *E. coli* demonstrating nucleoids and ribosomes. The dark dot-like areas around nucleoids (N) are ribosomes (R). CW = cell wall, CM = cytoplasmic membrane. (Courtesy of A. Ryter, Institute of Pasteur.)

causing disease and also producing endospores are *Bacillus* and *Clostridium*. *Bacillus anthracis,* for example, is the cause of anthrax, an invariably fatal disease in cattle that may also affect humans, while *Bacillus cereus* is a cause of food poisoning in humans. *Clostridium* species such as *C. botulinum, C. tetani,* and *C. perfringens* are the cause of human diseases such as botulism, tetanus, and gas gangrene, respectively. A knowledge of endospore-forming bacteria is important to allied health personnel because the spore is resistant to high temperatures, chemicals, and radiation that would normally kill nonsporeforming bacteria. The endospore is a highly refractile body that is difficult to stain but it can be observed easily in the unstained condition (Fig. 3-20). Once environmental conditions are suitable for growth the endospore can be induced to return to the vegetative state. The endospore

represents the bacterial cell's mechanism for surviving under unsuitable conditions.

The Sporulation Process

During endospore formation the following events occur (Fig. 3-21). The DNA material is extended along the entire length of the cell. The cell membrane invaginates, the DNA becomes compartmentalized, and a second membrane is formed around the unit, which can now be called a *forespore.* A peptidoglycan is synthesized and laid down between the two membranes of the forespore. This peptidoglycan layer, called the *cortex,* differs chemically from the peptidoglycan of the vegetative cell. Within the area surrounded by the cortex is a compound called *calcium dipicolinate,* which is found only in endospores. Thick coats of peptides that are impermeable to

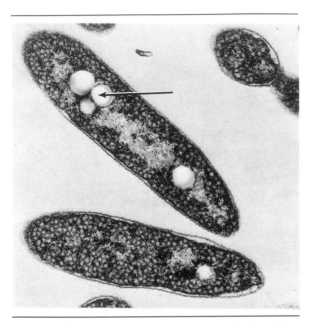

Fig. 3-19. Electron micrograph (× 43,000 before 23 percent reduction) of a species of *Rhodopseudomonas* containing membrane-bound inclusions of polyhydroxybutyrate (*arrow*). (From M. Madigan et al., *J. Bacteriol.* 150:1422,1982.)

water are laid down around the cortex. Completion of the spore coats signals the end of endospore formation. The spore may be located at the poles or at other various positions in the cell. The spore is released into the environment as soon as the vegetative portion of the cell disintegrates.

The mechanisms for resistance of spores to chemical and physical agents is not completely understood. For example, the degree of dehydration (loss of free water) is believed to be an important mechanism for resistance to heat. The greater the degree of dehydration, the greater the resistance to heat. Vegetative bacterial cells are usually killed at temperatures of 70°C and above, but spores can resist boiling temperatures for several hours. Only temperatures of 121°C for at least 15 minutes at 15 pounds of pressure per square inch will ensure destruction of the most heat-resistant endospores. Preventing spores from contaminating food, wounds, dressings, etc. and various medical objects that come into contact with the human body is of obvious importance to medical personnel. Once the spore ger-

Fig. 3-20. Electron micrograph (× 76,250 before 23 percent reduction) of ultrathin section of sporulating *Clostridium bifermentans*. The spore is the white refractile body in the cell. (From P. D. Walker, *J. Appld. Microbiol.* 33:1,1970.)

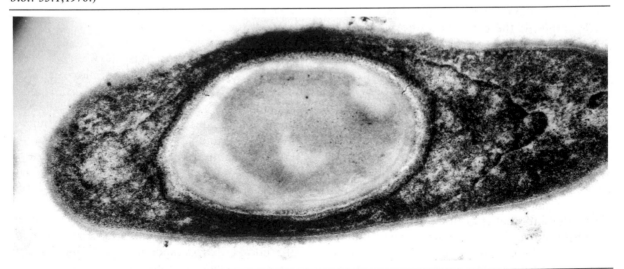

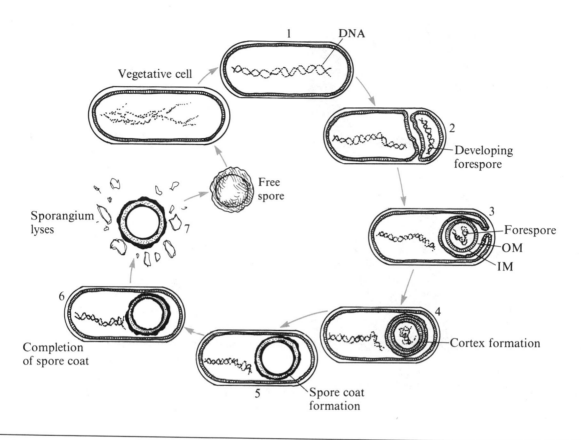

Fig. 3-21. Events in sporulation process. See text for details. (OM = outer membrane; IM = inner membrane.)

minates the vegetative cell may reproduce and cause disease.

The Germination Process

A spore may remain dormant for hundreds of years before becoming transformed into a vegetative cell. The transformation is related not to the age of the spore but to the need for certain environmental conditions. Before germination takes place, the spore must first be activated—for example, by heat in the presence of water, although other agents or conditions may also initiate activation. Once activated, the spore enters the stage of germination, in which portions of the spore coats become degraded. In the presence of growth-supporting nutrients the germinating spore swells and enters a period of biosynthetic activity in which vegetative cellular components are produced. This period ends with release of the spore coat and the initiation of vegetative growth (Fig. 3-22).

SUMMARY

1. The basic distinction between prokaryotes or bacteria and all other organisms is the nuclear membrane—present in eukaryotes and absent in

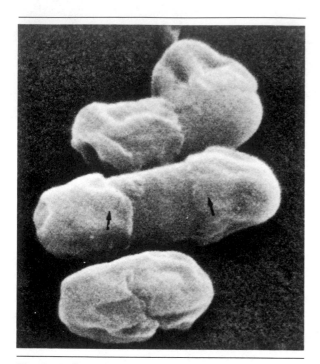

Fig. 3-22. Scanning electron micrograph of spores in the process of germination and loss of spore coat (*arrows*). (Courtesy Z. Yoshii.)

prokaryotes. Other characteristics separating prokaryotes from eukaryotes are outlined in Table 3-1.

2. Bacteria are given names (nomenclature) based on certain criteria. They are given Latin or Greek names that usually describe an important characteristic of the organism. Bacteria, like other organisms, are classified into various units, called taxa, based on the species, the fundamental unit of classification. The main purpose of classification is to distinguish one group of organisms from another, while nomenclature provides a convenient system of communication to define an organism without having to list all the characteristics of the species.

3. The most widely accepted scheme of bacterial classification is Bergey's Manual of Determinative Bacteriology. The various taxonomic groups have been arrived at on the basis of identification of specific characteristics, such as biochemical properties and physiological traits. Biochemical similarities and differences can be tested by determining DNA relatedness between two organisms.

4. Bacteria range in size from 0.2 to 60 μm in length, but those bacteria infectious for humans are usually 1.0 to 3.0 μm in length. There are four basic shapes of bacteria: spherical (coccus), rod-shaped (bacillus), spiral, and square.

5. Bacterial morphology, even in a single species, may vary depending on the growth conditions. Such morphological variation is referred to as pleomorphism, and this prevents taxonomists from using size as a criterion in classification.

6. All bacteria, except *Mycoplasma*, have cell walls and are divided into two basic groups: gram-positive and gram-negative. This separation is based on the chemical composition of the cell wall and its response to specific reagents during the Gram-staining procedure. In addition to the cell wall, other structures found in bacteria and their function are outlined in Table 3-3.

QUESTIONS FOR STUDY

Select the best response or responses for each of the following:

1. Which of the following group of characteristics describes a eukaryote?
   A. Any organism that possesses a nuclear membrane, has membranes containing sterols, can engage only in sexual or asexual activity, and possesses a cell wall.
   B. Any organism that possesses a nuclear membrane, can engage only in sexual ac-

Table 3-3. Summary of Prokaryotic Structure and Function

Structure	Chemical composition	Function
Cell wall		Cell shape and protection of cytoplasmic contents
Gram-positive	Mainly peptidoglycan plus teichoic acid	—
Gram-negative	Very little peptidoglycan: outer membrane multilayered, containing phospholipid, lipopolysaccharide, and protein	—
Cytoplasmic membrane	Phospholipid bilayer containing globular proteins	Controls movement of solutes into cell; site of respiratory enzymes; secretes cytoplasmic products; contains enzymes for cell wall synthesis; site of DNA synthesis
Extracellular polymeric substances	Single polysaccharides; mixed polysaccharides, or proteins	Adherence to substrates, inhibition of phagocytosis
Flagella	Protein	Movement
Pili	Protein	Conjugation in gram-negative bacteria; adherence to inanimate and animate surfaces
Nucleoid	DNA	Carries hereditary information
Ribosomes	RNA and protein	Protein synthesis
Inclusion bodies		
Glycogen	Polysaccharide (glucose)	Storage form of energy
Polyhydroxybutyrate	Lipid	Storage form of energy
Volutin (metachromatic granules)	Polyphosphate	?
Endospores	Complex peptidoglycan unit containing calcium dipicolinate; a dehydrated form of the vegetative cell	Protection from environmental stresses of a chemical or physical nature

tivity, has mitochondria associated with respiration, and may or may not possess a cell wall.

C. Any organism that possesses a nuclear membrane, has membranes containing sterols, has mitochondria associated with respiration, and possesses more than one chromosome.

D. Any organism that possesses a nuclear membrane, has membranes containing sterols, has mitochondria associated with respiration, and can engage in sexual or asexual activity.

2. Which of the following group of characteristics describes the staphylococci?

A. Gram-positive; thick peptidoglycan layer; appear in grape-like clusters; give rise to protoplasts in hypertonic medium plus lysozyme.

B. Gram-positive; thick peptidoglycan layer; produce long filaments in the presence of penicillin; give rise to protoplasts in hypertonic medium plus lysozyme.

C. Gram-positive; thin peptidoglycan layer; produce long filaments in the presence of penicillin; appear in grape-like clusters.

D. Gram-positive; appear in grape-like clusters; give rise to spheroplasts in hypertonic medium plus lysozyme; thick peptidoglycan layer.

3. Which of the following best describes active transport?
    A. Solutes move from an area of high concentration to an area of low solute concentration helped by carriers and an expenditure of energy.
    B. Solutes passively move from an area of high concentration to an area of low solute concentration.
    C. Carriers transport solutes from an area of low solute concentration to an area of higher solute concentration with an expenditure of energy.
    D. Solutes passively move from an area of low concentration to an area of higher solute concentration.

4. Which of the following group of characteristics best describes a gram-negative bacterium?

A. Possesses thin peptidoglycan layer; produces spheroplasts in hypertonic medium plus lysozyme; produces endotoxin; produces endospores
B. Possesses thin peptidoglycan layer; produces protoplasts in hypertonic medium plus lysozyme; produces endotoxin; does not produce endospores
C. Possesses thin peptidoglycan layer; produces spheroplasts in hypertonic medium plus lysozyme; produces endotoxin; produces endospores
D. Possesses thick peptidoglycan layer; produces spheroplasts in hypertonic medium plus lysozyme; produces endotoxin; produces endospores

5. Which of the following characteristics describes a stage or process in sporulation?
    A. A special peptidoglycan, called the cortex, is produced.
    B. Free water is absorbed by the developing spore.
    C. The DNA becomes compartmentalized.
    D. The synthesis of calcium dipicolinate.

Fill in the blank:

6. A member of a species that possesses a property distinct from another member of the same species is called a _____ of the species.

7. The _____, _____, and _____ of the bacterial cell can all help in adherence to substrates such as tissue.

8. The genus of bacteria that does not possess cell walls is the _____.

9. The area between the cell wall and cytoplasmic membrane in the gram-negative cell is called the _____.

10. The group of bacteria whose flagella are not in contact with their environment outside the cell are called the _____.

ADDITIONAL READINGS

Berg, H. C. How bacteria swim. *Sci. Am*. 250:36,1984.

Beveridge, T. J. Ultrastructure, chemistry and function of the bacterial cell wall. *Int. Rev. Cytol*. 72:229,1981.

Ferris, F. G., and Beveridge, T. J. Functions of bacterial cell surface structures. *Bioscience* 35:172,1985.

Ludish, H., and Rothman, J. E. The assembly of cell membranes. *Sci. Am*. 240:48,1979.

Rogers, H. J. *Bacterial Cell Structure*. Aspects of Microbiology. Washington, DC: American Society for Microbiology, 1983.

Stanier, R. Y., Rogers, H. J., and Ward, J. B. (eds.). *Relation between Structure and Function in the Prokaryotic Cell,* Twenty-eighth Symposium of the Society for General Microbiology. New York: Cambridge University Press, 1978.

4. MICROBIAL METABOLISM

OBJECTIVES

To explain how enzymes are able to speed up chemical reactions

To discuss the factors affecting enzyme activity

To explain the difference between substrate level phosphorylation and electron transport phosphorylation

To explain the relationship between electron transport, energy, and ATP formation

To explain the differences and similarities, if any, between fermentation and respiration

To explain the specific functions of the glycolytic pathway, Krebs cycle, and electron transport chain in aerobic respiration

To explain what cellular conditions are needed for biosynthesis to be initiated in the cell

To explain how allosteric enzymes control metabolic activity

To define: coenzyme, energy of activation, denaturation, dehydrogenation, beta oxidation, feedback inhibition

The primary function of all living material is to grow and reproduce. Both growth and reproduction rely on the outcome of chemical reactions in the cell. The sum of all cellular chemical reactions is referred to as *metabolism*. The metabolic process that involves the degradation of chemical components is called *catabolism*, while the synthesis of chemical components is called *anabolism* or *biosynthesis*. Catabolic processes are important because they result in the formation of molecules, such as adenosine triphosphate (ATP), which are immediate sources of energy. Energy is used to synthesize the necessary molecules that will become important components of the cell. In this chapter we will see the importance of enzymes in metabolic processes and then describe some of the more important metabolic processes that occur in the microbial cell.

ENZYMES: BIOLOGICAL CATALYSTS

GENERAL CHARACTERISTICS

Most metabolic processes in the cell would take forever if it were not for enzymes. Enzymes are proteins that have molecular weights ranging from 600 to 12,000. Their function is to speed up the various chemical reactions that occur in the cell. Molecules that speed up chemical reactions are called *catalysts*. Enzymes often cannot function alone and require additional molecules, called *cofactors*, to enhance activity. Some cofactors are organic molecules, such as vitamins, and are referred to as *coenzymes*. Inorganic co-factors are metal ions such as calcium, zinc, and magnesium. How cofactors enhance enzyme activity will be discussed shortly.

HOW ENZYMES SPEED UP CHEMICAL REACTIONS

In every cellular chemical reaction there is a molecule or molecules, called *substrates* (S), that interact with enzymes (E) and are converted to products (P). The reaction can be written:

$$S + E \rightleftharpoons ES \rightarrow P + E$$

$$\text{E-S complex}$$

Chemical reactions involve the making and breaking of bonds, and this requires energy, also called the *energy of activation*. In the example below an amino acid such as alanine can have its amino group (NH_2) removed (deamination), resulting in the formation of a product called pyruvic acid:

H—C—C—COOH → H—C—C—COOH + NH_2

Alanine   Pyruvic acid

The bond holding NH_2 to the remainder of the molecule must be broken for this reaction to occur, and this requires a certain amount of energy. The activation energy could be supplied in the form of heat, but the amount of heat required would literally burn up the cell. The cell, however, is supplied with enzymes that act as substitutes for heat energy. Enzymes lower the energy of activation. The question is, how do enzymes do this?

Enzymes, because they are proteins, are made up of a chain or chains of amino acids (also called polypeptide chain) that are folded in such a way as to resemble a globular shape. This folding produces specific arrangements in which certain amino acids are brought into close contact. For example, an amino acid at one end of the chain can be brought into close proximity to the amino acid at the opposite end of the chain by the way the enzyme is folded (Fig. 4-1). The folding of the protein and arrangement of various amino acids in the enzyme produces a specific conformational site, called the *active site*, where the substrates of a chemical reaction can bind (Fig. 4-1). Thus, there is a conformational specificity between substrate and enzyme—a lock-and-key relationship. There are about 1000 different enzymes in a microbial cell, and since the sequence of amino aids in each of them is different, the locks and keys are also different. The active site usually possesses amino acids that have a positively or negatively charged group, for example, an NH_3^+ or COO^- group. These charged groups help to bind substrate but it is the conformation of the active site that is the major determinant of specificity with a substrate. To simplify our discussion about how the active site is involved in bond breaking or bond making, we will use the following example. Suppose a substrate consists of a long chain of repeating units that we wish to cleave into smaller fragments. The fragments could be produced by heating the substrate in a test tube containing water. The heating process causes the molecules of water to collide with the substrate and bonds are broken—sometimes the broken bonds are the ones we want, and sometimes they are not. Enzymes can also break bonds, but with lower energy requirements, because they bring the substrate, and the specific bonds to be broken, to the active site. The active site possesses amino acids with charged groups that take part in bond breaking (Fig. 4-2). Inorganic factors, such as calcium, carry positive charges, which are believed to aid in the binding of substrate to active site, while many vitamins (Table 4-1) act as carriers of small chemical

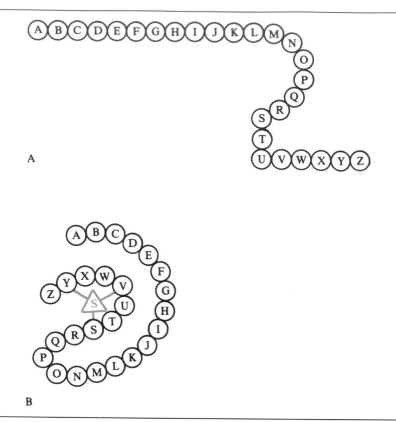

Fig. 4-1. How the polypeptide chain of a protein is folded to produce a globular shape. Each sphere in the chain represents an amino acid. A. Linear arrangement of amino acids in the polypeptide chain. B. Folding of polypeptide chain produces globular shape and close contact between amino acids B and X. The folding of the polypeptide produces a site where substrate (S) can bind by contact with amino acids S, V, and Y.

groups that are part of the enzymatic reaction. Since the enzyme itself is not altered in the chemical reaction, it is free to engage other substrate molecules once the product is released from the enzyme.

FACTORS AFFECTING ENZYME ACTIVITY

Enzymes are proteins subject to the same chemical and physical factors that affect other proteins. Conditions such as hydrogen ion concentration, temperature, etc. that alter the shape of the protein also affect its catalytic activity.

Hydrogen Ion Activity

The hydrogen ion concentration, or pH, greatly influences the activity of enzymes. The amino acids in enzymes can take up hydrogen ions (H^+) in acid solution and release them in alkaline (OH^-) solutions. For example, the COO^- group and the NH_2 group on an amino acid such as alanine take up H^+ in acid solution and become positively charged:

$$H\!-\!\overset{\overset{\displaystyle H}{|}}{\underset{\underset{\displaystyle H}{|}}{C}}\!-\!\overset{\overset{\displaystyle NH_2}{|}}{\underset{\underset{\displaystyle H}{|}}{C}}\!-\!COO^- + H^+ \rightarrow H\!-\!\overset{\overset{\displaystyle H}{|}}{\underset{\underset{\displaystyle H}{|}}{C}}\!-\!\overset{\overset{\displaystyle NH_3{}^+}{|}}{\underset{\underset{\displaystyle H}{|}}{C}}\!-\!COOH$$

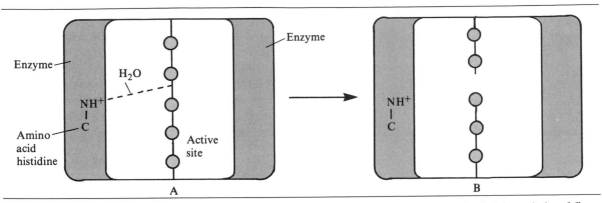

Fig. 4-2. Diagrammatic representation of mechanism of action of enzymes. Substrate (*color*) is a chain of five identical subunits that can be separated by breaking one of the bonds that hold them together. A. The active site possesses a charged group NH^+, belonging to the amino acid histidine, which in the presence of water (H_2O) breaks the bond, separating the subunits of the substrate. B. Substrate is cleaved into two fragments.

but release hydrogen ions in alkaline solution and become negatively charged:

$$H—\overset{\overset{\displaystyle H}{|}}{\underset{\underset{\displaystyle H}{|}}{C}}—\overset{\overset{\displaystyle NH_3{}^+}{|}}{\underset{\underset{\displaystyle H}{|}}{C}}—COOH + OH^- \rightarrow$$

$$H—\overset{\overset{\displaystyle H}{|}}{\underset{\underset{\displaystyle H}{|}}{C}}—\overset{\overset{\displaystyle NH_2}{|}}{\underset{\underset{\displaystyle H}{|}}{C}}—COO^- + HOH$$

In addition, sulfur-sulfur (S-S) bonds in proteins can also take on hydrogen ions to become sulfhydryl (SH) groups. (See Boxed Essay.) Most enzymes in the cell are active at pHs between 5 and 8 (Fig. 4-3).

Temperature

The most favorable temperature for enzyme activity in most biological systems is 37°C. In measuring enzyme activity as a function of temperature there is a doubling of activity for every 10°C increase in temperature. As the temperature increases, however, there is a point where the enzyme molecule begins to unfold and activity drops off very quickly. This unfolding process is called *denaturation* (*see* Fig. 4-4). As you will see

Table 4-1. Vitamins and Their Function in Microbial Metabolism

Vitamin	Function
Thiamine	A coenzyme involved in decarboxylation reactions
Riboflavin	As part of the flavin adenine dinucleotide molecule is a coenzyme involved in electron transport
Niacin	As part of the nicotinamide adenine dinucleotide (NAD) or NADP molecule is a coenzyme involved in electron transport
Pantothenic acid	As part of coenzyme A (CoA) molecule functions as carrier of acyl groups
Pyridoxal	Functions as coenzyme; important in amino acid metabolism, particularly in group transfer reactions involving the amino (NH_2) group
Biotin	Coenzyme important as carrier of CO_2
Folic acid	Acts as a carrier of formyl (HCHO) group. Very important in purine biosynthesis
Vitamin B_{12}	Coenzyme functioning as a carrier of alkyl groups

Sulfur and Enzymatic Activity

Sulfur is an element required by all living cells. It is a component of the amino acid cysteine, in which it can exist as a *sulfhydryl* (*SH*) group, i.e.,

$$SH-CH_2-\overset{\overset{\displaystyle H}{|}}{\underset{\underset{\displaystyle NH_3^+}{|}}{C}}-COO^-$$

Cysteine

Cysteine plays a particularly important role in protein structure because the sulfur of one cysteine can bond with the sulfur of another cysteine residue in the protein to form a disulfide (S-S) bond. For example, some enzymes have 8 cysteine residues that produce 4 disulfide bonds. When these disulfide bonds are formed the enzyme assumes a particular configuration. The activity of enzymes relies on specific configurations and if these configurations are disturbed enzyme activity is decreased or lost completely. Cysteine can exist in either a reduced or oxidized form. In the oxidized form (loss of hydrogen) the sulfurs of cysteines in the protein molecule are devoid of their hydrogens and they can form disulfide bonds. In a reduced form the sulfur of cysteine exists as a sulfhydryl (SH) group and disulfide bonds cannot form in the protein. For example, if an enzyme in its natural configuration contains 4 disulfide bonds, we can add a reducing agent that will break the disulfide bonds and the protein will assume a different configuration:

Active enzyme with
4 disulfide bonds

Reducing agent

Inactive enzyme (disulfide bonds broken and sulfhydryl groups produced)

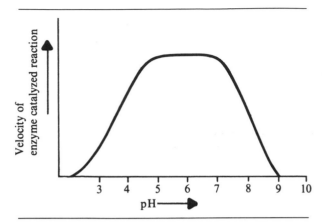

Fig. 4-3. Effect of hydrogen ion (pH) concentration on enzyme activity.

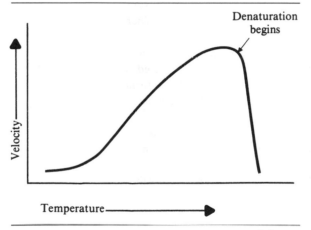

Fig. 4-4. Effect of temperature on enzyme activity.

later, heating is a technique for killing microorganisms.

Substrate Concentration

When substantial amounts of enzyme are present, the rate of the catalyzed reaction is directly proportional to the substrate concentration, provided all other factors, such as pH and temperature, have been standardized. As the substrate concentration is increased a point is reached at which all of the enzyme is in the form of an ES complex and the velocity of the reaction is at a maximum (Fig. 4-5) and independent of substrate concentration. Further increases in substrate concentration produce no further increase in activity, and only by adding more enzyme can the maximum velocity be increased.

Inhibitors

In medicine the control of some infectious diseases is generally based on the control of microorganisms. Agents that affect enzyme activity also affect the growth of microorganisms. Scientists are continually looking for chemical agents that selectively inhibit microbial enzymes without affecting host enzymes. Most of the chemical agents that show this selective inhibition are antibiotics, which are discussed in *Chapter 8*. Inhibitors of enzyme activity are of two types: *competitive inhibitors* and *noncompetitive inhibitors*. Competitive inhibitors compete with the normal substrate for the active site on the enzyme molecule. The competitive inhibitor has a structure similar to the natural substrate, which enables it to bind to the enzyme, but is different enough that it is not converted to the normal product. The inhibitor forms an enzyme-substrate complex just like the normal substrate. In competitive inhibition the velocity of the reaction is slowed, but the maximum velocity that is characteristic of the reaction in the absence of inhibitors can be obtained if the substrate concentration is increased (Fig. 4-6A). Noncompetitive inhibitors do not bind to the active site but at another site. The noncompetitive inhibitor affects the binding of substrate to the active site, probably by inducing some conformational change in the enzyme. Even if the substrate binds to the active site in the presence of inhibitor, a product may be formed very slowly or not at all. Increasing the substrate concentration will have no effect on enzyme activity in the presence of noncompetitive inhibitors, as it would for competitive inhibitors (Fig. 4-6B).

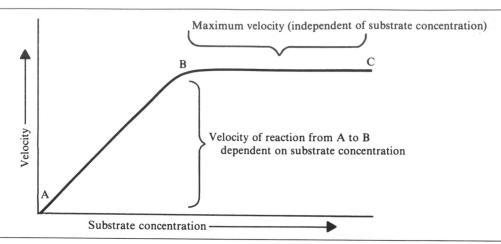

Fig. 4-5. Effect of substrate concentration on enzyme activity.

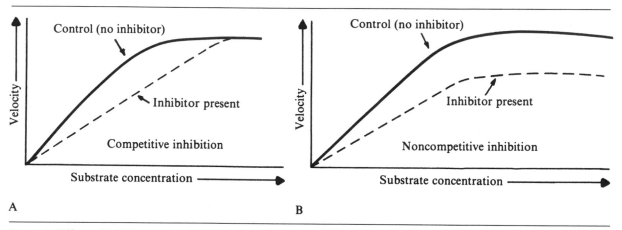

Fig. 4-6. Effect of inhibitors on enzyme activity. A. Competitive inhibitors. B. Noncompetitive inhibitors.

CLASSIFICATION OF ENZYMES

Based on Chemical Reactions

Except for enzymes such as pepsin and chymotrypsin, which were identified and named many years ago, enzymes end in the suffix *-ase*; for example, protease. The first part of the name usually indicates the type of substrate, chemical group, or type of chemical reaction that is catalyzed by the enzyme. Current nomenclature divides all enzyme-catalyzed reactions into the following groups:

1. *Oxidoreductases* are involved in electron (hydrogen) transfer reactions.
2. *Transferases* transfer specific groups such as aldehydes or phosphates from one substrate to another.
3. *Hydrolases* add water across chemical bonds to be cleaved or hydrolyzed.

4. *Lyases* remove chemical groups from substrates, forming double bonds, or add chemical groups to double bonds.
5. *Isomerases* rearrange certain compounds to produce molecules having the same groups of atoms, but in different arrangements.
6. *Ligases* produce bonds accompanied by the cleavage of adenosine triphosphate (ATP).

Based on Biological Activity

Some enzymes synthesized by the cell remain within the cell to carry out specific reactions and are called *endoenzymes*, while others are released from the cell into the surrounding environment and are called *exoenzymes*. Many microbial cells release exoenzymes that attack macromolecules and convert them into smaller units that can be selectively absorbed by the cell, for example, the conversion of the polysaccharide cellulose into units of glucose.

The prefixes *endo-* and *exo-* have also been used to describe the site of enzyme activity on macromolecules. Exoenzymes, for example, catalyze reactions involving the terminal residues on a macromolecule, while endoenzymes catalyze reactions involving residues found in the interior of the molecule.

APPLICATIONS OF MICROBIAL ENZYMES

Enzymes produced by microorganisms have a variety of uses, and some are commercially prepared on a large scale. Protease, an enzyme used to degrade protein by splitting peptide bonds, is obtained from the bacterium *Bacillus licheniformis*. Protease is used as a cleaning aid in detergents. Proteases obtained from other bacteria and from fungi can also be used as digestive aids in animal feeds and as meat tenderizers. Alpha-amylase, glucamylase, and glucose isomerase are bacterial enzymes used to convert starch into a sweetener (high-fructose corn syrup) that is rapidly replacing sucrose in soft drinks.

Proteolytic enzymes, such as streptokinase, are produced extracellularly by species of the bacterium *Streptococcus* and have been used clinically to dissolve fibrin clots because of their ability to convert blood plasminogen to active plasmin, the proteolytic component that breaks down fibrin molecules. Streptokinase is used in the treatment of deep venous thrombosis and massive pulmonary embolisms, conditions that ordinarily require surgical removal of vascular clots.

HOW MICROBIAL CELLS PRODUCE ENERGY

Some microorganisms use sunlight as a source of energy and convert this energy into chemical energy. These organisms are photosynthetic and are not infectious. Some bacteria found in the soil use inorganic elements such as sulfur, iron, etc. as sources of energy, and they too are not infectious. Microorganisms that infect humans must be able to utilize energy sources in a manner similar to that of their hosts. Infectious microorganisms obtain their energy from the degradation of organic molecules. Much of the time these organic sources of energy also provide the microbial cell with the necessary carbon skeletons it needs to synthesize organic molecules. For example, glucose (Fig. 4-7) is used as an energy source and during its degradation the carbons are used by the cell to produce other organic molecules.

ELECTRONS, OXIDATION, AND ENERGY

The release of energy from the degradation of organic molecules is associated with the release of electrons and their subsequent capture by other molecules in the cell. In chemistry the removal of electrons from a substance is called *oxidation*, while the gain of electrons by a substance is called *reduction*. Oxidation of organic molecules usually means the loss of an electron and

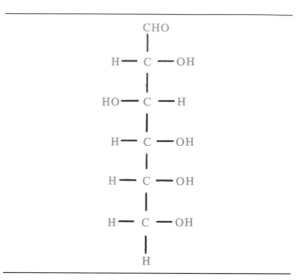

Fig. 4-7. Structure of glucose.

proton together that is a hydrogen atom (H). In the reaction below:

$$AH_2 + B \rightarrow BH_2 + A$$

AH_2 represents a compound (A) that contains hydrogen atoms (H_2) and in the reaction it loses them, that is, A is oxidized. B in the reaction becomes reduced to BH_2 by accepting the hydrogen atoms. In the reaction, AH_2 is considered the electron donor and B the electron acceptor. Oxidations in which H atoms are lost are called *dehydrogenations*.

Electron donors are molecules that release energy, while molecules that accept electrons are not sources of energy. If you observe the structure of glucose (*see* Fig. 4-7), a common source of energy for microorganisms, you see that it possesses many hydrogen atoms and is therefore a source of electrons; that is, it is an *electron donor*. Electrons released as part of hydrogen atoms are first transferred to carrier molecules. One of the most important carrier molecules is called *nicotinamide adenine dinucleotide*, or *NAD*. NAD takes the electrons, which are at a high energy level, and transfers them to a chain of molecules located in the cytoplasmic membrane called the *electron transport chain*. The electrons are transferred in the chain in a manner similar to running water that falls over a series of water wheels. The energy of the water at the top of the cascade (comparable to the energy in the electrons carried by NAD) is released in small increments as it tumbles over each wheel (comparable to the electron transport components). The last wheel might be considered the *final electron acceptor*. What happens to the energy generated during electron transfer?

ADENOSINE TRIPHOSPHATE: THE ENERGY MOLECULE OF THE CELL

The energy released during the transfer of electrons in the electron transport chain is conserved in the cell in the form of ATP. The energy trapped in ATP will be used to perform specific tasks, such as movement, nutrient transport, and biosynthesis. ATP is formed by the addition of phosphate to a molecule of adenosine diphosphate (ADP), a process called *phosphorylation*. Most of the energy in the ATP molecule is actually part of the last two phosphates and is represented as a squiggle (~), that is A-P~P~P. The reaction can be represented as:

$$A\text{-}P{\sim}P + PO_4 + energy \rightarrow A\text{-}P{\sim}P{\sim}P$$
(ADP)   (ATP)

while the reverse reaction releases energy:

$$A\text{-}P{\sim}P{\sim}P \rightarrow A\text{-}P{\sim}P + PO_4 + energy$$

ATP is not the only high-energy molecule used by the cell, but it is the most important one. Other high-energy molecules include acetyl phosphate, phosphoenol pyruvate, and acetyl coenzyme A. Later in the chapter we will see how energy is trapped in the molecule during the transfer of electrons.

Phosphorylation reactions in which ATP is produced can be divided into two types as they relate to infectious microorganisms: *substrate phosphorylation* and *electron transport phosphorylation* (also called *oxidative phosphorylation*). Substrate phosphorylation is a process in which the phosphate to be added to ADP is a high-energy phosphate that is part of a carbon compound in the cell:

$$C\sim PO_4^* + ADP \rightarrow ATP + C$$

*Carbon compound containing high-energy phosphate

Electron transport phosphorylation is a process in which energy released from electron transfer is trapped during the addition of phosphate to ADP. The term oxidative phosphorylation implies that the final electron acceptor is oxygen, but this is not always the case. We will see how substrate and electron transport phosphorylation operate when we discuss fermentation and respiration, metabolic processes that generate energy.

METABOLIC PROCESSES THAT GENERATE ENERGY

FERMENTATION

Fermentation is an oxidation process in which an organic electron donor gives up its electrons to an organic electron acceptor. Oxygen is not involved in fermentation, that is, it is an anaerobic process. A special fermentation process that occurs in most living cells is called *glycolysis* (also called the *Embden-Meyerhoff-Parnas (EMP) pathway*.

Glycolysis
Glycolysis is a metabolic process in which the electron donor is glucose, a six-carbon sugar. Glycolysis can be divided into two groups of reactions (Fig. 4-8). In the first group of reactions

glucose is cleaved, rearranged, and phosphorylated. The net result of this set of reactions is the formation of two 3-carbon molecules, dihydroxyacetone phosphate and glyceraldehyde 3-phosphate, and the consumption of two molecules of ATP. In the second set of reactions two molecules of glyceraldehyde 3-phosphate (dihydroxyacetone phosphate is converted to glyceraldehyde 3-phosphate) are rearranged to form two molecules of pyruvic acid. During the glycolytic oxidation, four molecules of ATP are produced by substrate phosphorylation and electrons are captured by the carrier NAD to form $NADH_2$. The final electron acceptor in glycolysis is *pyruvic acid*, which is converted to lactic acid:

$$\begin{array}{c} H \quad O \\ | \quad \| \\ H-C-C-COOH + NADH_2 \rightarrow \\ | \\ H \end{array}$$

Pyruvic acid

$$\begin{array}{c} H \quad OH \\ | \quad | \\ H-C-C-COOH + NAD \\ | \quad | \\ H \quad H \end{array}$$

Lactic acid

Lactic acid may be a major end product of fermentation for some microorganisms, such as the lactic acid bacteria. Other microorganisms, however, can produce a variety of products from the metabolism of pyruvic acid (Fig. 4-9). Pyruvate or lactate, as well as some of the other products of pyruvic acid metabolism, are incompletely oxidized and as a consequence some of the potential energy they possess is lost. The products of fermentation are excreted by the cell. In order to extract all the potential energy from a molecule such as glucose, it must be completely oxidized to carbon dioxide (CO_2) and water—a process we will discuss shortly.

In the overall process of glycolysis two molecules of ATP are consumed and four molecules of ATP are produced, leaving a net gain of two

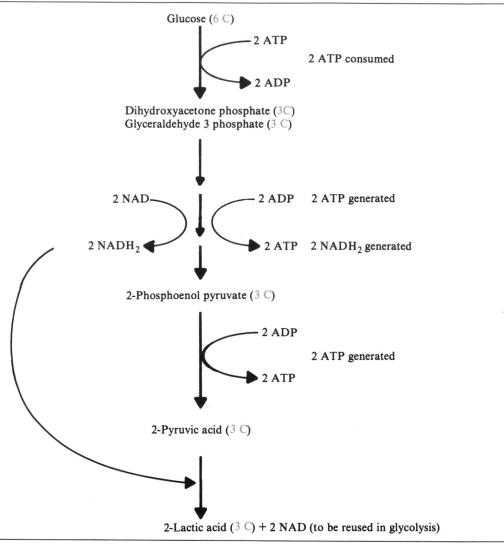

Fig. 4-8. Simplified scheme for glycolysis in which a molecule of glucose is converted to two molecules of pyruvic acid. The number of carbon atoms is indicated in parentheses. Note that dihydroxyacetone phosphate is converted to a molecule of glyceraldehyde 3-phosphate; thus, actually two molecules of glyceraldehyde 3-phosphate are oxidized. NAD is regenerated during the reduction of pyruvic acid to lactic acid by $NADH_2$.

molecules of ATP for every molecule of glucose fermented. Let us look at what happens when glucose is made available to *obligate aerobes, facultative anaerobes*, and *obligate anaerobes*:

1. Obligate aerobes. Obligate aerobes can grow only in the presence of oxygen. Glucose is oxidized to pyruvic acid, but the latter does not remain as the final electron acceptor. Instead, pyruvic acid is completely oxidized to carbon dioxide and water in a process called *aerobic respiration* (to be discussed later). Some microorganisms can use inorganic molecules other than oxygen, such as nitrate, as final electron acceptors.
2. Facultative anaerobes. Facultative anaerobes can grow either in the presence or absence of oxygen. The facultative anaerobe in the presence of oxygen completely oxidizes the organic molecule to carbon dioxide and water. When oxygen is absent, the organic electron donor is incompletely oxidized in the fermentation process to molecules such as lactic acid.
3. Obligate anaerobes. Obligate anaerobes can grow only in the absence of oxygen. In fact, oxygen often kills these microorganisms. Fermentation is one major mechanism used by obligate anaerobes to obtain energy; the other is anaerobic respiration. Obligate anaerobes can produce a variety of end products, such as organic acids from pyruvic acid metabolism (*see* Fig. 4-9). These organic acids form a species-specific profile that can be identified in the clinical laboratory by gas chromatography.

Other Pathways of Glucose Oxidation

In addition to the EMP pathway, other pathways of glucose catabolism are available to most microorganisms. They include the pentose phosphate pathway and the Entner-Doudoroff pathway.

The *pentose phosphate pathway* consists of a large number of reactions in which glucose is converted to a 5-carbon sugar, ribulose 5-phosphate. This pathway is significant for the following reasons (*see* Fig. 4-10):

1. A number of 3-, 4-, 5-, 6-, and 7-carbon sugars are produced. These sugars are phosphorylated and can be oxidized to pyruvic acid with the production of energy via substrate phosphorylation.
2. The sugars discussed in #1 can also be used as the framework for certain cellular components of the cell. For example, the genetic material of the cell, DNA and RNA, is made up of 5-carbon sugars, called deoxyribose and ribose, respectively.

Fig. 4-9. Some products of pyruvate metabolism. Carbon atoms in each molecule indicated in parentheses.

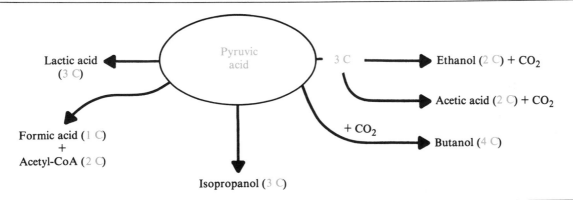

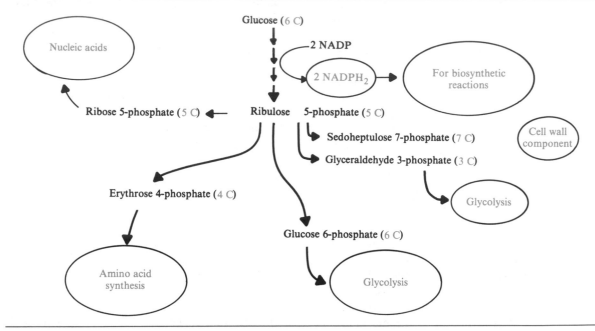

Fig. 4-10. Simplified scheme of pentose phosphate pathway.

3. Nicotinamide adenine dinucleotide phosphate (NADP) acts as a carrier of electrons and protons in the form of $NADPH_2$. Unlike $NADH_2$, $NADPH_2$ is used in biosynthetic processes. The hydrogens are fixed to carbon skeletons to produce organic molecules.

Another pathway of glucose oxidation is called the *Entner-Doudoroff* pathway (Fig. 4-11). In this pathway glucose is rearranged and cleaved to form the product glyceraldehyde 3-phosphate and pyruvic acid. Glyceraldehyde 3-phosphate can, as in glycolysis, be oxidized to release energy in the form of ATP but it can also be used to produce larger sugars.

Molecules Other Than Sugars Can Be Fermented

Amino acids, purines and pyrimidines, and organic acids can be fermented by some microorganisms. Of particular significance are the strictly anaerobic bacteria such as *Clostridium* whose species cause wound infections such as tetanus and gas gangrene.

RESPIRATION

Respiration is a cellular-energy-generating system in which the electrons released by oxidation are transferred to an *electron transport chain*. The electron transport chain is located in the cytoplasmic membrane of bacteria and mitochondrial membrane of eukaryotes. The final electron acceptor may be oxygen (aerobic respiration) or an inorganic molecule other than oxygen (anaerobic respiration).

Aerobic Respiration

Microorganisms that use aerobic respiration (or even anaerobic respiration) as a means of obtaining energy also utilize most of the reactions

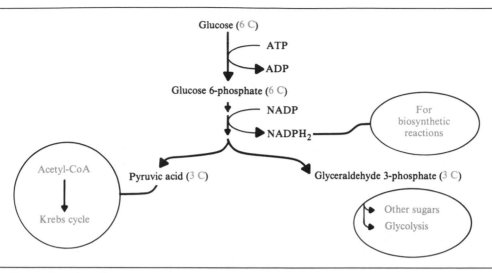

Fig. 4-11. Entner-Doudoroff pathway. Carbon atoms are in parentheses. How products are used in metabolism is indicated in color.

in glycolysis. The major difference is that in aerobic respiration pyruvate can be completely oxidized to carbon dioxide and water and the electrons and protons released are transported to an electron transport chain. Respiration occurs in the following way:

Electrons and protons captured by NAD during glycolysis are transported to the electron transport chain. Pyruvic acid loses a carbon, as carbon dioxide, and is converted to a two-carbon fragment (called an *acetyl group*) in the presence of two coenzymes: *coenzyme A (CoA)* and NAD. In the reaction the acetyl group binds to CoA to form acetyl CoA and NAD is reduced to $NADH_2$:

$$
\begin{array}{c}
\text{H} \quad \text{O} \\
| \quad \ \ || \\
\text{H—C—C—COOH} + \text{CoA} + \text{NAD} \rightarrow \\
| \\
\text{H}
\end{array}
$$

Pyruvic acid

$$
\begin{array}{c}
\text{H} \quad \text{O} \\
| \quad \ \ || \\
\text{H—C—C~CoA} + NADH_2 \\
| \\
\text{H}
\end{array}
$$

Acetyl CoA

The $NADH_2$ generated in the above reaction can transfer its electrons and protons to the electron transport chain while the acetyl CoA is ready to be oxidized in a series of reactions called the *Krebs* or *citric acid cycle*. The Krebs cycle is a pathway in which the remaining carbons of the acetyl group are converted to carbon dioxide and in the process electrons and protons are released. If we look at the Krebs cycle more closely (Fig. 4-12), the following intermediates and products are formed:

1. Acetyl CoA condenses with a four-carbon unit, *oxaloacetate*, to form the six-carbon *citric acid*.
2. Citric acid undergoes a series of reactions to form *isocitric acid*. Isocitric acid is oxidized to a 5-carbon molecule, *alpha-ketoglutaric acid*, with the release of a molecule of CO_2 and the reduction of NAD to $NADH_2$.
3. Alpha-ketoglutaric acid is further oxidized in the presence of CoA to a four-carbon unit, *succinyl-CoA*, with the liberation of one molecule of CO_2 and the reduction of NAD to $NADH_2$.
4. Succinyl-CoA loses the CoA unit, and energy is trapped by guanosine diphosphate (GDP) to

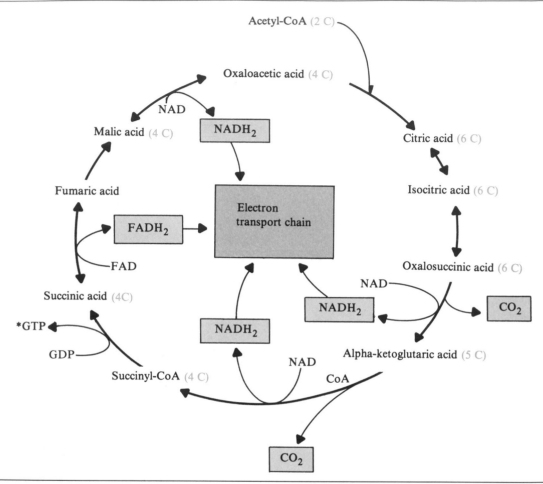

Fig. 4-12. The Krebs or citric acid cycle. Cycle oxidizes acetyl-CoA with the release of carbon dioxide and four pairs of electrons. Electrons picked up by NAD and FAD are carried to electron transport chain. *GDP (guanosine diphosphate) is converted to guanosine triphosphate (GTP). GTP is converted to ATP in the following reaction: $GTP + ADP \rightleftharpoons GDP + ATP$

form guanosine triphosphate (GTP). ATP is later produced from the reaction:

$$GTP + ADP \rightleftharpoons GDP + ATP$$

5. Succinic acid is oxidized to *fumaric acid* and another coenzyme, flavin-adenine dinucleotide (FAD) is reduced to $FADH_2$.
6. *Malic acid* is oxidized to oxaloacetic acid, and NAD is reduced to $NADH_2$.

What the Krebs cycle has accomplished is that it has: (1) oxidized a molecule of acetyl-CoA, producing two molecules of CO_2, (2) released four pairs of protons and electrons, which are capatured by NAD or FAD for transfer to the electron transport chain, (3) generated one molecule of ATP via GTP formation, and (4) produced a series of intermediates that, as we will see later, will be used in biosynthesis.

The potential energy of the electrons in re-

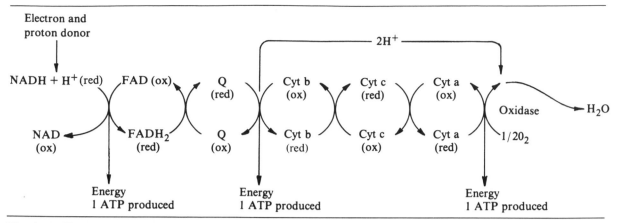

Fig. 4-13. Electron transport chain. NAD accepts electrons and protons from oxidized substrates and transfers them to the electron transport chain found in the cytoplasmic membrane of prokaryotic cells. These components include flavoproteins and their prosthetic group flavin-adenine dinucleotide (FAD), quinones (Q), and cytochromes (Cyt) b, c, and a. Hydrogens are transferred only as far as FAD, while electrons are used in the alternate reduction (red) and oxidation (ox) of all the respiratory transport components. The final product of oxidation is water. Energy is released in sufficient concentration at three places in the transport chain to produce a molecule of adenosine triphosphate (ATP). Three ATPs are produced for each pair of electrons transported the entire length of the chain. If reduced FAD is the original carrier (for example, FAD is used in the Krebs cycle) only two molecules of ATP are produced. The electron transport chain is believed to be a proton pump in which ATP synthesis is coupled to proton transfer.

duced NAD and FAD, formed in the Krebs cycle, is transferred to the electron transport chain. The chain is made up of coenzymes, proteins, and nonproteins that act as carriers (Fig. 4-13). The first components of the chain are *flavoproteins* called *NAD dehydrogenase* and *FAD dehydrogenase*, both of which carry protons and electrons. A nonprotein carrier called *quinone* also carries protons and electrons and is situated in the middle of the chain, while the remaining carriers are proteins called *cytochromes*. Cytochromes (abbreviated *cyt*) carry only electrons and are designated by letters (cyt b, cyt c, etc.). The electron transport chain is comparable to the water wheels described on p. 74. The dehydrogenase is the first wheel at the top of the chain, while at the bottom oxygen, the last wheel, is the final electron acceptor. Let us examine how electron and proton transfer occurs and where ATP is produced.

1. The electrons and protons generated during respiration are transferred by NAD and FAD from the cytoplasm to other electron transport components.

2. Each of the components in the chain becomes alternately reduced (if it picks up electrons from the previous carrier) and oxidized (if it releases electrons to the next carrier). The electrons picked up by NAD are at a very high energy level, and if they were transferred in a single step to oxygen (bypassing the intermediate carriers) a tremendous amount of energy would be released. The ATP molecule has a limited amount of energy it can trap and much of the energy released in a single oxidation would be lost as heat. Intermediate carriers provide a means of releasing small increments of energy.*

* This simplistic discussion of energy release and ATP synthesis is far from complete. We now know that electron flow is coupled to ATP synthesis by means of differences of electrical potential and differences of pH across the cytoplasmic membrane. This chemical and electrical difference is due to the movement of protons (*proton motive force*) across the cytoplasmic membrane. (See additional readings at the end of this chapter for a discussion of the proton motive force.)

3. Each oxidation step in the electron transport chain releases energy, and there are three sites where there is sufficient energy release for capture by ATP via electron transport phosphorylation. Thus, the transport of a pair of electrons from NAD to oxygen results in the release of 3 ATP. If the original electron carrier is FAD (as in the Krebs cycle) only 2 ATPs are produced:

$$NADH_2 + 3\ ADP + \tfrac{1}{2}O_2 + 3\ PO_4$$
$$\rightarrow NAD + 3\ ATP + H_2O$$
$$FADH_2 + 2\ ADP + \tfrac{1}{2}O_2 + 2\ PO_4$$
$$\rightarrow FAD + 2\ ATP + H_2O$$

4. The last carrier in the chain is called *cytochrome oxidase*, which transfers its electrons to oxygen. The hydrogen atoms that combine with oxygen to form water are those that were released by quinones during electron transport.

Energy Profile for Aerobic Respiration. The total amount of energy, in the form of ATP, that can be produced from the complete oxidation of one molecule of glucose will now be examined:

1. 2 $NADH_2$ produced during glycolysis	6 ATP
2. Substrate phosphorylation in glycolysis	4 ATP
3. $NADH_2$ produced during conversion of pyruvic acid to acetyl-CoA	6 ATP
4. 6 $NADH_2$ produced in Krebs cycle	18 ATP
5. 2 $FADH_2$ produced in Krebs cycle	4 ATP
6. Conversion of GTP to ATP in Krebs cycle	2 ATP
Total ATP gained	40
Subtract 2 ATP consumed in glycolysis	− 2
Net gain of ATP	38 per

molecule of glucose oxidized

As you can see, aerobic respiration results in the gain of substantial amounts of ATP (38 molecules) as compared to fermentation (2 molecules) when the latter is the only source of energy.

Anaerobic Respiration

Respiration does not always involve oxygen as the final electron acceptor. Alternative electron acceptors, such as nitrate (NO_3), sulfate (SO_4), and carbonate (CO_3) or organic molecules such as fumaric acid can be used by some bacterial species, especially the soil species. When the electron acceptor in respiration is a molecule other than oxygen, the process is called anaerobic respiration.

Sources of Electrons Other Than Carbohydrates

Carbohydrates are not the only source of electrons for energy formation. Organic molecules, such as lipids and proteins, can be metabolized to release electrons and produce intermediates that find their way into the Krebs cycle or glycolytic cycle. *Lipases* can cleave lipids into their component parts, glycerol and fatty acids (Fig. 4–14). Glycerol can enter the glycolytic cycle while fatty acids are oxidized in a process called *beta oxidation*. Beta oxidation brings about the release of two carbon fragments and their conversion of acetyl-CoA. Acetyl-CoA can directly enter the Krebs cycle.

Proteins are catabolized by *proteases* into their component amino acids. Amino acids lose their amino groups in a process called *deamination*,* and this can result in the formation of organic acids such as pyruvic acid, alpha-ketoglutaric acid, or others that make up the Krebs cycle.

BIOSYNTHESIS: A PROCESS THAT UTILIZES ENERGY

Many cellular components and enzymes are degraded during the life cycle of a cell and biosynthesis is needed to replenish them at normal lev-

---

* See page 67 for an example of a deamination reaction.

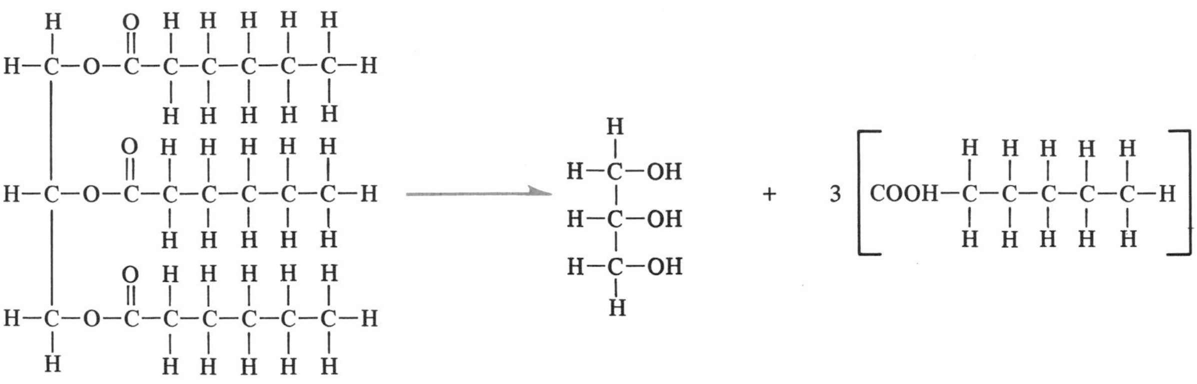

Fig. 4-14. Lipid degradation by lipases produces glycerol and fatty acids.

els. In order for biosynthetic pathways to become engaged, three processes or conditions must be operating. First, there must be a *source of carbon skeletons*; second, there must be a *source of reducing power* in the form of hydrogens; and, third, there must be a *source of energy*. Energy sources have already been discussed. We will now look at the other factors. In addition we will also discuss how these biosynthetic processes can be regulated.

THE NEED FOR CARBON SKELETONS

Very few molecules enter the cell and become directly incorporated into macromolecules, the components of cellular structures. Macromolecules are made up of basic building blocks: amino acids for proteins, purines and pyrimidines for nucleic acids, and simple sugars for polysaccharides. In addition, large molecules such as lipids are also made up of the building blocks glycerol and fatty acids. The building blocks are derived from carbon skeletons produced in pathways that are also involved in energy production. Let us look at the various metabolic pathways and see what they provide in the way of carbon skeletons.

Glycolysis

1. Glucose can be rearranged and converted to glucose 1-phosphate, which can be energized by ATP to form ADP-glucose:

Glucose 1-phosphate + ATP →
        ADP-glucose + P-P (pyrophosphate)

The glucose on ADP-glucose can be transferred to a growing polysaccharide chain to produce glycogen, a storage form of glucose in the bacterial cell.
2. Glucose-phosphate also serves as a precursor for the synthesis of other 6-carbon sugars.
3. Glyceraldehyde 3-phosphate is used in the synthesis of the amino acids serine, glycine, and cysteine.
4. Phosphoenolpyruvate is used in the synthesis of the amino acids tyrosine, phenylalanine, and tryptophan.
5. The carbons of pyruvic acid are used in the synthesis of the amino acids alanine, valine, and leucine.
6. Dihydroxyacetone phosphate is a precursor in lipid synthesis because it can be converted to glycerol.

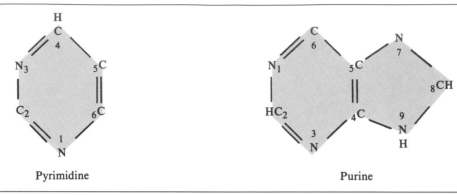

Fig. 4-15. Pyrimidine and purine, showing atom number and position.

Pentose Phosphate Pathway

1. A four-carbon sugar, erythrose 4-phosphate, is utilized in the synthesis of the amino acids tyrosine, phenylalanine, and tryptophan.
2. Five-carbon sugars, such as ribose phosphate, are used as the sugar component of the nucleic acids deoxyribonucleic acid (DNA) and ribonucleic acid (RNA).

Krebs Cycle

1. Alpha-ketoglutaric acid is a precursor to the amino acids lysine, glutamic acid, proline, and arginine.
2. Oxaloacetic acid is a precursor to the amino acids aspartic acid, threonine, isoleucine, lysine, and methionine.
3. Acetyl-CoA provides its carbons for the fatty acid components of lipids. Acetyl-CoA becomes bonded to a special carrier called *acyl carrier protein* (*ACP*). ACP acts as a primer by adding 2 carbon units to the growing fatty acid chain. Fatty acids may be up to 18 or more carbons in length.

So far we have not discussed the biosynthesis of the purines and pyrimidines (Fig. 4-15), which are the building blocks of nucleic acids. The principal precursor for them are the amino acids (Table 4-2). The replication of nucleic acids is discussed in Chapter 6.

THE NEED FOR REDUCING POWER

Once carbon skeletons have been supplied for biosynthesis, they must be reduced by adding hydrogen atoms. The source of these hydrogens is $NADPH_2$, which is generated in the pentose phosphate pathway discussed earlier (p. 78). One very important biosynthesis that requires considerable reduced NADP is the formation of fatty acids. Fatty acids consist of long chains of

Table 4-2. Origin of the Atoms of Purine and Pyrimidine Bases

Atom and position*	Molecule the atom is derived from	
	Purine	Pyrimidine
N-1	Aspartic acid (amino acid)	Aspartic acid (amino acid)
C-2	Formic acid	CO_2
N-3	Glutamine (amino acid)	NH_3
C-4	Glycine (amino acid)	Aspartic acid
C-5	Glycine	Aspartic acid
C-6	CO_2	Aspartic acid
N-7	Glycine	———
C-8	Formic acid	———
N-9	Glutamine	———

* The atom number and position are illustrated in Figure 4-16.

hydrocarbons and many of the hydrogens are supplied by $NADPH_2$.

CONTROL OF METABOLIC ACTIVITY

Since enzymes are the cells' mechanism for speeding up chemical reactions, it stands to reason that enzymes are involved in controlling the reactions in a positive or negative way. Controlling what reactions are to be used by the cell at any one time is a useful technique for conserving energy and producing only what the cell needs. There are two basic types of metabolic control:

1. Control of enzyme synthesis. This type of control involves mechanisms operating at the level of the gene. This aspect of control will be discussed later in Chapter 6.
2. Control of enzyme activity. This technique involves the turning on or turning off of enzyme activity and is associated with a special class of enzymes called *allosteric enzymes*.

ALLOSTERIC ENZYMES AND METABOLIC CONTROL

One of the distinguishing physical characteristics of allosteric enzymes is that they consist of subunits, often 4 or multiples of 4. The subunits can assume different conformations in response to the binding of molecules, such as substrates, to active sites. Each subunit may contain an active site and the binding of a substrate molecule to one subunit increases the binding of the second substrate molecule, etc. (Fig. 4-16). The subunits

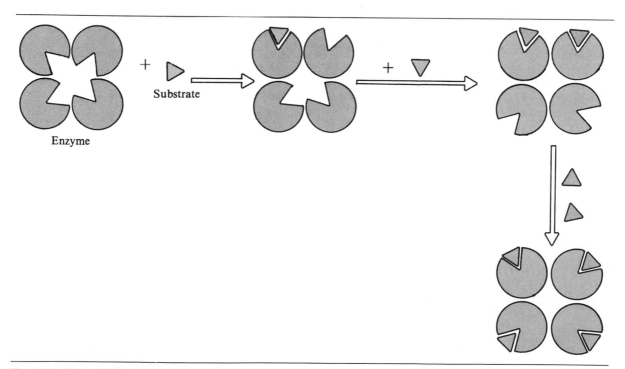

Fig. 4-16. How binding of substrate molecules to the active sites on the subunits of allosteric enzymes increases activity. Binding of one substrate molecule causes change in conformation of enzyme and results in an increase in the rate of binding of a second substrate molecule. The binding of two substrate molecules in turn increases rate of binding of substrate molecules to the remaining active sites.

of allosteric enzymes also possess *regulatory sites* that are distinct from the active site. Regulatory sites bind molecules, other than substrates, that change the conformation of the subunits and may cause an increase or decrease in the activity of the enzyme. Thus, the allosteric enzyme possesses sites that determine what products will be produced in the cell. The primary type of cellular control mechanism associated with allosteric enzymes is called *feedback inhibition*.

Feedback Inhibition

Feedback inhibition is the type of control most frequently associated with biosynthetic reactions, but catabolic reactions are also involved. This type of control assumes that when a product (or products) in a metabolic pathway begins to accumulate it can feed back on the first enzyme in the pathway and shut off not only the synthesis of the final product or products but also any intermediates in the pathway. In the following example, the final product D of the metabolic sequence feeds back and shuts off enzyme E_1. In the absence of product B, neither C nor D is produced. Enzyme E_1 in the sequence acts as the allosteric enzyme.

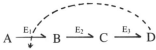

Some metabolic pathways are branched, and more than one product is involved in the control mechanism. The cell must control the amounts of all the different products. Under some environmental conditions, only one of the products may accumulate in the cell. Shutting down the first enzyme will prevent the formation of both products. In the following example the primary products are D, F, and H, and the allosteric enzymes are E_1, E_4, and E_6.

$$A \xrightarrow{E_1} B \xrightarrow{E_2} C \xrightarrow{E_3} D \underset{E_6}{\overset{E_4}{\lessgtr}} \begin{array}{c} E \xrightarrow{E_5} F \\ G \xrightarrow{E_7} H \end{array}$$

Control of branched pathways can take place in the following ways:

1. Cumulative feedback inhibition. In the preceding diagram neither product F nor product H alone could completely reduce the activity of the enzyme E_1; for example, each might reduce activity by 50 percent. Together, however, they totally shut off the activity of enzyme E_1.
2. Sequential feedback inhibition. Products F and H feed back on enzymes E_4 and E_6, causing accumulation of product D. Product D in turn feeds back on enzyme E_1, inhibiting its activity.
3. Multivalent feedback inhibition. Neither product F nor product H has any effect individually on the activity of enzyme E_1, but together they inhibit activity.

SUMMARY

1. Metabolism can be divided into two basic processes: catabolism, or energy production from the degradation of molecules, and anabolism, or the biosynthesis of molecules. Both processes require catalysts in the form of special proteins called enzymes.

2. Enzymes lower the energy of activation of a reaction. They exist in a special conformation that produces an active site for binding substrate. It is at the active site that bond breaking and bond making occur. Some enzymes require cofactors to be active and these may be in the form of vitamins or inorganic ions.

3. Enzymes are affected by pH, temperature, concentration of substrate, and inhibitors. Most enzymes exhibit maximum activity at pHs between 5 and 8 and at temperatures between 30 and 37°C. Very high temperatures can cause the protein to unfold or denature, with loss of activity. Inhibitors of enzymes are of two types: com-

petitive, in which the inhibitor competes with the normal substrate for the active site, and noncompetitive, in which the inhibitor does not bind at the active site but at another site that induces a conformational change affecting the active site.

4. The names of enzymes are written with the suffix "-ase." Enzymes can be classified into various groups depending on the type of reaction they catalyze. The major groups of enzymes are oxidoreductases, transferases, hydrolases, lyases, isomerases, and ligases. Enzymes are also classified according to their biological activity, that is, endoenzymes and exoenzymes. Enzymes can be recovered from microorganisms and used in commercial endeavors.

5. Infectious microorganisms obtain their energy from the oxidation of organic molecules. Energy is locked up in the electrons released during the oxidation process. Electrons can be transferred by carriers to the electron transport chain, which is located in the cytoplasmic membrane of prokaryotes and mitochondria of eukaryotes. During the movement of electrons in the electron transport chain, energy is released and is then captured during the phosphorylation of ADP to ATP.

6. In addition to electron transport phosphorylation, there is substrate phosphorylation. In this process energy is associated with a high-energy phosphate trapped in a substrate molecule. The high-energy phosphate is used to phosphorylate ADP to ATP.

7. Two metabolic processes that generate energy in the cell are fermentation and respiration. Fermentation is an anaerobic process that usually involves the oxidation of a sugar. The fermentation of glucose is referred to as glycolysis. During glycolysis energy is released in the form of ATP via substrate phosphorylation. The final electron acceptor in glycolysis is pyruvic acid, which can be converted to a multitude of products, depending on the species of microorganism.

8. Glucose can be oxidized to produce energy in two other pathways: the pentose phosphate pathway and the Entner-Doudoroff pathway. The pentose phosphate pathway also serves to pro-duce a variety of 3-, 4-, 5-, 6-, and 7-carbon sugars that can be utilized by the cell in various processes. In addition, $NADPH_2$ is produced that is required in biosynthetic reactions. The Entner-Doudoroff pathway produces glyceraldehyde-3 phosphate and pyruvic acid, as in glycolysis, but uses a different route.

9. Respiration is an oxidation process in which the energy of the electron is released during its transport in the electron transport chain. The final electron acceptor may be oxygen (aerobic respiration) or other molecules (anaerobic respiration). The electrons produced during respiration are derived from the oxidation of sugars, as in glycolysis, and in the Krebs cycle, but other organic molecules, such as lipids, can also be a source of electrons. Electrons are transported to the electron transport chain by carriers such as NAD and FAD.

10. The Krebs cycle represents a process in which the pyruvate molecule, generated during glycolysis, is completely oxidized to carbon dioxide. Many intermediates produced in the Krebs cycle, such as alpha-ketoglutarate, are also used in biosynthetic reactions especially in the synthesis of amino acids.

11. The electron transport chain consists of coenzymes, proteins, and nonproteins extended across the cytoplasmic membrane. NAD dehydrogenase and FAD dehydrogenase and quinone of the electron transport chain transport both protons and electrons, while the cytochromes, the last members of the chain, transport only electrons. The final electron acceptor in aerobic respiration, oxygen, is converted to water. Final electron acceptors in anaerobic respiration include such molecules as nitrate and sulfate. The net gain of ATP from aerobic respiration, using glucose, is 38, as compared to 2 for fermentation.

12. Biosynthesis in the cell requires energy, reducing power and carbon skeletons. The carbon skeletons give rise to various building blocks, such as amino acids, sugars, and purines and pyrimidines, which will be the foundation of macromolecules. The carbon skeletons are produced by the same pathways that were used to generate

energy in the cell. Reducing power is provided mainly by NADH$_2$ produced in the pentose phosphate pathway.

13. Metabolic processes can be controlled by regulating enzyme synthesis (see Chapter 6) or by controlling enzyme activity. Control of enzyme activity in the cell is brought about by allosteric enzymes, which consist of protein subunits that have regulatory sites in addition to active sites. Regulatory sites can bind molecules other than the substrate and they can increase or decrease enzyme activity.

14. Allosteric enzymes are especially evident in biosynthetic reactions, where they are usually found in the first reaction of a pathway that utilizes several enzymes to generate a product. One type of allosteric enzyme control is called feedback inhibition. In feedback inhibition the end product of the pathway inhibits the first enzyme of the pathway.

QUESTIONS FOR STUDY

Select the best response or responses for each of the following:

1. Which of the following statements about enzymes is *untrue*?
   A. Many enzymes require cofactors, such as metals, in order to become active.
   B. The temperature required to denature enzymes is called the energy of activation.
   C. Noncompetitive inhibitors of enzyme activity bind at the active site.
   D. Most enzymes exhibit maximum activity between pHs of 5 and 8.

2. Which of the following statements concerning microbial energy production is *true*?
   A. Energy formation or release follows biological oxidation and not reduction.
   B. Most of the energy generated by aerobic microorganisms is obtained by electron transport phosphorylation.
   C. The major electron or potential energy carriers in the cell are phosphorylated molecules such as ATP.
   D. Glycolysis is an anaerobic process that is used primarily by anaerobic organisms.

3. Which of the following statements concerning aerobic respiration is *true*?
   A. Most of the electrons supplied to the electron transport chain are derived from glycolysis.
   B. One of the functions of the Krebs cycle is to oxidize pyruvate generated during glycolysis.
   C. The cytochromes are engaged only in the transport of electrons and not hydrogen (protons).
   D. Microorganisms that lack many components of the Krebs cycle are unable to obtain energy by electron transport phosphorylation.

4. Which of the following statements concerning biosynthesis is *true*?
   A. Biosynthetic reactions are basically oxidation processes that generate energy.
   B. Many of the carbon skeletons required for biosynthetic reactions are obtained from the Krebs cycle.
   C. The sugars required for biosynthesis of nucleic acids are obtained from the pentose phosphate pathway.
   D. Much of the reducing power or hydrogen atoms required in biosynthetic reactions is provided by NADPH$_2$ generated in the Entner-Doudoroff pathway.

5. Which of the following statements concerning metabolic control is *untrue*?

A. Allosteric enzymes are involved in controlling the genes that code for metabolic enzymes.

B. Allosteric enzymes are composed of subunits that possess catalytic as well as regulatory activity.

C. Feedback inhibition refers to the mechanism in which the product of a metabolic pathway feeds back on the first substrate in the pathway.

D. Feedback inhibition refers to the mechanism in which the product of a metabolic pathway feeds back on the first enzyme of the pathway.

Fill in the blank:

6. An organism possessing only a glycolytic pathway for energy production would most likely excrete _____ into the medium.

7. The term beta-oxidation refers to a process that involves the release of two carbon fragments from _____ .

8. The last enzyme in the electron transport process is called _____ .

9. Adenosine triphosphate, acetyl CoA, and phosphoenolypyruvate are molecules that are similar in that they possess a _____ bond.

10. Enzymes are important in biological reactions because they lower the _____ .

ADDITIONAL READINGS

Gottschalk, G. *Bacterial Metabolism* (2nd ed.). New York: Springer-Verlag, Inc., 1985.

Hinkle, R. C., and McCarty, R. E. How cells make ATP. *Sci. Am.* 238:104,1978.

Jones, C. W. *Bacterial Respiration*. Aspects of Microbiology. Washington, DC: American Society for Microbiology, 1982.

Mandelstam, J., and McQuillen, K. *Biochemistry of Bacterial Growth* (3rd ed.). New York: Halsted Press, 1982.

Moat, A. G. *Microbial Physiology*. New York: Wiley, 1988.

Neidhardt, F. C., et al. (eds.). *Escherichia coli and Salmonella typhimurium: Cellular and Molecular Biology*. Washington, DC: American Society for Microbiology, 1987.

5. MICROBIAL GROWTH

OBJECTIVES

To briefly describe the stages of bacterial growth and the biochemical changes occurring in each stage

To list the chemical factors affecting growth and the function of each

To describe how oxygen is handled by the four groups of bacteria based on their oxygen requirements

To describe the physical factors affecting growth

To differentiate between: synthetic and nonsynthetic media; enriched and enrichment media; selective and differential media; to give examples of each type

To outline the various ways in which anaerobes can be cultivated

To discuss how pure cultures can be obtained in the laboratory

To discuss the various types of primary isolation media and their function

To outline the various ways in which microbial growth can be measured

To define: culture, logarithmic, nutrient, aerotolerant, plasmolysis, pure culture, lyophilization

Growth is the coordination of chemical and physical processes in the cell that ideally result in cell division. The cellular chemical and physical processes are also influenced by external chemical and physical forces. For laboratory technicians a knowledge of growth is important because they will be concerned with cultivating microorganisms for clinical and investigative purposes. Nurses, hygienists, and physicians may be concerned with microbial growth because under certain circumstances they utilize procedures that prevent microbial growth. The average citizen each day tries to prevent spoilage of foods or destruction of various articles susceptible to microbial attack. Industrial microbiologists are often concerned with enhancing microbial growth in order to provide increased synthesis of a commercially marketable microbial product such as vitamins or organic acids.

In this chapter we will examine the chemical and physical factors affecting growth and how a knowledge of microbial growth is utilized in the microbiological laboratory. Later in Chapter 9 we will discuss more specific aspects of microbial growth in relationship to infectious disease.

GROWTH OF BACTERIAL CELLS

Bacterial cells can be grown in various nutrient-containing preparations called *culture media*. The population of cells in the medium is called a *culture*. A microbial cell grows by increasing its cellular constituents and then dividing into two cells. Bacterial cells divide by an asexual process

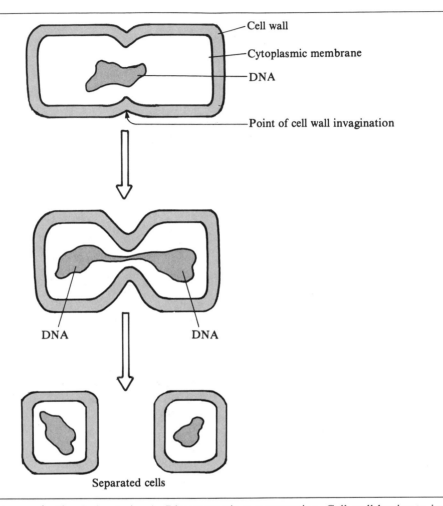

Fig. 5-1. Asexual reproduction in bacteria. A. Diagrammatic representation. Cell wall begins to invaginate while DNA duplicates. As cell wall invagination continues each side will possess a molecule of DNA. Cell wall invagination continues until the cell splits into two units or progeny of equal size.

called *binary fission* (Fig. 5-1). When the cell divides each of the progeny will possess a copy of the DNA, as well as other cellular components, that will enable them also to grow and divide. The division process continues in a geometric way, that is, after the first cell divides into two cells the population doubles: 4, 8, 16, 32, 64, etc. The time required for a single cell or population of cells to double is called the *generation time* or *doubling time*. The generation time can be calculated mathematically by determining the num-

ber of cells in samples taken from broth cultures at various time intervals during geometric growth. For example, suppose we remove one sample at time 0 and three samples each at 30-minute intervals. The number of bacteria found at each interval is found to be 100, 200, 400, and 800, respectively. We can see from these experimental results that the doubling time is 30 minutes. This type of data could be graphed by using an arithmetic scale but in the laboratory a culture containing 800 bacteria would not be visible to

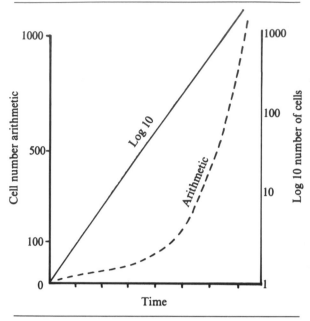

Fig. 5-2. Bacterial growth plotted logarithmically and arithmetically. One can see from the graph that measurements of growth at time intervals on the arithmetic scale are difficult to evaluate at early times and later when the cell number goes beyond 1000.

the naked eye and would be difficult to measure. Bacterial growth becomes visible as a turbid solution only when there are at least 1×10^7 (10 million) bacteria per ml. In the laboratory, cultures often contain up to 5×10^9 (5 billion) bacteria per ml. To graph this kind of data requires a logarithmic scale (Fig. 5-2).

THE GROWTH CURVE

A population of bacterial cells goes through a number of phases from the time it is introduced into a medium until it ceases growth. When these phases are graphed they produce a typical growth curve (Fig. 5-3). The growth curve includes the *lag, log, stationary*, and *death and decline phases.*

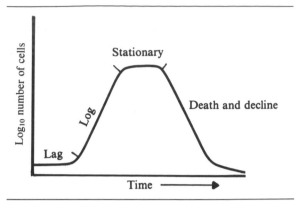

Fig. 5-3. Growth curve of bacterial culture.

Lag Phase

When microorganisms are introduced into a growth medium there is usually a period of adjustment to the new chemical and physical environment. There is a lag in cell division and the population does not divide at all or divides in a nongeometric fashion. This phase produces an almost horizontal line on the growth curve. Near the end of the lag phase the rate of cell division begins to accelerate.

Log Phase

The term *log* is an abbreviation for logarithmic, which means that the population of cells is dividing in a geometric or logarithmic fashion. During the log phase cell division is occurring at a constant rate, for example, every 30 minutes. The reason for this constancy in the log phase is that all components in the cell, such as DNA, RNA, protein, cell wall, etc., are doubling their mass at a specific rate just like cell division. The growth rate of bacterial species will vary and depends on:

1. The microbial species. Every species because of its genetic potential has a minimum and maximum rate of growth. In the log phase microorganisms are growing more efficiently than in any other phase of growth.
2. Temperature. An increase in temperature up

to a certain limit increases the rate of growth. For example, a culture of *Escherichia coli* grown at 30°C may have a generation time of 1 hour but at a temperature of 37°C may have a generation time of 30 minutes or less.

3. Growth-supporting ability of the culture medium. A medium containing a high concentration of preformed organic nutrients will support a faster growth rate than a nutritionally poor medium. Of course the nutrients must be ones than can be metabolized by the microbial species in question.

Stationary Phase

When bacteria are cultivated in a medium in which nutrients are not replenished, a point is reached during population growth at which the growth rate declines. Many bacteria in a nutrient-depleted medium will be dying while others will be dividing—the living ones using nutrients from dying cells. In the stationary phase there is a balance between the number of cells dying and the number dividing. This equilibrium is represented as a horizontal line in the growth curve when plotted on semi-log paper (Fig. 5-3). In addition to nutrient depletion, other factors are also responsible for the decline in growth and include:

1. pH changes. Acids are the common metabolic excretion product and cause a reduction in pH of the medium.
2. Accumulation of toxic waste products. Some of these toxic wastes may also be the acids described in 1.
3. Reduced concentration of oxygen (if the organism is aerobic) in the medium is usually due to overcrowding and rapid depletion of oxygen.

The chemical and physical changes occurring during the stationary phase can induce the formation of endospores by bacteria such as *Bacillus* and *Clostridium* and loss of vegetative cells.

Death and Decline Phase

The death and decline phase of growth is essentially the reverse of the logarithmic phase, that

is, the cells in the population are dying in a geometric fashion. Factors responsible for the death phase include those given for the stationary phase as well as the release of lytic enzymes by some groups of bacteria when they lyse or burst.

CHEMICAL REQUIREMENTS FOR GROWTH

Chemicals required for growth are called *nutrients*. Nutrients may be in the form of inorganic or organic compounds or a combination of both. Let us suppose that we wish to cultivate two species of bacteria, *Escherichia coli*, an inhabitant of the intestinal tract, and a species of *Streptococcus* from the oral cavity. Following cultivation we may wish to determine some of their growth characteristics. Our first task is to prepare a medium and determine what is needed. Most media used today are commercially prepared, but it is still important to understand why the constituents were chosen and their function in the cell.

WATER

We need water to dissolve the required nutrients. This will allow the nutrients to be transported across the cytoplasmic membrane into the cell. In addition, many biochemical reactions require water to break down (hydrolyze) certain compounds.

CARBON

Most microorganisms, including those infectious for humans, must be supplied carbon in an organic form (only a few bacteria can use inorganic carbon, such as carbon dioxide, as their carbon source). Organisms using organic molecules as a source of carbon are called *heterotrophs*. The organic carbon source one should use depends on the genetic potential of the bacterial cell—that is, can the bacterial cell produce enzymes that will metabolize the carbon source? The most common sources of carbon for bacterial cells are sugars, such as glucose, because they are easily degraded in glycolysis and because they can also serve as energy sources. When glucose is catabolized it provides the carbon skeletons for the various precursor materials (such as amino acids). *E. coli* can use glucose for all of its biosynthetic needs but this is not true for the *Streptococcus* species. Some biosynthetic reactions are absent in *Streptococcus* and the precursor material must be present in the medium. The organic precursor materials that must be supplied in the medium are called *growth factors* and may include amino acids, purines and pyrimidines, and vitamins. Vitamins are used as coenzymes (see p. 69).

The carbon source for some microorganisms could be a macromolecule such as the polysaccharide cellulose. However, the microorganism must be able to produce the enzyme cellulase that can be excreted from the cell (exoenzyme) to degrade the macromolecule into its constituent subunits, i.e., glucose. Macromolecules are not transportable through the cytoplasmic membrane, but their smaller subunits, such as glucose, are transportable.

NITROGEN

Nitrogen is a major element of proteins and is also found in the purines and pyrimidines. The microbial cells' nitrogen requirements are usually supplied via an inorganic molecule, such as ammonia (NH_3) or nitrate (NO_3), but nitrite (NO_2) and nitrogen gas (N_2) can also be used by some microorganisms. Inorganic forms of nitrogen are first converted by the cell into ammonia (Fig. 5-4), which then becomes the amino group in an amino acid. For an organism such as *Streptococcus*, with limited biosynthetic potential, inorganic nitrogen may be used to synthesize most

of the amino acids, but the various vitamins must be supplied in the medium (see Table 5-2 and discussion on page 101).

Proteins can be a source of nitrogen, as well as carbon and energy, provided the microbial cell produces exoenzymes, such as proteases, that degrade them. A partially digested protein called *peptone* is a component of several commercially available media and it serves these purposes.

Nitrogen gas (N_2) as a source of nitrogen is used primarily by organisms found in soil and water. They take up the gas and add hydrogens to it to make ammonia, a process called *nitrogen fixation*. This process can be utilized by only a few infectious microorganisms, such as *Klebsiella*, and then only when more normal nitrogen sources, such as nitrate, are absent. Neither *E. coli* nor *Streptococcus* can use nitrogen gas.

SULFUR AND PHOSPHORUS

Sulfur, which is an element found in some amino acids, is usually supplied to the microbial cell in the form of inorganic sulfate. The sulfate is converted to hydrogen sulfide (H_2S), which is used in the synthesis of the amino acid cysteine. Inorganic phosphate is the most widely used source of phosphorus for microorganisms. Phosphorus is important in the synthesis of the nucleic acids DNA and RNA. One of the components of these nucleic acids is adenosine triphosphate, which is the energy molecule of the cell (see Chapter 4). Phosphate in the medium is also important as a buffer when it is in the form of mono- or dipotassium phosphate (KH_2PO_4 and K_2HPO_4, respectively). Buffers absorb hydrogen ions generated during microbial metabolism when acids are produced. This buffering capacity enables the medium to support more growth since most bacteria are unable to grow at low or acid pHs.

OXYGEN

We have already observed in Chapter 4 that oxygen plays an important role in the growth of mi-

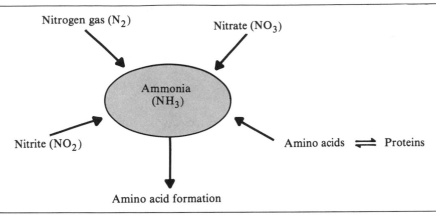

Fig. 5-4. The flow of nitrogen from inorganic to organic forms and vice versa within the cell. Ammonia (NH_3) is the central nitrogen compound because it is used in the synthesis of amino acids.

Table 5-1. Important Minerals and Their Function in Microbial Metabolism

Element	Function
Magnesium	Stabilization of nucleic acids and ribosomes; required in some enzymatic reactions
Potassium	Required in some enzymatic reactions. Important in protein synthesis
Iron	Important component of the cytochromes. Important in diphtheria toxin production by *Corynebacterium diphtheriae*. Important factor in bacterial disease (see Chapter 9).
Calcium	Cofactor for some enzymes. Required for attachment of some bacterial viruses to the bacterial cell. Important in spore formation by bacteria
Zinc	Cofactor for some enzymes
Molybdenum	An important component of the enzyme involved in nitrogen fixation
Cobalt	Component of vitamin B_{12}
Manganese	Cofactor for some enzymes and can substitute for magnesium
Sodium	Required primarily by marine microorganisms

croorganisms because it is a terminal electron acceptor in respiration. Although some organisms may not require oxygen for growth, they do respond to its presence in different ways. Let us see how and why microorganisms respond so differently to this element.

Products of Oxygen Metabolism

Many microorganisms possess enzymes that reduce oxygen not only to water, as in aerobic respiration, but to toxic products as well. Two of the most important of these toxic intermediates are *hydrogen peroxide* and *superoxide*. The oxygen atom in each of these molecules, in terms of electronic configurations, is different from molecular or atmospheric oxygen. These toxic molecules are also produced by mammalian white blood cells and are the basis of mammalian resistance to microbial invasion (see Chapter 11). Microorganisms have evolved enzymatic mechanisms for removing the toxic intermediates of oxygen metabolism and converting them to molecular oxygen. The enzymes involved are *catalase*,* which converts hydrogen peroxide to water and oxygen:

* Peroxidase can also break down hydrogen peroxide but oxygen is not produced.

$$H_2O_2 \xrightarrow{\text{catalase}} H_2O + O_2$$

and *superoxide dismutase*, which converts superoxide to hydrogen peroxide and molecular oxygen (the peroxide can be metabolized by catalase). Based on oxygen requirements, microorganisms are divided into four groups. We will see how each tolerates oxygen and its toxic intermediates.

1. *Obligate aerobes.* Obligate aerobes are totally dependent on oxygen for growth. The O_2 requirement is usually expressed as one atmosphere, or 20 percent, the concentration of oxygen in air at one atmosphere. Obligate aerobes produce hydrogen peroxide and superoxide but they also possess the enzymes catalase and superoxide dismutase, which enable them to tolerate high concentrations of oxygen.
2. *Microaerophiles.* Microaerophiles grow in the presence of oxygen but can tolerate only so much oxygen (about 0.2 atmospheres, or 4 percent). Microaerophiles produce the necessary enzymes to break down hydrogen peroxide and superoxide, but if too many toxic products are formed the enzymatic system of the bacterium becomes overloaded and growth is inhibited.
3. *Facultative anaerobes.* Facultative anaerobes can grow in the presence of oxygen or in its absence. In the presence of oxygen they use aerobic respiration for energy production but in its absence fermentation or anaerobic respiration is the major source of energy. Facultative anaerobes grow best under aerobic conditions and produce catalase and superoxide dismutase to break down hydrogen peroxide and superoxide that accumulate.
4. *Obligate anaerobes.* Obligate anaerobes can grow only in the absence of oxygen. Obligate anaerobes such as *Clostridium* are found in the soil, but anaerobes can also be found in certain environments in the human host. These anaerobic environments include the intestinal tract and areas such as the pockets lying between the teeth and gums (gingival crevice). The effect of oxygen on obligate anaerobes is variable. Oxygen can be lethal to some obligate anaerobes simply because the microorganisms possess enzymes that reduce oxygen to hydrogen peroxide and superoxide but lack enzymes that degrade them to nontoxic compounds. Other obligate anaerobes (called *aerotolerant* species) are tolerant of oxygen simply because they lack enzymes that reduce oxygen to water or any toxic intermediates.

MINERALS

Mineral requirements of microorganisms vary considerably. Some minerals, such as calcium, magnesium, potassium, and iron are needed by practically all bacteria. Other minerals, such as sodium zinc, molybdenum, cobalt, copper, and manganese are usually required in small or trace amounts. In most instances it is not necessary to add trace elements to laboratory media since many are normal contaminants of tap or even "distilled" water. The more important minerals and their function in microbial metabolism are summarized in Table 5-1. Iron plays a very important role in the infectious disease process; this is discussed in detail in Chapter 9.

PHYSICAL REQUIREMENTS FOR GROWTH

Many physical factors affect microbial growth, and manipulation of these factors can allow one to select specific microbial species. For the clinical microbiologist some of these physical factors are provided for in commercial media. Let us briefly examine how variations in some of these physical factors affect growth.

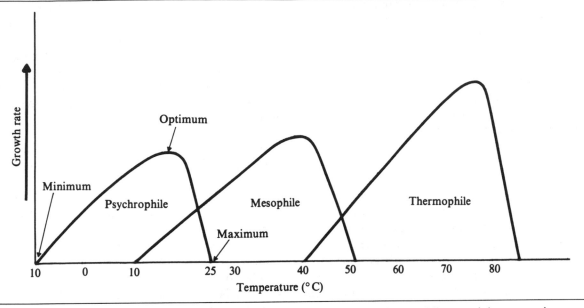

Fig. 5-5. Comparison of growth rates of psychrophiles, mesophiles, and thermophiles at minimum, optimum, and maximum temperatures.

HYDROGEN ION

Most bacteria grow best at pHs between 6 and 8 while fungi show optimum growth at pHs between 5 and 6. This is the principal reason that most microorganisms are unable to cause infections in the stomach, where the pH is approximately 2.0. Commercial media contain buffers to prevent a rapid drop in pH during bacterial growth on carbohydrates, such as glucose and other sugars. These buffers may be in the form of phosphates or organic molecules such as peptones or amino acids. The latter are often metabolized to alkaline products rather than acid products.

TEMPERATURE

Based on temperature requirements for optimal growth, microorganisms have been divided into three types: *psychrophiles, mesophiles,* and *ther-*

mophiles. When the growth rate of psychrophiles, mesophiles, and thermophiles is plotted, each group exhibits a characteristic minimum, optimum, and maximum temperature of growth (Fig. 5-5). The minimum temperature is the lowest temperature at which the organisms grow. The optimum temperature is the temperature at which growth is best. The maximum temperature is the highest temperature at which growth is possible and beyond which growth is not possible. At maximum temperatures of growth the enzymatic machinery of the cell is still operating but the enzymes are more rapidly inactivated than would occur at lower temperatures.

Psychrophiles

Psychrophiles have a temperature range for growth between −10°C and 20°C. They are found in many aquatic and soil environments of temperate regions as well as extremely cold regions of the earth. Food and dairy products are sometimes contaminated by psychrophiles, whose growth is stimulated when foods are refrigerated. Psychrophilic temperatures are usually not lethal to organisms that grow best above 25°C but they do inhibit growth.

Mesophiles

The microorganisms that cause disease in humans are characteristically mesophiles. They prefer growth at temperatures between 30° and 37°C, the latter being the normal body temperature.

Thermophiles

Thermophiles show a temperature range for growth between 45° and 70°C. They are found in hot sulfur springs and other areas where high temperatures are maintained. Thermophiles for the most part are incapable of growth at the usual temperatures of the body and are not involved in infectious diseases of humans.

PRACTICAL ASPECTS OF TEMPERATURE CONTROL

Low temperatures are used as a technique for preservation of foods by inhibiting microbial growth. Refrigeration temperatures (2–7°C) are suitable for the storage of a large number of perishable foods. Food-poisoning microorganisms, except for *Clostridium botulinum* type E, are prevented from growth at temperatures below 6°C. Still, many microorganisms can grow, albeit slowly, at temperatures from 0° to −34°. Several yeasts, for example, are capable of growth at temperatures between −18°C and −34°C. Generally speaking, gram-positive cocci such as *Staphylococcus* are more resistant to low temperatures than are gram-negative rod-shaped bacteria such as *Salmonella*.

The freezing of microorganisms that cannot grow at freezing temperatures is a method of preserving microorganisms in the laboratory. Once deep freezing temperatures (−50° to −95°C) have been reached, a great percentage of the microorganisms die. Those cells surviving the initial freezing die gradually in the frozen state. The rate

at which they die depends on (1) whether the freezing is slow or fast, (2) the composition of the medium in which the microorganisms were frozen, (3) the length of storage in the frozen state, and (4) the temperature at which the microorganisms were frozen. Several changes that contribute to the loss of viability occur in the cell during freezing:

1. Free water in the cell forms ice crystals, which lead to dehydration of the cell and an increase in the concentration of electrolytes.
2. The dehydration from ice crystal formation also changes the colloidal state of cytoplasmic proteins.
3. Some cellular proteins are denatured by freezing, apparently because of the removal of sulfhydryl groups.
4. There is a decrease in pH, as well as loss of gases such as carbon dioxide and oxygen, following freezing. Thus, metabolism and respiratory activity are suppressed. Once the frozen culture has thawed, many cells have increased nutritional requirements that remain for several generations. Apparently the freezing process has injured the cytoplasmic membrane and a restoration of normal activity does not occur until several generations have elapsed.

High temperatures, such as those between 62° and 71°C, are used in pasteurization processes while temperatures above 100°C are used in sterilization procedures, which are discussed in Chapter 7.

OSMOTIC PRESSURE

The concentration of solutes in a medium is an important factor controlling the growth of microorganisms. Maintaining a relatively constant ionic strength in the cell is important because the stability and activity of enzymes and other macromolecules are dependent on it. Several types of commercially available media contain sodium chloride (NaCl) to maintain the ionic strength of the medium. If the solute concentration outside the cell is higher than inside the cell, water will flow from the cytoplasm of the cell to the outside. This loss of water from the cell causes the cell protoplast to shrink, a condition called *plasmolysis*. Plasmolysis prevents growth. This technique is used in industry for curing hams and other meats by adding high concentrations of salt or sugar (sucrose).

CULTIVATION OF THE MICROBIAL SPECIES

In previous paragraphs we discussed what chemical and physical factors are required for the growth of microorganisms. Now we will examine the actual types of culture media used to cultivate a population of bacteria.

TYPES OF CULTURE MEDIA

The laboratory medium can be in the form of a liquid, in which instance it is called a *broth*, or in the form of a semi-solid, in which case *agar* is added to the broth. Agar, a carbohydrate isolated from seaweed, is not digested by bacteria and does not serve as a nutrient in the medium. Agar is added to the broth and the mixture is sterilized and then cooled. Cooling results in the formation of a semi-solid medium permitting the isolation and possible differentiation of bacteria on its surface. Laboratory media are classified according to their chemical content and laboratory use.

Media Based on Chemical Content

A medium in which the exact chemical composition is known is called a *synthetic* or *defined medium*. It may be a simple salts solution with a carbon source, or it may include many organic components (see Table 5-2). A medium in which the exact chemical composition is not known is

Table 5-2. Chemical Composition of a Defined and Complex Medium*

Defined medium (mg/liter)	Complex medium (mg/liter)
$CaCl_2$ (15)	Cysteine (15)
$MgSO_4$ (120)	Sodium glutamate (500)
$(NH_4)_2SO_4$ (1200)	$(NH_4)_2SO_4$ (1200)
Na_2HPO_4 (7000)	Sodium acetate (10,000)
NaH_2PO_4 (200)	Na_2HPO_4 (7000)
Glucose (10,000)	NaH_2PO_4 (1200)
	Folic acid (0.005)
	Biotin (0.0025)
	Para-aminobenzoic acid (0.1)
	Thiamine (0.5)
	Riboflavin (0.5)
	Pyridoxal (1.0)
	Pantothenate (0.5)
	Nicotinic acid (1.0)
	Glucose (10,000)

* The defined medium is a basal salts medium used to cultivate organisms such as *Escherichia coli*. The complex medium is used to cultivate bacteria such as some oral streptococci.

Table 5-3. Composition of a Complex Medium, Nutrient Broth

Component	Concentration (grams/liter)
Peptone	5.0
Beef extract	3.0
Sodium chloride	8.0
Water	1000 milliliters

called *nonsynthetic* or complex. *Nutrient broth* is an example of a complex medium (Table 5-3).

Most microbiological media are commercially available in the form of powder or crystals. The media are dissolved in water and sterilized to destroy any living organisms and then are cooled before laboratory use. A temperature is selected, usually 30° or 37°C, for cultivation of the bacteria. Because of the diverse requirements of some bacteria, it is sometimes necessary to add specific components to the commercial medium or adjust other factors. For this reason there now exists a classification of media based on specific laboratory use.

Media Based on Laboratory Use

An *all-purpose medium* is designed to support the growth of most microorganisms. Examples of all-purpose media are nutrient broth, nutrient yeast, and trypticase soy broth.

Enriched media contain a basal growth-supporting medium to which nutritive supplements are added. *Blood agar* is an enriched medium. Blood agar base contains an infusion of beef heart muscle, tryptose, salt, and agar. After sterilization this medium is allowed to cool to 50°C and to it is added 5% sterile defibrinated sheep or horse blood.

Some media can be *selective*, that is, they are used to select for wanted species of bacteria and select against unwanted species of bacteria. This selection is generally achieved in either a synthetic or nonsynthetic medium by the addition of specific chemical components. Many selective media incorporate dyes such as crystal violet or antibiotics to inhibit the growth of undesirable species. Other selective procedures include: (1) addition of specific energy or carbon sources, (2) adjusting the pH, (3) increasing the osmotic properties, and (4) adjusting the oxygen tension. Some bacteria, such as the *Neisseria*, require low levels of oxygen but increased concentrations of CO_2. Carbon dioxide incubators are available that electronically control the level of CO_2 for growth.

Some media are *differential*, that is, they enable one to distinguish between various genera and species of bacteria. Although two or more types of bacteria can grow on this medium, some agent in the medium allows them to be differentiated. Often the separation is based on color differences in the isolated colonies. An example of this kind of medium is eosin-methylene blue (EMB) agar, which differentiates *Escherichia coli* from *Enterobacter aerogenes*. The *E. coli* colonies on EMB agar are dark with a metallic sheen, while most *Enterobacter aerogenes* colonies are pink with a blue center and rarely have a metallic sheen. Most of the differential media are also selective and contain many kinds of growth-inhibiting agents.

An *enrichment medium* is used to inhibit the growth of an unwanted bacterial species that greatly outnumbers the wanted species in a specimen. For example, some fecal specimens containing the infectious agent *Salmonella* are outnumbered by the bacteria that are indigenous to the intestinal tract. An enrichment medium contains an agent such as selenite or tetrathionate that inhibits the growth of the unwanted species and favors the growth of the wanted species.

Transport media are especially designed to preserve microorganisms during their transit following isolation from the patient until they are cultivated in the laboratory. The medium is usually a buffered salts medium that prevents microbial growth. Some transport media contain agents that absorb oxygen, and these are used in transporting anaerobes to the laboratory.

CULTIVATION OF ANAEROBES

Obligate anaerobes grow only in the absence of air and some are sensitive to any level of oxygen. The cultivation of anaerobes, therefore, requires special precautions and the use of techniques that are not used in the cultivation of aerobic microorganisms. The most widely used and least expensive way to isolate anaerobes is by the *anaerobic jar method*. The jar, made of polycarbonate, is called the *GasPak* and is equipped with a removable lid that can form an airtight seal. The GasPak system (Fig. 5-6) is ordinarily used in clinical laboratories. A specified amount of water is added to the contents of a disposable aluminum foil envelope. The envelope is placed in the GasPak jar along with the inoculated cultures. The jar is sealed, and the water added to the envelope generates the production of hydrogen and carbon dioxide gases. With the aid of a catalyst (platinum) that is in the lid of the jar, any oxygen in the GasPak combines with hydrogen gas to

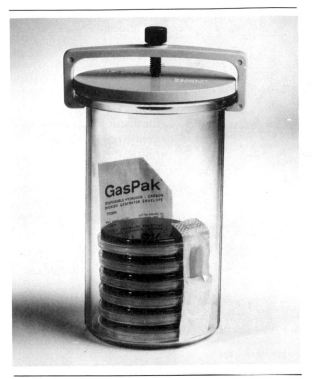

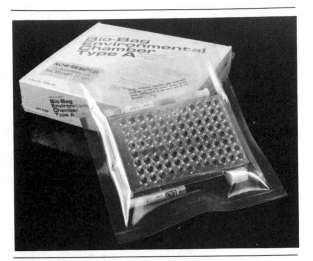

Fig. 5-7. Bio-Bag environmental chamber (type A), a disposable environmental system for the isolation of anaerobic bacteria. The chamber is sized to hold either a plate or the miniature identification systems currently used in clinical laboratories. (Courtesy Marion Laboratories, Inc., Kansas City, MO.)

Fig. 5-6. The GasPak for isolation of anaerobes. The GasPak is an anaerobic system consisting of a polycarbonate jar, lid holding a charged catalyst reaction chamber, GasPak disposable hydrogen-plus-carbon-dioxide generator envelope, and disposable anaerobic indicator. (Courtesy BBL Microbiology Systems, Division of Becton, Dickinson and Company, Cockeysville, MD.)

form water, thus producing an anaerobic environment.

Another simple technique for cultivating anaerobes is the *Bio-Bag* (Fig. 5-7). The Bio-Bag consists of a clear, gas-impermeable bag, an ampule containing an indicator, and a gas generator ampule. One or two plates are placed inside the bag and then the bag is sealed. The indicator ampule is crushed and the gas generator is activated. In about half an hour any oxygen in the bag is removed. The plates are easily observed and the organisms grow and remain viable for up to one week.

A technique for isolating anaerobes in labo-

ratories specializing in such procedures is the *anaerobic glove box*. The anaerobic glove box is made of a flexible vinyl plastic with openings for neoprene gloves (Fig. 5-8). The box may enclose up to 30 cubic feet. A mixture of nitrogen, hydrogen, and carbon dioxide gases fills the box and maintain its shape. Agar media are prepared outside the box and are placed in the box until the oxygen has been removed. Specimens are then inoculated onto the prepared agar plates within the box. An incubator may be placed in the box for incubation of the culture.

Isolation of anaerobes can be an important part of clinical microbiology because some anaerobes, such as species of *Clostridium*, are causes of fatal diseases. Nonsporeforming anaerobes, such as *Bacteroides*, *Fusobacterium*, and others, are more difficult to isolate than *Clostridium* species and special procedures are required for their isolation. These procedures may include special containers for transport of the clinical specimen and complex media containing blood and various supplements for cultivation, as well as special en-

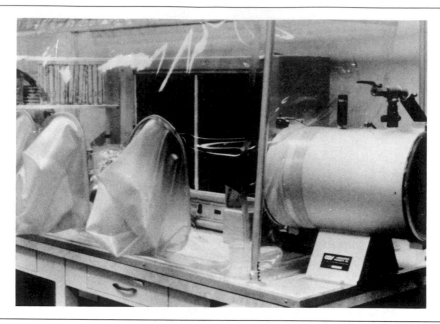

Fig. 5-8. The anaerobic glove box. (Courtesy Coy Laboratory Products, Inc., Ann Arbor, MI.)

vironments for cultivation such as those discussed above.

the basic mechanisms for isolating a pure culture and then look at types of isolation media.

TECHNIQUES FOR ISOLATING BACTERIA

PURE CULTURES

In medical microbiology the cultivation and isolation of a single species is a necessary prerequisite for identifying bacteria. The isolation of a single species from a mixed culture is called the *pure culture technique*. Several methods are available for obtaining pure cultures. In each case a culture or specimen containing microorganisms (called the *inoculum*) is introduced (*inoculated*) onto appropriate media for incubation at a specific temperature and time. We will first examine

Streak Plate

In the streak plate technique a small inoculum of the mixed population is streaked directly onto the surface of an agar medium. The streaking is performed with an inoculating loop. This procedure thins out the microbial population on the surface of the agar and where a single organism has been deposited a colony, which contains only one kind of bacterium, will develop after suitable incubation (Fig. 5-9). From one such colony an inoculum is streaked onto the surface of a second agar plate and the colonies that develop there are also examined. This subculture procedure ensures that only one kind of microorganism was present in the initially isolated colony. The pure culture can be used to conduct further laboratory investigations.

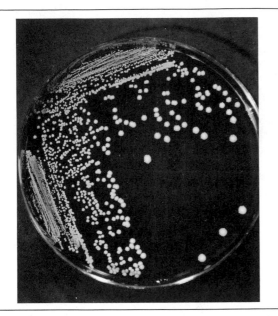

Fig. 5-9. The streak plate technique for isolation of colonies of bacteria. The area of heavy growth indicates the initial site of inoculation. A second streak was made at right angles to the first, and a third at right angles to the second. As the growth is thinned out, individual cells are deposited on the agar, giving rise to discrete colonies.

Pour Plate

In the pour plate procedure the mixed population is first diluted and a small quantity is transferred to the bottom of a sterile Petri dish. Melted agar (50°C) is then poured into the Petri dish to cover the bacteria. The dish is gently tilted to obtain uniform distribution of organisms. Colonies will develop on the surface of the agar as well as in the agar. This technique may be used for the isolation of anaerobes or microaerophiles tolerant of low levels of oxygen.

Membrane Filter

Membrane filters are thin porous sheets composed of cellulose esters or related materials. Once the sample is filtered, the filter can be placed on top of an agar medium, and after suitable incubation colonies will develop (Fig. 5-10).

In clinical microbiology the membrane filter technique has some applications when (1) the organism may be in small numbers in a large volume of fluid, (2) the fluid from which the organism is being isolated inhibits microbial growth (for example, spinal fluid or urine), and (3) total viable counts can be determined from urine samples and tedious dilution techniques are thereby avoided.

MEDIA USED FOR PRIMARY ISOLATION OF BACTERIA

Speed, specificity of the testing procedure, and economy of the test are three factors to be considered in diagnostic procedures in the clinical microbiology laboratory. When an organism can be identified quickly and with certainty, the patient can be treated more rapidly and the probability of cure is enhanced. The choice of the medium for isolation of the microbial species is,

Fig. 5-10. Colonies as they would appear on a membrane filter placed on an agar surface. (Courtesy Stanley Livingston.)

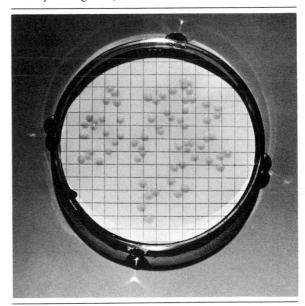

therefore, extremely important. It is usually dictated by the source of the specimen—feces, urine, etc.—and by the type of infectious agent suspected of causing the infection. A number of physiologically different microorganisms could conceivably be the cause of the infection. The clinical microbiologist will generally use more than one type of medium, as well as different environmental conditions for primary isolation: that is, the culture will be incubated both anaerobically and aerobically. The most commonly recommended primary isolation media are:

1. Thioglycolate. Thioglycolate contains, in addition to nutrients for growth, thioglycolyic acid and a small amount of agar. These components provide a reducing environment, that is, oxygen is depleted from the medium. Thus, some anaerobes can be cultivated without resorting to special anaerobic techniques.

2. Blood agar. Blood agar is an all-purpose medium that supports the growth of a wide range of pathogens, even those with very fastidious requirements. It also permits the evaluation of the hemolytic activity of microorganisms. Some microorganisms will completely lyse the red blood cells, and on blood agar the result is a clearing around the colony. This type of hemolysis is called *beta hemolysis*. Incomplete hemolysis or *alpha hemolysis* causes a greening around the colony. Absence of hemolysis is called *gamma hemolysis* (Fig. 5-11).

3. Phenylethyl alcohol agar. This agar medium is selective for the isolation of gram-positive cocci. The agents in this medium inhibit gram-negative species. Red blood cells may also be used in the medium for determining hemolytic activity of the coccal species.

4. Eosin-methylene blue (EMB) agar. EMB agar and MacConkey agar are selective media used in the isolation of gram-negative species, particularly those that infect the intestinal tract. Agents in these media inhibit gram-positive species; the inhibitors are often dyes that are toxic and interfere with electron transport.

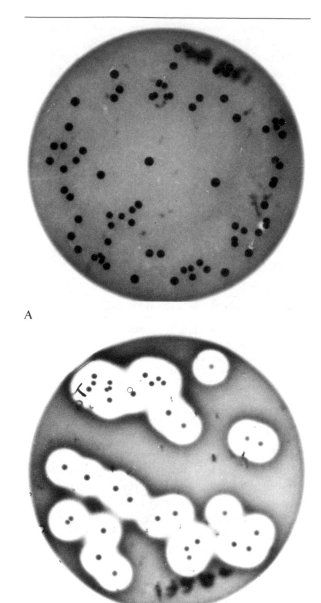

A

B

Fig. 5-11. Hemolytic activity. A. Colonies show no hemolytic activity (gamma hemolysis). B. Colonies show beta-hemolytic activity. (From J. LeBlanc and L. N. Lee, *J. Bacteriol.* 150:835, 1982.)

5. Chocolate blood agar. This agar medium contains blood that has been heated until the medium turns brown. It has been used for the isolation of *Haemophilus* and *Neisseria*. When antibiotics (vancomycin, colistin, and nystatin) are added to it, it is called Thayer-Martin medium and it becomes selective for the isolation of *N. gonorrhoeae* and *N. meningitidis*, the agents of gonorrhea and bacterial meningitis, respectively.

first frozen in a bath containing dry ice and acetone or some other mixture, the water in the cell can be removed by sublimation (as a gas) and damage to many of the cells can be prevented. This technique is commonly used for preservation of cultures and for shipment of cultures in the mail.

PRESERVATION OF ISOLATED MICROORGANISMS

Sometimes it is not possible to immediately perform tests on isolated bacteria and many bacteria do not survive for any length of time outside the host. Microorganisms can be preserved by a number of techniques, but the most widely used are freezing and freeze drying.

FREEZING

Most bacteria can be frozen in various types of media. The specimens are frozen rapidly to a temperature of $-20°$ to $-30°C$ to maintain the majority of cells in a viable state. Ultra-low temperatures obtained by using liquid nitrogen have been successfully employed for storage and preservation of all biological cell types, including fungi, viruses, and red blood cells.

FREEZE-DRYING (LYOPHILIZATION)

Ice crystal formation produced during the freezing process can damage cells. If the specimen is

LABORATORY MEASUREMENT OF MICROBIAL GROWTH

There are a number of ways to calculate microbial growth. In the research laboratory, for example, investigators can determine the concentration of macromolecules such as DNA, RNA, protein, etc. in a population of cells and these become parameters of growth. In the clinical laboratory, however, investigators are often more concerned with the actual number of bacteria in a specimen because this often relates to the intensity of infection in a patient. Two of the most commonly used techniques for determining bacterial numbers are cell count and cell density measurements.

CELL COUNT

Microscopic
Using the microscope, one can count bacterial cells directly when a small portion of the culture is spread on a calibrated slide called the *Petroff-Hauser counter*. This device is similar to the hemocytometer used to count red blood cells. Calibrated ruled areas are etched into a special glass slide (Fig. 5-12). An aliquot of bacteria is introduced under the coverslip that covers the ruled area. The ruled area is observed microscopically, and the microorganisms are counted.

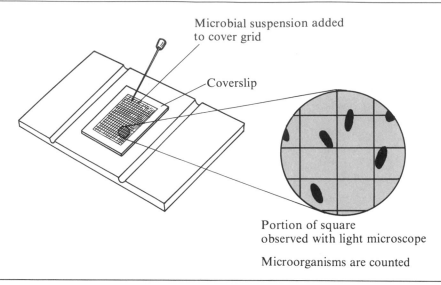

Microbial suspension added
to cover grid

Coverslip

Portion of square
observed with light microscope

Microorganisms are counted

Fig. 5-12. Petroff-Hauser counter. The large square is observed microscopically after the addition of an aliquot of a culture. The volume of fluid on the large square is known, and this number is multiplied by the number of bacteria observed times the original dilution factor. The product is the concentration of bacteria per milliliter present in the culture sample.

Since the depth of fluid above the calibrated area is known, the number of organisms per unit volume can be calculated. This method cannot, however, distinguish live from dead cells.

Standard Plate Count

Cells can be counted indirectly by determining the number of cells that, when spread on the surface of an agar medium, give rise to distinct colonies. The standard plate count technique usually involves some type of dilution that reduces the number of cells to a countable number (30 to 300 cells) before plating on suitable media. The colonies are counted, and that figure times the dilution factor will give the total number of viable bacteria per milliliter in the original culture before dilution (Fig. 5-13). This technique is one of the most widely used in microbiology laboratories. In addition to spreading directly onto the agar surface, the sample may also be filtered through a membrane filter that will retain the bac-

teria. The filter may then be placed over an agar surface and, after suitable incubation, the colonies may be counted (see Figs. 5 and 10).

CELL DENSITY

As the population in a culture increases, the turbidity or density of the broth culture also increases. Changes in turbidity can be detected by a device called a *spectrophotometer*, which records them in units called optical density (OD) units or absorbance (A) units (Fig. 5-14). When the measurements are correlated and graphed, they can save the researcher a considerable amount of time. In subsequent experiments, for example, an optical density reading alone is all that is required if the researcher wishes to know the population of cells. This technique can be applied only when one uses the same organism under the same environmental conditions and during logarithmic growth.

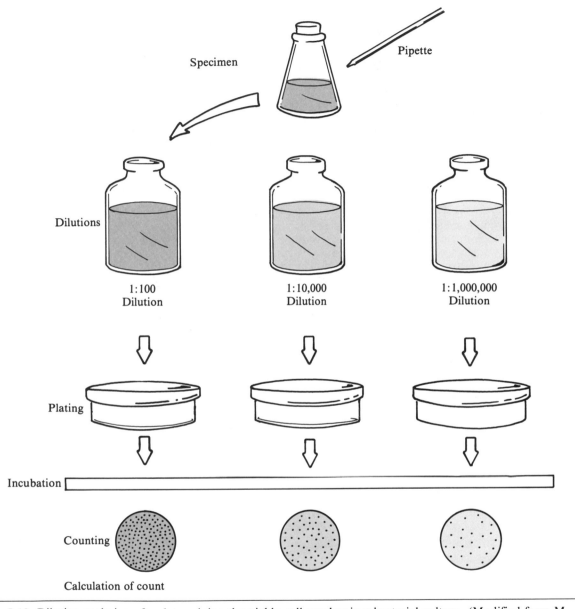

Specimen

Pipette

Dilutions

1:100
Dilution

1:10,000
Dilution

1:1,000,000
Dilution

Plating

Incubation

Counting

Calculation of count

Fig. 5-13. Dilution technique for determining the viable cell number in a bacterial culture. (Modified from M. J. Pelczar and R. D. Reid, *Microbiology*. New York: McGraw-Hill, 1972.)

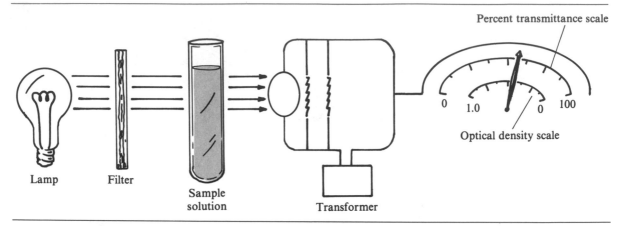

Fig. 5-14. Spectrophotometer. A sample of bacteria in solution acts as colloidal suspension that intercepts light passing through it. Some light is absorbed; the remainder, passing through, activates a photocell, which in turn registers percentage of transmittance on a galvanometer. The higher the percentage of transmittance, the fewer the cells in suspension. The amount of light absorbed by the suspension is reflected in the optical density. The greater the number of cells in suspension, the greater the optical density (OD).

SUMMARY

1. Bacteria reproduce asexually in a process called binary fission. They reproduce geometrically, with doubling times varying from a few minutes to several hours depending on the species.

2. Bacteria in culture exhibit a growth cycle that includes phases such as lag, log, stationary, and death and decline. The lag phase is a period of adjustment to the growth medium. The log phase is a period of constancy in which the rate of growth of a microbial species can be determined. The growth rate depends on the type of microbial species, temperature, and growth-supporting ability of the medium. The stationary phase is characterized by an equilibrium between the number of cells dying and the number dividing. The death and decline phase is a period of geometric decline brought about by toxic products and nutrient loss.

3. The major nutrients required for growth include water, carbon, nitrogen, sulfur, phosphorus, oxygen, and minerals. Water is needed for transport of nutrients and in the hydrolysis of molecules in the cell. Organic carbon serves both as a carbon and as an energy source in organisms referred to as heterotrophs. Organic molecules that cannot be synthesized from a carbon source and are required in the culture medium are called growth factors. Minerals are required only in trace amounts, and these are usually supplied in the water supply.

4. Nitrogen is most frequently utilized by bacteria in the form of inorganic molecules such as nitrate, nitrite, ammonia, and nitrogen gas. These forms are converted to ammonia, which is then incorporated into the organic phase as an amino acid. Sulfur and phosphorus are usually supplied to the cell in inorganic forms such as sulfate and phosphate, respectively. Phosphate also acts as a buffer against acids produced during growth.

5. Oxygen is required by aerobic, microaerophilic, and facultatively anaerobic bacteria but not by obligate anaerobes. Oxygen is a final electron acceptor that is usually converted to toxic products such as hydrogen peroxide and superoxide. Organisms that utilize oxygen, however, also produce enzymes, such as catalase and su-

peroxide dismutase, that inactivate the toxic products. For some obligate anaerobes oxygen is toxic but in other anaerobes oxygen can be tolerated because it is not reduced to toxic intermediates.

6. The major physical factors affecting growth are pH, temperature, and osmotic pressure. The pH of bacterial culture media is between 6 and 8, while fungi grow best at pHs below 6.0. Buffers, such as phosphate and proteins, are used in culture media to prevent rapid drops in pH due to accumulation of acids.

7. Bacteria can be classified as psychrophilic, mesophilic, and thermophilic based on their optimum temperatures for growth. Psychrophiles have an optimum temperature range between 0 and 20°C, mesophiles between 30 and 37°C, and thermophiles between 45 and 70°C. Temperatures between 62 and 71°C are used in pasteurization processes while temperatures at 100°C and above are used to sterilize. Low temperatures including freezing can injure and kill bacteria but some microorganisms can survive low temperatures for various lengths of time.

8. Osmotic pressure in culture media is usually supplied in the form of salt (NaCl). Some foods are prepared in high concentrations of salt or sugars to induce plasmolysis of bacteria and thus preserve food.

9. Culture media can be in the form of a liquid, called broth, or a semisolid produced by using the carbohydrate called agar. Media can be classified based on chemical content and laboratory use. On the basis of chemical content media may be synthetic, that is, the exact composition is known, or nonsynthetic, that is, the exact chemical composition is not known.

10. Media based on laboratory use are divided into all-purpose, enriched, selective, differential, enrichment, and transport. All-purpose media provide nutrients for growth of most microorganisms. Enriched media contain a basal growth medium plus additional nutrients, such as blood, for growth of more fastidious microorganisms. Selective media contain additives that select against some bacteria and for other bacteria. A differential medium contains additives that allow one to distinguish different species on an agar surface. An enrichment medium inhibits the growth of unwanted species that are in excess in a specimen and induces the growth of wanted species. A transport medium is used for specimens removed from patients that must be carried back to the laboratory without harming the microorganisms that are present.

11. Cultivation of anaerobes requires techniques that remove or replace oxygen. The anaerobic jar is a widely used device in which gases, such as hydrogen, are generated and combine with oxygen to form water. A smaller version of an anaerobic container is the Bio-Bag. For larger operations there is the flexible vinyl plastic glovebox, which contains gases that maintain the shape of the box and remove oxygen.

12. Pure culture techniques are used to isolate a single species from a mixed culture. There are three basic methods for obtaining a pure culture. The streak plate physically separates individual cells on an agar surface using an inoculating loop. In the pour plate technique bacteria are diluted and distributed in molten agar to effect their separation. Small numbers of bacteria in a fluid can be separated out of the fluid by use of the membrane filter technique. Bacteria retained on the filter can be cultivated on an agar surface.

13. The media for isolation of bacteria from laboratory specimens include: thioglycolate for some anaerobes; blood agar for detecting the hemolytic activity of bacteria; phenylethyl alcohol agar for isolating gram-positive cocci; eosin methylene blue agar for isolating gram-negative species; and chocolate blood agar for isolation of *Haemophilus* and *Neisseria* species.

14. Microorganisms can be preserved by freezing or freeze drying, but freeze drying is the more efficient technique.

15. Microbial growth can be detected in various ways. Microscopic cell counts using the Petroff-Hauser counter measure both live and dead cells. Standard plate counts measure only viable cells. Cell density is an indirect means of measuring growth by using a spectrophotometer.

QUESTIONS FOR STUDY

Select the best response or responses for each of the following:

1. Which of the following best describes the lag phase of growth?
   A. The bacterial cells are dividing in a geometric fashion.
   B. There is an accumulation of acids that reduce the pH of the medium.
   C. Most of the oxygen in the medium has been depleted.
   D. Cells are increasing in size but few are dividing.

2. The ability of species of *Klebsiella* to grow and divide in a sterile glucose solution, such as those used for intravenous nutrition, is probably related to the microorganism's ability to:
   A. Use carbon dioxide from the air as a source of oxygen
   B. Utilize ammonia, which is part of the glucose solution
   C. Use glucose as a carbon source and nitrogen gas as a source of nitrogen
   D. Use glucose as a source of carbon and nitrogen

3. Which of the following best explains the ability of obligate anaerobes to tolerate oxygen?

Fill in the blank:

6. The time required for a culture to double is called the_____.

7. If you have a culture containing 50 cells that has a doubling time of 20 minutes, the number of cells at the end of 3 hours will be:_____.

8. The stage of bacterial growth in which the growth curve is represented as a horizontal line is called the_____phase.

   A. They produce superoxide dismutase.
   B. They produce catalase and superoxide dismutase.
   C. They lack enzymes that reduce oxygen.
   D. They do not possess any Krebs cycle enzymes.

4. Enrichment media are designed to:
   A. Help distinguish between different species
   B. Increase the numbers of all species in the medium
   C. Increase the numbers of a species that is initially outnumbered by unwanted species
   D. Select for microbial species that can grow on media containing blood

5. Each of the media below contain glucose plus the listed inorganic and organic components. In which of the media would an organism such as *E. coli* be more likely to grow?
   A. Amino acids cysteine, alanine, and tryptophan; NaCl; $(NH_4)_2SO_4$; and KH_2PO_4
   B. $(NH_4)_2 SO_4$; KH_2PO_4; NaCl; and cysteine
   C. $(NH_4)_2SO_4$; $MgSO_4$; NaCl; KH_2PO_4
   D. Cysteine; $MgSo_4$; KCl

9. The enzyme produced by bacteria that enables them to break down hydrogen peroxide is called_____.

10. The mineral important in endospore formation is_____.

ADDITIONAL READINGS

Dawes, I. W., and Sutherland, I. W. *Microbial Physiology*. New York: Halsted Press, 1976.

Edwards, C. *The Microbial Cell Cycle*. Aspects of Microbiology. Washington, DC: American Society for Microbiology, 1981.

Higgins, M. L., and Shockman, G. R. Prokaryotic cell division with respect to cell wall and membranes. *CRC Crit Rev Microbiol*. 1:29, 1971.

Ingraham, J. L., Maaløe, O., and Neidhardt, F. C. *Growth of the Bacterial Cell*. Sunderland, ME: Sinauer, 1983.

Mandelstam, J., and McQuillen, K. *Biochemistry of Bacterial Growth* (3rd ed.). New York: Halsted Press, 1982.

Moat, A. G. *Microbial Physiology*. New York: Wiley, 1988.

6. MICROBIAL GENETICS

OBJECTIVES

To discuss the basic chemical structure of DNA and how it is physically arranged in the cell

To explain the relationship between DNA structure and replication

To list the enzymes associated with DNA replication and transcription and their specific functions

To outline the basic steps in protein synthesis

To describe the differences and similarities between a repressible and inducible operon

To explain what is meant by the genetic code and how mutations affect it

To explain how mutations may arise in the cell and how some of them can be repaired

To describe how mutants can be detected and isolated

To distinguish the three methods of DNA transfer: transformation, transduction, and conjugation

To describe the importance of plasmids to bacteria and how they are transferred

To briefly discuss the basics of genetic engineering and its potential importance to society and medicine.

To define: transcription, genotype, phenotype, plasmid, codon, anticodon, inducible, constitutive, insertion sequence, transposon, auxotroph, prototroph, sex factor, cloning, restriction endonuclease

A student might think that a discussion of microbial genetics and how microorganisms store and transfer genetic information would be boring and hardly worth the effort. Quite the contrary. The rapid development of molecular genetics, in conjunction with the ability of scientists to manipulate and transfer genes, has elicited considerable interest among physicians, scientists, and the public in general. Our ability to manipulate the hereditary material of microorganisms and even of our own species has far-reaching consequences.

The primary purpose of this chapter is to discuss the functions of the hereditary material in microorganisms and to examine how manipulation of the genetic material is being used to advance industrial and medical microbiology.

NUCLEIC ACIDS: THE BASIS OF HEREDITY

The characteristic traits that are expressed in one generation and are transferred to another gen-

eration have their origin in the nucleic acids of the cell, that is, deoxyribonucleic acid (DNA) and ribonucleic acid (RNA). All cellular organisms have DNA as the carrier of their heredity; however, acellular microorganisms, such as some viruses, substitute RNA for DNA.

The hereditary material consists of specific sequences of purine and pyrimidine bases (see Fig. 4–16, page 85) that are divided into units of information called *genes*. All the genes of the organism make up what is referred to as the *genotype* of the cell. The translation of the information in the genes leads to the expression of specific traits by the organism called the *phenotype*.

The genetic information of the bacterial cell can be carried on a single molecule of DNA, which is called a *chromosome*. Eukaryotes, however, require more than one chromosome or DNA molecule to carry all their hereditary information. Many bacteria also have smaller pieces of DNA, called *plasmids*, that are not part of the chromosome (extrachromosomal). Plasmid DNA confers traits that enable the bacteria to survive more efficiently in their environment.

The DNA molecule performs specific func-

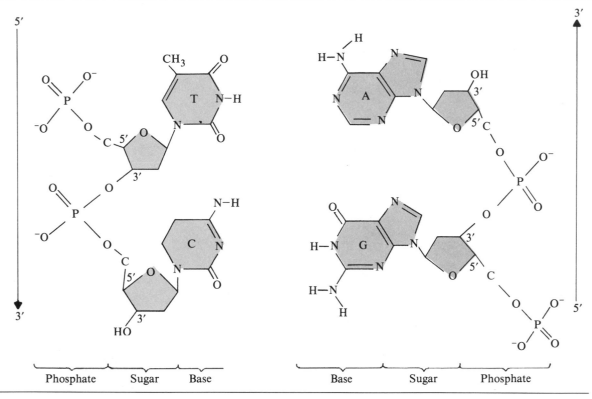

Fig. 6-1. Nucleotide arrangement as demonstrated in a portion of the DNA molecule. Each strand consists of a sugar phosphate backbone with purine (adenine and guanine) and pyrimidine (thymine and cytosine) bases attached to sugar group. Bases between strands are paired by hydrogen bonds (.....). The strands are antiparallel; strand on left is called the 5′ end, that is, it is arranged in the 5′ to 3′ direction. Strand on right is arranged in the 3′ to 5′ direction.

tions in the bacterial cell and includes the ability to:

1. Duplicate (replicate) itself for transfer to progeny (daughter cells) during cell division
2. Transcribe itself into a nucleic acid molecule that can be translated into protein
3. Control the synthesis of proteins
4. Mutate and change specific characteristics
5. Duplicate and transfer itself to other species in processes other than cell division

We will now examine each of these functions in more detail.

DNA STRUCTURE AND REPLICATION

The DNA molecule of bacteria consists of two chains of chemical units called *nucleotides*. A single molecule of bacterial DNA may contain from 10 to 40 million nucleotides. A nucleotide consists of a base, either a purine or pyrimidine, to which is attached a sugar phosphate group. Each chain consists of alternating sugar phosphates with a purine or pyrimidine base attached to each sugar group (Fig. 6-1). The bases in DNA are of four different types: adenine and guanine,

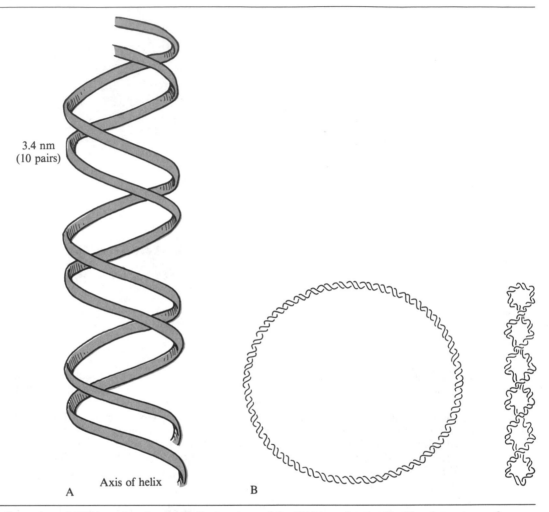

3.4 nm
(10 pairs)

Axis of helix

A   B

Fig. 6-2. Configuration of DNA molecule. A. Helical nature of the DNA molecule. B. Circular nature of DNA. Figure on left is a closed circle while figure on right shows how twisting of circle reduces circle size.

which are purines, and thymine (T) and cytosine, which are pyrimidines. The two nucleotide chains are attached to each other by virtue of the bonding of hydrogen atoms between a specific purine base on one strand and a specific pyrimidine base on the other strand. In DNA, adenine binds to thymine and guanine binds to cytosine. This is called a *base pair* arrangement, that is, adenine on one strand is *complementary* to thymine on the other strand and guanine on one

strand is complementary to cytosine on the other strand. If you look at Figure 6-1 you will notice that one strand appears to be upside down, that is, the strands are antiparallel. One strand has a free hydroxyl (OH) group attached to carbon 3 of the sugar, while on the opposite strand the free hydroxyl is on carbon 5 of the sugar. Each strand has a 3' and a 5' end.

Double-stranded DNA exists in the cell in the form of a helix with the two ends of the molecule

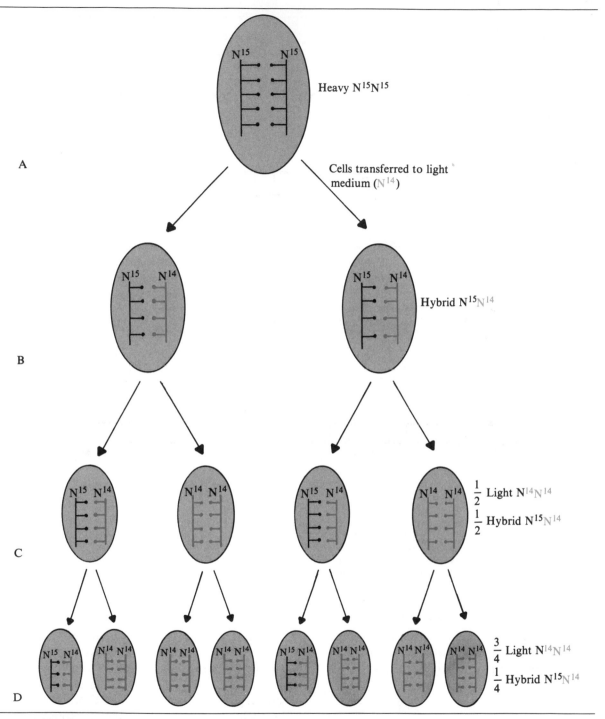

Fig. 6-3. Semiconservative replication of DNA. Microbial cells are grown in a medium containing heavy nitrogen (N^{15}). A. Both strands of DNA are labeled with heavy isotope. B. After transfer to a medium containing light nitrogen (N^{14}) this generation of cells contains DNA that has one light and one heavy strand. C. One-half of the progeny in this generation of cells contain hybrid DNA ($N^{15}N^{14}$). D. One-fourth of the progeny contain hybrid DNA while three-fourths contain light DNA.

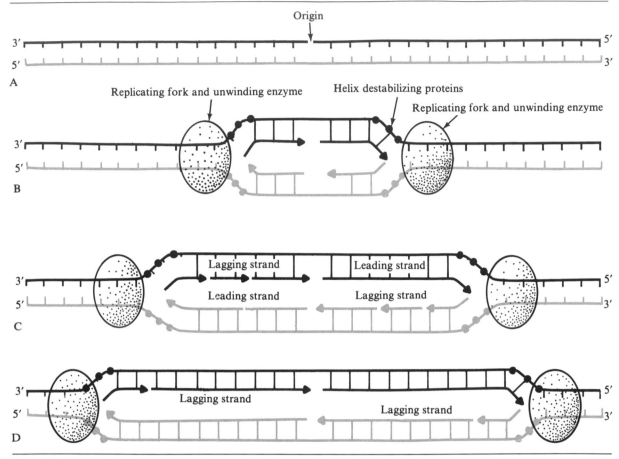

Fig. 6-4. Replication of DNA in bacteria. A. Double-stranded DNA molecule nicked by enzyme at origin. B. Unwinding enzyme produces two replicating forks. Single strands are prevented from unwinding by helix-destabilizing proteins. C. Behind each replicating fork one new DNA strand grows continuously (*leading strand*) and the other grows as a series of fragments (*lagging strand*). D. As DNA synthesis continues, those fragmented pieces of DNA nearest the origin become linked by DNA ligase. Please note that the RNA primers have been omitted for clarity.

joined to form a circle (Fig. 6-2). In its circular form the DNA molecule is much longer than the cell; therefore, the circle is folded on itself in order to fit into the bacterium.

MECHANISM OF DNA REPLICATION

The transmission of genetic material from parent to progeny requires an exact duplication of the original or parental DNA strands. Major errors in the duplication process could be disastrous, leading to conditions that prevent normal cell growth and development.

Because the bacterial chromosome is in a coiled state in the cell, it must be unwound to be duplicated. The DNA molecule replicates in a *semiconservative manner*. Each strand of the parent DNA serves as a template for the formation of a complementary strand (Fig. 6-3). The mechanism by which the DNA molecule undergoes this duplication process in the cell is believed to occur in the following way (see Fig. 6-4):

The bacterial chromosome possesses a site for unwinding DNA and for initiation of DNA replication, referred to as the *origin*. The origin is recognized and activated by specific proteins such as:

1. *Unwinding proteins*. One strand of the DNA molecule is nicked by an enzyme; thus, the tension in the circular helix is released. The unwinding of DNA is caused by unwinding proteins that promote separation of the two parental strands. Unwinding produces two *replicating forks*, one on either side of the origin (Fig. 6-4), which will move away from the origin during the replication process.
2. *Helix-destabilizing proteins*. Any unwound single-stranded DNA will be prevented from rewinding by the attachment of helix-destabilizing proteins.
3. *DNA polymerase*. The actual synthesis of new (daughter) DNA is catalyzed by the enzyme DNA polymerase. The substrates for the enzyme are the four deoxyribonucleotide triphosphates, that is, dATP (deoxyadenosine triphosphate), dGTP (deoxyguanosine triphosphate), dCTP (deoxycytosine triphosphate), and dTTP (deoxythymidine triphosphate). Just before DNA synthesis short RNA strands called *primer RNA* are laid down in the 5' to 3' direction.

DNA polymerase synthesizes DNA only in the 5' to 3' direction because the enzyme requires a free 3' hydroxyl group, that is, nucleotides are added to the free 3' end. Since the two strands are antiparallel, the continuous addition of deoxyribonucleotides to the RNA primer can occur only on one strand (Fig. 6-4). The DNA strand replicating continuously is called the *leading strand*. The 5' end of the leading strand is located at the origin and its 3' end at the moving replicating fork. The opposite or *lagging strand* is elongated by a different mechanism, because the

3' position is at the origin while the 5' end is at the replication fork. If nucleotides were sequentially added to the end of the lagging strand at the replication fork, then this strand's growth would proceed in a 3' to 5' direction. This does not take place. Instead, growth takes place by the synthesis of a number of short polynucleotide chains between the replication fork and the origin. Each short chain is laid down in the direction 5' to 3' and these are later linked together and to the 5' end of the lagging strand. Each short DNA chain is actually attached to the 3' ends of the individual primer RNA strands, which were laid down before DNA synthesis. Later the RNA primers are removed and the regions that are left vacant are filled in with deoxyribonucleotides. The smaller units of DNA synthesized on the lagging strand are united by the enzyme called *DNA ligase*. As a result, the overall direction of growth of the lagging strand is the same as that of the leading strand.

DNA TRANSCRIPTION

The information contained in the DNA molecule cannot be used by the cell until it is transcribed into a form that is translatable. *Transcription* is merely the process in which one strand of DNA serves as a template for the synthesis of a single-stranded RNA molecule, called *messenger RNA* (*mRNA*). RNA differs from DNA in that RNA possesses the sugar ribose instead of deoxyribose, and uracil takes the place of thymine. The base pairing between a DNA strand and an RNA strand is:

DNA	RNA
A	Ü
T	A
C	G
G	C

It is the information on the mRNA molecule that

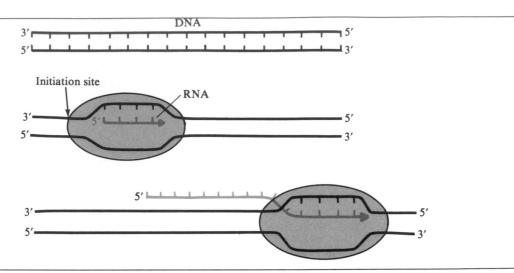

Fig. 6-5. Transcription of DNA into RNA. Transcription begins at an initiation site where the DNA unwinds and RNA polymerase binds. Only one strand is transcribed and this is in a 5′ to 3′ direction. RNA polymerase moves along the DNA with ribonucleotides being added to the 3′ end of the growing chain.

can be translated into usable information by the cell. This usable information is in the form of amino acids that are assembled into specific proteins. Thus the flow of information in the cell is: DNA → RNA → Protein.

The transcription of DNA into mRNA requires the enzyme *RNA polymerase*, which assembles the nucleotides adenosine triphosphate (ATP), uridine triphosphate (UTP), guanosine triphosphate (GTP), and cytosine triphosphate (CTP) into an RNA chain (Fig. 6-5). Bacteria may have a thousand or more genes and the transcription of each one is under the control of specific sites on the DNA, which will be discussed later under Control of Protein Synthesis. Keep in mind that a DNA strand can also be transcribed into RNA molecules other than mRNA, for example, ribosomal RNA (rRNA) and transfer RNA (tRNA), whose functions will be described shortly.

DNA AND THE GENETIC CODE

It is the particular sequence of nucleotides in a gene that determines the specific amino acid composition of the polypeptide* for which it codes. The nucleotides on the mRNA are arranged as a linear sequence of coding units or *codons* (also called *triplets*). Each codon consists of three successive purine or pyrimidine bases. The sequence of codons on the mRNA contains the necessary information to (1) initiate polypeptide synthesis, (2) designate the sequence of amino acids in the polypeptide, (3) terminate the synthesis of the polypeptide, and (4) release the completed polypeptide.

Since there are four different purine or pyrimidine bases and the code is a triplet code, the total number of possible code words is 64 (4 × 4 × 4). The maximum number of different amino acids in the polypeptide is 20; thus, each amino acid can have at least 3 code words. Codons that specify amino acids are referred to as *sense codons*. Three of the codons do not code for an amino acid and are referred to as *nonsense codons* (see Table 6-1).

---

* Proteins are made up of amino acids linked together by bonds called *peptide bonds*; hence the name *polypeptide*. Most proteins are made up of more than one polypeptide molecule. .

Table 6-1. The Genetic Code

First letter	Second letter				Third letter
	U	C	A	G	
U	Phe	Ser	Tyr	Cys	U
	Phe	Ser	Tyr	Cys	C
	Leu	Ser	Nonsense	Nonsense	A
	Leu	Ser	Nonsense	Trp	G
C	Leu	Pro	His	Arg	U
	Leu	Pro	His	Arg	C
	Leu	Pro	Gln	Arg	A
	Leu	Pro	Gln	Arg	G
A	Ileu	Thr	Asn	Ser	U
	Ileu	Thr	Asn	Ser	C
	Ileu	Thr	Lys	Arg	A
	Met	Thr	Lys	Arg	G
G	Val	Ala	Asp	Gly	U
	Val	Ala	Asp	Gly	C
	Val	Ala	Glu	Gly	A
	Val	Ala	Glu	Gly	G

U = uracil; C = cytosine; A = adenine; G = guanine; Phe = phenylalanine; Ser = serine; Tyr = tyrosine; Cys = cysteine; Leu = leucine; Trp = tryptophan; Pro = proline; His = histidine; Arg = arginine; Gln = glutamine; Ileu = isoleucine; Thr = threonine; Asn = asparagine; Lys = lysine; Met = methionine; Val = valine; Ala = alanine; Asp = aspartic acid; Gly = glycine; Glu = glutamic acid.

TRANSLATION OF THE GENETIC CODE: PROTEIN SYNTHESIS

Messenger RNA is translated into polypeptides in a process that takes place on the ribosome. *Ribosomes* are small structural components in the cell that are composed of RNA molecules, called ribosomal RNA, and a variety of proteins. Bacterial ribosomes are composed of 2 subunits 50S and 30S (S refers to *Svedberg*, which is a relative size unit derived from sedimentation studies). Before polypeptide synthesis begins each amino acid is *activated* and brought to the ribosome by means of another RNA called *transfer RNA* (tRNA). There are 20 different tRNA molecules, one for each amino acid. The amino acid is attached to one end of the tRNA and in this form is called *aminoacyl tRNA* while the other end of the tRNA possesses a sequence of bases called the *anticodon* (Fig. 6-6). If, for example, the tRNA carried the amino acid phenylalanine and the code word on the mRNA for phenylalanine was UUU, then the anticodon on the tRNA carrying the amino acid would be AAA. Thus, the anticodon sequence is complementary to the codon sequence and this provides a potentially errorless translation. The process of protein synthesis occurs in a series of steps referred to as *initiation, elongation*, and *termination*.

The synthesis of the polypeptide takes place by the linear movement of ribosomes along the mRNA so that each codon is translated in sequence. The first aminoacyl tRNA attaches to an *initiation site* on the mRNA and with a ribosome forms an initiation complex. The ribosome moves to the next codon and a second aminoacyl tRNA, with the proper anticodon, attaches to the ribosome. The two amino acids are joined by a bond called a *peptide bond* (Fig. 6-7). The peptide becomes attached to the second aminoacyl tRNA while the first tRNA is released and is free to go

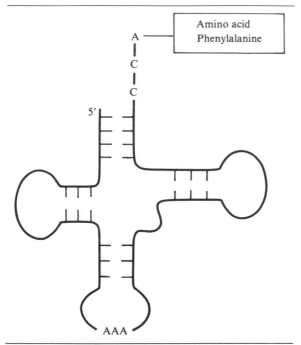

Amino acid
Phenylalanine

Fig. 6-6. Basic structure of transfer RNA (tRNA). Transfer RNA is single-stranded but the molecule folds and some hydrogen bonding (———) occurs between bases that give the molecule the appearance of a clover leaf. One end of the tRNA chain ends in CCA and this is the site for attachment of an amino acid (in this example, it is phenylalanine). One of the loops on the RNA molecule contains a triplet base called the anticodon (in this example, it is AAA that is complementary to one of the codons for phenylalanine, which is UUU; see Table 6-1).

back into the cytoplasm and pick up another amino acid. This process continues in a sequential manner until the last codon on the mRNA is reached and the complete polypeptide has been synthesized. After the first ribosome has moved away from the initiation site, another ribosome can attach to the initiation site and the synthesis of a second molecule of the polypeptide is begun. Thus, each ribosome on the mRNA is carrying a polypeptide of varying length. Termination and release of the polypeptide is due to the presence of nonsense codons (see Table 6-1). When the polypeptide is released into the cytoplasm the ri-

bosome separates from the mRNA and it (ribosome) can be used again to initiate polypeptide synthesis.

CONTROL OF PROTEIN SYNTHESIS

The metabolic potential of most microbial cells is vast, and synthesis of all of the enzymes used in metabolism is not necessary. The cell will coordinate its genetic potential with the availability of nutrients to determine which enzymes are needed for growth. Protein synthesis is therefore not an unrestricted metabolic process but is under the control of a genetic mechanism subject to induction and repression.

INDUCTION AND REPRESSION

The concentration of many enzymes in the cell is directly associated with specific nutrients in the cell's environment. Enzymes that show an increase in concentration in the presence of specific nutrients are called *inducible enzymes*. The enzyme beta-galactosidase, for example, is an inducible enzyme that is produced when its substrate, lactose, a disaccharide (carbohydrate composed of two sugars), is present in the cell's environment. If lactose is not present the cell produces a protein that represses the synthesis of beta-galactosidase. Not all enzymes are subject to this dual induction-repression response. Some enzymes in the cell, called *constitutive enzymes*, are produced whether the natural substrate is present or not. Constitutive enzymes can be controlled by mechanisms that affect enzyme activity; this type of control is discussed in Chapter 4. Much of our knowledge concerning induction and repression is the result of work by two French microbiologists, Jacob and Monod. They were instrumental in developing the operon theory of control.

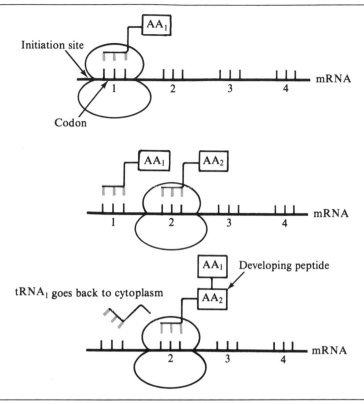

Fig. 6-7. Mechanism of protein synthesis. Ribosome binds to mRNA initiation site along with aminoacyl tRNA(AA$_1$) possessing an anticodon that is complementary to codon I. Ribosome moves to second codon and anticodon of aminoacyl tRNA(AA$_2$) binds to it. A peptide bond is formed between amino acids 1 and 2 and peptide becomes attached to second tRNA, while first tRNA is free to return to the cytoplasm. Process continues until termination triplet is reached and polypeptide is released.

THE OPERON

The operon consists of a cluster of genes and nucleotide sequences (they do not code for any polypeptide) that control the synthesis of proteins in the cell. For example, the formation of some molecules in the cell may require from 2 to 10 different enzymes. The genes that code for these enzymes are clustered together in the operon. The synthesis of these enzymes can be genetically turned on or turned off to suit the particular needs of the cell. The operon and associated areas consist of the following component (Fig. 6-8):

1. *Structural genes*. Genes coding for enzymes involved in the formation of a specific molecule in the cell are called structural genes.
2. *Operator*. The operator is not a gene but a sequence of nucleotides that are adjacent to the structural genes. The operator is able to bind a protein called the *repressor protein* and this prevents transcription of the structural genes.
3. *Promoter*. The promoter is not a gene but a special sequence of nucleotides lying outside the operator. The promoter is the site for binding RNA polymerase, which is required for transcription of the structural genes.
4. *Regulator gene*. The regulator gene lies out-

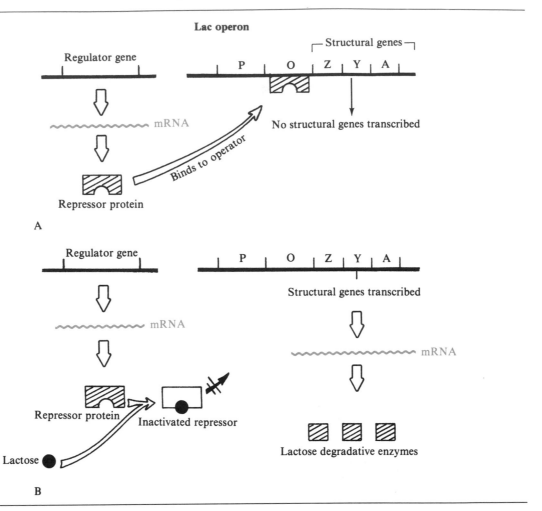

Fig. 6-8. Inducible operon. A. Lactose operon in absence of the inducer lactose. Repressor protein is synthesized and binds to operator (O). Structural genes are not transcribed. B. Lactose operon in presence of inducer. Lactose binds to repressor and inactivates it. Inactivated repressor is unable to bind to operator and structural genes are free to be transcribed.

side the operon. It codes for the synthesis of the *repressor* protein molecule, whose site of action is the operator.

Let us examine each type.

Inducible Operons
Inducible operons are primarily involved in controlling enzymes that are associated with degradative systems in the cell, that is, processes that

release energy. The lactose(*lac*) operon is an example of an inducible operon. The lac operon possesses three structural genes: the *beta-galactosidase gene* (*Z*), which codes for the enzyme that cleaves lactose into glucose and galactose sugars; the *permease gene* (*Y*), which codes for a protein that transports lactose into the cell; and the *transacetylase gene* (*A*), which is involved in utilization of galactosides other than lactose.

In the absence of lactose (a condition in which

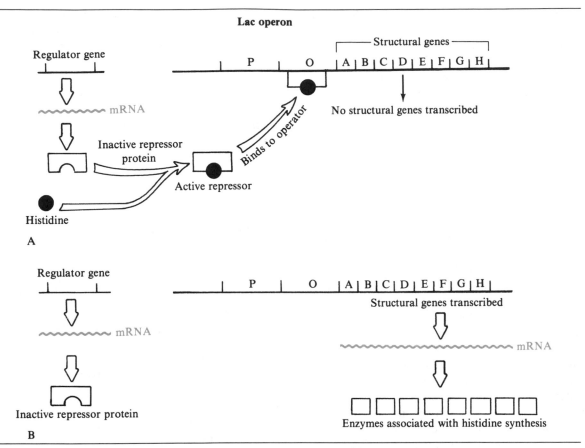

Fig. 6-9. Repressible operon. A. Operon involved in controlling enzymes associated with synthesis of the amino acid histidine. In this example histidine is in excess. Histidine acts as a co-repressor and activates repressor, which prevents transcription of structural genes. B. Histidine operon in absence of histidine in the cell. Inactive repressor has no effect on operator and structural genes are transcribed.

the bacterial cell does not need beta-galactosidase), the regulator gene produces a repressor protein that binds to the operator and transcription of structural genes by RNA polymerase is prohibited (Fig. 6-8A). When lactose is present the repressor protein attaches to this sugar and the complex is unable to bind to the operator. Under these circumstances RNA polymerase is free to transcribe the structural genes (Fig. 6-8B).

Repressible Operons

Repressible operons are involved primarily in biosynthetic systems, for example, pathways as-

sociated with amino acid synthesis. In this system the repressor protein does not bind to the operator until it first complexes with a *co-repressor* molecule. The co-repressor molecule is the end product of biosynthesis. For example, the tryptophan operon controls the synthesis of enzymes involved in tryptophan formation in the cell. If tryptophan is already present in the culture medium the bacterial cell does not need to synthesize its own tryptophan. Tryptophan acts as a co-repressor and binds to the repressor protein, forming a complex that binds to the operator and prevents transcription of the tryptophan structural genes (Fig. 6-9).

Inducible and repressible operons help the cell conserve energy by preventing the unnecessary synthesis of enzymes at a particular time in the bacterial cell cycle. Recall that another form of control, called feedback inhibition, also helped conserve energy by reducing the activity of enzymes that were already present in the cell (see Chapter 4).

MUTATION

The term *mutation* refers to change or modification in a specific characteristic of the organism. These changes or modifications are the result of alterations in the base sequence of the hereditary material. Mutation may bring about advantages or disadvantages to the cell. Some mutations may be lethal, while others may help the organism to survive in its environment. The induction of mutations is called *mutagenesis* and the agents involved are called *mutagens*. Mutations play an important role in many fields of microbiology. They are used by research scientists to delve into the various aspects of structure and function, metabolism, and reproduction of microorganisms. The results from such studies have been helpful in understanding the genetic systems of higher organisms, including humans. Mutation is also important in areas of applied microbiology. Increased synthesis of industrially useful products resulting from microbial metabolism is due to the ability of microbiologists to select naturally occurring mutants or to induce mutations.

Mutations may arise in two general ways: they may arise spontaneously or they may be induced. The probability of a mutation arising spontaneously may be only one in a million, that is, the mutation rate is 1×10^{-6}. For example, if the mutation rate for "inability to metabolize lactose" is 1×10^{-6}, this means that in a population of one million bacteria that are able to metabolize lactose there is the probability that one of them will be a mutant and unable to metabolize lactose.

Some areas of the DNA are more susceptible to mutation than others and are called *hot spots*. Thus, the mutation rate for a hot spot may be one in 10,000 (1×10^{-4}) while in another gene the mutation rate may be one in every 10 million (1×10^{-7}). The frequency at which mutations may arise can be increased substantially by inducing them with a mutagenic agent. Mutagens include both physical and chemical agents.

SPONTANEOUS MUTATIONS

Spontaneous mutations occur in the absence of human intervention. For example, purine and pyrimidine bases can temporarily exist in different electrochemical forms, which results in mispairing. Adenine instead of pairing with thymine can pair with cytosine. Guanine, which normally pairs with cytosine, can pair with thymine. When DNA duplicates, the mispairing leads to a permanently altered base pair in the bacterial cell (Fig. 6-10). When this altered base pair is transcribed as part of a gene, the mRNA may be transcribed incorrectly, thus producing an altered polypeptide.

Spontaneous mutations may also occur by a biological mechanism. It has been observed that specific nucleotide sequences or elements, called *insertion sequences* (IS), are present in the DNA molecule. Insertion sequences are usually less than 2000 nucleotide sequences in length and are capable of moving from one location to another. IS elements do not confer any known phenotype on the cell, but they can insert themselves within or between genes and thus affect the activity of genes at the site of insertion or distal to it (Fig. 6-11). IS elements are known to prevent transcription of structural genes or to reduce the rate of their transcription.

INDUCED MUTATIONS

Physical Agents
Physical agents that induce mutations include x-rays, gamma rays, and ultraviolet (UV) light. X-

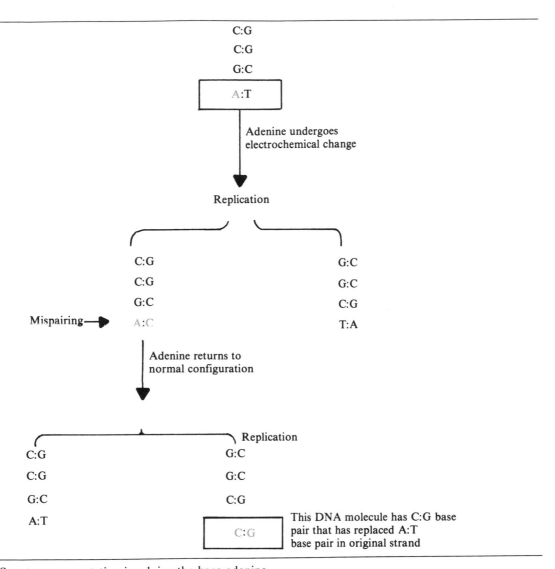

Fig. 6-10. Spontaneous mutation involving the base adenine.

rays and gamma rays are extremely energetic and when they bombard cells impart this energy to various molecules. The impact of these rays causes the discharge of electrons from molecules (called ionization) and the latter become very reactive (ions) and damage the DNA. For example, water struck by x-rays changes to a reactive form (the hydroxyl radical) that breaks the sugar phosphate backbone of DNA.

Ultraviolet light is not so energetic as x-rays or gamma rays but it is readily absorbed by molecules such as proteins and nucleic acids. Pyrimidines in particular absorb UV light and form abnormal bonds with adjacent pyrimidines on the DNA strands. This abnormal bonding produces what are referred to as *dimers* (Fig. 6-12) of thymine (thymine-thymine) and cytosine (cytosine-cytosine). Dimers are very inflexible and have a

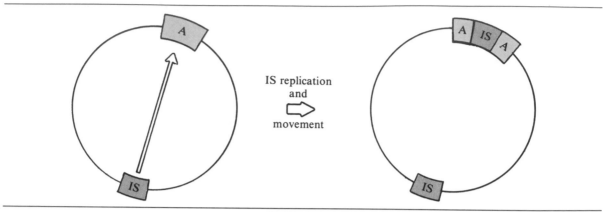

Fig. 6-11. Movement of insertion sequence (IS). IS element replicates and inserts a copy within the A gene.

tendency to become obstacles to normal DNA replication.

Chemical Agents

A variety of chemicals, from simple molecules such as nitrous acid (HNO_3) to more complex molecules such as acridines, can react with DNA to cause changes in the sequence of bases. The altered purine or pyrimidine bases have a tendency to mispair with other bases. For example, nitrous acid removes the amino group (deami-

Fig. 6-12. Thymine dimer formation. Ultraviolet light causes covalent bonding between adjacent thymines on the same DNA strand.

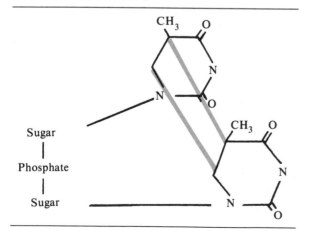

nation) from purine and pyrimidine bases. Deamination of cytosine leads to cytosine pairing with adenine instead of guanine.

Some chemical agents, such as 5-bromouracil, are structurally similar to the normal DNA bases (Fig. 6-13) and are incorporated into the DNA in place of the normal base during replication. These structurally similar compounds are referred to as *analogues*; they can mispair with other bases and this leads to mutations.

Another group of chemical agents are those like the *acridines* (proflavin, for example) that because of their chemical and physical properties can slip in between bases on the DNA strand. This activity distorts the DNA molecule and produces large gaps between normal bases. The outcome is that following replication deletions or insertions of bases can occur in the DNA.

Fig. 6-13. Structural similarity between 5-bromouracil and thymine.

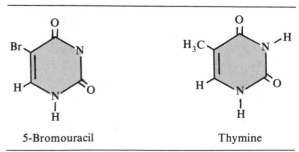

5-Bromouracil   Thymine

HOW MUTATIONS AFFECT THE GENETIC CODE

When mutations are produced they affect the coded information on the DNA. Transcription of altered DNA leads to the formation of an altered messenger RNA. Finally, translation of the affected mRNA affects the polypeptide product in a variety of different ways, depending on the mutation (see Fig. 6-14):

1. No effect. Mutation may result in a change to an alternate code word. Recall that there are at least three different code words for a single amino acid.
2. Missense mutation. A single base pair change leads to a change in the codon and its translation into a different amino acid. The activity of the polypeptide may or may not be affected, depending on the type of amino acid and its location in the peptide chain.
3. Nonsense mutation. A single base change in the DNA can occasionally lead to premature chain termination on the mRNA if nonsense codons are formed.
4. Frameshift mutation. The deletion or addition of a single base can cause the reading frame of the message to be shifted one base. The message distal to the insertion or deletion will code for a new set of amino acids. This usually leads to the formation of a nonfunctional polypeptide, but, again, this depends on the site of mRNA alteration.

REPAIR OF MUTATIONS

Even in the absence of mutagens, mutations can occur in the DNA during the replication process. Damage to DNA is repaired by a variety of different enzymatic mechanisms. When DNA damage does occur a series of cellular changes takes place called the SOS (international distress signal) response. One of the changes is that cell division is inhibited. The other is that the activities of the bacterial cell are focused on repairing the DNA damage. Some enzymes are induced by the cell to remove specific altered purine or pyrimidine bases. This excision event is followed by the use of enzymes such as DNA polymerase and DNA ligase to insert the correct bases and zip up the sugar phosphate backbone, respectively. A common repair mechanism induced by UV damage is called *excision repair* (Fig. 6-15). In this process an enzymatic incision is made on one side of the thymine-thymine or cytosine-cytosine dimers. A second enzyme removes the dimer as well as several adjacent bases. All the bases are replaced with the help of DNA polymerase and the sugar-phosphate backbone is zipped up by DNA ligase.

Despite the various mechanisms for DNA repair, mutations do occur and sometimes it is the repair process that is faulty.

MUTANT ISOLATION AND DETECTION

Some mutations result in visible changes that are easily detected. In bacteria these changes may involve colony pigmentation, colony size, and colony texture. Other mutations affect the growth of microorganisms. Many microorganisms are capable of synthesizing all their organic material using a simple carbon source and basic salts (see Chapter 5). Mutants in which the phenotypic change involves the requirement of a growth factor are called *auxotrophs*, while the parent organisms that have no such requirements are called *prototrophs*. Auxotrophic mutants can be isolated by using a technique called *replica plating* (Fig. 6-16). In this technique a sample of cell culture is spread on an agar plate (master plate) that is supplemented with nutrients that will permit the growth of auxotrophs and prototrophs. Colonies will appear on the plate after suitable incubation, and the pattern of these colonies on the plate can be transferred to a velveteen cloth. Each tuft of the velveteen cloth acts like an inoculating needle. The velveteen cloth is pressed onto an agar surface that has a minimal medium, that is, it will support the growth of pro-

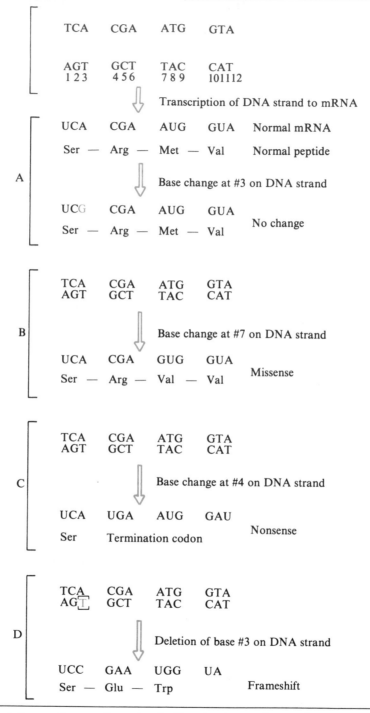

Fig. 6-14. Effects of mutation on the genetic code. A. Genetic change that produces no change in the peptide. B. Mutation that causes missense or change in the amino acid. C. Mutation that results in the formation of a nonsense or terminating codon. D. Mutation in which a base is deleted, resulting in a frameshift or change in all the amino acids distal to the initial mutation. (Ser = serine; arg = arginine; Met = methionine; Val = valine; Glu = glutamic acid; trp = tryptophan.)

totrophs but not auxotrophs. By comparing the colony distribution on the master plate with those on the plate containing minimal medium the auxotroph can be isolated. If one wishes to determine the specific requirement of the auxotroph, one can replica plate from the master plate to minimal media plates containing specific amino acids, vitamins, etc.

DETECTION OF CHEMICAL CARCINOGENS

Scientists as well as the general public are very aware of the need to detect chemicals that can cause cancer (*carcinogens*). It is believed that mutations induced by chemical agents can lead to cancer. Bruce *Ames* devised a *test* (that bears his name) that is used to screen compounds that may be potential carcinogens. The basis of the test is whether or not a chemical compound can cause the reversion of a well characterized mutation in one of the histidine genes in the bacterial species *Salmonella typhimurium*. The tester bacterial strain is added to a mixture containing rat liver extract plus the suspected chemical carcinogen (Fig. 6-17). Rat liver extract is used because many potentially carcinogenic chemical compounds that enter the body must be activated by mammalian enzymes to exhibit mutagenic or carcinogenic effects. The mixture is allowed to incubate and is then inoculated onto a medium devoid of histidine. The auxotrophic *Salmonella* will grow on the medium only if the suspected carcinogen has caused a reversion of the original mutation in the tester strain.

DNA TRANSFER OTHER THAN IN CELL DIVISION

In the previous paragraphs we have spoken of how mutations cause a change in the phenotype of the cell. In the following paragraphs we will show how microorganisms can change their ge-

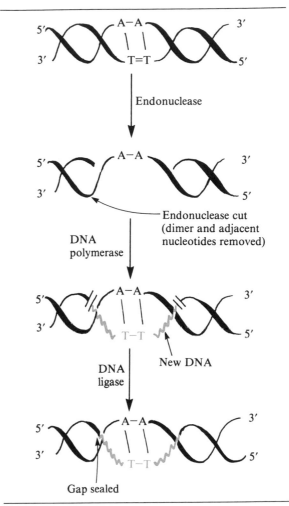

Fig. 6-15. Excision repair of DNA damaged by ultraviolet light. (Adapted from E. M. Witkin, *Bacteriol. Revs.* 40:869,1976.)

netic constitution when genes are transferred in processes other than cell division. There are three general mechanisms for gene transfer: transformation, conjugation, and transduction. In each of these processes there is a transfer of genes from the donor to recipient DNA. This genetic exchange is called *recombination*. Most recombination occurs between two DNA segments that are homologous; that is, they have similar nucleotide sequences (the sequence of events

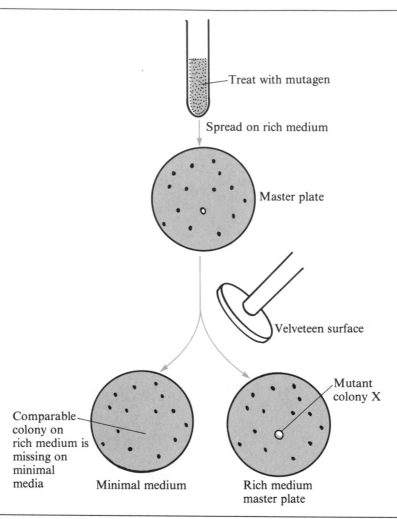

Treat with mutagen

Spread on rich medium

Master plate

Velveteen surface

Comparable colony on rich medium is missing on minimal media

Minimal medium

Mutant colony X

Rich medium master plate

Fig. 6-16. Replica plating technique. A culture may be treated with a mutagen to produce mutants or an un-treated culture may be used for recovery of spontaneous mutants. An aliquot of the culture is spread on an agar medium that supports the growth of mutants as well as nonmutants. Only enough culture medium is added so that fewer than 100 colonies are distributed over the surface of the agar. A velveteen pad is used to press over the colonies (master plate) and they are transferred to an agar surface containing minimal medium (which will not support the growth of mutants). Colony X does not grow on this plate. Cells from the mutant colony can be tested by setting up a new master plate and replica plating to medium that is deficient in specific nutrients such as amino acids. Thus specific amino acid mutants can be recovered.

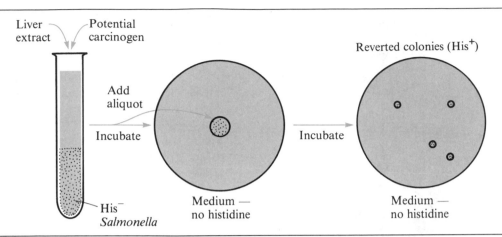

Fig. 6-17. Ames test for carcinogenicity. A mixture containing liver extract, potential carcinogen, and *Salmonella* species with a specific mutation in the histidine operon (his⁻) are incubated. An aliquot is transferred to an agar medium that does not contain histidine. The plate is incubated, and any bacteria that have reverted to his⁺, because of the mutagenic effect of the carcinogen, will grow on the plate and produce colonies. Liver extract contains enzymes that are normally involved in the biochemical transformation of a chemical to an active mutagen.

Fig. 6-18. How recombination takes place between homologous DNA strands.

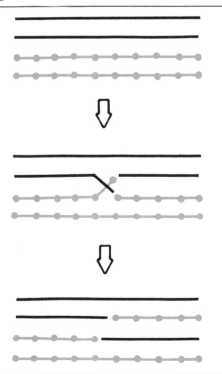

that leads to formation of recombinant DNA is diagrammed in Fig. 6-18). The central feature of this model is that recombinant DNA molecules are formed by breaking and rejoining of intact DNA molecules of similar genotype. Let us now examine the three mechanisms in which genes can be transferred.

TRANSFORMATION

Transformation is the most primitive of the mechanisms for gene transfer among bacteria and is known to occur in only a few genera. The probability that transformation has contributed much to genetic variety is very small for most microorganisms. Transformation involves the taking up of cell-free fragmented DNA by a recipient cell and the recombination of genetic elements. Experimentally, DNA is extracted from the donor cell and fragments of DNA are mixed with a population of viable recipient cells of a related species. The recipient cell will take up pieces of the DNA. Transformation has been studied primarily in gram-positive organisms such as *Ba-*

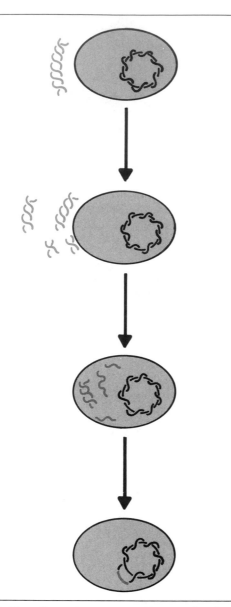

Fig. 6-19. Transformation process. See text for details of this process.

1. Development of competence. *Competence* refers to the ability of a cell to take up DNA. Transformable bacteria become competent only under certain growth conditions. Log phase cultures of streptococci, for example, release a protein competence factor that induces competence for the entire cell population.
2. Binding of DNA. Competent cells are believed to carry receptor sites for binding DNA. Only double-stranded DNA is bound; single-stranded DNA or RNA is not bound. DNA from the same or different bacterial species can be taken up by the recipient cell.
3. Uptake of DNA. DNA is taken up by the cell and converted to single-stranded DNA of specific lengths.
4. Integration of DNA. Single-stranded donor DNA with sequences homologous to recipient DNA can enter into a recombination event. The donor single strand physically displaces a homologous strand of the recipient chromosome. Donor DNA that is not homologous does not engage in recombination and is eventually degraded by enzymes (nucleases).

CONJUGATION

Conjugation is an important means of gene transfer, especially among gram-negative bacteria. Only a few gram-positive species are known to be involved in conjugation. Conjugation involves the interaction of two cell mating types, referred to as the *donor* and *recipient*. The genetic transfer between donor and recipient is mediated by an extrachromosomal piece of DNA known as the *sex factor*, or fertility factor (also called *F factor*) found in the donor cell. The donor cell is called F^+; the recipient cell, which does not contain the sex factor, is called F^-. The sex factor is double-stranded DNA that is about one-fortieth the size of chromosomal DNA. The sex factor is not under control by the bacterial chromosome and

cillus subtilis and species of *Streptococcus*. The overall process of transformation may be divided into the following steps (Fig. 6-19) (these apply only to gram-positive bacteria; there are some variations in gram-negative species).

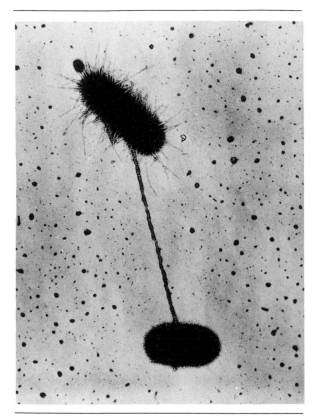

Fig. 6-20. Electron micrograph showing conjugation between donor cell containing the sex factor (F⁺) and recipient cell (F⁻). The highly piliated cell (top) is the donor. (Courtesy of C. C. Brinton.)

it can replicate autonomously. The F-factor possesses several genes that code for the formation of sex pili that aid the donor in attaching to a recipient cell (Fig. 6-20). The sex pili are believed to retract into the donor cell, thereby bringing the donor and recipient closer together. How the channel for transfer of donor DNA is produced is not known. During the conjugation process (Fig. 6-21) a copy of the sex factor is made and one of its single strands is transferred to the recipient. The complementary strand of the donor single strand is synthesized in the recipient, which is now converted to an F⁺.

HFR Cell Formation

The fertility factor does not always exist outside the chromosome but occasionally is integrated into the bacterial chromosome (Fig. 6-22). In an

Fig. 6-21. Sex factor transfer during conjugation between F⁺ and F⁻. A conjugation bridge is formed between the donor (F⁺) and recipient (F⁻) cells. A single DNA strand of the donor F factor is cleaved and transferred to recipient. Complementary DNA synthesis occurs on the strand that is transferred as well as on the strand remaining in the donor. Once the F factor has been transferred, the cells separate.

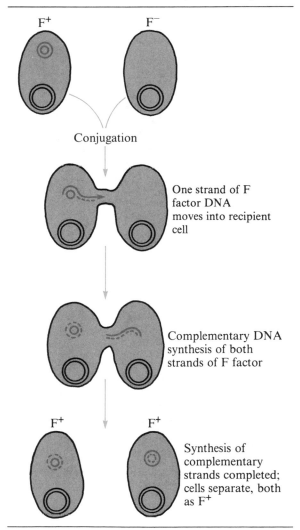

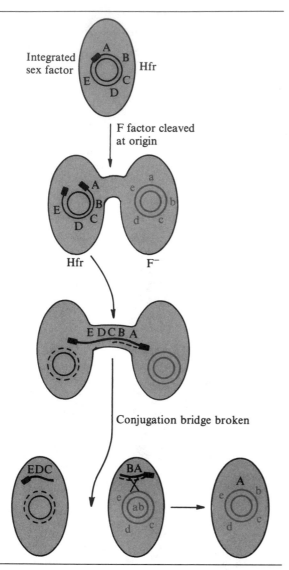

Fig. 6-22. Conjugation process involving Hfr and F⁻. Conjugation bridge is formed between donor (Hfr) and recipient (F⁻) cells. Sex factor on Hfr chromosome is cleaved, and single-strand transfer is initiated. There is complementary synthesis of transferred DNA strand as well as remaining single strand in Hfr cell. The conjugation bridge is broken, and only genes A and B are transferred to recipient, Recombination between homologous genes results in the incorporation of Hfr gene A into the recipient chromosome.

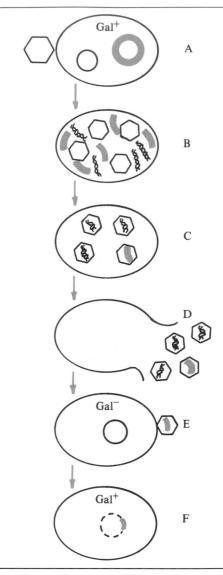

Fig. 6-23. Generalized transduction. A. Bacterial cell with a functional galactose gene (gal⁺) is infected by a virus (bacterial DNA is red; viral DNA is black). B. Bacterial DNA is degraded. C. Bacterial cell lyses, releasing virus, one of which carries bacterial gal⁺ gene. E. Another bacterial cell that carries a nonfunctional galactose gene (gal⁻) is infected by the transducing virus. F. The transduced gal⁺ gene engages in recombination with gal⁻ gene of bacterial chromosome, converting the cell to gal⁺. The bacterial cell does not lyse because there was no viral information in the infecting viral particles.

integrated state the sex factor is under control of chromosomal replication. The cells possessing the integrated form of the sex factor are called *Hfr* (*high frequency of recombination*). During conjugation and chromosome transfer most of the sex factor genes are not transferred. The reason for this is that they represent some of the last genes to be transferred, and because the conjugation bridge is very fragile and is broken before they can be transferred.

Once the donor DNA is transferred recombination can take place and again involves an exchange between homologous DNA sequences. DNA that is not involved in recombination is degraded by nucleases.

TRANSDUCTION

Transduction involves the transmission of DNA from donor bacterium to recipient bacterium but, unlike conjugation and transformation, the DNA is transferred by a bacterial virus called a bacteriophage. To understand transduction we must first discuss how bacterial viruses operate (Fig. 6-23). Viruses infect bacterial cells by injecting viral DNA into the bacterial cytoplasm. The virus takes over the machinery of the cell and produces more virus. After so many virus particles have been produced the bacterial cell lyses and the progeny virus are released and are capable of infecting other bacteria. During the formation of virus the bacterial DNA is eventually broken up into smaller pieces, and some of them become accidentally packaged into the virus particle in place of viral DNA. The virus carrying the bacterial DNA is called a *transducing virus*. When the transducing virus infects a bacterial cell the bacterial DNA it carries can exchange with the DNA of the infected bacterial cell, provided the sequences are homologous. Since any bacterial gene can be carried by the transducing virus, the transduction process is called *generalized transduction*. Another type of transduction called *specialized transduction* can also take place and this is discussed in Chapter 30.

PLASMIDS

Plasmids are circular double-stranded molecules of DNA that are found outside the bacterial chromosome. They are from one-tenth to one-ten-thousandth the size of the bacterial chromosome. Plasmids are autonomous and are not controlled by the bacterial chromosome. As few as one or as many as 100 plasmid molecules may be present in the cell. Plasmids can be divided into two classes: *conjugative* and *nonconjugative*. A conjugative plasmid possesses the genes for pilus formation and this permits transmission of copies of itself to a recipient during conjugation. Nonconjugative plasmids do not possess the information that can affect their own transfer. Nonconjugative plasmids can be transferred by such processes as transduction or transformation or by conjugation, but in the latter instance only if the bacterial cell also contains conjugative plasmids.

CHARACTERISTICS ASSOCIATED WITH PLASMIDS

Both conjugative and nonconjugative plasmids contain information that confers important characteristics to the bacterial cell. Plasmid-associated characteristics, although not indispensable, are important for helping the bacterium to cope in its particular environment. We will discuss only those characteristics that have medical significance.

R Plasmids
R plasmids possess information for resistance to antimicrobial compounds such as antibiotics. R plasmids are readily dispersed because of two important features: they are conjugative and they carry genetic elements called *transposons*. There is little difference between a transposon and an insertion sequence (IS) element except that transposons possess information for antibiotic resis-

tance while IS elements do not. A transposon can replicate and transfer a copy of itself to other genetic elements (other plasmids, chromosomal DNA). This promiscuity is one of the reasons that bacteria quickly become resistant to antimicrobials. The conjugative ability of R plasmids resides on a segment called the *resistance transfer factor* or *RTF*. RTF carries information for pilus formation and is similar to the F factor. The antimicrobial resistance genes (designated *r*), of which there may be one or several on the R plasmid, are usually clustered together.

R plasmids can be transferred from nonpathogenic bacteria to pathogenic bacteria and vice versa because conjugation can be between the same or different species of bacteria. When antimicrobials, such as penicillin or tetracycline, are administered to patients over a long period of time there is a selection process that favors the emergence and growth of drug-resistant strains. These drug-resistant strains can be transferred to individuals who do not harbor drug-resistant strains—a situation that occurs repeatedly in the hospital.

Resistance to Heavy Metals

Heavy metal ions such as cobalt and mercury are inhibitory to the growth of bacteria. There are plasmids, found primarily in the gram-positive staphylococci, that code for resistance to heavy metals. Heavy metals ions are in such antimicrobial preparations as silver nitrate. Metal ion plasmid resistance is often associated with antibiotic resistance factors. Thus, the transfer of metal ion resistance via plasmids from one cell to another is often accompanied by antibiotic resistance as well.

Virulence Determinants

The ability of some microorganisms to cause disease (referred to as virulence) is associated with special determinants carried on plasmids. These determinants often code for toxins that are det-

rimental to the host, but not always. Some of the principal virulence determinants coded by plasmids are found in the following bacteria:

1. *E. coli.* Some E. coli strains produce two types of toxins that affect the intestinal tract: heat-labile (LT) and heat-stable (ST). Both toxins are plasmid-associated.
2. *Staphylococcus aureus.* An affliction of the skin of newborns called scalded skin syndrome is caused by certain strains of *S. aureus*. The toxin is plasmid-associated.
3. *Clostridium perfringens.* One type of diarrheal disease in domestic animals is caused by *C. perfringens* type C. The disease is associated with a toxin that is encoded on a plasmid.
4. *Streptococcus* species. Several species of *Streptococcus* produce *hemolysins* (lyse red blood cells) that are encoded on plasmid DNA.

GENETIC ENGINEERING AND RECOMBINANT DNA

We have previously discussed the genetic mechanism of recombination; however, the term *recombinant DNA* has a slightly different meaning. Recombinant DNA refers to the creation of DNA molecules by the association of DNA molecules from different biological sources. Recombinant DNA technology is commonly called *gene splicing* or *genetic engineering*. The basis of recombinant DNA technology is *restriction endonucleases* found in bacteria and other organisms. The term *restriction* refers to the fact that the enzymes are capable of degrading specific sequences in a DNA molecule. This type of recognition is illustrated in Figure 6-24. As you can see from the figure, these particular restriction enzymes open up the DNA, producing "sticky tails" on each strand that are complementary to each other. In other words, they will be able to

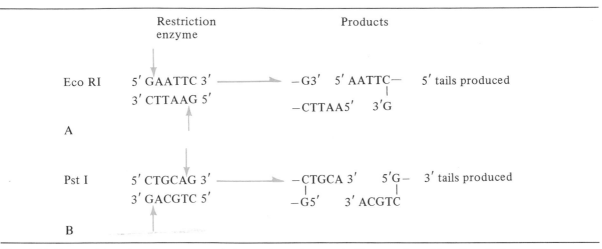

Fig. 6-24. Recognition sites for two restriction endonucleases. A. Enzyme from *E. coli*, called EcoRI, cuts DNA to produce DNA with 5′ tails B. Enzymes from *Providencia stuarti*, called PstI, cuts DNA to produce 3′ tails.

reattach (a process also called annealing). Regardless of the DNA molecule, each restriction enzyme is specific, and the same "sticky" ends are always produced. Thus, if you had DNA from bacteria, yeast, or plant and each was treated with the same restriction enzyme, the recognition sites would be the same. If restriction endonuclease–treated DNA from different sources is placed together, recombinant DNA molecules can be produced. A sequence of steps is used in recombinant DNA technology. For our example we will assume that we wish to produce a recombinant DNA molecule that contains eukaryotic and prokaryotic information. The recombinant DNA will then be inserted into a bacterial cell (see Fig. 6-25):

1. Eukaryotic DNA is treated with a specific restriction endonuclease, and the sticky segments are isolated. These segments are called *passenger DNA*.
2. Plasmid DNA will serve as the *vehicle* or *vector* for carrying the eukaryotic DNA segments. The vehicle DNA is usually a bacterial plasmid, but a bacteriophage could also be used. The vector DNA is treated with the same restriction endonuclease as the passenger DNA. We have now produced a vector with sticky tails that can bind (hybridize) with the sticky tails of eukaryotic DNA segments.
3. Once the eukaryotic DNA segments are inserted into the vector a DNA ligase seals the open ends and a circular hybrid plasmid is produced.
4. The hybrid plasmid or recombinant can now be inserted into a host cell. In our example the host cell is the bacterium *E. coli*. The insertion is actually a transformation event. The information on the recombinant DNA will be converted into a specific product in the host cell. This process is called *cloning*.

IMPORTANCE OF RECOMBINANT DNA TECHNOLOGY

Recombinant DNA technology has tremendous application to basic science as well as applied areas of science. Gene cloning has provided geneticists with a tool for the mutation and manipulation of organisms. The applications of recombinant DNA technology are practically limitless.

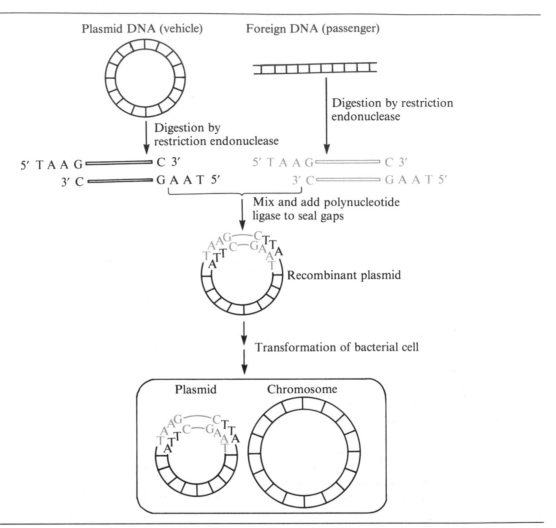

Fig. 6-25. Recombinant DNA experiment. Plasmid DNA (bacterial source) plus foreign DNA (eukaryotic source, for example) are digested by endonuclease. DNA fragments are produced with complementary "sticky" ends. Some foreign DNA will bond with plasmid DNA. The plasmid circularizes and can be used to transform a bacterial cell. The foreign DNA (gene) can be expressed in the bacterium. (From R. F. Boyd, *General Microbiology* [2nd ed.]. St. Louis: Mosby, 1988.)

Gene manipulation is being exploited to create products such as hormones, vaccines, enzymes, and pharmaceuticals that can be produced within microorganisms. Animal products like insulin and growth hormone are now produced in bacterial cells and are commercially available. Some commercial waste products are being converted to useful products such as single-cell protein that can be used as animal feed or can be converted to sources of energy. Genetic engineering may some day play a role in therapy for humans (see Boxed Essay).

Genetic engineering is also playing a very important role in the infectious disease clinical laboratory. When large outbreaks of disease occur it is important to determine the source of infection and the specific strain or species that is causing the disease. Differentation can be made in tests using DNA as a diagnostic reagent. The basis of these tests is that there is an inherent specificity of DNA and if one can select and clone a DNA sequence that is found in only one strain, species, or genus, then this DNA will hybridize with DNA from organisms containing the same sequence and not others. The cloned sequences are usually virulence determinants such as genes that code for toxins. The known sequence can be cloned by using restriction endonucleases and labeled with a material such as radioactive phosphorus (^{32}P). The labeled DNA, which is now called a "*DNA probe*," is denatured into single strands and then bound to filter paper such as nitrocellulose filters (Fig. 6-26). The microorganisms to be examined for the presence of the gene (for example, from clinical material such as pus), are lysed and their DNA is denatured into single strands. This DNA is not labeled. The unlabeled DNA is passed over the same filter. Double-stranded DNA, containing labeled and unlabeled strands, will form on the filter if the specific sequence is present in the DNA of the microorganisms from the clinical material. Unreacted single-stranded DNA can be removed from the filter by washing. The presence of radioactive material on the washed filter indicates the presence of the gene in the DNA of the microorganisms from the clinical specimen.

SUMMARY

1. DNA, the basis of heredity, performs specific functions in the bacterial cell: (a) duplication for transfer during cell division, (b) transcription into mRNA, which can be translated into protein, (c) control of protein synthesis, (d) ability to mutate, and (e) transfer of genes in processes other than cell division.

2. Bacterial DNA is a double-stranded molecule in which a sequence of nucleotide bases on one strand is complementary to the sequence of nucleotide bases on the opposite strand. In the cell the DNA exists in the form of a circle that is folded on itself.

3. The DNA molecule is replicated in a semiconservative manner in which each strand acts as a template for synthesis of a complementary strand. Replication of DNA begins at the origin and involves both strands. DNA synthesis proceeds in opposite directions from the origin. Replication is initiated by an enzyme that nicks one strand at the origin while other proteins, such as unwinding proteins and helix destabilizing proteins, unwind the DNA and prevent it from rewinding, respectively.

4. Synthesis of DNA is catalyzed by the enzyme DNA polymerase, which adds nucleotides in the 5' to 3' direction. Since the two strands are antiparallel, one strand adds nucleotides continuously. The other strand lags behind because short RNA primers must first be produced along the lagging strand.

5. One of the DNA strands is transcribed into mRNA by the enzyme RNA polymerase. The nucleotides in the mRNA are arranged as a linear

GENETIC ENGINEERING AND GENE THERAPY: WHAT ARE ITS IMPLICATIONS?

The ability of scientists to manipulate genes has brought great excitement to the medical community because the potential to cure disease by gene therapy is now within sight. Gene therapy is defined as the insertion into an organism of a functional gene that corrects a genetic defect. Gene therapy cures have been performed in mice and are now awaiting experimentation in humans. At present the only human tissues that can be used for gene transfer are bone marrow and skin cells because they can be extracted from the body, grown in culture, and reimplanted into the patient. Most clinical work has been done with bone marrow.

At present, injecting a functional gene into the bloodstream in order to correct a defect would not be efficient with our present state of technological development. Functional genes can be efficiently transferred to cells if they are part of a virus. For example, a gene therapy experiment might be carried out in the following way:

1. The functional gene is inserted into the hereditary material of a virus that is allowed to replicate.
2. Defective bone marrow cells are removed from the patient and infected with virus containing the functional gene. The functional gene slips into the chromosome of the defective cell.
3. The repaired bone marrow cells are reinfused into the patient. Since most of the bone marrow cells will differentiate into erythrocytes, lymphocytes, etc., these descendants will also possess the functional gene.

So far, this type of technique is suitable for disease in which the defect is in the patient's bone marrow, for example, a disorder in which there is a missing enzyme or protein. If gene therapy can eventually be applied to somatic (body) cells, what about its application to germ (sex) cells? Will society accept manipulation of sex cells that would permit the "new" gene to be passed on to the patient's children? The technology that will bring this issue to the forefront is not far off.

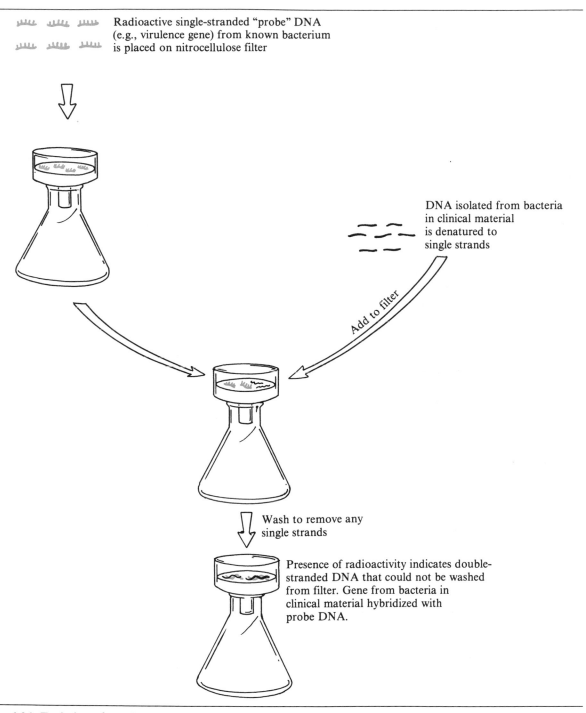

Fig. 6-26. Technique for using probe DNA to identify genes from clinical material.

sequence of coding units or triplets called co-dons. There are 64 possible codons, a minimum of three for each of the 20 different amino acids. Three triplets do not code for amino acids and are called nonsense.

6. Information on the mRNA is translated into a polypeptide when it engages a ribosome and the first aminoacyl tRNA is brought to it to form an initiation complex. As the ribosome moves down the mRNA, amino acids are brought by tRNA molecules whose anticodons are complementary to the codons. When each amino acid arrives a new peptide bond is formed. The message is ter-minated when a nonsense triplet has been reached. The completed polypeptide is released into the cytoplasm.

7. Some enzymes in the cell are inducible and are under the control of genetic mechanisms. The genetic unit controlling inducible enzymes is called an operon. The operon, which consists of structural genes, an operator, and promoter, is itself under the control of a repressor protein en-coded by the regulator gene.

8. Operons are of two basic types: inducible and repressible. Inducible operons are turned off by an active repressor protein but in the presence of inducer the repressor becomes inactive and the structural genes of the operon are turned on. In a repressible operon the repressor molecule be-comes active only in the presence of a corepres-sor molecule, which is usually the end product of a biosynthetic pathway.

9. Mutations may arise spontaneously without human intervention or they may be induced. Spontaneous mutation may involve electrochem-ical changes in a base that permit it to mispair during replication. Many spontaneous mutations are caused by short units of DNA called insertion sequences (IS). IS elements can replicate and in-sert themselves into other DNA molecules and interfere with normal gene transcription.

10. Induced mutations may be caused by phys-ical or chemical agents. Physical agents such as x-rays or gamma rays can energize molecules in

the cell that damage DNA. UV light is absorbed by pyrimidines to form dimers that interfere with replication.

11. Chemical mutagens cause changes in the DNA that usually involve mispairing events. Some chemicals alter the purine or pyrimidine base while others are analogues and are incor-porated into the DNA in place of the normal base. Some chemicals can insert themselves between bases, and this ultimately results in the addition or deletion of bases following DNA replication.

12. The effect of mutation on the genetic code may be (a) no effect, (b) to change a codon that causes missense, (c) to produce a nonsense triplet that terminates the message, and (d) to insert or delete a base that causes a shift in the reading frame of the message. These effects may or may not affect the polypeptide, depending on their lo-cation in the message.

13. Mutations can be repaired by enzymes that are induced following an SOS response. There are repair enzymes that can remove specifically damaged bases and replace them with the correct base. UV light damage can be repaired by en-zymes that remove the dimer and additional bases in a process called excision repair.

14. Some bacterial mutants can be detected visually but mutants with growth requirements are detected by replica plating techniques. Mu-tants of *Salmonella typhimurium* are used com-mercially to determine the potential of chemicals to be carcinogenic. The test (Ames test) is based on the ability of the potential carcinogen to pro-duce mutations in *S. typhimurium* that reverse the effects of the original mutations.

15. Bacteria can transfer copies of their genes to other bacteria in processes other than cell di-vision. After the gene is transferred it enters into a recombination event with the host gene and ho-mologous sequences are exchanged. Transfor-mation is a process in which cell-free DNA is taken up by the cell. Conjugation is a process in which there is DNA transfer from a donor that contains a fertility factor (F^+) to a recipient that

does not contain the sex factor (F^-). If the sex factor is outside the chromosome (F^+) only the sex factor is transmitted, but if the sex factor is integrated into the chromosome (Hfr), all or part of the chromosome is transferred. Transduction is a process in which a bacterial virus picks up bacterial DNA from an infected host and transfers it to a new bacterial host.

16. Plasmids are small extrachromosomal pieces of DNA carrying traits that are not indispensable to the bacterium. Some plasmids can affect their own transfer (conjugative) while others cannot (nonconjugative). Some of the characteristics encoded in plasmids are antibiotic resistance, heavy metal resistance, and virulence determinants.

17. Genetic engineering is a technology that removes genes from a variety of different sources and clones them in a microbial host. The cloned genes are carried on a vector DNA molecule and the hybrid is called recombinant DNA. Recombinant DNA technology has many applications in pure and applied science and may someday be used in gene therapy for humans.

QUESTIONS FOR STUDY

Select the best response or responses for each of the following:

1. Which of the following statements concerning DNA replication in bacteria is *untrue*?
   A. Each strand of the bacterial DNA serves as a template for producing a complementary strand.
   B. Unwinding of the bacterial DNA produces a single replicating fork.
   C. Helix-destabilizing proteins help prevent rewinding of any unwound single-stranded DNA.
   D. Both strands of DNA are replicated in a continuous manner.

2. Which of the following statements concerning the operon is *untrue*?
   A. The regulator is a gene that codes for the synthesis of a repressor.
   B. The promoter is a gene that serves as a site for binding of RNA polymerase.
   C. The operator is a sequence of nucleotides that binds the repressor protein.
   D. Inducible operons contain genes that exert control primarily over catabolic processes in the cell.

3. Which of the following statements concerning transformations involving gram-positive bacteria is *untrue*?
   A. Only double-stranded DNA is bound to the cell being transformed.
   B. Only double-stranded transforming DNA is integrated into recipient DNA.
   C. Competence is a factor or molecule released by bacteria that can induce competence in other bacteria.
   D. Only single-stranded transforming DNA is integrated into recipient DNA.

4. Which of the following statements concerning conjugation involving F^+ and F^- cells is *true*?
   A. F^- cells carry sex factors.
   B. Sex factor genes in the F^+ cell cannot replicate in the absence of chromosome replication.
   C. Only double-stranded sex factor DNA is transferred from F^+ to F^-.
   D. All sex factor genes are transferred to the recipient F^- cell.

5. Which of the following statements concerning plasmids is true?
    A. All plasmids possess the information for their own transfer.
    B. Much of the information coded in the plasmid is absolutely essential to the survival of the bacterial cell.
    C. R plasmids may possess both transposons and insertion sequences.
    D. R plasmids cannot be transferred to other bacterial cells.

Fill in the blank:

6. The conjugative ability of R plasmids is associated with an element called the_____.

7. Bacteriophage can transfer bacterial genes to another bacterium in a process called_____.

8. Mutant bacterial cells that have a requirement for a specific growth factor are called_____.

9. A mutation that can lead to the premature termination of mRNA translation is called_____.

10. The triplet nucleotide on the transfer RNA molecule that recognizes a specific triplet on the mRNA is called a(n)_____.

ADDITIONAL READINGS

Bainbridge, B. W. *Genetics of Microbes* (2nd ed.). New York: Chapman and Hall and Methuen, 1987.

Birge, E. A. *Bacterial and Bacteriophage Genetics* (2nd ed.). New York: Springer-Verlag, 1988.

Dulbecco, R. *The Design of Life*. New Haven: Yale University Press, 1987.

Hawkins, J. D. *Gene Structure and Expression*. New York: Cambridge University Press, 1985.

Primrose, S. B. *Modern Biotechnology*. Palo Alto, CA: Blackwell Scientific, 1987.

Smith, J. E. *Biotechnology Principles*. Aspects of Microbiology. Washington, DC: American Society for Microbiology, 1985.

Watson, J., Hopkins, N. H., Roberts, J. W., Steitz, J. A., and Weiner, A. M. *Molecular Biology of the Gene* (4th ed.). Menlo Park, CA: Benjamin Cummings, 1987.

II. CONTROL OF MICROORGANISMS

7. STERILIZATION AND DISINFECTION

OBJECTIVES

To define the commonly used sterilization/
disinfection terms and use them in specific
contexts, and especially to differentiate between
antisepsis and disinfection

To appraise conditions or factors that affect
sterilization/disinfection procedures and agents

To name the commonly used modes of attaining
sterility; to point out the advantages and the
limitations of each; for each mode, to state the
minimum conditions that must be applied to
assure the attainment of sterility

To give the mechanisms of action, the good and bad
features, and the typical applications of moist and
dry heat, cold, filtration, ultrasound, and radiation
as they pertain to the control of microorganisms

To comment on sterilization indicators as to their
composition, rationale for use, interpretation of
readouts, and reliability

To give the good and the bad features and the
typical applications of representative disinfectants
from each of the major chemical disinfectant
groups; specifically, include hexachlorophene,
70% alcohol, bleach, tincture of iodine, iodophors,
cationic detergents, ethylene oxide,
glutaraldehyde, and chlorhexidene

Infectious disease agents are controlled in four ways: by public sanitation measures, by sterilization and disinfection procedures, by chemotherapeutic agents, and by the body's defensive mechanisms. Public sanitation methods are used to control the sources of microorganisms by such measures as proper disposal of wastes and purification of water. Sterilization and disinfection procedures seek to destroy microorganisms before they have an opportunity to enter the body. Chemotherapeutic measures (see Chapter 8) are used to affect microorganisms once they have entered the body. The body's nonspecific resistance mechanisms and its immune system (see Chapters 11 and 12) either prevent microorganisms from entering or, once they have entered, remove, inactivate, or destroy them.

TERMINOLOGY

Sterilization/disinfection terms are given in Table 7-1. Additional explanatory comments follow.

Sterility indicates *freedom from viable forms* of microorganisms. It is an absolute state—there are no degrees of sterility. Either an object is sterile or it is not sterile. There may be billions of killed bacteria present, as in some vaccines, but

Table 7-1. Sterilization and Disinfection Terminology

Process	Noun		Verb	Adjective	Action, agent, or state
	Agent	State or condition			
Sterilization	Sterilant (if a chemical)	Sterility	Sterilize	Sterile, sterilized	Completely destroys or removes all microorganisms; renders treated microorganisms permanently incapable of reproducing
	-cide			-cidal	Kills the form of microorganism named in the prefix: bactericide, sporicide, tuberculocide, fungicide, etc.
	-stat	-stasis		-static	Prevents multiplication of the type of microorganism named in the prefix without necessarily killing it: bacteriostat, fungistat, etc.
		Asepsis		Aseptic	"Without sepsis": the absence or the exclusion of sepsis
	Antiseptic	Antisepsis	Antisepticize		"Against sepsis": the application of nonchemotherapeutic agents to living tissue with the objective of at least preventing the multiplication of pathogenic microorganisms (does not ordinarily include spores)
Disinfection	Disinfectant		Disinfect	Disinfected	Prevents infection: carried out with chemical agents (disinfectants) or by physical means (e.g., boiling, pasteurization) on inanimate objects with the objective of at least killing (with the exception of spores) all harmful forms (e.g., pathogens)
	Germicide			Germicidal	Kills all types of microorganisms but not spores necessarily; used on body surfaces and on inanimate objects
Degermation			Degerm		Removes microorganisms, especially transients on the skin, by chemical (antiseptics/soaps) and mechanical (scrubbing) means
Sanitization			Sanitize		Reduces the number of microorganisms on inanimate objects (tableware, garments) to a safe level as judged by public health standards

if not a single viable bacterium is present the preparation is sterile. A preparation may be sterile and yet be harmful because of microbial products. Injection fluids, for example, may be sterile but contain fever- or shock-inducing pyrogens (endotoxins) that are derived from microorganisms.

The breakdown of living tissue by the action of microorganisms is known as *sepsis*. It is accompanied by an acute inflammatory reaction. Pus formation is a prominent feature of bacterial sepsis. Toxic microbial products may contribute to the septic process. The host has an intense, overwhelming infection, toxemia, or both when sepsis exists.

Disinfection at the very least destroys harmful (pathogenic) microorganisms that are in the vegetative state. The expected action of a disinfectant or of disinfection depends on the purpose for which the agent or process is employed and the species or types of microorganisms that are likely to be present. The target microorganisms in the health fields, for example, are the microorganisms that can cause an infection, whereas in an industrial situation the target microorganisms are those that might spoil or alter a product. A disinfected object should not be expected to be sterile; it may harbor viable nonpathogens and spores of pathogens. According to the strict interpretation of the term, disinfection is carried out on inanimate objects, not on living tissue. The skin and mucosa are antisepticized.

GENERAL CONSIDERATIONS

PROBLEM MICROORGANISMS

The specific population of microorganisms present on or in any surface or article to be sterilized or disinfected is not usually known. The assumption is made, therefore, that the most resistant microbial forms are present—the ubiquitous bacterial endospores. Among the types of microorganisms there is a somewhat arbitrary descending order of relative resistance to sterilization procedures and disinfecting agents: bacterial endospores, mycobacteria, fungal spores, small or nonlipid viruses, fungi in the vegetative form, enveloped (lipid) viruses, and vegetative bacterial cells.

Bacterial Endospores
The bacterial endospore is the most resistant form of microbial life. Some soil spores withstand as much as 16 hours of boiling. That being the case, if sterility is the objective, a procedure must be used that is sporicidal.

Mycobacteria
The mycobacteria, of which the bacterium causing tuberculosis is the most important, are noted for their resistance to the disinfectants, especially the aqueous disinfectants. The mycobacterial cell surface is hydrophobic because the cell wall is rich in wax-like lipids. The mycobacteria do, however, have about the same level of susceptibility to heat as do the other bacteria that are in the vegetative state.

Hepatitis Viruses
The hepatitis B virus (HBV) and the hepatitis C virus (HBC) are regarded as problem agents because it is difficult to control the situations in which transmission most frequently occurs. The durability of the viruses, the infinitesimal quantities that can initiate infection, the commonness of contact with blood, and the carrier rate in the general population—all contribute to the control problems that accompany the disease. The viruses are not cultivable, so there is no easy way to check the effects of disinfectants. The modes of transmission for the HBV and the human immunodeficiency virus (HIV or AIDS virus) are similar. Both can be transmitted in occupational settings by percutaneous inoculation, by contact with an open wound, by non-intact mucous mem-

branes or skin (chapped, abraded, weeping, dermatitic), by blood-contaminated body fluids, and by concentrated virus. *Blood is the single most important source of HBV and HIV in the workplace setting.*

Certain Vegetative Bacteria

Staphylococci and enterococci are among the more resistant of the gram-positive bacteria. Among the gram-negative bacilli, *Pseudomonas, Serratia, Enterobacter,* and *Klebsiella* species appear to be comparatively more resistant to certain disinfectants than are other vegetative bacteria. These genera are being found more and more as hospital-associated pathogens (see Chapter 34). *Pseudomonas* species are noted for causing infections in burned patients and in patients with acute leukemia and cystic fibrosis. Pseudomonads proliferate well in distilled and deionized water, and in low-level disinfectants such as iodophors and cationic detergents when used in dilute concentrations.

INTERFERING MATTER

A major consideration in sterilization and disinfection procedures is that of interfering matter, which protects microorganisms, especially from disinfection. In the health-related fields, the *interfering matter is largely organic matter derived from the body*: blood, pus, saliva, perspiration, urine, feces, and skin oils. Lubricants, soil, or other debris can also interfere with sterilization and disinfection. In processing reusable soiled instruments and other such items, a necessary step is proper cleansing to remove the interfering matter. Aesthetic considerations are an added reason.

NO UNIVERSAL METHOD

No given sterilization or disinfection procedure is applicable to every situation. The biological or physical nature of the object being subjected to an antimicrobial procedure differs and dictates the mode to be employed. Heat is the surest, most practical, and most widely applicable means of controlling microorganisms. In some situations, however, heat is not appropriate because of the thermolability or thermosensitivity of the object to be treated. What may be an excellent way to control microorganisms on an instrument may be totally inapplicable on the oral mucosa. Generally speaking, in the health-related fields as much overkill is provided as conditions will permit.

PRINCIPAL MODES OF ACHIEVING STERILITY

The routinely used methods for obtaining sterility are *autoclaving* with saturated steam under pressure; *elevated dry heat* (hot air); and exposure to the *gas ethylene oxide* (ETO). This is not to say that other devices or chemical agents do not produce sterility. It is possible, for example, to sterilize by using filtration, irradiation, or chemicals such as glutaraldehyde, but such methods are applicable in limited situations.

CRITICAL, SEMI-CRITICAL, AND NONCRITICAL ITEMS

Items and equipment that are used in patient care are categorized as critical, semi-critical, and noncritical. Critical items are those that are introduced into the body and therefore must be sterile: surgical instruments, intravenous and irrigation fluids and their delivery devices, catheters, and implants. Semi-critical items make contact with mucous membranes but do not penetrate into tissues that normally are sterile. Preferably these items should be sterilized, but high-level disinfection is adequate so that at least vegetative bacteria are destroyed. Noncritical items may or may not make contact with the skin: crutches, bedpans, carafes, floors, furniture, bed linens, and electrodes used for electrocardiograms. Such articles should at least be thoroughly cleansed with hot soapy water and/or treated with low-level disinfectants.

chemical methods. Physical methods include moist and dry heat, cold, filtration, ultrasonics, and irradiation.

PHYSICAL METHODS

Sterilization and disinfection procedures are customarily divided into physical methods and

HEAT

Rate of Thermal Death Determination

It is useful to determine the heat susceptibility of a given microorganism so that the extent of treatment to be applied in a given situation is under-

Fig. 7-1. Determination of decimal reduction time (D). A sample of cells, for example, 1×10^7 cells per milliliter, is exposed to a given temperature over a specified period of time. The culture is measured at various times (minutes) for the number of microorganisms that have been killed. The data are plotted and a straight line is obtained. By drawing lines from the ordinate corresponding to one log unit (between 10^5 to 10^6 in the example) to the curve and then extrapolating to the abscissa, the decimal reduction time can be determined. In the above example, D is approximately 5 minutes, that is, it takes 5 minutes to reduce the population by a factor of 10. Theoretically, the population is reduced by a factor of 10 every five minutes.

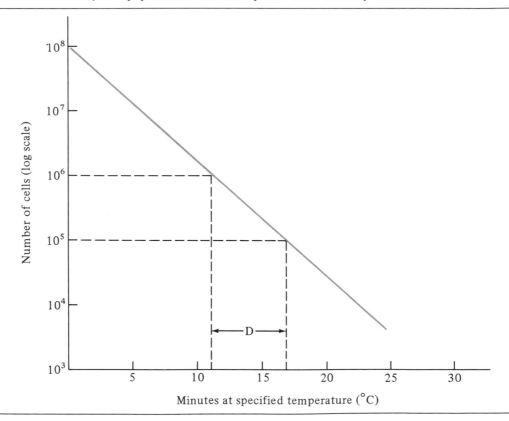

stood. Establishing the rate of kill lends the element of predictability to the heating process and can be determined from the *decimal reduction time (D value)*. The D time is the time in minutes that is required to kill 90 percent (one log unit) of the population at a given temperature. If the D time values are plotted for the most part a straight line is obtained (Fig. 7-1). Thus, if 90 percent of a population dies in one minute, then 90 percent of the remaining 10 percent dies in the next minute, and 90 percent of the remaining 1 percent dies in the next minute, and so on.

Moist Heat

Most mesophilic bacteria in the vegetative form are killed by the comparatively low moist heat temperature of 60°C applied for 30 minutes. Vegetative forms of bacteria, yeasts, and molds are killed in 5 to 10 minutes at 80°C. Mold spores require 30 minutes at 80°C. The heat resistance of most viruses is similar to that of the vegetative forms of other microorganisms. Bacterial spores have a much greater thermoresistance, and so a moist heat temperature of at least 121°C is applied for at least 15 minutes to destroy the most resistant of spores.

The mode of action of moist heat is generally stated to be via the *coagulation* of proteins. Coagulation undoubtedly occurs when overkill conditions are attained, but thermal death probably results from subtler changes that take place before coagulation. Less drastic changes such as inactivation of enzymes, changes in nucleic acids, and cytoplasmic membrane alterations probably kill the microorganisms before coagulation occurs.

Boiling. Boiling is *not reliably sporicidal* and so it cannot be relied on to achieve sterility within a practical period of time if the population of microorganisms is unknown. It is, however, an efficient means of physical disinfection. Vegetative forms of infectious agents are readily killed by boiling in a matter of minutes.

Steam at Atmospheric Pressure. Steam contains latent heat that is generated during vaporization. Steam at 100°C has 540 calories of heat, as compared with the 80 calories of boiling water at that temperature. The latent heat is released when steam condenses on a colder surface. The condensation releases not only heat but moisture, which is necessary for protein coagulation to occur. The shrinking in volume of the steam during condensation creates a negative pressure, thereby drawing in more steam. As the heated object reaches the temperature of the steam, condensed water returns to the vapor phase. Steam under pressure is used in the process of autoclaving.

Steam Under Pressure—Autoclaving. A temperature of 121°C of moist heat applied for 15 minutes is known to kill the spores of virtually every species. To obtain a moist heat temperature of 121°C, saturated steam is placed under pressure of 15 pounds per square inch (psi). The pressure as such has no deleterious effect on microorganisms, but it is needed to raise the moist heat temperature to 121°C. The value generally quoted for achieving sterility by using steam under pressure is 15 psi applied for 15 minutes, or, more correctly, *121°C* applied for *15 minutes*. The value changes according to time–temperature relationships (Table 7-2). As the temperature is raised (via a rise in pressure), the required time of exposure diminishes. Thus, at 20 psi, the temperature becomes 126°C and the sterilization time is 10 minutes. At 30 psi, 134°C is obtained and the time is reduced to 3 minutes.

Moist heat sterilization ordinarily is performed in a sealed chamber, an *autoclave*. It is the preferred method of sterilization if it is applicable. To request that something be autoclaved is tantamount to requesting that it be sterilized. The home pressure cooker in essence is an autoclave but it lacks the double-walled construction and the control devices of commercial autoclaves.

STERILIZATION INDICATORS. Since saturated steam autoclaving is the principal mode of achieving sterility, it is fitting to describe steri-

Table 7-2. Minimum Sterilization Exposure Period—Wrapped and Unwrapped Goods, Gravity Cycle Only

Items	Autoclave setting	
	(121°C) (250°F) (minutes)	(132°C) (270°F) (minutes)
Dressings, wrapped in muslin or equivalent	30	15
Glassware, empty, inverted	15	3
Instruments, metal only, any number (unwrapped)	15	3
Instruments, metal, combined with suture, tubing, or other porous materials (unwrapped)	20	10
Instruments, wrapped in double thickness muslin or equivalent	30	15
Linen packs (maximal size 12″ × 12″ × 12″, maximal weight 12 pounds)	30	—
Treatment trays, wrapped in muslin or equivalent	30	15
Utensils, unwrapped	15	3
Utensils, wrapped in muslin or equivalent	30	15

Source: Courtesy of American Sterilizer Co., Erie, PA.

lization indicators at this juncture. *The two likely causes of sterilization failures are malfunctioning equipment and inadequate treatment* because of the size, nature, or positioning of the load. The saturated steam autoclave is prone to malfunctions. The elevated heat, electrolysis, and deposition of minerals contribute to the degradation and encrusting of valves, gauges, discharge lines, and so on. Loads differ in size and nature (e.g., hard-surfaced items vs. absorbent items), and these in turn affect the length of time that is required to attain sterilizing conditions in the innermost regions.

The commonly used indicators and checks are chemicals that undergo a color change and/or spores of selected bacterial species (biological monitors). The chemical indicators that exhibit a color change have the chemical imprinted on tapes and wrappers for surface exposure indication and on tabs that are used for insertion into the interior of items. The former are less satisfactory, for they merely indicate the conditions that prevailed on the package surface. The chemical *color-change indicators offer the advantage of immediate readout*, and they bear the evidence of exposure directly on the exposed article. *They are not accurate indicators of sterilization* but they are useful for evaluating that the proper temperature has been attained.

The *culture test* (biological monitor) is regarded as the most reliable of the sterilization indicators. *The major disadvantage is the requirement for an incubation period.* The spores of several species of bacteria with a known thermoresistance or a known resistance to ETO are commercially available in ampules or impregnated in filter paper strips (Fig. 7-2). The species whose spores are commonly used are *Bacillus stearothermophilus* for moist heat, *B. subtilis var globigii* for ETO, and *B. subtilis var niger* for dry heat. The Joint Commission on Accreditation of Hospitals and the Communicable Disease Center recommend that *steam autoclaves and ETO sterilizers be tested at least once a week* with appropriate spore indicators.

Pasteurization. Pasteurization may be regarded as a physical method of achieving disinfection. Mild heat is used in pasteurization to destroy pathogenic vegetative forms while preserving the palatability of the liquid. In the beer and wine industries, the process is expected to kill contaminants and the microorganisms that produced the fermentation. The pasteurization of milk is expected to kill vegetative pathogens that are derived from infected cattle and from human and environmental contamination. Infectious diseases that are associated with transmission via raw milk include tuberculosis, brucellosis, streptococcal and *Campylobacter* infections, typhoid fever, dysentery, diphtheria, and Q fever.

With all microbial control processes that use

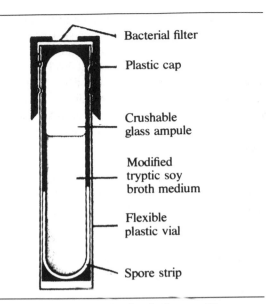

- Bacterial filter
- Plastic cap
- Crushable glass ampule
- Modified tryptic soy broth medium
- Flexible plastic vial
- Spore strip

Fig. 7-2. Biological sterilization indicator. The capsule contains a strip impregnated with bacterial spores, a pH indicator, and culture medium in a crushable ampule. After removal from the sterilizer the ampule is crushed, releasing the culture medium onto the spore strip. A yellow color after incubation indicates incomplete sterilization. (The capsule is part of the ATTEST system manufactured by the 3M Co., St. Paul, MN.)

heat, the higher the temperature the shorter the time the process must be applied. This point is nicely illustrated in the two milk pasteurization extremes. In the *holding* or *batch method*, milk in vessels such as vats is pasteurized at a temperature of 62.0°C applied for 30 minutes. In the *flash method* or *continuous flow method*, thin films of milk stream over pipes or plates that are held at 71.7°C. An exposure of only 15 seconds is required to pasteurize in the latter *high-temperature, short-time (HTST process)* pasteurization method.

Dry Heat

Biomolecules exhibit less thermosensitivity to dry heat than to moist heat. Damaging alterations of proteins by dry heat are the result of oxidation, desiccation, and changes in osmotic pressure owing to the evaporation of moisture. Dry heat is slower and requires temperatures higher than those used in moist heat sterilization. For example, a temperature of 170°C must be applied to anhydrous egg albumin to denature it while an aqueous solution of egg albumin is coagulated in 30 minutes at 56°C.

Dry Heat Sterilization. Dry heat is customarily used at 160°C for at least 2 hours or 170°C for at least 1 hour. Dry heat temperatures below 140°C do not destroy spores within a reasonable period of time. Mechanically convected ovens are used to provide evenly distributed heat. Use of dry heat is the method of choice for sterilizing powders, oils, and thermostable materials that are adversely affected by moisture. Heat convected to the surfaces of the items to be sterilized penetrates by conduction.

Incineration. Discardable, combustible items such as masks, gloves, wipes, and surface covers that are soiled with blood or body fluids should be disposed of in sturdy, impervious plastic bags. The exterior of the bags must not be contaminated to avoid infection to handlers. Flaming is a convenient way to kill microorganisms or to sterilize inexpensive heat-tolerant implements.

COLD

The effect of cold, which is not a method of sterilization, on microorganisms varies, depending on the species of microorganism and the level of cold at which the microorganisms are maintained. Ordinary refrigerator temperatures (2°C to 8°C) have a microbiostatic effect on most microorganisms. Their metabolic rate is greatly reduced, so that they neither reproduce nor shed products in this quiescent state. Psychrophilic microorganisms (those that grow at low temperatures) sometimes multiply in refrigerated intravenous fluids and foods. Freezing gradually destroys parasites such as the trichinella larva and the *Toxoplasma* protozoon found in meats (Chapter 33).

FILTRATION

A number of porous materials are used to remove microorganisms from liquids and from the air. There are many applications of filters in microbiology: sterilization of liquids and air; separation of microorganisms of different sizes (viruses from bacteria); preparation of cell-free solutions of toxins, antigens, and enzymes; clarification of solutions; and determination of the size of viruses.

Membrane filters are the principal filters used in today's laboratories. Membrane filters are paper-thin, sieve-like elements composed of inert cellulose esters and other polymeric materials. The pores are comparatively uniform in size, and the flow rate is much superior to that of the formerly employed depth filters because of the numerous pore openings. The pore sizes range down to sizes that retain the smallest viruses and some of the larger protein molecules (Fig. 7-3). They are disposable, can be autoclaved (they can also be purchased as single-use sterilized de-

vices), and are compatible with many chemicals. Some can be made transparent so that the materials collected on the surface can be stained and examined under the microscope. Body fluids can be run through a filter and the filter then aseptically placed on an agar medium. Organisms present in the fluid—for example, in a urine specimen—grow on the filter surface and can be enumerated.

A popular application of filters is in air control systems for the purpose of removing particles, including microorganisms. High-efficiency particulate air filters (HEPA filters) remove particles as small as 0.3 μm with 99.97 percent efficiency. They are used in "clean room" installations (where the intent is to avoid the alighting of particles on delicate instruments) and in biohazard hoods.

ULTRASONIC CLEANERS

High-frequency sound waves, above the human auditory level, have several applications in microbiology and in the health-related fields. They are used in the laboratory for cell disintegration and in sterilization and disinfection procedures for cleansing purposes.

Fig. 7-3. Reference guide to pore size of membrane filters. (Courtesy Gelman Sciences, Inc., Ann Arbor, MI.)

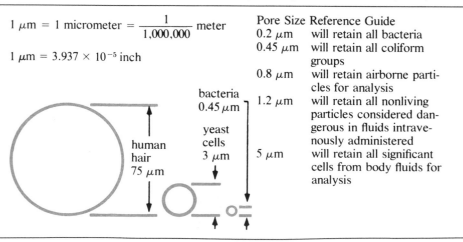

$$1 \ \mu m = 1 \ \text{micrometer} = \frac{1}{1,000,000} \ \text{meter}$$

$$1 \ \mu m = 3.937 \times 10^{-5} \ \text{inch}$$

human hair 75 μm

bacteria 0.45 μm

yeast cells 3 μm

Pore Size Reference Guide
0.2 μm   will retain all bacteria
0.45 μm   will retain all coliform groups
0.8 μm   will retain airborne particles for analysis
1.2 μm   will retain all nonliving particles considered dangerous in fluids intravenously administered
5 μm   will retain all significant cells from body fluids for analysis

Ultrasonic cleaners are used as a *presterilization mode* to remove interfering matter. They consist of tanks filled with specially designed detergents through which sound waves are propelled. Ultrasonic cleaners are very efficient for removing blood, pus, and other organic soil from instruments and glassware. In comparison, brush cleaning is not nearly so efficient, tends to damage delicate instruments, and creates additional risks of injury to the operator. Ultrasonic cleaners effectively clean hinged, serrated, and recessed areas where bristles do not readily reach.

Modern ultrasonic cleaners have individual removable polycarbonate baskets that allow separation of instruments by task. Models are available with cassettes that are filled with soiled instruments after use on a patient. The cassettes are then placed directly into ultrasonic cleaners and from there are removed to the sterilizer without being opened.

RADIATION

Electromagnetic energy affects cells in varying ways, depending on the wavelength, intensity, and duration of the energy. The absorbed energy may produce fluorescence (infrared), heat (infrared), and photochemical changes in which the absorbing molecules of the cell are internally rearranged and decomposed (ultraviolet and ionizing radiation).

Ultraviolet (UV) Radiation

The practical application of UV radiation in the control of microorganisms is primarily that of reducing the population of microorganisms in the air. UV lamps are referred to as *germicidal lamps*. Most germicidal lamps are low-pressure mercury-vapor lamps that generate UV rays with a predominant wavelength of 2537 Å.

Irradiation of Room Air. There are UV barrier installations by which incoming ducted air of buildings is irradiated with germicidal lamps. The air and room surfaces of hospital rooms, operating rooms, entryways, nurseries, gymnasiums, and cafeterias can be irradiated by louvered or shielded ceiling fixtures. The fixtures are designed in such a manner that the UV energy is reflected through a maximum distance without striking the occupants of the room. Warmed air normally rises to the ceiling, carrying with it the microorganism-bearing droplet nuclei (minute particles of mucus that are aerosolized during talking, sneezing, and coughing).

Limitations of Ultraviolet Radiation. There are two major drawbacks associated with UV irradiation when it is used in the control of microorganisms. UV rays have low penetrability. Organisms must be rather directly exposed to the incident rays. Organisms within solids or organisms protected or shielded by any covering material such as ordinary glass, paper, or textiles remain unaffected. Precautions must be taken to avoid prolonged exposure of humans to intense UV radiation. Overexposure to UV lamp irradiation causes skin erythema and conjunctivitis. There have been cases in which persons who attended or played basketball games in gymnasiums suffered conjunctivitis, which gives the sensation of "sand in the eyes" and is accompanied by itching, burning, tearing, and swollen eyelids. Investigations traced the cause of the conjunctivitis to overhead mercury lamps whose outer protective globes or casings had been damaged by basketballs.

Ionizing Radiation

Electromagnetic rays have profound effects when directed at microorganisms. When passing through matter the energy of the rays causes the ejection of electrons, leaving the atoms with a positive charge. The dislodged electrons attach to other atoms to render them electronegative. Short-wavelength electromagnetic rays include x-rays, which are produced by electron accelerators, and gamma rays, which are produced by decay of radioactive substances.

Ionizing radiation, when used in sterilizing, offers the advantages of avoiding both heat and moisture, of having great penetrability (gamma rays, for example, penetrate 2 feet of water), and of allowing prepackaging and sealing of the items to be sterilized. The disadvantages are the special expensive equipment installations, the required safety measures, and the effects on the materials that are exposed. The effects on materials include loss of tensile strength in fabrics, discoloration, chemical changes in certain pharmaceuticals, and organoleptic (e.g., taste) changes in food.

Ionizing radiation is especially useful for sterilizing pharmaceuticals and disposable medical, dental, and laboratory supplies, such as syringes, catheters, surgical gloves, blood transfusion sets, suturing materials, and the many other plastic supplies and devices used in health-related fields.

CHEMICAL METHODS

Chemical agents used for the control of microorganisms on body surfaces and on inanimate objects are grouped under the general heading of disinfectants or germicides. They include antiseptics and sanitizing, degerming, and disinfecting agents. In certain contexts, then, the word *disinfectant* or *germicide* represents all the chemical agents that are used in sterilization or disinfection.

There are a number of situations in which it is not possible to achieve sterility or in which sterility is not really necessary. In many instances, all that is required is to reduce the population of microorganisms to a safe level or to rid an object of the habitually pathogenic vegetative forms.

Sterility can be attained with certain chemicals when they are used under prescribed conditions. Such chemicals are referred to as chemosterilizers or sterilants. They include ethylene oxide (ETO), betapropriolactone, some phenolics and

halogens, strong acids and alkalis, formaldehyde and glutaraldehyde, and peracids. Situations in which chemosterilizers are applicable (with the exception of ETO) are very limited.

QUALITIES OF A UNIVERSAL DISINFECTANT

Just as no single physical method is applicable to every sterilization or disinfection problem, no one chemical agent is able to contend with the many variables that are part of differing control problems. An ideal disinfectant would have the following qualities:

1. It would be able to destroy all forms of microorganisms, including bacterial spores, within a practical period of time.
2. Soil would not interfere with its actions. Most disinfectants interact as well with the reactive chemical groups of organic matter, such as body proteins, as with the chemical groups of microorganisms.
3. It would be nonirritating to tissues, nonallergenic, and nontoxic.
4. It would be noncorrosive, nondiscoloring, nondegradative; it would leave no unsightly or toxic residues on inanimate objects.
5. It would make effective contact because of wettability and penetrability.
6. It would be soluble in readily available solvents, preferably in water.
7. It would be chemically stable; neither it nor the solvent would evaporate and thus lead to a too-concentrated solution that would be damaging to tissues or objects.
8. Its effective range would not be easily bypassed as a result of reasonable diluting factors.
9. It would not have a disagreeable odor, leave stains, or be inordinately expensive.

No disinfectant meets all these qualifications. Disinfectants must be chosen on the basis of their intrinsic properties and on the basis of the job at hand.

LEVELS OF GERMICIDAL ACTIVITY

Germicides may be categorized as high-, intermediate-, and low-level. High-level germicides kill vegetative bacteria, the TB bacillus, fungi, lipid and medium-sized viruses, nonlipid and small viruses, and spores. Sterility is achievable but it should be noted that the killing of bacterial endospores may require as long as 24 hours. Six to ten hours is the more likely exposure time to achieve sterility with high-level germicides. Intermediate-level germicides are expected to kill all but spores and nonlipid small viruses. They exhibit some sporicidal activity but they cannot be relied on to be completely sporicidal. Low-level germicides kill vegetative bacteria, lipid and medium-sized viruses, and some fungi.

It should be emphasized that these categories are arbitrary. There are exceptions with respect to individual species within the broad microbial groups; there sometimes are differing formulations of a germicide; and application situations vary.

CLASSES OF DISINFECTANTS

We cannot describe the properties, applications, advantages, and disadvantages of the thousands of disinfectants on the market. It is customary to divide the disinfectants into several major classes based on chemical relatedness: phenol and phenolics, alcohols, halogens, surfactants, alkylating agents, and heavy metals (Table 7-3). Brief general commentaries are made about the salient features of the members of each class.

Phenol and Phenolics

Phenol, formerly called carbolic acid, figured in a medical classic. Lister used sprays of phenol and phenol-soaked dressings to markedly lessen infections in surgical and traumatic wounds. Dilutions of pure phenol are not used today as antiseptics because of phenol's irritant and anesthetizing qualities.

Phenol is the parent compound of a large number of disinfectants referred to as phenolics, phenol derivatives, phenol-related compounds, and phenol homologues. Since phenol and phenolics are among the more active compounds in the presence of organic matter, they are suitable agents for disinfecting saliva, feces, and similar matter. They are stable and persist on surfaces for long periods after application. Dried residues again become active when rehydrated. They thus have a combination of desirable features lacking in many other disinfectants: they are tuberculocidal, and they are comparatively active in the presence of organic matter.

Hexachlorophene. Chemically, hexachlorophene (HCP) is a bisphenol; that is, two molecules of phenol are joined together (Fig. 7-4). Hexachlorophene at one time was especially valuable in controlling hospital nursery staphylococcal infections, a continually worrisome problem of the hospital nursery. Since 1972 there has been a change in the use of hexachlorophene. It is absorbed through the intact skin. According to experimental studies, it causes gross brain damage in rats. Studies of newborn infants who received three or more daily baths in 3% HCP for more than three days revealed that a percentage of premature infants suffered brain damage. The FDA has directed that hospitals restrict 3% HCP to prescription use. It is not to be used in hospital nurseries unless a staphylococcal epidemic is flourishing.

Other Phenolics. Other effective phenol-related compounds are chlorophene and orthophenylphenols (Fig. 7-5). Commercial preparations include the products Amerse, O'Syl, Dettol, Multicide, Omni II, and Amphyl. Cresols and xylenols are phenolic-related compounds that are coal tar derivatives. They are generally used for sanitation.

Alcohols

Alcohols are bactericidal, tuberculocidal, and fungicidal but not sporicidal. Enveloped viruses

Table 7-3. Disinfectants and Antiseptics[a]

Class	Disinfectant[b]	Antiseptic	Other properties
GAS			
Ethylene oxide	+2 to +4	0	Toxic; good penetration; requires relative humidity of 30% or more; bactericidal activity varies with apparatus used; absorbed by porous materials. Dry spores highly resistant; moisture must be present, and presoaking is desirable.
LIQUID			
Glutaraldehyde, aqueous	+3	0	Sporicidal; active solution unstable; toxic.
Formaldehyde + alcohol	+2	0	Sporicidal; noxious fumes; toxic; volatile.
Formaldehyde, aqueous	+1 to +2	0	Sporicidal; noxious fumes; toxic.
Phenolic compounds	+3	±	Stable; corrosive; little inactivation by organic matter; irritate skin.
Chlorine	+1	±	Flash action; much inactivation by organic matter; corrosive; irritate skin.
Alcohol	+2	+3	Rapidly -cidal; volatile; flammable; dries and irritates skin.
Iodine + alcohol	0	+4	Corrosive; very rapidly -cidal; causes staining; irritates skin; flammable.
Iodophors	+1	+3	Somewhat unstable; relatively bland; staining temporary; corrosive.
Iodine, aqueous	0	+2	Rapidly -cidal; corrosive; stains fabrics; stains and irritates skin.
Quaternary ammonium compounds	+1	+2	Bland; inactivated by soap and anionics; absorbed by fabrics.
Hexachlorophene	0	+2	Bland; insoluble in water, soluble in alcohol; not inactivated by soap; weakly -cidal.
Mercurial compounds	0	+1	Bland; much inactivated by organic matter; weakly -cidal.

± = some compounds may or may not be effective antiseptics.
[a] More detailed information must be obtained from descriptive brochures, journal articles, and books. Selection of the most appropriate germicide should be based on whether it is to be used as a disinfectant or as an antiseptic and on the estimated level of antimicrobial action needed.
[b] Maximal usefulness is denoted by +4.
Source: From E. H. Spaulding, *Manual of Clinical Microbiology* (2nd ed.). Washington, DC: American Society for Microbiology, 1974.

are susceptible to the alcohols because of the lipid components of the viral envelope. The mode of action of alcohols is primarily that of denaturation of proteins. Ethyl and isopropyl alcohols are the only alcohols that are extensively used. The recommended concentration is 70% even though concentrations from 60 to 95% seem to kill as fast. Alcohols appear to be underrated as

antimicrobial agents. A study reported in 1989 (see Suggested Readings: Christensen, R. P., et al.) that tested 39 products under a variety of test conditions showed that ethyl alcohol alone or products containing high ethyl alcohol concentration had consistently high antimicrobial activity on environmental surfaces regardless of the test method, test organism, or contact time used

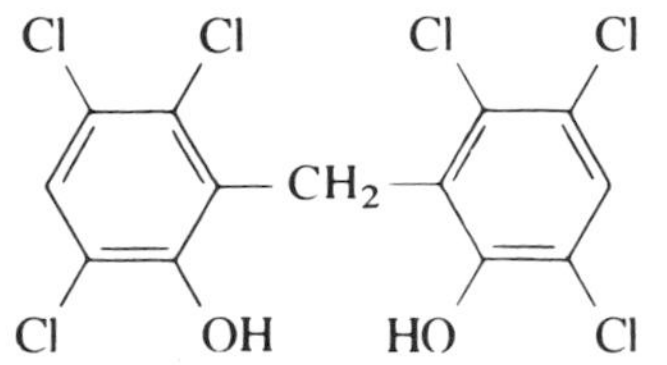

Fig. 7-4. Hexachlorophene.

both in the absence and presence of bioburden. A disadvantage of the alcohols is that the effective concentration is easily bypassed. Once the concentration falls below 45%, the antimicrobial activity is slow and uncertain.

Halogens

Most disinfectants categorized as halogens are inorganic halogen compounds. The mode of action is due to oxidation and to direct halogenation of proteins. The commonly used halogens are chlorine and iodine. All halogens are, furthermore, important as substituents in other disinfectants, in which they play a contributory antimicrobial role. Chlorine is especially important as a substituent in other disinfectants.

Chlorine Elemental chlorine and inorganic chlorine compounds are employed principally in sanitation, purification, and disinfection. Elemental chlorine is used for water purification. Hypo-

Fig. 7-5. Phenol and two popular phenol-related compounds.

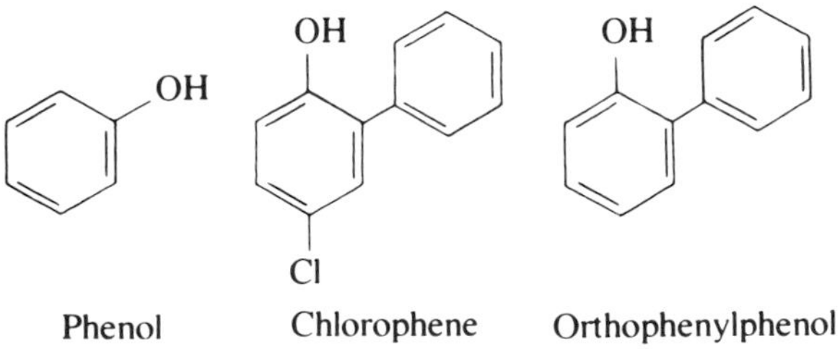

chlorites and other chlorine-releasing compounds serve as bleaching agents and as sanitizing agents in dairies, abattoirs, and swimming pools, and in housekeeping. Organic matter interferes with the antimicrobial activity of the chlorine compounds to a considerable extent. *Household bleach* is an effective and inexpensive germicide. The active ingredient is *sodium hypochlorite (NaOCl)* at 5.25 percent concentration. It is diluted 1:10 to 1:100, depending on the amount of organic matter present on the surface to be disinfected. It is corrosive to some metals, especially to aluminum. Dilutions should be prepared fresh daily.

Iodine Iodine compounds currently are the most popular for wound and skin antisepsis and for preoperative skin antisepsis. They are also used as general disinfectants for thermometers and surgical appliances and for purification of water.

TINCTURES OF IODINE. The early popular iodine formulations were tinctures of iodine. Molecular iodine is not readily soluble in aqueous solution. Therefore it is usually dissolved in alcohol (hydroalcoholic solutions). The ready evaporation of alcohol creates problems because strong iodine concentrations can cause tissue necrosis. Tinctures of iodine formulations contain differing percentages of elemental iodine and of alcohol; 1, 5, and 7 percent tincture formulations destroy 90 percent of skin bacteria in 90, 60, and 15 seconds, respectively.

IODOPHORS. The disadvantages of the tinctures were largely overcome by the development of a group of compounds collectively called the iodophors. Iodophors are composed of complexes of iodine and surface-active organic carrier molecules. The complexed iodine is released gradually from the carrier molecule. The activity is not so great as with the tinctures because of the lowered available iodine content. Iodophors are nonstaining, nonallergenic, water-soluble, and relatively nonirritating, and thus have an advantage over the inorganic iodine formulations. Proprietary iodophors include Wescodyne, Iosan,

Virac, Hi-Sine, Betadine, Surgidine, Prepodyne, Biocide, Surf-A-Cide, and Promedyne.

Surfactants

Surfactants are surface-active agents that have the property of concentrating at interfaces. They lower surface tension. They are good wetting and solubilizing agents. Surfactants include the soaps and detergents.

Soaps. Cosmetic soaps are usually sodium and potassium salts of long-chain fatty acids. They are invaluable in controlling microorganisms even though many of them have no direct antimicrobial activity. Their usefulness resides in their ability to degerm the skin by mechanically removing microorganisms. They emulsify the oily layer of the skin, where most of the transient and cross-infecting microorganisms are enmeshed. The lipid layer with its contents of microorganisms is broken up and vanishes down the drain in the rinse water. In addition to the emulsifying and degerming action, about 50 percent of the cosmetic soaps are designed to have some direct antimicrobial activity. They contain bacteriostatic or bactericidal compounds that potentially reduce cross-contamination, body odor, and superficial cutaneous infections (Fig. 7-6).

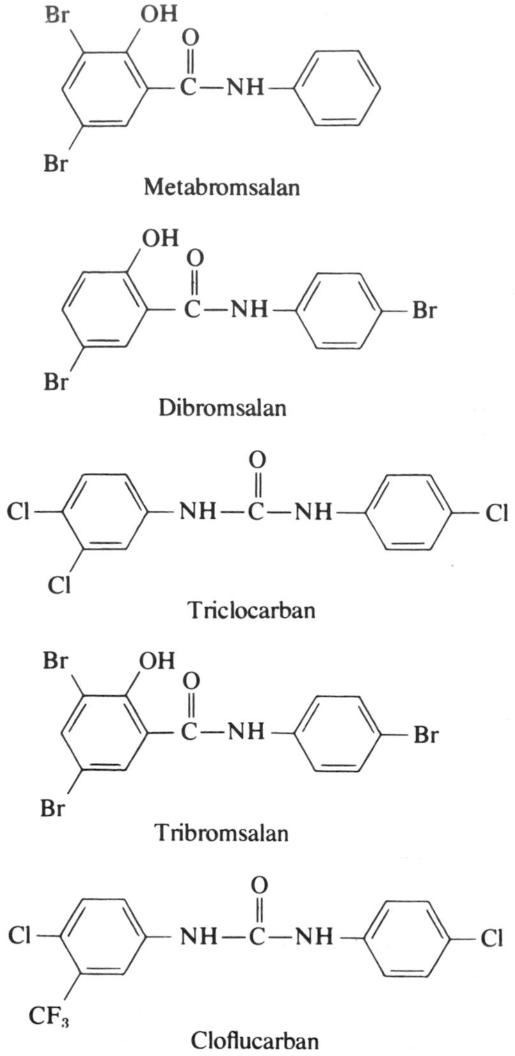

Detergents. Detergents are synthetic surfactant cleansing agents. They are regarded as superior to the soaps as cleansing agents because they do not form precipitates and deposits with water minerals as the soaps do. They are divided into the *anionic, cationic,* and *nonionic* detergents on the basis of the polarity and activity of their polar groups.

Anionic detergents are used in laundry powders and liquids. They are not disinfectants. Like soaps they remove microbial contaminants with the grime and dirt of soiled articles.

Members of the *cationic detergent* group have been among the most popular disinfectants, antiseptics, and sanitizers. The lipid-containing, negatively charged membrane of the bacterial cell attracts the positively charged component of

Fig. 7-6. Bacteriostatic agents used in soaps such as Lifebuoy, Gamophen, Dial, Palmolive Gold, and Phase III.

the lipophilic alkyl chain portion of the cationic detergent molecule. The lethal action of the cationic detergents is primarily ascribed to cell membrane disruption. Enveloped viruses, because of their lipid content, are inactivated by cationic detergents.

Hundreds of cationic detergents have been synthesized and tested, but only three main types

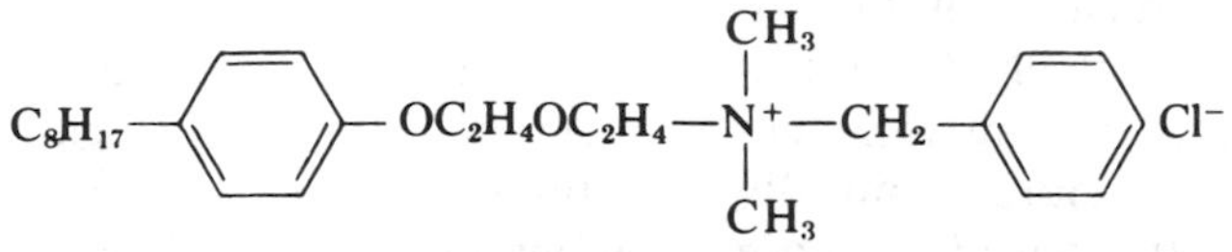

Benzethonium chloride

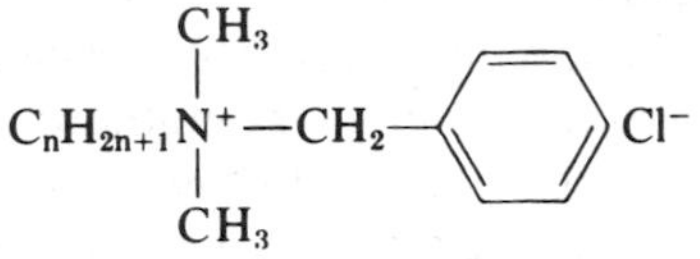

Benzalkonium chloride

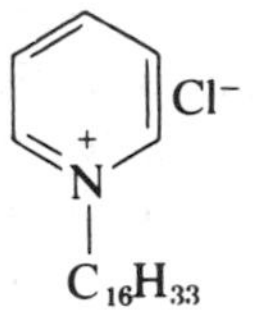

Cetylpyridinium chloride

Fig. 7-7. Three popular cationic detergents.

are popularly used as antimicrobial agents: *benzalkonium chloride* (Zephiran), *benzethonium chloride* (Phemerol), and *cetylpyridinium chloride* (Ceepryn) (Fig. 7-7). The words in parentheses are the proprietary names of some of the better-known commercial products.

Cationic detergents are bland (colorless, tasteless, odorless), very stable, nontoxic, and inexpensive, and remain active at high dilutions. These good qualities have to be weighed against a number of shortcomings. They are not sporicidal or tuberculocidal. Pseudomonas organisms appear to be refractory to them at low-level concentrations. Cationic detergents are readily absorbed by surfaces such as gauze and cotton, which are sometimes used to cushion instruments being decontaminated or being kept sterile in disinfectant solutions. Organic matter interferes with their action. They are readily neutralized by soaps and anionic detergents. If soap is used to remove gross contamination or soil from the skin or from an object, follow-up use with a cationic detergent may be self-defeating and deceiving if a soap residue remains. The cationic detergent loses its antimicrobial activity because it chemically interacts with the soap.

Alkylating Agents

Alkylating agents exert their antimicrobial effects by substituting alkyl groups for the hydrogen of reactive groups of enzymes, nucleic acids, and proteins. Labile reactive hydrogens are available on carboxyl groups ($-COOH$), sulfhydryl groups ($-SH$), amino groups ($-NH_2$), and hydroxyl groups ($-OH$). Some of the alkylating agents are used in the gaseous or vapor phase, some as liquids, and some in either the gaseous or the liquid state.

Formaldehyde. Formaldehyde is sometimes employed in the gaseous state as a fumigant. In solution as formalin, it is known for its uses as a fixative for anatomical and pathological tissue specimens, as an inactivator in vaccines, and as a component of embalming fluids. Sterilization and disinfection applications are limited because it is a tissue irritant.

Fig. 7-8. Alkylating agents.

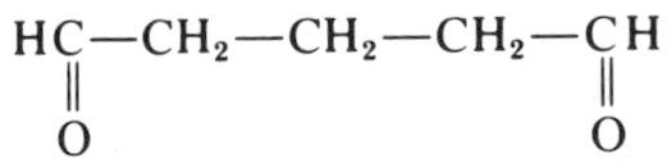

Glutaraldehyde

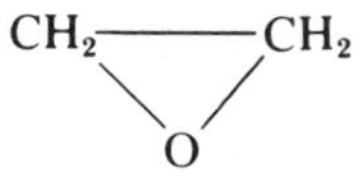

Ethylene oxide
(ETO)

Glutaraldehyde. A chemical relative of formaldehyde, glutaraldehyde has two aldehyde groups, one at either end of a five-carbon chain (1,5-pentanedial) (Fig. 7-8), and it is therefore chemically categorized as a *dialdehyde*. It is one of the more recent additions to the disinfectant and sterilant armamentarium and is highly rated as a disinfectant. It has a wide spectrum of activity. When used in a 2% solution, it is bactericidal, tuberculocidal, and virucidal in 10 to 90 minutes and sporicidal in 10 hours. Glutaraldehyde disinfectants along with iodine compounds and bleach are recommended for use against hepatitis viruses in situations in which sterilization is not feasible. There are both alkaline formulations and acid formulations. Since glutaraldehyde is irritating to the skin and mucous membranes and very irritating to the eyes, it is not used as an antiseptic. Commercially available glutaraldehyde preparations include Cidex, Sporicidin, Glutarex, Banacide, and Wavicide.

Ethylene oxide (ETO). The gas ETO is a cyclic ether (Fig. 7-8). The major advantage of ETO is that this penetrative gas is able to sterilize in the absence of high levels of heat or moisture. A wide range of articles that are affected by elevated heat are sterilized with ETO: catheters; disposable medical, dental, and laboratory items; dental handpieces; textiles; sutures; and heart-lung machines.

ETO forms explosive mixtures with air. ETO is, therefore, diluted with inert gases such as carbon dioxide, nitrogen, or halogenated hydrocarbons. ETO is toxic if inhaled, and it is a vesicant (i.e., it can cause blisters) on contact. It is slow-acting, requiring 4 hours at 50 to 56°C or 6 to 12 hours at room temperature to produce sterility. Special equipment is necessary. Many hospitals now have ETO autoclaves as part of their standard sterilizing equipment. Items treated with ETO that are to be used in patient contact must first be aerated to remove the residual ETO. Also, educational materials must be provided to all workers who use ETO because of the hazards.

Heavy Metals

Most of the heavy-metal disinfectants contain mercury or silver. Inorganic and organic preparations are available, but metal-containing disinfectants have been largely replaced by more effective compounds. They are slowly bactericidal, their action being principally bacteriostatic and reversible. Organomercurial antiseptics have lost the popularity they once had and have been superseded by iodine compounds, cationic detergent formulations, and alcohol. The one silver compound to be noted is silver nitrate. It is the law in most states that a 1% prophylactic silver nitrate solution or certain antibiotics be instilled into the eyes of all newborns to prevent the development of gonococcal conjunctivitis. A recent burn treatment technique also incorporates silver nitrate.

Chlorhexidene

Special mention is due an antiseptic with the generic name chlorhexidine. A 4% chlorhexidine preparation (the commercial product is called Hibiclens or Hibitane) is used for surgical scrubs, for hand washing by health care personnel, and as a skin wound cleanser. Chlorhexidine persists on the skin whereas iodophors do not; it is not appreciably absorbed into the blood from the skin as hexachlorophene is; it is generally nonirritating; and it is active against gram-positive and gram-negative bacteria.

PRACTICAL RECOMMENDATIONS

To prevent self-infection, the cross-infection of patients, and contamination of the environment, it is important to keep these suggestions in mind:

1. Make liberal use of soap and water.
2. Keep immunizations current.

3. Keep contaminated fingers from the mouth and nose for they are the major portals of entry of microorganisms into the body.
4. Use germicides according to the manufacturers' instructions and for their intended use. Allow the prescribed time for them to act.
5. Be especially wary of needlestick injuries. Wear heavy-duty gloves when processing needles and sharp instruments.
6. Use the recommended barrier techniques when they are called for: face masks, disposable gloves, protective eyewear, gowns.
7. Most important, "think through" or "see in the mind's eye," as Lister phrased it, how transmission of microorganisms might occur.

Imagine that the contaminating material is stained with a fluorescent, eye-catching dye. The contamination from a wound dressing might show up on the hands of the nurse, on the instruments that were used to remove the dressing, on the hospital bedstand, the bedclothes, the floor, the patient's gown, the nurse's clothing—anywhere in the room. With this mental picture should come the realization that every move must be made in such a manner as to provide the fewest opportunities for disseminating microorganisms. Asepsis procedures should not be performed in a perfunctory, indifferent manner. All efforts should be made to utilize available methods to prevent or minimize infection.

SUMMARY

1. An understanding of the basic principles of sterilization and disinfection begins with an understanding of the commonly used terms of sterile, -cide, -stasis, sepsis, asepsis, antisepsis, disinfection, sanitization, and germicide.
2. The composition of the population of microorganisms to be controlled usually is unknown, and, therefore, the assumption is made that highly resistant forms are present.
3. Rarely is the level of kill in the population tested and, therefore, sterilization or disinfection procedures should be carried out as prescribed.
4. Certain microorganisms pose special problems, notably, bacterial endospores because of their resistance to heat and disinfectants, mycobacteria because of their resistance to disinfectants, pseudomonad bacteria because of their ubiquity and resistance to antimicrobial agents, and the hepatitis and human immunodeficiency viruses because of the mode of transmission.
5. Interfering matter, especially that derived from the body (for example, blood), and environmental conditions affect the activity of antimicrobial procedures and agents.
6. The principal modes of attaining sterility are autoclaving in saturated steam, use of elevated dry heat, and exposure to ethylene oxide.
7. Because sterilizing devices are subject to physical stresses and because sterilizing conditions vary, use of sterilization indicators is advised.
8. The physical methods of controlling microorganisms include the moist heat methods of boiling, saturated steam autoclaving, and pasteurization; the dry heat methods of elevated hot air temperatures and incineration; filtration of liquids and air; ultrasonic cleaning for the purpose of removing interfering matter; irradiation with ultraviolet (germicidal) lamps for surface sterilization or disinfection; and irradiation of the ionizing type for the sterilization of disposable supplies.
9. There is no all-purpose disinfectant that has all the properties of the ideal disinfectant; the disinfectant to be used must be chosen on the basis of its properties and the characteristics of the job at hand.
10. The major classes of disinfectants are phenol and its derivatives, alcohols, halogen compounds, surfactants (soaps and detergents), alkylating agents, and heavy-metal compounds.

QUESTIONS FOR STUDY

Select the best response or responses for each of the following:

1. Some disinfectants/antiseptics have a bacteriostatic effect. This means that they:
   A. Kill bacterial cells that are in the vegetative state
   B. Kill bacterial spores
   C. Are toxic and corrosive
   D. Destroy tissue cells
   E. At least prevent the multiplication of bacteria that are in the vegetative state

2. The method that is regarded as the most reliable to achieve sterility of instruments is:
   A. Immersion for 30 minutes in buffered glutaraldehyde
   B. Dry heat (hot air) at 121°C for 2 hours
   C. Saturated (air-free) steam at 121°C for at least 15 minutes
   D. Irradiation with ultraviolet rays for 3 minutes with a germicidal lamp
   E. Exposure to ethylene oxide for 15 minutes

3. The main purpose of cleansing (sonication, brushing) soiled instruments prior to sterilizing them is:
   A. To make them aesthetically acceptable to the patient
   B. To prevent corrosion
   C. To reduce the number of microorganisms on the instruments
   D. To remove the "soil" (organic matter or grease and oil) that protects entrapped microorganisms
   E. To activate bacterial spore germination

4. The principal disadvantage of using the endospores of members of the genus Bacillus as the biologic standard for testing the efficacy of a sterilization procedure is:
   A. The unexposed spores unpredictably convert into the vegetative form after about a two-week storage period
   B. The delay in the readout because an incubation period is required after exposure
   C. The spores are obtained from pathogenic species and breakage or spillage could lead to infections of the handlers
   D. Breakage during sterilization could permanently contaminate the interior of the sterilizing equipment

5. The primary value of soap in controlling microorganisms lies in its:
   A. Sporicidal action
   B. Bactericidal action
   C. Bacteriostatic action
   D. Removal of microbes from skin surfaces
   E. Virucidal action

6. Preparations of iodine compounded with non-ionic detergents and other organic "carrier" molecules circumvent some of the undesirable features of hydroalcoholic iodine compounds. Collectively, these compounds are termed:
   A. Iodotrophs
   B. Iodophors
   C. Halophors
   D. Surfactants
   E. Alkylating agents

Match each term on the left with the correct definition on the right:

7. Saturated steam
   autoclaving

8. Tincture of iodine

9. Ethylene oxide
   exposure

10. Glutaraldehyde
    preparation

11. Ultrasonication

A. Routinely used mode for attaining sterility
B. Removal of interfering matter from contaminated instruments
C. Potent antiseptic formulation
D. Requirement for post-sterilization aeration of certain articles
E. Potent disinfectant used for immersed articles

ADDITIONAL READINGS

Benenson, A. S. (ed.). Control of Communicable Diseases in Man (14th ed.). American Public Health Association. Springfield, VA: John D. Lucas, 1985.

Block, S. S. (ed.). Disinfection, Sterilization, and Preservation (3rd ed.). Philadelphia: Lea & Febiger, 1983.

Christensen, R. P., et al. Antimicrobial activity of environmental surface disinfectants in the absence and presence of bioburden. J. Amer. Dental Assn. 119:493,1989.

Dental Asepsis Review. #1 Gloving: some additional comments; #2 Improving the performance of the office sterilizer; #3 Notes on eye protection; #4 Tetanus—an old and persistent problem; #8 Hepatitis B vaccination; #11 Using an ultrasonic cleaner; #12 Disinfection of surfaces and equipment. Indianapolis, IN: Sterilization Monitoring Service, Indiana University School of Dentistry. vol. 9, 1988.

Favero, M. S. Sterilization, Disinfection, and Antisepsis in the Hospital. Chapter 13 in E. H. Lennette, et al., Manual of Clinical Microbiology (4th ed.). Washington, DC: American Society for Microbiology, 1985.

Palmer, M. B. Infection Control: A Policy and Procedure Manual. Philadelphia: Saunders, 1984.

Perkins, J. J. Principles and Methods of Sterilization in Health Sciences (2nd ed.). Springfield, IL: Charles C Thomas, 1983.

8. CHEMOTHERAPY

OBJECTIVES

To describe the characteristics of certain drugs that make them suitable as chemotherapeutic agents

To list the major chemotherapeutic drugs that are inhibitors of cell wall synthesis, cytoplasmic membrane function, protein synthesis, nucleic acid synthesis, and cell metabolites

To briefly describe the mechanism of action of penicillins on the cell wall

To describe the various ways in which protein synthesis can be inhibited by chemotherapeutic agents

To outline those factors that a physician must consider when deciding on a drug for chemotherapy

To describe how microorganisms are able to develop resistance to an antimicrobial

To describe what types of tests are used to measure a microorganism's susceptibility to antimicrobials

To define: antibiotic, chemotherapeutic agent, beta-lactamases, penicillin-binding proteins, prophylaxis, antimetabolite, minimal inhibitory concentration (MIC), transposon-associated resistance, Kirby-Bauer method

Chemotherapeutic agents are a class of compounds used in the treatment of disease. They fall into two general categories: those produced synthetically by chemists and those produced biologically by microorganisms, that is, *antibiotics*. This separation is rather imprecise because scientists can also produce semisynthetic chemotherapeutic agents. To do this the nucleus of a biologically synthesized compound is recovered from the producing organism and various chemical groups are synthetically added to it.

Chemists began synthesizing antimicrobial agents in the late 1800s and early 1900s but antibiotics were not discovered until the 1930s. Antibiotics were shown to be produced by soil bacteria and fungi but only in small amounts. Microbiologists seized on this natural metabolic process and began manipulating the growth characteristics of the microorganisms in order to increase antibiotic production. Today the commercial production of antibiotics and other antimicrobials is on a large scale. The scale of antibiotics produced by American companies alone is between 1 and 1½ billion dollars per year.

This chapter will describe the various characteristics of antimicrobials and the factors that influence the choice of antimicrobials for therapy. We will also discuss the mechanisms of antimicrobial resistance among microorganisms and how the clinician uses various tests to determine what antimicrobial can be used by the physician.

GENERAL CHARACTERISTICS OF CHEMOTHERAPEUTIC AGENTS

A chemotherapeutic agent is one that is selectively toxic, that is, it is toxic to the microbial cell but relatively nontoxic to the host cell. Selective toxicity is possible because of differences in the biochemistry of the host and the microbial cell. For example, penicillin inhibits the synthesis of bacterial cell wall, a component that is not present in mammalian cells. In addition, even though some biochemical activities are similar in the two types of cells, a chemotherapeutic agent has a greater affinity for the bacterial component. For example, protein synthesis occurs in all biological systems but the ribosomes of eukaryotes differ from those of bacteria. Thus, an antibiotic is likely to have a different effect on the two types of cells if the ribosome is the target of the drug. Some drugs have a *low selective toxicity*, that is, they are almost as toxic to the mammalian cell as they are to the infectious microbe. For this reason a measure of this selective toxicity of drugs, called the *therapeutic index*, was developed. The therapeutic index represents the ratio between the minimum toxic and maximum therapeutic concentrations of a drug. A high therapeutic index indicates that the concentration of drug that is therapeutic is virtually nontoxic to host tissue. A low therapeutic index indicates

that the concentration of drug that is therapeutic is also harmful to host tissue.

Chemotherapeutic agents have been classified according to their *spectrum of activity*, that is, which group(s) of microorganisms they inhibit. A *broad-spectrum* drug is one that has activity against gram-positive as well as gram-negative species. A *narrow-spectrum* drug affects only one group of microorganisms or perhaps only one species.

HOW TO DETERMINE ANTIMICROBIAL ACTIVITY

The antibiotic activity of a microbe isolated from the soil can be measured in a number of ways. In the *plate diffusion method*, agar blocks containing a culture of the microorganism producing the antibiotic are placed on an agar surface seeded with a test microorganism. Following incubation, antibiotic activity is noted as a clear zone around the agar block. A second test involves the use of a culture filtrate from an antibiotic-producing microorganism or a synthetic agent made in the laboratory. The potential chemotherapeutic agent can be put into regularly spaced holes punched into the agar, or it may be introduced into cylinders placed on the surface of an agar plate seeded with the test microorganism. Antibacterial activity is again noted as a clear zone around the agar well or the cylinder (Fig. 8-1).

FACTORS DETERMINING THE POTENTIAL OF A CHEMOTHERAPEUTIC AGENT

Antimicrobial activity is not the only factor that must be considered in selecting a drug for com-

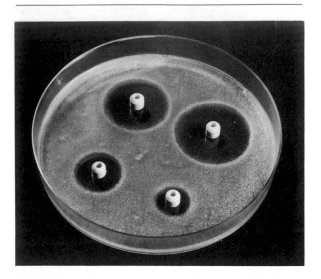

Fig. 8-1. Cylinder method for determining bacterial sensitivity to drugs. Cylinders are placed on agar plates and filled with a specified quantity of antibiotic. Antibiotic is considered effective if a zone of inhibition develops. Note the variation in the width of zones of inhibition. The width may be due to the type of antibiotic placed in the cylinders or to a variation in the concentration of one antibiotic. (From L. P. Garrod and F. O'Grady, *Antibiotic and Chemotherapy* [5th ed]. London: Churchill Livingstone, 1973.)

mercial use. A variety of tests must be performed that will measure the following:

1. Spectrum of activity
2. Stability to heat
3. Solubility in water
4. Toxicity
5. Rate of excretion of drug from the host

The two most important criteria for the use of a drug as a chemotherapeutic agent are that (1) it must exert antimicrobial activity at very low concentrations and (2) it should be relatively nontoxic.

CHEMOTHERAPEUTIC AGENTS

Chemotherapeutic agents either kill (*-cidal*; for example, *bactericidal*) the infectious agent or arrest (*-static*; for example, *bacteriostatic*) its growth. In very life-threatening situations a chemotherapeutic agent that quickly kills the infectious agent may be required. Chemotherapeutic agents that arrest growth are also useful because they enable the host to utilize his defensive arsenal. These defenses are in the form of phagocytes and antibodies. If antibodies can be stimulated, future infections from the same infectious agent may in many instances be handled by the host without the intervention of antimicrobials. This is the principle of the vaccination process. In general, the antimicrobial activity of chemotherapeutic agents relates to their ability to affect metabolism in several ways.

INHIBITORS OF CELL WALL SYNTHESIS

The most important drugs that inhibit cell wall synthesis are the penicillins, the cephalosporins, bacitracin, and vancomycin. These drugs are effective only in bacterial cells that are actively synthesizing cell wall peptidoglycan precursors. All these drugs are bactericidal.

Penicillin
Penicillin comes as close as any drug to being the model antibiotic because of its low toxicity and the minimal concentration required for antibacterial activity. Penicillins and cephalosporins belong to a class of compounds called *beta-lactams*. This designation is based on the common nucleus of these antibiotics, which contains a beta-lactam ring (Fig. 8-2). Except for penicillin G (benzyl penicillin) all penicillins are semisynthetic (Fig. 8-2). The laboratory synthesis of the side chains has resulted in three classes of penicillins that (1)

Penicillin nucleus

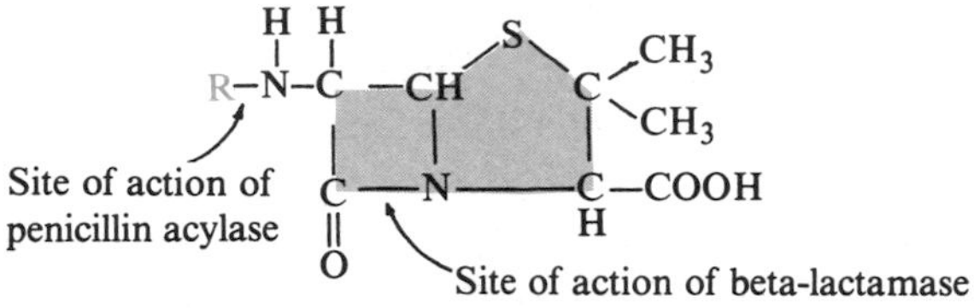

Site of action of penicillin acylase

Site of action of beta-lactamase

NAME OF DERIVATIVE	SIDE CHAIN	CHARACTERISTICS
Penicillin G (benzyl penicillin)	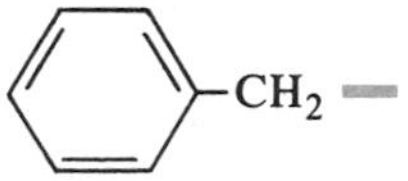	Inexpensive, acid labile, susceptible to beta-lactamases of gram-negative and gram-positive bacteria; ineffective orally
Penicillin V (phenoxymethyl penicillin)	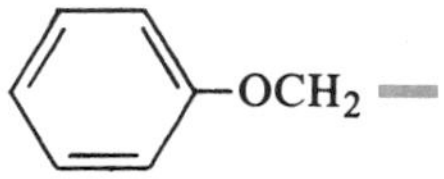	Acid resistant; can be taken orally; narrow spectrum
Oxacillin	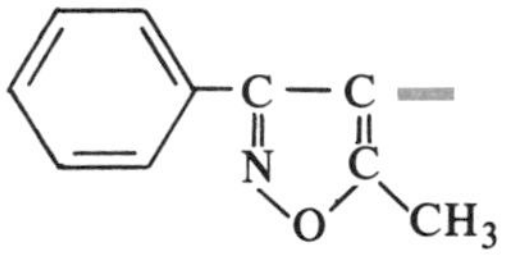	Can be taken orally; not susceptible to beta-lactamases; narrow spectrum
Ampicillin	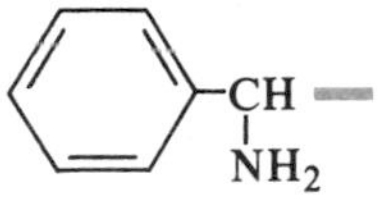	Sensitive to beta-lactamases; broad spectrum; acid resistant
Piperacillin	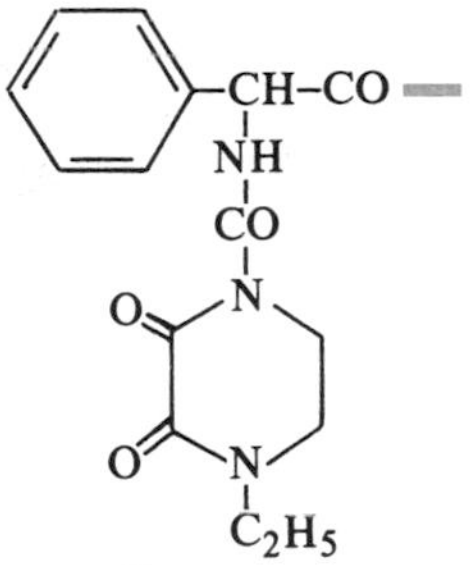	Similar to ampicillin in activity; inhibits *Klebsiella* resistant to carbenicillin; inhibits *Pseudomonas;* more resistant to cephalosporinases than other beta-lactam antibiotics
Carbenicillin	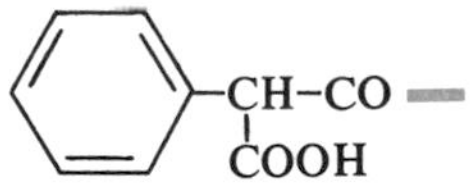	Cannot be administered orally; resistant to gram-negative beta-lactamases; active against *Pseudomonas*
Ticarcillin	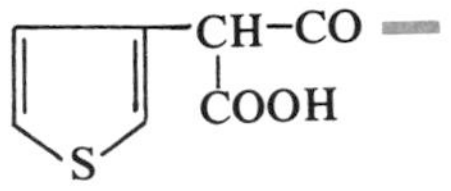	Similar to carbenicillin
Methicillin	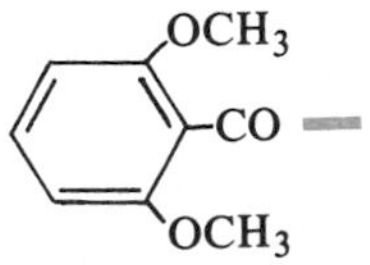	Relatively resistant to beta-lactamases; most effective against *S. aureus* resistant to penicillin G

Fig. 8-2. Structure of the penicillin nucleus (6-amino-penicillamic acid) and some of its more clinically useful derivatives.

are resistant to acid, such as in the stomach, (2) are resistant to degradation by microbial enzymes, and (3) have a broad spectrum of activity.

Special dosage forms of penicillin are often used in treatment. The potassium salt of penicillin G is dissolved very rapidly in body fluids. Even with intramuscular injections penicillin is quickly absorbed from the site of injection into the bloodstream. The rate of dissolution of penicillin can be reduced if the penicillin is combined with *procaine*. A single intramuscular injection of procaine-penicillin can produce a therapeutic level of drug for 24 hours in the bloodstream, whereas the same dose of penicillin in water is effective only for 4 to 5 hours. In its aqueous form penicillin is rapidly excreted from the kidneys. A preparation called benzathine penicillin is used to circumvent this problem. Benzathine penicillin consists of two molecules of benzyl penicillin bound to dibenzylmethylenediamine. Given intramuscularly, this preparation produces high levels of the drug in the serum for several days.

Penicillin and its derivatives are the least toxic of all the drugs used in chemotherapy. When doses approach 40 to 50 million units, however, neurotoxicity can result. The most adverse effect caused by administration of penicillin is an allergic response, observed in up to 8 percent of the population who receive the drug. All persons are at potential risk of such allergic reactions because penicillins are found everywhere in the environment as a result of agricultural, industrial, and medical contamination.

Mechanism of Action. The mechanism by which penicillin is lethal to bacteria has been a subject of controversy for many years. The exact mechanism is still not known, and more than one mechanism may actually be involved. The discovery of *penicillin-binding proteins (PBPs)* and the identification of a transpeptidase as the lethal target of beta-lactam antibiotics have shed some light on the mechanism. PBPs are located in the cytoplasmic membrane and there are three to eight distinct types in a given microorganism. PBPs are involved in the synthesis of cell wall.

When beta-lactams enter the cytoplasmic membrane they bind to PBPs and form a complex. The affinity of PBPs for beta-lactams is variable and is related to the type and concentration of the beta-lactam as well as the type of PBP affected. The binding of beta-lactams to different PBPs affects certain morphological responses associated with cell wall synthesis (Fig. 8-3). PBP 1 is associated with the enzymes involved in cell elongation, PBP 2 with cell shape, and PBP 3 with septum formation. The addition of a penicillin to a culture of rod-shaped bacteria will sometimes cause immediate lysis, while with other penicillins the cells may round up, forming ovoid cells, and with yet other penicillins there may be the formation of filaments (Fig. 8-4). It now appears that the initial action of beta-lactams is to inhibit bacterial growth by affecting the activity of an enzyme involved in peptidoglycan metabolism. The most likely candidate for this is a transpeptidase, that is, the enzyme that links peptides in the peptidoglycan strands. Breakage of strand linkages is believed to be followed by an irreversible response in which a hydrolytic enzyme acts autocatalytically and breaks the covalent bonds in the peptidoglycan strands, thus exposing the cytoplasmic membrane to the environment. This ultimately leads to lysis of the cell (Fig. 8-3).

Beta-Lactamases and Resistance to Penicillin. Resistance to antibiotics is discussed in more detail on page 196; however, penicillin resistance is discussed here because penicillin and its derivatives are the most widely used antimicrobial agents and the least toxic. The major reason many microorganisms are resistant to penicillins and other beta-lactams is a microbial enzyme called *beta-lactamase*. There are several classes of beta-lactamases and each splits the beta-lactam ring, thereby inactivating the antibiotic (see Fig. 8-2). Beta-lactamases are found primarily in the periplasmic space, where they are believed to be responsible for the assembly of peptidoglycan. They have been found in almost all gram-positive and gram-negative bacteria but their ability to in-

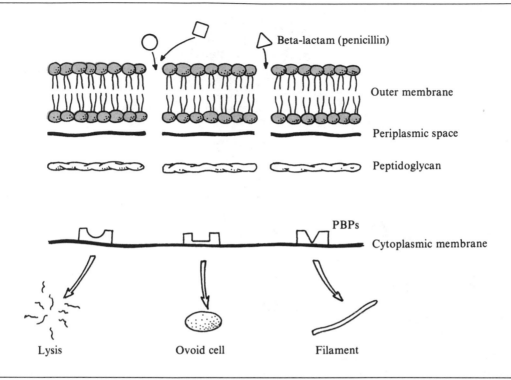

Fig. 8-3. Movement of beta-lactams through the cell envelope and their effect on the bacterial cell. The affinity of a beta-lactam for penicillin-binding proteins (PBPs) varies depending on the structure of the beta-lactam antibiotic. The effect on the bacterial cell is associated with the type of PBP.

activate penicillin can vary from one penicillin derivative to another. The genetic determinants for beta-lactamase may be chromosome- or plasmid-associated. Sensitivity to beta-lactamases is now the single most important consideration in the development of new penicillins. One solution to the problem has been to use combinations of beta-lactams to broaden the scope of antibacterial activity. Another solution is the use of beta-lactamase inhibitors in conjunction with beta-lactams. Experimental results indicate that treatments in which inhibitors, such as *clavulanic acid* and *sulbactam*, are administered with a beta-lactam may be a valuable therapeutic regimen.

Cephalosporins
Cephalosprins are beta-lactam antibiotics similar in structure and activity to the penicillins (Fig. 8-

5). The naturally occurring cephalosporins (cephalosporin C) were first isolated from a fungus in 1945, and all had minimal antimicrobial activity. Semisynthetic derivatives have since been prepared with cephalothin, the first marketed derivative of cephalosporin C. One of the most important properties of many of the cephalosporins is their resistance to the beta-lactamases of gram-positive bacteria. Cephalosporins are useful alternatives to the penicillins, particularly in the treatment of disease caused by gram-positive species resistant to penicillin and in situations in which the patient is allergic to penicillin. There are now second- and third-generation cephalosporins (Fig. 8-5), including cefamandole, cefazolin, cefoxitin, cefotaxime, and cefoperazone. Some of these new cephalosporins such as cefamandole have activity against gram-negative

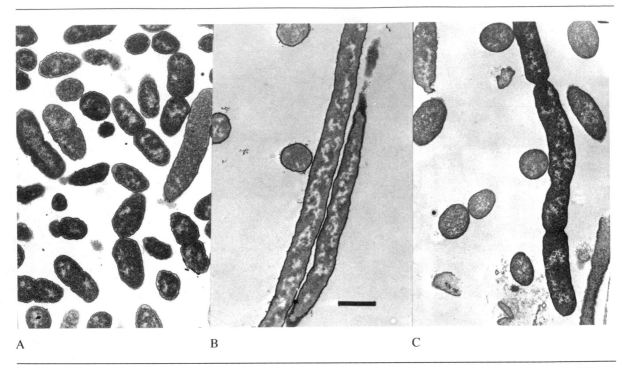

A   B   C

Fig. 8-4. Effect of subinhibitory concentrations of ampicillin on the gram-negative bacillus *Proteus mirabilis*. A. Control. B. *P. mirabilis* exposed to subinhibitory concentrations of ampicillin. C. *P. mirabilis* filaments from B after transfer to drug-free agar. (Courtesy Barbara Atkinson.)

bacteria and are resistant to the beta-lactamases of this group of bacteria.

A group of cephalosporins called *cephamycins* are also unusually resistant to beta-lactamase of gram-negative bacteria. A semisynthetic cephamycin called *cefoxitin* has a broad spectrum of activity that includes gram-negative anaerobes such as *Bacteroides fragilis*.

The third generation cephalosporins, such as cefotaxime, cephtizoxime, and ceftriaxone, appear to have excellent activity against gram-negative rods causing meningitis, which include the agents *Hemophilus influenzae*, *Neisseria gonorrhoeae*, and *E. coli*.

The mechanism of action of the cephalosporins is similar to that of the penicillins since it is the beta-lactam ring that exhibits specificity for the penicillin-binding proteins.

Bacitracin

Bacitracin is a peptide antibiotic originally isolated from the bacterium *Bacillus subtilis*. It is active against gram-positive bacteria but not gram-negative species. The drug is not absorbed from the intestinal tract and is very toxic to the kidneys (nephrotoxicity). Its primary use has been as a topical agent in combination with other topical agents such as polymyxin, neomycin, or both.

Bacitracin inhibits cell wall synthesis by preventing the transfer of peptidoglycan precursors to the growing cell wall.

Vancomycin

Vancomycin is a drug with limited usefulness in the clinical situation. Its use has been restricted

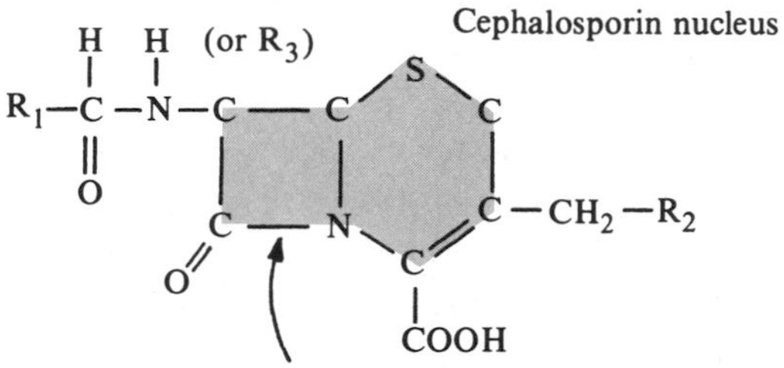

Cephalosporin nucleus

Site of action of beta-lactamase (cephalosporinase)

NAME OF DERIVATIVE	SIDE CHAIN R_1	SIDE CHAIN R_2	CHARACTERISTICS
Cephalothin	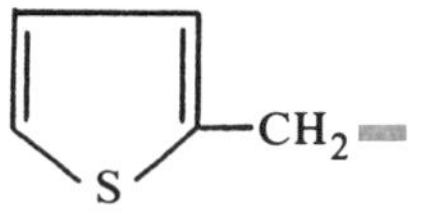	$OCOCH_3$	Can be given only IM or IV; used for severe staphylococcal infections
Cefazolin	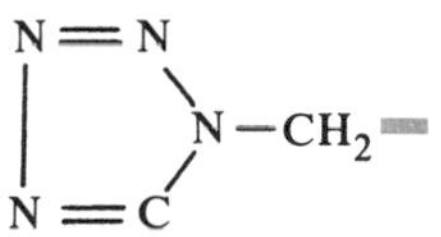	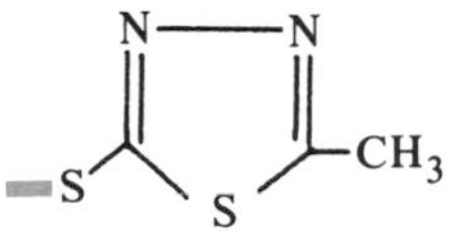	Can be given only IM or IV; more active than cephalothin against *E. coli* and *Klebsiella;* more susceptible to beta-lactamase than cephalothin
Cefamandole	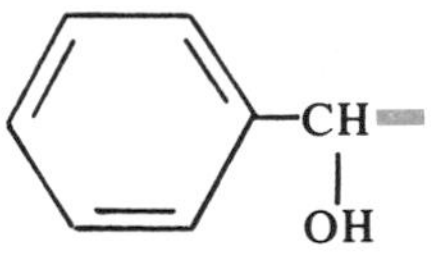	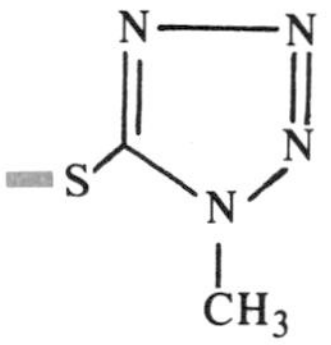	Inhibits enterobacteriaceae to greater degree than cephalothin; active against *Hemophilus influenzae;* administered parenterally
Cefoxitin*	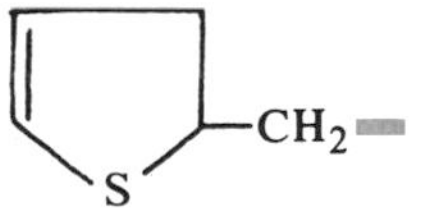	$OCONH_2$	Diminished activity against gram-positives but greater activity against gram-negative organisms than cefamandole; administered primarily IV
Cefotaxime	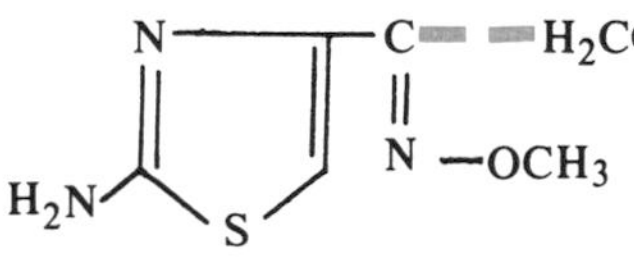	$H_2COCOCH_3$	Marked resistance to beta-lactamases of certain gram-negative bacteria such as *Hemophilus influenzae;* active against *Pseudomonas*

*Cefoxitin has an R_3 side chain of $^-OCH_3$

Fig. 8-5. Structure of the cephalosporin nucleus (7-aminocephalosporanic acid) and some of its more important derivatives. (IM = intramuscularly; IV = intravenously.)

to the treatment of staphylococcal infections in which the infectious agent is resistant to methicillin or oxacillin. Almost all strains of *Staphylococcus aureus* resistant to these penicillins are sensitive to vancomycin. Vancomycin is also used in the treatment of antibiotic-associated pseudomembranous colitis (see Chapter 18).

The exact site of action of vancomycin during cell wall synthesis is not known, but it does block the synthesis of peptidoglycan with the accumulation of cell wall intermediates. Vancomycin is also believed to alter the permeability of the cytoplasmic membrane.

The most common adverse effects of vancomycin include a group of signs and symptoms known as *red man syndrome* or RMS. RMS is characterized by pruritus, erythema, and in severe cases angioedema, hypotension, and cardiovascular collapse. The severity of the reaction, which is usually associated with rapid administration of the drug, correlates with the amount of histamine released into the plasma.

INHIBITORS OF CYTOPLASMIC MEMBRANE FUNCTION

Polyenes

Polyenes are antibiotics that are used primarily as antifungal agents and are produced mainly by Streptomycetaceae. The principal polyenes are amphotericin B (Fig. 8-6) and nystatin, but minor ones include candicidin, pimaricin, trichomycin, and hamycin. The mechanism of action of these drugs is similar. They have an affinity for lipids and bind irreversibly to cytoplasmic membrane sterols such as ergosterol. Large pores are produced in the cytoplasmic membrane when polyenes bind, and this results in permeability changes. There is leakage of potassium ion, sugar, and other compounds plus impaired uptake of nutrients such as amino acids. The membranes surrounding the various fungal organelles are similarly affected by these antibiotics.

Amphotericin B, like other polyenes, has a low solubility in water, and most preparations are

Fig. 8-6. Structure of amphotericin B.

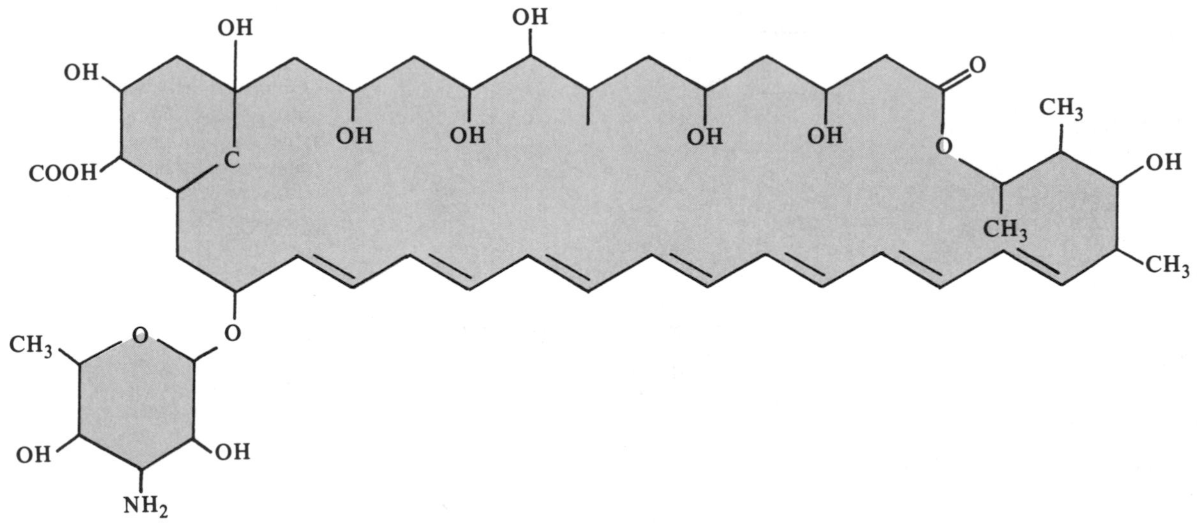

made up in sodium deoxycholate. The polyenes are relatively toxic drugs and most adverse effects involve the kidney. Except for amphotericin B the polyenes are seldom administered parenterally. Amphotericin B is used in the treatment of serious systemic fungal diseases such as candidiasis, histoplasmosis, and blastomycosis. The concentration of drug that is effective in treatment is very close to the dosage that is also very toxic. Amphotericin B is often administered with flucytosine—a combination that permits the use of smaller doses of amphotericin B.

Nystatin, the second most widely used polyene, is used primarily as a topical agent in the treatment of disease caused by the yeast *Candida*.

Imidazoles

The imidazoles are primarily antifungal agents but some show antibacterial activity. They are synthetic drugs that have a broad spectrum of fungal activity and are active against yeasts and molds. The major imidazoles are miconazole, clotrimazole, and econazole. Most are used as topical agents. Clotrimazole induces formation of liver enzymes that destroy the antifungal activity of the drug. Miconazole is also toxic when administered for systemic infections, but systemic use is indicated if the patient fails to respond to amphotericin B or other drugs such as ketoconazole (see below).

One of the newest imidazoles is ketoconazole. This drug has a broad spectrum of activity and can be taken orally. It is fairly well tolerated by patients and can be administered over long periods of time. These attributes make it an important alternative to amphotericin B in the treatment of systemic disease. Ketoconazole can be toxic to those treated over a prolonged period of time. Adverse effects include nausea, vomiting, and some liver dysfunction but not hepatitis.

A recent addition to the imidazole arsenal is itraconazole, an orally active drug. It is less toxic than other azole drugs. Clinical trials indicate it is effective against superficial fungal infections.

A new oral imidazole, fluconazole, can penetrate the blood-brain barrier. This drug was approved in 1990 for use in the treatment of cryptococcal meningitis and candidiasis (thrush). These two fungal diseases have been devastating particularly in patients with AIDS. Fluconazole can also be administered intravenously.

The imidazoles affect the permeability of the cytoplasmic membrane. These permeability changes appear to be due to interference with lipid biosynthesis in the fungal cell, especially the synthesis of sterols. The effect of these drugs on bacteria and protozoa suggests that imidazoles may also influence the biosynthesis of lipid triglycerides.

Polymyxins

The polymyxins are polypeptide antibiotics produced by *Bacillus polymyxa*. Only polymyxin B and polymyxin E (colistin) are used clinically. The polymyxins are antibacterial agents and are active against gram-negative bacteria. They interact with phospholipids in the cytoplasmic membrane, thereby disrupting it and causing leakage of cellular contents. These drugs are nephrotoxic and are used primarily as topical agents. Polymyxin B is not absorbed from the intestinal tract. Occasionally the drug is administered for intestinal infections.

INHIBITORS OF PROTEIN SYNTHESIS

Aminoglycosides

The major class of inhibitors of protein synthesis are the aminoglycosides. They consist of an amino ring structure to which are attached amino and non-amino sugars. The aminoglycosides are bactericidal and bacteriostatic against a wide variety of bacteria including staphylococci and the facultative and aerobic gram-negative bacilli. Some of the important aminoglycosides are streptomycin, amikacin, gentamicin, kanamycin, tobramycin, and others. The aminoglycosides are uniformly nephrotoxic and bring about morphological as well as functional alterations of the proximal renal tubules. With rational administration nephrotoxicity is minimal and is usually reversible. The aminoglycosides are also toxic to the hearing mechanism, but this varies considerably depending on dosage and the aminoglycoside being used. Despite some of these toxic effects the aminoglycosides are nonallergenic, and do not interfere with immunologic processes. Microbial resistance to the aminoglycosides has increased dramatically in the past 10 years and the use of these antimicrobials has also dramatically waned.

Our understanding of the mechanism of action of the aminoglycosides is not yet complete. Their primary microbial inhibiting action is due to attachment of the drug to the ribosome and subsequent disruption of protein synthesis. There are different ways in which the aminoglycosides can affect the process of protein synthesis, but ribosomal RNA is the principal target. Protein synthesis may also be affected by the effects of increased or decreased binding of aminoacyl tRNA to the ribosome or by various effects of the drugs on initiation, elongation, or termination. Aminoglycoside-treated bacterial cells also show considerable membrane damage and it is now believed that several steps are involved in the bactericidal action of these drugs (see reference B. Davis at the end of this chapter). The effect of the drug is believed to occur in the following way:

1. A small amount of antibiotic penetrates the bacterial cell and binds to ribosomes. Ribosome binding causes misreading of the mRNA and formation of abnormal protein occurs.
2. Some of the abnormal protein is incorporated into the cytoplasmic membrane, producing pores that enable more antibiotic to enter the bacterial cell. This results in an increase in the rate of abnormal protein formation.
3. The concentration of antibiotic reaching the cytoplasm is so high that it totally blocks the binding of ribosomes to mRNA and protein synthesis is shut off.
4. The binding of antibiotic to all of the ribosomes is irreversible and the bacterial cell dies.

A variety of naturally occurring and some semisynthetic aminoglycosides have been discovered and developed. The activities of the newer aminoglycosides as well as the characteristics of the older drugs are outlined in Table 8-1.

Tetracyclines

Tetracyclines (Fig. 8-7) are bacteriostatic agents that inhibit protein synthesis by binding to the 30S ribosome and blocking the binding of aminoacyl tRNA to the A site. Tetracyclines have the broadest spectrum of activity of all antibiotics. They inhibit gram-positive and gram-negative bacteria, the rickettsiae, mycoplasmas, spirochetes, chlamydiae, and some protozoa. Although tetracyclines are relatively nontoxic, there are situations in which their use is not appropriate. Continued use of tetracyclines eliminates the bacterial flora and predisposes the patient to disease by indigenous fungi, such as species of *Candida*, a condition called *superinfection*. Tetracyclines stain developing teeth, and the drug should not be administered to children under 5 years of age. Tetracyclines also cause fatty degeneration of the liver in pregnant women; other drugs should be considered to treat infections of this group. Tetracyclines are the drug of choice for infections caused by rickettsiae and chlamydiae and are frequently used in the treatment of upper respiratory diseases. Doxycycline and minocycline are absorbed more efficiently than are other tetracyclines. Minocycline is active against some bacteria resistant to other tetracyclines.

Chloramphenicol

Chloramphenicol is a bacteriostatic agent that inhibits protein synthesis by binding to the 50S ri-

Table 8-1. Characteristics of the Aminoglycosides

Aminoglycoside	Principal clinical use	Comments
Streptomycin	Treatment of tuberculosis but always with other drugs; treatment of tularemia and plague; combined with penicillin in treatment of endocarditis caused by enterococci and viridans streptococci	Most microorganisms develop resistance to drug when used alone; therefore it is used only under special circumstances
Kanamycin	Used primarily as a topical drug or for oral therapy	Lacks activity against pseudomonads; susceptible to inactivation by a number of aminoglycoside-modifying enzymes
Gentamicin	Widely used in treatment of infections caused by facultative and aerobic bacilli, for example, the Enterobacteriaceae	Effective against pseudomonads and most Enterobacteriaceae; resistant strains found primarily in hospitals
Tobramycin	Spectrum of activity similar to gentamicin's	More active against *Pseudomonas aeruginosa* than is gentamicin; resistant strains primarily in hospitals
Sisomicin	Spectrum of activity similar to gentamicin's	Similar to tobramycin in its activity against *P. aeruginosa*
Amikacin	Has broadest spectrum of activity of aminoglycosides; particularly effective against *Pseudomonas* species	Produced from the acylation of kanamycin; resistant to aminoglycoside-modifying enzymes; no major resistant strains detected
Neomycin	Used primarily as a topical agent because of toxicity; activity spectrum similar to kanamycin	Occasionally administered orally as an antiseptic before bowel surgery
Fortimicin A	Activity parallels that of amikacin but has greater activity against *Serratia marcescens*	Resembles kanamycin in its poor activity against *P. aeruginosa*
Netilmicin	Resistant to enzymes that modify gentamicin and sisomicin; effective against more strains of enteric bacilli than is gentamicin	A semisynthetic derivative of sisomicin
5-Episisomicin	More active against *P. aeruginosa, S. marcescens, Providencia* species than is gentamicin	A semisynthetic derivative of sisomicin

bosome and blocking peptidyl transfer. It has a broad activity spectrum similar to that of the tetracyclines but is more toxic and is used only under special circumstances. Toxicity is associated with inhibition of protein synthesis in bone marrow cells of the host. The drug gives rise to conditions such as anemia and leukopenia, and repeated administration may result in fatal aplastic anemia. It is still a drug of choice for typhoid fever, and for cases of meningitis in which the patient is allergic to penicillin.

Erythromycin

Erythromycin is most active against gram-positive species and is one of the least toxic of all antibiotics. It is a frequent alternative drug when other drugs are too toxic or when an individual is allergic to drugs such as the penicillins. It is

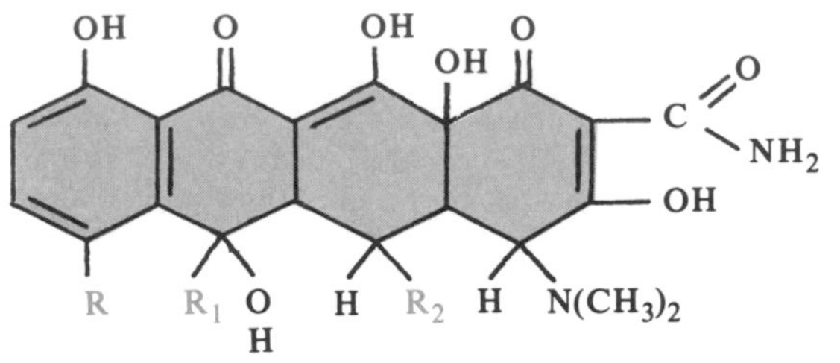

Fig. 8-7. Structure of the tetracycline nucleus and some of its derivatives.

the drug of choice in the treatment of infections caused by *Legionella pneumophila* and *Mycoplasma pneumoniae*.

Erythromycin affects protein synthesis by binding to free ribosomes but not polysomes. The ribosome-bound drug allows the formation of a small peptide but then prevents further elongation of the peptide.

Lincomycin and Clindamycin

Lincomycin and clindamycin resemble erythromycin in spectrum of activity and pharmacologic characteristics. Clindamycin is a derivative of lincomycin. Clindamycin is the drug of choice in the treatment of serious anaerobic pulmonary infections. Lincomycin is used in treating staphylococcal and streptococcal infections that do not respond to penicillin therapy or when the patient is allergic to penicillin. One of the toxic side effects of clindamycin and lincomycin is diarrhea and *pseudomembranous colitis*. These toxic effects are controllable (see Chapter 18).

Clindamycin has a greater spectrum of activity than lincomycin, with activity against many gram-positive and gram-negative anaerobic bacteria as well as protozoal organisms such as *Toxoplasma* and *Plasmodium*.

Lincomycin and clindamycin are similar to chloramphenicol in inhibiting protein synthesis, that is, they inhibit peptidyl transfer.

Spectinomycin

Spectinomycin is not a true aminoglycoside but is very similar structurally. It inhibits protein synthesis much as chloramphenicol does. Its principal use is in the treatment of gonorrhea when the agent of disease is resistant to penicillin.

INHIBITORS OF NUCLEIC ACID SYNTHESIS

Inhibitors of nucleic acid synthesis include antibacterial drugs such as nalidixic acid and rifampin, the antifungal drug flucytosine, and several antiviral agents.

Rifampin

Rifampin is a semisynthetic derivative of the antibiotic rifamycin B. Rifampin inhibits RNA synthesis by affecting the DNA-dependent RNA polymerase of the bacterial cell. Mammalian RNA polymerases are not affected by the drug. Rifampin has activity against mycobacteria and gram-positive species but is less active against gram-negative species. It is used primarily in the treatment of tuberculosis, being combined with other drugs such as streptomycin and ethambutol. Most of the undesirable side effects of rifampin therapy are minor gastrointestinal symptoms.

Nalidixic Acid

Nalidixic acid is a synthetic *quinolone* that is chemically unlike all other antimicrobial agents (Fig. 8-8). It is most effective against gram-negative organisms but not anaerobes. Its use is restricted to very specific situations. It has been used in combination with other drugs to prevent infections in cancer patients undergoing therapy. The drug selectively suppresses those bacteria in the intestinal tract that are major causes of urinary tract infection in the compromised cancer patient but does not affect the anaerobic population.

The bacteriostatic activity of the drug is associated with its ability to hinder DNA replication, presumably because of its effect on one of the DNA-binding proteins, DNA gyrase.

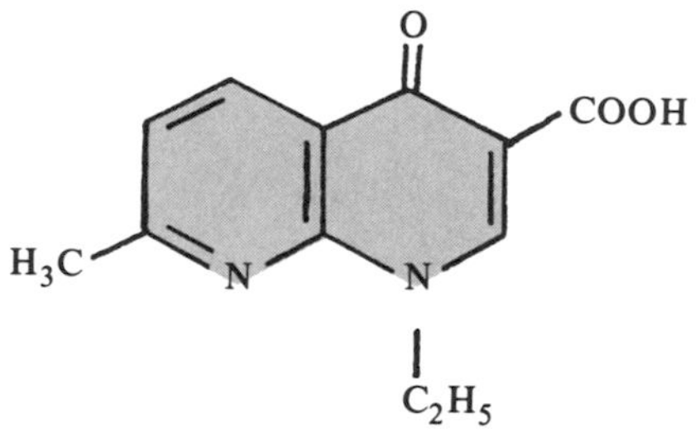

O
‖
COOH

H₃C   N   N

C₂H₅

Fig. 8-8. Structure of nalidixic acid.

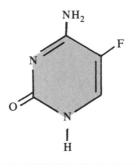

Fig. 8-9. Structure of flucytosine (5-fluorocytosine).

Recently, derivatives of nalidixic acid have been synthesized and used in clinical trials. Some of the most clinically effective quinolones now possess fluorine residues. These *fluoroquinolones* show increased potency, greater spectra of antimicrobial activity, and decreased frequency of selection of resistant mutants than nalidixic acid. Resistance to quinolones is usually at a low frequency because the resistance determinants are on the chromosome and not on a plasmid. Thus, resistance is not spread by mobile genetic elements.

The quinolones appear to be important substitutes for aminoglycosides in the treatment of gram-negative infections and possibly gram-positive infections as well. *Ciprofloxacin* is one example of a fluoroquinolone that appears to be a breakthrough in the treatment of *Pseudomonas aeruginosa* and other gram-negative infections.

Flucytosine

Flucytosine is a fluorinated pyrimidine (Fig. 8-9) originally developed as an antimetabolite for use in cancer chemotherapy. It has a narrow spectrum of activity that is limited to yeast infections such as candidiasis. When used alone it induces the development of resistant microbial species. It is frequently combined with amphotericin B for the treatment of systemic mycoses. It is rapidly absorbed from the intestinal tract and can be administered orally.

Flucytosine is deaminated in the cytoplasm of the fungal cell to 5-fluorouracil, which is subsequently phosphorylated and incorporated into RNA. This fluorinated derivative interferes with normal protein synthesis. Flucytosine can also interfere in DNA synthesis (Fig. 8-10).

Toxic effects from flucytosine therapy are minimal and include nausea, vomiting, and diarrhea.

Amantadine Hydrochloride

Amantadine hydrochloride (α-adamantanamide hydrochloride) inhibits the primary transcription process in the influenza A virus and thus prevents the uncoating of the capsid. Amantadine hydrochloride is used for the prevention of influenza A, but it is not a substitute for the influenza vaccine. Maximum effectiveness can be obtained only when the drug is administered at the start of the influenza season and is maintained daily as long as virus exposure is certain (usually 6–8 weeks). The drug is used more extensively in the Soviet Union than in the United States, where it is administered only to high-risk groups. The drug can cause side effects such as dizziness, depression, and drowsiness, particularly in the elderly.

Rimantadine is an analog of amantadine that has been used with considerable success in the prophylaxis of influenza. The drug has been used for years in eastern Europe but only recently has it been studied in the United States. The drug appears to present fewer side effects, particularly for the elderly, than amantadine.

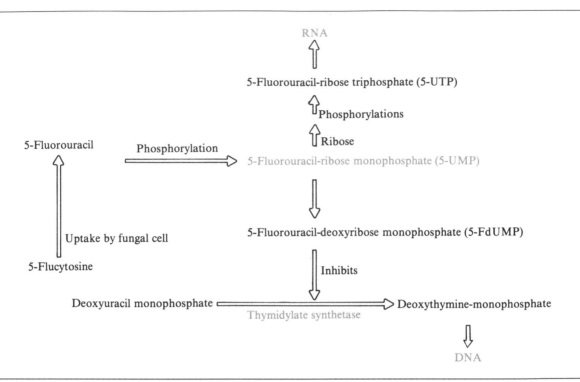

Fig. 8-10. Action of flucytosine in fungi. Flucytosine is taken into cytoplasm of fungal cell, where it is converted to 5-fluorouracil ribose monophosphate (5-UMP). The latter can be phosphorylated and incorporated into RNA and interfere with normal protein synthesis or it can be converted to a deoxy form (5-FdUMP), which is an inhibitor of thymidylate synthetase.

Fig. 8-11. Structure of idoxuridine (IDU).

Ribavirin

Ribavirin (virazole) is a synthetic nucleoside resembling guanosine that is active against both RNA and DNA viruses. The drug appears to inhibit an early viral replication step that leads to the synthesis of viral nucleic acids. Ribavirin has been approved by the FDA for use in treatment of respiratory syncytial virus and influenza virus infections. Aerosolization of the drug is effective in treatment of both viral infections.

Idoxuridine (5'-iododeoxyuridine or IDU)

Idoxuridine is a halogenated analog of thymidine (Fig. 8-11). It is incorporated in place of thymidine into cellular as well as viral DNA. IDU is

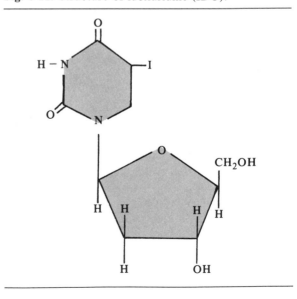

used for localized herpesvirus infections of the eye. Since the infected cells of the eye do not divide, only viral DNA incorporates IDU and host toxicity is avoided.

Vidarabine (Adenine Arabinoside, ara-A)

Vidarabine has a spectrum of activity similar to that of IDU. Vidarabine is effective in the treatment of life-threatening herpesvirus infections. It has been used in the treatment of herpes zoster infections, herpes simplex encephalitis, and chickenpox in immunocompromised patients.

Acyclovir

Acyclovir (9-[(2-hydroxyethoxy) methyl] guanine) (Fig. 8-12) is an antiviral agent that has been demonstrated to be effective in the treatment of herpes simplex virus infection. Acyclovir is a unique antiviral agent in that it is selectively metabolized by virus-infected cells. To be effective this drug must be phosphorylated and this occurs efficiently only in virus-infected cells (Fig. 8-13). The phosphorylation is carried out only by a

Fig. 8-12. Structure of acyclovir.

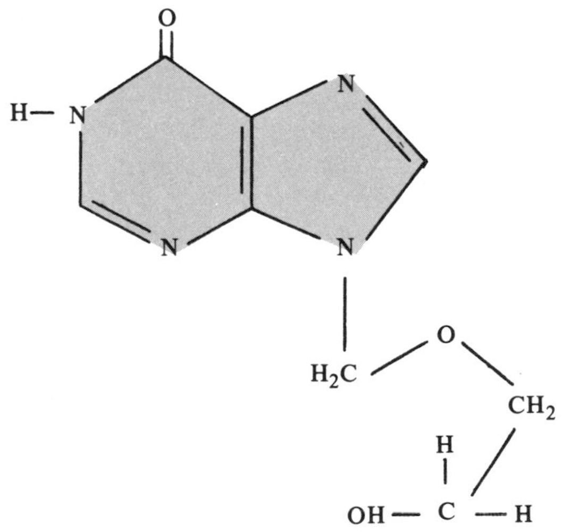

virus-coded thymidine kinase. The phosphorylated acyclovir is further phosphorylated to acyclovir triphosphate, which is a potent inhibitor of herpes simplex–induced DNA polymerase but has little or no effect on host cell DNA polymerase. Acyclovir triphosphate is also incorporated into replicating viral DNA and this results in chain termination during DNA synthesis. Acyclovir can be administered intravenously in small doses for the treatment of mucocutaneous herpes simplex virus infections in immunocompromised patients. It is used more frequently, however, in a topical or oral form in the treatment of primary genital herpes virus infections.

Zidovudine (Azidothymidine [AZT])

AZT was initially synthesized for use as an anticancer drug in 1964. Like acyclovir, AZT is converted into an active triphosphate (AZT-TP) by cellular kinases. AZT-TP inhibits the virus (human immunodeficiency virus [HIV]), causing acquired immune deficiency syndrome (AIDS). The site of inhibition is the HIV reverse transcriptase, which is the enzyme that converts viral RNA into viral DNA. AZT is toxic but it nevertheless prolongs survival from advanced HIV infection 12–30 months. The major adverse effects are anemia and granulocytopenia. (See Chapter 31 for further discussion of AZT in AIDS patients.)

ANTIMETABOLITES

Compounds that are structurally similar to normal cellular metabolites and may compete with them for attachment to an enzyme surface are called *antimetabolites*.

Sulfonamides

The sulfonamides were among the first synthetic agents used successfully in the treatment of disease. Important derivatives of the sulfonamides are sulfanilamide, sulfadiazine silver, sulfame-

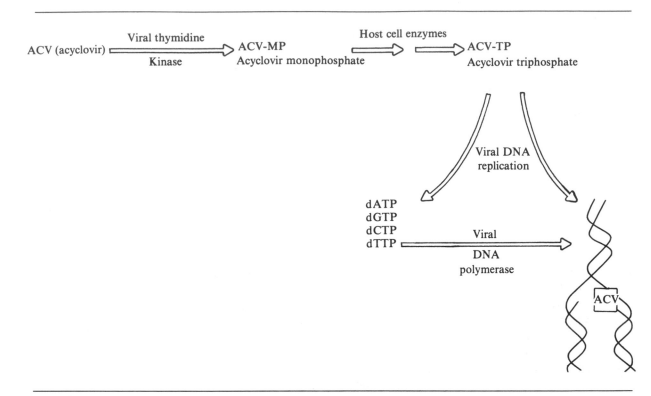

Fig. 8-13. Mechanism of action of acyclovir (ACV).

thoxazole, and sulfamerazine. On account of their broad antibacterial activity these drugs were in earlier times used almost exclusively in the treatment of a wide assortment of diseases. It is most fortunate that other drugs have replaced the sulfonamides as antimicrobial agents because all pathogenic bacteria are capable of developing resistance to the sulfonamides. The bacteriostatic action of the sulfonamides is related to their similarity in structure to para-aminobenzoic acid (PABA) (Fig. 8-14). PABA is a component of the vitamin folic acid, one of the B vitamins. Sulfonamides prevent the synthesis of bacterial folic acid, which is a coenzyme important in amino acid metabolism and purine nucleotide synthesis (Fig. 8-15).

The sulfonamides are not administered so frequently as they were before the discovery of antibiotics. Some sulfonamides such as sulfisoxa-

zole are still used in the treatment of acute urinary tract infections because of their solubility in urine. Oral sulfonamides are sometimes recommended as a prophylaxis for "travelers' diarrhea" caused by *E. coli*. Other agents such as sulfadiazine silver are used topically for burn patients. More recently the combination of sulfamethoxazole and trimethoprim has proved particularly effective against many intestinal and urinary tract pathogens. The reason for this effectiveness is the apparent inhibition of two reactions in the synthesis of folic acid (Fig. 8-15).

The sulfonamides are for the most part readily tolerated; however, they do have some undesirable side effects. The drugs can bind to plasma proteins that are normally occupied by bilirubin. In the newborn, bilirubin can penetrate the blood-brain barrier, causing encephalopathy (kernicterus). Sulfonamides should therefore not be ad-

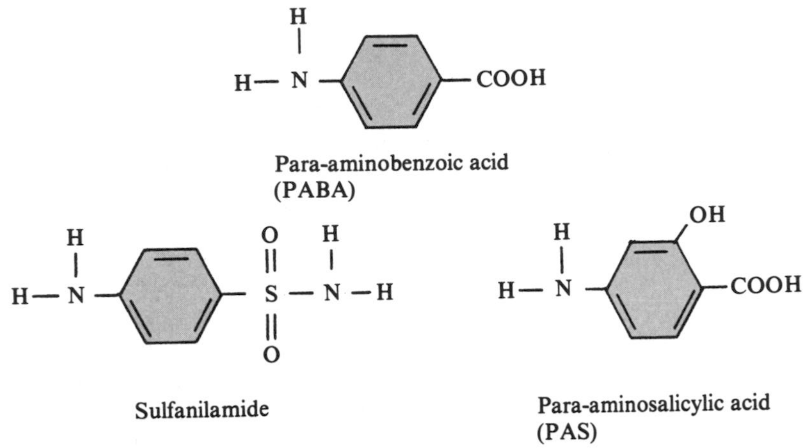

Fig. 8-14. Structural relationship between the antimetabolites sulfanilamide and para-aminosalicylic acid and the metabolite para-aminobenzoic acid.

ministered to pregnant women. Approximately 1 to 3 percent of patients receiving sulfonamide therapy exhibit hypersensitivity to the drug. Persons with glucose 6-phosphate dehydrogenase deficiency experience a minor anemia caused by the instability of red blood cells. The anemia is severely exaggerated if they are treated with sulfonamides or nitrofurans.

Para-aminosalicylic Acid and the Sulfones

Both para-aminosalicylic acid (PAS) and the sulfones are analogues of PABA. PAS shows little activity against most organisms except *Mycobacterium tuberculosis*. It was once used in combination with other drugs for the treatment of tuberculosis, but today drugs such as ethambutol and rifampin have replaced it in treatment. The sulfones are used almost exclusively in the treatment of leprosy. *Dapsone* is the most commonly prescribed sulfone. Since sulfones are known to cause hemolytic and nonhemolytic anemia, careful monitoring of patient response to the drugs is required during treatment.

Trimethoprim

Trimethoprim is a structural analogue of pteridine, a component of the folic acid molecule. It is a potent inhibitor of the enzyme dihydrofolate reductase in bacteria and interferes competitively with the conversion of dihydrofolic acid to tetrahydrofolic acid (see Fig. 8-15). Trimethoprim interferes with normal amino acid and purine and pyrimidine synthesis. The drug is not used alone but in combination with sulfamethoxazole, the combination abbreviated TMP-SMZ. This combination is bactericidal and is used most frequently in the treatment and prophylaxis of hospital-associated diseases. Some of the advantages of TMP-SMZ to the clinician include long half-life in the blood, excellent tissue penetration, ability to use oral and parenteral preparations, and relatively low toxicity. TMP-SMZ is especially useful in the treatment of urinary tract and respiratory infections as well as gastrointestinal diseases caused by gram-negative bacteria. The drug is also useful in treating infections in which the microbial agent is resistant to the newer third-generation cephalosporins and penicillins. TMP-SMZ is used in the treatment of *Pneumocystis*

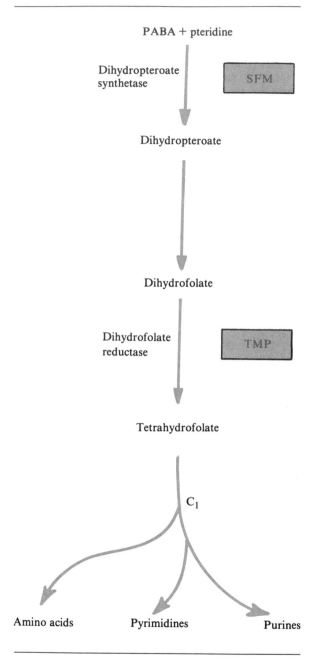

PABA + pteridine

Dihydropteroate
synthetase

SFM

Dihydropteroate

Dihydrofolate

Dihydrofolate
reductase

TMP

Tetrahydrofolate

C_1

Amino acids   Pyrimidines   Purines

Fig. 8-15. Reaction pathway in which para-amino-benzoic acid (PABA) is involved in the synthesis of amino acids, pyrimidines, and purines. The drugs that act as antimetabolites in the pathway are enclosed in boxes. C_1 = one carbon unit. (SFM = sulfonamide; TMP = trimethoprim.)

carinii pneumonia in patients afflicted with AIDS. Serious toxicity is a rare event, but when it occurs the most likely complications are severe skin lesions and the combination of thrombocytopenia and leukopenia.* TMP-SMZ should not be administered to pregnant women or those known to be sensitive to sulfonamides.

Ethambutol

Ethambutol is used exclusively in the treatment of tuberculosis. It affects only growing microorganisms and is believed to interfere with RNA synthesis. It is beneficial in combination with other drugs for the treatment of tuberculosis because it helps delay the emergence of drug-resistant strains. At high dosage it can affect visual acuity.

Isoniazid

Isoniazid (INH) is important in the treatment of tuberculosis. It is employed in combination with other drugs such as streptomycin or rifampin. Isoniazid is particularly effective in treatment of tuberculosis because it is readily absorbed from the intestinal tract and is only mildly toxic to the host in low dosages. It resembles nicotinamide (Fig. 8-16) in structure and competes with it for incorporation into nicotinamide-adenine dinucleotide (NAD), an important coenzyme in metabolism.

Isoniazid is relatively nontoxic when administered in small doses. In 50 percent of the population (only 15 percent in Orientals) it is inactivated very slowly in the body and can result in a cumulative toxicity causing neuritis. The latter can be prevented by simultaneous administration of pyridoxine.

Nitrofurans

Nitrofurans have various antibacterial, antiprotozoal, and antifungal activities. They are bac-

---

* Thrombocytopenia is a condition in which there is a decrease in the number of blood platelets. Leukopenia is a condition in which there is a decrease of leukocytes below normal blood levels.

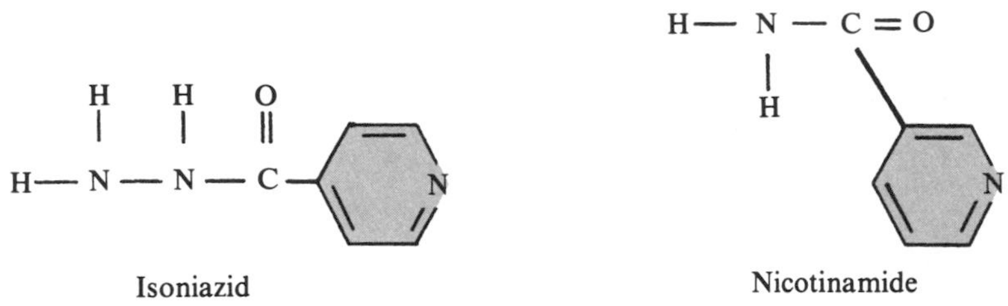

Fig. 8-16. Structural relationship between isoniazid and nicotinamide.

tericidal and bacteriostatic and are used primarily in the treatment of urinary tract infections. Nitrofurantoin is the most widely prescribed of the nitrofurans. It is frequently used for hospitalized patients to prevent urinary tract infections following catheterization. Nitrofurantoin administration does not result in the development of antimicrobial resistance by the patient's fecal flora. Although its exact mechanism of action is not known it is believed to affect carbohydrate metabolism in the bacterial cell by interfering with acetyl coenzyme A activity.

FACTORS IN SELECTING A DRUG FOR CHEMOTHERAPY

The choice of a drug is dictated primarily by the kind of microorganism (or microorganisms) involved in the infection. In some instances a direct relationship exists between the disease and the microorganism involved. Diphtheria, for example, is always caused by *Corynebacterium diphtheriae*. In other diseases, such as pneumonia, there may be more than one causal agent. The following factors must be considered before a drug is administered.

DOSAGE

The dosage of drug to be given to the patient may be affected by many factors, including the rate of excretion or inactivation of the drug, its toxic potential, the age of the patient, and the presence of underlying organic illness. Selecting the correct dosage depends on a knowledge of the *minimal inhibitory concentration (MIC)* of the drug (the smallest amount of antibacterial agent that still inhibits growth; see under Broth Dilution Test, later in this chapter) and the amount that will produce the MIC in the serum of the patient. The general recommendation is that the concentration of the drug in the serum be three to five times the MIC to ensure effective therapy. In very serious infections the ratio of serum level to MIC may be as much as 100:1—for example, in penicillin therapy in meningitis infections caused by species of *Neisseria*.

ROUTE OF ADMINISTRATION

Many drugs are not absorbed from the intestinal tract, and others are destroyed by acids in the gut. This knowledge is important in determining whether a drug is to be given orally or parenterally (injection by a route other than oral). In severely ill patients the parenteral route is preferred because the drug will appear more rapidly at the site of infection and at higher concentrations than with the oral route. A great percentage of drug is excreted in the feces if it is given orally. Drugs not absorbed from the intestinal tract are effective in the treatment of gastrointestinal disorders when high concentrations of the drug are required.

DRUG COMBINATIONS

Drugs used in combination can produce a number of different results (see Fig. 8-17). (1) *Indifference* is a situation in which the combined effect of the two drugs is no greater than the effect of either one administered separately. (2) *Synergism* is a condition in which the activity of the two drugs together exceeds the combined activity of each drug administered separately. Synergism occurs frequently when two bactericidal agents are administered. In the treatment of bacterial endocarditis, for example, penicillin and streptomycin have an effect that neither drug alone can accomplish. (3) In *addition* the effect of the combined drugs is equal to the sum of the effects of each drug administered separately, and (4) in *antagonism* the combined effect is less than that of either drug administered separately. Antagonism is often incurred when a bactericidal and bacteriostatic agent are given together; the bacteriostatic agent inhibits growth, and microbial growth must be present before some bactericidal agents (such as penicillin) are effective.

Combination drug therapy can be expensive and increase the risk of toxicity and superinfection. Still, combinations of drugs are of important clinical value. Enhanced bactericidal effects may result when (1) a cell wall–active agent is combined with an aminoglycoside, (2) a beta-lactam is combined with inhibitors of beta-lactamase, and (3) the combined drugs inhibit separate steps in a critical metabolic pathway. The use of combinations of drugs, when resistance to one drug may readily develop, has been applied in the treatment of tuberculosis. Tuberculosis is a chronic disease in which the offending pathogen replicates slowly. Chemotherapy must therefore be applied over a long period of time. The use of one drug for treatment invariably selects for resistant microbial strains.

Toxicity from a single drug can sometimes be reduced by using a smaller dose in combination with another chemotherapeutic agent. For example, amphotericin B dosage can be reduced by using it in combination with flucytosine in the treatment of fungal disease. Drug combinations are used primarily (1) in mixed infections, (2) to prevent emergence of drug-resistant strains, and (3) as a stopgap measure in bacteriologically obscure illness.

The inappropriate use of drug combinations can lead to serious consequences. One of the drugs may select for an organism carrying the drug resistance factor on a plasmid. The plasmid may also carry other antibiotic resistance genes, thus complicating chemotherapy.

PROPHYLAXIS

The prophylactic administration of drugs can sometimes be detrimental to patients, especially if prophylaxis is continued for several days. Continued exposure of the host's microbial flora to antimicrobials often selects for resistant strains, and this can lead to superinfection, that is, infection by the host's own microflora. Prophylaxis is recommended when the host is subjected to a treatment or therapy, not involving antimicrobials, that can lead to serious disease, as in some of the following circumstances:

1. Dental extraction. Chemotherapy is considered before dental extractions only if the patient has a history of rheumatic fever, subacute bacterial endocarditis, or congenital heart defect. Extraction leads to displacement of oral microorganisms, particularly species of streptococci, into the circulation. These microorganisms can be implanted on heart tissue and can lead to serious disease.

2. Rheumatic fever. Penicillin is given prophylactically to rheumatic fever patients to prevent recurrence of streptococcal infection in heart tissue.

3. Tuberculosis. Isoniazid is administered prophylactically to individuals who are closely associated with persons with tuberculosis. It is also used to prevent the development of progressive tuberculosis.

4. Tonsillectomy. Prophylaxis is indicated for

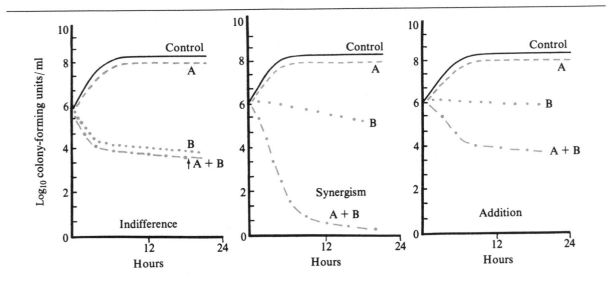

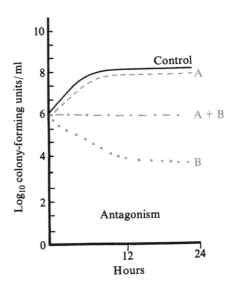

Fig. 8-17. Growth curves for microorganisms in which combinations of drugs (A and B) produce different effects.

patients with a history of rheumatic fever, bacterial endocarditis, or congenital heart disease.

5. Surgical procedures. Antibiotic prophylaxis appears to be necessary only when there is a penetrating wound of the abdomen (for example, in bowel surgery, which presents a high probability of contamination) and in vaginal hysterectomy. Prophylaxis is usually directed in preventing staphylococcal infection. In surgical techniques that are considered "clean" (not likely to be contaminated), antibiotics are not recommended. Antibiotics should never be considered a substitute for careful surgical procedures.

TOXICITY

The toxic potential of a drug is a major factor in the selection of a chemotherapeutic agent, especially if the drug is to be administered to children, pregnant women, the elderly, and persons suffering from organic diseases. In patients with underlying renal disease antibiotics may persist in the body for extensive lengths of time because of the inability of the kidneys to excrete them. Drugs such as polymyxin, amphotericin B, and bacitracin should be used with extreme caution since they are directly toxic to kidney tissue.

DRUG RESISTANCE

Since the first antibiotics were discovered over 50 years ago, there has been a continual race to find new antibiotics or derivatives of them. These efforts are required because of the ability of microorganisms to develop resistance to drugs and the growing medical problems such resistance presents. Data indicate that mortality, likelihood of hospitalization, and length of hospital stay are likely to be twice as great for patients infected with drug-resistant strains as for those infected with drug-sensitive strains of the same bacteria.

Increases in the number of drug-resistant bacterial strains may be due to the following:

1. Indiscriminate antibiotic use by physicians
2. Feeding of subtherapeutic levels of antimicrobials to farm animals, a practice that increases the pool of drug-resistant species (*Salmonella* species, for example) that can spread to humans)
3. Inappropriate use of antibiotics by nonphysicians in developing countries (for example, in some countries antibiotics can be purchased without a prescription)
4. Patient apathy toward the antimicrobial regimen prescribed by the physician

HOW DRUG RESISTANCE DEVELOPS

Drug-resistant populations of bacteria develop because of mechanisms of gene transfer between them, that is, *transformation*, in which cell-free DNA can induce heritable changes in another strain; *transduction*, in which bacteriophages act as vectors of genetic material; and *conjugation*, which involves direct cell-to-cell contact. Conjugation may involve chromosomal transfer or transfer of R genes (see Chapter 6 for discussion of these mechanisms).

Most antibiotic resistance genes are located on small pieces of DNA called *transposons* (also called jumping genes). Transposons are equipped with the information that allows them to independently move a copy of themselves, not only to another site on the bacterial chromosome, but also to bacterial plasmids, such as transmissible R factors and into bacteriophage. The transposon is, therefore, the major fundamental unit of drug resistance because it allows drug resistance genes to be spread from one generation to another within a strain and to other bacterial species. The genetic exchanges between different bacterial species allows the development of the multiple drug-resistant strains that have become so prevalent in hospital-associated epidemics.

MECHANISMS OF DRUG RESISTANCE

Four major mechanisms are responsible for the ability of microorganisms to resist the action of antimicrobials: interference with transport across the cell wall or cytoplasmic membrane, enzyme modification of the drug, alteration of the antimicrobial target in the microbe, and synthesis of resistant metabolic pathways. It is important to note that more than one mechanism may be available to a single microbial species and that is why treatment of some infections is so difficult.

Interference with Transport

Interference with antimicrobial transport is frequently associated with chromosomal mutations. Such mutations result in alterations of the structure of cell wall or cytoplasmic membrane components or changes in certain sugar transport systems. Antimicrobial resistance in some species of *Salmonella*, for example, is related to the reduction in size or change in chemistry of porin channels in the cell wall.

Aminoglycosides have no effect on obligate anaerobes or facultative anaerobes that are growing in the absence of oxygen. Apparently transport of the drug across the cytoplasmic membrane requires energy that is not sufficiently generated under anaerobic conditions.

Some drugs reach the periplasmic space but cannot be transported across the cytoplasmic membrane because they are modified by enzymes. These modifying enzymes also inactivate the drug—a characteristic discussed in the next section.

Enzymatic Inactivation

The most important antimicrobial resistance mechanism in bacteria is plasmid-mediated enzymatic inactivation (Table 8-2). Most of the enzyme inactivators are located in the periplasmic space. They include the beta-lactamases (beta-lactamases of *S. aureus* are excreted extracellularly; the same enzymes of gram-negative organisms are found in the periplasmic space) and enzymes that acetylate, adenylate, or phosphorylate various aminoglycosides. The only drug-inactivating enzyme located in the cytoplasm is chloramphenicol transacetylase. Modification occurs at a specific amino or hydroxyl group on the drug. Some drug-modification sites are common to many of the aminoglycosides, and thus cross resistance is common. The manner in which modification of aminoglycosides renders them inactive is not known but may be the result of (1) competition with unmodified aminoglycosides for the drug's target site, (2) ineffective binding to ribosomes, or (3) inability to interfere with ribosome function. A number of aminoglycoside resistance determinants are found on transposable elements. In some instances the transposon resistance factor is associated with as many as four or five resistance determinants. Thus a wide spectrum of cross resistance can be found in microorganisms when these transposons have been disseminated. It is the promiscuity of the transposon that makes antimicrobial therapy so difficult.

Table 8-2. Modifying Enzymes of the Aminoglycosides

Enzyme	Antibiotic substrate
Acetyltransferase	Kanamycin, tobramycin, amikacin, sisomicin, neomycin, gentamicin
Adenyltransferase	Tobramycin, amikacin, kanamycin, neomycin, gentamicin, streptomycin, spectinomycin
Phosphotransferase	Neomycin, kanamycin, streptomycin, gentamicin

Alteration of the Microbial Target

Alteration of the microbial target is usually associated with a chromosomal mutation, but plasmids may also be involved. Two of the most widely examined instances involving alteration of a microbial target are penicillin-binding proteins and the 30S ribosome.

The catalytic actions associated with the various PBPs have already been discussed. If PBPs are absent or are altered in such a way that their affinity for beta-lactams is decreased then penicillin resistance may ensue.

Streptomycin resistance is associated with the loss or alteration of a single protein in the 30S ribosomal subunit. These mutations result in decreased ribosomal binding of streptomycin.

Other targets whose alteration results in resistance include DNA gyrase, resistance to nalidixic acid; RNA polymerase, resistance to rifampin; and methylated 23S RNA, resistance to erythromycin and lincomycin.

Synthesis of Resistant Metabolic Pathways

Synthesis of resistant metabolic pathways is associated with resistance to sulfonamides and related antimetabolites. An altered enzyme allows the organism to bypass the competitive inhibition of these drugs (see Fig. 8-15). This type of resistance has been observed in the Enterobacteriaceae during treatment with trimethoprim. These organisms are known to contain plasmid-coded dihydrofolate reductases or dihydropteroate synthetases that are resistant to the drug.

QUANTITATIVE AND QUALITATIVE DETERMINATION OF ANTIBIOTIC ACTIVITY

Both qualitative and quantitative measurements of potential antibiotics must be made to deter-mine their usefulness as chemotherapeutic agents in the treatment of human infections. In these procedures the unknown antibiotic is tested against microbial species such as *Escherichia coli*, *S. aureus*, and *Pseudomonas aeruginosa* that are fast growers and are known to be sensitive to antibiotics. The same tests are applied in the clinical setting to determine the susceptibility of an unknown pathogen, recently isolated from an infected patient, to known antibiotics. Susceptibility tests are important for evaluating which antibiotics can be used by the physician in the treatment of the disease.

QUANTITATIVE TESTS

Broth Dilution Test

In the broth dilution test the minimal inhibitory concentration (*MIC*) and minimal bactericidal concentration (*MBC*) of the drug can be determined. A standard inoculum of the test organism is seeded into tubes of sterile broth containing decreasing concentrations of the antibiotic (Fig. 8-18). After 24 hours of incubation at 35°C the MIC is determined by finding the lowest concentration of drug inhibiting bacterial growth. The MBC can be found by subculturing those tubes showing no visible growth into broth tubes that contain no antibiotic. Subculturing dilutes out the antibiotic. The lowest concentration of drug in the original culture that leads to no growth is the MBC. Major disadvantages of the broth dilution technique are that (1) only one organism can be run in a single series of tubes, (2) contamination is difficult to detect in broth, and (3) the test is expensive if large numbers of bacterial strains are being surveyed. The development of *microdilution trays* in frozen or dried form and *automated dispensing devices* has reduced the cost and time required to carry out these procedures. In some commercially available systems an automated photometric device is available to read the results of microdilution tests.

Most clinical laboratories do not use the broth dilution test as a routine method for determining

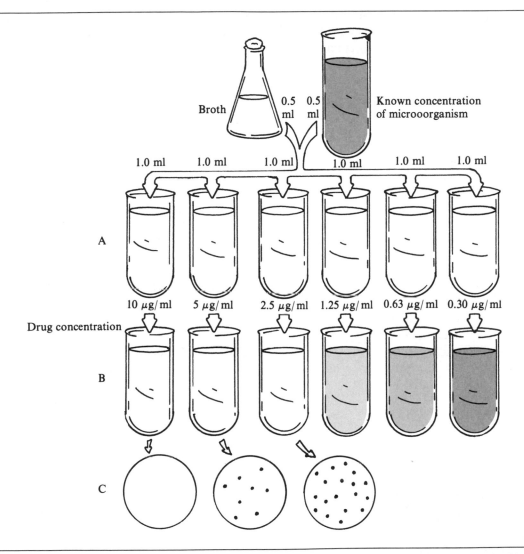

Fig. 8-18. Broth dilution test used to determine minimal inhibitory concentration (MIC) and minimal bactericidal concentration (MBC) of antimicrobial compounds. A. Each broth tube contains 9.0 ml of sterile broth with a different concentration of antimicrobial. To each tube is added 0.5 ml of broth and 0.5 ml of a known concentration of microorganisms. The concentration of microorganisms in each broth tube is so small that there is no visible turbidity. Tubes are incubated at 35°C for 12 to 18 hours. B. Tubes are examined for macroscopic growth. Lowest concentration of drug showing no growth is the MIC. In this case it is 2.5 μg/ml. C. To determine MBC, loopfuls are removed from tubes showing no visible growth and are streaked on agar plates. Those plates showing no growth indicate drug concentrations that destroy the microorganisms (10 μg/ml).

antimicrobial susceptibility but as a supplemental procedure to the disk diffusion method. Broth dilution is used primarily for determining the MICs of test organisms at several concentrations of drug. These data are then used in determining the dosage that will be effective in treating human infections and will be correlated with results obtained with the disk diffusion technique (discussed below).

Agar Dilution Method

The agar dilution method is a simplified procedure for testing the effect of an antibiotic against many bacterial strains. In the test the antibiotic at various concentrations is mixed with molten agar, poured into Petri dishes, and allowed to harden. Standard aliquots of the test microorganisms are transferred to each of the agar plates by an inoculum-replicating apparatus. As many as 36 different bacterial isolates can be seeded on one plate (Fig. 8-19). Three areas on the plate are reserved for the control cultures, *S. aureus*, *E. coli*, and *P. aeruginosa*. All the plates containing the various concentrations of antibiotic

Fig. 8-19. Steers inoculum-replicating device. Plate on left contains 36 reservoirs for bacterial inocula. Bottom plate on right contains antibiotic-containing medium on which bacteria will be seeded. (From J. A. Washington, II, *Mayo Clin. Proc.* 44:811, 1969.)

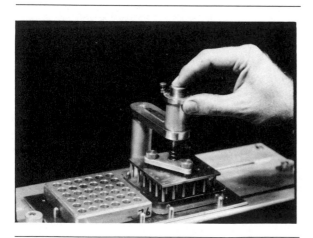

are read after 18 to 24 hours of incubation. The MIC is read as the lowest concentration of antibiotic that inhibits growth. Both the broth and agar dilution techniques yield more precise results, but because of heavy work loads most laboratories use the disk diffusion test.

QUALITATIVE TESTS

Disk Diffusion Test

The disk diffusion test is an agar diffusion technique and is the most widely used procedure for determining bacterial susceptibility to antimicrobials. In the disk diffusion test, paper disks impregnated with known amounts of antibiotics are placed on an agar medium seeded with a known species of bacteria. As the antibiotic diffuses into the medium, it produces a gradient of antibiotic concentration. After suitable incubation antibiotic activity is determined by the width of the zone of no growth around the antibiotic disk (Fig. 8-20).

The size of the zone of inhibition can be correlated with the clinical susceptibility of the microorganism to the antibiotic, provided standardized conditions are maintained. One standardized test is called the *Kirby-Bauer* method. In this technique, Mueller-Hinton agar, a standard inoculum, and a single antibiotic disk of standardized potency (usually 30 μg for many antibiotics) are used. Zones of inhibition are described as susceptible, intermediate, and resistant. The breakpoint between the zones for each antibiotic is obtained from published tables. The Kirby-Bauer tables have taken into account the MIC of the organism obtained from broth or agar dilution techniques, the blood levels obtained with normal dosage of the antibiotic, and the distribution of zone sizes among species with known responsiveness to the antibiotic (Table 8-3).

The disk diffusion test provides information that is adequate for guiding the therapy of most infections. Disk diffusion is not applicable for slowly growing organisms, obligate anaerobes, or microorganisms requiring higher than usual lev-

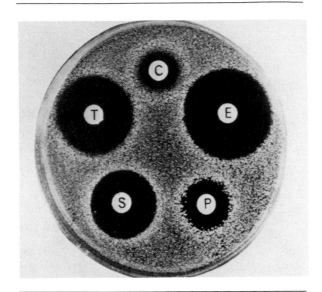

Fig. 8-20. Disk diffusion test. An agar medium is inoculated with a strain of *Staphylococcus aureus*. Disks containing specified amounts of antibiotic are placed on the agar. The type of antibiotic in each disk is indicated by the letter: *T*, tetracycline; *C*, chloramphenicol; *E*, erythromycin; *P*, penicillin; *S*, streptomycin. Inhibition of growth of *S. aureus* is evidenced by a clear zone around the antibiotic disk. (From L. P. Garrod and F. O'Grady, *Antibiotic and Chemotherapy* [5th ed.]. London: Churchill Livingstone, 1973.)

els of CO_2 because the test has been standardized for fast-growing aerobic and facultatively anaerobic organisms.

ANTIBIOTIC CONCENTRATIONS IN THE PATIENT'S SERUM

An estimate of the concentration of an antibiotic in the patient's serum or other body fluids is necessary when very toxic antimicrobials are being administered. Depending on the health of the patient and the condition of various organs such as the kidneys, the concentration of the drug in the serum may be at or above toxic levels during the course of therapy. Under these circumstances

the serum should be assayed periodically. One commonly employed technique for serum assay is the agar diffusion technique, used often for gentamicin assay. In this procedure a patient's serum is removed at times when the antimicrobial will be at maximum and zero levels. An agar plate seeded with *B. subtilis* spores is prepared. Normal serum (not from the patient) is placed on disks containing standard amounts of the antimicrobial. The test serum from the patient is then placed on disks. The standard and the test disks are placed on the agar plate, which is incubated. After 2 to 3 hours zones of inhibition around the disks containing the antimicrobial are observed. A standard curve is produced relating concentrations of antibiotic to zones of inhibition. The zones of the unknown samples are also determined, and by extrapolation from the standard curve the concentration of the antimicrobial in the patient's serum is found. Other methods available for assay of antimicrobials include immunological assays, enzymatic assays, chromatographic assays, and chemical assays.

SUMMARY

1. Chemotherapeutic agents are drugs that are selectively toxic. This selectivity may be due to the fact that the target of the drug is not present in mammalian cells or to microbial targets that are biochemically different from their mammalian counterparts. Selective toxicity can be expressed as a ratio between the minimum toxic level and the maximum therapeutic level.

2. Chemotherapeutic agents can be synthesized totally or partially in the laboratory or they may be produced biologically by microorganisms, that is, antibiotics. Chemotherapeutic agents may have a broad or narrow spectrum of activity and they inhibit growth (-static) of microbes or they may kill (-cidal) them.

3. Antimicrobial activity of newly isolated

Table 8-3. Examples of Zone Size Interpretative Standards for Some Antimicrobial Agents Used in the Treatment of Infectious Disease

Antimicrobial agent	Disk content	Inhibition zone diameter (to nearest mm)		
		Resistant	Intermediate*	Susceptible
Amikacin	30 μg	≤14	15–16	≥17
Ampicillin				
Gram-negative enterics	10 μg	≤13	—	≥17
Staphylococci	10 μg	≤28	—	≥29
Carbenicillin				
Enterobacteriaceae	100 μg	≤19	—	≥23
Pseudomonas	100 μg	≤13	—	≥17
Cefoxitin	30 μg	≤14	—	≥18
Chloramphenicol	30 μg	≤12	13–17	≥18
Clindamycin	2 μg	≤14	15–20	≥21
Erythromycin	15 μg	≤13	14–22	≥23
Gentamicin	10 μg	≤12	13–14	≥15
Moxalactam	30 μg	≤14	—	≥23
Nalidixic acid	30 μg	≤13	14–18	≥19
Penicillin G				
Staphylococci	10 units	≤28	—	≥29
Sulfonamides	250 or 300 μg	≤12	—	≥17
Tetracycline	30 μg	≤14	15–18	≥19
Trimethoprim	5 μg	≤10	—	≥16
Vancomycin	30 μg	≤9	10–11	≥12

* *Intermediate* indicates that the test result be considered equivocal or indeterminate.
Source: Adapted from Table 2, in *Performance Standards for Antimicrobial Disk Susceptibility Tests* (4th ed.), M2-A4, by the National Committee for Clinical Laboratory Standards. The interpretive data are valid only if M2-A4 methodology is followed. Used with permission.

chemotherapeutic agents can be determined by using a plate diffusion technique with test microorganisms. Several factors must be considered in evaluating the potential of a chemotherapeutic agent but the two most important are that (1) the drug is active at very low concentrations and (2) the drug is relatively nontoxic to mammalian tissue.

4. The characteristics of the various chemotherapeutic agents are outlined in Table 8-4.

5. Several factors must be taken into account before the physician prescribes a drug regimen: (1) selecting the correct dosage based on the minimal inhibitory concentration (MIC) of the drug, (2) route of administration of the drug, (4) toxicity of the drug, and (5) whether the drug can be used prophylactically.

6. Drug resistance in bacteria is related primarily to transfer of resistance determinants via conjugation, transformation, and transduction. Most antibiotic resistance genes are located on transposons, which can be transferred to future generations of the same species or to different species.

7. The mechanisms that permit bacteria to resist antimicrobials are: (1) interference with transport of the drug, (2) enzymatic inactivation of the drug, (3) alteration of the drug's target site, and (4) synthesis of resistant metabolic pathways.

Table 8-4. Characteristics of Some Important Chemotherapeutic Agents

Drug and site of inhibition	Microbial group involved and specific clinical use
Cell Wall Inhibitors	
Penicillins (see also Fig. 8-2)	Bacteria; effective against gram-positive and gram-negative, depending on preparation used
Cephalosporins (see also Fig. 8-5)	Bacteria; effective against gram-positive and gram-negative, depending on preparation used
Bacitracin	Bacteria; used primarily in topical preparations because of tissue toxicity
Vancomycin	Bacteria; for staphylococcal infections that do not respond to penicillins, treatment of antibiotic-associated pseudomembranous colitis
Cytoplasmic Membrane Inhibitors	
Amphotericin B	Fungi; treatment of systemic fungal infections by *Candida, Histoplasma,* and *Blastomyces*; combined with flucytosine to reduce potential toxicity to kidney
Nystatin	Fungi; topical agent in treatment of *Candida* infections
Imidazoles (ketoconazole, miconazole, etc.)	Fungi; ketoconazole for systemic fungal infections but others used primarily as topical agents
Polymyxins	Bacteria; because of toxicity to kidneys, used primarily in topical preparations
Protein Synthesis Inhibitors	
Aminoglycosides (streptomycin, amikacin, etc.; see Table 8-1)	Bacteria; see Table 8-1
Chloramphenicol	Bacteria; toxicity reduces its use to treatment of typhoid and meningitis in which the patient is allergic to penicillins
Erythromycin	Bacteria; absence of toxicity makes it suitable alternative to other drugs that are toxic or cause allergic reactions; drug of choice in Legionnaires' disease and pneumonia caused by *Mycoplasma pneumoniae*
Lincomycin	Bacteria; used to treat staphylococcal and streptococcal infections that do not respond to penicillins
Clindamycin	Bacteria and some protozoa; anaerobic pulmonary infections
Spectinomycin	Bacteria; treatment of gonorrhea when microbe is resistant to penicillin
Nucleic Acid Synthesis Inhibitors	
Rifampin	Bacteria; treatment of tuberculosis combined with other drugs
Nalidixic acid	Bacteria; primarily in preventing gram-negative urinary tract infections in compromised patients
Flucytosine	Fungi; yeast infections (*Candida*) but also combined with amphotericin B to reduce toxicity in treatment of systemic infections
Ribavarin	Virus; respiratory syncytial virus and influenza virus infections
Amantadine	Virus; influenza A virus infections
Idoxuridine	Virus; herpes simplex virus type 1 infections of the eye
Vidarabine	Virus; herpes zoster (shingles), herpes simplex encephalitis, and chickenpox in immunocompromised patients
Acyclovir	Virus; genital herpes infections
Rimantadine	Virus; influenza virus infections
Antimetabolites	
Sulfonamides	Bacteria, some urinary tract infections; topical forms for burn patients; oral preparations to prevent travelers' diarrhea
Para-aminosalicylic acid	Bacteria; only in tuberculosis
Ethambutol	Bacteria; used exclusively in treatment of tuberculosis
Trimethoprim	Bacteria; used primarily in combination with a sulfonamide, sulfamethoxazole, for treatment of hospital-associated diseases of respiratory, urinary, and gastrointestinal tracts; also used in treatment of *Pneumocystis carinii* pneumonia in AIDS patients
Isoniazid	Bacteria; tuberculosis
Nitrofurans	Bacteria, fungi, protozoa; nitrofurantoin used to prevent urinary tract infections following catheterization

8. Quantitative and qualitative tests are used in the clinical laboratory to determine what antimicrobial will be effective in treatment. The most widely used test is a qualitative one called the disk diffusion test, which provides zones of microbial inhibition described as susceptible, intermediate, and resistant.

9. Quantitative determinations of antibiotic activity are provided by two types of tests called broth and agar dilution. They are used primarily to determine the minimal inhibitory concentration of various drugs.

10. Quantitative determinations of antibiotic levels in the serum are also important if antimicrobials accumulate to toxic levels in the blood. Various techniques such as agar diffusion, enzymatic assays, etc. can detect the serum concentrations of various antimicrobials.

QUESTIONS FOR STUDY

Select the best response or responses for each of the following:

1. The activity of chloramphenicol and tetracycline are similar in that
   A. Both are bactericidal agents.
   B. Both are inhibitors of protein synthesis.
   C. Both have a broad spectrum of activity.
   D. Both are inhibitors of DNA synthesis.

2. The most important antimicrobial resistance mechanism used by bacteria is associated with
   A. Alteration of the antimicrobial target site
   B. Synthesis of resistant metabolic pathways
   C. Alteration of cytoplasmic membrane permeability
   D. Plasmid-mediated enzymatic inactivation of the drug

Match each antimicrobial on the left with one or more of the characteristics on the right.

3. Penicillin

4. Acyclovir

5. Erythromycin

6. Amphotericin B

7. Quinolones

8. Bacitracin

A. Antiviral agent used in treatment of herpes virus infections
B. Derivatives of nalidixic acid that have been used as substitutes for aminoglycosides
C. Used primarily as a topical drug in the treatment of bacterial infections
D. Used primarily in the treatment of superficial fungal infections
E. Bactericidal at very low concentrations
F. Very toxic drug used in the treatment of systemic fungal infections
G. An inhibitor of protein synthesis, primarily in gram-positive species, that is relatively nontoxic
H. Used primarily in the treatment of tuberculosis

9. The principal target of the aminoglycosides is _____.

10. The procedure most widely used in the clinical laboratory to determine bacterial susceptibility to antimicrobials is the _____ test.

11. The principal target of penicillin in the cell wall of bacteria is an enzyme called _____.

12. The group of enzymes produced by bacteria that enable them to resist the action of penicillins and cephalosporins are called _____.

13. The condition in which the activity of two drugs together exceeds the combined activity of each drug administered separately is called _____.

ADDITIONAL READINGS

Bush, K. Beta-lactamase inhibitors from laboratory to clinic. *Clin. Microbiol. Revs.* 1(1):109,1988.

Davis, B. D. Mechanism of bactericidal action of aminoglycosides. *Microbiol. Revs.* 51(3):341,1987.

Eliopoulos, G. M., and Eliopoulos, C. T. Antibiotic combinations: Should they be tested? *Clin. Microbiol. Revs.* 1(2):139,1988.

Fromtling, R. A. Overview of medically important antifungal azole derivatives. *Clin. Microbiol. Revs.* 1(2):187,1988.

International symposium on new quinolones. *Rev. Infect. Dis.* 10(1):1988.

Lacey, R. W. Evolution of microorganisms and antibiotic resistance. *Lancet* 2:1022,1984.

Lorian, V. (ed.). *Antibiotics in Laboratory Medicine* (2nd ed.). Baltimore: Williams & Wilkins, 1986.

Lupski, J. R. Molecular mechanisms for transposition of drug resistance genes and other movable genetic elements. *Rev. Infect. Dis.* 9(2):357,1987.

New developments in resistance to beta-lactam antibiotics among nonfastidious gram-negative organisms. *Rev. Infect. Dis.* 10(4),1988.

O'Brien, T. F. Resistance of bacteria to antibacterial agents. *Rev. Infect. Dis.* 9(Suppl. 3):244,1987.

Peterson, P. K., and Verhoef, J. (ed.). *Antimicrobial Agents Annual.* Amsterdam: Elsevier Science Publishers B.V., 1986.

Stratton, C. W. Serum bactericidal test. *Clin. Microbiol. Revs.* 1(1)19,1988.

III. HOST-PARASITE INTERACTION

9. INTERACTION BETWEEN HOST AND INFECTIOUS AGENT

OBJECTIVES

To differentiate between a commensal and a parasite; an intracellular and extracellular parasite; an infection and a disease; pathogenicity and virulence; exotoxin and endotoxin

To describe the various chemical and physical characteristics of the skin, mucosal surfaces, respiratory tract, intestinal tract, genitourinary tract, and epithelial and subepithelial surfaces that resist invasion by microorganisms

To briefly explain how the immunological state of the host, nutrition, occupation, and underlying conditions affect the host's resistance to disease

To explain what microbial factors contribute to initiation of the infectious disease process

To explain how some microorganisms avoid host defense mechanisms

To define: indigenous, attenuation, invasive, siderophore, enterotoxin, toxoid, adhesin, fibronectin

One of the most important areas of microbiological research involves the molecular biology of the host–parasite relationship. The initial step in this relationship often is the binding of microbe to host tissue. A knowledge of the chemistry and molecular biology of the components involved in this process will eventually lead to the development of vaccines to prevent disease. The purpose of this chapter is to describe those factors, both microbial and host-related, that are associated with the disease process.

MICROORGANISMS AS COMMENSALS AND PARASITES

The human body is a shelter and source of nutrients for many microorganisms, primarily bacteria and secondarily fungi. Microorganisms that benefit from this association without harming the host are referred to as *commensals*. A *parasitic* relationship is one in which the microorganism benefits at the expense of its host. Let us look more closely at these two associations.

COMMENSALISM

Before birth the fetus is essentially in a sterile environment, but at delivery microorganisms come into contact with the host. Some of these microorganisms are derived from the mother or others who come into contact with the infant. Most microorganisms are transient passersby that are destroyed by conditions in the host, but others establish themselves and produce microcolonies. This latter group has therefore colonized the host. As several types of microorganisms colonize a particular body site the *microflora* are established. The factors that influence the kind and number of microorganisms at any body site are (1) the availability or unavailability of oxygen, (2) the availability of appropriate receptor sites for attachment, (3) the pH of the host site, (4) the availability of nutrients, (5) the influence exerted by other microorganisms at the site, and (6) the immunological response of the host to the presence of the microorganism.

Not all areas of the body are occupied by commensal species. There are appreciable numbers of microorganisms in the upper respiratory tract, lower intestinal tract, and skin (see Tables in Appendix B). Areas such as the esophagus, urinary tract, and stomach contain few microorganisms while the blood, spinal fluid, urine, and endothelial tissues are normally sterile.

The indigenous microflora will remain with the host for life, with only minor changes resulting from disease, dietary alterations, or hormonal changes. Many of the indigenous microorganisms appear to be important in maintaining the health of the host. For example, in some animals microorganisms of the intestinal tract are capable of synthesizing vitamins such as pantothenic acid, riboflavin, and vitamin B_{12}. It has been suggested that certain vitamin deficiencies in the human diet can be remedied by bacterial vitamin synthesis in the intestinal tract. Experiments on germ-free animals have also demonstrated that without intestinal microflora there is a reduction in the size and plasticity of the digestive tract, compared with that in conventional animals. In addition, some commensals produce metabolic products that are effective in preventing invasion by parasites. For example, commensals in the intestinal tract produce fatty acids that inhibit ingested bacteria that attempt to colonize the host.

There is a dynamic interrelationship among commensals that make up the microflora of any particular body site. In general terms, the gram-positive bacteria control the number of gram-negative bacteria and vice versa, while both groups of bacteria control the concentration of yeasts. Any established member of the normal microflora is recognized as such and the host's immune system does not respond to it as a foreign body.

PARASITISM

Any microorganism that can inhabit the human body is a potential parasite and this includes commensals. Parasitism may or may not result in damage to the host. Many parasites, such as the AIDS virus, bring about devastating changes in the host. If the host dies one chain of transmission of the parasite to other hosts is lost. A successful parasite is one that obtains enough nutrients to multiply without causing major damage

to its host. In this way the parasite can be maintained indefinitely within its population of hosts.

Most successful parasites are able to colonize the host because the host has been compromised by some condition or disease and/or the parasite possesses such potent weapons that it is able to overcome the host's normal defense mechanisms. Once the parasite enters its host, it may take up residence within various cells of the body (*intracellular parasite*) or it may remain attached to the surface of host tissue (*extracellular parasite*) to cause disease. Let us examine both options.

Extracellular Parasites

Extracellular parasites are exposed to many of the host's defensive forces that are exerted at cell or tissue surfaces. An important characteristic of many extracellular parasites is their ability to produce potent toxins or other proteins that enable them to colonize and damage tissue. Many of these microbial products quickly induce an inflammatory response, which helps the host recover from the disease. Extracellular parasites usually cause diseases referred to as *acute*, that is, the symptoms of disease appear for only a short period and then quickly subside. Recovery from diseases caused by extracellular parasites often occurs within a few days.

Intracellular Parasites

Only a few microorganisms (except viruses) are able to carry out their life cycle within the environment of a host cell. The host cell is not an entirely peaceful environment when invaded by a microbial cell. Many host cells, such as macrophages found in the bloodstream, are equipped with molecules that can degrade and kill invading microorganisms. The intracellular parasite must be equipped with special attributes that enable it to defend itself against the environment of the cell. Even as important, the parasite must not destroy any host functions that are essential to its (the parasite's) own survival and multiplication. For example, the protozoan *Plasmodium vivax*, which causes malaria, must remain in the red blood cell of its host in order to use certain coenzymes that it (the parasite) cannot produce. A quickly killed red blood cell is of no use to the parasite.

Despite the potential pitfalls for microorganisms living within host cells there are advantages to intracellular living. As we have already mentioned, some microorganisms are totally dependent on certain metabolic products found only in the intracellular environment. In addition, the intracellular parasite is not directly exposed to various immune forces such as antibodies, immune cells, and other immune factors found in the bloodstream.

Intracellular parasites are of two types (Table 9-1): those that can live inside or outside host cells (*facultative intracellular parasites*) and those that can replicate only inside host cells (*obligate intracellular parasites*).

Diseases caused by intracellular parasites (except viruses) are usually *chronic* in nature. In other words, disease symptoms appear over an extended period of time (weeks to months) be-

cause the immune factors found in the bloodstream are not in direct contact with the parasite.

TERMINOLOGY ASSOCIATED WITH THE INFECTIOUS DISEASE PROCESS

The terms *infection* and *disease* are often used synonymously in discussing the host–parasite relationship. When microorganisms make contact with a host there are three things that can happen: (1) the host does not respond to the presence of the microorganism and the latter acts as a *colonizer*; (2) the host responds to the microorganism by producing antibodies—thus an *infection* takes place; and (3) the host produces antibodies in response to the microorganism and the latter causes tissue damage, that is, a *disease* occurs.

Terms that also deserve explanation are *pathogenicity* and *virulence*. Microorganisms that are able to cause disease are said to be pathogenic (noun, pathogen). As you have probably surmised, some microorganisms are more pathogenic than others. For example, a strain of *Streptococcus pneumoniae* (strain A) that does not produce a capsule is unable to cause the type of disease that is associated with a capsule-producing strain (strain B). In other words, strain B is more pathogenic than strain A. Pathogenicity is a very qualitative term that describes a microorganism's disease-producing potential. A more quantitative measurement of a microorganism's disease-producing abilities is termed *virulence*. Virulence determinations, for example, measure the number of microorganisms or amount of microbial product, such as toxins, that can cause death or disease in 50 percent of the test animals (Fig. 9-1). These measurements are referred to as LD_{50} or ID_{50}, respectively.

Virulence is a property that can be modified in the laboratory. A highly virulent microorganism may lose its virulence on serial passage of the

Table 9-1. Some of the Major Intracellular Parasites

Parasite	Obligate (O) or facultative (F)
VIRUS	
All viruses	O
BACTERIA	
Mycobacterium tuberculosis	F
Neisseria gonorrhoeae	F
Salmonella typhi	F
Legionella pneumophila	F
Brucella species	F
Listeria monocytogenes	F
Francisella tularensis	F
Rickettsia species	O
Chlamydia species	O
	O
PROTOZOA	
Plasmodium vivax	O

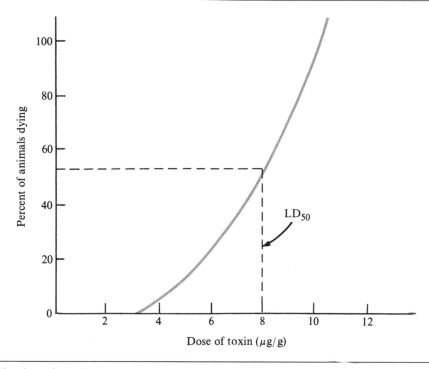

Fig. 9-1. Determination of the 50 percent lethal dose (LD_{50}) for a toxin. Various doses of toxin are injected into animals. The percentage of animals that die is plotted and the LD_{50} is extrapolated. In this figure 8 μg of toxin per gram of animal is the LD_{50}.

microbe in unnatural hosts. Growing the microorganism in laboratory media devoid of certain compounds may also cause it to lose its virulence. The loss or substantial reduction of virulence is referred to as *attenuation*. Our ability to attenuate microorganisms enables us to produce vaccines. Many vaccines (for example, polio, measles, and mumps vaccines) are merely attenuated microbial agents that when injected into the body do not cause disease but do stimulate the formation of antibodies that can ward off future infections. The virulence of microorganisms is related to their capacity either to invade tissue (*invasiveness*) or to produce *toxins* that affect host tissue. Among the literally thousands of microbial species, probably no more than 300 can cause disease in humans.

There are situations in which a highly pathogenic microorganism may not be pathogenic. For example, some individuals, because of certain inherited genetic traits, can be infected by a pathogen but not show symptoms of disease. Individuals who harbor these pathogens and show no disease symptoms are called carriers (see Chapter 10).

The diseases caused by microbial agents are not always the same in terms of location or host response. The following terms explain the various types of disease:

LOCAL   a disease that is restricted to a confined area

FOCAL   a localized site of disease from which bacteria and their products are spread to other parts of the body

SYSTEMIC   a disease in which the microorganism or its products can spread throughout the body, not necessarily from a localized site

PRIMARY   a disease caused by one microbial species

SECONDARY   a primary disease complicated with a second pathogen (for example, pneumonia following primary influenza)

MIXED   a disease caused by two or more microorganisms

INAPPARENT OR SUBCLINICAL   a disease that does not give rise to any detectable overt symptoms

LATENT   a disease in which the microbial agent persists in the tissues in a dormant state and later becomes activated to induce symptoms

BACTEREMIA   a transitory disease in which bacteria present in the blood are usually cleared from the vascular system with no harmful effects. Other microbial agents, as fungi (fungemia) and viruses (viremia), may also be present in the blood.

SEPTICEMIA   a condition in which the blood serves as a site of bacterial multiplication as well as a means of transfer of the infectious agent from one site to another.

PYEMIA   the presence of pyogenic (pus-forming, such as staphylococci and streptococci) bacteria in the blood as they are being spread from one site to another in the body.

TOXEMIA   the presence of microbial toxins in the bloodstream

The properties of pathogenicity and/or virulence are not stable and are influenced by host as well as microbial factors. In the following paragraphs we will discuss how these factors affect the outcome of host–parasite interactions.

HOST FACTORS AND THE DISEASE PROCESS

PORTAL OF ENTRY

The body surface presents various sites for the entry of microorganisms. Each site offers resistance to the establishment of microorganisms not indigenous to the host. Moreover, microorganisms that make up the normal microbial flora release metabolic products that prevent colonization by potential pathogens acquired from the environment.

Skin

The tough, thick outer layer of the skin (Fig. 9-2) is a natural barrier to invading microorganisms. In addition, fatty acids secreted by the glands of the skin can inhibit the growth of microorganisms. If one swabs the surface of the skin or removes material from sebaceous glands, a number of microorganisms can be cultured, among them species of *Staphylococcus* and *Corynebacterium*. These resident microorganisms are not pathogenic unless the skin becomes abraded and the individual's natural immune mechanisms become depressed. Microorganisms may enter the host through skin abrasions, or they may be transferred by the bite of animals or insects. The rabies virus, for example, can be transmitted to humans by the bite of dogs, carnivorous wild animals (especially skunks, raccoons, foxes, and coyotes), and bats. Other infectious agents, including the causal agents of plague, malaria, and Rocky Mountain spotted fever, are transmitted by insect bites.

Mucosal Surfaces

The mucosal surface is one of the first surfaces on which microorganisms make contact with the host. The gastrointestinal tract, respiratory tract, salivary and lacrimal glands, biliary system, and portions of the genitourinary tract all have mucosal surfaces. Many of these surfaces are in contact with the external environment. A variety of host defense mechanisms are available at the mucosal surface to prevent parasite colonization and prevent damage by microbial products such as toxins:

1. Immunological defenses. The most important immunological defense at the mucosal sur-

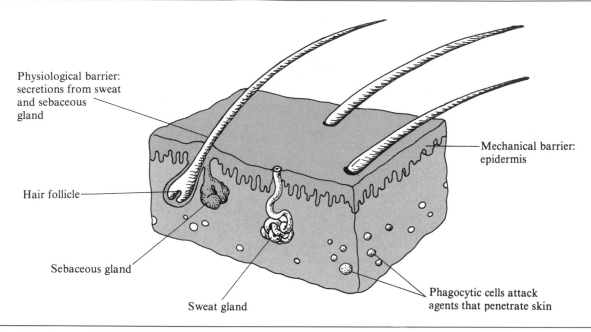

Physiological barrier:
secretions from sweat
and sebaceous
gland

Mechanical barrier:
epidermis

Hair follicle

Sebaceous gland

Sweat gland

Phagocytic cells attack
agents that penetrate skin

Fig. 9-2. Cross-section of the skin demonstrating the barriers to infectious agents.

face is the immunoglobulin called secretory IgA (sIgA). Plasma cells located beneath the mucosal epithelia produce sIgA (see Chapter 12 for further details on this immunoglobulin). sIgA antibodies have been shown to prevent the binding of certain pathogenic microorganisms to the mucosal surface. Binding is an important property of most pathogenic microorganisms. Microbial species such as *Vibrio cholerae, Streptococcus mutans, Streptococcus salivarius*, and *Neisseria gonorrhoeae* will not bind to epithelial surfaces in the presence of sIgA. Local sIgA has also been shown to neutralize virus and thus play a role in protecting the host from reinfection by respiratory viruses. It should be pointed out that some pathogenic bacteria, such as species of *Neisseria, Haemophilus*, and *Streptococcus*, produce a protease that cleaves sIgA. Protease production may therefore be considered a virulence factor for some bacteria

2. Microflora. The sites at which an invading microorganism may enter the host (skin, respiratory tract, digestive tract) are usually colonized by an indigenous population of microorganisms (see Appendix B). The metabolic products of some commensal microorganisms can directly or indirectly affect the ability of noncommensal species to colonize a body site. The antagonistic effects on invading microbial species are usually due to one or all of the following: (1) change in the pH or oxidation-reduction potential, (2) production of an antagonistic product, or (3) depletion of essential nutrients. Fatty acid production by anaerobes in the intestinal tract is responsible for inhibiting potential pathogens such as species of *Shigella* and *Salmonella*. Viridans streptococci indigenous to the pharynx inhibit the growth of pneumonocci, while *Staphylococcus epidermidis* retards the colonization of *Staphylococcus aureus* in the nasal cavity. The mechanisms involved in these interactions are not known, and much of the evidence is circumstantial, since only in vitro experiments have been performed.

3. Mucins. Mucins are hydrophilic glycoproteins that form a film in the intestinal tract and a

partial coat in the respiratory tract. They lubricate and waterproof the mucosal surface, but they have also been shown to prevent adherence in some microorganisms and/or their toxic products. Microorganisms bound by mucins may be removed via ciliary action in the respiratory tract or by peristalsis in the intestinal tract.

4. Lysozyme, lactoferrin, and peroxidase. Lysozyme, lactoferrin, and peroxidase are three substances found on the mucosal surface that aid in defense against microbial invasion. Lysozyme is found in most normal secretions, including tears, nasal secretions, breast milk, and genital fluids. Its activity on the bacterial cell wall was discussed in Chapter 3. Lactoferrin is an iron-binding protein whose importance is discussed later in this chapter. Peroxidase is found in saliva and, in combination with thiocyanate and hydrogen peroxide, is active against several bacteria, fungi, and viruses (see Chapter 11).

Respiratory Tract

Inhaled air contains suspended particles of various sizes. The inhaled particles may include dust; epithelial cells shed from the skin, which may contain microorganisms; freely suspended molds or bacterial spores; and suspended aerosols from sneezing and coughing, which may also contain microorganisms. Particles that are 10 μm in diameter or more seldom reach the lungs because of the mucociliary blanket that covers the respiratory tract (Fig. 9-3). Cilia lining the nasal cavity trap particles and sweep them to the throat, where they are swallowed. The lower part of the respiratory tract contains macrophages that aid in resistance. These cells of the immune system can ingest and digest microorganisms. When host defense mechanisms for the respiratory tract become defective, some microorganisms are equipped to adhere strongly to the respiratory epithelium (Fig. 9-4) and may be the cause of serious infection such as whooping cough and bacterial and viral pneumonias. Other agents, the causative agent of tuberculosis, for instance, can be ingested by macrophages but are

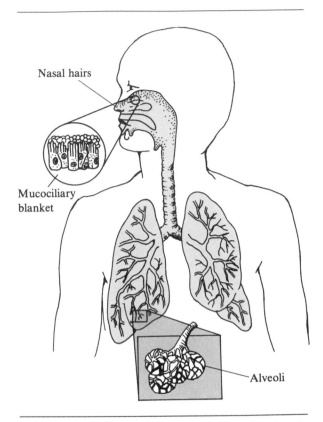

Fig. 9-3. Diagram of the respiratory tract showing the barriers to infectious agents. Alveoli contain phagocytic cells that engulf parasites.

still capable of infection because immune responses are defective (see Chapter 14).

Oropharynx

Microorganisms in the oral cavity are numerous (see Appendix B). Gingival fluid has as many as 1×10^{10} microorganisms per milliliter. Saliva is responsible for flushing out microorganisms from the oral cavity, and when salivary flow is impeded, for example, by anesthesia, the numbers of microorganisms increase. Saliva also contains such microbial inhibitors as lysozyme and secretory antibodies.

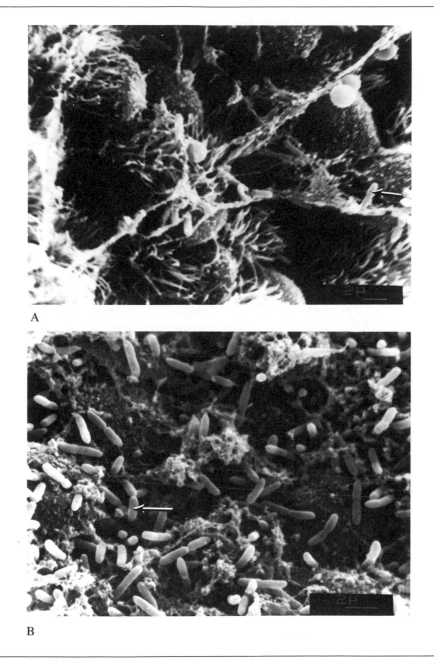

Fig. 9-4. Effect of an environmental factor on the adherence of microorganisms to respiratory epithelium. A. Normal tracheal cells, in which a few rare bacteria (*arrow*) can be found adhering to cilia. B. Tracheal cells that have been injured with acid. Many bacilli (*arrow*) can be seen to adhere. (From R. Ramphal and M. Pyle, *Infect. Immun.* 41:345, 1983.)

Intestinal Tract

Many microorganisms can enter the intestinal tract via the ingestion of food and drink. Those that are indigenous to the oral cavity are also swallowed. Organisms that survive the acid conditions of the stomach enter the intestinal tract and encounter acids, bile salts, and enzymes. Although the mucus lining the epithelial cells acts as a mechanical barrier to microbial colonization, some pathogenic species such as the causal agents of typhoid fever and plague resist these physiological barriers. Microorganisms indigenous to the intestinal tract (see Appendix B), because of their metabolic activities, prevent colonization by pathogenic species, as is discussed later.

Genitourinary Tract

Under normal conditions urine in the bladder is a sterile fluid. When it contains large numbers of microorganisms, serious infection is often indicated. Infections of the urogenital tract occur more frequently when structural abnormalities prevent the normal flow or flushing action of urine. Women are more prone to such infections because of the shortness of the urethra and its close proximity to the anus with its indigenous microflora. In women the normal acidity of the vagina is due to the presence of lactic acid, which inhibits many microbial species. Lactic acid is produced by bacterial degradation of glycogen, a major component of the vaginal epithelium.

SUBEPITHELIAL FACTORS

Once past the chemical and physical barriers at the sites of entry into the host, infecting microorganisms seek a site for multiplication and protection from the host's other defense mechanisms. The latter are directly or indirectly associated with the immune response of the host—interferon production and the production of antibodies and cells of the immune system will immobilize or destroy the invading microbial species. The battle between microbe and host is influenced by both microbial and host factors but finally boils down to the state of the host's immune system.

Many microbial species colonizing the epithelial surface remain on the epithelium because they do not possess invasive factors for penetration into subepithelial tissue or because they are readily destroyed by antimicrobial factors in the subepithelial tissue of the host. Respiratory viruses such as those causing the common cold and viruses causing warts are examples of parasites that remain on the epithelium. It is not always necessary that the microorganism invade tissue to cause serious disease. The causal agent of diphtheria (*Corynebacterium diphtheriae*), for example, multiplies on the epithelial surface of the respiratory tract and produces a toxin that penetrates to the bloodstream and is carried to various organs and tissues.

Once the epithelial surface has been penetrated there are three host antimicrobial defense mechanisms: (1) tissue fluids, (2) the lymph system, and (3) phagocytic cells. Tissue fluids contain antimicrobial factors including antibodies and various serum factors such as properdin (see Chapter 12). A complex system of lymphatics, particularly near the skin and the intestinal wall, can carry microorganisms to lymph nodes, where phagocytic cells are present. Phagocytic cells are ready and able to ingest and kill microorganisms. Local phagocytic cells are also present at the subepithelial surface at the time of penetration or when inflammatory conditions have taken place. Sometimes the microorganisms can evade these antimicrobial mechanisms. A few microorganisms, such as the agent of tuberculosis (*Mycobacterium tuberculosis*), are engulfed by the phagocyte but are resistant to phagocytic digestion. This provides the organism with a habitat for avoiding the host's remaining defense mechanisms. This is one reason why some diseases, such as tuberculosis and brucellosis, are chronic and sometimes difficult to cure. A more detailed discussion of the cellular and fluid elements of the blood and their role in host resistance to disease appears in Chapter 12.

FACTORS INFLUENCING HOST RESISTANCE TO INFECTION

Immunological State of the Host

As stated previously, the major factor that determines the outcome of microbial infection is the immunological state of the host. Today diseases such as measles are not nearly as devastating as they were several hundred years ago because people have developed a more benign relationship with the microorganisms causing them. Repeated infections in a community have resulted in the selection of more resistant individuals. That this process has taken place is evident from studies of infectious diseases that have recently occurred in isolated communities for the first time. In Greenland, as well as among some jungle tribes in South America, first infections from smallpox ravaged the populations. In developed countries, where smallpox has existed for a long time, a more benign relationship exists between the host and pathogen. This long-term interaction has reduced the morbidity and mortality for other diseases as well. Resistance to infections is also influenced by factors such as race, nutrition, occupation, and underlying conditions. The influence of the immunological state of the host will be discussed in more detail in Section IV, Immunology.

Race

Some races of humans are more susceptible to diseases than others. The fungal disease coccidioidomycosis is found more predominantly in dark-skinned individuals such as Hawaiians, Mexicans, and American Indians than in light-skinned persons. The reason for this is not known. A biochemical basis for racial immunity to malaria is known. In persons with sickle cell anemia, which affects blacks almost exclusively, there is resistance to malaria. The malaria parasite grows and develops in the erythrocyte. In persons with sickle cell, the conformation of the hemoglobin molecule has changed because of mutation, and parasite development in the erythrocyte is impeded.

Nutrition

The nutrition of the individual may also contribute to the disease process. In general, one can say that if the state of health of the host is seriously impaired by inadequate nutrition infections are more likely to occur. Considerable evidence has shown that iron plays an important role in the host's susceptibility to disease. Iron is required by most living organisms. It is a component of cytochromes and is therefore involved in electron transport. Iron is found in high concentrations in the host (approximately 4.5 gm in an adult human), but most of this is unavailable to an infecting microorganism. Iron in host tissue is complexed with iron-binding glycoproteins such as transferrin or lactoferrin that are found in most body fluids. Host iron is also part of the heme molecule in red blood cells. Any free iron in the host is in an insoluble ferric form (Fe^{3+}), and this creates a condition in which the pathogen must compete with the host for available iron. Some microorganisms have evolved special mechanisms for accumulating iron and transporting it into the cell. These bacterial iron transport systems are associated with low molecular weight iron-binding compounds called *siderophores*. Bacterial siderophores are able to remove iron from transferrin and other iron-binding molecules. They also remove iron from the heme molecule following lysis of erythrocytes.

Four types of siderophores have been found in *Escherichia coli* (Fig. 9-5). They are regulated by the iron content in the microorganism's immediate environment. Siderophores are synthesized when the bacterial growth medium in which they are growing is iron deficient. Siderophores are released into the environment where they remove iron from host complexes or heme and transport it into the bacterial cytoplasm. The mechanism by which the bacterial cell removes iron from the siderophore is not known.

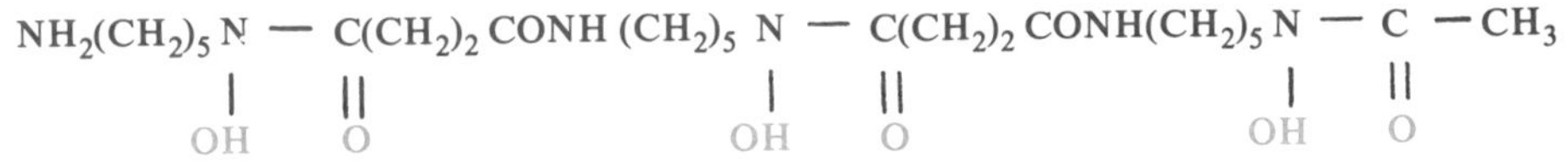

$$NH_2(CH_2)_5 \underset{\underset{OH}{|}}{N} - \underset{\underset{O}{||}}{C}(CH_2)_2 CONH(CH_2)_5 \underset{\underset{OH}{|}}{N} - \underset{\underset{O}{||}}{C}(CH_2)_2 CONH(CH_2)_5 \underset{\underset{OH}{|}}{N} - \underset{\underset{O}{||}}{C} - CH_3$$

Fig. 9-5. Structure of one type of siderophore. Sites of iron binding are in color.

Transferrin and lactoferrin exhibit bacteriostatic effects in the host, but this activity is lost when these molecules become saturated with iron. Lactoferrin is present in high concentrations in human milk and is probably responsible, along with antibody, for inhibiting microorganisms such as *E. coli* that cause gastroenteritis in infants. Several studies have shown that breast-fed babies are more protected against enteritis caused by *E. coli* and other microorganisms than are non-breast-fed babies. Breast milk has occasionally been used to stop outbreaks of enteritis when all other methods of treatment have failed. Microorganisms whose virulence has been associated with excess iron include *Yersenia pestis* (plague), *Neisseria meningitidis* (meningitis), and *N. gonorrhoeae* (gonorrhea).

Occupation

Occupation is an important factor in susceptibility to infection. One would expect more infections of tularemia (rabbit fever) and brucellosis in persons who are exposed to animals and animal hides—hunters, stockyard workers, veterinarians. Hepatitis, which can be acquired through infected blood or blood products, is more prevalent among surgeons, nurses, and others who work in hospitals than in the general population.

Underlying Conditions

Underlying conditions or diseases are major predisposing factors to infection. Individuals who produce no immunoglobulins or abnormal ones are susceptible to repeated microbial infections. Diabetics whose disease is not under control by insulin or diet are particularly prone to tuberculosis and staphylococcal infections. Many viral infections can reduce patients' resistance to the point at which secondary bacterial infections are common. For example, viral influenza is sometimes followed by a staphylococcal infection that may be worse than the original viral infection.

Numerous conditions that predispose to disease can be induced in the host. For instance, corticosteroid treatment and ionizing radiations used in cancer therapy reduce antibody formation and interfere with the normal inflammatory response. Under these circumstances the patient is at the mercy of what are normally mild infectious agents such as the chickenpox virus and many gram-negative bacteria of the intestinal flora. The advent of transplants has necessitated the use of immunosuppressive drugs to prevent rejection of the foreign tissue or organ by the host. As a result of immunosuppressive therapy, patients often survive the transplant only to succumb to microbial infection. The patient with heart disease is also susceptible to infections of heart tissue. Some streptococci in the oral cavity, for example, may be displaced into the bloodstream during oral surgery. In the healthy person these microorganisms are rapidly cleared from the circulation. In the patient with heart disease they lodge in the heart tissue and set up foci of infection.

MICROBIAL FACTORS AND THE DISEASE PROCESS

ADHERENCE TO HOST TISSUE

In order to gain a foothold in the host, microorganisms must be able to adhere to host tissue.

This necessity applies to both commensals as well as potential parasites. Unattached microorganisms are usually removed from potential sites of infection by host forces (for example, cilia in the respiratory epithelium). The surface components that enable microorganisms to adhere to host tissue are called *adhesins*. Microbial adhesins bind to specific sites on the host cell called *receptors*, which are made up of glycoproteins. Microbial adhesins may be composed of proteins or carbohydrates; for example, most gram-positive bacteria use the carbohydrate teichoic acid as an adhesin while gram-negative bacteria can utilize carbohydrates in the outer membrane or surface proteins. The proteins are surface projections called *pili* (fimbriae).

In some instances microorganisms may be able to select a desirable environment for attachment. For example, flagellated bacteria possess receptors in the cytoplasmic membrane that act as sensing devices. These sensors can combine with molecules such as oxygen, amino acids, sugars, etc. When these complexes form, the flagella are induced to propel the microorganism in the direction of the desired substrate or away from an undesirable one. This microbial property called *chemotaxis* was discussed in Chapter 3.

The chemistry of host–parasite interactions is known for only a few species of bacteria and includes among them the following:

1. At least two surface components of *Neisseria gonorrhoeae* are believed to be associated with attachment to epithelial cells in the genitourinary tract: *protein II (PII)* and *pili*. Piliated *N. gonorrhoeae* attach in greater numbers to human fallopian tube mucosa than do nonpiliated gonococci. However, it has also been demonstrated that nonpiliated organisms attach more readily to the same tissue than do commensal species. This indicates that factors other than pili are probably involved in this selective attachment process. Protein II is an outer membrane protein of the gram-negative organism. Protein II is believed to promote either the attachment of the microorganisms to nonciliated cells of the fallopian tube

or the aggregation of the microorganisms at the attachment site.

2. *Streptococcus pyogenes* adheres to epithelial cells of the skin and nasopharynx of the human host. One of the surface components, *lipoteichoic acid (LTA)*, plays an important role in attachment. LTA, which consists of a backbone of polyglycerolphosphate attached to a glycolipid, is secreted through the cytoplasmic membrane. Some of the LTA molecules join with the M protein on the surface of the microorganism. This leaves the lipid ends exposed near the surface of the microorganism (Fig. 9-6). The host cell receptor is believed to be a glycoprotein called *fibronectin*. Fibronectin is thought to be a major receptor for adhesion of many other microbial pathogens, including viruses.

3. Strains of *E. coli* cause a variety of diseases from diarrhea to diseases involving the urinary tract. In each case pilial (fimbrial) adhesins appear to be important factors contributing to disease (Fig. 9-7). Most strains of *E. coli* possess only *type I pili*, which enable them to bind to host

Fig. 9-6. Lipoteichoic acid (LTA) attachment process. LTA associated with the cytoplasmic membrane of the bacterial cell is negatively charged. Positively charged M protein binds to LTA at the surface, leaving exposed lipid ends that bind to receptors on the host cell.

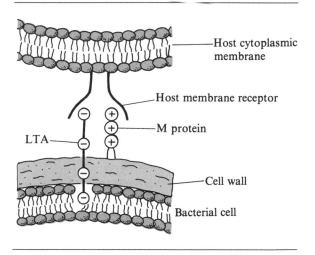

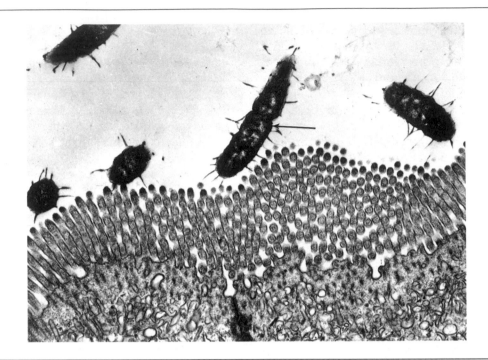

Fig. 9-7. Electron micrograph demonstrating attachment of *Escherichia coli* (*arrow*) to the intestinal epithelium. The pili can be seen to project from the surface of the bacterial cells and are in contact with host cell surface. (From H. W. Moon, B. Nagy, and R. E. Isaacson, *J. Infect. Dis.* 136 [Suppl.]:124, 1977.)

cell surfaces containing the sugar mannose. They do not appear to be associated with the disease-causing potential of the microorganism. The presence of other pili, however, has been found to be correlated with pathogenicity. Specific pili confer on pathogenic strains the ability to adhere to and colonize specific epithelial surfaces.

INVASIVENESS

Once pathogenic microorganisms adhere to host tissue, they multiple at or near the surface and then attempt to penetrate the surface. This ability to penetrate is called *invasiveness*. Invasiveness is not always a prerequisite for virulence. For example, *Clostridium tetani*, the causative agent of tetanus, is not an invasive organism but it is extremely virulent, because of the release of a

potent toxin once it has infected the host. Many viruses are also capable of invading tissue but are not pathogenic to humans.

Some virulent microorganisms such as *C. diphtheriae* are restricted to the type of tissue that is suitable for their multiplication. *C. diphtheriae* organisms invade only the superficial cells of the upper respiratory tract. Some fungi, however, can multiply and invade a variety of host tissue and organs. The reason for these differences in tissue affinity has not been clearly defined. Many may be due to the chemical environment of the host tissue. The fact that *Proteus mirabilis*, for example, produces more severe and persistent infections in the kidney than elsewhere is perhaps related to its production of urease, an enzyme that splits urea into carbon dioxide and ammonia, thereby promoting the growth of this microorganism. *Brucella abortus*, which causes abortion in cattle, localizes in the placenta, the only area containing erythritol, a polyhydric alcohol that *B. abortus* can rapidly metabolize.

The invasiveness of bacteria is associated with their ability to produce certain extracellular enzymes (Table 9-2). These enzymes are discussed at more length in connection with the bacterial diseases with which they are associated. A great deal of controversy has been raised concerning the role, if any, of these enzymes in the pathogenic process. For example, the virulence of *S. aureus* was at one time attributed to the ability of the microbe to produce the extracellular enzyme coagulase. Coagulase has been shown in vitro to cause the deposition of fibrin around the bacterial cell, presumably protecting it from antibacterial substances in the blood. Virulent strains of *S. aureus* have been found, however, that produce no coagulase. Although no single enzyme has been unequivocally associated with virulence, it is certain that enzymes play some role in the pathogenic process.

TOXINS

Toxins may be one of the major causes of tissue damage during the infectious disease process. Two types of toxins are produced by bacteria: exotoxins and endotoxins. The major distinctions between the two types are outlined in Table 9-3. Toxins are not characteristically found in microorganisms other than bacteria.

Exotoxins

Exotoxins are heat-labile proteins released by the bacterial cell into the surrounding environment. Most exotoxins are produced by gram-positive bacteria. They include some of the most potent poisons known, such as the diphtheria, tetanus, and botulism toxins. Exotoxins whose site of action is the intestinal tract are called *enterotoxins*.

Most exotoxins are highly antigenic; that is, they can stimulate the formation of antibodies (*antitoxins*) when injected into appropriate hosts. For this reason exotoxins can be used to induce

Table 9-2. Microbial Products Associated with Invasiveness and Spread of Microorganisms in the Host

Invasive fiber	Organism	Function
Coagulase	Staphylococci	Causes formation of fibrin, which may deposit on surface of microorganism and inhibit phagocytosis
Streptokinase (fibrinolysin)	Streptococci	Transforms plasminogen to plasmin, an active proteolytic enzyme that digests fibrin; importance in disease not totally understood
Hyaluronidase	Streptococci, staphylococci, and clostridia	Splits hyaluronic acid, a component of connective tissue
Hemolysins	Many bacteria, especially streptococci, staphylococci, and clostridia	Lyse red blood cells
Lecithinase	Clostridia	Splits lecithin, a component of cytoplasmic membranes
Collagenase	Clostridia	Digests collagen, a component of connective tissue
Extracellular polymeric substances (capsules and slime layers)	Several bacteria, including pseudomonads, staphylococci, streptococci, and others	Inhibits phagocytosis and in some instances may be important in adhering to host tissue

Table 9-3. Characteristics Differentiating Exotoxins from Endotoxins

Exotoxins	Endotoxins
Most are polypeptides with molecular weights between 1×10^4 and 9×10^5	Low-molecular-weight component of lipopolysaccharide complex; lipid A is toxic component
Excreted by living cells	Part of the cell wall of gram-negative bacteria and can be released when the cell lyses or during vegetative growth
Relatively unstable to temperatures above 60°C	Relatively stable to temperatures above 60°C for several hours with no loss of activity
Antigenic (stimulates formation of antibodies)	Lipid A is not antigenic
Can be converted to a toxoid	Cannot be converted to a toxoid
Does not produce fever in the host	Produces fever in the host
Very toxic in microgram quantities to laboratory animals	Weakly toxic; hundreds of microgram quantities required to be lethal for animals

active immunity against toxin-caused diseases such as diphtheria and tetanus. However, because many toxins are potent and lethal poisons, they cannot be injected into the human body without some modification of the toxin molecule. Exotoxins can be modified chemically by phenol, formaldehyde, betapropiolactone, and various acids. In its modified form the toxin is called a *toxoid*. When injected into the body, toxoids have the ability to stimulate the formation of antibodies that neutralize the specific exotoxins from which they were derived. Toxoids are not toxic to the host. Toxoids or inactivated virulent microorganisms used in immunization are referred to as *vaccines*. (The term *vaccine* was previously reserved for killed or attenuated micro-

organisms and not their products. A more complete definition of *vaccine* must now include specific microbial components. For example, a surface antigenic component on the hepatitis virus is now used as a vaccine.) The major exotoxins produced by pathogenic bacteria and their activities are listed in Table 9-4. Most exotoxins are composed of two subunits; one is nontoxic but binds to specific cell surface receptors and facilitates the entry of the second subunit, which is the toxic component (Fig. 9-8). The exotoxins of enteropathogenic *E. coli* and *V. cholerae* exert their activity in the intestinal lumen. Both of these species cause diarrhea via the action of toxin on the enzyme adenyl cyclase in the mammalian cytoplasmic membrane. The enzyme catalyzes the following reaction.

Adenosine triphosphate (ATP)

$$\xrightarrow[\text{cyclase}]{\text{adenyl}} \text{adenosine } 3',5'$$

cyclic monophosphate (cAMP)

The increase in cAMP causes a change in the electrical potential of the mammalian cytoplasmic membrane, and this results in a leakage of fluids and electrolytes (Boxed Essay, p. 225). *C. diphtheriae* and *Pseudomonas aeruginosa* produce exotoxins whose mechanism of action is similar. They inhibit protein synthesis by preventing the transfer of amino acids to the growing polypeptide chain. This is accomplished by inactivation of the translocating enzyme. The diphtheria toxin is synthesized as a single polypeptide that is fragmented by a bacterial protease. Only the fragmented polypeptide shows toxic activity. Although the mechanisms of action like *C. diphtheriae* and *P. aeruginosa* toxin are alike, they are specific to different tissues and are also structurally different.

Endotoxins

As discussed in Chapter 3, an endotoxin is a complex found in the gram-negative cell wall. The complex is made up of a core of oligosaccharides

ADENYL CYCLASE AND BACTERIAL VIRULENCE

Mammalian adenyl cyclases are the targets of various hormones and neurotransmitters that control the levels of cyclic AMP in the cell. Cyclic AMP activates specific protein kinases in the cell and the kinases in turn phosphorylate different proteins. Phosphorylated proteins are involved in a variety of cellular responses involving growth and metabolism. We now know that the activity of a number of microbial toxins is associated with the regulation of cyclic AMP of host cells. This group includes toxins from *Vibrio cholerae*, *E. coli*, *Bacillus subtilis*, *Bordetella pertussis*, and *Bacillus anthracis*.

In the above examples, except for *B. pertussis* and *B. anthracis*, the toxins interact with host adenyl cyclases. With *B. pertussis* and *B. anthracis*, however, the adenyl cyclase is provided by the microorganism and is found on the microbial surface. When the bacterium makes contact with host cells the bacterial enzyme penetrates the host cell membrane. Inside the host cell the bacterial adenyl cyclase is activated by a host protein called *calmodulin*. The subsequent increase in cyclic AMP can result in different effects on the host cell including increased secretory activity. In skin cells, for example, *B. anthracis* toxin (the cause of anthrax) causes edema but in phagocytic cells, such as alveolar macrophages, the toxin impairs phagocytic activities. More will be said about the specific activities of microbial toxins in later chapters.

Table 9-4. Important Exotoxins Associated with Disease in Humans

Toxin or disease	Microorganism	Mechanism of action
Exotoxin A	*Pseudomonas aeruginosa*	Inhibits peptide chain elongation
Enterotoxin	*Bacillus cereus*	Similar to cholera toxin
Enterotoxin (travelers' diarrhea, infant diarrhea)	*Escherichia coli*	Same as cholera toxin
Scalded skin syndrome	*Staphylococcus aureus*	Separation of the epidermis
Erythrogenic toxin (scarlet fever)	*Streptococcus pyogenes*	Produced only by strains of streptococci carrying a bacteriophage that is nonvirulent; toxin causes a rash
Enterotoxin (food poisoning)	*Staphylococcus aureus*	Neurotoxin that affects motility of the gut
Diphtheria toxin	*Corynebacterium diphtheriae*	Inhibits peptide chain elongation during protein synthesis
Cholera enterotoxin	*Vibrio cholerae*	Stimulation of adenyl cyclase and increase in cAMP, leading to fluid and electrolyte loss from the gut
Tetanus or lockjaw	*Clostridium tetani*	Neurotoxin blocks function of inhibitory synapses in the spinal cord, thus causing muscular spasms
Botulism (types A, B, and E toxins)	*Clostridium botulinum*	Neurotoxin that blocks release of acetylcholine or blocks its production at synapses or neuromuscular junctions
Enterotoxin	*Clostridium perfringens*	Causes hypersecretion of electrolytes and water in the intestine
Alpha toxin (gas gangrene)	*Clostridium perfringens*	Splits lecithin, a component of cytoplasmic membranes

cAMP = adenosine 3′,5′-cyclic monophosphate.

to which a lipid, called lipid A, is bound. The toxic component of the endotoxin complex is believed to be *lipid A*. Also bound to the core are the O-specific side chains, polymers of oligosaccharide units, that carry the antigenic determinants responsible for the serological specificity of the bacterium (Fig. 9-9). Endotoxin is released usually when the cell is lysed, but can also be released during vegetative growth.

Endotoxin has been isolated from gram-negative bacteria, and its biological properties have been determined through studies of a number of susceptible animals. The effects of endotoxin on the cardiovascular, respiratory, and blood-clot-ting mechanisms have been known to lead to intravascular coagulation, septic shock, and death. Evidence of the role endotoxin plays in gram-negative septicemia in humans is circumstantial even though people are very sensitive to intravenous injections of purified endotoxin. What happens when endotoxin is released during infection by gram-negative bacteria is not completely understood. The clinical features of fever, intravascular coagulation, and depression of the reticuloendothelial system that appear in animals injected with endotoxin are sometimes duplicated in human gram-negative bacteremia. These features are explained as follows:

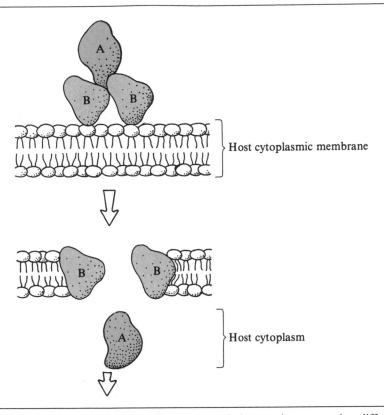

Fig. 9-8. Possible mechanism for entry of exotoxins, such as cholera toxin, possessing different subunits A and B. B subunits of toxin bind to cytoplasmic membrane of host cell and insert themselves across it. This provides an avenue for diffusion of A, or toxic subunit, into the cell cytoplasm.

1. Fever. Endotoxin has the ability to induce fever in susceptible animals. Endotoxin causes macrophages and other cells to release endogenous pyrogens. The pyrogen is a protein and acts on the temperature-regulating center, that is, the anterior hypothalamus. Fever is discussed at more length in Chapter 10.

2. Activation of the coagulation mechanism. Intravascular coagulation is one of the manifestations of gram-negative bacteremia, although it also occurs in other types of infections. Endotoxin activates components of the clotting mechanism and thus leads to the formation of fibrin. If fibrin becomes trapped in the small blood vessels, intravascular coagulation and shock can follow.

3. Depression of the reticuloendothelial system. Macrophages make up the reticuloendothelial system, and endotoxin prevents the macrophages from clearing the fibrin polymers that become trapped in the small blood vessels.

4. Vascular collapse. In animals endotoxin is known to cause the release of biologically active substances from the cells of the immune system. Some of these active substances affect the circulatory system; they can cause increased vascular permeability and dilatation. The circulatory changes lead to impaired blood flow to vital organs—kidneys, liver, brain, and lung—and ultimately to shock and possibly death. These vascular reactions are also seen in gram-negative bacteremia in humans.

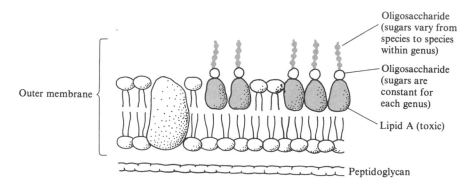

Fig. 9-9. Relationship of endotoxin to gram-negative cell wall. Endotoxin represented in color is a lipopolysaccharide (LPS). Lipid A, the toxic component of endotoxin, is inserted into membrane and is complexed with two types of oligosaccharides. The outermost oligosaccharide is sometimes called the 0 or somatic region. Variations in the sugars of this region enable microorganism to differentiate into specific serological groups.

It is currently believed that interaction of endotoxin with the macrophage may be the primary event in initiating all of the biological effects of endotoxin. Several in vitro and in vivo studies with endotoxin have demonstrated that these biological effects can be produced by endotoxin-stimulated macrophages. The stimulated macrophages release two potent molecules called *tumor necrosis factor* and *interleukin-I*. Tumor necrosis factor, for example, is believed to be the primary mediator of endotoxic shock.

AVOIDING HOST DEFENSE MECHANISMS

Antiphagocytic Factors

Once microorganisms have penetrated beneath the surface of the skin they are exposed to cellular elements of the blood, lymph, and tissues. These cellular elements are the host's major line of defense against foreign bodies such as microorganisms. Cellular elements, such as macrophages, engage in a process called *phagocytosis,* that is, they ingest and kill microorganisms. Several microorganisms are virulent because they are able to prevent ingestion by phagocytes or,

if they are ingested, are able to prevent digestion and killing. One of the most important microbial antiphagocytic devices is the *capsule*. Capsule formation by bacteria such as *Streptococcus pneumoniae, Klebsiella pneumoniae, Bacillus anthracis*, and *Yersinia pestis*, is an important device for preventing phagocytic ingestion (Fig. 9-10). Other surface components, such as the cell wall protein of *Staphylococcus aureus*, called *protein A*, also inhibit ingestion by phagocytic cells. Still other microorganisms such as species of *Mycobacterium* and *Salmonella* are resistant to digestion by phagocytic enzymes once they are ingested. For a more detailed explanation of phagocytosis, please see page 268.

Changing Surface Chemistry

Some microorganisms avoid host defenses by altering the chemistry of surface components. It is the surface components of microbial agents that cause the host's immune system to respond to them as foreign agents. Species of *Borrelia*, a spirochete, on infection of the host are able to bring about changes in a protein on the cell surface. *Borrelia* species cause relapsing fever, and once in the bloodstream induce antibodies that re-

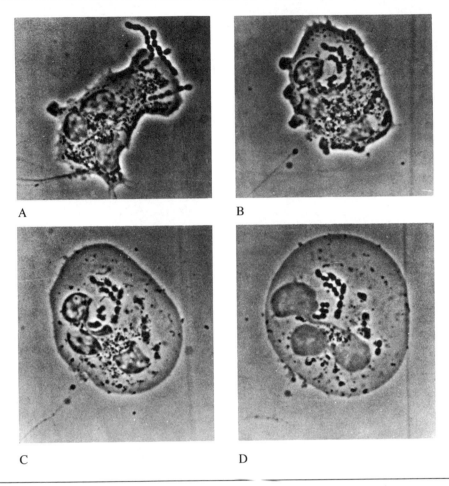

Fig. 9-10. Phase-contrast micrograph demonstrating leukotoxic action of streptococci on human neutrophils. A. Neutrophil is seen to engulf three streptococcal chains. B. Neutrophil has ceased moving and has begun to round up. Cytoplasmic blebs are seen to emanate from its surface. C. Neutrophil is swollen and immobile. D. Most internal structures of neutrophil have disappeared, and nucleus appears swollen. (From G. W. Sullivan and G. L. Mandell, *Infect. Immun.* 30:272, 1980.)

spond to a specific surface protein. As the number of borrelia are being destroyed some strains change the chemistry of their surface proteins. Once the change has been made the host's circulating antibodies do not recognize the new protein and require time to respond to it. Eventually, after several changes in surface proteins, the host's immune system becomes overtaxed.

Other microorganisms, such as the helminth *Schistosoma*, can also change their surfaces, but in a way different from *Borrelia*. *Schistosoma*, after invading the host, assumes residence in the veins of the bladder and intestine. It avoids detection by the host's immune system by coating itself with the proteins that coat red blood cells and other host cells. Thus, the parasite goes unrecognized because its surface does not contain foreign molecules.

SUMMARY

1. Microorganisms can inhabit many sites in the human body. Some of the microorganisms become permanent residents (commensals) but others can be parasitic. Factors determining the fate of microbial species in the body include: presence or absence of oxygen, presence of receptors for attachment, availability of nutrients, and immunological response of the host.

2. The most successful parasites merely live off their hosts without causing major damage to tissue. Parasites colonize the host either because the host has been compromised by some underlying condition or because the parasite possesses mechanisms for overcoming host defenses.

3. Parasites can live outside or inside host cells. Extracellular parasites usually produce toxins or release products that enable the host to respond quickly to infection. Extracellular parasites usually produce acute infections.

4. Intracellular parasites may be of two types: those that can survive only intracellularly and those that can live intracellularly as well as extracellularly. Intracellular parasites use the host cell for important metabolites and/or as a mechanism for evading immune products in the bloodstream. Many intracellular parasites produce chronic disease.

5. Microorganisms that inhabit the host but do not induce an immune response are merely colonizers, but if antibodies are produced the microorganism causes an infection. If tissue is destroyed during infection the microorganism causes disease.

6. The disease-producing potential of microorganisms is referred to as *pathogenicity*. A more quantitative term is *virulence*, which refers to the number of microorganisms or amount of microbial product that can cause disease in 50 percent of the animals tested. Microbial virulence can be attenuated in the laboratory and this is the mechanism for producing some vaccines.

7. The host defense mechanisms are initiated at the site of entry, the epithelium, as well as in subepithelial tissue, including the bloodstream. The skin is a thick epithelial covering that offers physical resistance to microbial penetration. The skin also contains chemical antimicrobial factors such as fatty acids.

8. The mucosal surface is an important defense against infection because it contains secretory IgA, has a resident microflora, has a film of mucin, and contains substances such as lysozyme, lactoferrin, and peroxidase. All of them help in preventing attachment of microorganisms or help destroy microorganisms that come in contact with the mucosal surface.

9. The respiratory tract is a barrier to infection primarily because of its mucociliary blanket. The flushing action of saliva helps to reduce the microbial content in the oropharynx. The acidity of the stomach and the acids, bile salts, and enzymes present in the intestinal tract help prevent microbial colonization. In the genitourinary tract the acidity of the vagina inhibits microbial activity while the flushing action of urine deters microbial colonization.

10. Three host defense mechanisms exist below the epithelial surface: tissue fluids, which contain antimicrobial factors such as antibodies and various chemical factors; the lymph system, with its channels that carry microorganisms to lymph nodes for destruction; and phagocytic cells in the bloodstream and at tissue surfaces.

11. The host's resistance to infection can also be influenced by factors such as the immunological state of the host and the race, nutrition, occupation, and underlying condition of the host.

12. Microorganisms are equipped to invade host tissue through the release of various enzymes and other proteins. Much of the damage to host tissue is due to toxins, which are of two types: exotoxins and endotoxins.

13. Exotoxins are proteins released by the bacterium into the surrounding environment. Most exotoxins are made up of two subunits, one used to bind to the host cell and to facilitate the entry of the second subunit. The second subunit is the

toxic component. Exotoxin activities are described in Table 9-4.

14. Endotoxins are part of the lipopolysaccharide of the outer membrane of the gram-negative cell wall. Lipid A is the toxic component. Endotoxin released during bacteremia can affect the host by (1) inducing fever, (2) activating the coagulation mechanism and causing intravascular coagulation, (3) depressing the reticuloendothelial system, and (4) causing vascular collapse.

15. Some microorganisms can avoid host defense mechanisms by preventing phagocytosis. The bacterial capsule and some surface proteins are the major antiphagocytic factors. Other microorganisms can also alter their surface chemistry so that the host's immune system has problems in recognition.

QUESTIONS FOR STUDY

Select the best response or responses for each of the following:

1. The following statements about endotoxins are true except
   A. They are heat labile.
   B. They cannot be converted to a toxoid.
   C. They do not produce fever in the host.
   D. They are also referred to as lipopolysaccharide.

2. Two bacterial toxins that have the same mechanism of action are produced by
   A. Enteropathogenic *E. coli* and *Cornyebacterium diphtheriae*
   B. *C. diphtheriae* and *Clostridium perfringens*
   C. *Vibrio cholerae* and enteropathogenic *E. coli*
   D. *Bacillus cereus* and *Pseudomonas aeruginosa*

3. Siderophores are important in bacterial pathogenesis because
   A. They inhibit phagocytosis.

B. They help to extract iron from the host for use by the bacterium.
C. They enable the bacterium to adhere to host tissue.
D. They are enzyme-like products that enable the bacterium to invade red blood cells.

4. The two major components of microbial virulence are
   A. Invasiveness and toxigenicity
   B. Adhesins and capsule formation
   C. Spreading factors and antiphagocytic factors
   D. Intracellular and extracellular parasitism

5. Which of the following are components of mucosal surfaces that aid in preventing infection?
   A. Secretory IgA
   B. Mucins
   C. Microflora
   D. Lysozyme

Fill in the blank:

6. The process in which microorganisms lose their virulence is called _____ .

7. _____ are bacterial invasive factors associated with lysis of red blood cells.

8. Microorganisms that benefit from their habitation of the body but cause no harm are called _____ .

9. A disease that does not give rise to overt symptoms is called _____ .

10. _____ is an enzyme found primarily in normal secretions that attacks the cell wall of bacteria.

ADDITIONAL READINGS

Dinarello, C. A., Canon, J. G., and Wolff, S. M. New concepts on the pathogenesis of fever. *Rev. Infect. Dis.* 10(1):168,1988.

Fibronectin and the pathogenesis of infections. *Rev. Infect. Dis.* 9 (Suppl. 4),1987.

Isenberg, H. D. Pathogenicity and virulence: Another view. *Clin. Microbiol. Revs.* 1(1):40,1988.

Kingston, M. E., and Mackey, D. Skin clues in the diagnosis of life-threatening infections. *Rev. Infect. Dis.* 8(1):1,1986.

Mims, C. A. *The Pathogenesis of Infectious Disease* (2nd ed.). New York: Academic Press, 1986.

Perspectives on bacterial pathogenesis and host defense. *Rev. Infect. Dis.* 9 (Suppl. 5):1987.

Roth, J. A. *Virulence Mechanisms of Bacterial Pathogens.* Washington, DC: American Society for Microbiology, 1988.

Roth, R. R., and James, W. D. Microbial ecology of the skin. *Annu. Rev. Microbiol.* 42:441,1988.

Russell, M. W, and Mestecky, J. Induction of the mucosal immune response. *Rev. Infect. Dis.* 10 (Suppl. 2):440,1988.

Salzman, R. L., and Peterson, P. K. Immunodeficiency of the elderly. *Rev. Infect. Dis.* 9(6):1127,1987.

Thomas, E. L., Lehrer, R. I., and Rest, R. F. Human neutrophil antimicrobial activity. *Rev. Infect. Dis.* 10 (Suppl. 2):450,1988.

10. EPIDEMIOLOGY

OBJECTIVES

To describe the various stages and symptoms associated with acute disease

To understand the mechanisms that enable microorganisms to persist in the host

To differentiate between reservoirs and sources of disease

To list those diseases that are transmitted from animals to humans

To list those diseases that are transmitted to humans from contaminated water or food

To describe how microorganisms can be transmitted by air

To briefly explain the laboratory techniques used to identify the source of a disease

To define: chronic disease, subclinical infections, pyrogen, carrier, zoonoses, vector, droplet nuclei, fomite, epidemic, endemic, herd immunity, morbidity, index case, biotype, serotype, DNA probe

In the previous chapter we discussed the one-on-one relationship between host and parasite. Epidemiology (from the Greek *epidemios*, which means "among the people") is concerned with disease as it applies to populations of individuals. The science of epidemiology may be involved with infectious as well as noninfectious disease. The role of the epidemiologist is to gather statistics that will indicate the prevalence or frequency of disease. Our discussion of epidemiology will be directed at how infectious diseases are spread, how they are controlled, and how they may be identified, as well as their frequency and prevalence in a population.

CLINICAL STAGES OF DISEASE IN THE HOST

To understand the various aspects of disease in a population we should first have some knowl-edge of the clinical stages of infectious disease in the individual.

ACUTE VS. CHRONIC DISEASE

Individuals infected by a pathogenic microorganism will respond to it in various ways. Sometimes the host's immune system will inhibit the pathogen before it can elicit symptoms or the symptoms will be so slight as to be almost imperceptible. Such infections are called *subclinical* or inapparent. When the pathogen overcomes the host's defense mechanisms, the manifestations of disease may ensue and proceed in an acute or chronic manner.

Acute Disease
Acute disease is characterized by symptoms that usually appear quickly, become very intense, and then subside when the host's immune system has

overwhelmed the pathogen or its toxic products. Acute disease is the type of disease with which most of us are acquainted, for example, the childhood diseases such as measles and chickenpox and the various types of influenza. One can always determine the approximate length of time it will take to recover from such diseases. Both acute and chronic diseases proceed in such a way that they can be divided into various stages: *incubation, prodromal, acute*, and *convalescent*. These stages in chronic disease, however, cannot be as precisely identified as in acute disease.

Incubation Period. The incubation period is that period of time from the moment the infectious agent enters the host until the first symptoms of disease appear. This period may be as short as a few hours or as long as several years. The time interval is influenced by how fast the infectious agent can multiply and how quickly the microorganisms or the microbial products affect host tissue. Food poisoning caused by the ingestion of preformed toxin in contaminated food often produces symptoms within 8 to 24 hours. Other diseases, in which the infectious agent is taken into the body, may have incubation periods of one to several weeks. Many of the fungal pathogens, for example, have long incubation periods in the host. One must remember that the incubation period is greatly influenced by the virulence of the microorganism, the antigenic potential of the microorganism or its products, and the immunological state of the host. Measles affecting a normal healthy child in the community may have an incubation period of 7 to 10 days, but the same virus infecting a hospitalized patient could have an incubation period of 1 to 2 days. The average incubation period for most diseases is between 10 and 21 days.

Prodromal Period. The term *prodromal* is derived from the Greek word that means "running before." In terms of the infectious disease cycle *prodromal* refers to the warning symptoms that indicate the onset of disease. This is the period in which the individual characterizes his or her general state of health as "not feeling well." The technical term for this symptom is *malaise*. It may include such symptoms as headache, upset stomach, or slight fever. The infectious agent during the prodromal period has multiplied only to the extent that its products have induced a slight response by the host.

Acute Period. The acute period is the stage in which the symptoms of disease are at their peak. During this period the infectious microorganisms have reached a population level that induces the host to respond with immunological intensity. The intensity of this immunological response as well as the intensity of the symptoms are related to the number of host–parasite encounters. If the encounter is the first of its kind then the symptoms of disease are usually very intense and the maximum immunological response takes longer to develop. A rapid immunological response and less intense symptoms will develop if the disease represents a repeat encounter between host and parasite.

The types of symptoms associated with the acute disease period vary from disease to disease, but some symptoms are more prevalent in most diseases than others. *Fever* is one of the most common symptoms of disease and is mediated by endogenous pyrogens (*pyro* = heat) produced by leukocytes. Endogenous pyrogens are released into the arterial blood. They act on the body's thermostat, the anterior hypothalamus of the brain, which contains thermosensitive nerve cells. The hypothalmus in turn releases molecules called *prostaglandins* (arachidonic acid, for example), which become metabolized. The metabolized prostaglandins cause the hypothalmic thermostat to be raised to a higher level. The new thermostatic reading signals various efferent nerves, for example, those innervating peripheral blood, to constrict blood vessels and this conserves heat. The increased heat of the body from vasoconstriction continues until the temperature of the blood supplying the hypothalmus matches the elevated thermostat reading. The thermostat can be reset to normal when the concentration of endogenous pyrogens falls.

Endogenous pyrogens are produced primarily by macrophages. The principal endogenous pyrogen is a protein called *interleukin I (IL-1)*; however, interferon and tumor necrosis factor (cachectin) can also induce fever. Endogenous pyrogens are induced primarily by molecules such as microbes, toxins, or other products that are not indigenous to the body (Fig. 10-1).

Fever enhances the inflammatory response and at the same time interferes with microbial growth as well as replication of tumor cells. This positive response must be weighed against the detrimental aspects of fever. Fever may result in increased heart rate, which would be deleterious to those with compromised cardiovascular function. Fever also increases the basic metabolic rate by 7 to 8 percent for each degree Fahrenheit of temperature elevated. This usually results in

Fig. 10-1. Mechanism of fever induction following infection.

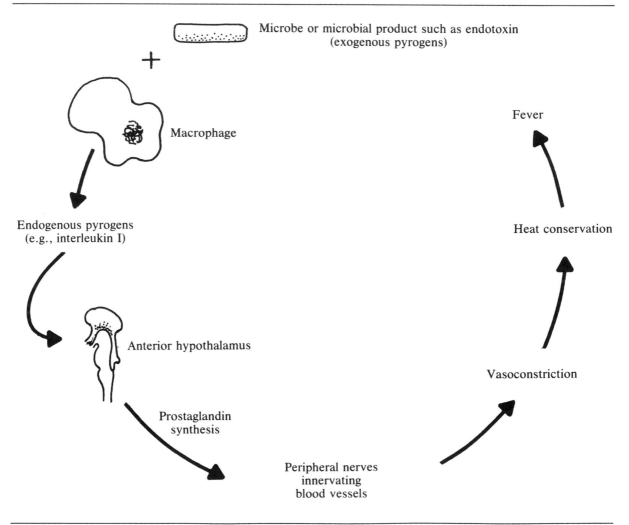

increased caloric demand and mild to severe dehydration.

Skin or epithelial lesions are a frequent response to infection by many microorganisms and result from (1) localization of the microorganisms near the body surface, (2) the effects of a microbial toxin near the body surface, or (3) an inflammatory response (hypersensitivity) to a microbial antigen. Multiple lesions that appear on the body surface are called *rashes*. The rashes produced by viruses often go through a succession of forms such as the following:

Macule. A macular lesion is flat and usually red.
Papule. A papular lesion is firm and elevated.
Vesicle. A vesicular lesion contains fluid.
Pustule. A pustular lesion contains pus, often a result of secondary bacterial infection.

Rashes that are localized on the body surface can be of diagnostic importance.

Other symptoms of disease may include cough, which is associated with respiratory disease. Intestinal diseases are usually characterized by the symptoms of vomiting, diarrhea, or dysentery (bloody diarrhea).

Convalescent Period. *Convalescence* refers to the recovery period from a disease. Convalescence is associated with a sharp decline in symptoms such as fever or headache associated with the disease in question. The subsiding of symptoms is correlated with maximum antibody levels in the host and usually means the pathogen is being eradicated.

Chronic Disease

Some microorganisms are capable of persisting in the host for long intervals because they can avoid the normal immunological responses of the host. Persistent infections can be divided into chronic, latent, and slow. We will concern ourselves with chronic infections since latent and slow infections are more characteristic of viruses, discussed in Chapter 32. Chronic infec-

tions are those in which the symptoms of disease are expressed over a long period of time. Many times in chronic disease the infectious agent is an intracellular parasite that localizes in phagocytes. The organism can, therefore, be transported to various organs and body sites where microbial multiplication or even lysis of microorganisms releases products that give rise to the original symptoms of disease or new symptoms. The symptoms arising during relapses are often due to hypersensitivity reactions by the host. Chronic diseases such as brucellosis and tuberculosis are believed to be due to the inability of the host to respond with any immunological efficiency. Apparently the microbial antigens are not sufficiently immunogenic to make the host produce antibodies that can eliminate the pathogen.

RESERVOIRS AND SOURCES OF DISEASE

Pathogenic microorganisms, if they are going to retain their potential to cause disease, must have a place where they can maintain themselves and replicate. This place of survival and replication is called the *reservoir*, and it may be animate or inanimate. Viruses, which are obligate intracellular parasites, replicate only in living cells and are harbored in a variety of living hosts. Animate reservoirs are also required for bacterial species such as the streptococci and staphylococci, even though they are not obligate parasites. Reservoirs may also be inanimate. Many microorganisms replicate in soil, water, and food, provided nutrients are available. Many bacterial species that cause disease in the hospital, such as *Pseudomonas* and *Klebsiella* species, may be found in both inanimate and animate reservoirs.

Sources of disease are those objects or places, either animate or inanimate, from which the infective agent passes to the host. Sometimes the reservoir and source are one and the same. The organism that causes pneumonia (*Streptococcus pneumoniae*), for example, is harbored by humans in the oral cavity. If the infected individual comes into direct contact with another individual (by kissing, for example) and causes disease, the reservoir and source are the same. There are also many examples in which the reservoir and source are not the same. If the reservoir of disease is the kidney of an animal, the infectious microorganism may infect a human in two ways. Humans may eat the kidneys of the diseased animal, in which case the reservoir and source are the same. The live animal may also contaminate a water supply through urination. Ingestion of the contaminated water by humans could also lead to disease, and in this instance the source of the disease would be water. The length of time that the microorganism remains viable in the source depends on environmental as well as microbial factors.

ANIMATE RESERVOIRS

Human

Humans not only represent the most important reservoir of microbial agents but in many instances they are the only reservoir. Many viral agents, such as the measles, rubella, mumps, influenza, and poliomyelitis virus, and bacterial agents, such as those causing sexually transmitted disease, whooping cough, and diphtheria, are maintained only in human reservoirs.

As stated previously, humans also harbor microorganisms that cause *persistent* infections. The two most important consequences of persistence is that (1) the microorganisms remain in the community for extended periods of time and (2) there can be reactivation of disease when the immunological state of the host becomes temporarily or permanently impaired. Two diseases that illustrate persistence are typhoid fever and tuberculosis, caused by the bacteria *Salmonella typhi* and *Mycobacterium tuberculosis*, respectively. During recovery from typhoid fever the

host may harbor bacteria in the gall bladder and disease symptoms are not apparent. Periodically (over months to years), bacteria multiply and are shed from the gall bladder into the intestinal tract and hence into the environment via feces. The individual shedding the microorganisms is a *carrier*. The carrier can shed microorganisms that may contaminate food or water. Thus, the carrier becomes a permanent source of infections for others. In tuberculosis the infecting bacteria can be walled off in calcified lesions (such as in the lung) that are not affected by the host's immune system. The bacteria remain viable in the lesions for many years. The lesions can rupture at any time, releasing viable bacteria that multiply in tissue and thus cause a reactivation of disease. Reactivation also makes the host a new source of infection.

Even though the carrier state may be a result of microbial persistence, not all carriers are alike. *Convalescent carriers*, for example, are those who are recovering from the disease and in whom the infectious agent remains and multiplies without causing overt symptoms (as in typhoid fever, for example). *Healthy carriers* are those who do not have the disease but still carry infectious microorganisms. Those who carry strains of *Staphylococcus aureus*, which are causes of food poisoning, are examples of healthy carriers. The carrier harbors the staphylococci in the nares (nostrils) and, when he or she handles food, contaminates it with staphylococci. Detection of the carrier state is very important in severing the chain of transmission that may involve hundreds or even thousands of individuals.

Animal

Animals, particularly domestic animals, are important reservoirs and sources of disease to humans. A disease that occurs primarily in animals and is secondarily transmitted to humans is called a *zoonosis*. *Salmonella* species are normally found in the intestinal tract of animals such as poultry or cattle. When they contaminate food ingested by humans the salmonellae can cause disease (salmonellosis). Table 10-1 describes the zoonoses. Many times when animals are reservoirs the human represents a dead end in terms of disease transmission because the disease cannot be transferred from human to human. For example, Q fever and brucellosis are diseases of animals that can be acquired through contact with the animals or animal products. There are exceptions, of course, such as in the case of the disease salmonellosis. Salmonellosis may be acquired from animals but the infected human can also serve as a source of disease to other humans.

Insect

Two classes of arthropods, Insecta and Arachnida, are important in the transfer of infectious agents from one host to another. Arthropods are therefore called *vectors* in the disease process. The class Insecta includes flies, mosquitoes, fleas, lice, and true bugs; Arachnida includes ticks and mites. Insect vectors may be divided into two types: mechanical and biological. *Mechanical vectors* are invertebrate animals that carry the infectious agent on their appendages and are not involved in the life cycle of the in-

Table 10-1. Diseases of Animals (Zoonoses) That are Transmissible to Humans

Disease	Transmission to humans	Animal reservoir
BACTERIAL		
Salmonellosis	Ingestion of contaminated food or water	Dogs, cats, farm animals, poultry, reptiles, rodents
Brucellosis	Drinking raw milk or direct contact with animal	Dogs, farm animals, rodents
Tularemia	Ingestion of or contact with contaminated meat and arthropod vectors	Rodents and rabbits
Anthrax	Contact with contaminated animal hides or products	Farm animals
Leptospirosis	Contact with contaminated water	Dogs, cats, wild rodents, farm animals
Bubonic plague	Rat flea but human-to-human transmission in pneumonic plague	Rodents such as ground squirrels, rats, chipmunks
Rickettsial disease (scrub typhus and murine typhus)	Ticks, fleas, mites	Primarily wild rodents
Q fever	Ingestion of raw milk, inhalation of contaminated dust, or contact with contaminated animal	Farm animals (cattle, sheep, goats)
Cat-scratch fever	Scratch or bite of cat	Cats
VIRAL		
Rabies	Bite of animal or contact with infectious saliva or tissue, inhalation of aerosols	Dogs, cats, farm animals, and wild animals, particularly skunks and raccoons
Equine encephalitis	Horses to mosquitoes to humans	Horses, pheasants, domestic pigeons
PARASITIC (HELMINTHS)		
Echinococcosis	Ingestion of eggs deposited on raw fruit	Fox, dogs, cats are principal hosts, but life cycles in nature completed in voles and mice
Trichinosis	Ingestion of contaminated meat, usually pork	Pigs and bears are most important reservoirs

fectious agent. Flies, for example, may pick up *Salmonella* organisms from animal feces and transmit them to humans via contaminated food. Thus the fly is not a true reservoir of the infectious agent. *Biological vectors* are invertebrate animals that serve as host and reservoir of the microbial agent. Many arthropods feed on animals and humans and during the blood feast acquire the infectious microorganism. The infected arthropod can feed on other hosts, which may include humans, and thus transmit the infectious microorganisms from one host to another. Occasionally the arthropod is required in the developmental cycle of the microbial agent. The protozoal agent that is the cause of malaria requires the mosquito to undergo its sexual cycle. In the epithelial cells of the mosquito stomach the protozoan matures and then migrates to the salivary glands. When the mosquito bites a human the pathogen is injected into the human host. The insect vectors and the diseases with which they are associated are outlined in Table 10-2.

INANIMATE RESERVOIRS

Inanimate reservoirs or sources of disease are soil, water, and food. Many microorganisms can carry out their life cycle in soil and water, and, fortunately for us, most are not pathogenic for humans. Most fungal species, for example, exist in the soil as spores. When some of these spores are inhaled by a susceptible host, they germinate and engage in vegetative growth and produce disease. Bacteria that produce the deadliest toxins known to humans are indigenous to the soil. Species of *Clostridium* such as *C. botulinum* and *C. tetani* exist in the soil as spores. *C. botulinum* may contaminate food and under anaerobic conditions produces the toxin associated with food poisoning (botulism). If *C. tetani* spores contaminate a wound they germinate and produce a toxin responsible for the symptoms of the highly fatal disease called *tetanus*. Animal parasites such as the parasitic worms (helminths) are usually

passed as eggs from the intestinal tract of the animals they parasitize. These eggs may remain in an infective state until they are picked up by another host. Very few microorganisms pathogenic for humans are capable of vegetative growth or a free-living existence in the soil.

Pure water is unable to support the growth of microorganisms, but most water contains minerals and organic nutrients that have been derived from the surrounding soil or air. Humans also contaminate waters either directly or indirectly via raw or processed sewage. Pathogenic as well as nonpathogenic microorganisms may find their way from humans or animals into water supplies. Some potential pathogens for humans live in the fish and shellfish that inhabit inland and coastal waters. Thus water supports their existence and also contributes to their potential for infecting humans.

Food is an important reservoir for microorganisms infectious for humans. Human disease may result from ingestion of the meat of the infected animal or ingestion of originally uninfected meat that has been contaminated. Several bacterial and animal parasite diseases can be acquired by humans from the ingestion of meat from diseased animals. Eggs may be infected with *Salmonella* and when eaten raw can cause human disease. Cows carry several microorganisms infectious for humans. Ingestion of infected meat or milk may cause disease in humans. Tuberculosis, brucellosis, and Q fever are the most frequently encountered diseases resulting from the ingestion of infected meat or milk; however, diseases caused by species of *Campylobacter and Streptococcus* can also occur. These diseases are associated with drinking raw milk. Pasteurization ordinarily destroys these organisms. Some worms infect animals and are encysted in muscle. Ingestion of uncooked pork, for example, can lead to the disease called *trichinosis*.

Foods may be accidentally contaminated with potentially infectious microorganisms. Shellfish such as oysters, for example, may be harvested from waters that are polluted with human sewage. Ingestion of such foods uncooked can lead

Table 10-2. Major Vector-borne Diseases of Humans

Vector	Disease	Microbe classification
Mosquito	Animal parasite diseases	
Culex, Anopheles, and *Aedes* species	Filariasis	*Wuchereria* and *Brugia* species
Anopheles species	Malaria	*Plasmodium* species
	Viral diseases	
Aedes species	Dengue fever	Flavivirus
	Yellow fever	Flavivirus
	St. Louis encephalitis	Flavivirus
Culex species	Eastern equine encephalitis	Alphavirus
	Western equine encephalitis	Alphavirus
	St. Louis encephalitis	Flavivirus
Tick	Bacterial diseases	
	Relapsing fever	*Borrelia recurrentis*
	Rocky Mountain spotted fever	*Rickettsia rickettsii*
	Q fever	*Coxiella burnetii*
	Tularemia	*Francisella tularensis*
	Lyme disease	*Borrelia burgdorferi*
	Viral diseases	
	Colorado tick fever	Orbivirus
	Crimean hemorrhagic fever	? (ungrouped)
Mite	Bacterial diseases	
	Q fever	*Coxiella burnetii*
	Rickettsialpox	*Rickettsia akari*
Flies	Animal parasite diseases	
Deerfly	Eye worm	*Loa loa*
Tsetse flies	Sleeping sickness (African)	*Trypanosoma* species
Blackflies	Leishmaniasis	*Leishmania* species
	Onchocerciasis	*Onchocerca volvulus*
	Bacterial diseases	
Deerfly	Tularemia	*Francisella tularensis*
Muscoid flies	Yaws	*Treponema pertenue*
	Viral diseases	
Sandfly	Sandfly fever	?
	Vesicular stomatitis	Vesiculovirus
Lice	Bacterial diseases	
	Epidemic typhus	*Rickettsia prowazekii*
	Trench fever	*Rochalimaea quintana*
Fleas	Bacterial diseases	
	Endemic typhus	*Rickettsia typhi*
	Bubonic plague	*Yersinia pestis*
True bugs (reduviids)	Animal parasite diseases	
	Chagas' disease (American trypanosomiasis)	*Trypanosoma cruzi*

Source: From R. F. Boyd, *General Microbiology* (2nd ed.). St. Louis: Mosby, 1988.

to such diseases as viral hepatitis. Carriers may contaminate food and be a source of disease to humans. Diseases such as salmonellosis, shigellosis, amebiasis, and cholera can be acquired in this way. Some microorganisms that contaminate foods produce toxins that when ingested cause gastrointestinal symptoms (see Transmission of Infectious Microorganisms). When properly refrigerated, smoked, canned, or pasteurized, however, foods are safe to eat and will not cause disease.

TRANSMISSION OF INFECTIOUS MICROORGANISMS

Disease transmission refers to the method of transfer of infectious microorganisms from the source (which may or may not be the same as the reservoir) to the host. Transmission may occur by contact, through the air, or by means of a vector. (Transmission by vectors was discussed under Reservoirs and Sources of Disease.) Sometimes an organism may have more than one route of transmission.

CONTACT

Spread of microorganisms by contact occurs when the potential victim has contact with the source of the microorganisms. This contact may be either direct or indirect.

Direct

Direct contact refers to transmission of microorganisms from person to person by close personal association. Handshaking, kissing, sneezing, coughing, and sexual contact represent the most usual ways that microorganisms are transferred by direct means (Fig. 10-2).

Sexually transmitted diseases have become rampant in many parts of the world, especially in developed countries like the United States. To most people, sexually transmitted diseases are represented by the traditional diseases syphilis and gonorrhea. Greater sexual freedom, as well as changes in sexual practices, has resulted in recent years in an increasing number of sexually transmitted diseases of unusual types. For example, chlamydial infection is now more common than gonorrhea, and the incidence of genital herpes is believed to be as high as one million or more cases per year. Homosexual activity can also lead to diseases usually considered to be primarily enteric. Enteric diseases such as giardiasis, salmonellosis, and shigellosis are now frequently encountered in the gay community. A list list of the sexually transmitted diseases is presented in Table 10-3. The complications of sexually transmitted disease, especially in women, have created great concern. Increased health expenditures, loss of productivity, and human suffering have resulted from sexually transmitted disease complications such as pelvic inflammatory disease. These complications have led to loss of fertility as well as detrimental effects in the newborn.

Sneezing and coughing may also be considered a method of direct spread, provided the individuals are within a few feet of each other. The microorganisms are expelled in droplets that are carried only a few feet and then drop to horizontal surfaces. Direct spread of this kind is characteristic of measles, a viral disease.

Direct contact may also be responsible for the transmission of those diseases that are caused by the patient's own microbial flora These infections, sometimes referred to as *endogenous*, are frequently encountered in the hospital environment. Patients, because of either examination or treatment procedures, can have indigenous microbial species transferred from one body site to another. During surgery, for example, intestinal microorganisms may be accidentally displaced from the intestinal tract into the bloodstream, where they replicate rapidly and cause disease (see Chapter 34).

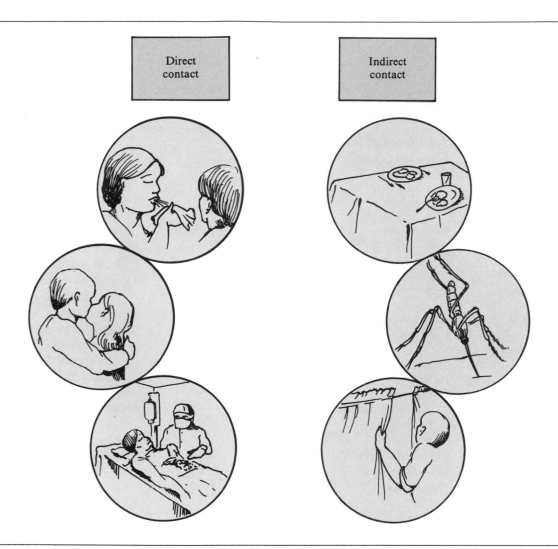

Fig. 10-2. Routes of transmission for infectious agents. On the left are direct routes of transmission. A. Sneezing disperses microorganisms that will directly infect an individual within 3 feet of its origin. B. Kissing or direct contact between individuals, as in sexual intercourse. C. During surgery an individual's indigenous microflora can be transferred by the surgeon to another body site and this may result in infection. On the right are indirect routes of transmission. D. Food, water, or eating utensils may be contaminated with microorganisms that can be acquired by a person coming in contact with them. E. A mosquito can transfer infectious microorganisms from a source such as an animal to a new host. F. Microorganisms may be in particles that contaminate articles such as curtains. Handling the curtain can disperse the microorganisms, which can be inhaled or come into contact with other open tissue.

Indirect

Indirect transmission occurs when the infectious microorganism is carried from one person to another on various intermediate objects such as food, dust, water, or *fomites* (inanimate objects other than food or water). The intermediate objects may be contaminated from an animate or inanimate source (Fig. 10-2).

Table 10-3. Characteristics of the Sexually Transmitted Diseases

Disease	Causal agent	Type of parasite	Cause of infertility, abortion, or infection to fetus	No. of cases reported to CDC, 1989	Estimated no. of infections per year
Gonorrhea	*Neisseria gonorrhoeae*	Bacterium	Yes	733,151	2.5 million
Syphilis	*Treponema pallidum*	Bacterium	Yes	44,540[a,b]	340,000
Nongonococcal urethritis	*Chlamydia trachomatis, Ureaplasma urealyticum*	Bacteria	No	NR	4–5 million
Trichomoniasis	*Trichomonas vaginalis*	Protozoan	No	NR	1.0 million
Venereal warts	Human papilloma virus	Virus	No	NR	12–24 million
Genital herpes	Herpes simplex virus	Virus	Yes	NR	30 million
Lymphogranuloma venereum	*Chlamydia trachomatis*	Bacterium	No	189[b]	?
Soft chancre (chancroid)	*Hemophilus ducreyi*	Bacterium	No	4,692	?
Granuloma inguinale	*Calymmatobacterium granulomatis*	Bacterium	No	7	?
Candidiasis	*Candida albicans*	Fungus	Yes	NR	?
Scabies	*Sarcoptes scabiei*	Arachnid (mite)	No	NR	?
Pediculosis pubis	*Phthirus pubis*	Insect (louse)	No	NR	?
Enteric disease	*Salmonella* species	Bacterium	No	NR	?
	Shigella species	Bacterium	No	NR	?
	Campylobacter fetus subspecies *jejuni*	Bacterium	Yes	NR	?
	Entamoeba histolytica	Protozoan	No	NR	?
	Giardia lamblia	Protozoan	No	NR	?
AIDS (acquired immune deficiency syndrome)	Human T-lymphocyte virus type III	Virus	No	33,722	?

CDC = Centers for Disease Control; NR = not reportable.
[a] Primary and secondary cases only.
[b] Civilian cases only.

Water. Water is a common vehicle for the transmission of infectious microorganisms. An outbreak of waterborne disease is defined as an incident in which two or more persons experience similar illness after consumption or use of water intended for drinking and epidemiological evidence implicates water as the source of the illness. Community as well as noncommunity water systems may be involved. Many outbreaks occur in recreational areas where wells or other water sources become fecally contaminated. From 40 to 50 outbreaks, involving about 4000 to 5000 cases, occur each year in the United States. The most frequently recovered pathogen is *Giardia lamblia*, a protozoan that causes gastrointestinal disease. The infectious agents associated with waterborne disease are outlined in Table 10-4.

Water is also an important vehicle for extraintestinal infection. A number of pathogens can be acquired through occupational, recreational, and even therapeutic contact with water. Waterborne pathogens can enter the human through intact or abraded skin, for example, hot tub–associated dermatitis; inhalation and aspiration, for example, contaminated aerosolized medications or humidifiers; or simply application of water to eyes, ears, nose, oral cavity, and mucosa of the genitourinary tracts. Extraintestinal infections are primarily superficial infections involving the skin but severe systemic disease may occur in those who are immunologically deficient. The spectrum of microbial agents that can cause such water-related diseases include bacteria, fungi, viruses, and protozoa. Two of the most important recognized agents of water-related extraintestinal infections are bacteria, that is, *Legionella pneumophila*, the cause of Legionnaires' disease, and marine *Vibrio* species that cause wound infections.

Food. A foodborne disease outbreak is defined as an incident in which two or more persons experience a similar illness, usually gastrointestinal, after ingestion of a common food and epi-

Table 10-4. Infectious Agents Associated with Waterborne Disease*

Causal agent	Incubation period	Clinical syndrome
BACTERIAL		
Escherichia coli	6–36 hr	Gastrointestinal syndrome, usually diarrhea
Salmonella species	6–48 hr	Gastrointestinal syndrome, usually diarrhea
Shigella species	12–48 hr	Gastrointestinal syndrome, usually diarrhea
Campylobacter jejuni	2–5 days	Gastrointestinal syndrome, usually diarrhea
Yersinia enterocolitica	3–7 days	Gastrointestinal syndrome, usually diarrhea
PARASITIC		
Giardia lamblia	1–4 weeks	Gastrointestinal syndrome, usually chronic diarrhea, cramps, fatigue, and weight loss
Entamoeba histolytica	2–4 weeks	Gastrointestinal syndrome, variable from acute fulminating dysentery with fever, chills, and bloody stools to mild diarrhea and abdominal cramps
Cryptosporidium	5–21 days	Cholera-like diarrhea, abdominal cramps
VIRAL		
Hepatitis A	2–4 weeks	Fever, nausea, vomiting, dark urine
Norwalk and Norwalk-like agents	24–48 hr	Gastrointestinal syndrome, vomiting, watery diarrhea, abdominal cramps, often headache
Rotavirus	24–72 hr	Gastrointestinal syndrome, vomiting, watery diarrhea, abdominal cramps, often with dehydration
Enterovirus	5–10 days	Other syndromes than gastrointestinal: poliomyelitis, aseptic meningitis, and herpangina

* Heavy metals may also be associated with waterborne disease, but they are not included here.

demiological analysis implicates the food as the source of the illness. Over 60 percent of foodborne disease outbreaks are associated with restaurants; the remainder are associated with foods eaten at home (Table 10-5). Factors that contribute to foodborne illness are (1) improper holding temperatures for food, (2) poor personal hygiene, (3) contaminated equipment used in the processing of food, (4) inadequate cooking, and (5) food obtained from an unsafe source. The microbial agents most frequently implicated in foodborne illness are *Salmonella* species, *Campylobacter* species, *S. aureus*, and *Clostridium perfringens*. They are responsible for nearly 80 percent of the outbreaks in the United States.

Table 10-5. Confirmed Microbial Foodborne Disease Outbreaks, United States, 1987*

Etiological agent	Outbreaks	Cases	Deaths
BACTERIAL			
Bacillus cereus	2	9	0
Brucella	0	0	0
Campylobacter	3	39	0
Clostridium perfringens	2	290	0
Clostridium botulinum	11	18	2
Escherichia coli	0	0	0
Salmonella	52	1846	2
Shigella	9	6494	0
Staphylococcus aureus	1	100	0
Streptococcus group A	1	123	0
Vibrio cholerae 01	0	0	0
Vibrio cholerae non-01	0	0	0
Vibrio parahemolyticus	2	9	0
Yersinia enterocolitica	0	0	0
PARASITIC			
Trichinella spiralis	4	15	0
VIRAL			
Hepatitis A	9	187	0
Norwalk virus	1	365	0

* Note that several agents associated with foodborne disease are listed even though they were not involved in outbreaks in 1987. Foodborne disease may also be caused by chemicals, for example, heavy metals, mushrooms, and contaminated fish, which are not included in this table.
Source: *Foodborne Disease Outbreaks, CDC Surveillance Summaries*, Atlanta: Centers for Disease Control, March 1990.

Campylobacter species are now considered the most frequent cause of bacterial diarrhea in the United States. A major factor responsible for some outbreaks is improper holding temperature. Foodborne disease may be divided into two types: *food infections* and *food poisonings*. Food infections result from the ingestion of microorganisms, such as *Salmonella*, found in the food. Salmonellae produce a toxin in the victim's intestine that causes gastrointestinal symptoms. Food poisonings are the result of ingestion of toxins that were liberated during growth of microorganisms in the food. Microbial growth occurs because the contaminated food was left at an improper holding temperature. *S. aureus*, for example, may be transmitted by food handlers, and if the food is left at a temperature that supports microbial growth the microorganisms multiply and produce a toxin that, if ingested, causes gastrointestinal disease.

In recent years *Listeria monocytogenes* has become established as a foodborne pathogen. This organism is psychrophilic and capable of growth at refrigeration temperatures. *L. monocytogenes* is especially virulent in compromised patients, for example, in those with underlying malignancy or in pregnant women. Neonatal or adult disease can result in meningitis. Stillbirths may also occur in the neonate. Major outbreaks of listeriosis have occurred since 1981 and case-fatality ratios have been high in each outbreak.

Fomites. Inanimate objects (fomites) are also involved in disease transmission. Contamination of inanimate objects is a frequently encountered means of disease transmission in the hospital. Catheters, needles, and other objects may be contaminated by hospital personnel. When these devices come into contact with the patient the contaminating microorganisms may initiate disease (see Chapter 34).

AIR

Microorganisms cannot use air as a reservoir, but they can use it as means of dissemination. Airborne transmission implies that the organisms travel longer distances than in the direct type of transmission between individuals, which usually involves distances of only a few feet. Wind currents, humidity, and other environmental factors influence the distance microorganisms can travel in the wind currents or as vegetative forms that have been aerosolized and carried by currents of air. Many of the fungal diseases, for example, result from the inhalation of spores that contaminate the environment and are carried in the air.

Indoors, microorganisms are also disseminated either in dust or as droplet nuclei. *Dust* is material that has settled to surfaces and is subject to dissemination by air currents or various physical actions (shaking a dust mop, for example). The dust particles may remain suspended in the air for various lengths of time. Some microorganisms such as staphylococci and streptococci can remain viable in dust for up to three months. This is a characteristic that is more common among the gram-positive bacteria than gram-negative bacteria. The cell envelope of gram-positive bacteria is considerably thicker and more resistant to drying and ultraviolet radiation than that of gram-negative bacteria. *Droplet nuclei* are particles of mucus that have been expelled from humans by sneezing or coughing. These mucus particles contain microorganisms and because of their small size (5 μm or smaller) remain suspended in air for long periods of time. Tuberculosis is a disease that is transmitted by droplet nuclei.

Aerosols generated by spraying water into the air (e.g., at water treatment facilities or in humidifiers or water coolers) may also contain microorganisms that are infectious for humans. Legionnaires' disease, for example, is caused by a microorganism whose primary habitat is water and is transmitted to humans by aerosols.

HORIZONTAL VS. VERTICAL TRANSMISSION

Microorganisms must spread from one individual to another if they are to persist and cause disease.

If an individual infected with the measles virus, for example, does not make contact with other individuals, the virus will die in the host. Microorganisms can be spread horizontally or vertically. *Horizontal spread* is the transfer of disease by everyday contact, that is, by air, water, food, contact, or vectors. *Vertical spread* involves transfer of infectious agents from parent to offspring via sperm, ovum, placenta, milk, or direct contact.

Vertical Transmission

The vertical transmission of infectious agents may occur after birth (postnatal), before birth (congenital), or during birth (perinatal). Congenital transmission involves transfer of the microbial agent across the placenta; perinatal infection occurs during passage through the birth canal. The microbial agents associated with congenital and perinatal infections are outlined in Table 10-6. Transmission across the placental membrane results in deposition of the microbial agent into the fetal blood. The infectious agent can then be disseminated to any organ or tissue of the fetus. Transmission during passage through the birth canal results initially in infection of the skin, eyes, or respiratory tract of the infant. Depending on its virulence, the microbial agent may later invade the bloodstream. The infant, after infection, often sheds the microbial agent because of immune tolerance. The infected host may produce antibodies to the infectious agent, but they are not sufficient to neutralize the microorganism. Infections can be devastating to the newborn, resulting in malformations, damage to various organs or tissues, and even death.

Transmission after birth (postnatal) occurs when the parent (1) experiences a primary infection at or just after the birth; (2) experiences a reactivation of a latent infection (some persistent viruses, for example, are activated during pregnancy); or (3) has been shedding virus continuously during pregnancy. Hepatitis virus, for example, is carried in the blood of the mother and is transmitted during or shortly after birth. A

Table 10-6. Microbial Agents Associated with Congenital or Perinatal Disease in Infants

Agent	Consequences of infection
CONGENITAL INFECTION	
Cytomegalovirus	Hepatitis, jaundice, congenital heart disease, mental retardation
Rubella virus	Abortion, congenital malformation, deafness, cataracts, heart defects, encephalitis
Poxvirus (smallpox)	Abortion, stillbirth, congenital smallpox
Varicella-zoster virus	Low birth weight, bilateral cataracts, atrophic limbs, mental retardation, congenital varicella
Vaccinia virus	Abortion, generalized vaccinia
Poliovirus	Congenital poliomyelitis
Measles virus	Stillbirth, congenital measles
Mumps virus	Abortion, endocardial fibroelastosis
Herpes simplex virus	Abortion, excessive brain damage, hepatoadrenal necrosis
Hepatitis B virus	Neonatal hepatitis, stillbirth, abortion
Echovirus	Hydrocephalus and neurological sequelae, jaundice (most infections are asymptomatic or mild)
Coxsackievirus B	Myocarditis and central nervous system involvement
Arbovirus	Congenital encephalitis
Treponema pallidum (bacterium)	Stillbirth, abortion, saddle nose, notched teeth, central nervous system involvement
Toxoplasma gondii (protozoan)	Stillbirth, hydrocephalus, mental retardation
PERINATAL INFECTION	
Herpes simplex virus	Localized infection of oral cavity, skin, eye
Neisseria gonorrhoeae (bacterium)	Infections of the eye (ophthalmia neonatorum)
Chlamydia trachomatis (bacterium)	Inclusion conjunctivitis
Streptococcus group B (bacterium)	Pneumonia, septicemia, meningitis

mother who sheds microorganisms in the milk during lactation represents one of the most common means of postnatal transmission. Other vehicles of transmission include feces, urine, saliva, blood, and contact with skin and mucosa.

Transmission to the offspring via the germ line is also possible. Ova and sperm may be infected with microbial agents such as viruses. These agents, provided they do no harm to ova or sperm, could conceivably be transferred to the developing embryo. This type of transmission has been observed in animals. The mouse mammary tumor virus, for example, is transmitted via sperm in some laboratory strains. Viruses, such as the herpes simplex virus, cytomegalovirus, hepatitis virus, Marburg virus, and Ebola virus, have been found in human semen although they

have not been found to be involved in germ-line transmission. The established examples of germ-line transmission are the oncoviruses, whose genome becomes part of the host's genome during infection. Human sex cells can transmit the virus to the offspring.

PATTERNS OF DISEASE IN THE COMMUNITY

ENDEMIC, EPIDEMIC, AND SPORADIC DISEASE

Infectious diseases occur in a population with a particular frequency, which may be defined as *endemic*, *epidemic*, or *sporadic*. To determine which term applies to the disease in question one must have some idea of the history of the disease in the community. The history of the disease can be evaluated by noting when the disease has occurred and the number of persons involved. *Endemic* disease implies that the disease continues in a specified population without interruption. Cholera, for example, is a disease endemic to Southeast Asia. Diseases become endemic when an equilibrium has been established between the host and the parasite. One characteristic of endemic disease is that many individuals in the community have clinically inapparent disease. An influx of persons, for example, from a geographical area where the disease is not endemic represents a highly susceptible population. Endemic disease may also be associated with animal populations, where it is referred to as *enzootic disease*. An outbreak of 2 to 3 cases of diphtheria every 8 to 10 years exemplifies a sporadic disease.

When the number of new cases of disease in a defined period of time rises above its normal endemic level, we speak of the disease as being *epidemic*. The epidemic usually begins with a sudden occurrence of disease in those who are susceptible and who come into contact with an infected source. Epidemics involve specific populations that may vary from a single site such as a hospital, to a city, to large geographic areas that may encompass the globe. The term *pandemic* is used to denote world-wide epidemics.

Sporadic diseases are those that occur in such an irregular pattern that their frequency cannot be calculated. For example, an individual may develop a disease after the fracture of a limb.

INCIDENCE AND PREVALENCE

The occurrence of disease in a population may be quantified by determining its incidence and prevalence. *Incidence* refers to the number of new cases in a particular population within a specifically defined time period. For example, the incidence may be expressed as the number of new cases per 10,00 or 100,000 individuals in the population per year. The incidence may also be referred to as *morbidity rate*. The number of individuals who have died as a result of disease in a specific time is referred to as the *mortality rate*. A constant check on morbidity and mortality rates by epidemiologists helps health care officials to ward off future outbreaks and to warn the public of how to avoid disease. *Prevalence* refers to the total number of cases (both new and old) of disease in a defined population within a specified time. It includes newly detected cases of disease as well as those earlier cases whose symptoms are still clinically apparent. If an individual had a disease that lasted eight weeks, he or she would be counted once in an incidence survey. If two prevalence studies were performed in that eight-week period the infected patient would be counted both times.

HERD IMMUNITY

The rate at which an epidemic spreads and the number of individuals involved is determined by the factors that affect the communicability of the disease and the immunity of the population. Many diseases are highly communicable because of the manner in which they are spread. Respiratory diseases, for example, often spread rapidly, particularly in confined populations, such as in classrooms, military barracks, hospitals, and institutions for the infirm. Foodborne and waterborne diseases occur with great rapidity and involve large numbers of individuals because the victims have been exposed to a common source and because the incubation period is often very short. There are instances when exposure to a common source does not reveal itself as an epidemic because the incubation period for the disease is long and variable. Hepatitis B, for example, has an incubation period of several weeks. Thus the number of cases of hepatitis that have been defined are spread out over several weeks.

With this type of disease it is difficult to identify the source and thus control the spread of disease.

The number of individuals who develop disease during an epidemic is also related to the immunity of the host. An individual who, by either passive or active means, is immune to the disease removes himself or herself as a potential source of infection to others (unless the person is a carrier). When many immune individuals are present in a community there exists what is called *herd immunity*. The herd immunity concept is based on the relative number of immune and susceptible individuals in a population. Immune individuals act as a barrier to the spread of infectious agents from infected persons to susceptible individuals. Even though a highly communicable disease may cause an epidemic, many nonimmune individuals will be protected because of the unlikelihood of their coming in contact with an infected person. One of the values of vaccine immunization is that enough individuals will be protected from disease to prevent its rapid spread to those in the population who have not received the vaccine.

DESCRIPTIVE EPIDEMIOLOGY

The routine surveillance of disease in a community to show its distribution is called *descriptive epidemiology*. Descriptive epidemiology takes into account (1) host factors that may contribute to susceptibility to disease, (2) the geographical areas where the host came in contact with the infectious agent, and (3) the time of the appearance of disease.

Host Factors

Many host factors, including age, sex, race, underlying disease, and immunization status, contribute to the susceptibility to disease. These variables are discussed in Chapter 9. All of them must be considered in evaluating the development of disease in a community.

Place

Knowing the place where contact between host and infectious agent occurs is very important in evaluating diseases in a community. If one is able to determine the site where contact has been made, measures can be taken to break the chain of transmission. Determining the place of contact between host and infectious agent is usually much easier in a confined environment such as a hospital than in the community, where infected individuals may be spread out.

Time

Time in relationship to the disease process can be viewed from different perspectives. One may observe seasonal trends, month-to-month variations, or long-term trends that span several years. Seasonal patterns are important for determining in which seasons diseases are more likely to occur. Respiratory diseases, for example, are at a considerably higher level in the fall and winter than in the summer months. Foodborne diseases, on the other hand, occur more frequently during the summer months because the ambient temperatures are higher, which permits microorganisms contaminating food to multiply rapidly. Long-term evaluations of epidemiologic patterns have been important in determining the periodicity of diseases such as influenza A. Influenza A reaches epidemic proportions every two to three years. One strain of the influenza A virus is able to bring about sufficient immunity in a community after an epidemic, but then the virus spontaneously changes the chemical nature of its surface molecules (antigenic drift). The new strain is not recognized by the immune system of those who developed immunity to the first strain. Thus the entire population becomes susceptible to the new strain of virus (see Chapter 31 for more details on viral surface changes during infection).

An epidemic can be represented graphically by plotting the number of cases of disease against time. The time scale will vary according to the incubation period of the disease. The epidemic curve begins with the *index case*, that is, the first case observed in the disease outbreak. The upslope of the curve is influenced by the incubation period, the number of exposed individuals, and the rapidity with which transmission occurs. The downslope of the curve is usually more gradual than the upslope because of the decreasing numbers of individuals susceptible to disease. Epidemics that are the result of contact with a contaminated material such as food or water are called *common-source epidemics*. In a common-source epidemic the epidemic curve rises sharply and then gradually falls off (Fig. 13-1). Epidemics that arise from person-to-person contact are called *propagated* or *contact-spread epidemics*. The epidemic curve in propagated epidemics rises slowly, has a flatter peak than the common-source epidemic, and then falls off gradually (Fig. 10-3).

LABORATORY TECHNIQUES IN EPIDEMIOLOGY

Epidemiological investigations, as we now know, provide us with valuable information that can lead to the breaking of the chain of transmission of disease and reduce its incidence. During an epidemiological investigation the symptoms of disease are often sufficient to establish the cause of disease. The causal agent of disease is also isolated in many epidemics to determine the

Fig. 10-3. Comparison of common-source epidemic and a propagated epidemic. Food poisoning resulting from contamination of a food eaten by a group is an example of a common-source epidemic. Influenza, which is spread by contact between individuals, is an example of a propagated epidemic.

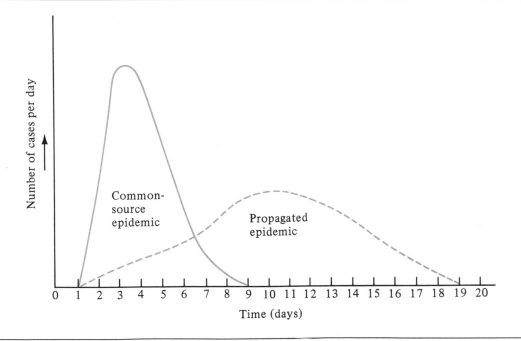

source of disease. Many strains of an organism may exist in a community—some strains may be involved in the epidemic, but others may be non-epidemic. The problem is to separate the epidemic strains from the nonepidemic ones. *Escherichia coli*, for example, may be involved in an epidemic of urinary tract infections. The *E. coli* strains isolated from the infected patients may be identified by several laboratory procedures. Since *E. coli* is harbored by all humans we must find a property that is unique to the epidemic strains and not to the strains found in the healthy population. A biochemical, serological, or other type of test may differentiate the two types of strains. These differentiating characteristics are extremely important not only for determining the source of the epidemic; they also have practical value. The bacterium causing pneumonia, *Streptococcus pneumoniae*, for example, produces a capsule. Many strains of *S. pneumoniae* exist; these can be separated on the basis of the antigenic characteristics of the capsule. Only a few strains, however, are regularly found during epidemics. To produce an effective vaccine using capsular antigens it is necessary to know which strains are the most frequently associated with disease in the community.

The principal laboratory techniques employed in epidemiological investigations are biotyping, serotyping, bacteriocin typing, antibiograms, and bacteriophage typing. Sometimes more than one technique must be used to obtain suitable results.

BIOTYPING

Biotyping refers to laboratory techniques used to identify a biological property, usually a biochemical property. The normal biochemical tests used in the clinical laboratory to identify a microorganism are sufficient for determining genus and species. Additional tests, however, may be required to separate the epidemic from nonepidemic strains. There may not be sufficient biochemical tests to differentiate strains, and tests based on nonbiochemical properties may therefore be required.

SEROTYPING

Serotyping makes use of antigenic differences between strains. These differences may be flagellar, cell wall, or capsular antigens, depending on the organism. Serotyping is commonly used for identifying *Salmonella* and *Shigella* strains and enteropathogenic strains of *E. coli* associated with diarrhea. M protein serotyping is also useful in the epidemiology of glomerulonephritis caused by strains of *Streptococcus pyogenes*. Capsular swelling (quellung reaction) has been useful in the serotyping of *Klebsiella* species. Many laboratories do not have the antisera for typing some species, so the specimens must be sent to a reference laboratory.

ANTIBIOGRAMS

Antibiograms are tests used to determine a microorganism's susceptibility to antibiotics or other antimicrobials. Antibiograms are particularly useful in evaluating hospital epidemics because the overall susceptibility patterns of hospital-associated microorganisms are known. Antibiograms are more reliable when the acquired resistance of the organism is due to a chromosomal trait. Chromosomal traits are more stable than plasmid-associated traits since the latter can be easily transferred to other microorganisms via conjugation. The susceptibility patterns for members of the Enterobacteriaceae are generally less reliable because of the ease with which gram-negative enteric bacilli transfer R plasmids by conjugation. Antibiograms are also more useful in common-source outbreaks than in propagated epidemics because in the former each patient receives the infectious agent from the same source and there is less likelihood of the infectious agent's acquiring new resistance traits. When there is person-to-person spread there is a greater chance for conjugational transfer among microorganisms and thus the acquisition of new resistance traits.

PHAGE TYPING

Bacterial viruses are very specific in respect to the hosts they infect, and this specificity can be used as an epidemiological tool. The basis of the test is to determine the susceptibility of the isolated clinical bacterial strains to infections by various bacteriophage sets. Phage typing systems have been internationally standardized for some bacterial species. Phage typing has one of its widest applications in the identification of strains of *Staphylococcus aureus*. The laboratory procedure involves spreading the staphylococcal strain onto an agar plate surface so as to produce confluent growth (Fig. 10-4). The plate is marked off into small squares—a grid—and a drop of each phage type is placed in an individual square that is appropriately identified. Plaques (holes) in the bacterial lawn appear on the squares, where the applied phage type caused lysis of the staphylococcal strain. A phage typing investigation of this sort might reveal that the staphylococci, for example, which are isolated from a surgical wound, have the same phage pattern as staphylococci isolated from the attending physician, from surgical technicians, or from attending nurses.

Phage typing has also been used in epidemiological studies involving *Pseudomonas aeruginosa*, *Vibrio cholerae*, *Salmonella typhi*, and mycobacteria.

Fig 10-4. Phage typing of staphylococci. An agar plate is marked off in squares. The plate is then streaked with *S. aureus* and allowed to dry. Specific phage suspensions, corresponding to the strains indicated on the right are placed in the appropriate squares. After being allowed to dry again, the plate is incubated for 12-18 hours. The plate on the left shows confluent growth except where plaques appear in the squares corresponding to phage preparation 7, 42E, and 47.

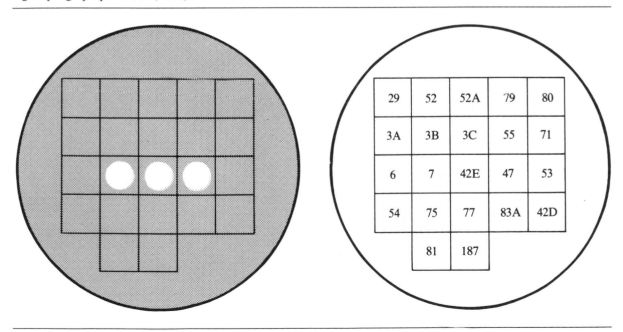

BACTERIOCIN TYPING

Bacteriocins are antimicrobial-like proteins produced primarily by strains of gram-negative enteric species. The bacteriocins are active against strains of the same or closely related species. The test is usually performed by making a single streak of a known bacteriocin-producing strain on an agar plate. The clinical isolates (about six per plate) are then streaked at right angles to the known bacteriocin-producing strain. The plate is incubated overnight, and during this period bacteriocin diffuses into the agar. The plate is then read for growth inhibition (Fig. 10-5). Bacteriocin

Fig. 10-5. Bacteriocin typing. Colicin sensitivity of strains of *Escherichia coli*. The macrocolony of *E. coli* in the center of the plate is an active colicin producer. As it is produced, the colicin diffuses out from the colony into the medium. This colony was grown for 24 hours, after which each of the four quarters of the plate was seeded with strains of *E. coli* with various degrees of sensitivity to the colicin. After incubation, zones of inhibition proportional to the sensitivity of the strain developed. Within the zones, growth of colicin-resistant colonies can be seen. (From L. E. Hawker and A. H. Linton [Eds.], *Microorganisms: Function, Form and Environment* [2nd ed.]. London: Edward Arnold, 1979.)

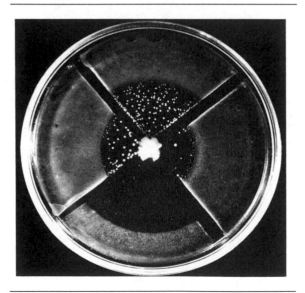

typing has been used to identify *Serratia marcescens*, *E. coli*, *Shigella* species, and *Proteus mirabilis*. Bacteria may also be typed by their ability to inhibit indicator strains. This is a procedure used for typing *Pseudomonas aeruginosa* strains.

OTHER METHODS

Plasmid Profiles

Sometimes the more routinely used typing systems are not applicable to the identification of some microbial species or, when used, do not provide results suitable for differentiation. Under these circumstances the epidemiologist must use other techniques. One of the newly developed techniques for epidemiologic investigation is plasmid characterization. Plasmids are infectious and carry many important bacterial determinants, including antibiotic resistance, toxin formation, bacteriocin production, heavy metal resistance, and metabolic enzyme activity. Techniques involving plasmids fall into two categories, direct and indirect.

Direct plasmid analysis involves hybridization of plasmid DNA from different strains, which allows the quantitative assessment of base sequence homology. Indirect techniques include agarose gel electrophoresis and restriction endonuclease analysis. In the agarose gel technique the clinical isolates are cultivated and lysed, and then the supernatant is electrophoresed on agarose gel. The gel is washed and stained by ethidium bromide, transluminated with ultraviolet light, and photographed. Plasmid size is determined by comparing gel migration distances (Fig. 10-6) of unknown plasmids with those of plasmids of known molecular size. Plasmids of the same size may have entirely different base sequences, and these differences can be detected by using restriction endonucleases. Restriction endonucleases cleave double-stranded DNA at specific recognition sites and produce a number of plasmid fragments. If two plasmids are of the same size and yield identical patterns of fragments on

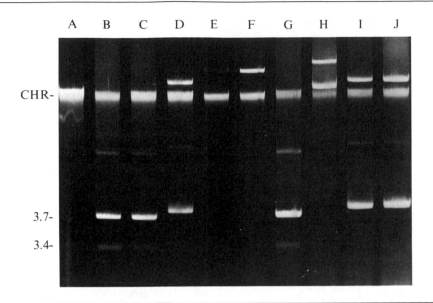

Fig. 10-6. Agarose gel electrophoresis of *Salmonella newport* from isolated cases in Pennsylvania and New Jersey, June–August 1981. Lanes B, C, and G represent the epidemic strains. (CHR = chromosome band.) (From L. W. Riley et al., *J. Infect. Dis.* 148:12, 1983.)

restriction endonuclease analysis, they are assumed to be identical or nearly so. If the plasmids of equal size have different sequences, then different fragments will be produced from endonuclease digestion.

Restriction endonuclease-fingerprinting can also be applied to chromosomal DNA. This technique has been used to differentiate strains of some bacteria such as *Vibrio cholerae* and *Campylobacter* species. Typing of herpes simplex viruses is now performed by using restriction endonuclease fingerprinting.

DNA Probes

DNA probes are specific single-stranded DNA sequences derived from one microorganism (*the probe*). The probe DNA represents a specific microbial feature that distinguishes it from other microorganisms. Once the DNA probe is isolated it is reproduced in large quantities by cloning it in *E. coli* (Fig. 10-7). The DNA sequences are re-isolated from *E. coli* and then labeled (with iso-

tope or enzyme). The labeled probe is now capable of hybridizing with either a DNA or RNA strand of complementary sequences. The DNA from the sample or clinical material is denatured to isolate single-stranded DNA and attached to a filter. The DNA probe is passed over the filter and this allows hybridization between DNA single strands to occur with the formation of double-stranded duplexes. Unreacted single-stranded DNA is washed off the filter. The specificity of DNA probes has been used to differentiate toxin-producing *E. coli* strains from strains that do not produce toxin. Many new developments are occurring in DNA probe technology and the student is referred to the readings at the end of the chapter.

Polymerase Chain Reaction

One of the outgrowths of in vitro gene amplification has been the development of the polymerase chain reaction (PCR). PCR can be used to amplify genes and culture may not be required.

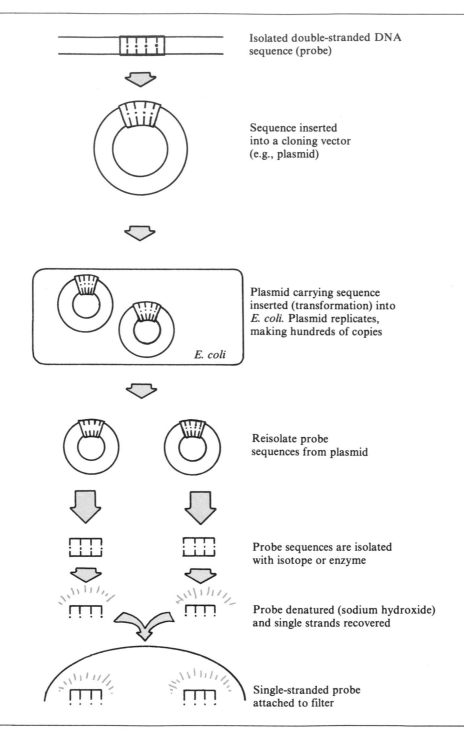

Isolated double-stranded DNA
sequence (probe)

Sequence inserted
into a cloning vector
(e.g., plasmid)

Plasmid carrying sequence
inserted (transformation) into
E. coli. Plasmid replicates,
making hundreds of copies

Reisolate probe
sequences from plasmid

Probe sequences are isolated
with isotope or enzyme

Probe denatured (sodium hydroxide)
and single strands recovered

Single-stranded probe
attached to filter

Fig. 10-7. Cloning and isolation of DNA probes.

It allows amplification of a single copy of a DNA sequence by more than a millionfold. PCR is based on the repetition of 3 steps that are conducted in sequence (Fig. 10-8).

Step I   Denaturation of the target double-stranded DNA (the template). Denaturation is accomplished by high temperatures that dissociate the complementary DNA strands. Known primers that flank the target sequence are then produced. The primers constitute a pair of synthetic oligonucleotides that flank the DNA segment to be amplified. The primers are complementary to opposite strands of the target sequence. The sequence of the primers is determined by the sequence of the DNA to be amplified. The primers are usually 20 to 30 bases in length and are not complementary to each other.

Step II   The primers are annealed to the template when the temperature is lowered to 40 to 50°C. Because the primers are in excess, the formation of primer-template duplexes occurs in preference to the reassociation of two complementary template strands.

Step III   By adding DNA polymerase to the reaction there is extension of the annealed primers. Primer extension doubles the number of DNA molecules that were present initially.

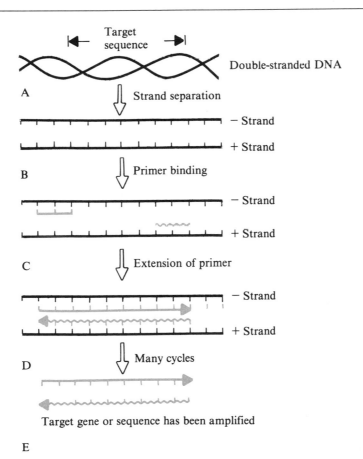

Fig. 10-8. Polymerase chain reaction (PCR). See text for details.

The combination of these three steps (denaturation, annealing, and extension) makes up a cycle. As each cycle is repeated the amount of DNA doubles. Usually the cycle is repeated 20 to 40 times before the amplified product can be detected by gel electrophoresis or DNA hybridization with a ^{32}P-labeled probe.

PCR has provided a revolution in genetic sequencing and will have profound effects on the work of genome mappers (for example, the human genome mapping and sequencing project recently initiated), forensic scientists, AIDS researchers (detecting the DNA of HIV in infants), medical diagnosticians, and others. It is currently being evaluated for detecting human papilloma virus in order to determine the relationship of virus to cervical cancer. Another important role of PCR will be in detecting genes associated with genetic diseases in humans, that is, beta-thalassemia, hemophilia, Tay-Sachs disease, phenylketonuria, Duchenne muscular dystrophy, and cases of cystic fibrosis.

SUMMARY

1. Epidemiology is the study of determinants, occurrence, and distribution of health and disease in a population.

2. Humans respond to infectious agents in different ways depending on the traits of the microorganism and the immunological state of the host. Some infections are subclinical or inapparent. Most human infections are acute, that is, the symptoms are intense but quickly subside and the microbe is eliminated.

3. Acute diseases can be divided into stages: (1) incubation period, (2) prodromal period, (3) acute period, and (4) convalescent period. One of the most frequent characteristics of infection is fever. Fever helps to enhance the inflammatory response and prevent microbial multiplication, but fever also has detrimental effects to the host.

4. Another characteristic of many infections is rash formation. Rashes can be divided into four major types: macular, papular, vesicular, and pustular. Other symptoms of disease include cough in respiratory infections and diarrhea or dysentery in intestinal infection.

5. Chronic diseases represent a type of persistent infection in which the microbe avoids the normal immunological responses of the host.

6. In order for microorganisms to survive and gain access to a host they must have a site for multiplication, that is, a reservoir, and they must have a site for transmission to the host, that is, a source. Sources may be animate or inanimate objects.

7. Reservoirs may be animate and include humans, animals, and insects. Inanimate reservoirs include soil, water, or food. Some human reservoirs act as carriers, that is, they shed infectious microorganisms without showing symptoms. Carriers may be of two types: convalescent and healthy.

8. Diseases that occur primarily in animals but can be transmitted to humans are called zoonoses. Insects behave as vectors in the transmission of infectious agents to humans. Mechanical insect vectors are not involved in the life cycle of the infectious microbe but biological vectors serve as host and reservoir of the infectious agent.

9. Microorganisms can be spread by direct or indirect contact. Direct contact includes handshaking, kissing, sneezing, coughing, and sexual contact. Indirect contact implies transmission of microbes from human to human via objects such as food, water, or inanimate objects (fomites).

10. Waterborne diseases in the United States are frequently associated with community and noncommunity water systems. *Giardia lamblia* is the most frequently recovered pathogen. Most foodborne diseases are associated with restaurants, with *Salmonella* species, *Staphylococcus aureus*, and *Clostridium perfringens* the most frequently implicated microbial agents.

11. Air acts as an avenue for transmission of infectious microorganisms. Spores from the soil are easily disseminated by air and many fungal diseases are spread by this means. Indoors, microorganisms are disseminated in dust or as droplet nuclei. Aerosols generated by humidifiers, etc. also carry infectious microorganisms.

12. Microorganisms can be spread horizontally or vertically. Horizontal transmission implies spread by everyday contact, that is, air, food, water, direct or indirect contact, and vectors. Vertical transmission implies spread from parent to offspring via sperm, ova, etc. Vertical spread may occur after birth (postnatal), before birth (congenital), or during birth (perinatal).

13. The patterns of disease in a community may be referred to as endemic, epidemic, or sporadic. *Endemic* implies continuous presence of the disease. *Epidemic* refers to levels of disease above the endemic level. Global epidemics are referred to as pandemics. *Sporadic* diseases do not occur with any regularity.

14. Occurrence of disease in a population may be quantified by determining the incidence and prevalence. *Incidence,* or morbidity, refers to the number of new cases of disease in a specific population within a defined time period. *Prevalence* refers to the number of new and existing cases of disease in a certain time frame.

15. The rate at which a disease spreads is to some extent influenced by the number of immune individuals at the time of the epidemic. They represent a barrier to spread of disease, a concept called *herd immunity*.

16. Descriptive epidemiology uses surveillance measures that take into account (1) host factors that affect the spread of disease, (2) the place of contact with the infectious agent, and (3) the time of the appearance of disease.

17. Several laboratory techniques can be used to differentiate epidemic from nonepidemic strains of microbial species: biotyping, serotyping, bacteriophage typing, bacteriocin typing, antibiograms, plasmid profiles, DNA probes, and polymerase chain reactions.

QUESTIONS FOR STUDY

Match the various periods or conditions associated with the disease process on the left with their definitions on the right.

1. Chronic disease

2. Convalescent period

3. Incubation period

4. Acute disease

5. Macular rash

6. Prodromal period

7. Papular rash

A. Symptomatic period warning the onset of disease

B. Time required for infectious agent to cause symptoms in the infected host

C. Persistence of the infectious agent in the host

D. A disease that runs its symptomatic course and ends with total recovery

E. A flat red lesion

F. Period of recovery from disease

G. A firm, elevated rash

H. A lesion containing pus

Select the best response or responses for each of the following:

8. All of the following are considered reservoirs of infectious agents except
   A. Food
   B. Water
   C. Soil
   D. Air

9. Which of the following would be considered a mechanism of horizontal transmission?
   A. Infectious agent is transmitted from mother's milk to infant.
   B. Infectious agent is transmitted to infant in utero.
   C. Infant acquires infection by inhalation of contaminated aerosol generated by the father.
   D. Infectious agent is transmitted to infant following ingestion of contaminated bottle formula.

Fill in the blank:

10. _____ are diseases of animals that are transmitted to humans.

11. Microorganisms that cause persistent infections are often characterized by their ability to live as _____ parasites.

12. Invertebrate animals that serve as host and reservoir of infectious agents are referred to as _____.

13. Inanimate objects other than food or water that may be important in transmission of infectious agents are called _____

14. A disease that is permanently present in a population without interruption is called a(an) _____ disease.

15. Tests that determine a microorganism's susceptibility to antibiotics are called _____.

16. The first case observed in a disease outbreak is called the _____ case.

ADDITIONAL READINGS

Archer, D. L., and Young, F. E. Contemporary issues: Diseases with a food vector. *Clin. Microbiol. Revs.* 1(4):377,1988.

Advances in molecular epidemiology (several articles devoted to epidemiologic methods). *Rev. Infect. Dis.* 8(5):681,1986.

Cliff, A., and Haggett, P. Island epidemics. *Sci. Amer.* 250(5):138,1984.

Henneken, C., and Buring, J. *Epidemiology in Medicine.* Boston: Little, Brown, 1988.

Mayer, L. W. Use of plasmid profiles in epidemiologic surveillance of disease outbreaks and tracing the transmission of antibiotic resistance. *Clin. Microbiol. Revs.* 1(2):228,1988.

Rothman, K. J. *Modern Epidemiology.* Boston: Little, Brown, 1986.

Tenover, F. C. Diagnostic deoxyribonucleic acid probes for infectious disease. *Clin. Microbiol. Revs.* 1(1):82,1988.

Zinsser, H. *Rats, Lice, and History.* Boston: Bantam Books, 1935.

IV. IMMUNOLOGY

11. NONSPECIFIC RESISTANCE

OBJECTIVES

To differentiate between nonspecific host resistance, innate immunity, and acquired immunity by comparing specificity, effectiveness, and duration of protection

To describe the systems, cell types, and soluble factors involved in nonspecific resistance and to explain their roles in resistance

To describe the mononuclear phagocyte system with emphasis on the important functional roles of macrophages

To discuss phagocytosis with reference to the types of cells involved, the structures involved in the process of destruction of the ingested material, and the oxidative and nonoxidative mechanisms involved in the killing and digestion of the ingested material; to identify in the discussion phagosome, phagolysosome, respiratory burst, myeloperoxidase

To discuss the features of inflammation, especially as they pertain to resistance, and to distinguish between acute and chronic inflammation

To discuss the interferons, particularly in their role of nonspecific resistance to virus infection

In Chapter 9 host resistance and immunity were cited as factors that determine whether an individual who had been exposed to an infectious agent would suffer an infection. Resistance and immunity to infectious agents and other foreign substances take three forms (Table 11-1) described below.

1. Nonspecific host resistance. The principal elements here are the integumentary system, which protects the body surfaces, and the tissue elements such as the phagocytes, which protect against those agents that have penetrated the integument and have entered the tissues.

2. Innate immunity. In innate immunity, there

Table 11-1. Types of Protection Against Microorganisms

Type of protection	Source of protection	Protection available	Specificity	Level of protection
Non-specific host resistance	Integumentary factors; tissue elements (e.g. phagocytes, antibacterial substances)	Immediate	None (non-antigen specific)	Variable
Innate immunity (nonsusceptibility)	Hereditarily governed factors (e.g., lack of appropriate receptors for microorganisms)	Immediate	High (non-antigen specific)	Absolute
Acquired (adaptive) immunity	Antibodies; effector T cells	Days to weeks—induction period required in primary immune response; prompt—in secondary immune response	High (antigen specific)	Variable

is a species-specific nonsusceptibility to certain microorganisms. Humans, for example, suffer natural infections of meningococcal meningitis or gonorrhea, whereas other animals do not; humans do not contract canine distemper. Species specificity is determined by anatomical and physiological properties governed by heredity—such as body temperature and the availability of appropriate cell receptors for microorganisms—and not by antigenic specificity; that is, the immune system proper is not involved. Alternative terms for innate immunity are genetic immunity, constitutional immunity, and natural immunity.

3. Acquired (adaptive) immunity. Acquired immunity results from the interactions between the immune system and antigens. Antigens are agents such as bacteria or substances that mostly are foreign to the body and that have certain characteristics to be described in the next chapter. The interactions result in immune system products, namely, antibodies and effector lymphocytes, which are specific for the antigens. The immune system products, when they subsequently react with the same antigen, are instrumental in destroying, eliminating, or neutralizing the antigen in most cases; the reaction, however, may be harmful, as occurs in allergies. The immune system proper is the subject of the three following chapters.

INTERNAL NONSPECIFIC DEFENSES

Once foreign agents penetrate the first-line external barriers such as the skin and the mucosal surfaces, as described in Chapter 9, containment is largely through the interactions of certain elements of the blood and the reactions of the blood vascular system, the lymphatic system, the mononuclear phagocyte system, and tissue factors. The reactions of these elements are best evident in the inflammatory response, which can be evoked by almost any foreign substance. Phagocytic cells of the blood and tissues have the crucial defensive function of ingesting and destroying foreign substances. It should be understood that most of the systems, factors, cells, and responses that are to be described here under nonspecific resistance are also involved in the acquired immune responses that will be described in the next chapters.

THE BLOOD

Besides distributing oxygen and nutrients and channeling wastes, the blood serves as a source, and a means of conveyance, of cellular and fluid elements that are important in nonspecific resistance and in immunity. The cellular and fluid elements are not only operative in the blood but also readily enter the tissues under a variety of conditions, for example, in response to the presence of microorganisms in the tissues.

Cellular Elements of the Blood

The cellular elements of the blood include *erythrocytes, granulocytes, lymphocytes, monocytes*, and *platelets (thrombocytes)* (Fig. 11-1). The blood granulocytes are subdivided into *neutrophils, eosinophils*, and *basophils*. The differentiation is based on developmental, morphological, and staining characteristics. The granules are aggregates of hydrolytic enzymes and other active degradative factors (see under Phagocytes).

Neutrophils. The neutrophils, also referred to as microphages or *polymorphonuclear cells* (the latter abbreviated to *PMNs* or *PMNLs*), are the most numerous of the white blood cells. They and the macrophages are the principal phagocytic cells of the body. Neutrophils appear to have a few major functions other than phagocytosis. They reach and attack foreign materials first. They are incapable of a sustained effort because they have little renewable energy and so they soon succumb in battle. Recently, neutrophils

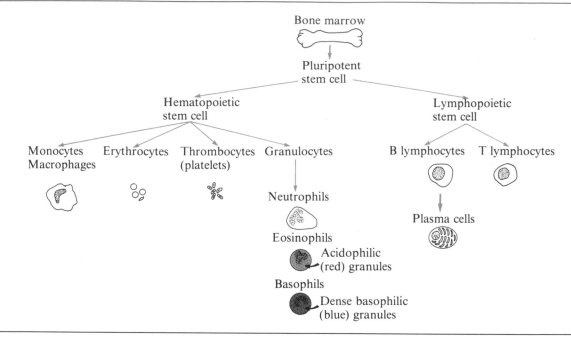

Fig. 11-1. Cell types involved in resistance and immunity.

have been described as a source of endogenous mammalian peptide antibiotics (see Boxed Essay, p. 267).

Eosinophils. Eosinophils are abundant in certain allergic reactions and in some infections that are caused by animal parasites. The granules in the cytoplasm contain basic proteins that are implicated in diverse biological activities. *Major basic protein* (MBP) and eosinophil cationic protein (ECP) are toxic to parasites. It was believed for many years that eosinophils moderated allergic reactions. Indications now are that the basic proteins are the principal mediators of damage to the respiratory epithelium in asthma and that they are involved in the pathophysiology of other hypersensitivity diseases.

Basophils. Basophils resemble mast cells (see later, this chapter) because both have receptors on their surfaces for the Fc portion of the IgE class of immunoglobulin. Both contain mediators

that affect blood vessels and smooth muscles and mediators that intensify inflammation.

Lymphocytes. Lymphocytes are the second most numerous cell type of the blood. They are the circulating cell type in the lymph, and they densely populate the thymus, the spleen, and lymph nodes. The role of lymphocytes in nonspecific resistance is not clearly understood, even though they are a prominent cell type in chronic inflammation. Lymphocytes have the central role in immunity and hypersensitivity, as the next three chapters will show.

Monocytes. Blood monocytes are immature macrophages that migrate from the circulation into the tissues, where they enlarge and differentiate into macrophages.

Platelets (Thrombocytes). Platelets are small, cell-like structures that do not contain a nucleus. They have several roles in hemostasis (the stop-

DEFENSINS: NATURAL PEPTIDE ANTIBIOTICS PRODUCED BY HUMANS AND ANIMALS

Antibiotics generally are thought of as being produced by fungi and bacteria. Defensins are a newly defined family of broad-spectrum antibiotic peptides found in the leukocytes of humans and other mammals. Defensins comprise a group of similar carbohydrate-free peptides, containing 29 to 34 amino acids. Each defensin includes six cysteine residues that form three characteristic intramolecular disulfide bonds. Human neutrophils contain four defensins: human neutrophil protein (HNP)-1, -2, -3, and -4. Together, these four defensins constitute 30 to 50 percent of the total protein in the human neutrophil's azurophilic granules, where they are strategically located for extracellular secretion or for delivery to phagocytic vacuoles. Defensin-positive neutrophil cells, for example, are found within blood capillaries adjacent to the air spaces in human lung tissue. Macrophages constitute the lung's first line of cellular defense against inhaled microorganisms, but neutrophils readily enter air spaces to protect the lung when infection occurs.

Although defensins are most prominent in neutrophils, at least two rabbit defensins are synthesized in alveolar macrophages. Defensin-like molecules are abundant in preparations of murine small intestine and are not limited to mammals. Certain insect larvae contain defensin-like molecules in their hemolymph (body fluid).

The microbial targets susceptible to mammalian defensins include a variety of gram-positive and -negative bacteria, fungi, and certain viruses. Experimentally human defensin HNP-1 kills a smooth strain of *Escherichia coli* by sequentially affecting the permeability of the outer and inner membranes. The bacteria have to be under conditions that support growth or active metabolism to be susceptible to HNP-1.

Defensins express biological properties other than antimicrobial activity. They exert potent but nonselective cytotoxic activity in vitro against various actively metabolizing human and mouse tumor cells. They may play an important role in cell differentiation and function. They exert selective in vitro chemotactic activity for blood monocytes.

Perhaps future therapeutic agents will be patterned after endogenous antibiotics such as defensins.

Excerpted from R. I. Lehrer, T. Ganz, and M. E. Selsted, *ASM News* 56:315, 1990.

ping of bleeding). They seal off breaks in blood vessels by aggregating where the continuity of the endothelium (the cell layer that lines blood vessels) has been broken. Platelets help collect the 13 blood clotting factors and facilitate their interactions. Once a clot is formed, platelets cause contraction of the clot to prevent obstruction of the vessel. Like basophils and mast cells, platelets contain mediators that are important in allergic reactions.

FLUID ELEMENT OF THE BLOOD— PLASMA

The fluid portion of uncoagulated blood is called *plasma*. Plasma contains many substances: proteins, carbohydrates, lipids, water, hormones, salts, and gases. The principal proteins are albumin, fibrinogen, and globulins. Fibrinogen is converted into fibrin in blood coagulation and in inflammation. Globulins have their greatest relevance in acquired immunity; as immunoglobulins, they function as the antibodies of the so-called humoral immunity. Various complement (see Chapter 12) components also are globulins. When plasma exits from the bloodstream into the tissues in an inflammatory response, it leads to *edema* (swelling). Edema fluid facilitates the emigration and mobility of phagocytes, conveys antibodies into the tissues, and dilutes toxic elements. Edema fluid in the tissues may lead to blockage and blanching because of the swelling.

THE LYMPHATIC SYSTEM

The lymphatic system consists of lymph vessels, lymph, and lymph nodes.

Lymphatic Vessels and Lymph
The lymphatic vessels are widely distributed in the body, especially in loose connective tissue near blood vessels. The capillaries of the system flow into larger collecting vessels. The largest of the collecting vessels, the left and right thoracic ducts, empty into veins in the base of the neck. The fluid in the system, lymph, transports foreign materials such as bacteria to lymph nodes. The lymph vessels also absorb and transport ingested fats, and they recover fluids that have escaped from blood vessels into the tissues and return the fluids to the blood. Lymphocytes are the principal cell type of the system.

Lymph Nodes
Lymph nodes are ovoid, encapsulated structures that are strategically located throughout the body. Lymphocytes are the most numerous cell type found in lymph nodes. Other cell types that are present are arranged on a network of reticular fibers and reticular cells (collectively called a reticulum). Phagocytic cells such as macrophages are plentiful, and they increase in numbers and activity as needs arise. Functionally, lymph nodes carry out major defensive and immunological functions as they filter the lymph fluid. It is primarily in the lymph nodes (and spleen) that immune responses are initiated.

THE MONONUCLEAR PHAGOCYTE SYSTEM (MPS)

Developmentally, cells of the MPS originate as *stem cells* in the bone marrow and differentiate there from *promonocytes* to *monocytes* (Fig. 11-2). Monocytes enter the blood, remain there for about three days, and emigrate into the tissues, where they develop into *macrophages*. These cells are widely deployed throughout the body. Some are *fixed* primarily along the blood vessels of the spleen, lymph nodes, liver, and bone marrow. Others are motile and are called *wandering* or *free macrophages*. Depending on their location and their histological appearance, macrophages are given more specific designations, such as Kupffer cells in the liver, microglia in the brain, and alveolar or ''dust'' cells in the lung.

Bone marrow	Peripheral blood	Tissues
Promonocyte → Monocyte →	Monocyte →	Macrophages
		Liver (Kupffer cells)
		Lung (alveolar macrophages)
		Spleen (fixed and wandering)
		Bone
		Lymph nodes
		Central nervous system (microglial cells)
		Connective tissue (histiocytes)
		Granulomatous tissue (epithelioid and giant cells)
		Freely migrating cells of peritoneal and pleural cavities
		Germinal center cells of reticuloendothelial system

Fig. 11-2. Mononuclear phagocytes—maturation and compartmentalization.

Irrespective of location, they are all macrophages.

Morphologically, macrophages assume a wide variety of shapes, which are usually determined by their habitats. In suspension they are round, about 14 to 20 μm in diameter. The nucleus may be round or elongated and bean-shaped. The peripheral cytoplasm is usually clear and constantly forming and reforming veil-like ruffles.

Functionally, macrophages are incredibly talented (Table 11-2). The two major functions are *phagocytosis* and *antigen processing*. In their capacity as phagocytes they engulf foreign materials, kill microorganisms if those are the engulfed material, and then break down the trapped material for excretion and reutilization. Macrophages are long-lived, being replaced at a rate of about 1 percent per day; hence they are capable of sustained activity.

The second major function is that of antigen processing. They are referred to as *antigen-presenting cells* or *accessory cells* in this capacity (Chapter 12). Briefly, macrophages reside primarily in the lymph nodes and spleen, ingest antigens, process them, and present fragments of the antigen on their surface to lymphocytes. This initiates the immune response.

PHAGOCYTES

Phagocytes are cells that are specialized for ingesting, killing, degrading, and disposing of microorganisms (Fig. 11-3), damaged substances and debris of host origin, foreign cells and substances, and circulating immune complexes (Chapter 14).

Cell Types

Although there are other cell types that are phagocytic (e.g., eosinophils), most of the phagocytic activity is carried out by neutrophils and macrophages—in fact to such a degree that they are referred to as the "professional phagocytes."

Dynamics of Phagocytosis

Vacuole Formation. The locomotion of phagocytic cells to the foreign substance frequently is directed by chemotactic factors such as molecules released by infectious microorganisms as well as plasma proteins called complement. Contact also occurs as a random encounter. The adsorption of the foreign substance to the phagocytic cell may be facilitated by antibodies, com-

Table 11-2. Some Functions of Macrophage Cells (Mononuclear Phagocytes)

ROLES IN RESISTANCE AND SCAVENGING

Ingestion and destruction of microorganisms and foreign particles without the involvement of antibodies or effector T cells

Production of complement components and interferons

Elimination of foreign tissue cells

Antitumor activity (e.g., production of tumor necrosis factor)

Clearance of debris of host origin

ROLES IN IMMUNE REACTIONS*

Roles in afferent (inductive) arc of an immune response
  Processing of antigen (ingestion, degradation)
  Presentation to T cells of processed antigen in association with MHC-coded surface glycoprotein
  Secretion of Interleukin I (activates T cells and stimulates T cell proliferation)
Roles in efferent (effector) arc of an immune response
  Ingestion and degradation of immune complexes
  Destruction of antigens through mechanisms involving:
    Opsonins—Fc portion of an immunoglobulin and complement fragment C3b bind antigens to macrophages as a prelude to ingestion and destruction
    Lymphokines—T cell (primarily) products that promote the attraction, activation, and proliferation of macrophages at the site of antigen incursion

MHC = Major histocompatibility complex; Fc = crystallizable fragment of immunoglobulins.
* To be described in Chapter 12.

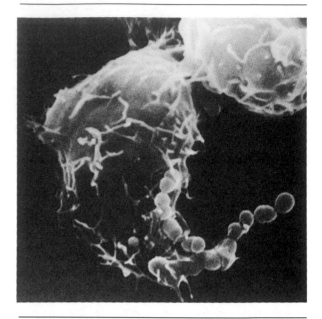

Fig. 11-3. A scanning electron micrograph of a neutrophil polymorphonuclear granulocyte ingesting a chain of streptococci (original magnification ×5,000). From I. R. Tizard, *Immunology* (2nd ed.). Philadelphia: Saunders, 1988.

plement fragments, and receptor sites on the phagocyte surface (see under Biological Activities of Complement, Chapter 12). In the phase of phagocytosis called *endocytosis* the contacted portion of the cytoplasmic membrane of the phagocyte engulfs (surrounds) the particle, and the involved segment of the membrane is pinched off (Fig. 11-4). This action creates an internalized vacuole that contains the particle. The membrane-surrounded vacuole with the contained particle is termed a *phagosome*. Killing, if re-

quired, and digestion of the ingested particle take place by nonoxidative or oxidative mechanisms.

Nonoxidative Killing and Digestion. The cell organelle called the *lysosome* contains the principal factors involved in the digestion of ingested substances and of killed microorganisms. Lysosomes are membrane-enclosed granules that are also called *primary* or azurophilic *granules.* They hold a collection of about 60 enzymes, many of which are hydrolytic enzymes such as proteases, lipases, carbohydrases, and nucleases. The enzymes act under slightly acid conditions and are referred to by the collective term *acid hydrolases.* Following phagocyte activation, lysosomes move rapidly to, and fuse with, the phagosome to form a new structure, now called a *phagolysosome. Degranulation* occurs, releasing

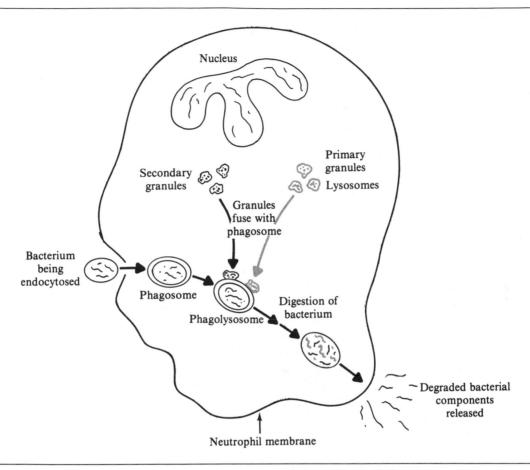

Fig. 11-4. Phagocytosis—structures and activities in nonoxidative killing and digestion.

degradative enzymes and antimicrobial proteins. The enzymes and proteins, walled off from the normal constituents of the phagocytic cell by the phagolysosomal membrane, contribute to the killing of ingested microorganisms and they digest the killed microorganisms or other ingested substances.

Not all cytoplasmic granules are lysosomes. *Secondary* or *specific granules* contain antibacterial substances such as lysozyme and lactoferrin (Chapter 9). They also contain substances crucial to the inflammatory response (e.g., complement activators) and receptors that move to the cell surface, allowing neutrophils to approximate their targets and adhere to them. Macrophages usually contain only a few granules until lymphocytes activate them.

Oxidative Killing—The Respiratory Burst. At the time of phagocytosis there is an increase in metabolic activity referred to as the *respiratory burst.* Within seconds after stimulation, phagocytes activate a specialized pathway that results in a one hundred-fold increase in oxygen consumption. The purpose of the respiratory burst is to generate reactive, toxic oxygen compounds that kill microorganisms. This oxidative mechanism is more important for killing microorganisms than is the nonoxidative mechanism.

The chain of chemical events involved in the generation of the toxic oxygen products is presented in Figure 11-5. The enzyme responsible for initiating the respiratory burst is a pyridine nucleotide oxidase (NADPH oxidase). *Superoxide anion* ($.O_2^-$) and *hydrogen peroxide* are the major products of the respiratory burst. They, however, are relatively nonmicrobiocidal. Phagocytes have two pathways to convert these products to more toxic forms. One pathway employs hydrogen peroxide and *myeloperoxidase* (found in lysosomes) to form the *hypochlorite ion* (OCl^-), a strong oxidizing agent that is effective against many bacteria, fungi, mycoplasmas, and viruses. The second pathway generates hydroxyl ($.OH$) radicals and singlet oxygen ($^1O_2$) (from hydrogen peroxide and superoxide anion), which are used to form microbiocidal peroxides. Inherited defects occur in this chain of events (see under Immunodeficiencies in Phagocytes, Chapter 14). Individuals with such defects experience serious infections even with organisms of low virulence. The defects are found in chronic granulomatous disease of children, in Chediak-Higashi disease, and in myeloperoxidase deficiency.

Neutrophils and macrophages differ somewhat in their phagocytic activities. Neutrophils, usually first at the scene of an infection, do not survive long. Dying neutrophils attract macrophages and it is the macrophages that scavenge the battle remnants. Macrophages, however, are perfectly capable of destroying microorganisms in a manner similar to neutrophils except that the respiratory burst is not so intense as it is in neutrophils.

Secretion. Destruction by phagocytes is not always confined to the interior of the phagocytic cell. The contents of lysosome granules and of specific granules, and toxic oxygen products, can be released into the tissues. This may occur if the materials are too large, too numerous, or too inaccessible to be endocytosed. The released cell products can affect normal body components, resulting in serious tissue damage. This is a major factor in immune-complex diseases such as streptococcal glomerulonephritis and rheumatoid arthritis (Chapter 14).

Intracellular Survival of Some Microorganisms. Neutrophils rarely serve as hosts for intracellular parasites. Many different kinds of intracellular parasites, however, survive and thrive within macrophages and may be transported to other parts of the body to spread the infection. Among the intracellular survival mechanisms of microorganisms are escape from the phagosome, resistance to lysosomal enzymes, and prevention of phagosome-lysosome fusion.

TISSUE FACTORS

Chemical Substances

There are certain less well defined antimicrobial chemical substances that contribute to nonspecific host resistance (Table 11-3). The long-chain fatty acids of the skin and lysozymes found in saliva, tears, and nasal secretions have already been mentioned. Others reside in phagocytic cells and bear such names as *phagocytin* and *leukin*. A polyamine named *spermine*, found in semen, is bactericidal. Gram-positive bacteria are killed by *betalysin*, which is produced during clot formation. Basic polypeptides high in lysine and arginine content are present in animal tissues. These compounds have antibacterial activity.

Mast Cells

Mast cells are tissue cells that can be regarded as "sentinel" cells because of their distribution on or near the body surfaces and because they react with foreign substances. They are found primarily in the mucosa and submucosa, in the dermis, and around venules. Their recognition sys-

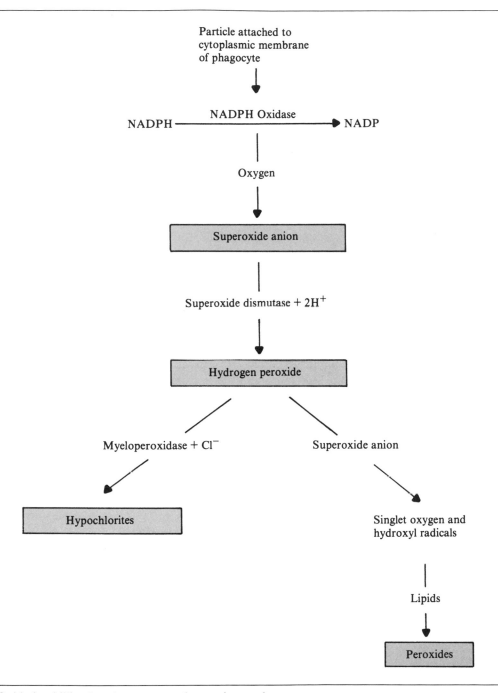

Fig. 11-5. Oxidative killing by phagocytes—the respiratory burst.

Table 11-3. Some Nonimmunological Protective Factors

Name	Major sources	Type of activity
Fatty acids	Ubiquitous; skin glands	Gram-negative
Transferrin, lactoferrin	White blood cells, milk, serum	Gram-positive and gram-negative
Spermine, spermidine	Pancreas, prostate	Gram-positive
Lysozyme	Serum, white blood cells, saliva, tears	Gram-positive and gram-negative, some viruses
β-lysin, plakin	Platelets	Gram-positive
Phagocytin, leukin	Neutrophils	Gram-positive
Complement (alternative pathway)	Serum	Bacteria, viruses, protozoa
Interferon	Most cells except neutrophils	Viruses, some intracellular protozoa
Myeloperoxidase; xanthine oxidase	Neutrophils, milk	Bacteria, viruses, protozoa

tem allows them to recognize "nonself" substances as soon as the substances penetrate mucosal or cutaneous surfaces. Through the release of chemotactic factors they attract phagocytes to the foreign substances that have entered the body surfaces, they facilitate the importation of antibodies and complement to the affected site, and they release proteases that apparently serve to debride (remove) damaged tissue. Mast cells are known mostly for their role in the types of immediate hypersensitivity known as local and systemic anaphylaxis (see Chapter 14) and not for their role in nonspecific immunity.

INFLAMMATION

Inflammation is primarily a protective response wherein interacting defensive factors are focused at a localized site of injury, infection, or irritation (Table 11-4). The protective actions seek to contain, to destroy, and to remove the cause of the intrusion, followed by repair of the damaged tissues (Fig. 11-6). Inflammation is divided into two major categories, acute and chronic. The categories are based primarily on the time stage of the inflammation and on the principal cell types involved.

Table 11-4. Types of Substances That Incite an Inflammatory Response*

ENDOGENOUS

1. Nonimmunogenic cell and tissue debris of self origin—"worn-out,' devitalized, traumatized cells and tissues
2. Immunogenic substances of self origin—involved in autoimmune disease

EXOGENOUS

1. Nonimmunogenic inert physical materials—talcum, asbestos fibers, splinters, pieces of metal
2. Nonimmunogenic chemical agents—drugs, various organic and inorganic chemicals
3. Immunogenic substances
   a. Nonmultiplicative (innocent) immunogens—foreign proteins (as in foreign serum), transfused and transplanted cells and tissues, pollens, drugs
   b. Multiplicative immunogens—microorganisms

* Substances that are immunogenic elicit responses by the immune system.

Acute inflammation starts immediately after the tissue insult and is characterized by the neutrophil cell type. The cardinal or classic signs and symptoms of acute inflammation as it progresses are pain, redness, heat, swelling, and loss of function. The initial events of inflammation are dilation of blood vessels and capillary permeability.

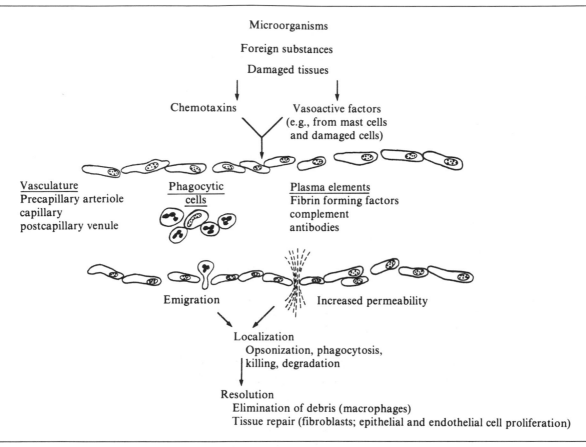

Microorganisms

Foreign substances

Damaged tissues

Chemotaxins   Vasoactive factors
                     (e.g., from mast cells
                     and damaged cells)

<u>Vasculature</u>   <u>Phagocytic</u>   <u>Plasma elements</u>
Precapillary arteriole   <u>cells</u>   Fibrin forming factors
capillary   complement
postcapillary venule   antibodies

Emigration   Increased permeability

Localization
Opsonization, phagocytosis,
killing, degradation

Resolution
Elimination of debris (macrophages)
Tissue repair (fibroblasts; epithelial and endothelial cell proliferation)

Fig. 11-6. Inflammation. Phagocytic cells and plasma elements, influenced by chemotaxins and vasoactive factors, escape from the vasculature to the site of irritation in the tissues. Localization, destruction, elimination, and repair follow.

These are mediated by vasoactive (affecting blood vessels) agents such as histamine and prostaglandins that derive from injured cells and later from cells that infiltrate the area. The vascular responses facilitate the emigration of neutrophils and monocytes from the blood into the tissues, and the passage of blood fluid (edema fluid) with its content of immune system products (antibodies and effector T lymphocytes), complement factors, and blood-clotting factors. The phagocytes, assisted by the immune products (if they have already been formed) and by complement factors carry out their functions as previously described. Activated clotting factors provide fibrin to help

localize the irritant. *Pus formation* is a common feature of acute inflammation. It results primarily from the accumulation of dying and disintegrating dead neutrophils. Macrophages arrive later, signalled by the dying neutrophils. The macrophages help eliminate microorganisms, phagocytose damaged cells and tissues, including neutrophils and fibrin deposits, and attract fibroblasts. *Fibroblasts* synthesize collagen and proteoglycans that restore connective tissue. Proliferation of the endothelial cells of the small vessels restores local microvasculature. Proliferation of the epithelial cells results in wound closure.

If the offending microorganisms or materials persist, the inflammatory process progresses into the chronic state. The cell types characteristic of *chronic inflammation* are macrophages, lymphocytes, and plasma cells. Persisting microorganisms and materials include bacteria of the genus mycobacterium, fungi, eggs of parasites, and inorganic substances such as talc and asbestos. The continuous arrival of macrophages and fibroblasts can lead to the formation of epithelioid cells (macrophages that form groups of epithelium-appearing cells) and multinucleated giant cells (macrophages that coalesce to form a large cell with many nuclei). Fibroblasts may deposit excessive collagen and form dense fibrous scar tissue. The formation of *granulomas* (chronic inflammatory lesions characterized by epithelioid and giant cells, and extensive fibrosis) often is an undesirable outcome. In syphilis, tuberculosis, and some worm and fungus infections, there may be extensive tissue destruction due to granuloma formation. Chronic inflammation usually is accompanied by immune responses if the irritant is immunogenic. This probably accounts for the presence of lymphocytes and plasma cells at the inflammatory focus.

Excessive inflammation, both acute and chronic, and serious tissue injuries, many of which stem from immune responses, characterize a wide variety of human diseases, as shall be seen, for example, in the description of hypersensitivities in Chapter 14.

OTHER NONSPECIFIC RESISTANCE FACTORS

Interferons

Interferons are a family of low-molecular-weight proteins synthesized by cells in response to virus infection, to immune stimulation, to a variety of molecules such as endotoxins, to polysaccharides, and to certain bacterial species. Interferons (IFN) are classified as IFN-α, IFN-β, and IFN-γ. The primary natural sources are leukocytes for IFN-α, fibroblasts for IFN-β, and T cells for IFN-γ.

The interferons were first discovered when it was determined that infection with one virus interferes with infection by another virus. This phenomenon of virus interference is probably the most important of the nonimmunological antiviral defense mechanisms that serve as an early protective device while the immune response is still relatively ineffective. Infected cells release interferons a few hours after viral infection, and higher levels are attained within a few days. The released interferons bind to receptors on other nearby cells. Interferons are not virus-specific but they are relatively species-specific. Interferon induced in response to one virus may be equally effective against an unrelated virus. Human interferon is most effective in humans, bovine interferon is most effective acting on bovine cells, and so on.

The antiviral action of interferon is believed to develop in this way (Fig. 11-7): Small amounts of double-stranded RNA are formed by the virus-infected cells. The RNA induces the cell to produce interferon. The produced interferon is secreted and binds to nearby uninfected cells. The interferon does not affect viruses directly but stimulates the host cell to activate latent enzymes. Two new enzymes are formed. One is 2'5'-oligoadenylate synthetase. It acts on ATP to generate 2-5A, an adenine trinucleotide; 2-5A activates an endoribonuclease that preferentially cleaves the mRNA required for the synthesis of viral protein. The second enzyme is a protein kinase. Protein kinase phosphorylates initiation factor (IF-2) and inactivates it. This prevents the elongation of viral double-stranded RNA and so acts to inhibit viral protein synthesis. Maturation of viruses is therefore interfered with in two ways: through cleavage of viral mRNAs and through inhibition of viral protein synthesis.

Interferons also inhibit multiplication of cells. The molecular basis of this activity is unknown. The inhibitory activity often is greater against cancer cells than against normal cells. Interferons are produced in small amounts in hosts. They are

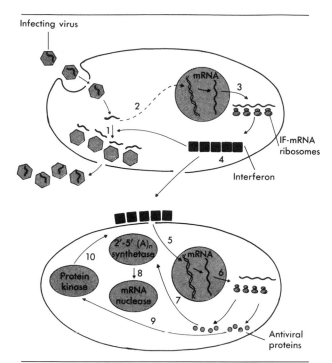

Infecting virus

mRNA

IF-mRNA
ribosomes

Interferon

2'-5' (A)ₙ
synthetase

Protein
kinase

mRNA
nuclease

mRNA

Antiviral
proteins

Fig. 11-7. Proposed mechanism of interferon action. Infecting virus (1) produces new viral particles but also (2) induces cell to produce interferon mRNA (IF-mRNA), which (3) is translated into interferon molecules. (4) Interferon released by cell may inhibit development of virus in same cell, or it may bind to adjacent cells and (5) induce cell to produce antiviral proteins (6) such as $2'\text{-}5'$ $(A)_n$ synthetase (7), which activates (8) an mRNA endonuclease that cleaves viral mRNAs. A second enzyme, protein kinase (9) phosphorylates and thus inactivates a factor, IF-2, required for protein synthesis. (From R. F. Boyd, *General Microbiology* [2nd ed.]. St. Louis: Mosby, 1988.)

now produced in quantity by tissue-culture cell lines utilizing recombinant DNA technology. Clinical trials in which interferon has been used for treatment of virus infections and cancer have been disappointing. Interferon does seem to be able to inhibit the growth of certain warts and of hairy cell leukemia. A new human interferon-based topical gel appears to reduce the symptoms of recurrent genital herpes infections significantly.

An equally important role for the interferons, especially IFN-γ, is as a modulator of immune reactivity. This is described in the next chapter with the cytokines.

The Complement System

The complement system is a complex of serum proteins that act in a sequence once they are activated by antigen-antibody complexes or by high-molecular-weight carbohydrates (polysaccharides). The complement system is described in greater detail in Chapter 12. Complement has a number of biological activities, among which is a key role in nonspecific resistance. When the complement system is activated, as the sequence moves along its pathway, fragments are generated that have biological activities. The activities promote inflammation, chemotaxis, phagocytosis, and lysis of foreign cells.

SUMMARY

1. First-line nonspecific host resistance is provided by the intact integument (skin and mucous membranes) and by substances, cells, and structures on its surface such as mucus, keratin, enzymes, fatty acids, normal microflora, and cilia.

2. Once foreign agents or materials penetrate the first-line barriers, nonspecific containment occurs largely through the interactions of elements of the blood; through the reactions of the vascular, mononuclear phagocytic, lymphatic, and complement systems; and through tissue factors.

3. The mononuclear phagocyte system consists of multifunctional macrophages. Two important functions are elimination of foreign materials and the debris from inflammatory reactions, and processing and presentation of antigens.

4. Phagocytic cells have the crucial defensive

functions of ingesting and destroying foreign substances. In the nonoxidative mechanism, particles ingested by phagocytes are surrounded by a piece of cytoplasmic membrane that coalesces with lysosomes to form a phagolysosome. Hydrolytic enzymes of the lysosomes digest the particles. In the oxidative mechanism, toxic oxygen products destroy ingested microorganisms.

5. Other internal defenses include antimicrobial chemical substances such as phagocytin, leukin, spermine, betalysin, and several basic polypeptides. Mast cells, most of which reside near body surfaces, attract phagocytes and facilitate the importation of antibodies and complement.

6. Infection, injury, and irritants evoke a series of interdependent reactions that seek to contain, destroy, and remove the intruder. The various defensive elements are focused on the intruder or injury and produce responses that collectively are called inflammation.

7. A family of proteins called interferons are produced by lymphocytes, fibroblasts, and macrophages. The first known and a prominent function of interferons is the nonspecific prevention of virus infections. Interferons stimulate the formation of an endonuclease that cleaves viral mRNA and the formation of a protein kinase that interferes with the initiation factor required for viral protein synthesis.

8. Fragments generated by the cascading serum complement system promote inflammation, phagocytosis, and cell lysis.

QUESTIONS FOR STUDY

Select the best response or responses for each of the following:

1. Mice lack cell-surface receptors specific for poliovirus and, consequently, are resistant to poliovirus infections. Such resistance exemplifies
   A. Innate immunity
   B. Naturally acquired immunity
   C. Passive immunity
   D. Nonspecific host resistance
   E. Artificial immunity

2. The sequential formation of the superoxide anion, hydrogen peroxide, hypochlorite, and peroxides represents the principal products that are involved in: (1) The intraphagocytic oxidative killing of bacteria; (2) The leukoattraction of phagocytes to the site of antigen location; (3) The activation of T_H cells by Interleukin-2 (IL-2); (4) What is known as the respiratory burst; or (5) The activation of the alternative pathway of the complement sequence.
   A. 1,2,3,5

B. 1,4
C. 2,3,5
D. 3,4
E. 4,5

3. Eosinophils:
   A. Are fixed cells of the mononuclear phagocytic system (MPS)
   B. Are a source of basic proteins that are toxic to some parasites
   C. Are a primary source of histamine in the inflammatory response
   D. Are a source of secondary pharmacological mediators in chronic inflammation
   E. Are neutrophils

4. Which of the following is an important factor in nonspecific host resistance?
   A. Opsonization mediated by the Fc receptor expressed on macrophage cells
   B. Antigen processing and presentation by macrophage cells

C. Formation of memory B cells following antigenic stimulation

D. Complement activation via the alternative pathway

E. IgE-stimulated release of histamine by mast cells

5. Macrophage cells:
   A. Are dependent on the gut-associated lymphoid tissue for development and maturation
   B. Are differentiated monocytes
   C. Are a class of granulocyte
   D. Do not possess lysosomes
   E. Are also known as thrombocytes

6. The cytoplasmic vacuoles where killing and degradation of phagocytosed microorganisms occur are called
   A. Lysosomes
   B. Episomes
   C. Phagolysosomes
   D. Phagosomes
   E. Granulomas

7. Which of the following cell types are the principal phagocytic cells of the body?
   A. Mast cells and basophils
   B. Lymphocytes and plasma cells
   C. Macrophages and neutrophils
   D. Eosinophils and platelets
   E. Bone marrow stem cells and erythrocytes

True or false:

8. Interferon inhibits viral replication by activating enzymes that cleave viral mRNAs and that inhibit viral protein synthesis.
   A. True   B. False

9. The neutrophil is the characteristic cell type of acute inflammation.
   A. True   B. False

10. Monocytes evolve from macrophage cells.
    A. True   B. False

11. Eosinophils are a primary source of histamine.
    A. True   B. False

12. Myeloperoxidase is involved in the intracellular oxidative killing mechanism that occurs in phagocytes.
    A. True   B. False

13. Lymphocytes play a major role in nonspecific host resistance.
    A. True   B. False

14. Basophils functionally most closely resemble mast cells.
    A. True   B. False

ADDITIONAL READINGS

Christensen, G. D., and Beachy, E. H. The molecular basis for the localization of bacterial infections. *Adv. Intern. Med.* 30:79, 1985.

Gabig, T. G., and Babior, B. M. The killing of pathogens by phagocytes. *Annu. Rev. Med.* 32:313, 1981.

Gleich, G. J. Current understanding of eosinophil function. *Hosp. Pract.* 23:97, 1988.

Ho, M. Interferon for the treatment of infections. *Annu. Rev. Med.* 28:5, 1987.

Horowitz, M. A. Phagocytosis of microorganisms. *Rev. Infect. Dis.* 4:104, 1982.

Larsen, G. L., and Henson, P. M. Mediators of inflammation. *Annu. Rev. Immunol.* 1:335, 1983.

Robbins, S. L., and Kumar, V. Inflammation and Repair. In *Basic Pathology* (4th ed.). Philadelphia: Saunders, 1987.

Van Furth, R. Current view on the mononuclear phagocyte system. *Immunobiology* 161:178, 1982.

Weiss, L. (Ed.). *Cell and Tissue Biology: A Textbook of Histology* (6th ed.). Baltimore: Urban and Schwartzenberg, 1988.

12. ACQUIRED IMMUNITY: COMPONENTS AND FUNCTIONS OF THE IMMUNE SYSTEM

OBJECTIVES

To discuss the scope of immunology

To describe the physical, biochemical, and biological characteristics of an antigen: to differentiate among antigens, antigenic determinants, haptens, and carrier molecules, and between immunogenicity and reactivity

To describe the general structure of immunoglobulins and differentiate between the specific structures

To discuss the origin and importance of antibody diversity and heavy chain switch

To discuss the stages of B cell maturation from bone marrow stem cells; to characterize the cell at each stage of differentiation

To explain the concept of clonal selection as it applies to the humoral response to antigenic determinants

To describe T cell differentiation in the thymus gland, including description of cell surface antigens and T cell antigen receptor

To discuss the biological activities of the various T cell subpopulations, their mechanisms of action, and the role of cytokines

To describe the classic and alternative pathways of complement activation in general terms; to describe the biological activities of complement

To discuss the biological importance of histocompatibility antigens and the major histocompatibility complex (MHC), emphasizing the role of histocompatibility antigens in the recognition of foreign antigenic determinants by T cell populations

To describe how the major components of the immune system interact in producing an immune response

To differentiate between active and passive immunity and between naturally acquired and passively acquired immunity

To discuss the dynamics of an active humoral response, emphasizing the differences between primary and secondary responses and the effects of adjuvants on the dynamics observed

INTRODUCTION TO THE CONCEPTS OF IMMUNOLOGY

Immunology is concerned with the specific responses of the body to foreign substances and with the responses to substances from the body that it fails to recognize as "normal self." Non-specific resistance alone often is inadequate, as is revealed in persons with defective immune systems (see Chapter 14). They have increased susceptibility to disease, especially infectious disease.

The immune system is set in motion during the early nonspecific resistance encounters with certain kinds of substances (antigens). Many of the cell types and systems associated with nonspecific resistance are involved in acquired immunity (specific resistance), especially as the mediators of the final effects on the foreign substance. On entrance of the foreign antigenic substance into the body, the immune system "recognizes" the foreign substance as not being "self," processes the substance, and gradually produces antibodies or lymphocytes that subsequently interact specifically with it. Usually at least one week is required after the first contact for the immune system to deal effectively with the substance in terms of being able to neutralize, destroy, or remove it. Once the immune system is primed by the first encounter, it reacts more quickly and forcefully in subsequent engagements with the same substances (antigen).

THE RELATIONSHIP OF IMMUNOLOGY TO MICROBIOLOGY

Immunology is an integral part of microbiology for these reasons:

1. The immune system provides protection against many microorganisms and their products.
2. Immune system products are essential ingredients of the serological tests that are used extensively in microbial identification procedures.
3. Some allergic conditions are directly or indirectly related to microorganisms or their products.
4. Some antimicrobial chemotherapeutic agents incite hypersensitivities.

The preceding points indicate the linkages of microbiology and immunology. It is customary in medical microbiology courses also to cover other clinical aspects of the immune system: the immunology of the red blood cell, especially as it relates to blood transfusion and the Rh factor; allergy; organ and tissue grafting; control of cancer; fetal-maternal relationship.

MAIN FEATURES OF THE IMMUNE SYSTEM

Several of the main features and factors of the immune system are briefly described here and will be discussed in more detail in this chapter.

1. The major players in an immune response are antigens, macrophages, B lymphocytes, T lymphocytes, the complement system, cytokines, and MHC antigens.
2. There are two distinct complementary lymphocyte populations, namely, B cells, which are responsible for humoral immunity, and T cells, which are responsible for cell-mediated immunity.
3. B cells produce antibodies, which belong to one of five immunoglobulin classes.
4. Functionally, T cells are categorized as regulator T cells (helper T cells and suppressor T cells) and effector T cells (cytotoxic or killer T cells and delayed-type hypersensitivity T cells).
5. Antigens, which usually are high-molecular-weight, chemically complex foreign substances, induce specific responses from the immune system. The specific responses by the B cells and T cells really are not to the entire antigen itself but to discrete regions of the antigen called *antigenic determinants*.
6. Each mature B or T cell has the hereditarily determined ability to display membrane-embedded receptor molecules that are specific only for the small regions of the antigen called antigenic determinants. A given lymphocyte and its progeny specifically recognize and react with only that region. There is established, then, around the time of birth, before any antigen is ever encountered, the capability to respond specifically to virtually every antigen to be encountered during a lifetime.
7. To initiate an immune response, antigen-presenting cells such as macrophages present fragments of the antigen on their cell surface membrane. The antigenic determinants of the antigen fragments are recognized by the spe-

cific membrane receptors of lymphocytes. Chemical messengers, especially originating from the now activated helper T cells, signal antigen-specific B cells and effector T cells to proliferate.

8. The proliferated B cells (and their products, antibodies) and the proliferated effector T cells, frequently in conjunction with biologically active factors generated by the activated complement system, eliminate the remaining molecules or cells associated with the recognized antigen.

We shall at the same time provide some answers to the following important questions: How is it that an individual has the potential to produce millions and millions of diverse antibodies when there are a limited number of genes available to code for antibodies? How does the immune system recognize antigens, and how does it route and adapt the responses to different antigen types? How do the components involved in an immune response communicate so that the responses are properly regulated?

ANTIGENS

IMMUNOGENICITY AND REACTIVITY

An *antigen* (abbreviated Ag) is a molecule with attributes such as foreignness, high molecular weight, and chemical complexity that induces the immune system to form specific products, namely, antibodies and activated T lymphocytes; the same antigen subsequently reacts in vivo or in vitro with the products. The preceding statements imply two features of antigens—immunogenicity and reactivity. *Immunogenicity* refers to the quality of being able to stimulate an immune response. *Reactivity* refers to the capacity to combine with the formed immune products, namely, with the antibodies or with the activated T cells. Some scientists prefer the term *immunogen* rather than the term antigen in contexts in

which the reference is to the stimulation property of an antigen.

Typical foreign antigens that the immune system responds to include the various types of infectious disease agents and their products (e.g., toxins), proteins of foreign serum, mismatched transfused red blood cells, transplanted tissues, capsular and other polysaccharides, and vaccines.

What are frequently called antigens—for example, bacterial cells—in actuality are a composite of many diverse antigenic molecules. The various structural and molecular components of a bacterial cell—capsules, flagella, pili, lipopolysaccharide, teichoic acid, and subfractions thereof—all are antigens. Disassembly of the native antigen such as a bacterial cell occurs in vivo during the phagocytic process in the afferent (input) phase of the immune response.

ATTRIBUTES OF ANTIGENS

The three main requirements for immunogenicity are foreignness, high molecular weight, and chemical complexity.

1. *Foreignness*. The immune system of necessity ordinarily does not react to its own molecules. Serum albumin, for example, obtained from a rabbit and injected back into that same rabbit elicits no immune response. Rabbit albumin, however, injected into a guinea pig induces the formation of anti-rabbit albumin antibodies in the guinea pig. Generally, the greater the chemical and structural disparities between the antigen and similar molecules in one's own body, the more immunogenic the foreign material.

2. *Molecular weight*. The molecular weight usually needs to be higher than 10,000 for a molecule to be immunogenic. Large molecules usually are better antigens than small molecules.

3. *Chemical complexity*. Simple repetitive polysaccharides such as starch and repeating polymers such as the glutamic acid polymer of the capsular material of *Bacillus anthracis*, despite

high molecular weights, are poorly immunogenic or nonimmunogenic. Heteropolymers, on the other hand, which consist of several different amino acids or of complexed polysaccharides, are good immunogens. Lipids and nucleic acids by themselves usually are poorly immunogenic or nonimmunogenic. In general, the best antigens are native proteins composed of one or more polypeptide chains, each of which folds into a specific three-dimensional structure.

ANTIGENIC DETERMINANTS (EPITOPES)

We shall see later that in the immune response, the mechanisms by which lymphocytes recognize an antigen, and by which the immune products react with the antigen, really involve only restricted portions of the antigen molecule and not the entire molecule. On the antigen molecule there are small, discrete sites of specific chemical composition and physical configuration, which are called *antigenic determinants* or *epitopes*. It is against these areas of unique molecular configuration or composition that the immune response is directed and with which the antigen-binding sites of antibodies react.

A single antigen molecule may possess multiple antigenic determinants that differ from each other. Such an antigen is said to be multideterminant, and because of the variety of determinants it probably is a good antigen. An antigen that has multiple antigenic determinants that are all alike is said to be unideterminant and multivalent. *Multivalent* signifies that there are multiple combining sites that are all identical. Each different determinant reacts only with a specific lymphocyte and its progeny.

Most antibodies are formed against antigenic determinants that project from the surface of the antigen molecule or exist on terminal parts of polymers. Many antigenic determinants result from conformational folding of proteins. In the folded condition distant amino acids (residues) are brought close together; in the unfolded con-

dition these amino acid residues would be far apart (see formation of globular proteins, Fig. 4-1). The sequence of amino acids that exists where the folds are joined together and the resulting conformation very often comprise an *antigenic determinant*. Thus, if the amino acid sequence in the unfolded condition were numbered 88, 89, 90 . . . all the way through to 147, 148, 149, in the folded condition 97, 98, 99 might lie next to 133, 134, 135 and that combination of amino acids 97, 98, 99, 133, 134, 135 would comprise the antigenic determinant projecting from the antigen surface. B cells recognize antigenic determinants mainly by their shape. T cells respond to the distinctive sequence of the amino acids regardless of how the molecule is folded.

HAPTENS

Certain molecules or substances cannot by themselves induce antibody formation. This inability is usually due to their small size. When coupled with carrier molecules, however (and coupling can be achieved artificially in the laboratory or can occur naturally), small molecules can serve as antigenic determinants. In this capacity they are called *haptens*. They are said to be *partial* or *incomplete antigens*. They interact specifically with homologous antibodies. Haptens do not incite antibody production unless coupled with a carrier protein. As will be described later, many of the naturally occurring allergenic substances of allergic contact dermatitis are haptens (Chapter 14).

IMMUNOGLOBULINS (ANTIBODIES)

THE FIVE CLASSES OF IMMUNOGLOBULINS

Immunoglobulins (abbreviated Ig) are glycoproteins that are responsible for humoral immunity, which is also called antibody-mediated immunity. Immunoglobulins are produced by B cells. Immunoglobulins have a twofold role, *receptors for antigen* and *effectors against antigen*. As receptors located on B cell membranes, they recognize incoming antigen. The recognition initiates proliferation and differentiation of B cell clones. The clones secrete large amounts of immunoglobulins (antibodies) that are specific for the antigen. The secreted immunoglobulins effect the elimination of the remaining antigen. There are five immunoglobulin classes—IgM, IgG, IgA, IgE, and IgD—the basis of the classification being differences in the composition of the heavy chains (H chains) of the Ig molecule (Table 12-1).

STRUCTURE OF THE BASIC IMMUNOGLOBULIN MOLECULE

Heavy Chains and Light Chains

Immunoglobulins have a basic pattern of four polypeptide chains (Fig. 12-1). Two of the chains are of a higher molecular weight and are called the *Heavy* (*H*) *chains*. They are identical. The two *Light* (*L*) *chains* have a lower molecular weight and are approximately one-half the length of the H chains. L chains are of two types, kappa or lambda. The kappa is always paired with an identical kappa in a given Ig molecule, and a lambda with another lambda. Each L chain is linked to an H chain by disulfide bonds. Two such identical halves are joined together by disulfide bonds and by noncovalent forces to form the basic four-chain polypeptide unit. A schematic representation of the Ig molecule depicts it as a Y-shaped structure. The terminal of each arm of the *Y* (called the N-terminal) has two variable amino acid sequences, one on the L chain, the other on the H chain. Each variable region is linked to a constant region (domain) of its respective chain. The two identically composed arms comprise the Fab (fragment, antigen-binding) portion of the immunoglobulin molecule. The tail part of the *Y* has a constant (C) amino acid

sequence, and its terminal is referred to as the *C-terminal* or *carboxy terminal*. The tail part is called the *Fc* (from *fragment, crystallizable*).

Domains

Each H and L chain consists of several repeating loops that are held together by intrachain disulfide bonds. Each loop comprises a domain. L chains have one variable (V_L) domain and one constant (C_L) domain. The H chains of IgG and IgA have one variable domain (V_H) and three constant domains—C_H1, C_H2, and C_H3. IgM, IgD (probably), and IgE have an additional H chain domain, C_H4.

Variable Region of the Fab Portion

The *variable regions* of the H and L chains are across from each other and form an antigen-binding site (Fig. 12-2). The variableness is due to differences in amino acid composition and sequences. The variable regions have two principal subregions: the hypervariable subregions and the framework subregions. The *hypervariable regions* are the areas actually involved in antigen binding. There are three such subregions on V_L and four on V_H.

The flexible framework regions flank the hypervariable regions and mold the V_H and V_L into a three-dimensional cavity-like structure that accommodates an antigenic determinant that comprises as few as five to seven amino acids or glucoses. An antibody molecule has an identical antigen-binding site at each arm of the *Y*, making the molecule divalent.

Hinge Region

The H chains have a flexible hinge region between the C_H1 and C_H2 domains where the two arms of the *Y* join the tail part of the Ig molecule. This region demarcates the Fc from the Fab when the Ig molecule is digested with the enzyme papain. This region, because it swings through a 30-degree arc, allows the distance between the two

Table 12-1. Selected Physicochemical and Biological Properties of Immunoglobulins

	IgG	IgM	IgA	IgE	IgD
H-chain class	Gamma (γ)	Mu (μ)	Alpha (α)	Epsilon (ε)	Delta (δ)
Physicochemical properties					
Sedimentation (rate)	7	19	7–11	8	7
Molecular weight (daltons)	146,000	900,000	160,000	200,000	180,000
Serum concentration (mg/ml)	8–6	0.4–2.0	1.4–4.0	trace	0.03
Half-life in serum (in days)	21–23	5	6	2.5	3
Number of four-chain units	1	5	1–3	1	1
Antigen-binding sites	2	10	2–6	2	2
Biological properties					
Types of antibody	Agglutinin Precipitin Opsonin Neutralizing	Agglutinin Precipitin Opsonin Neutralizing	Secretory antibody on mucous surfaces Aggregates activate complement through the alternative pathway.	Reagin; skin-sensitizing Aggregates activate complement through the alternative pathway.	?
Fixes complement	+	+	−	−	−
Crosses placenta	+	−	−	−	−
Binds to Fc receptors on neutrophils and macrophages	+	−	−	−	−
Other distinct properties	Blocking antibody of atopic allergy hyposensitization; RH isoagglutinin; prominent in secondary response	First Ig formed; ABO antibodies; receptor on B cell membrane	Found in serum and external secretions; provides local/topical immunity	Reaginic antibody of anaphylaxis and atopic allergies; attaches to mast cells	Receptor on B cell membrane

+ = positive; − = negative.

antigen-binding sites to vary, thereby improving efficiency of adjusting to antigenic determinant location and of *cross linking* (binding antigenic determinants on neighboring antigens). The hinge region contains disulfide bonds that join the two H chains together.

Constant Region (Fc Region)

The tail part of the Ig molecule, the part that contains only constant regions of the paired heavy chains, is composed of amino acid sequences that are the same for all chains of the same immunoglobulin class or for the same subclass. It is

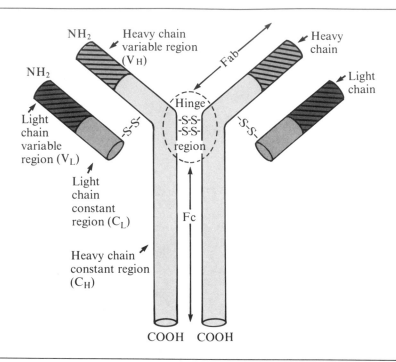

Fig. 12-1. Basic structure of immunoglobulin. (S—S = disulfide bonds; Fab = antigen-binding fragment; Fc = crystallizable fragment; NH_2 = amino terminal; COOH = carboxy terminal.)

responsible for a variety of effector biological functions. The Fc region binds to specific receptors on macrophages and neutrophils, thereby facilitating the capture and ingestion of antibody-coated antigens such as bacteria. The Fc region may also bind to other cell types such as mast cells and eosinophils. Antibodies that are bound to cells via the Fc region are said to be *cytophilic* or *cytotropic*. The Fc region of IgG and IgM also binds and thereby activates the first component of the complement system (which is described later in this chapter). Maternal IgG antibodies are the only antibodies that cross the placenta into the fetus, and that passage is mediated by the Fc portion of the IgG molecule.

Immunoglobulin Polymers

The basic immunoglobulin molecule exists as a monomer, that is, a single structural unit composed of two H and two L chains. Some of the immunoglobulin classes occur as polymers, namely, as dimers, trimers, and pentamers, which are, respectively, two, three, or five basic immunoglobulin molecules joined together (Fig. 12-3). Polymers have a *J chain* (*joining chain*), which is believed to initiate the assembly of the polymer. IgM is a monomer when it is serving as a receptor on the B cell surface and is a pentamer as a secreted immunoglobulin. IgA can exist as a monomer, a dimer (usually), and a trimer (occasionally). IgG, IgE, and IgD do not polymerize and therefore exist only as monomers.

BIOLOGICAL PROPERTIES OF THE FIVE IMMUNOGLOBULIN CLASSES

1. IgG. Beginning about the age of two years and into the fourth decade of life, IgG makes up

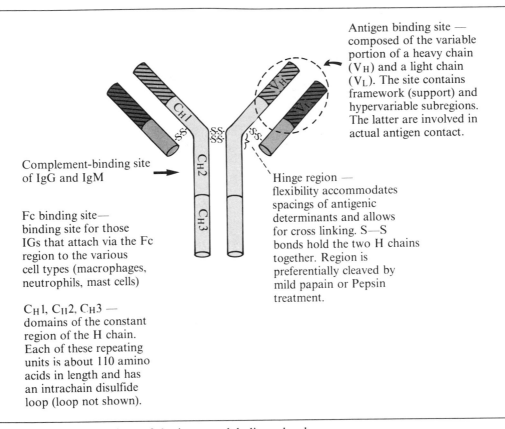

Antigen binding site — composed of the variable portion of a heavy chain (V_H) and a light chain (V_L). The site contains framework (support) and hypervariable subregions. The latter are involved in actual antigen contact.

Complement-binding site of IgG and IgM →

Fc binding site— binding site for those IGs that attach via the Fc region to the various cell types (macrophages, neutrophils, mast cells)

Hinge region — flexibility accommodates spacings of antigenic determinants and allows for cross linking. S—S bonds hold the two H chains together. Region is preferentially cleaved by mild papain or Pepsin treatment.

C_H1, C_H2, C_H3 — domains of the constant region of the H chain. Each of these repeating units is about 110 amino acids in length and has an intrachain disulfide loop (loop not shown).

Fig. 12-2. Major functional regions of the immunoglobulin molecule.

about 75 to 80 percent of the immunoglobulin in normal human serum (Table 12-1). It is also found extravascularly in tissue spaces. It is the only immunoglobulin that crosses the placental barrier, thereby protecting the newborn child temporarily against certain infectious diseases to which the mother has antibodies (Fig. 12-4). Functionally, IgG neutralizes toxins, inactivates extracellular viruses and bacteria, and coats antigens in preparation for phagocytosis in the process known as *opsonization*. IgG serves as the blocking antibody in hyposensitization of atopic allergies (see under Atopy in Chapter 14). When IgG reacts with tissue cell surface antigens and complement is activated, cytotoxic immune injury results (Chapter 14, Type II hypersensitivity). When IgG combines in certain proportions

with soluble antigen, complement is activated and immune complex disease develops (Chapter 14, Type III hypersensitivity).

2. IgM. IgM is the largest of the immunoglobulin molecules. Secreted IgM is primarily found intravascularly, where it constitutes about 7 to 10 percent of the immunoglobulin in normal adult serum. The IgM pentamer (having five units) has ten antigen-binding sites. IgM antibodies are the first to be synthesized in life. The human fetus is capable of forming IgM. In fact, its presence is indicative of fetal infection or exposure to antigens. IgM is the first class of antibody synthesized by adults in response to an antigen. Functionally, IgM antibodies are similar to IgG antibodies. They protect against extracellular antigens, and they form harmful complexes. Most

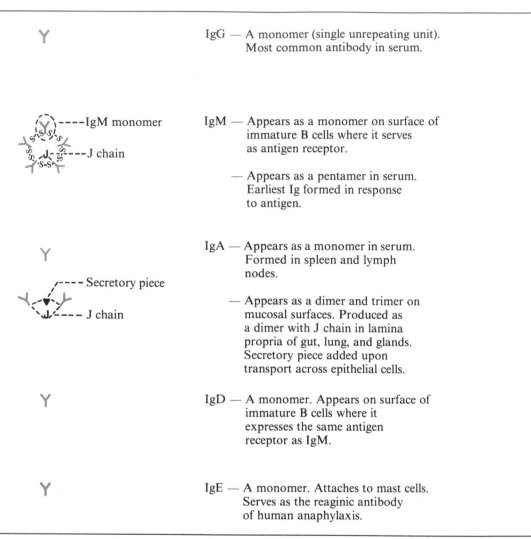

IgG — A monomer (single unrepeating unit). Most common antibody in serum.

IgM — Appears as a monomer on surface of immature B cells where it serves as antigen receptor.

— Appears as a pentamer in serum. Earliest Ig formed in response to antigen.

IgA — Appears as a monomer in serum. Formed in spleen and lymph nodes.

— Appears as a dimer and trimer on mucosal surfaces. Produced as a dimer with J chain in lamina propria of gut, lung, and glands. Secretory piece added upon transport across epithelial cells.

IgD — A monomer. Appears on surface of immature B cells where it expresses the same antigen receptor as IgM.

IgE — A monomer. Attaches to mast cells. Serves as the reaginic antibody of human anaphylaxis.

Fig. 12-3. Structures of the immunoglobulin classes.

of the naturally occurring antibodies (i.e., those that develop in the absence of known antigenic stimulation) belong to the IgM class. The cold agglutinins (which react only at temperatures below body temperature) and ABO red blood cell agglutinins are in this latter category.

3. IgA. Although a considerable percentage (about 40 percent) of IgA appears intravascularly, its greatest importance derives from its presence on the epithelial surfaces in external secretions. It is found in saliva, tears, colostrum (the milky fluid secreted by the mammary gland around the time of birth), and secretions on the surfaces of the intestinal, respiratory, and genital tracts. It is called *secretory IgA* (*sIgA*) when it appears in the exocrine secretions. sIgA as a dimer has four components: two IgA molecules, a polypeptide J chain, and a polypeptide trans-

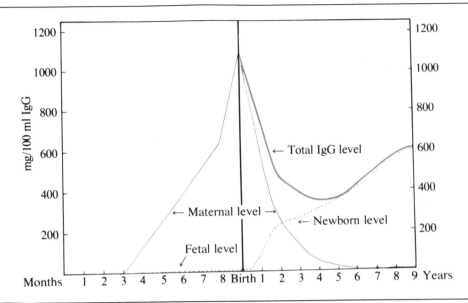

Fig. 12-4. Probable IgG levels in the fetus and newborn (From M. R. Allansmith. In F. Falkner [ed,]. *Human Development*. Philadelphia: Saunders, 1966.)

port piece called secretory component or secretory piece. Two cell types are involved in the formation of sIgA (Fig. 12-5).

Secretory IgA is resistant to enzymatic digestion, evidently because of the molecular conformational characteristics of the dimer. Secretory IgA functions as a topical, local immune system. Most of the microorganisms and foreign antigens that enter the body do so through the mucosa. They apparently must attach to the mucosa before they are able to harm the host. Secretory IgA prevents that attachment and subsequent penetration.

4. IgE. The principal importance of IgE antibodies is in their pathogenic role in the classic clinical allergies (atopic allergies) and in systemic anaphylactic hypersensitivity (see Chapter 14). IgE is cytotropic to mast cells and basophils. The protective role of IgE is open to speculation. IgE acts primarily just below the integumentary surface, where its function may be to set off a beneficial inflammatory response against an irritant that penetrates the integument. IgE-mediated re-

actions can also cause an outpouring of mucus, which is thought to provide a flushing action on the intestinal mucosa, as appears to occur in certain intestinal worm infections.

5. IgD is found only in very small amounts in the serum, but it occurs on the surface of mature immunocompetent B lymphocytes. Along with monomeric IgM it serves as a specific membrane receptor for its "intended" antigenic determinants.

ANTIBODY DIVERSITY

VDJ Deletion/Recombination

It was believed for many years that there is a separate gene in germ cells that codes for each protein molecule an individual synthesizes, including antibody molecules. Immunologists were puzzled by this because they knew that there were many millions of antibodies with different specificities, yet there were no more than an estimated total of one million genes in animals that

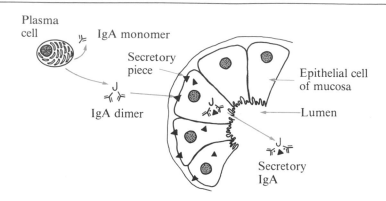

Fig. 12-5. IgA dimers (two units of IgA and a J chain) are formed in submucosal plasma cells. The secretory piece initially is located across the cell membrane (the piece is termed a *transmembrane glycoprotein*) of mucosal epithelial cells, where it serves as a receptor for the IgA dimer. The IgA dimer-secretory piece complex is transported through the cytoplasm of the epithelial cell and secreted through the opposite side of the cell. The secreted IgA provides local, topical immunity on the mucosal surface.

coded for all the proteins of the body, not just for the Igs. It was furthermore known that the amino acid sequences in the constant part of each Ig class were identical, whereas the variable part of the molecule had differing amino acid sequences. What could be the genetic explanation for this diversity? Dreyer and Bennett in the 1960s reasoned that it would have required an impossible number of mutations to account for the diversity. They proposed that separate gene sequences in a germ cell encoded for multiple variable (V) regions and for the constant (C) region. This implied that there are two genes for a single protein chain (i.e., for an Ig chain), and that there must be a mechanism for joining the two genetic components in the somatic cell to form a single transcription unit. Evidence obtained in animal studies using modern DNA manipulation methods of restriction endonucleases, recombinant DNA, cloning, and rapid DNA sequencing proved the proposal correct.

The studies originally conducted in mice showed that the V and C genes are far apart in the germ line (embryonic DNA) and move closer together in the DNA of lymphocyte precursor cells (somatic cells) (Fig. 12-6). There are also genes that code for J (junctional) sequences of portions of the V_L and V_H domains. The V, J, and C region gene sequences are separated by non-coding sequences (introns) that serve as "spacers." During the development of the B cell, a V gene segment is translocated through intrachromosomal recombination to a site next to a J segment, thereby forming a contiguous J sequence with intervening introns. Any of the multiple V gene segments can be joined to any of the J gene sequences. Once this recombination has taken place, the cell is committed to synthesizing an antibody whose antigen-binding specificity is encoded by that VJ sequence. The DNA that originally was located between the chosen V segment and the chosen J segment is deleted. Thus, if there were 200 V gene segments and the sixth was the chosen segment, V segments 7 to 200 would be deleted (the Vs are on the 5′, "up-stream" end of the gene) and segments 1 to 6 would remain. Likewise with the J segment—if J3 were chosen, then J1 and J2 would be deleted and J3, J4, and J5 would remain. The resulting gene, which would contain V segments 1 to 6, J segments 3 to 5, introns, and the constant segment, would be transcribed into high-molecular-

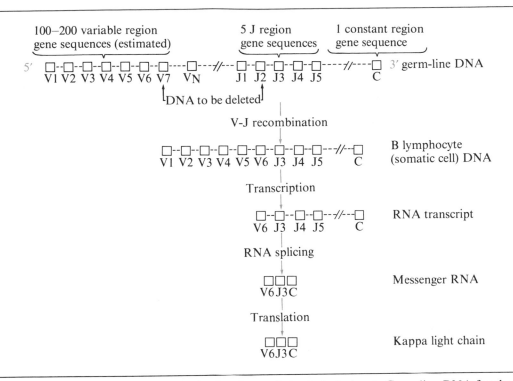

Fig. 12-6. The generation of antibody diversity in a kappa light chain (human). Germ-line DNA for the light chain contains multiple variable (V) and joining (J) gene sequences and a single constant (C) region gene sequence. There is a long intervening DNA sequence (intron) between the V and J segments and a shorter sequence between the J and C segments. During recombination in the somatic cell (the B cell), segments of DNA are deleted as the chosen V gene sequence comes to be translocated next to one of the J segments. The entire gene is transcribed. The intervening sequences and the extra J's then are spliced out to yield the messenger RNA that is to be translated into the kappa light chain. (Not illustrated: A leader segment accompanies these steps; the leader is cleaved away as the chain exits through the B cell membrane.)

weight RNA, which would subsequently be processed to form a functional message that would be translated into an Ig light chain.

Heavy chain recombination events in the Fab portion of the Ig molecule are like those just described for the light chain, but with one difference. The variable region of the heavy chain has an additional gene segment, called the D (diversity) gene segment, and V and J recombinations with alternative sequences in this segment afford additional chances for variability.

This capability of recombining selected sequences of germ-line DNA into a single active sequence in somatic cells explains how a large

repertoire of antibodies can be generated without having to have a germ-line gene for each antibody specificity. In humans, for example, each light chain is thought to have between 50 and 200 separate V genes and 5 J genes, and each heavy chain between 100 and 200 V genes, 4 J genes, and 12 D genes. If we assume that $200 V_L + 5 J_L$ genes plus $200 V_H + 4 J_H + 12 D_H$ genes randomly associate, the total number of different antibody molecules that could be synthesized from this gene pool would be 9.6×10^6. This illustrates how a limited amount of DNA (421 genes) can generate a potential 10 million antibody specificities. Additionally, gene mutations occur during

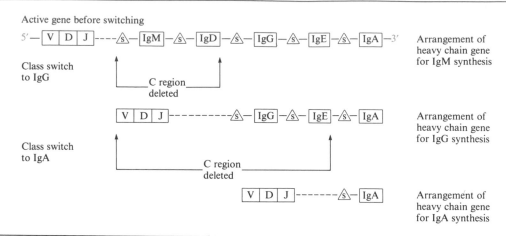

Fig. 12-7. Heavy chain switch (S/S recombination). The recombinational steps on the 5' (left) side of the active gene that produced the V, D, and J sequence (the variable region) are shown in Fig. 15-11. The D (diversity) gene segment is found only in heavy chains. The constant (C) region gene sequences are lined up in the order of IgM, IgD, IgG, IgE, and IgA. Each constant region gene is preceded by a switching signal (*S*). This arrangement leads to IgM synthesis if there is no gene switching. The switch to IgG secretion involves deletion of the S, IgM, S, IgD sequence and the translocation of the VDJ transcription unit to a position next to the IgG gene sequence. The switch to IgA secretion involves deletion of the S, IgM, S, IgD, S, IgG, S, IgE sequence and the translocation of VDJ to a position next to the IgA sequence.

the lifetime of B cells, and that increases the variety of antibodies that B cells produce.

Heavy Chain Switch During Antigen-Driven Maturation of B Cells: S/S

Recombination. A type of diversity that involves the biological functions of the antibody molecule occurs at the heavy chain end of the immunoglobulin molecule through a mechanism that is known as the *heavy chain switch* (Fig. 12-7). The antibody diversity that takes place in the variable region exists by the time the B cell membrane has receptor Ig molecules and before antigen recognition ever occurs. The cell does not go on to secrete antibodies unless the appropriate antigen binds to the preordained (according to the clonal selection theory) receptor. Upon antigen recognition, the cell is driven ("antigen-driven") along its developmental pathway to form a clone of lymphocytes that produce an antibody of a single specificity. B cells begin their antibody-secreting

functions by first making IgM. They are able to switch, however, to make the other Ig classes, while retaining the same antigen-binding sites on the Fab. The switch involves a second recombinational event, called *S/S recombination.* The switch from one class to another is accomplished through recombination of switching sequences (S) that exist in the introns between the exons of each H-chain class.* Starting from the VJ region, the DNA sequences for the constant region of the heavy chains of the Ig classes are lined up in the order of IgM, IgD, IgG_3, IgG_1, IgA_1, IgG_2, IgG_4, IgE, and IgA_2. (There are four subclasses of IgG and two subclasses of IgA.) If the heavy chain switch is to IgG (the most frequent switch), IgM and IgD sequences encoding the constant regions are deleted. If the switch is to IgA_2, then the sequences encoding the constant regions of IgM, IgD, IgG, and IgE are deleted. The functional implication of the switches is that the antigen-

* Introns are noninformational areas in DNA; exons are informational areas in DNA.

binding sites of a particular Ig molecule can associate with any of the five Ig classes and thereby acquire the biological functions characteristic of each Ig class.

B LYMPHOCYTES

DIFFERENTIATION AND MATURATION OF B CELLS

A central lymphoid organ for B cells was first discovered in birds. It is the cloaca-associated organ known as the bursa of Fabricius—hence the term B cell (Fig. 12-8). The bone marrow of mammals is regarded as the principal central lymphoid organ for B cells. The peripheral or secondary lymphoid tissues are the lymph nodes, red pulp spleen, bone marrow, and lamina propria of secretory glands. During differentiation and maturation, a B cell undergoes a succession of changes in location, morphology, immunocompetence, and function.

The differentiation of a bone marrow B cell stem cell into a mature, antibody-producing cell can be divided into stages (Fig. 12-9).

1. Stem cell. The first indication of differentiation is in the rearrangement of the V, D, and J

Fig. 12-8. Schematic representation of ontogeny of immune response, showing differentiation of non-lymphoid stem cells into blood cells and lymphoid stem cells into T lymphocytes or B lymphocytes. (From J. A. Bellanti, *Immunology III*. Philadelphia: Saunders, 1985.)

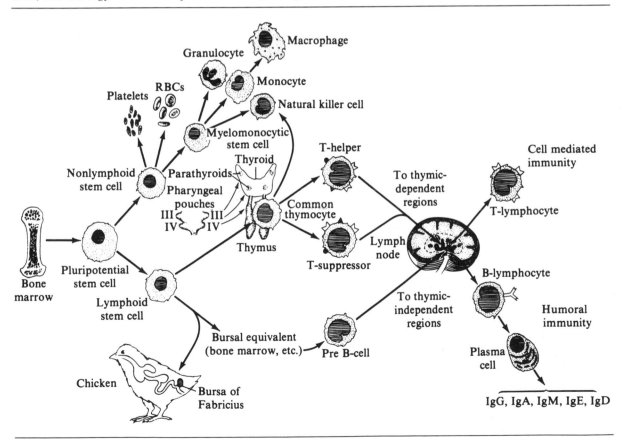

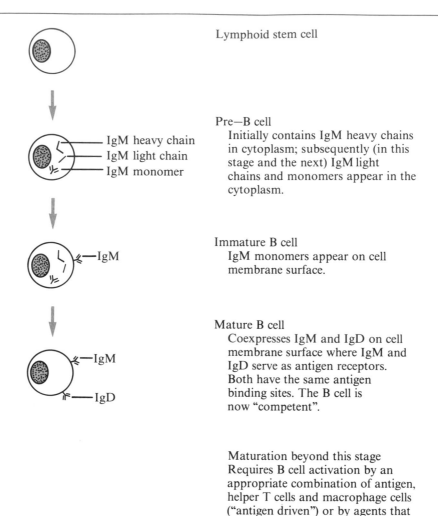

Lymphoid stem cell

IgM heavy chain
IgM light chain
IgM monomer

Pre—B cell
Initially contains IgM heavy chains
in cytoplasm; subsequently (in this
stage and the next) IgM light
chains and monomers appear in the
cytoplasm.

—IgM

Immature B cell
IgM monomers appear on cell
membrane surface.

—IgM

—IgD

Mature B cell
Coexpresses IgM and IgD on cell
membrane surface where IgM and
IgD serve as antigen receptors.
Both have the same antigen
binding sites. The B cell is
now "competent".

Maturation beyond this stage
Requires B cell activation by an
appropriate combination of antigen,
helper T cells and macrophage cells
("antigen driven") or by agents that
induce mitosis.

Fig. 12-9. Stages of B cell differentiation.

genes that code for the formation of the heavy
chain of IgM.

2. Pre-B cell. Heavy chains of IgM appear in
the cytoplasm.

3. Immature B cell. Following rearrangement
of V and J genes, IgM light chains are formed,
and monomers of IgM appear in the cytoplasm.
IgM monomers can now be inserted into the cell
membrane, where they function as surface receptors. The cell can now recognize and bind an-

tigen. Contact with antigen at this point, however, does not lead to cell proliferation and antibody formation. The antigens encountered at
this stage are self-antigens, not foreign antigens.
The immature B cells that contact self-antigens
at this stage are deleted, so that the organism
becomes tolerant of its own antigens.

4. Mature B cell. IgD is formed and is inserted
into the cell membrane along with IgM. The IgD
and IgM receptors have identical specificities and

are now ready to respond to the antigen for which they are specific.

All this has taken place in the absence of foreign antigen. A pool, however, of B cells has built up and continues to be restocked. There is a great variety of specificities but *an individual B cell can respond to only one antigen, the one for which it has the specific receptor.* The organism is now ready to respond to a diverse array of antigens.

Clonal Selection Theory

We interrupt the description of B cell differentiation to introduce the Clonal Selection Theory. Over the years several theories were developed to explain how antibodies are produced in response to induction by specific antigens. The postuates of the Clonal Selection Theory, proposed by Burnet in 1954, have been amply confirmed and accepted. According to this theory and its corollaries:

a. In every person there is a large array of previously genetically programmed clones of lymphocytes, each one bearing specific surface receptors capable of reacting only with specific antigenic determinants.
b. Theoretically, a person possesses a fixed repertoire of receptors, which can recognize all the antigens that the individual will encounter.
c. Incoming antigen selectively stimulates only that clone of lymphocytes to proliferate that exhibit the preordained complementary antigen-specific receptors (Fig. 12-10).
d. The specificity of the antibodies produced by the proliferated B lymphocytes is identical to that of the antigen receptor immunoglobulins.

5. Plasma cells and memory cells. When foreign antigen is contacted, a B cell undergoes proliferation and further differentiation, usually with the assistance of signals from helper T cells (Fig. 12-11). Most of the cells of the expanded clone differentiate into plasma cells. Plasma cells are the end-cells of B cell differentiation. The plasma cells secrete antibodies at a high rate, as many as 300 per second. Some of the cells of the expanding clone (or possibly they develop from a special subclass of B cells) form a reserve of cells called *memory cells.* The reserve of lingering cells contains more antigen-sensitive cells than were present in the original clone. These cells are "dormant" until a second dose of the same antigen comes along in what is termed a secondary immune response. The already primed B memory cells produce a much greater level of antibody than occurred in the primary immune response and in a much shorter period of time.

T LYMPHOCYTES (T CELLS)

DIFFERENTIATION AND MATURATION

Precursor T cells from the bone marrow migrate as prothymocytes to the thymus gland, guided by a chemotactic peptide, thymotaxin, and a homing receptor (Fig. 12-8). Here they gradually mature into immunocompetent cells. As the T cells differentiate in the thymus gland, they diverge into four functionally different subsets. Two of the subsets, *helper T cells* (T_H) and *suppressor T cells* (T_S), are referred to as *regulator T cells.* The other two subsets, *cytotoxic* or *killer T cells* (T_C or T_{CTL}) and *delayed-type hypersensitivity cells* (T_D or T_{DTH}), are referred to as *effector T cells.* It is also during the sojourn of lymphocytes through the thymus toward maturity that MHC restriction originates (see MHC or genetic restriction) and antigen receptors appear (Fig. 12-12). The thymus-conditioned cells are exported as post-thymic cells into the peripheral lymphoid compartments, mainly the lymph nodes and spleen, from whence some enter the circulation (the vascular compartment). The T cells preferentially locate in the corticomedullary junctions of the lymph nodes and appear as cuffs of lymphocytes around arterioles of the spleen.

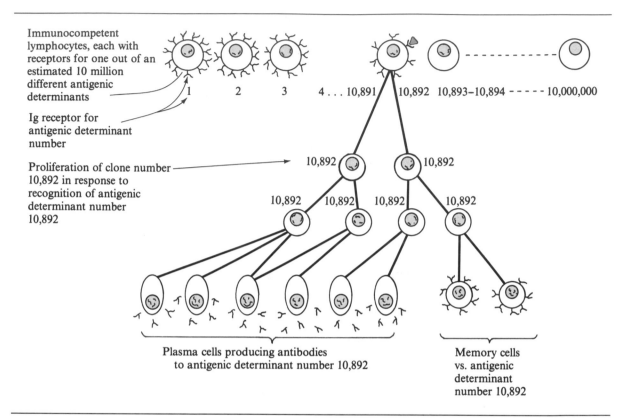

Immunocompetent lymphocytes, each with receptors for one out of an estimated 10 million different antigenic determinants

Ig receptor for antigenic determinant number

Proliferation of clone number 10,892 in response to recognition of antigenic determinant number 10,892

1   2   3   4 ... 10,891   10,892   10,893–10,894 - - - - - 10,000,000

10,892   10,892

10,892   10,892   10,892   10,892

Plasma cells producing antibodies to antigenic determinant number 10,892

Memory cells vs. antigenic determinant number 10,892

Fig. 12-10. Clonal selection. When a specific antigenic determinant—for example's sake, called number 10,892 here—enters the body, it is recognized only by a small group (a clone) of B lymphocytes—those that have the membrane Ig receptors for antigenic determinant number 10,892. That clone of B lymphocytes, "selected" by antigenic determinant number 10,892, forms plasma cells that secrete antibodies against antigenic determinant number 10,892. Memory cells for that same antigenic determinant are formed.

T CELL SURFACE ANTIGENS

T cells exhibit a succession of cell surface glycoprotein antigens as differentiation progresses. The antigens are symbolized by the letters CD (cluster designation) and a number or by the letter T and a number. Highly specific antisera produced via the hybridoma technique (see the discussion of monoclonal antibodies in the next chapter) were used to detect at least 11 glycoprotein cell surface CD antigens, which are numbered CD1 to CD11. Some of the earlier surface antigens disappear as maturation progresses, and others appear, making it possible to trace the stages of T cell differentiation. Different combinations of the surface antigens can be related to the T cell subsets that are found in peripheral lymphoid compartments. Thus T lymphocytes with CD7, CD2, CD3, and CD4 markers (abbreviated to just CD4) represent the circulating T cells that have the helper (inducer) and delayed-type hypersensitivity functions; lymphocytes with CD7, CD2, CD3, and CD8 markers (abbreviated to CD8) are T cells with cytotoxic and suppressor functions.

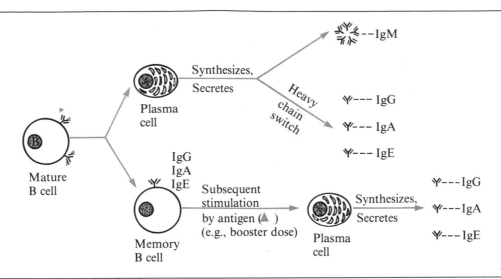

Fig. 12-11. Differentiation of mature B cell on antigen stimulation.

T CELL ANTIGEN RECEPTOR

As T cells differentiate they acquire antigen-specific receptors analogous to the immunoglobulin receptors on the B cell surface. The T cell receptor of humans is called *TCR* (*T cell receptor*). The originally discovered receptor has an antigen-specific, antigen-binding, variable part that is composed of two peptide chains, an alpha chain (T_α) and a beta chain (T_β). This receptor is referred to as TCR-$\alpha\beta$. There are striking similarities between the B cell immunoglobulin receptor and the T cell receptor. Like immunoglobulin molecules, the alpha and beta chains have V regions formed by rearrangement of V, D, J genes that differ among clones of T cells of different specificities.

The T cell receptor appears to be part of a receptor complex that is composed of TCR, CD3, and CD4. TCR is joined to the T cell through the CD3 surface marker described in the preceding topic. The CD3 molecule is required to transfer a signal from TCR to the cell interior. The CD4 is believed to cooperate with the TCR in binding to MHC-II molecules of antigen-presenting cells (see Major Histocompatibility Complex and the Immune System).

A second T cell receptor was subsequently discovered, TCR-$\gamma\delta$. This receptor is found on only 1 to 10 percent of T cells in the blood. Its function is enigmatic.

Cells bearing autoreactive TCRs are eliminated in the thymus during development. This clonal deletion is a major mechanism for the maintenance of self-tolerance.

FUNCTIONAL ROLES OF T CELLS

Helper T Cells (T_H Cells)

T_H cells have the crucial functions of recognizing antigen at the early stage of an immune response and of inducing antigen-specific B cells and effector T cells to proliferate and differentiate. These actions will be explained more fully under The Immune Response. It is the T_H cell (the "on" switch for most immune responses) that the AIDS virus destroys. The CD4 molecule on the surface of T_H cells provides the port of entry for the virus. Efforts are being made to copy the mol-

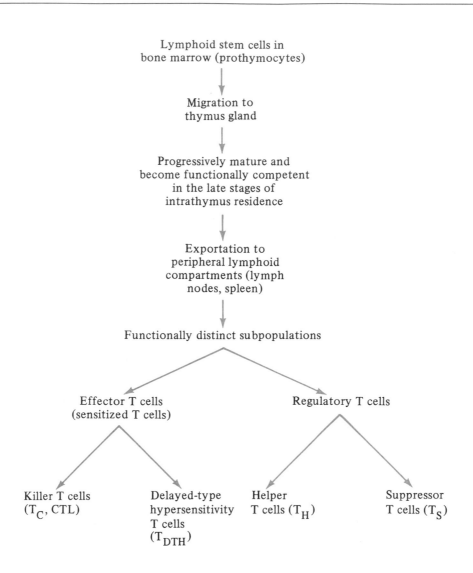

Fig. 12-12. T cell differentiation.

ecule in pharmacological amounts so that it can be injected into patients as a molecular decoy.

The regulatory role of T_H cells in relation to B cells requires explanation. Antigens that elicit a B cell response are divided into thymus-dependent antigens and thymus-independent antigens.

Thymus-dependent antigens are so named because they can evoke an immune response by B cells only when thymus-processed lymphocytes, namely, helper T cells, participate in the response. Most B cell antigens are thymus dependent. Some antigens are *thymus independent*, meaning that they can elicit a B cell response in the absence of help from T_H cells. T-independent antigens usually are protein-free, high-molecular-weight polymers such as certain lipopolysaccharides, dextrans, and pneumococcal capsular polysaccharides that require high concentrations to activate B cell clones. The multivalent binding of these antigens to Ig molecules on the surface of B cells primarily induces IgM antibodies. They do not incite memory cell formation.

Suppressor T Cells (T_S Cells)

T_S cells, by interacting with T_H cells, can prevent the induction of an immune response, or they can down-regulate the magnitude of an ongoing response. T_S may also directly act on effector T cells by regulating their activation. A number of observations support the concept that T_S cells suppress the response of B cells; but the mechanisms by which this occurs are unclear.

Cytotoxic T Cells (T_C or T_{CTL} Cells)

T_C are effector T cells that bear the CD8 surface antigen marker. Cytotoxic T cells directly destroy antigen-bearing target cells (Fig. 12-13). A T_C must first recognize the foreign antigen complexed with Class I-MHC antigen (see Major Histocompatibility Complex and The Immune System, this chapter) on the target cell surface (MHC restriction) in order to react to the foreign-antigen–bearing cell and in order subsequently to bind to and destroy the cell. Recognizing the antigen-Class I MHC complex, however, does not stimulate the T_C to multiply. An additional signal is required, namely, interleukin-2 (IL-2), which is released by a helper T cell before the antigen-responding T_C can be activated and proliferate. Once the T_C cell has been activated, it binds to a target cell and the death of the target cell follows rapidly. The T_C can disengage from a dying target cell and proceed to attack other target cells. Virus-infected host cells are typically killed in this manner.

One way in which cytotoxic T cells destroy target cells is through complement-like proteins known as *perforins*. Perforins are stored in cytoplasmic granules of the T cells. Upon T_C-target cell contact, the granules are released and form tubular transmembrane structures in the target cell. This causes target cell disruption because of osmotic lysis. Other mechanisms of killing appear to include fragmentation of target cell DNA through the activation of endonucleases, and activation of an endogenous suicidal pathway of the target cell.

Other Killer Cells. There are other killer cells that are non-T, non-B cells (Fig. 12-13). It is convenient to portray them here with the cytotoxic T cells.

Natural Killer (NK) Cells. Natural killer (NK) cells are effector cells of nonspecific immunity. They are sometimes referred to as members of the "third population" of lymphocytes. They are large, granular cells that comprise about 5 percent of human peripheral blood lymphoid cells. Through contact-dependent mechanisms like those of T_C cells, they lyse certain types of tumor cells and normal cells without manifesting classic immunological specificity or memory. Since they appear "naturally," they (along with macrophages) provide a first-line defense against malignancies. Other effector roles that are being ascribed to NK cells include rejection of bone marrow transplants, regulation of cellular development, and protection against infection.

K Cells. K cells are responsible for antibody-dependent cell-mediated cytotoxicity (ADCC). *K cells or ADCC cells* actually are not a single cell type but include cells such as macrophages, neutrophils, and NK cells. Cells with ADCC function have surface receptors that bind the Fc portion of IgG. When a host cell is coated with IgG (the Fab portion is bound to the host cell), the cell becomes a target for killing by K cells. Complement is not required, nor does MHC restriction apply.

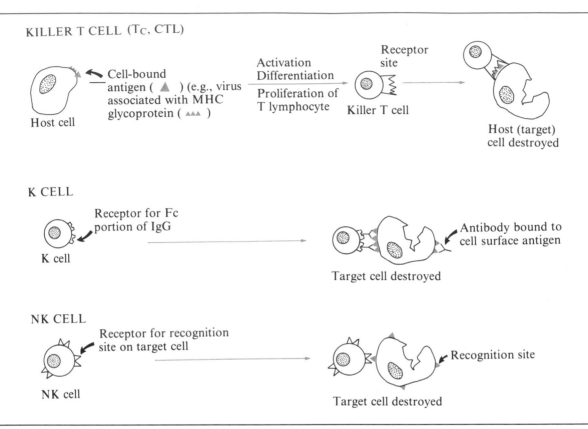

KILLER T CELL (Tc, CTL)

Cell-bound antigen (▲) (e.g., virus associated with MHC glycoprotein (▲▲▲)

Host cell

Activation
Differentiation

Proliferation of T lymphocyte

Receptor site

Killer T cell

Host (target) cell destroyed

K CELL

Receptor for Fc portion of IgG

K cell

Antibody bound to cell surface antigen

Target cell destroyed

NK CELL

Receptor for recognition site on target cell

NK cell

Recognition site

Target cell destroyed

Fig. 12-13. Top: Killer T cells. Before they become sensitized, killer T cells must be exposed to the antigens of the target cell surface. The target cell must bear the class I glycoprotein of the major histocompatibility complex (MHC). Middle: K cells. When a tissue cell has cell surface antigens to which IgG antibodies are bound via the antigen-binding sites, the cell becomes a target for destruction by K cells. K cells have receptors for the Fc portion of the IgG molecule. Bottom: Natural killer (NK) cells. NK cytotoxic activity does not require antibodies. The receptors on the NK cells and the recognition site on the target cell have not been characterized.

Delayed-Type Hypersensitivity T Cells (T$_{DTH}$, or T$_D$)

T$_{DTH}$ cells are involved primarily in slowly developing immunologically mediated tissue inflammation. Some immunologists no longer regard T$_{DTH}$ as a separate subset of T cells but regard them as T$_H$ (CD4) cells that have an effector function in delayed-type hypersensitivity (DTH) reactions. The phenomena underlying DTH reactions are not well understood. DTH reactions are mediated by small populations of specifically sensitized T$_{DTH}$ cells that alone are unable to

cope with the sensitizing antigen. T$_{DTH}$ cells usually do not directly destroy the antigen themselves. Their activities are greatly expanded through their ability to recruit macrophages, neutrophils, and other cells to the site of antigen confrontation. They do this by secreting soluble, short-range messenger substances called *lymphokines*, which recruit other cell types, especially macrophages, and it is cells of this other type that finally destroy or dispose of the antigen.

Some properties that differentiate B cells from T cells are listed in Table 12-2.

Table 12-2. Some Properties of B and T Cells

Property	B Cell	T Cell
Site of pluripotent stem cells	Fetal yolk sac (to about 60 days) → liver (days 50 to 150) → bone marrow (day 79)	Same
Site of maturation	Bone marrow, peripheral lymphoid compartments	Thymus
Percentage of lymphocytes in blood	20	80
Surface markers	Immunoglobulins	CD or T 1-11
Antigen receptors	IgM, IgD	TCR-$\alpha\beta$, TCR-$\gamma\delta$
Inactivation by radiation	High sensitivity	Low sensitivity
Agents that cause in vitro proliferation	Lipopolysaccharide, purified protein derivative	Concanavallin A; phytohemagglutinin
Products/functions	As plasma cells, produce antibodies that neutralize/opsonize/destroy (with complement) antigens	T_H cells initiate and promote expansion of an immune response; T_S cells control expansion of an immune response; T_{CTL} cells destroy antigens; T_{DTH} cells via lymphokines activate macrophages to eliminate antigens

CYTOKINES: LYMPHOKINES, MONOKINES, INTERLEUKINS

There is an array of proteins involved in intercellular communication and regulation in response to antigens and injury. They are produced primarily by T cells, and also by other cells, such as antigen-presenting cells. The proteins are small molecules that act at short ranges through a hormone-receptor-like mechanism. Ways that these proteins regulate immune responses include: as *mitogens* (substances that stimulate cells to multiply), they signal B and T cells to proliferate; as chemotaxins they attract phagocytes and eosinophils to the site of an infection; as mediators of differentiation they cause antigen-stimulated proliferating B cells, for example, to convert into antibody-producing plasma cells; as cytotoxins and growth inhibitory factors they are involved in the killing of tumor cells or in the inhibition of their growth.

Originally it appeared that all these chemical messengers were produced by lymphocytes. They were named *lymphokines*. Eventually it was shown that other cell types such as monocytes (*monokines*) also produced some of these factors and so the collective term *cytokine* came to represent all these communication/regulation factors.

There are over one hundred named lymphokines and monokines. They are named for their biological properties—for example, lymphocyte activation factor (LAF), B cell growth factor (BCGF), and eosinophil chemotactic factor (ECF). Biochemical characterization was elusive for many years because only small amounts of these compounds appeared in vivo on antigen stimulation and they quickly disappeared.

The use of lymphocyte- or monocyte-conditioned culture media for the propagation of lymphocytes made possible the exact biochemical characterization of many of the compounds. Successful cultivation yielded large enough amounts of the lymphokines and monokines that they could be analyzed in the laboratory. Amino acid sequences were determined, genes were isolated, and gene-cloning technology made possible virtually unlimited quantities of some cytokines.

All this led to adoption of the term *interleukin* (IL), a term that conveys the meaning of a mediator that serves as a communication link between leukocytes. At the Sixth International Congress of Immunology, held in 1986, it was agreed that communication/regulatory factors initially would be named according to their biological activity and would be designated an interleukin (IL) and assigned a number once the amino acid sequence had been determined. Specific interleukins usually affect more than one target cell type, and a specific interleukin may have several effects on the cells of a single target cell population (Table 12-3). Actually it had already been realized in the past that there was an overlap, that the number of actual lymphokines was smaller than the one hundred-plus named lymphokines, since many of the actual lymphokine molecules had more than one biological action. Interleukin 5 (IL-5), for example, was found to be one and the same molecule that had formerly been known as T cell replacing factor, B cell growth factor—II, eosinophil colony stimulating factor, eosinophil differentiation factor, and IgA enhancing factor. Interleukins may still be referred to as lymphokines or monokines, depending on the source cell type.

Interleukins hold great promise as therapeutic agents. Studies are under way using interleukins to enhance an immune response to cancers and

Table 12-3. Interleukins (IL)[a]

Type of interleukin	Produced by (sources)	Synonyms or previously termed	Cell types (targets) that respond	Functional properties
IL-1	Macrophages in immune response; Nucleated cells in response to injury	Lymphocyte activating factor (LAF) Endogenous pyrogens	T_H, neurons of hypothalamus, NK, CTL	With accessory cells, activates T_H cells to produce IL-2 and gamma interferon (IFN-γ) Enhances or is required for IL-4, IL-5, IL-6 production by T_H cells As endogenous pyrogen stimulates thermoregulatory center of brain
IL-2	T cells	T cell growth factor (TCGF)	T_H, CTL, NK	Promotes increase in cell size (blastic transformation), DNA replication, and cell growth of mature T cells and thymocytes Promotes autocrine (self-stimulated) growth of T_H cells Induces cytotoxicity of T cells Stimulates NK cell activity
IL-3	Antigen-activated T cells	Colony-stimulating factor (CSF)	Bone marrow hemopoietic stem cells	Regulates the growth and differentiation of bone marrow stem cells
IL-4	T_H cells	B cell growth factor (BCGF) B cell differentiation factor (BCDF) Macrophage-activating factor (MAF)	B, T, monocytes	Promotes heavy chain switch to production of IgE or IgG$_1$ by B cells Increases MHC-II expression by resting cells Activates macrophages and B cells

Table 12-3. (continued)

Type of interleukin	Produced by (sources)	Synonyms or previously termed	Cell types (targets) that respond	Functional properties
IL-5	T cells	T cell replacing factor (TRF)	B, thymocytes	Stimulates growth and differentiation of B cells to especially produce IgM and IgA
IL-6	Monocytes, T cells, fibroblasts	B cell stimulating factor-2 (BSF-2) or B cell differentiation factor (BCDF) Interferon-β (IFN-β)	B, T, bone marrow stem cells	Induces expanded B cell clones to differentiate into plasma cells Stimulates T cell IL-2 or IL-4 production Preferentially stimulates granulocyte and macrophage colony formation
IL-7	Stromal cells of thymus, spleen, kidney	Lymphopoietin-1 Pre-B cell growth factor	Thymocytes, pre-B cells	Involved in the development of pre-B cells and thymocytes
IFN-γ[b]	T, NK	Macrophage-activating factor (MAF)	Macrophages, B, NK	Activates macrophages to increase phagocytic and tumor destroying capability Activates and promotes growth of cytolytic T cells and NK cells Induces MHC-II and Fc receptor expression on macrophages and other cell types With IL-2 and IL-4, augments B and T cell responses

[a] This table contains only some of the sources, targets, and activities of interleukins.
[b] Interferons fall within the definition of an interleukin.

intractable infections. T cells or NK cells obtained from patients are stimulated by IL-2 to proliferate in large numbers in vitro, and they are infused back into the patient. Selective suppression of immune responses to organ transplants or to the antigens in autoimmune diseases may be feasible someday by inhibiting production of the interleukins that promote T cell proliferation.

Examples of a few of the better-known cytokines follow. It should be realized that the terminology applied to these intercellular messengers is in a transition period.

1. Migration inhibition factor (MIF). A factor produced by activated lymphocytes that causes blood monocytes to adhere to the endothelial lining of venules and causes the monocytes after they have exited through the vessel wall to remain at the site of the antigen intrusion.

2. Macrophage activating factor (MAF). MAF induces blood monocytes to convert into mature macrophages. The effects include increased size, greater content of lysosome granules, and increased ability to endocytose and ingest microorganisms, particles, and debris.

3. Gamma interferon (IFN-γ). IFN-γ has multiple effects in cellular immunity (Table 12-4). It is sometimes referred to as immune interferon. It is produced by antigen-stimulated T_H and T_S cells and by activated NK cells. It helps activate T_C cells, enabling them to destroy infected host cells, and it increases the ability of B cells to produce antibodies. In vitro studies using IFN-γ synthesized by use of recombinant DNA show that immune interferon has virtually the same effects on macrophages as MAF described just above. It can also increase the level of Class II MHC antigens on cells other than macrophages.

4. Interleukin-1 (IL-1). IL-1 is derived from macrophages. It is an important signal released by antigen-presenting macrophages to helper T cells during the initiation of an immune response. This signal initiates the production of interleukin-2 (IL-2) by helper T cells. IL-1, aside from other functions in an immune response, has the function of endogenous pyrogen (internal fever inducer) in inflammation (see Chapter 10).

5. Interleukin-2 (IL-2). IL-2 and its receptors are produced by helper T cells on receiving the IL-1 signal from macrophages. It is a signal required by antigen-exposed effector T cells (T_C and T_D) and, to a lesser extent, by B cells in order for them to proliferate. At one time this lymphokine was called T cell growth factor (TCGF).

THE COMPLEMENT SYSTEM

The complement system is frequently involved in acquired immunity and in nonspecific resistance (Fig. 12-14). It is comprised of a group of 30 proteins recognized to date that on activation participate in a regulated, orderly sequential or cascade fashion. Biologically active products are formed at various stages of the cascade, products that mediate chemotaxis, phagocytosis, cell lysis, and acute inflammation. The complement proteins, produced primarily by macrophages and the liver, comprise about 10 percent of the globulin portion of the serum. Some of the proteins are proenzymes that convert to enzymes.

The complement system has two pathways, the *classical pathway* and the *alternative pathway*. There is a basic series of factors that are numbered C1 through C9. Factors C1, C4, C2 are involved only in the classical pathway. The factors involved in the alternative pathway are designated by capital letters B, H, D, I, and P. Split products of these factors are represented by lowercase letters a, b, c, d, g, i.

The pivotal factor of the complement sequence is C3. It is the most abundant complement protein present in the serum. The crucial step for both the classical and alternative pathways is the generation of C3 convertase. For the classical pathway, C4b2a is the split product that serves as the C3 convertase; for the alternative pathway, it is the split product C3b,Bb,P. The action of C3 convertase on C3 leads into the terminal sequence (some speak of this as the terminal pathway), where most of the biologically active fragments are formed.

Table 12-4. Some Effects of Gamma Interferon (IFN-γ)

Enhances cell killing by killer cells (CTL, NK, K cells)

Enhances suppressive activity of suppressor T cells (T_S cells)

Inhibits migration of macrophages

Activates macrophages and promotes phagocytosis and intracellular destruction by macrophages

Enhances expression of F_C receptors or macrophages

Increases expression of histocompatibility antigens (class I and class II MHC antigen) on various cells, including macrophages, tumor cells, endothelial cells

With B cell differentiation factor (BCDF), stimulates B cell differentiation and increases antibody production by B cells

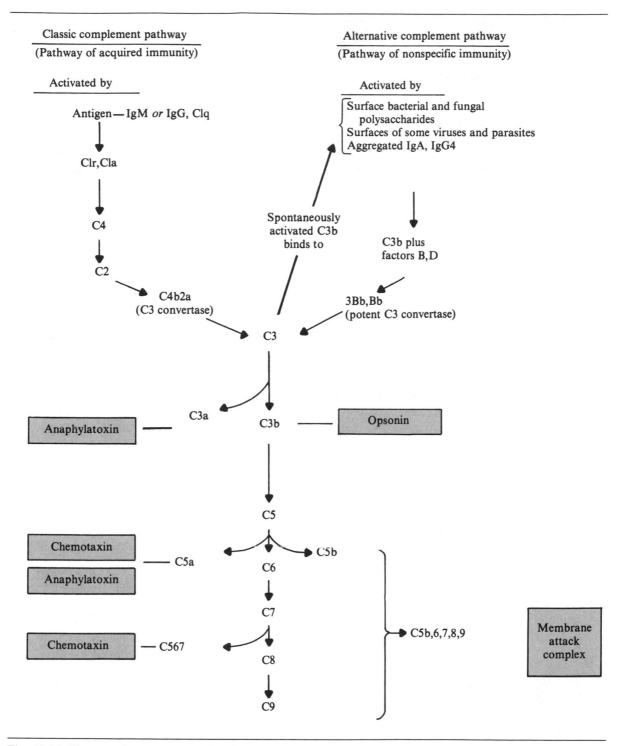

Fig. 12-14. The complement system showing the classical pathway and the alternative pathway leading into the pivotal C3 complement component. The biologically active fragments generated during the terminal sequence are shown in boxes.

THE CLASSICAL PATHWAY

This is the pathway that is involved in acquired immunity. It is activated when a single IgM antibody or two closely spaced IgG antibodies that are bound to homologous antigen bind complement factor C1q. IgG and IgM are the only immunoglobulins that have binding sites (on the CH_2 domain of the Fc portion of the molecule) for C1q. The antigen-antibody-C1q union sets of the sequential involvement of C1r, C1s, C4, and C2 leads to the formation of C4b2a, which serves as the crucial C3 convertase.

THE ALTERNATIVE PATHWAY

The alternative pathway is an important element of nonspecific resistance. Antibodies are not required. C1, C4, and C2 are bypassed. Activation is at the C3 level through the action of C3b,Bb,P, which serves as C3 convertase. Activation of the alternative pathway occurs mainly when there are surfaces present that are deficient in *sialic acid*. Normally, the presence of sialic acid on the surfaces of the host's own cells prevents C3 from forming a deposit on self surfaces and keeps the complement system in a holding pattern. Surfaces that are deficient in sialic acid and on which deposits of C3b readily accumulate include the cell walls of many bacteria, bacterial lipopolysaccharide of gram-negative bacteria, most fungi, some parasites, and aggregated immunoglobulins of classes IgA and IgG4. Enzymes from phagocytes and platelets at the sites of inflammation or of clots can also activate the alternative pathway.

BIOLOGICAL ACTIVITIES OF COMPLEMENT

The better-known, biologically active fragments and their activities are summarized as:

C3b. *Acts as an opsonin*. Opsonins coat bacteria and other materials. Phagocytes have receptors for C3b and so C3b acting as a ligand or bonding agent enhances ingestion of the coated bacteria. Antibodies of classes IgG and IgM also function as opsonins.

C5a, C5a,6,7. Act as *chemotaxins*. Chemotaxins attract phagocytic cells, causing them to migrate from an area of lesser concentration to an area of higher concentration. C5a is extremely potent as a chemotaxin for neutrophils. It also stimulates their metabolism, especially their respiratory burst.

C3a, C4a, C5a. Act as *anaphylatoxins*. Anaphylatoxins intensify inflammation by inducing degranulation of mast cells and basophils, thereby causing, among other things, increase of vascular permeability and smooth muscle contraction.

C5b,6,7,8,9. Act as *cytolysins*. This complex is referred to as the *membrane attack complex (MAC)*. Although several stages in the formation of this complex are cytolytic, it is polymerized C9 that causes most lysis. Polymerized C9 forms ring-shaped channels ("holes") in cell membranes. The net effect is that the integrity of the cell membrane is disrupted and the exchange of solutes and the influx of water lead to cell lysis.

The biologically active complement fragments help to maintain normal host defenses, but they are also capable of mediating tissue injury (Chapter 14).

THE RELATIONSHIP BETWEEN HISTOCOMPATIBILITY ANTIGENS AND THE IMMUNE SYSTEM

BACKGROUND—TRANSPLANTATION ANTIGENS

Tissue and organ transplantation studies led to the discovery that there are certain antigens on transplanted tissues that figure prominently in the rejection or acceptance of transplants by the immune system. The antigens, genetically determined, were found to be glycoproteins that are inserted into the cell membrane. All mammalian species studied thus far have a single chromosome region where the genes that encode the major tissue antigens are located. This region is referred to as the *major histocompatibility complex*. The MHC is more specifically designated as the H-2 system in mice and as the HLA system in humans. HLA stands for *human leukocyte antigen* (the antigens were first demonstrated on leukocytes), a term internationally agreed on to represent the MHC of humans. The multiple HLA genes are located in close proximity to each other on the sixth chromosome of humans.

There are two principal classes of MHC glycoproteins. Class I MHC antigens appear on virtually all nucleated somatic cells. Class II, not nearly so widely distributed as Class I, are expressed on antigen-presenting macrophages, dendritic cells, most B cells, and some T cells.

MAJOR HISTOCOMPATIBILITY COMPLEX AND THE IMMUNE SYSTEM

Immunologists in the 1970s came to realize that the normal or primary immunologic function of MHC proteins was something other than their role in graft rejection. Grafts in nature are rare. It was found that T cells, in order to respond to a foreign antigen, had to recognize both the self cell-surface MHC proteins and the foreign antigen. T cells, in other words, can recognize and respond to foreign antigens only in the context of a self marker or self reference point. This limitation during antigen recognition by T cells is called *genetic* or *MHC restriction*.

As part of their thymic "education" to recognize self MHC proteins and foreign antigens, immature T cells undergo a two-stage selection process as they differentiate. In stage one, T cells that can recognize self MHC proteins are allowed to propagate; those that do not are eliminated. In stage two, those cells that bind too avidly to self MHC proteins are eliminated, or at least inacti-

vated, to avoid self-destructive autoimmune reactions (Chapter 14).

After this selection process in the thymus there should remain T cells that recognize self MHC markers but are not activated by self-recognition alone. To the latter point, in order for an immune response to proceed the T cell needs to recognize not only the self-MHC antigen but the foreign antigen combined with the self-MHC antigen.

We shall return to the subject of MHC restriction when we discuss the sequence of events that take place in an immune response.

THE IMMUNE RESPONSE

We have considered the major elements involved in an immune response, namely, antigens, macrophages, immunoglobulins, B lymphocytes, T lymphocytes, and their subsets (T_H, T_S, T_C, T_D), MHC restriction, cytokines, and the complement system. Let us now see how these elements interplay in the sequence of events of an immune response (Fig. 12-15). It is important to recall that before an immune response takes place—before there is antigen recognition—there already exist millions of lymphocytes, each of which possesses receptors only for small regions of the antigen for which they are specific.

A precise event initiates the immune response. A receptor molecule on the surface of a B cell or a T cell recognizes the antigen to which the cell is programmed to respond and binds to some small part of it. It is the nature of the antigen that determines whether it is the B cells or the T cells that will have the effector function; how the antigen is presented to trigger the immune response; and the pathway of the immune response. The proliferation of B cells and T cells that leads to the production of antibodies and effector T cells does not result simply by binding of antigen with receptor. Cross-linking of several receptors usually is required, as is collaborative cellular inter-

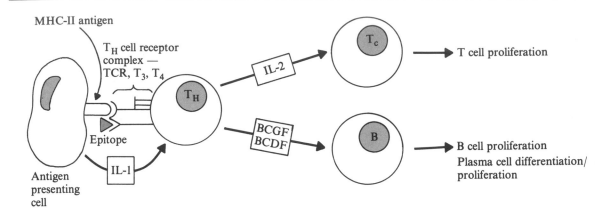

Fig. 12-15. Cellular interactions involved in an immune response.

actions and regulation under the control of cytokines.

The triggering event of an immune response most often involves protein antigen recognition by T_H cells. The most common sequence of events when the antigen is one that elicits a cell-mediated immune response or when the antigen is a T-dependent antigen for B cells is (see Helper T Cells, this chapter, for T-dependent antigens):

1. The production of antibodies or of effector T cells involves three cell types: (a) antigen-processing/presenting macrophages called accessory cells (dendritic cells and B cells also function as antigen-presenting cells); (b) helper T cells; and (c) either B cells or effector T cells.

2. The macrophages ingest, process, and present on their cell membrane antigen fragments (e.g., peptides), which contain antigenic determinants composed of a cluster of some 10 to 20 amino acid residues.

3. In order for a given T_H cell to recognize and respond to its specific small part of the antigen presented on the macrophage surface: (a) the macrophage has to have on its surface a self-marker, a Class II-MHC glycoprotein. The requirement for this marker is called MHC restriction. This marker forms a complex with the antigen fragment and that antigen fragment-MHC complex can be regarded as signal 1 to the appropriate T_H cell; (b) the T_H has a receptor on its surface, symbolized by TCR, that is specific for a small part of the antigen; and (c) a second signal is given by the macrophage in the form of a chemical messenger called interleukin-1 (IL-1).

4. The T_H cell, activated by the two signals from the macrophage, produces interleukin-2 (IL-2). IL-2 initiates clone formation of the activated T_H cell in an autocatalytic manner and the cells of the clone produce more IL-2 and other lymphokines (interleukins).

5. If the antigen that incited the immune response is one that evokes response by a B cell: (a) the B cell must have the specific IgM/IgD receptors for the involved antigenic determinant; (b) the T_H cell and the B cell actually recognize different antigenic determinants of the same antigen molecule, in what is termed cognate interaction or cooperation; and (c) the activated T_H cell and its clone, which recognizes the appropriate antigenic determinant on the same antigen that the B cell responds to, produces two lymphokines that particularly affect the B cell. One lymphokine, IL-4, or B cell growth factor (BCGF), is mitogenic for B cells—that is, it induces the B cell to form an expanded population

of itself. The other lymphokine, IL-6, or B cell differentiation factor (BCDF), induces the expanded B cell population to differentiate into plasma cells and it is the plasma cells that now go on to produce antibodies that are all of the same specificity.

6. If the antigen that initiated the immune response is one that calls for response by effector T cells (T_C or T_D), IL-2 from the T_H clone cited in 4 above stimulates clone formation in the appropriate T effector cell that has recognized its specific antigenic determinant.

What has been discussed so far pertains to the afferent arc or input phase of an immune response. Now let us consider the effects of the formed immune products on the remaining antigen (e.g., bacteria that are causing an infection) during what is called the efferent arc or output phase of an immune response. Immune system products destroy, neutralize, or eliminate antigens either directly or through the assistance primarily of macrophages, an inflammatory response, and the complement system. Antitoxins directly neutralize toxins; T_C cells destroy virus-producing host cells by direct contact. T_{DTH} cells indirectly destroy antigens by inducing a buildup of activated macrophages at the antigen site and it is the macrophages that confine or destroy the antigens. Antibodies with opsonic activity bind via antigen-binding sites to the antigenic determinants of a bacterial cell and by the other end of the antibody molecule, the Fc end, bind to Fc receptors on the surfaces of phagocytic cells. It is the phagocytes that destroy the antigen. Destruction by phagocytes is the ultimate fate of most antigens. Immune products usually affect the intact native antigen such as a bacterial cell or a foreign cell but recognition and binding is via the antigenic determinants.

The outcome of immune responses is not always beneficial. When we consider the hypersensitivities in Chapter 14 we shall see that the emphasis is not on what happens to the antigen but on what happens to the tissues of the host as a consequence of an immune response.

TYPES OF IMMUNITY

The prime function of the immune system is to provide protection. One of the major harmful antigens that enters the body is the infectious disease agent. Special terms are employed to describe an individual's state and type of protection, especially as related to protection against infectious agents and their products.

INNATE IMMUNITY

The immune status is customarily divided into two major categories, innate immunity (see Chaper 11) and acquired immunity.

ACQUIRED (ADAPTIVE) IMMUNITY

The acquired immune state depends on antibodies and the cell-mediated immune mechanisms. Most of the time, when an individual's immunity is being discussed, it is the acquired immune state that is being referred to. It may be artificially acquired immunity or naturally acquired immunity, an active or a passive immune state.

Types of Acquired Immunity

1. Artificially acquired. In artificially acquired immunity the antigens or the antibodies are introduced by artificial means, ordinarily involving the use of a vaccine or an antiserum, respectively.

2. Naturally acquired. In naturally acquired immunity the antigen, usually an infectious agent, or antibodies are transmitted to the individual under natural circumstances. Exposure to antigen or contact with antigen is unintentional.

3. Active. If the individual whose immune state is being described produced the antibodies, the immunity is said to be an active one. It can be naturally acquired as the result of an infection

or artificially acquired as the result of the introduction of immunizing materials such as vaccines and toxoids.

4. Passive. If the individual whose immune state is being described did not produce the antibodies, the immunity is said to be passive. The antibodies may have been injected in the form of an antiserum or immune globulins that were obtained from animals or from other humans (artificially acquired passive immunity). The antibodies may have been transmitted under natural circumstances, as in the transfer of maternal antibodies across the placenta to the fetus or the transmission of antibodies via colostrum (naturally acquired passive immunity). The passive immune state is of short duration—weeks to months. The proteins of administered serum are foreign, and the body may react to them as to foreign antigens.

IMMUNIZATION PRACTICES

ACTIVE IMMUNIZATION

The material that is deliberately introduced to evoke the active immune state is referred to as a *vaccine*, *immunogen*, *immunizing material*, or *antigen*. More specifically, it may be designated *toxoid* when it is a modified toxin, or *bacterin* when it is a suspension of modified bacteria. The ability of an immunogen to elicit an immune response that is protective is governed by the composition of the immunogen, the immune responsiveness of the individual being immunized, and the manner in which the immunogen is presented.

The composition of immunogens may be divided as follows:

1. Toxoids. The exotoxins of some bacteria, notably of the tetanus and diphtheria bacteria, are converted in the laboratory to a nontoxigenic form by treatment with formalin or with other modalities.

2. Whole-cell killed vaccines. Some vaccines consist of suspensions of inactivated intact microorganisms. The whooping cough, typhoid fever, and plague vaccines are whole-cell vaccines. Whole-cell vaccines sometimes produce serious side effects, so there are ongoing efforts to define a subunit of the whole cell that confers immunity and avoids unwanted side effects.

3. Attenuated vaccines. A number of effective vaccines consist of living microorganisms that, through laboratory processing, have lost their virulence (or their virulence has been greatly reduced). The genetically stable attenutated microorganisms can still multiply in the host but lack the ability to cause disease. It is a general tenet of immunization practices that living microorganisms induce a higher and longer-lasting level of immunity than do nonliving microorganisms. The need for booster doses furthermore may be lessened. The attenuation process commonly involves adapting microorganisms to conditions that they do not face in the host so that they lose their ability to multiply unrestrictedly in the host. For virus attenuation the method often involves prolonged growth of the virus in cells of a species that the virus normally does not infect. Thus, poliovirus is grown in monkey tissue culture, yellow fever and influenza viruses in embryonate hens' eggs, German measles virus in duck embryo cells.

4. Purified antigens, subunit vaccines. Intact microorganisms are a composite of various antigens. The bacterial envelope, for example, has structures or molecular components such as the capsule, the slime layer, pili, LPS, flagella, and teichoic acid, which of themselves are antigenic and sometimes also harmful. The immunity an individual develops against a given microorganism very often is directed only against a predominating antigen ("protective" antigen) and, more specifically, against only one or a few antigenic determinants of that antigen. Once that antigen is identified, the vaccine, whenever feasible, is made of the isolated purified antigen. A *subunit vaccine* then is composed of that fraction or a part of the whole microorganism that is known to contain the antigenic molecules that stimulate immunity. Antibodies against the capsular anti-

gens of a number of pathogenic bacteria protect against disease caused by the pathogens. Vaccines containing purified capsular polysaccharides are available against strains of *Streptococcus pneumoniae*, *Neisseria meningitidis*, and *Hemophilus influenzae*. Some vaccines, incidentally, are polyvalent—meaning that the vaccine is composed of several to many variants of the antigen. The current vaccine against *S. pneumoniae*, for example, contains polysaccharides from 23 of the more than 80 capsular types of this organism. The 23 strains represented in the vaccine account for the majority of cases of pneumococcal lobar pneumonia.

5. Recombinant vaccines. If the protective antigen of a microorganism is known, it can be refined beyond the subunit stage by isolating the genetic material of the microorganism. Segments of nucleic acid, including those that code for the antigen, are inserted into bacteria, yeasts, or animal cells. Large quantities of purified antigen can be produced in this way. The gene that codes for the surface antigen of the hepatitis B virus, for example, has been cloned in yeast cells. This vaccine seems to have immunogenicity as great as, if not greater than, the vaccine that is prepared from hepatitis B surface antigen obtained from human plasma. Pure preparations of antigen as obtained by recombinant technology may have limited immunogenicity, however, because the antigens are not effectively processed in the host to be delivered to antigen-responsive cells. A way around this difficulty is to insert the genes into a nonvirulent carrier organism such as the vaccinia virus. The gene for the glycoprotein antigen of the rabies virus, for example, has recently been inserted into the vaccinia virus. Edible bait containing the virus is being tested for its ability to confer protection against rabies in wild and domesticated animals.

6. Synthesized immunogens. Future vaccines may consist of synthesized immunogens. Monoclonal antibodies (described in Chapter 13) are precisely specific for epitopes (antigenic determinants) and so they can be used to identify the epitopes responsible for protection among the sites on the entire antigen molecule. Once the

isolated epitope is analyzed for amino acid composition and sequence it can be synthesized. A pure preparation of the synthesized sequence alone usually is nonimmunogenic, so it would be coupled to a carrier molecule or inserted into a nonvirulent carrier microorganism.

In 1990, the Immunization Committee of the American College Health Association provided recommendations (Table 12-5) to colleges and universities to use as guidelines for establishing and implementing a comprehensive Prematriculation Immunization Requirement (PIR). Universities have protected their students from vaccine-preventable disease outbreaks by requiring them to have proof of vaccination prior to entrance and, in the process, have protected themselves from costly tracking procedures and emergency immunizations.

Prolongation and Intensification of the Immune Response

The antibody level attained and its persistence are enhanced by the addition of adjuvants to the antigen preparation. Adjuvants are believed to prolong the antigenic stimulus, thereby elevating the antibody response. Alum-precipitated toxoids, for example, produce higher antibody titers and longer-lasting immunity than do toxoids alone. Freund's complete adjuvant, consisting of mycobacteria in a water-in-oil emulsion, is used experimentally by immunologists especially to heighten the CMI response.

DYNAMICS OF THE IMMUNE RESPONSE

Primary Immune Response

The first exposure to the antigen, whether through infection or vaccination, leads to the *primary immune response* (Fig. 12-16). A readily detectable level of antibodies does not develop immediately. There is a lag period, or induction period, of days before detectable protective levels of antibody are formed. Artificial active immunization would not be needed if a protective

Table 12-5. Prematriculation immunizations recommended by the American College Health Association, 1990.

Vaccine	Age indicated	Major indications[a]	Major precautions[a]
MMR (if given instead of individual vaccines)	First dose at 12 months[b]; second dose at school entry or later	All entering college students born after 1956 should have two doses of live measles vaccine; susceptible travelers	Pregnancy; history of anaphylactic reaction following egg ingestion or receipt of neomycin; immunosuppression; appropriate for HIV-antibody-positive persons
Measles vaccine	First dose at 12 months[b]; second dose at school entry or later	All entering college students born after 1956 should have two doses of live measles vaccine; susceptible travelers	Pregnancy; history of anaphylactic reaction following egg ingestion or receipt of neomycin; immunosuppression; appropriate for HIV-antibody-positive persons
Rubella vaccine	12 months[b]	Both males and females without verification of live vaccine on or after first birthday or laboratory evidence of immunity; susceptible travelers	Pregnancy; history of anaphylactic reaction following receipt of neomycin; immunosuppression; appropriate for HIV-antibody-positive persons
Mumps vaccine	12 months[b]	All entering college students born after 1956 should have had one dose of live mumps vaccine or a history of mumps	Pregnancy; history of anaphylactic reaction following egg ingestion or receipt of neomycin; immunosuppression; appropriate for HIV-antibody-positive persons
Tetanus-diphtheria toxoid	Primary series in childhood, booster 14–16, booster every 10 years	All persons	History of a neurologic hypersensitivity reaction following a previous dose
Polio vaccine: killed vaccine (E-IPV), live vaccine (OPV)	Primary series in childhood, booster only if needed for travel after age 18	Persons traveling to areas where wild poliovirus is endemic or epidemic; OPV not indicated for persons over 18 years unless previously immunized with OPV	OPV should not be given to immunocompromised persons or to HIV-antibody-positive persons

[a] Refer to appropriate Immunization Practices Advisory Committee (ACIP) recommendations for more details.
[b] Public health authorities recommend that a first dose of MMR be given at 15 months of age; however, vaccine administered at 12 months of age is still accepted as a first dose.

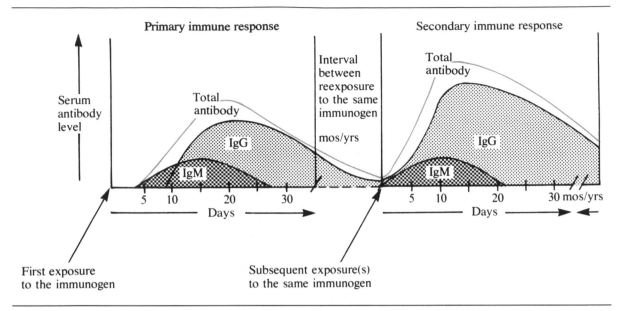

Fig. 12-16. Primary and secondary immune responses. In the primary response IgM is the first to appear in the serum. It appears on the fifth to seventh day and peaks at about 14 days. IgG appears about the tenth day and peaks several weeks later. In the secondary immune response, both IgM and IgG appear to increase within 2 to 3 days. In the secondary immune response, the lag period is shorter, the total antibody level far surpasses that of the primary immune response, antibody is formed over a longer period of time, and much more IgG is formed than IgM.

level were reached in hours. The antibodies first produced are typically of the IgM class and have low affinity for the antigen. As the response progresses there is a selective expansion of B cells that have switched from production of IgM to IgG and there is expansion of B cells that have an increased affinity for antigen because of somatic mutations in their V domains. With a single antigen exposure the antibody titer frequently drops after a comparatively short time, sometimes to a level that is no longer protective.

Secondary Immune Response

With a number of immunogens it is the practice to give additional exposures to the antigen at appropriately spaced intervals. These ensuing stimuli are commonly termed *booster doses*. The additional antigenic stimulus elicits prompt antibody formation, and the antibody level is higher,

persists longer, and is primarily of class IgG. The prompt, elevated response to additional antigenic stimuli is due to the *anamnestic response*, also termed the *recall phenomenon*. The selectively accumulated B cells (memory cells) from the primary immune response are poised to produce high-affinity IgG antibodies to the same antigen. The number and spacing of booster doses differ according to the requirements of different age groups and populations, and for the various disease agents. An antigen may be given in combination with other antigens because the antibody-forming mechanism responds to each antigen of the preparation. The foremost example of active immunization is that of the DTP series. Preschool children are protected against diphtheria (the *D* of DTP), tetanus (*T*), and pertussis (*P*) in a series of spaced immunizations that contain all three antigen preparations.

PASSIVE IMMUNIZATION

It is sometimes necessary to protect an individual with antibodies that have been developed in an animal or that are obtained from another human. The patient may have suffered exposure to an infectious agent to which he or she has not been actively immunized or for which active immunization is not routine practice (infectious hepatitis) or perhaps against which it is not feasible to immunize actively (botulism). In the first instance, even if active immunizing material were available, it is not possible for the patient to produce a sufficient level of his or her own antibodies to fight off the current infection. Antisera developed in animals or gamma globulins obtained from humans are used to provide temporary, immediate protection. Passive immunization is also referred to as *passive immunotherapy* or, when serum is used, as *serotherapy*.

The use of animal (foreign or heterologous) antisera for humans has declined. Foreign antisera in vivo have a short half-life, between 7 and 23 days. The level diminishes through four phases: dilution, catabolism, immune complex formation, and elimination. Foreign antisera can cause anaphylactic reactions on second exposure, and serum sickness (painful joints, fever, rash). Animal antisera still used in humans are equine diphtheria antitoxin, polyvalent botulinum antitoxin, and equine anti-lymphocyte serum.

Human gamma globulin has few side effects and is not eliminated so rapidly as animal antisera. Gamma globulin preparations are of two types. *Immune serum globulin (ISG)* is prepared from pooled plasma or serum obtained from a group of donors irrespective of their infection or immunization history (with certain precautions). When gamma globulin from a number of individuals is pooled, it is likely to contain antibodies to the common infectious diseases. ISG is used for pre- and post-exposure hepatitis A; for *hypogammaglobulinemia*, that is, individuals at risk who have low levels of gamma globulin; and for measles in nonimmunized children who have

been exposed to measles or who are immunosuppressed. The second type of gamma globulin is obtained from individual donors who have been deliberately actively immunized against a given disease agent or who have recovered from the disease. These preparations are specifically named—for example, tetanus immune globulin (TIG), hepatitis B (HBIG), rabies (RIG), and varicella-zoster (chickenpox-shingles) (VZIG), to name some of the better-known preparations.

Gamma globulin is administered intramuscularly. Intravenous administration is contraindicated because of anaphylactoid (anaphylaxis-like) reactions. In preparing gamma globulin, alcohol fractionation of the serum produces aggregates of immunoglobulins. IgG and IgM aggregates bind and activate complement, leading to the formation of anaphylatoxins, which in turn cause intense inflammation and tissue damage. Recently there has been renewed interest in using immunoglobulin preparations on a broader scale to provide protection to patients with life-threatening or debilitating illness. Newer preparative methods prevent immunoglobulins from aggregating. The immunoglobulins consequently can be intravenously infused and much higher doses provided. Immune serum globulin, to start with, already contains about 14 times more IgG than whole serum. Patients with intractable infections, transplant recipients, and cancer patients on chemotherapy are candidates for this type of *immunoprophylaxis* or *immunotherapy*.

SUMMARY

1. The immune system specifically recognizes foreign substances with certain characteristics (antigens), forms immune products (antibodies and activated T lymphocytes) against the substances, and through memory lymphocyte cells is prepared to react swiftly in the next encounter with the same substances.

2. Antigens stimulate the formation of immune products (the property of immunogenicity) and react with immune products (the property of reactivity).

3. Antigens possess small discrete chemical groups on their surfaces called antigenic determinants. The chemical and physical nature of the determinants confers specific characteristics on the antigen molecule, and it is against these determinants that immune products are formed.

4. Lymphoid stem cells differentiate into two separate but largely interdependent lymphocyte populations. The B lymphocyte (B cell) population, which differentiates in the bone marrow, is responsible for the production of antibodies that give rise to humoral immunity. The T lymphocyte (T cell), which differentiates in the thymus gland, is responsible for the production of effector lymphocytes that give rise to cell-mediated immunity (CMI).

5. B cells produce five classes of immunoglobulins—namely, IgM, IgD, IgG, IgE, and IgA. The classes differ in amino acid composition and sequences, in their biological activities, and antigenically.

6. A basic Ig molecule is composed of two heavy (H) chains and two light (L) chains. The Fab portion of the molecule contains variable (V) and constant (C) regions of H and L chains. The V regions form the antigen-binding site of an antibody molecule.

7. The other end of the Ig molecule, the Fc portion, is composed of constant (C) regions of H chains. The biological functions of the Fc include binding of Igs to host cells (e.g., mast cells, macrophages, and neutrophils), binding of complement by IgG and IgM, and facilitation of the transplacental passage of IgG.

8. Antibody diversity is due to intrachromosomal recombination in somatic cells of selected V, J, D, and C gene sequences to form a single transcription unit. This mechanism allows the generation of a large repertoire of immunoglobulin receptors of differing specificities without requiring an individual germ-line gene for each antibody specificity.

9. Another recombinational event, the heavy chain switch, occurs at the other end of the Ig molecule after antigen recognition. Through S/S recombination, an antigen-binding site can associate with any of the five Ig classes and thereby acquire the biological functions characteristic of that class.

10. Immunoglobulins serve as receptor molecules in the membranes of mature B cells before antigen recognition. On antigen recognition B cells differentiate into plasma cells and secrete antibodies.

11. According to the Clonal Selection Theory, there are small clones of B cells, each cell of which is specific for a given antigen, before antigen recognition occurs. On recognition of its specific antigen each cell of the clones expands to produce antibodies of the same original specificity.

12. T cells are functionally divisible into subpopulations of effector T cells (killer T cells and T_{DTH} cells) and regulator cells (helper T cells and suppressor T cells).

13. Helper T (T_H) cells are essential for most B and other T cells to respond to antigens. Suppressor T (T_S) cells regulate the responses of B and other T cells.

14. Killer T cells (T_C or T_{CTL}) directly destroy host target cells that express foreign antigens on their surfaces. NK and K are other types of killer cells that are non-T cells. T_{DTH} cells secrete messenger substances called lymphokines, which involve uncommitted cells in dealing with an antigen.

15. The complement system is frequently involved in nonspecific resistance and in acquired immunity. The biologically active factors that are serially generated when the complement system is activated facilitate the localization and destruction of foreign substances. Complement's biological roles include cell lysis, chemotaxis, opsonization, and stimulation of inflammation.

16. In most cases, for an immune response to be initiated a T_H cell must specifically recognize an antigen in combination with the Class II–MHC marker (MHC restriction) on the surface of an

antigen-presenting accessory cell. The T_H cell subsequently signals, via lymphokines, B cells and other T cells to proliferate.

17. Intercellular messengers called cytokines have a key role in regulating the responses of lymphocytes and their supporting cast of phagocytes, the complement system, and inflammatory reactions.

18. Immune states are described by the terms innate vs. acquired, natural vs. artificial, and active vs. passive.

19. The level of the attained active immune state is related to such considerations as the type of immunogen, the frequency and spacing of exposure to the immunogen, the use of adjuvants, and the role of memory cells. Types of immunogens include toxoids, whole-cell vaccines, vaccines with attenuated microorganisms, subunit vaccines with purified antigens, and recombinant vaccines.

20. Passive immunization practices in humans include the administration of animal antisera and human gamma globulin prepared either from pooled sera (ISG) or from serum obtained from an individual donor who has been deliberately immunized with, or who has recovered from, a specific infectious disease agent.

QUESTIONS FOR STUDY

Select the best response or responses for each of the following:

1. The only known function of this class of antibody is to serve as an antigen receptor on the surface of mature immunocompetent B lymphocytes.
   A. IgA
   B. IgD
   C. IgE
   D. IgG
   E. IgM

2. Substances, administered along with an immunogen, that enhance the immune system response to the immunogen are called
   A. Reagins
   B. Releasins
   C. Toxoids
   D. Adjuvants
   E. Attenuators

3. The immune status acquired by a child who has been immunized with the oral polio vaccine (OPV—an attenuated strain) is described as
   A. Naturally acquired passive immunity
   B. Artificially acquired passive immunity
   C. Naturally acquired active immunity
   D. Innate immunity
   E. Artificially acquired active immunity

4. Interleukin-2:
   A. Is a monokine
   B. Is an activated component of complement
   C. Stimulates the proliferation of antigen-stimulated T cells
   D. Is a lymphotoxin secreted by T_{DTH} cells
   E. Is a pharmacological mediator of immune complex-type hypersensitivity reactions

5. Oleoresin, the allergen associated with poison oak and poison sumac, is a small-molecular-weight compound that is unable to elicit an immune response unless first complexed with proteins in the skin. Thus, oleoresin is a(n)
   A. Hapten
   B. Opsonin
   C. Monomer
   D. Antigenic determinant
   E. Petite molecule

6. In order for a molecule to be antigenic it must be
   A. A hapten
   B. Initially contacted in high concentrations
   C. Recognized as foreign or "non-self"
   D. Particulate in nature

7. Following V/J and V/D/J recombination in the early stages of differentiation, a clone of B cells
   A. Is committed to synthesizing antibody of a single antigen-binding specificity
   B. Is no longer dependent on helper T-cell function in order to respond to thymus-dependent antigens
   C. Switches from the synthesis of IgM to the synthesis of some other class of antibody
   D. Loses its ability to respond immunologically to an antigenic determinant
   E. No longer expresses both IgM and IgD on its surface

8. The S/S recombination event:
   A. Occurs on T cells during maturation in the thymus
   B. Pertains to the switch by plasma cells from synthesis of one class of immunoglobulin to another
   C. Commits B cells to a response to a single antigenic determinant
   D. Precedes V/D/J recombination

9. Vaccines that contain living (infective) microorganisms are often developed from microorganisms that originally were virulent. Such strains that have a lost or greatly diminished virulence are said to be
   A. Passive immunogens   D. Noninfective
   B. Secondary pathogens   E. Derepressed
   C. Attenuated

10. Mature B cells:
    A. Usually require helper T cell function in order to respond optimally to an antigen
    B. Have only IgG receptor molecules on their surfaces before antigen recognition
    C. As individual cells, each responds to many different antigenic determinants
    D. Respond to antigenic determinants presented on the surface of a neutrophil
    E. Must have matured in the thymus gland in order to gain immunocompetence

11. One means of destruction of bacteria in the body is by antibodies or complement fragment C3b coating the bacterial cells. The bacteria as a consequence are now much more readily ingested by phagocytes. The antibodies or C3b in this role are called
    A. Opsonins   D. Chemotaxins
    B. Epitopes   E. Cytolysins
    C. Agglutinins

12. Which of the following is not an antibody?
    A. Agglutinin   D. Complement
    B. Precipitin   E. Immune cytolysin
    C. Antitoxin

13. Antibodies are contained in which protein fraction of the serum?
    A. Alpha globulins   D. Albumen
    B. Beta globulins   E. Fibrinogen
    C. Gamma globulins

14. The chemical groups on the surfaces of antigens that represent the groups against which antibodies are formed are collectively referred to as
    A. Phagosomes   D. Lymphokines
    B. Complementary sites   E. Reagins
    C. Antigenic determinants

15. The part of the antibody molecule that combines with the antigenic determinant is found in the
    A. C (constant) domains of the H chains
    B. C (constant) domains of the L chains
    C. The hypervariable region of the H and L variable domain of the Fab
    D. Terminal Fc domains of both H chains
    E. Hinge region of the Ig molecule

16. An antibody that has the composition of two basic immunoglobulin molecules joined by a J chain, and a secretory piece (that is added on in glandular epithelial cells), is most likely to be found
    A. In the thymus

B. On the mucosa where it provides topical, local immunity
C. In the serum
D. Associated with atopic allergies
E. Attached to the surface membrane of uncommitted B lymphocytes

17. According to the clonal selection theory:
    A. Lymphocytes acquire specific receptors for antigen only after contact with antigen.
    B. Lymphocytes bear receptors that have genetically determined specificities before contact with foreign antigen is ever made.
    C. Macrophages make RNA copies of ingested antigen and transfer the copies to T_{CTL} cells.
    D. Every mature B cell has IgM and IgD receptor molecules and can be activated by two different antigenic determinants.

18. Genetic or MHC (major histocompatibility) restriction means that
    A. Allografts are rejected only when the graft donor and recipient are genetically identical.
    B. The degree of antibody diversity is governed by the product of the total number of gene sequences that code for the respective VDJ regions of the antibody molecule.
    C. Rh incompatibilities are restricted to

those situations in which the father is Rh positive and the mother is Rh negative.
    D. T cells are unable to recognize (respond to) antigenic determinants unless the determinants are associated with self-MHC glycoproteins on the surface of the host's own cells.

19. The functionally distinct subsets (subpopulations) of T cells include (1) helper T cells; (2) suppressor T cells; (3) cytotoxic T lymphocytes; (4) pre-thymocytes; or (5) delayed-type hypersensitivity T cells.
    A. 1,2,3,5
    B. 1,2,4
    C. 2,3,4
    D. 4
    E. 1,2,3,4,5

20. The development of immunological tolerance is primarily dependent upon
    A. Activation of the classical complement pathway
    B. Degradation of self antigens in the phagolysosomes of neutrophils
    C. Clonal abortion (or deletion) of self-reactive clones of B and T cells during maturation
    D. Sequestering (compartmentalization or hiding) of self antigens
    E. Presentation of foreign antigens on the surface of antigen-presenting cells

True or false:

21. IgM as a receptor molecule on a B cell exists as a pentamer whereas as a secreted immunoglobulin it exists as a monomer.
    A. True   B. False

22. The antibody specificity of a particular B cell is induced by interactions with an antigenic determinant rather than being genetically determined.
    A. True   B. False

23. When activated effector T cells proliferate, some differentiate into plasma cells while others remain as memory cells.
    A. True   B. False

24. Live attenuated microorganisms rather than killed microorganisms stimulate a greater primary humoral response by proliferating, thus providing a source of antigen over a prolonged period of time.
    A. True   B. False

25. The categorization of immunoglobulins into five basic classes is determined by the amino acid composition of their light (L) chains.
    A. True   B. False

Match each cell type on the left with each set of characteristics on the right.

26. Plasma cells

27. Macrophages

28. Helper T cells

29. Mast cells

30. Neutrophils

A. Granulocytic, phagocytic cells characteristically found at sites of acute inflammation
B. Have receptor sites for immunoglobulins of class IgE
C. Process antigens and present antigen fragments on their surface
D. Antibody producers
E. Specifically recognize foreign antigen complexed with self Class II MHC glycoproteins on accessory cell surface

ADDITIONAL READINGS

Barrett, J. T. *Textbook of Immunology* (5th ed.). St. Louis: Mosby, 1988.

Benjamini, E., and Leskowitz, S. *Immunology: A Short Course*. New York: Alan R. Liss, 1988.

Centers of Disease Control. General recommendations on immunization. *M.M.W.R.* 28:13,1989.

Dillman, R. O. Monoclonal antibodies for treating cancer. *Ann. Intern. Med.* 111:592,1989.

Frank, M. M. Complement: A brief review. *J. Allergy Immunol. Clin.* 84:411,1989.

Grey, H. M., Sette, A., and Buus, S. How T cells see antigen. *Sci. Am.* 259:56,November, 1989.

Jaret, P. Our immune system: The wars within. *National Geographic* 169(6):702,1986.

Leder, P. Genetic control of immunoglobulin production. *Hosp. Pract.* 18(2):73, 1983.

Nossal, G. J. V. Immunologic tolerance: Collaboration between antigen and lymphocytes. *Science* 245:147,July, 1989.

Nossal, G. J. V. Immunology: The basic components of the immune system. *N. Engl. J. Med.* 316:1320,1987.

Smith, K. A. Interleukin-2. *Sci. Am.* 259:50,March, 1990.

Snell, G. D. The major histocompatibility complex: Its evolution and involvement in cellular immunity. *Harvey Lect.* 74:49, 1980.

Strominger, J. L. Developmental biology of T cell receptors. *Science* 244:943,1989.

Tizard, I. R. *Immunology* (2nd ed.). Philadelphia: Saunders, 1988.

Young, J. D., and Cohn, Z. A. How killer cells kill. *Sci. Am.* 258:38,January, 1988.

13. IMMUNODIAGNOSIS

OBJECTIVES

To cite the two features of antigen–immune product interactions that make serological testing feasible

To explain the role and the value of serological tests in diagnosis, identification, and monitoring

To describe the principles and the qualitative and quantitative aspects of representative serological tests, including especially agglutination, complement fixation, immunodiffusion, radioimmunoassay, fluorescent antibody, and enzyme immunoassay

To discuss monoclonal antibodies; explain how they are developed; compare monoclonal antibody preparations and conventionally produced antisera; evaluate their importance; and give examples of their diagnostic and therapeutic applications

To discuss the ABO system of red blood cells as it pertains to transfusion reactions and to discuss the Rh system as it pertains to hemolytic disease of the newborn

An important application of immune system products (antibodies and effector T cells) is their use in identification, diagnosis, and monitoring. The fact that the interactions between antigens and immune system products are essentially highly specific and that these interactions produce detectable reactions makes possible a great variety of valuable in vitro and in vivo tests. The subdiscipline of immunology that uses these interactions is variously entitled *serology, immunoserology, serodiagnosis, immunodiagnosis*, or *immunoidentification*. The term *serology* implies the use of serum or components thereof in the tests. Serum is commonly used as a test ingredient because the most frequently used immune product—antibodies—is most accessible in serum. It should not be concluded, however, that every immunodiagnostic test involves serum.

THE VALUE OF SEROLOGICAL TESTS IN MEDICAL MICROBIOLOGY

The information obtained from serological tests is valuable for the following reasons:

1. Sometimes the only way, or the only practical way, to identify the causal agent of an infection is via serological testing. This is the situation with diseases in which the isolation of the causative agent is not feasible or is impractical because of cost–benefit considerations.
2. Serological tests are frequently used to confirm a diagnosis that was made on clinical grounds or by other laboratory findings.
3. It may be important to know the immune status of a person or of a population. A dentist may wish to know if he or she has antibodies to the hepatitis B virus. a woman of childbearing age may wish to know if she is immune to the rubella (German measles) virus.
4. The course or severity of a disease can be followed and the treatment or prognosis or both indicated by such determinations.
5. Sometimes it is important to know the serogroup or serotype or immunotype of a causal agent. Most species of microorganisms through mutation and selection develop strains that differ in antigenic composition. These strains also frequently differ in immunogenicity and drug susceptibility. Their identification may affect patient therapy and appropriate immunization of a population at risk.

There are many applications of serological tests outside the realm of medical microbiology: cancer detection, diagnosis of allergies, identification and localization of tissue components (immunohistochemistry), immunodetection in forensic pathology, and assessment of the compatibility of donor-recipient transplant tissues and organs.

THE GENERAL PRINCIPLES OF IMMUNODIAGNOSIS

Most routinely employed immunodiagnostic tests involve antibodies, and so the descriptions and the tests to follow pertain almost entirely to antibodies.

How can antibodies be detected? How is it determined that an individual has antibodies to a given antigen as a result of immunization or in consequence of infection? Such determinations are valuable for diagnosis.

One of the components, either the antigen or the antibody, in a serological test is known. Thus, if the identity of an infectious agent (an antigen) recovered from a patient is unknown or is to be confirmed, or if its serotype is to be determined, it is tested against an antiserum that has a known antibody content. Conversely, the antibody content of a patient's serum may be the unknown component of the test, in which case the serum is tested against known antigens. A patient with an infection, for example, after a suitable induction period has usually produced antibodies against the infecting microorganism. Blood is drawn, the serum is collected after the blood is allowed to clot, and the serum is tested against known antigen. The antigens and antisera that are used as the known component of a serological test are usually commercially available. They are stable preparations that can be kept in the refrigerator for long periods of time.

Serological tests have a qualitative aspect, and most tests also have a quantitative aspect. The qualitative aspect is to answer one of the following questions: Are there antibodies in this serum for this known antigen? Or: Does this unidentified microorganism react with this serum, which has a known antibody content? Since the antigen–antibody relationship is specific, a positive reaction usually identifies the antigen or antibody—the qualitative aspect. Not only can it be determined that the antigen and antibody interact, however, but the relative quantities of one or the other can be established; that is, a *titer* can be determined. This is the quantitative aspect of serological tests. To determine a titer, either the antigen preparation or the serum is serially diluted in uniform increments. In a typical titration a series of tubes containing doubling dilutions of the test serum is set up. A constant amount of antigen is added to each tube (Fig. 13-1). The reciprocal of the highest dilution (i.e., of the last tube of the series) to give a detectable reaction in the form of a precipitation, agglutination, or other reaction is the titer. In the course of an illness it is frequently meaningful to discover that a change in titer has occurred between an early, acute-phase serum specimen and a convalescent or recovery-phase specimen.

THE TRADITIONAL SEROLOGICAL TESTS

For many years, six kinds of antibodies have been designated: *agglutinins, precipitins, antitoxins, cytolysins, opsonins,* and *virus-neutralizing antibodies.* These terms were chosen because they are descriptive of what happens when an antigen interacts with its homologous antibody under the conditions of the test system. The earlier serological test procedures were rather straightforward and uncomplicated, compared with today's refinements. In the earlier procedures straight serum was used without fractionation or conjugation. The tests were conducted primarily in tubes and on slides. This is not to say that such an approach is no longer used or useful. These still are basic serological tests in clinical serodiagnosis. Refinements, however, have increased the sensitivity and the applications of serological tests, especially as investigative tools.

Before antigen–antibody interactions are described it is important to know the difference between *particulate test antigens* and *soluble test antigens.* Antigens may be particulate, that is, particle-sized, as are intact bacterial cells, red blood cells, white blood cells, and particles and cells artificially coated with soluble antigens. Antigens may also be soluble, consisting of molecules in solution.

PRECIPITATION

Precipitation occurs when a soluble antigen reacts with its homologous antibody in appropriate relative proportions. Antibody molecules cross-link antigen molecules to form a lattice. Two well-known techniques for demonstrating precipitating antibody are the ring test and the capillary tube test.

Ring Test

The ring test is carried out in small-diameter tubes. A column of antiserum is placed in the lower half of the tube with a capillary pipette. A column of soluble antigen is gently superimposed. Precipitation occurs at the interface in the form of a ring.

Capillary Tube Test

In the capillary tube test, antigen and antiserum are sequentially drawn into a capillary tube by capillary action (Fig. 13-2). Precipitates form at the interface where the two solutions meet in positive reactions.

AGGLUTINATION

The antigen in agglutination reactions is particulate. In the presence of homologous antibody, antigens (such as intact bacterial cells or red blood cells) or uniform particles (as of latex or bentonite onto which soluble antigens have been absorbed or conjugated) clump together to form visible aggregates. Agglutination reactions are

Procedure:

1. Add 1.0 ml saline (diluent) to each tube.

2. Starting with a 1:4 dilution of the antiserum, serially transfer 1.0 ml of each succeeding dilution to each tube except the control tube.

3. Add 1.0 ml of antigen suspension (no serial dilution) to each tube including the control tube.

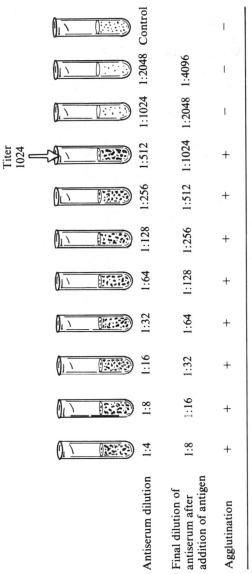

Antiserum dilution	1:4	1:8	1:16	1:32	1:64	1:128	1:256	1:512	1:1024	1:2048	Control
Final dilution of antiserum after addition of antigen	1:8	1:16	1:32	1:64	1:128	1:256	1:512	1:1024	1:2048	1:4096	
Agglutination	+	+	+	+	+	+	+	+	−	−	−

Titer 1024

Fig. 13-1. Titration series (agglutination).

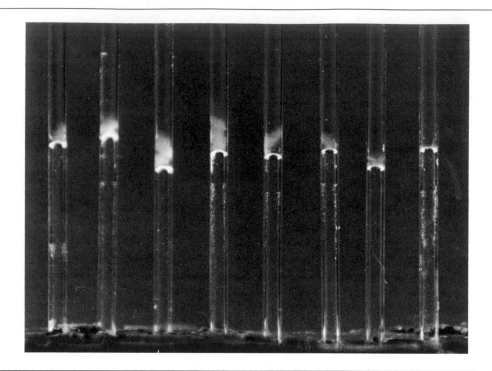

Fig. 13-2. Capillary tube precipitin test. Dilutions of soluble antigen and constant amount of specific antiserum were drawn into capillary tubes. Tubes 3 and 4 show greatest amount of precipitate. White semicircle in each tube is due to light reflection from interface where antiserum and antigen dilution meet. Final tube is negative control. (Courtesy William Krass. From J. T. Barrett. *Textbook of Immunology* [4th ed.]. St. Louis: Mosby, 1983.)

widely used for the diagnosis of certain bacterial diseases and in human blood grouping and typing. The reaction can be carried out on a slide by mixing serum with a suspension of the antigen. Most bacterial agglutination tests are serial tube tests in which a titer is determined (Fig. 13-1).

Agglutination of red blood cells is called *hemagglutination*. Tests employing red blood cells that are coated with a soluble antigen are called *passive hemagglutination tests*.

Viral Hemagglutination-Inhibition

Viral Hemagglutination. Influenza, mumps, rubella, and other viruses naturally bind to red blood cells of various animal species. Each virus particle is multivalent and so it can simultane-

ously attach to more than one blood cell. Binding is between protein spikes (called viral hemagglutinins) on the surface of the virus and receptors on the red blood cell membrane. If enough virus is present, cross-linking takes place and lattice-like aggregates form. Viral hemagglutination is a rapid, accurate method of quantitating viruses. A hemagglutinating titer (HA titer) is obtained by serially diluting the virus and finding the highest virus dilution that will just agglutinate a standardized suspension of red blood cells that is added to each tube of the test. The test is referred to as the HA test.

Viral Hemagglutination-Inhibition. The HA test is used not only to quantitate viruses but as the basis for identifying viruses in the hemagglutination-inhibition test (HAI test) (Fig. 13-3). A standardized suspension of virus, as determined in an HA test, is incubated with the antiserum, followed by the addition of red blood cells. In a positive reaction antibodies in the antiserum are specific for the virus and hemagglutination is prevented. The test set-up usually is such that a titer can be determined.

VIRUS NEUTRALIZATION

Because of their small size, viruses generally do not give readily visible reactions with their homologous antibodies. Viruses with known effects in animals or on tissue culture are mixed with serum to determine the neutralizing effect of the serum. If specific antiviral antibodies are present in the serum, the effect of the virus on the test animal or the tissue culture cells is neutralized.

IMMUNE CYTOLYSIS

The combination of cell-associated antigen, specific IgG or IgM antibodies, and complement can effect the lysis of cells on which the antigens are located. Lesions created in the cell membrane by

Fig. 13-3. Viral hemagglutination—inhibition test (HAI test).

Procedure:

1. Add patient's serum to virus suspension.

2. Add standardized suspension of red blood cells to serum-virus mixture.

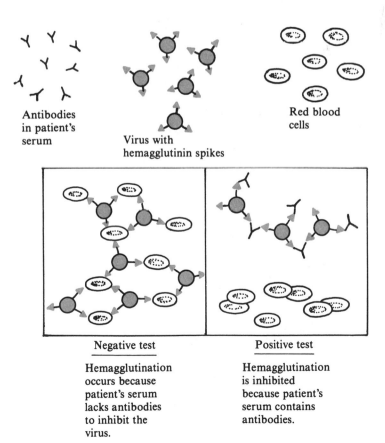

Antibodies in patient's serum

Virus with hemagglutinin spikes

Red blood cells

Negative test

Hemagglutination occurs because patient's serum lacks antibodies to inhibit the virus.

Positive test

Hemagglutination is inhibited because patient's serum contains antibodies.

the late-acting complement components (membrane attack complex) bring about lysis of the cell. The antigens involved in the reaction may be part of the affected cell itself, such as those on bacterial cells, or the antigens may be soluble antigens that have combined with the cell membrane, for example, of red blood cells.

COMPLEMENT FIXATION

The phenomenon of immune cytolysis involving complement serves as the basis of the complement fixation (CF) test (Fig. 13-4). The test has two distinct components, the indicator system and the test system. The systems vie for complement, which is one of the ingredients of the test.

Indicator System
The indicator system consists of sheep red blood cells (SRBC) as the antigen and an antiserum

(commercially available) that contains antibodies against SRBC. The SRBC of the indicator system lyse when exposed to the antiserum of the indicator system in the presence of complement. Lysis is a visible reaction because the hemoglobin released from lysed red blood cells produces a pink-to-red color in the otherwise clear, uncolored supernatant fluid.

Test System
In the other component, the test system, either the antigen is unknown or, as is most often the case, the patient's serum is being tested for unknown antibody content. The combination of the antigen with antibody must be able to fix complement. Not all antigen–antibody combinations bind complement.

Test Procedure
The first step in the CF test is to inactivate any residual complement in the test serum by heating

Fig. 13-4. Complement fixation (CF) test. (SRBC = sheep red blood cells; C = complement.)

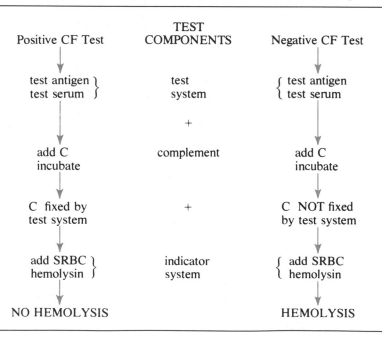

TEST COMPONENTS

Positive CF Test		Negative CF Test
test antigen ⎱ test serum ⎰	test system	⎰ test antigen ⎱ test serum
	+	
add C incubate	complement	add C incubate
C fixed by test system	+	C NOT fixed by test system
add SRBC ⎱ hemolysin ⎰	indicator system	⎰ add SRBC ⎱ hemolysin
NO HEMOLYSIS		HEMOLYSIS

the test serum for 30 minutes at 56°C. The order of the test procedure is as follows: The test antigen and the inactivated test serum are mixed. A measured amount of complement is added. The complement source is fresh guinea pig serum, which is available commercially in the lyophilized form. After the mixture of the test antigen, test serum, and complement has been incubated, the indicator system is added to the test system tube. If there is antibody in the test system that is specific for the test antigen, complement is fixed or bound to the antigen–antibody combination. In a positive CF test the complement that is fixed by this combination is not available to the indicator system when it is added. Lysis of SRBCs therefore does not occur. In a negative CF test, in which the test antibody is not specific for the test antigen, complement is not bound by the test system and remains available to the indicator system. Lysis occurs. The test is not only qualitative, as described, but can also be quantitative; that is, a titer can be determined.

Applications of Complement Fixation

The CF test is especially useful when the test antigen and antibody combination alone does not give a visible reaction. Lysis of SRBC serves as the visible, detectable reaction. The diagnosis of many viral and fungal diseases and of immunological disorders is made or confirmed by this means.

MORE RECENT IMMUNODIAGNOSTIC TECHNIQUES

Refinements in testing have led to giving serological tests names that reflect the nature of the testing technique. The same kinds of antibody are involved, but the reactions are not those typical of precipitation, agglutination, cytolysis, and neutralization.

The more recent techniques are of three major types:

1. There are techniques *for separating out the different antigens* that may be present in the antigen material and techniques *for separating out the different components of serum*. The separations are performed in or on support media such as agar gel and polymeric membranes. Separations take place under the influence of diffusion, osmosis, electrical charge, or combinations of these modalities. The separated components are then detected/identified by additional steps that may include additional diffusion and attachment of marker chemicals to antibodies.
2. Techniques for *attaching soluble antigens or antibodies to cells* (e.g., red blood cells) *or to particles* (e.g., latex, bentonite, beads) allow a visible reaction such as lysis or agglutination to occur when antigen and antibody unite.
3. In some techniques *marker chemicals* (also called *labels*) *are conjugated to immunoglobulins* (usually) *or to antigens*. Marker chemicals include dyes that fluoresce on ultraviolet irradiation, radioactive materials that are detected by radioactivity-sensing devices, and enzymes whose presence is detected when appropriate substrate is added to the preparation.

Most of these techniques have numerous modifications. Gel precipitation, for example, may take the form of simple diffusion, double diffusion, single radial diffusion, immunoelectrophoresis, or rocket immunoelectrophoresis.

IMMUNODIFFUSION

Immunodiffusion is a form of precipitation test that makes use of agar gel and other support media. Completed reactions are "fixed" in the support medium. In agar gel immunodiffusion, wells are formed in agar gel according to a predetermined pattern (Fig. 13-5). Solutions of antigen and antiserum are placed in the respective wells. Antigens and antibodies diffuse toward each other in a radial pattern. Where homologous antibody reacts in proper proportions with antigen, lines of precipitate form within the agar. This *double-diffusion method* is named the *Ouchterlony technique*.

This method has many good features. One is the stability of the precipitate; that is, once the precipitate is formed, it will remain fixed in that position in the agar over a long period of time. In addition, more than one antigen or antibody can be tested because the different antigenic molecules in the solution diffuse and aggregate separately on the basis of their size, configuration, and other properties. And, further, unknown antigens can be identified when known control antigens in a neighboring well form continuous lines of precipitate with the unknown. A continuous line (fusion) indicates identity; crossed lines indicate nonidentity. The major disadvantage of the immunodiffusion procedure is the length of time (days to weeks) it takes for the lines of precipitate to develop.

IMMUNOELECTROPHORESIS

The separation of different antigens in a solution and their identification can be refined by first *subjecting the solutions within a support medium to electrical current* (electrophoresis) (Fig. 13-6). On the basis of their charges, molecular size, and other properties, the various antigens in a solution or proteins of a serum are separated in or on a support medium such as thin layers of agar gel, cellulose acetate, or starch. Electrophoresis is combined with immunodiffusion in immunoelectrophoresis. After electrophoretic separation, troughs for antiserum (or other means of application) are placed parallel to the lines of migration of the electrophoresed solution. Arcs of antigen–antibody precipitate form. Human serum, as antigen, has been extensively investigated by this technique. As many as 37 zones of precipi-

Fig. 13-5. Immunodiffusion in agar gel. Antigen–antibody recognition results in a readily visible, opaque band of precipitate in the zone of equivalence of antibody and antigen (*Ag*). A. Reaction of identity. The continuous precipitation band is termed a *line of identity* and indicates that the antigen in both wells contains the identical antigenic determinant *a*. B. Reaction of *nonidentity*. The crossed lines of precipitation indicate that the antigen in one well does not possess common antigenic determinants with the antigen in the other well. C. Reaction of *partial identity*. The continuous precipitation band as in A indicates that the antigens in both wells contain a common antigenic determinant, *a*. The spur-like projection in the direction opposite the Ag *a,b* well indicates that the antigen in that well possesses an antigenic determinant (*b*) that is not present on the antigen of the other well.

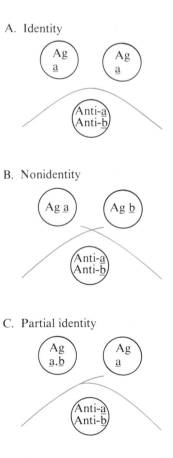

A. Identity

B. Nonidentity

C. Partial identity

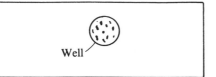

1. Antigen preparation containing four different antigens is placed in well. The well was cut in an agar film that covers the slide.

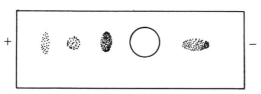

2. The agar is electrophoresed and the four antigens separate.

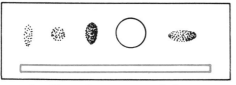

3. Electrodes are removed. A trough is cut in the agar and antiserum is placed in the trough.

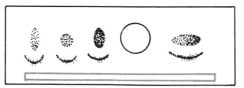

4. The four antigens and their homologous antibodies diffuse toward each other and arcs of precipitate develop where they meet.

tate, representing different proteins or subgroups of a protein class of the serum, have been distinguished (Fig. 13-7).

COUNTERIMMUNO-ELECTROPHORESIS

Counterimmunoelectrophoresis (CIE) is so named because *the antigen and antibody are made to flow toward each other in opposite directions*. The antiserum is placed in a well on the anode side with the antigen in a well on the cathode side. Antibodies move toward the cathode swept there by positively charged buffer ions due to a phenomenon called electroendosmosis. Negatively charged antigens move toward the anode. A precipitin line appears after as little as 30 minutes of electrophoresis.

FLUORESCENT ANTIBODY TECHNIQUE

Fluorescent antibody (FA) and its microscopical detection were discussed briefly in Chapter 2 under Fluorescent Microscope. Described here are the two ways the FA technique can be utilized: the direct method and the indirect (sandwich) method.

Direct Method

In the direct method the fluorescent dye is conjugated with the antibody that is specific for the antigen (Fig. 13-8). Example: A throat specimen suspected of containing group A streptococci is affixed to a slide. An antiserum containing fluorescent anti-group A antibody is applied to the smear for a brief incubation period. After being

Fig. 13-6. Immunoelectrophoresis. One method of separating molecules or particles in a solution is to apply current to the support medium. The charged molecules or particles move toward the oppositely charged electrode.

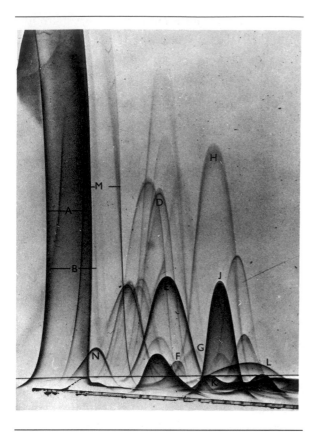

Fig. 13-7. Crossed immunoelectrophoresis of human serum. A strip of agarose that contains electrophoretically resolved human serum proteins is placed along the bottom edge, and molten agarose that contains goat antiserum is poured over the plate. When the plate has gelled, the antigens in the human serum are forced into the antibody-containing gel layer by electrophoresis. Thirty-seven precipitation zones can be seen. Some of the antigens identified in the human serum are albumin (*A*), cerulo-plasmin (*D*), hemopexin (*H*), and gamma globulin (*L*). (From H. Michin Clarke, in C. Z. Williams and M. W. Chase [eds.], *Methods in Immunology and Immunochemistry,* Vol. 3. San Diego: Academic, 1971.)

rinsed, the slide is placed on the microscope stage, irradiated, and viewed. Foci of fluorescence where antibodies have united with bacterial cells indicate the presence of group A streptococci.

Indirect Method

In the indirect method an additional step is required (Fig. 13-8). Antisera can be produced against globulins of another species. If human gamma globulin is injected into a goat, the animal produces antibodies to it. The goat antibody formed against gamma human globulin will interact with human immunoglobulin (antibodies).

The major application of the indirect FA technique is in the situation in which the antibody is the unknown component of the serological test. Example: Does the patient have antibodies to the syphilis organism? The patient's serum cannot be specifically labeled for syphilis antibody because it is not practically possible to separate the syphilis antibody immunoglobulins from the other globulins of the serum. Instead, the patient's unlabeled serum is reacted with the syphilis antigen on the slide. If there are antibodies to the antigen, the reaction is not visible at this time. The patient's serum is rinsed off and the labeled goat antihuman globulin is added. It will attach to bound human globulin (syphilis antibody) and on irradiation there will be foci of fluorescence wherever there is antibody from the patient attached to the syphilis antigen on the slide.

ENZYME IMMUNOASSAY

A popular type of label employs enzymes that have been conjugated with antibody. Enzyme immunoassay (EIA) tests are highly specific, versatile, accurate, reproducible, and relatively inexpensive. When the antibody with the attached enzyme reacts with its specific antigen, the antigen or the antigen location can be detected by adding the substrate that the enzyme attacks. In a positive immunoperoxidase test, for example, a colored reaction is produced when peroxidase substrates, such as benzidine, alphanaphthol, 3,3-diaminobenzidine, or 3-amino-9-ethylcarbazole, are added.

EIA tests have replaced some of the time-honored but nonspecific histologic staining methods

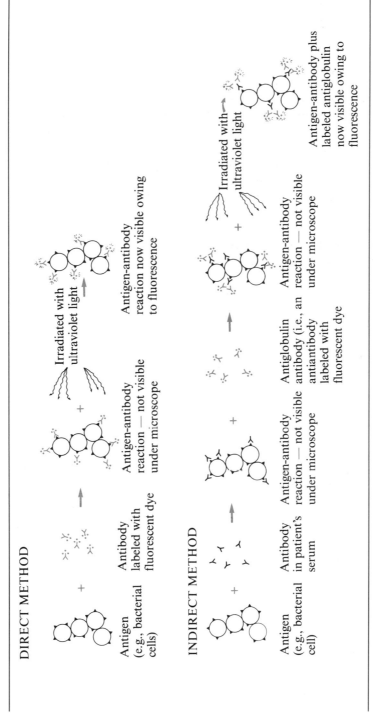

Fig. 13-8. Fluorescent antibody techniques.

and as such are referred to as immunohistochemical or immunostaining methods.

A very popular EIA test is the *enzyme-linked immunosorbent assay (ELISA)* (Fig. 13-9). In ELISA tests the antigen (or antibody) is passively or chemically attached to a solid support such as plastic microtiter plates (plates with series of small wells) or to small beads. When the test serum is added, any specific antibody present will attach to the antigen anchored to the solid support. Next added is antiglobulin that has been labeled with an enzyme. The antiglobulin will attach to the antibody of the test serum that has bound to the antigen. Thorough washing with buffer follows each of these steps. Finally, substrate specific for the enzyme is added. The enzyme-labeled antiglobulin adheres if there is specific antibody in the test serum and so hydrolysis of the enzyme substrate with the accompanying color change occurs. Color development is either detected visually or spectrophotometrically measured.

RADIOIMMUNOASSAY

Radioimmunoassay (RIA) is a highly sensitive microtechnique that detects trace amounts of antigens such as drugs, hormones, and biologically active molecules in a patient's serum. This very complex assay can be performed in several ways. A common form of RIA is a competition test, in which stock radio labeled antigen and unlabeled antigen from the patient's serum vie for specific antibody. The test components are a measured amount of known, purified labeled antigen, a measured amount of antibody that is specific for the labeled antigen, and a serum sample from the

Fig. 13-9. Positive ELISA test.

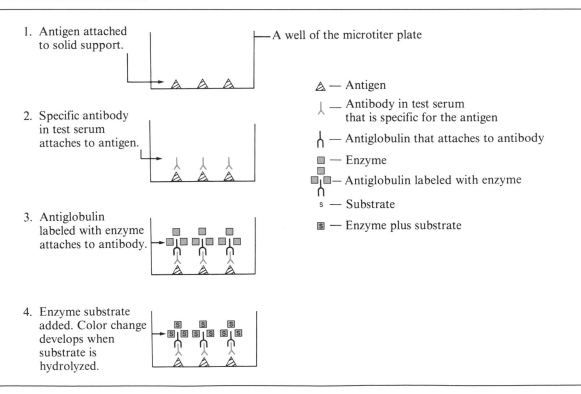

1. Antigen attached to solid support.

   A well of the microtiter plate

2. Specific antibody in test serum attaches to antigen.

3. Antiglobulin labeled with enzyme attaches to antibody.

4. Enzyme substrate added. Color change develops when substrate is hydrolyzed.

△ — Antigen

⊥ — Antibody in test serum that is specific for the antigen

⋔ — Antiglobulin that attaches to antibody

▢ — Enzyme

▢▢ — Antiglobulin labeled with enzyme

s — Substrate

▣ — Enzyme plus substrate

patient that may or may not contain the same antigen as the known labeled antigen. The patient antigen is unlabeled.

There are two reaction mixtures. Reaction mixture one, which provides a baseline, contains labeled antigen and only enough antibody to complex with about 70 percent of the labeled antigen. The labeled antigen-antibody complex is separated out from reaction mixture one by one of several techniques. The radioactivity remaining in the supernatant fluid (or, alternatively, the radioactivity in the antigen-antibody complex) is determined. This now provides a measure of the unbound known antigen. Reaction mixture two contains the patient's serum with the unlabeled antigen, plus the same components in the same measured amounts as used in mixture one. If the unlabeled antigen in the patient's serum is the same antigen as the unlabeled antigen, there will be less labeled antigen bound in mixture two because the unlabeled antigen of the patient's serum has competed for, and has been bound by, the antibody. Consequently there is more labeled antigen in the supernatant fluid than in mixture one. A standard curve is constructed by using known amounts of unlabeled antigen in reaction mixture two. The amount of antigen in the patient's serum can now be determined by referring to the standard curve.

Radioallergosorbent Test (RAST)

This is a widely employed radioimmunoassay that tests for antibody rather than for antigen. The test is most frequently used to detect IgE antibodies in the serum of patients who suffer common clinical allergies such as hay fever, asthma, and insect sting allergies. The antigen that is suspected to be causing the allergy—for example, pollen extract or bee venom—is impregnated into a cellulose (paper-like) disc. The patient's serum is applied to the disc. After the disc has been washed, radioactively labeled antiglobulin that is specific for human IgE is applied to the disc. After several washings the antibody activity of the patient's serum is determined by

counting the radioactivity associated with the disc.

WESTERN BLOT OR IMMUNOBLOT

Analysis of the many proteins in a complex mixture can be accomplished by the technique called Western blotting or immunoblotting. Proteins are transferred from a gel matrix to a membrane surface. Protein detection in the gel is limited because probes (identifying markers) do not easily penetrate the gel matrix. There are three steps to the procedure.

Step 1 The protein mixture is placed in a polyacrylamide gel slab and electrophoresed. This separates the proteins into invisible bands in the gel.
Step 2 The bands from the gel are transferred to an immobilizing paper (a nitrocellulose membrane) by means of a blotting technique. The nitrocellulose sheet is placed onto the agar and the two are sandwiched between buffer-saturated sponges. The sandwich is held together by plastic sheets, immersed in a buffer-filled chamber, and electrophoresed to effect the transfer of the bands from the gel to the nitrocellulose sheet.
Step 3 Enzyme-labeled or isotope-labeled antibodies (as described under the ELISA and RIA techniques) with known specificities are applied to the nitrocellulose sheets and identification of the protein bands is made.

One of the most important Western blot applications is in finding antibodies to HIV (human immunodeficiency virus, or AIDS virus) antigens. This is a multi-step indirect ELISA.

AVIDIN-BIOTIN TECHNIQUE

This technique is regarded as four to five times more sensitive than the other labeling procedures. The biotin-avidin complex may be conjugated to antibodies and other labels. Since only one conjugate preparation is required for many different assays, the biotin-avidin system is very attractive for use in immunological procedures. It can also be used in the absence of antibody, as is described next.

Biotin is a small protein molecule that binds readily to other proteins without changing the biological activities of the other proteins. Avidin, obtained from egg-white, binds avidly and specifically to biotin. The avidin may be conjugated to an enzyme, for example, horseradish peroxidase. The "sandwich" involved in identifying an unknown protein may consist of:

1. The protein that is being identified
2. Biotin bound to the protein
3. Avidin, which specifically and strongly binds to the biotin
4. Horseradish peroxidase, which is conjugated to the biotin

One important application of the avidin-biotin system is in the detection and identification, or in the classification, of bacteria and viruses. The technique involves nucleic acid hybridization and *nucleic acid probes*. A nucleic acid probe is an extracted strand of nucleic acid that has a sequence unique to the organism sought. The biotin-avidin–labeled enzyme becomes attached to the probe through biotin, which readily binds to free amino groups of the nucleic acid cytosine bases. If the labeled probe hybridizes (by complementary base pairing) with the extracted DNA of the unknown bacterium or virus, identification is made. The enzyme-labeled avidin substitutes for enzyme-labeled antibodies in this application of the avidin-biotin technique.

MONOCLONAL ANTIBODIES PRODUCED BY HYBRIDOMAS (FUSED CELLS)

An immensely important technique that lends a high degree of specificity, uniformity, and rapidity to immunodiagnosis involves applications of monoclonal antibodies (MABs). Monoclonal antibodies initially are produced in vitro by a hybrid cell. *The hybrid cell results from the fusion of a cancerous plasma cell* (called a myeloma cell) *and an antibody-producing lymphocyte* obtained from the spleen.

C. Milstein and G. Kohler fused myeloma cells and spleen cells and the resulting hybridoma produced the first monoclonal antibody of predefined specificity. This monumental biotechnical advance, for which Milstein and Kohler were awarded the Nobel Prize, has launched a multitude of actual and anticipated applications, not only for *immunodiagnosis and immunoidentification*, which is our interest here, but also for *immunotherapy*.

Hybridomas—The Source of Monoclonal Antibodies

Myeloma Cells as the Source of Vast Quantities of Immunoglobulins and "Immortality." The hybridoma consists of two cell types that are experimentally fused. One of the cell types is a malignant plasma cell whose clones produce vast quantities of whole immunoglobulin molecules, or fractions of immunoglobulin molecules that are all of the same kind and type. Plasma cell cancer is called myeloma or plasmacytoma and the condition it produces is termed monoclonal gammopathy. The immunoglobulins that are formed are either nonspecific, that is, they have no defined antibody function or their function is against specific antigens, only a few of which have been identified. The study of monoclonal gammopathies has contributed much to the fundamental knowledge about the immune system. The monostructural immunoglobulins produced by myeloma cell strains have been especially important in the determination of the basic structure of the immunoglobulin molecule and in distinguishing the five immunoglobulin classes.

The contribution of the myeloma cell to the hybrid resides in its vigorous, continuous growth both in vitro and in vivo and in the virtually endless supply of immunoglobulins it is capable of producing. The permanent and robust growth has caused some to say that the myeloma half of the hybrid imparts "immortality."

Spleen-Derived Lymphocytes as the Source of Specific Antibodies. The other half of the hybridoma cell is an antibody-producing lymphocyte usually obtained from the spleen of an animal that has been deliberately immunized with a given antigen.

Technique of Creating Hybridomas. Since only a small proportion of the total spleen cell lymphocyte population is responding to the antigen, it is necessary to bring together a large number of spleen (1 to 3×10^8) and myeloma (1 to 10×10^7) cells to increase the likelihood of contact between antibody-producing cells and myeloma cells. Fusion occurs slowly and spontaneously, but it can be enhanced by the addition of polyethylene glycol or by electrofusion (Fig. 13-10). Fusion takes place between spleen cell and spleen cell, myeloma cell and myeloma cell, and spleen cell and myeloma cell. It therefore becomes essential to be able to select out the spleen cell-myeloma cell hybrid. Spleen cells that are unfused or that are fused to each other are no problem because they soon die in culture. Unfused and fused myeloma cells are eliminated when they are transferred to a growth medium that contains hypoxanthine, aminopterin, and thymidine (HAT medium). Myeloma cells are deficient in hypoxanthine phosphoribosyl transferase (HRPT). Spleen cells provide HRPT. A mixture of spleen cell-myeloma cell hybrids remains that produces antibodies and grows well in vitro.

Selection of the Hybrids to be Cloned

The number of hybrids that remain after two to six weeks in the HAT medium may be in the range of 150 to 500 cells. The hybridoma cell mixture is diluted so that individual clones can be grown and sorted to find and identify the cells that are producing antibody for specific antigenic determinants. Transient antibody secretion by the spleen cells becomes a stable and permanent property of an established cell line, the hybridoma.

Advantages of Monoclonal Antibodies over Conventionally Obtained Antibodies

Over the years the conventional method of obtaining antibodies for immunodiagnostic and immunotherapeutic applications consisted of immunizing an animal and harvesting the antibody-containing serum (an antiserum). By comparison with monoclonal antibodies, animal antisera are not very "clean" preparations. To begin with, antigen preparations that are used to immunize the animal usually contain many antigens. The antiserum from the animal therefore is a very heterogeneous mixture of antibody specificities. Even though each B cell makes only one specific antibody, there are hundreds of B cells making different antibodies and their products are mixed in the serum. The "specificity" of a given antiserum, for the most part, is determined by those antibodies that are present in highest concentration; those of lower activity are usually masked.

Monoclonal antibodies, by contrast, have precisely defined characteristics. They are specific for a single antigenic determinant. The hybridomas can be grown continuously in culture, where they yield 10 to 100 micrograms of antibody per milliliter. The yield can be increased by inoculating the hybridoma cells into the peritoneal cavity of a syngeneic (genetically identical to the hybrid cell) animal.

Applications of Monoclonal Antibodies

The list of already prepared monoclonal antibodies of differing specificities, many of which are commercially available, is long and will continue to expand because of the many actual and anticipated applications in diagnosis, investigation, and therapy (Table 13-1). A major advantage that derives from the high degree of specificity of

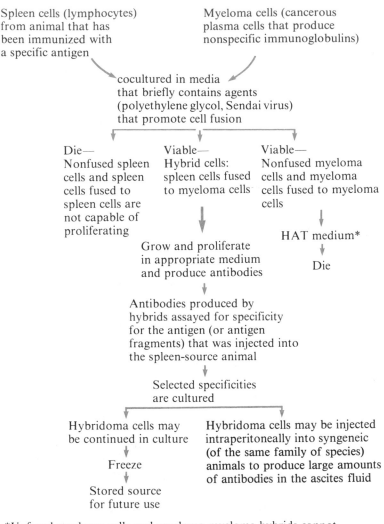

Spleen cells (lymphocytes) from animal that has been immunized with a specific antigen

Myeloma cells (cancerous plasma cells that produce nonspecific immunoglobulins)

cocultured in media that briefly contains agents (polyethylene glycol, Sendai virus) that promote cell fusion

Die— Nonfused spleen cells and spleen cells fused to spleen cells are not capable of proliferating

Viable— Hybrid cells: spleen cells fused to myeloma cells

Viable— Nonfused myeloma cells and myeloma cells fused to myeloma cells

HAT medium*

Die

Grow and proliferate in appropriate medium and produce antibodies

Antibodies produced by hybrids assayed for specificity for the antigen (or antigen fragments) that was injected into the spleen-source animal

Selected specificities are cultured

Hybridoma cells may be continued in culture

Freeze

Stored source for future use

Hybridoma cells may be injected intraperitoneally into syngeneic (of the same family of species) animals to produce large amounts of antibodies in the ascites fluid

*Unfused myeloma cells and myeloma-myeloma hybrids cannot survive in HAT (hypoxanthine, aminopterin, thymidine) medium because myeloma cells are selected that lack the enzyme HPRT (hypoxanthine phosphoribosyl transferase).

Fig. 13-10. Hybridoma technique.

monoclonal antibodies is that the time interval for the identification of infectious disease agents is shortened to 15 to 20 minutes, a great improvement over the conventional time-consuming methods of cultivation, staining, and biochemical testing. Therapeutically, monoclonal antibodies hold great promise for treating cancers through such means as immunotoxins. Being investigated are immunotoxins that are composed of a monoclonal antibody that is specific for antigens of the patient's cancer cells and toxins that are covalently bound to the antibody. The antibody

Table 13-1. Actual and Anticipated Applications of Monoclonal Antibodies

DIAGNOSTIC APPLICATIONS

In vitro diagnosis of infectious disease agents

In vivo diagnosis or localization with labeled (e.g., radioactive) antibodies; specific imaging of tumor metastases, organs, infectious agents, hormone receptors, neuron receptors, etc.

As standardized diagnostic antibodies available in limitless quantities for world-wide distribution

As standardized antibodies for tissue typing or organ transplants

INVESTIGATIVE APPPLICATIONS

Analyses of single antigenic determinants of a complex antigen

Discernment of cell subtypes, e.g., T lymphocyte subtypes

THERAPEUTIC APPLICATIONS

Highly specific passive immunization against infectious agents, toxic drugs, cancers

As carriers of covalently bound drugs against pathogens

As carriers of toxic substances (immunotoxins) that can be precisely focused on cancer cells

As toxin or virus captors for the extracorporeally circulated blood of patients

specifically attaches to the cancer cell, and the attached toxin enters the cancer cell and poisons it.

SPECIAL SEROLOGIC TESTS

C-REACTIVE PROTEIN   an antibody test for a protein that appears in the serum as a consequence of acute inflammation.

OPSONOPHAGOCYTIC INDEX   a test that measures the increased ability of phagocytes to ingest encapsulated bacteria in the presence of antibody that is specific for the capsule.

TPI TEST   a test for antibodies that immobilizes live *Treponema pallidum* (syphilis) bacteria.

QUELLUNG (CAPSULAR SWELLING) TEST   a test in which the capsule of bacteria enlarges in the presence of specific antibody.

IMMUNOFERRITIN TECHNIQUE   an electron microscopy technique in which ferritin molecules that are attached to antibody appear as uniform-shaped spheres that indicate the location of antigens.

IN VIVO IMMUNODIAGNOSTIC TESTS

In vivo tests are generally not called serological tests unless they are neutralization tests. Instead, in vivo tests are variously named after the mode of application of the test antigen, the disease in question, or the person who devised the test: skin test, histoplasmin test, tuberculin Mantoux test, Schick test, Frei test, to name a few. Most in vivo tests are qualitative tests, with only one dilution of antigen being used. The size and intensity of the reaction does, however, lend a quantitative aspect.

Radio-labelled antibodies are now being developed as in vivo diagnostic aids to help uncover otherwise undetected sites of infection and cancer metastases in patients.

IMMUNOLOGY OF RED BLOOD CELLS

Immunology of the blood, *immunohematology*, is a broad, complex subject. There are hundreds of antigens associated with the human red blood cell alone. The antigens of the red blood cells are grouped into antigenic systems or factors: ABO, Rh, MNSs, Duffy, Kell, Kidd, Lewis, and Lutheran. These antigens can have a bearing on transfusion, but fortunately most of them, except the ABO and Rh antigens, are weak and do not incite a major antibody response or are of limited occurrence. The ABO system will be described because of its importance in that type of transplantation known as blood transfusion, and the Rh system will be described because of its role in hemolytic disease of the fetus and newborn.

THE ABO SYSTEM

Two major antigens are involved in the ABO system: A and B. There are *four major blood groups*, A, B, AB, and O, in which humans are placed according to the presence or absence of A or B antigen or combinations of those antigens on their red blood cells. The antigens are termed hemagglutinogens. The antibodies are referred to as hemagglutinins. More specifically, they are called *isohemagglutinogens* and *isohemagglutinins*. Actually it is more correct to use the prefix *allo-* in place of *iso-* but the term *isohemagglutinin* has retained general acceptance (see Transplantation Terminology, Chapter 14).

ABO System Genetics
The antigens A and B are genetically determined co-dominants. Transmission follows mendelian inheritance patterns. The blood group that a person belongs to represents the phenotype. The genotypes of groups O and AB are automatically

known when the phenotype is known. The genotype of a group O person is OO; of group AB, it is AB. Group AB individuals can transmit the A or the B gene to offspring; group O transmits neither. Group A and group B individuals may be genotypically homozygous (AA, BB) or genotypically heterozygous (AO, BO). Table 13-2 shows selected parental phenotypes and genotypes and possible offspring types. There are subgroups to the A and B antigens, of which antigenic variants A_1 and A_2 are the most frequently encountered.

ABO Antibodies
Antibodies (isohemagglutinins or allohemagglutinins) to the A and B antigens are "naturally" occurring. The antibodies belong predominantly to class IgM. They develop spontaneously without a known specific stimulus. Thus, an individual who belongs to blood group A automatically has anti-B antibodies, one in group B has anti-A antibodies, one in group AB has no antibodies to the A and B antigens, and one in group O has anti-A and anti-B antibodies.

ABO Blood Group Typing
Commercially prepared antisera are used in a slide or tube agglutination procedure to determine the ABO phenotype of the patient's red blood cells.

Table 13-2. ABO Blood Group System

ABO pheno-types	Serum anti-bodies	Percent of population	Possible genotypes	Possible phenotypes when mated with					
				AA	AO	BB	BO	OO	AB
A	Anti-B	42	AA	A	A	AB	A, AB	A	A, AB
			AO	A	A, O	B, AB	A, B, AB, O	A, O	A, B, AB
B	Anti-A	10	BB	AB	B, AB	B	B	B	B, AB
			BO	A, AB	A, B, AB, O	B	B, O	B, O	A, B, AB
O	Anti-A, Anti-B	44	OO	A	A, O	B	B, O	O	A, B
AB	None	4	AB	A, AB	AB, A, B	B, AB	AB, A, B	A, B	AB, A, B

The ABO System and Transfusion

The major consideration in blood transfusion is based on the recipient's antibodies versus the donor's cells. Incorrectly matched cells are destroyed by the recipient's antibodies and complement. The donor's antibodies, unless a large amount of whole blood is being transfused, are diluted by the recipient's volume of blood. Blood group O individuals are termed *universal donors* because their red cells do not have the A and B antigens and so, even if the recipient has antibodies, no reaction normally occurs in respect to the ABO system. AB individuals, who do not have anti-A and anti-B antibodies, are termed *universal recipients*. In routine practice people are transfused as far as possible with blood of their own ABO groups and Rh compatibility. It is not safe to tranfuse a patient solely on the basis of information obtained in the routine ABO and Rh typing procedures. Those are merely preliminary tests to identify the blood group of the cells. Additional testing is explained later.

The ABO System and Disputed Parentage

The ABO blood group system may be of value in determining disputed parentage. It is sometimes possible to exclude an individual accused of fathering a child on the basis of the ABO blood group testing. Thus, an O male could not father an AB child. This technique does not, however, prove that a male is the father just because the blood group of the child is compatible with the blood group of the putative father.

THE RH SYSTEM

The Rh system is particularly crucial in the situation of an Rh-positive fetus borne by an Rh-negative mother. Notable differences from the ABO system are that the Rh antibodies involved in hemolytic disease of the newborn belong to immunoglobulin class IgG (they cross the pla-

centa) and that Rh antibodies are not naturally occurring. For Rh antibodies to develop, there has to be an opportunity for stimulation by the Rh factor or factors.

Determination of Rh Type

In preliminary general testing, individuals are designated Rh-positive if their red blood cells have Rh factor D. They are Rh-negative if they do not have that factor, symbolized by the lowercase letter d. An individual can also be Rh-positive on the basis of other Rh factors, C and E, but these are of much lower incidence. About 85 percent of the population is Rh-positive. Persons who are Rh-positive are homozygous (D/D) or heterozygous (D/d) for the major factor. Thus, a prospective father who phenotypically is Rh-positive may be heterozygous (D/d), and in that case there is a 50 percent chance that the child will be Rh-negative if the mother is Rh-negative.

Rh Isoimmunization (Alloimmunization)

Transfusion of an Rh-negative individual with Rh-positive blood leads to the production of anti-Rh antibodies. If these are formed in sufficient amounts, a subsequent transfusion with red blood cells with the corresponding Rh antigen will cause a transfusion reaction.

Rh incompatibility problems, however, develop primarily because of isoimmunization during pregnancy. An Rh-negative mother carrying an Rh-positive fetus produces anti-Rh antibodies when the fetus's Rh-positive cells enter the mother's circulation (Fig. 13-11). The best opportunity for the fetus's cells to enter the mother is during the perinatal period, when "major bleeds" occur. Late in pregnancy the epithelium that covers the placental villi atrophies, rendering the villi more fractious and therefore more vulnerable to penetration by the fetal cells. The antigenization by the fetal red blood cells stimulates the production of anti-Rh antibodies by the mother.

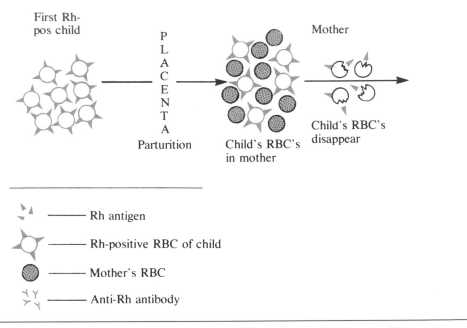

Fig. 13-11. Development of Rh hemolytic disease of the newborn. (RBC = red blood cell.)

Hemolytic Disease of the Newborn

The titer of anti-Rh antibodies generally does not reach a level high enough to be damaging to fetal red blood cells until about the third Rh-incompatibility pregnancy. The disease results when the mother's antibodies cause the lysis of the child's red blood cells. The degree of lysis is governed by the titer of the mother's antibodies. In hemolytic disease of the fetus and newborn (erythroblastosis fetalis and erythroblastosis neonatorum) the maternal antibodies destroy red blood cells of the child late in fetal life or in the neonatal period (Fig. 13-11). Immature, nucleated red blood cells (erythroblasts) increase in number to replace the lysed red blood cells. Three clinical conditions (listed in order of decreasing severity) can follow: *hydrops fetalis* (extensive pouring out of blood fluid into the tissues), *icterus gravis neonatorum* (jaundice), and *congenital anemia*.

Management of Rh Disease

1. The anti-Rh antibody level of women can be monitored during pregnancy if an Rh incompatibility exists between the mother and the father, or when there has been previous hemolytic disease in offspring of multiparous women. Serious fetal disease is not likely to occur if the mother's titer is less than 1:8. A good indication of impending disease is discerned by Coombs' test (see the following section), carried out on cord blood. Serum bilirubin levels in the child reflect the severity of the child's condition.

2. If an exchange transfusion of blood, which is a slow-dilution procedure, is required for the newborn child, the Rh-positive child is transfused with Rh-negative blood. The mother's anti-Rh antibodies in the child's system would destroy transfused Rh-positive red blood cells.

3. It is possible to prevent or to minimize the isoimmunization of a mother who does not al-

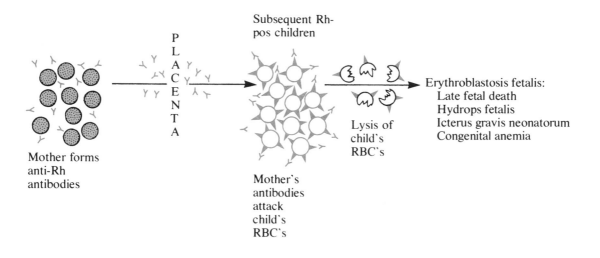

Subsequent Rh-pos children

PLACENTA

Mother forms
anti-Rh
antibodies

Mother's
antibodies
attack
child's
RBC's

Lysis of
child's
RBC's

Erythroblastosis fetalis:
Late fetal death
Hydrops fetalis
Icterus gravis neonatorum
Congenital anemia

Fig. 13-11. (Continued)

ready have Rh antibodies by injecting anti-Rh antibodies into the mother within 72 hours after the birth of an Rh-positive child. The anti-Rh antibodies are in the form of a gamma globulin preparation called RhIG. Passive immunization suppresses the antigenization by the fetal cells in the postpartum period. Preventing antibody formation at this juncture forestalls the development of an Rh incompatibility problem in the next pregnancy.

TECHNIQUES FOR DETERMINING ANTI-RED BLOOD CELL ANTIBODIES

It is important to be able to detect incompatibilities in vitro for monitoring purposes and to prevent transfusion reactions. The antibodies, either the naturally occurring ones or those that result from isoimmunization or idiosyncrasies (self-peculiarities), are not all of the same type. Several techniques therefore are employed so as not to overlook the presence of incompatible antibodies. Positive reactions are in the form of hemagglutination or hemolysis.

Cross-matching

After routine ABO and Rh slide and tube tests are carried out with commercial antisera, cross-matches are performed before transfusion. Cross-matching detects incompatibilities that are not discovered in the routine typing and picks up typing procedure errors. In the major crossmatch the donor's cells are tested against the recipient's serum. In the minor crossmatch the donor's serum is tested against the recipient's cells.

Coombs' Test

Antibodies do not always give a detectable reaction in the cross-matching procedure. Certain particulate antigens such as red blood cells have a net negative charge on their surfaces. When such charged particles are suspended in saline, an electrical potential called the zeta potential is created between the particles. The potential prevents the cells from getting close to each other. While one antigen-binding site of an antibody molecule is attached to one red blood cell, the other antigen-binding site cannot extend far enough to bind to another red blood cell because of the zeta potential, and so hemagglutination does not occur. The principle of Coombs' test lies in providing a divalent immunoglobulin bridge between the functionally monovalent antibody molecules. The immunoglobulin bridge is an antibody against human immunoglobulin. It is produced by injecting human gamma globulin into goats or rabbits. The animal forms antibodies to the human gamma globulin. When the animal serum is added to antibody-coated cells, the divalent animal molecule joins two human immunoglobulin molecules together, leading to the visible reaction.

SUMMARY

1. Immunodiagnosis is a subdiscipline of immunology in which immune system products (antibodies and sensitized T cells) are used, mostly in vitro but also in vivo, for purposes of identification, diagnosis, and monitoring. Reactions between antigens and immune system products essentially are specific and detectable; these facts make possible a great variety of valuable tests.

2. Serological tests are used to identify pathogenic microorganisms, to confirm diagnoses made by other means, to determine the immune status of an individual or of a population, to follow the course of a disease, and to type or group members of the same species of microorganism on the basis of antigenic differences.

3. Serological tests may be as simple as placing an antigen and a serum on a slide or in a single tube and observing whether a reaction occurs. In many instances, however, a single concentration of both components is not satisfactory because a single positive reaction with little or no dilution may represent former disease or cross-reactivity. In addition, a positive reaction may not be obtained because a disproportionately high concentration of antigen or antibody may prevent the development of visible aggregates.

4. Serological tests frequently have a quantitative aspect. Either the serum (the antibodies) or the antigen preparation is subjected to a series of measured dilutions for the purpose of determining a titer. The titer is expressed as a numerical value that signifies the highest dilution of the serum (usually) or of the antigen that gives a detectable reaction.

5. The more recent serological techniques are of three major types: techniques for separating out the different molecular components of an antigen preparation or of an antiserum; techniques for attaching soluble antigens or antibodies to cells or to particles; and techniques in which marker chemicals (labels) are conjugated to immunoglobulins (usually) or to antigens.

These basic techniques are performed in numerous ways. Gel precipitation tests, for example, may take the form of simple diffusion, double diffusion, single radial diffusion, immunoelectrophoresis, counterimmunoelectrophoresis, or rocket immunoelectrophoresis.

6. Monoclonal antibodies lend a high degree of specificity, uniformity, and rapidity to immunodiagnosis. Monoclonal antibodies are produced by a hybrid cell that results from the fusion of a cancerous plasma cell and an antibody-producing lymphocyte. They are being marketed commercially for a variety of clinical diagnostic and investigative procedures.

QUESTIONS FOR STUDY

Select the best response or responses for each of the following:

1. Which of the following serological techniques always involve markers (labels) that are conjugated to an immunoglobulin (usually) or to an antigen? (1) radioimmunoassay (RIA); (2) agglutination; (3) fluorescent antibody (FA); (4) enzyme immunoassay (EIA, e.g., ELISA); or (5) toxin neutralization.
   A. 1, 3, 4, 5
   B. 1, 3, 4
   C. 2, 5
   D. 3, 4

2. The indirect method of immunofluorescence analysis involves
   A. A soluble antigen
   B. A labeled antibody specific for a particulate antigen
   C. The use of an electron microscope to detect antigen–antibody recognition
   D. A fluorescein-conjugated antiglobulin (secondary) antibody specific for the (primary) antibody that is bound to the antigen
   E. A fluorescein dye coupled to a particulate antigen

3. The radioallergosorbent test (RAST):
   A. Is a skin test in which a wheal-and-erythema response is indicative of the presence of IgE antibodies in the patient's serum for a test allergen
   B. Measures the amount of histamine released from an allergic person's cultured mast cells
   C. Measures the amount of radio-labelled allergen in the patient's serum
   D. Employs a radio-labelled secondary antibody to indicate the presence of IgE antibody in a patient's serum for a test allergen that has been adsorbed to beads or to a paper disc

4. The ring test:
   A. Is an immunoprecipitation test used to quantitate particulate antigen
   B. Is the serological test most often used to determine the sensitivity of an individual to an allergen
   C. Is an immunodiffusion assay
   D. Is judged to be positive when a precipitate forms at the antigen–antibody interface

5. A positive complement fixation test is indicated by
   A. Agglutination of sheep red blood cells (SRBCs)
   B. Lysis of SRBCs
   C. Formation of a soluble antigen–antibody complex
   D. The failure of SRBCs to lyse
   E. Precipitation of antigen–antibody complexes

6. In an agglutination series, the fourth tube was the last tube to show a positive reaction. The starting dilution of the serum in the first tube of the series was 1:10 and doubling dilutions were made of the serum in the remaining tubes of the series. Since the addition of the antigen again halved the concentration of the serum, the titer (fourth tube) would be reported as
   A. 320   D. 40
   B. 160   E. 20
   C. 20

7. The combination of these three—antibacterial antibody, homologous bacterial cells, and complement—leads to a reaction known as
   A. Immunodiffusion   D. Immune hemolysis
   B. Neutralization   E. Agglutination
   C. Bacteriolysis

True or false:

8. An intact bacterial cell is an example of a soluble antigen.
   A. True   B. False

9. The precise specificity of a monoclonal antibody antiserum for a single antigenic determinant depends on the fact that a given B cell produces antibodies of only a single specificity.
   A. True   B. False

10. The titer of an antiserum is a numerical expression of the highest dilution of the antiserum that gives a detectable reaction with the test antigen.
    A. True   B. False

11. Monoclonal antibody is a cytophilic antibody bound to the surface of monocytes.
    A. True   B. False

12. The antibodies involved in hemolytic disease of the newborn are of class IgM.
    A. True   B. False

ADDITIONAL READINGS

Milstein, C. Monoclonal antibodies. *Cancer* 49:1953, 1982.

Payne, W. J., Jr., Marshall, D. L., Shockley, R. K., and Martin, W. J. Clinical laboratory application of monoclonal antibodies. *Clin. Microbiol. Revs.* 1:313,1988.

Rose, N. R., and Friedman, H. (eds.). *Manual of Clinical Immunology* (2nd ed.). Washington, DC: American Society for Microbiology, 1980.

Stansfield, W. D. *Serology and Immunology.* New York: Macmillan, 1981.

Thaler, M. S., Klausner, R. D., and Cohen, H. J. *Medical Immunology.* Philadelphia: Lippincott, 1977.

Turgeon, M. L. *Immunology and Serology in Laboratory Medicine.* St. Louis: Mosby, 1990.

14. IMMUNOLOGICAL DISORDERS

OBJECTIVES

To differentiate between primary and secondary immunodeficiency diseases and to give examples of such diseases, including a description of the type of defect and the associated clinical manifestations.

To explain the basis for categorizing hypersensitivities into the immediate or delayed types or into types I to IV

To discuss the basic differences between anaphylactic, immune complex, and cytotoxic hypersensitivity reactions; to identify the antibodies, cells, mediators, and mechanisms involved in each reaction

To discuss delayed-type hypersensitivity reactions with respect to the role of T cells, lymphokines, other influential factors, and the tissue events

To define autoimmune disease, noting current concepts of how it is thought to arise

To describe the role of the immune system in graft rejection and discuss maneuvers that serve to enhance the probability of graft acceptance

To comment on the role of the immune system in cancer surveillance and the potential for cancer immunotherapy

Disorders of the immune system stem from *genetically determined or developmental defects (primary immunodeficiencies), from malignancies, and from infections and drugs (secondary immunodeficiencies)*. Parts of the system or the entire system may fail to function, depending on the nature of the defect. There are also disorders of what is basically a normal immune system. In the hypersensitivities, the normal immune system responds to antigens in an exaggerated way that falls outside the normal response range. A number of clinical diseases result from immune disorders.

IMMUNODEFICIENCIES

Immunodefective diseases have served as "experiments of nature" that, on analysis in the laboratory, have greatly increased understanding of the lymphoid immune system. In turn, this understanding is leading to clinical maneuvers that can be undertaken to correct immunodeficiencies. In some clinical immunodeficiency diseases it is feasible to reconstitute the individual immunologically by injecting bone marrow and lymphocytes or by transplanting thymus tissue, fetal liver, or both. The study of immunodefects has shown which component of the dual immune system is instrumental in overcoming certain infectious diseases (Table 14-1).

PRIMARY IMMUNODEFICIENCIES

Genetically determined or developmental defects of the lymphoid system may affect the B cell component (humoral immunity), the T cell component (cell-mediated immunity), or both. There is a multitude of diseases associated with these immunodeficiencies. Following are brief descriptions of representative primary immunodeficiency diseases.

Infantile X-linked Agammaglobulinemia

Male infants with infantile X-linked or sex-linked agammaglobulinemia (also called Bruton's agammaglobulinemia) *form virtually no plasma cells*

or antibodies and serum immunoglobulins are almost entirely lacking. They have a normal CMI response; that is, they are able to reject grafts and to respond to antigens that regularly elicit the CMI response. Starting at approximately 5 to 6 months of age, when maternally derived passive immunity wanes, the patient begins suffering a repeated succession of infections with pyogenic cocci, *Haemophilus influenzae*, *Pseudomonas aeruginosa*—infections that humoral immunity normally controls. Immunological reconstitution is not available for this disorder. Bacterial infection can be controlled by the injection of gamma globulin preparations at approximately one-month intervals and antibiotics. Nonetheless, chronic respiratory and gastrointestinal symptoms may persist.

DiGeorge's Syndrome

In DiGeorge's syndrome (also called congenital thymic aplasia), the thymus fails to develop;

Table 14-1. Infection as Clue to Immune Dysfunction

Type of infection	Possible dysfunction of
Severe and/or recurrent infection with pyogenic bacteria	B cells (except in IgA deficiency)
	Phagocytic system (neutrophil killing defect, splenic dysfunction)
	Complement (deficiency of C1, C2, C3, C5, C6, C7, or C8)
Severe infection with	
Herpesvirus, cytomegalovirus, chickenpox, live vaccine	T cells (SCID, treated malignancy)
Hepatitis, echovirus, vaccine-strain poliomyelitis	B cells (deficiency of IgG, IgM, or IgA)
Resistant superficial candidiasis	T cells (SCID, thymic hypoplasia, chronic mucocutaneous candidiasis, steroid therapy)
Systemic infection with opportunistic fungi (e.g., *Nocardia, Aspergillus, Candida*)	T cells (Hodgkin's disease)
	Phagocytic system (neutrophil killing defect)
Pneumonia caused by *Pneumocystis carinii*	T cells (SCID, treated leukemia)
	B cells (very rare)
Giardiasis	B cells (deficiency of IgG, IgM, or IgA)
Sudden severe sepsis	B cells (deficiency of IgM)
	Spleen
	Complement

SCID = severe combined immunodeficiency disease.
Source: H. Meuwissen. Evaluating patients with suspected immunodeficiency. *Postgrad. Med.* 66:116, 1979.

hence the *failure of the thymus-dependent CMI component*. The B cell population is comparatively normal. The lymphoid organs have a changed morphology. Patients with DiGeorge's syndrome do not reject foreign grafts and do not develop delayed hypersensitivity responses. They are likely to die of infections caused by organisms such as enteric bacteria, fungi, certain viruses, and atypical mycobacteria—infections that normally are controlled by the CMI component of the immune system. Transplants of fetal thymus glands no older than 14 weeks' gestation have resulted in prolonged survival of DiGeorge syndrome patients. Fetal thymus glands older than 14 weeks contain immunocompetent T cells, which can recognize the recipient's antigens and destroy them in what is known as a graft-versus-host reaction (GVHR) (see Graft-vs.-Host Reaction, this chapter). DiGeorge patients unfortunately have an array of other defects such as hypoparathyroidism and cardiac and vascular anomalies, some of which can be lethal. Neonatal tetany caused by hypoparathyroidism may signal the immunodefect.

Severe Combined Immunodeficiency Diseases

Severe combined immunodeficiency diseases (SCID) represent a number of syndromes. They have in common *defects in both humoral and cell-mediated responses*. Usually there is a marked deficiency of both B and T cells. *Some patients also have a defective gene for the production of adenosine deaminase (ADA)*. Lack of ADA leads to a build-up of a metabolite that is toxic for T and B cells (see Boxed Essay, p. 353).

Infants afflicted with SCID fail to thrive. They are susceptible to infections by virtually every microorganism that comes along. Attempts at immunization by using live vaccines often end fatally. Patients face certain death unless they are isolated from contact with microorganisms or are constantly monitored and treated for infections, or are immunologically reconstituted with bone marrow from at least a partially HLA-matched donor.

Early attempts at reconstitution with transplanted bone marrow frequently led to graft-versus-host reaction (GVHR) unless donor and recipient were closely MHC matched. There is a recently employed technique that eliminates mature T cells from donor bone marrow by using complement and monoclonal antibodies that are specific for T cell surface antigen CD3. The transplantation of the treated bone marrow has been highly successful in providing a functioning immune system in the recipient. The lymphocytes in the recipient are entirely of donor orgin.

Immunodeficiencies in Neutrophils

Chronic granulomatous disease (CGD) is a childhood illness caused by a *lack of surface oxidase of the neutrophils*, in consequence of which the phagocytes are unable to generate the superoxide ion (see Oxidative Killing, Chapter 11). In most cases, CGD is inherited as an X-linked trait. Boys, starting at about the age of one year, show a greatly increased susceptibility to recurrent infections with pyogenic cocci and with organisms that normally are of low virulence, such as organisms from the skin and GI tract. Staphylococcus species are the most common. Recurrent disseminated abscesses and pneumonia, often accompanied by enlargement of lymph nodes, spleen, and liver, and chronic dermatitis are common findings. Tissue biopsies reveal granuloma formation in virtually every organ. Although at one time the prognosis was poor, early diagnosis, aggressive chemotherapy, and surgery have improved the long-term prognosis. Another defect, similar to CGD but at a different point in the chain of chemical events that lead to oxidative intracellular killing, is *myeloperoxidase deficiency*. Patients apparently form normal amounts of hydrogen peroxide but they lack the enzyme myeloperoxidase, which is required for the generation of hypochlorite from hydrogen peroxide. In *Chediak-Higashi disease*, part of the defect rests

TREATMENT FOR SCID PATIENTS WHO ARE ADA DEFICIENT

Severe combined immunodeficiency disease (SCID) affects about 1 out of 100,000 babies. SCID is also known as the boy-in-the-bubble disease, after David, a patient who survived with SCID until the age of 12 by living in a sterile plastic bubble. David died in 1984 of blood cancer after he underwent bone marrow treatment that was designed to free him from life in the bubble. Most SCID patients do not live in circumstances so extreme as those of the boy in the bubble.

One form of SCID is due to an inherited lack of the enzyme ADA. All mammalian cells contain ADA but its deficiency appears to be deleterious only for lymphocytes. Children with the ADA deficiency constantly have infections and fevers, spend much time in isolation at a hospital, and require frequent blood transfusions. The Food and Drug Administration in 1990 gave the first-ever approval of the treatment for human disease using gene therapy. Approval was given for experimental gene-therapy treatment for two diseases, SCID due to ADA deficiency and the cancer, malignant melanoma. The process involves inserting curative genes into human T lymphocytes. T lymphocytes are removed from patients and cultured. In ADA deficiency normal genes that code for ADA will be inserted into the lymphocytes of SCID patients. After the treated lymphocytes have multiplied in culture they will be returned to the patient. The ADA-engineered lymphocytes will have to be replenished periodically. Patients will also be treated with a purified preparation of ADA that is bound to polyethylene glycol. The preparation prolongs the lifetime of ADA in the body.

If experimental gene therapy is successful, it will initiate a revolution in medical treatment for a number of serious human diseases.

in the inability of lysosomal granules to discharge their usual battery of hydrolytic enzymes.

SECONDARY (ACQUIRED) IMMUNODEFICIENCIES

Defects may arise secondarily as a result of malignancies, age, infections, and drugs that adversely affect the lymphoid system.

Malignancies that specifically affect the immune system are monoclonal gammopathies, leukemias, and lymphomas. Monoclonal gammopathies develop when plasma cell cancers called myelomas or plasmacytomas produce great excesses of whole immunoglobulin molecules or of immunoglobulin chains. The immunoglobulins have no defined antibody function. There are numerous kinds of monoclonal gammopathies, some of which are more specifically designated—for example, Waldenstrom's macrogammaglobulinemia, multiple myeloma, and heavy or light chain disease. *Malignant myeloma* is the most common. When fully developed, the disease affects the bone marrow, the skeletal and nervous systems, and the kidneys. *Leukemias* are (usually) blood-borne malignancies of various types of white blood cells, all of which in some way affect immunity. *Lymphomas* grow as isolated tumors, often in lymph nodes and other lymphatic tissue.

A secondary immunodeficiency disease caused by an infectious disease agent and of great current interest and concern is acquired immune deficiency syndrome (AIDS) (Chapter 32). The AIDS virus (HIV) selectively destroys helper T cells, which are the"on" switch for most immune responses.

HYPERSENSITIVITIES—ALLERGIES

The responses of the body to antigens are not always beneficial, as the term *immune* implies.

The immune system may respond to an antigen in an altered way (the word *allergy* means "altered reactivity"), a way that represents a departure from its normal range of responses. In most instances this is an overresponse, an excess reactivity; hence the word *hypersensitivity*. In the hypersensitivities the concern is not with what happens to the antigen as a consequence of an antigen–antibody reaction but with what happens to the body tissues as a consequence of such a reaction.

Hypersensitivities are categorized on the basis of the schema proposed by Gell and Coombs. This schema is reflective of the underlying mechanisms of allergic response. According to this schema, allergic reactions are divided into four types:

Type I—anaphylactic, reagin dependent
Type II—cytotoxic
Type III—immune complex
Type IV—delayed type, cell-mediated

Descriptions in the literature refer to hypersensitivity reactions as a Type I reaction, a Type II reaction, and so on, on the basis of the above categorization.

Types I, II, III are antibody mediated. Type IV is T cell mediated. Type I hypersensitivities are referred to as immediate-type hypersensitivities. Sensitized individuals respond within seconds to minutes on subsequent exposure to the same antigen. Type IV hypersensitivities are referred to as of the delayed type. The reaction is slow in developing and does not reach the maximum for 24 to 72 hours. The terms *hypersensitivity* and *allergy* have been used more or less interchangeably to imply any adverse immunologic reaction. In recent years the term *allergy* has been applied primarily to immune diseases involving IgE antibodies (Type I hypersensitivities). See Table 14-2 for a summary of humoral (antibody) and cell-mediated immune injury (hypersensitivities).

Table 14-2. Principal Characteristics of Humoral and Cell-Mediated Immune Injury

	Type of allergy	Examples of antigens	Coupler: Ig class or T cells	Principal effector cells and their mediators	Principal pathophysiological effects
HUMORAL HYPERSENSITIVITY Antibody-mediated Passively transferable via serum	*Type I* Systemic anaphylaxis	Penicillin Hymenoptera venoms Foreign serum	IgE	Mast cells: Histamine Leukotrienes Kinins	Capillary permeability (edema); smooth muscle contraction; exocrine secretions
	Atopic allergies (localized anaphylaxis)	Pollens House dust Animal epidermoids Mite feces	IgE	Mast cells: Histamine Leukotrienes Kinins	Exocrine secretions; edema; urticaria
	Type II Cytotoxic	Foreign RBCs; drugs that resemble, adhere to, or alter self antigens	IgG or IgM plus complement	MAC of complement; neutrophils	Lysis of RBCs; destruction of host cells and platelets
	Type III Immune (toxic) complex	Soluble antigens	IgG or IgM plus complement	Mast cells: neutrophils (degranulate)	Intense inflammation; tissue necrosis
CELL-MEDIATED HYPERSENSITIVITY Passively transferable via lymphocytes and transfer factor	*Type IV* Tuberculin (infectious allergy)	Tuberculin Fungi	T cells	Lymphocytes: lymphokines Macrophages	Antigen lysis or isolation Destruction of host cells and tissues that surround antigen
	Allergic contact dermatitis	Poison ivy Industrial chemicals Cosmetics	T cells	Lymphocytes: lymphokines Macrophages	Antigen lysis or isolation Destruction of host cells and tissues that surround antigen
	Graft rejection	Foreign tissues, organs, cells	T cells	Lymphocytes: lymphokines	Antigen lysis or isolation Destruction of host cells and tissues that surround antigen
	Cancer surveillance	Cancer cells	T, NK cells	Macrophages	Antigen lysis or isolation Destruction of host cells and tissues that surround antigen
	Autoimmune disease	"Self" antigens	T cells and antibodies	Lymphokines and immune complexes	Antigen lysis or isolation Destruction of host cells and tissues that surround antigen

355

TYPE I—ANAPHYLACTIC, REAGIN-DEPENDENT DISEASES

The Greek word *phylaxis* signifies "guarding" or "protection." Combined with the negative *ana-*, the word *anaphylaxis* is translated to mean "unguarded," or the reverse of protecting. Individuals can be "unguarded" in respect to an antigen. They are "sensitized" to the antigen. If in this anaphylactic, unguarded condition they encounter the same antigen under certain conditions, an anaphylactic reaction develops within seconds to minutes. The response may be so extreme that the person undergoes a life-threatening or even fatal systemic reaction called *systemic anaphylaxis*. The response may remain localized, as in the clinical allergies that are referred to as *atopy*.

The antibody in Type I reactions belongs to immunoglobulin class IgE. The antibody is also called *reagin*. IgE binds to mast cells and basophils by the Fc end of the molecule. There is a hereditary predisposition to form IgE antibody (see Incidence and Familial Distribution).

Systemic Anaphylaxis in Humans

Clinical Manifestations. Essentially, there are three syndromes of *systemic anaphylaxis* in humans: extensive swelling of the upper respiratory tract, which leads to airway obstruction and asphyxiation; spasms of the bronchioles in the lower respiratory tract, which lead to asphyxiation; and vascular collapse (shock) without respiratory distress. The following are some of the signs and symptoms present in a systemic anaphylactic reaction in humans: reactions of the skin in the form of a diffuse *erythema* (reddening), or raised, blanched areas known as *urticaria* (*hives*), and *pruritus* (intense itching); *hypotension* (i.e., shock resulting from increased vascular permeability and collapse); obstruction of the upper respiratory tract, especially as the result of laryngeal edema; pulmonary involvement, usually manifested as an asthma-like syndrome but sometimes owing to fluid (edema); and smooth muscle spasms, evidenced particularly in the genitourinary and gastrointestinal tracts as abdominal pain, diarrhea, vomiting, or incontinence. Itching of the scalp and the effects on the gastrointestinal tract are among the early warning signs and symptoms.

Agents of Human Anaphylaxis. The administration of *therapeutic agents*, *antibiotics*, *and antisera* and natural exposure to certain antigens such as the *venom of Hymenoptera* (bees, wasps, hornets, yellow jackets) may at a given unknown time lead to the unguarded status in respect to the antigen (see Boxed Essay, p. 357). A subsequent direct exposure to the same antigen in an exquisitely sensitized individual may lead to a fatal or life-threatening reaction. The need to take histories, to conduct appropriate tests, to heed warnings from previous reactions, and to know the conditions that are likely to produce such reactions should be apparent to those who are responsible for giving injections to patients. Six illustrative cases of fatal systemic anaphylaxis in humans are summarized in Table 14-3.

Cellular and Tissue Events. The sensitizing dose or doses of soluble antigen evoke the production of antibodies of the IgE class (see Fig. 14-1, Type I). When the same antigen later makes contact with two adjacent IgE molecules of the same specificity (the union of the antigen with two neighboring IgE antibodies is called antigen bridging) on the mast cell surface, there are essentially two responses by the mast cell. One response is cytoplasmic: mast cell granules fuse with the cell membrane and release their contents. The contents of the granules that are released are primary (preformed) mediators such as histamine, chemotactic factors such as eosinophil chemotactic factor and phagocyte chemotactic factor, and proteins, many of which are of the neutral protease class. The principal effects of histamine are the altering of vascular permeability and the contraction of smooth muscle.

In addition to the primary cytoplasmic response, there is a concomitant response that takes place in the cell membrane, with the re-

THE IMPORTED FIRE ANT AND ANAPHYLACTIC REACTIONS

Local and systemic anaphylactic reactions to *Hymenoptera* venoms usually are associated by the public with the stings of bees, wasps, hornets, and yellow-jackets. Imported fire ants, however, are a major cause of such reactions in all or parts of the states of Texas, Louisiana, Mississippi, Alabama, Georgia, Florida, South Carolina, and North Carolina. Surveys indicate that as high as 58 percent of the population in some areas are stung by imported fire ants and that up to 1 percent of those suffer hypersensitivity reactions. The ants will attack humans or animals that disturb their nests. Each ant will attack repeatedly if left undisturbed.

The fire ant is so named because its venom elicits a sharp, burning sensation. The venom contains chemically unique alkaloids that cause allergic and toxic reactions. The toxic reaction is an intense, necrotizing inflammatory reaction that produces a characteristic sterile pustule within 24 hours at the sting site. The hypersensitivity reactions include diffuse erythema, pruritus, and hives manifested in the skin, respiratory distress due to laryngeal edema and bronchospasms, nausea, shock, coma, and death. Treatment of an ongoing reaction is the same as for any anaphylactic reaction. Skin testing with whole body extract (WBE) of fire ants or venom and the RAST test (Chapter 13) are used for diagnosis. Immunotherapy (desensitization) with WBE is recommended for selected patients who have had a systemic reaction.

From R. F. Lockey, The imported fire ant: Immunopathologic significance. *Hosp. Pract.* 25(3):109, 1990.

Table 14-3. Clinical Data from Six Cases of Human Anaphylaxis

Case no.	Sex	Age (yr)	Agent	Dose (ml)	Route of administration	Estimated time from challenge to death (min)	Symptoms and signs	Known prior exposure	"Allergic history"
1	F	39	Penicillin	1.5	Intramuscular	60	Generalized warmth; tightness of throat; respiratory distress; cyanosis; convulsion; respiratory failure	Yes	"Hives" 2 weeks before death; allergen unknown
2	F	21	Guinea-pig hemoglobin	0.2	Subcutaneous	16	Headache; wheezing; cyanosis	No	"Asthma"; skin sensitivity to dog hair, kapok, shellfish, ragweed, timothy, orris root, and house dust
3	M	52	Bee venom	—	Subcutaneous	20	Unknown	Yes	Severe local reaction to bee sting 20 years previously
4	M	45	Penicillin	—	Intramuscular	60	Dyspnea	Unknown	Unknown
5	M	56	Hay-fever desensitization vaccine	1/16	Subcutaneous	45	Difficulty breathing	Yes	"Hay fever"—injection was 11th in series of weekly desensitization injections
6	F	38	Penicillin and streptomycin	—	Intramuscular	120	Chest pain; cough; collapse; hypotension; cardiac arrest	Unknown	Unknown

Source: L. P. James and K. F. Austen. Fatal systemic anaphylaxis in man. *N. Engl. J. Med.* 270:598, 1964.

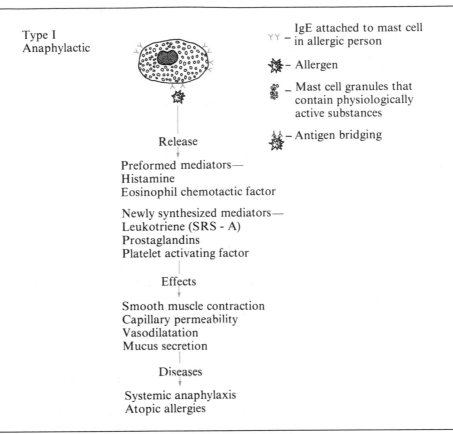

Type I
Anaphylactic

Release

Preformed mediators—
Histamine
Eosinophil chemotactic factor

Newly synthesized mediators—
Leukotriene (SRS - A)
Prostaglandins
Platelet activating factor

Effects

Smooth muscle contraction
Capillary permeability
Vasodilatation
Mucus secretion

Diseases

Systemic anaphylaxis
Atopic allergies

YY – IgE attached to mast cell
in allergic person

– Allergen

– Mast cell granules that
contain physiologically
active substances

– Antigen bridging

Fig. 14-1. Type I hypersensitivity—anaphylaxis.

sultant formation and release of secondary mediators (i.e., they are not preformed) that are lipids. Antigen bridging of adjacent specific IgE molecules triggers a sequence of changes of the phospholipids in the mast cell's membrane. *Prostaglandins, thromboxanes, and leukotrienes* are formed through the oxidation of *arachidonic acid*. Prostaglandins and thromboxanes mediate bronchial muscle contraction, platelet aggregation, and vasodilation. The leukotrienes (LTA4 to LTE4) were for many years called SRS-A—the slow-reacting substance of anaphylaxis. They are potent chemotactic, vasoactive, and spasmogenic agents.

When there is a great abundance of these effects—in other words, if many blood vessels become "leaky"—fluid from the blood vessels pours out into the tissues, leading to shock and blockages in blood vessels. When many key smooth muscles are contracted, as, for example, in the lung, the affected organ is compromised and ceases to function adequately.

Management of a Systemic Anaphylactic Reaction. Increased permeability of blood vessels and smooth muscle contraction are the principal effects of the mediators of an anaphylactic reaction. Top priority is accorded to *epinephrine* as a countermeasure to control an ongoing systemic anaphylactic reaction. Epinephrine is a physiological antagonist of histamine; that is, it counteracts the effects of histamine. It dilates bronchioles, has a vasoconstricting influence, and aids in the resorption of edema fluid. It also blocks the release of mediators of allergy. If shock is severe, drugs must be administered *to maintain blood pressure*. Upper airway obstruction owing to laryngeal edema may necessitate some form of *airway maintenance*.

Atopy

In 1923 Coca applied the term *atopy* to the *common clinical allergies*, recognizing that there is a hereditary predisposition of family members to develop allergies. Allergies are *naturally or spontaneously occurring* and are due to the everyday inhalation of, ingestion of, or contact with the antigen. The atopic hypersensitivities are largely those associated by the layperson with the term *allergy*: asthma, hay fever, hives (urticaria), and food allergies. Most of the atopic allergies are clinical allergies—those for which the patient goes to see the physician for diagnosis, treatment, and control (Table 14-4).

Atopy and Systemic Anaphylaxis. When IgE was discovered, it was recognized that the mechanism of systemic anaphylaxis and of the atopic allergies was the same from the standpoint of the antibody type involved, the general mechanism of release of physiologically active substances as a result of antigen–antibody combination, and the pharmacological effects of those mediators. The atopic allergies differ from systemic anaphylaxis in degree. Systemic anaphylaxis affects the smooth muscles and blood vessels on a grander scale and in a more violent manner. The antigen in systemic anaphylaxis generally enters the body by a more direct route—by injection (e.g., penicillin shots) and by penetration through the skin, as in insect stings.

Incidence and Familial Distribution. It is estimated that 10 percent of the population have minor allergies that are detected when the individuals are appropriately tested. A history of allergy among close relatives can be obtained among a majority of allergic patients. The allergic syndrome in the offspring is not necessarily the same as that of the parents. The allergic substance may well be different, and the clinical type may be different. Indeed, the target organ within the same individual may change. The first allergic disease experienced in infancy may be a food allergy with gastrointestinal involvement, progressing through allergic dermatitis in childhood, and eventually developing into asthma in young adulthood.

The Antigen of Atopic Allergies. The routes of sensitization are primarily through the respiratory mucosa (Table 14-5, center column), the gas-

Table 14-4. Common Clinical Allergies

Allergic respiratory disease (ARD)
Pollinosis—seasonal allergic rhinitis. Pollens are from trees and grasses in spring and early summer, weeds in late summer. Pollens are mostly wind-borne but also insect-borne.
Perennial allergic rhinitis (PAR)—year-round. Common allergens are house dust and animal epidermals (hair, feathers, dander). Among the many allergens of house dust are mold spores, animal epidermals, and mites.
Bronchial asthma. Common allergens are those cited under ARD and PAR. The air sacs are overdistended, plugs of mucus fill bronchial passages, smooth muscles enlarge (hypertrophy) to thicken and narrow the walls of the bronchi. Symptomatic relief is obtained by bronchodilators that relax the muscles of the bronchi, and by expectorants and liquefacients that dissolve and expel the mucous plugs and the other accumulations.
Gastrointestinal allergies—colic and possibly ulcerative colitis
Allergic skin disorders
Atopic dermatitis. This can be divided into stages: infant, childhood, and adolescent-adult.
Allergic contact dermatitis (ACD). A variety of allergens (contactants), many serving as haptens, elicit nonatopic skin allergies via the delayed hypersensitivity mechanism.

Table 14-5. Allergens and Other Stimuli Provoking Bronchopulmonary Disease

Provoking stimuli in bronchial asthma	Allergens of importance in bronchial asthma	Organic dusts of hypersensitivity pneumonitis

Immunological reactions
  Immediate hypersensitivity (type I)
  Immune complex (type III)
Infection
  Viral (in upper or lower respiratory tract)
  Acute bacterial sinusitis or bronchitis
  Chronic sinusitis
Aspirin intolerance
Isoproterenol abuse
Inhalation of irritant smoke, fumes
Exercise
Atmospheric change
Emotional upset
Associated disease states
  Chronic obstructive pulmonary disease
  Cardiac failure
  Esophageal disorder
	Inhalants
	  Tree, grass, weed pollens
	  Mold spores
	  Animal danders, feathers
	  House dust (mites, cotton linters, etc.)
	  Pyrethrum (insecticide spray)
	  Orris root (cosmetics)
	  Insect parts (moths, cockroaches, etc.)
	Ingestants
	  Foods (grains, nuts, eggs, etc.)
	  Drugs (penicillin)
	Injectants
	  Hymenoptera stings (bee, wasp, hornet, yellow jacket)
	  Drugs (penicillin, allergy extracts, adrenocorticotropic hormone)
		Mold growths in
		  Hay
		  Redwood dust
		  Maple bark dust
		  Oak bark dust
		  Mushroom dust
		  Wheat flour weevil
		Contaminated humidifiers and air conditioners
		Vegetable dusts
		  Sisal
		  Coffee
		Enzyme detergents
		Pituitary snuff

Source: D. A. Mathison and D. D. Stevenson, Bronchopulmonary diseases, immunologic perspectives. *Postgrad. Med.* 54:105, 1973.

trointestinal tract mucosa, and the skin; hence the allergic substances are spoken of as *inhalants*, *ingestants*, *contactants*, *or injectants*. The antigen or allergic substance is usually called an *allergen*.

Allergy Testing. Allergy testing is usually in the form of skin testing or a laboratory test known as the *radioallergosorbent test* (*RAST test*—see Chaper 13). Many of the antigen preparations for allergic testing are commercially available, but some may have to be tailored by the allergist to the patient's history or idiosyncrasies.

SKIN TESTS. The introduction of the allergen to which the patient is allergic leads within minutes (immediate) to the *wheal-and-erythema reaction*, which is also referred to as the triple-response reaction (Fig. 14-2). The site first reddens (erythema); as edema fluid collects in the area, the central portion becomes raised and blanched while the periphery becomes erythematous. In the *scratch test* the surface of the skin is abraded

with a dull needle or implement, and a droplet of allergen is instilled. Skin testing may be intradermal, measured amounts of allergen being injected between the layers of the skin. The *intradermal test* is the most sensitive of the two tests. In the *patch test* the suspected allergen is either directly taped to the skin or applied to gauze or cotton that is taped to the skin.

Nonallergic Asthma and Urticaria. The symptom complex that is seen in asthma and urticaria (hives) is not always allergic in origin (see Table 14-5, left column). The mediators of the atopic allergies can also be discharged without the involvement of antibodies in response to emotions (neurogenic mechanism), heat, cold, and other triggering agents.

Management and Treatment of Clinical Allergies. The order of preference is *avoidance* of the allergen, *reduction of the patient's sensitivity* by hyposensitization as applicable, and *relief of the*

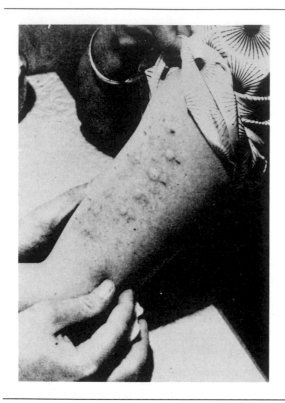

Fig. 14-2. Whealing reactions following intradermal testing. (From B. F. Feingold, *Introduction to Clinical Allergy,* 1973. Courtesy of Charles C Thomas, Publisher, Springfield, Illinois.)

symptoms with drugs, medications, and applications.

Hyposensitization. It is possible to lessen (hyposensitize) certain allergic states by parenteral injections of the corresponding allergen. Good success has been attained, for example, in hay fever and insect sting allergies. The parenterally introduced antigen ("allergy shots" to the patient) elicits the formation of IgG antibodies. They are termed *blocking antibodies* because they are believed to interfere with the action of the reagins. The IgG antibodies are believed to have a greater affinity for the allergen, thereby forestalling the stimulation of more homologous IgE antibodies and preventing the allergen from interacting with the IgE antibodies already formed.

Drugs, Medications, and Applications. Drugs used to relieve or manage common allergic reactions and states fall into the general categories of antihistamines, decongestants, bronchodilators, vasoconstrictors, expectorants, and corticosteroids. Antihistamines, of little value in systemic anaphylaxis because of the extent of the reaction, are mainstays in allergic rhinitis and urticaria.

TYPE II—CYTOTOXIC DISEASES

The targets of the reactions in Type II hypersensitivities *are foreign blood cells or the patient's own cells* (Fig. 14-3). The antigens may be part of the patient's own cells or they may be soluble foreign antigens or antigen–antibody complexes that have attached to the cells. They may be cross-reacting antigens, that is, self antigens that are identical or sufficiently similar to foreign antigens to react with antibodies formed against the foreign antigen. They may be normal self antigens that have been altered by drug-induced changes. The target cells are mostly red blood cells, platelets, and leukocytes. The antibodies that bind to the cell surface antigens are of classes IgG and IgM, classes that bind complement. Target cell destruction occurs in one of two ways, both involving complement. Either the membrane attack complex (MAC) of activated complement induces lysis of the antibody-coated target cells, or phagocytes, especially neutrophils, drawn to the target cells by complement-derived chemotactic factors destroy the cells, abetted by complement-derived opsonins.

Clinically, Type II reactions include transfusion and Rh incompatibility reactions (Chapter 13), autoimmune hemolytic anemia, and drug-induced reactions. In autoimmune hemolytic anemia the patient's erythrocytes are destroyed as a consequence of certain infections or because of unknown patient idiosyncrasies (idiopathic ane-

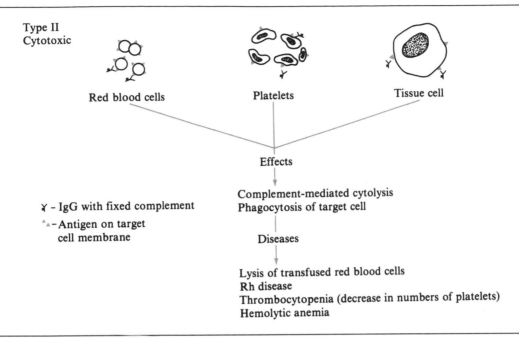

Fig. 14-3. Type II hypersensitivity—cytotoxic.

mia). Drugs sometimes act as haptens and attach to blood cells. Agranulocytosis (decrease in granulocytes) may develop when an antibiotic such as chloramphenicol attaches to granulocytic leukocytes. Hemolytic anemia may develop when phenacetin (an analgesic) binds to erythrocytes.

TYPE III—IMMUNE COMPLEX DISEASES

The cardinal feature of immune complex diseases is *intense, immunologically mediated, destructive inflammation* (Figs. 14-4 and 14-5). *The deposition of complexes composed of soluble antigens and antibodies of classes IgG or IgM on cells or tissues activates complement.* The cells or tissues on which complex deposition most frequently occurs are endothelial cells (cells that line blood vessels), basement membranes of kidney glomeruli and blood vessels, and synovial tissue (membranes that secrete viscid fluid into

joints). Activation of complement produces anaphylatoxin and chemotactic factors. Mast cells and platelets activated by anaphylatoxins release vasoactive amines and prostaglandins that cause, among other effects, vascular permeability. Phagocytes accumulate at the site of complex deposition in response to the complement-derived chemotactic factors. The neutrophils and macrophages recognize the immune complexes via their surface Fc receptors for IgG and IgM and normally ingest and eliminate the complexes. If the amount of complexes, however, is large, or if the complexes are enmeshed in the tissue, say, in a basement membrane, the phagocytes are unable to completely ingest the antigen–antibody deposit. Rather, they degranulate (discharge lysosomes and specific granules) and release toxic oxygen products via the activated respiratory burst mechanism (Chapter 11). These actions interrupt the integrity of blood vessels and basement membranes, and lead to hemorrhagic necrosis and other forms of local tissue destruction.

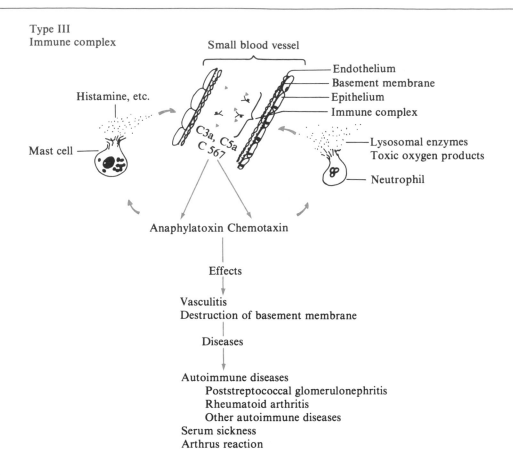

Fig. 14-4. Type III hypersensitivity—immune complex.

The Arthus reaction and *serum sickness* are prototypes of immune complex disease. In the Arthus reaction the repeated injection of a soluble antigen into the skin of an experimental animal such as a rabbit, at intervals of about one week, progressively leads to the formation of an ever-increasing inflammatory focus that ultimately becomes necrotic. In serum sickness the administration of a single large dose of a soluble antigen, such as an antiserum or a chemotherapeutic agent designed to persist in the body, brings about a systemic condition in 6 to 12 days. The patient experiences arthralgia (painful, swollen joints), fever, rash, and enlargement of the lymph nodes. The large or persisting dose of antigen allows enough antigen to remain and form complexes when sufficient antibody has been formed.

The tissue pathology and clinical manifestations of the Arthus reaction and of serum sickness were known for many years before the underlying immune events were understood. Gradually a number of heretofore poorly understood diseases were found to be attributable, at least partially, to reactions to immune complexes: rheumatoid arthritis, systemic lupus erythematosus, acute

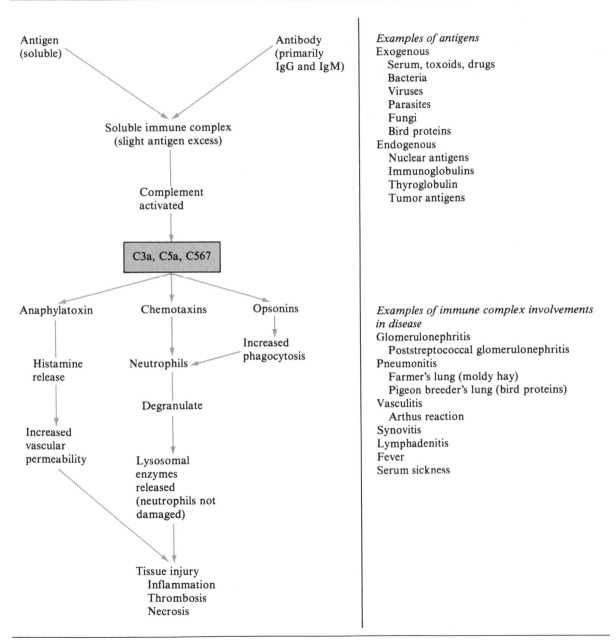

Fig. 14-5. Immune complex disease. The antigen-antibody complexes (microprecipitates) are formed in the blood and tissue spaces and deposited in the walls of blood vessels, in basement membranes, and in joint synovia.

viral hepatitis, Hashimoto's thyroiditis, scleroderma, poststreptococcal glomerulonephritis, and other diseases. Some immune complex diseases are attributable to dirty environments that exist at the workplace or that are associated with hobbies. Occupational or lifestyle diseases of this type include farmers' lung, maple bark strippers' disease, bagassosis (caused by contact with sugar cane fiber), and pigeon breeders' lung.

TYPE IV—DELAYED, CELL-MEDIATED DISEASES

Delayed-type hypersensitivities involve effector T cells, especially T_{DTH} cells (Fig. 14-6). When activated through antigen recognition and interleukins released by T_H cells, *T_{DTH} cells release*

an array of lymphokines at the site of antigen incursion. *Lymphokines* such as macrophage chemotactic factor and macrophage activating factor *attract and activate monocytes, macrophages, and other cell types.* It is the actions of the attracted cells and of cooperating T_{CTL} cells that lead to tissue damage, as described under Chronic Inflammation in Chapter 11.

Tuberculin Hypersensitivity; Hypersensitivity of Infection

Delayed Hypersensitivity and Tuberculosis. Tubercle formation (i.e., areas of cell and tissue necrosis), as occurs in tuberculosis (TB), is due largely to the delayed hypersensitivity mechanism. TB bacteria are located intracellularly and so a cell-mediated response is required to elimi-

Fig. 14-6. Type IV hypersensitivity—delayed (cell-mediated).

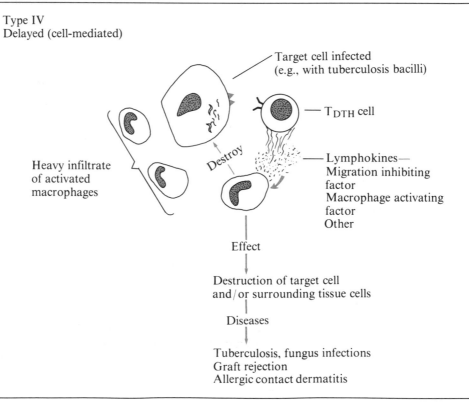

Type IV
Delayed (cell-mediated)

Target cell infected
(e.g., with tuberculosis bacilli)

T_{DTH} cell

Heavy infiltrate
of activated
macrophages

Destroy

Lymphokines—
Migration inhibiting
factor
Macrophage activating
factor
Other

Effect

Destruction of target cell
and/or surrounding tissue cells

Diseases

Tuberculosis, fungus infections
Graft rejection
Allergic contact dermatitis

nate them. Their cell envelope, furthermore, contains abundant wax-like materials that are not easily degraded. Elimination therefore is a prolonged process because of the persisting antigen. The "sensitizing" dose of the initial infection merges into what is equivalent to the second exposure of a sensitized individual to the same antigen. Under these circumstances many macrophages and other cell types accumulate at the site of infection and die. Necrotic material forms, probably including surrounding healthy tissue that was sacrificed in order to contain the infection. The reaction basically is that of chronic inflammation.

Other Infectious Hypersensitivities. Other infectious agents that incite delayed hypersensitivities are persisting types that take up cellular abode and/or are not easily destroyed and degraded. Fungi especially and certain parasites, bacteria, and viruses are of this type.

Diagnostic Skin Tests. The delayed hypersensitivity that develops in certain infectious diseases serves as the basis for diagnostic skin tests. Circulating sensitized T cells respond to skin test antigens in a positive test reaction. There are no live multiplying organisms in the test antigen and so the lesion at the challenge site resolves in time. Commercially prepared extracts of the various infectious agents are used for skin testing. Among preparations available are *histoplasmin* for fungus infections with *Histoplasma capsulatum*, *brucellergen* for infections with bacteria of the genus *Brucella*, *lepromin* for leprosy, and *Ly-granum* for the venereal disease lymphogranuloma venereum (the Frei test).

The best-known and most widely applied of the delayed hypersensitivity skin tests is the *tuberculin test*. A purified preparation of tuberculoprotein, referred to as *purified protein derivative*, is used in TB skin testing. In a positive reaction an indurated inflammatory reaction begins to appear after 6 to 12 hours, reaches its greatest intensity in 24 to 72 hours, and gradually subsides. The degree of sensitivity of the patient and the amount of tuberculin applied in the skin test are related to the size of the reaction and the amount of tissue damage in the skin test site.

Allergic Contact Dermatitis

Allergic contact dermatitis (ACD) ordinarily results from exposure to simple chemical allergens via the skin. Clinical allergists categorize ACD as a "non-atopic" allergy to distinguish it from the immediate, hereditarily predisposed atopic clinical allergies.

The Allergens of Allergic Contact Dermatitis. The most common causes of ACD are simple chemicals: ingredients of soaps and cosmetics, industrial chemicals, ointments, chemotherapeutic agents (especially those that are topically applied), and plant substances, to mention a few. The classic example of ACD involves plants in the genus Rhus—poison ivy, poison oak, and poison sumac—in which the active allergenic factor is an oleoresin.

Allergic Contact Dermatitis Allergens as Haptens. ACD allergens often are substances of relatively simple chemical composition. The point was emphasized in an earlier chapter that antigens are usually large molecules, with a molecular weight of at least 10,000. How then can simple chemicals such as nickel, mercury, and the catechols of Rhus plants be allergenic? The commonly accepted theory is that they act as partial antigens, that is, as haptens. They conjugate with proteins of the skin. The complete antigen consists of the haptens of the allergenic substances as the determinant groups and the proteins of the skin as the carrier molecules.

Allergic Manifestations. An acute ACD reaction, occurring on the average 18 to 24 hours after a sensitized individual encounters the allergen, may range from a well-defined erythematous area to extensive areas of vesiculation (bullae). The vesiculated (blistered) lesions may ooze, crust, and become infected (Fig. 14-7). Pruritus (intense itching) is almost always present. The oleoresin of the Rhus plants may be spread by rubbing or contact before the vesicular reaction occurs.

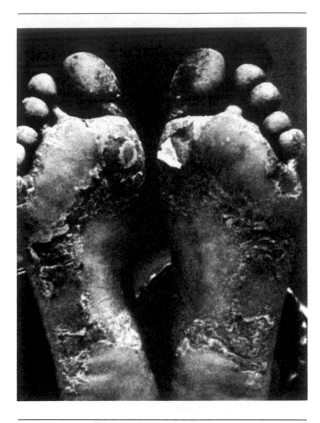

Fig. 14-7. Pruritic scaly eruption caused by delayed hypersensitivity reaction to adhesive in lining of tennis shoes. (From S. M. Connolly, *Postgrad. Med.* 74:227, 1983. By permission of Mayo Foundation.)

Mode of Contact. Usually there is a history of a repeated direct contact with the allergen. But a sensitized person experiencing a reaction may not have a history of direct contact. With poison ivy, for example, pets and clothing may be the indirect bearers of the stimulus. Burning of the plants may vaporize the allergenic components, and the smoke, coming in contact with exposed parts of the body, may elicit a violent exacerbation.

Testing and Treatment. The customary mode of testing for hypersensitivity is the patch test method, as described under Atopy. Treatment is usually in the conservative form of compresses and soaks. Steroids are used in severe cases.

AUTOIMMUNE DISEASES

The Nature of Autoimmune Diseases

Autoimmune diseases, or autoallergies, are *diseases in which the body's own molecules/cells/ tissues are the targets for attack by the immune system.* Autoimmune diseases occur inTypes II, III, and IV hypersensitivities. We discuss autoimmune diseases separately to emphasize special features of the diseases and to summarize pertinent information that has been noted previously.

Autoimmune diseases develop when self antigens have become altered by drugs, chemicals, or infectious disease agents; self antigens and foreign antigens share identical or similar antigens (*cross-reacting antigens*); self antigens that normally are sequestered (separately compartmentalized, hidden) or that develop later become exposed to the immune system; and the immune system self-recognition mechanism fails. Anatomically separated sequestered antigens as a result of injury, infection, or surgery become exposed to the immune system. The immune products formed against them lead to conditions such as aspermatogenesis, thyroiditis, or uveitis (inflammation of the middle coat of the eye).

The normal situation with most self antigens (we are not speaking about MHC antigens here) is that they are recognized by the immune system as self early in development. Self recognition is a cardinal feature of the immune system and it is expressed by the term *immune tolerance.* As lymphocytes mature, they get to "see" the body's antigens before they are immunocompetent to respond to foreign antigens. Those clones of lymphocytes that react to self antigens at this juncture are eliminated (clonal abortion). Studies show, however, that not all autoreactive T cells are eliminated. They may be responsible for, or associated with, some cases of autoimmunity.

Those that escape clonal deletion may do so because they fail to transit the thymus or because the self antigens they react with were not presented in the usual manner with the appropriate components.

Human Autoimmune Diseases

Numerous human diseases are regarded as having autoimmune disease components: Hashimoto's chronic thyroiditis, systemic lupus erythematosus, rheumatoid arthritis, Sjogren's syndrome, scleroderma, autoimmune hemolytic anemia, and myasthenia gravis, to name a few. Two diseases for which the probable mechanisms are known and which shall serve as examples are myasthenia gravis and rheumatoid arthritis.

Myasthenia Gravis. Myasthenia gravis autoantibodies develop against acetylcholine receptors at neuromuscular junctions. This action blocks muscle contraction that normally occurs when acetylcholine released from neurons binds to the acetylcholine receptor. Victims experience extreme muscle weakness. There may be difficulty in chewing, swallowing, and breathing that eventually leads to respiratory failure.

Rheumatoid Arthritis. Antibodies predominantly *of class IgM* (these antibodies are referred to as *rheumatoid factor) are formed against the Fc portion of the patient's own IgG molecules.* IgG, in other words, serves as an antigen. The IgM-IgG immune complexes are deposited in the synovia of joint spaces. *Complement is activated* by the complexes *and intense inflammation ensues*, progressively breaking down collagen and cartilage in the joints.

GRAFT REJECTION

The immunology of transplantation is usually discussed under Type IV hypersensitivity because *the principal mechanism of tissue immunorejections is T cell mediated.* Immunorejection by the immune system is regarded as a disservice. In actuality, immunorejection under normal circumstances is a beneficial reaction; without it the body could serve as a culture medium for any cell or tissue it contacts.

Transplantation Terminology

Certain prefixes (*auto, iso-, allo-, xeno-*) and certain suffixes (*-graft, -antigen, -antibody, -geneic*) are used to form terms that are part of transplantation parlance (Table 14-6). Autografts and isografts are not immunorejected because their antigens are identical with the recipient's antigens. *Most grafts between humans are allografts* (formerly called homografts). The donor and recipient are allogeneic; that is, they are members of the same species, but they are not genetically identical. The tissues of the donor are foreign to the recipient and are therefore antigenic. The antigens of the graft involved in immunorejection are called *transplantation antigens.* They are controlled by histocompatibility genes of the major histocompatibility complex, as described in Chapter 12.

Maneuvers to Prevent Graft Immunorejection

There are two general approaches used to increase the survival of grafts: (1) *tissue typing*, to select donors with as few MHC mismatches with the recipient as possible, and (2) reducing the immune responses (*immunosuppression*) of the recipient.

1. Tissue typing. The purpose of tissue typing is to match the tissue antigens of the donor and recipient as closely as conditions allow. The genes for HLA (human leukocyte antigens) are located on a small segment of human chromosome 6. The products of some of the gene loci on this segment can be serologically identified. In kidney grafting, long-term survival of the graft occurs in a high percentage of cases when there is a sibling donor who is serolog-

Table 14-6. Transplantation Terminology

Prefix	Meaning	Combining suffixes	Transplantation parlance
Auto-	Self	-graft -geneic -antigen -antibody	An autograft is a self graft, e.g., skin from one site of the patient's body moved to another site on the patient's body
Iso-	Equal; identical with another	-graft -geneic -antigen -antibody	An isograft is a graft between isogeneic individuals, i.e., between genetically identical individuals such as identical (uniovular) twins
Allo- (homo-)	Similar; like another	-graft -geneic -antigen -antibody	An allograft is a graft between allogeneic individuals, i.e., between nonidentical members of the same species
Xeno- (hetero-)	Dissimilar; unlike another; foreign	-graft -geneic -antigen -antibody	A xenograft is a graft between xenogeneics, i.e., between members of different species, as a graft from ape to human

ically matched with the recipient at both the HLA-A and HLA-B loci and when appropriate immunosuppression accompanies the grafting. Once the donor has been selected on the basis of the HLA matching, the donor's lymphocytes and the recipient's lymphocytes are cultured together for several days. The test is called *the mixed leukocyte reaction (MLR)*. The object is to detect lymphocyte proliferation. The greater the proliferation, the greater the disparity between donor and recipient. The important proliferation is that of the recipient's lymphocytes, because that reflects the degree of immunorejection. The MLR test, therefore, usually is modified by first treating the donor's lymphocytes with drugs that inhibit donor cell multiplication.

2. Immunosuppression. The purposes of immunosuppressive procedures are to destroy lymphocytes before they recognize antigen, to prevent antigen-stimulated lymphocytes from proliferating, to reduce the immunogenicity of the graft, and to reduce inflammation. Immunosuppressive modalities include:

a. Immunosuppressive drugs. Azathioprine, mercaptopurine, and cyclophosphamide functioning as antimetabolites interfere with RNA or DNA synthesis. Proliferating lymphocytes, and, regrettably, other proliferating cells of the body, such as bone marrow cells and intestinal epithelial cells, are nonspecifically affected by these drugs. Cyclosporine A, a more recent addition to the immunosuppressive drug armamentarium, appears to have a greater specificity for lymphocytes than for other cell types. Its primary action is to inhibit the production of interleukin-2 (IL-2) and the IL-2 receptor, thereby preventing T cells from receiving the signal to divide. Corticosteroids have a similar action, and so they are frequently used, very effectively, in combination with cyclosporine A.

b. Anti-inflammatory agents. Adrenocortical hormones depress phagocyte chemotaxis. They stabilize lysosome membranes, thereby affecting the ability of lysosomes to release graft-destroying hydrolytic enzymes.

c. Immunological measures. Equine anti-lymphocytic serum (ALS) is administered to graft recipients specifically to destroy T cells. The procedure is of variable effectiveness. Already proven effective in experimental animals is an anti-IL-2 monoclonal antibody that is covalently linked to the cytotoxic part of the diphtheria toxin molecule. The anti-IL-2 antibodies bind to T cells that were activated by recognition of donor MHC antigens. The attached toxin enters and selectively kills the T cells. Other measures that are of a theoretical or investigational nature include efforts to block recognition of the MHC antigens of the donor cells through the application of antibodies specific for donor MHC-II antigens or for the CD3 and CD4 components of the T cell receptor complex.

d. X-radiation. X-radiation destroys lymphoid tissue. Irradiation has largely been replaced by other immunosuppressive modalities. Furthermore, it must be done several days prior to transplanting to be effective. It usually is not possible, however, to know beforehand that a suitable organ will be available when cadaver organs are used.

Since most of these suppressive procedures affect the whole immune system, the immunocompromised patient has lowered resistance to infectious agents, including many opportunistically pathogenic microorganisms. However, the rate of infections has declined greatly in recent years because transplant specialists have learned that patients do not require so intensive antirejection therapy as was once thought necessary.

Graft-vs.-Host (GVH) Reaction

A serious anti-host reaction can occur when the recipient of a graft has a defective immune system or response and the allograft contains sufficient immunocompetent cells (lymphocytes) to attack the recipient's cells and tissues. The graft literally rejects the recipient. GVH reaction was a major deterrent in the early efforts to immunologically reconstitute immunodefective individuals with stem cell (bone marrow, fetal thymus, fetal liver) transplants. The advent of HLA matching techniques and the use of bone marrow from which mature T cells have been eliminated (see Severe Combined Immunodeficiency Diseases) have reduced GVH reactions.

Immunologically Privileged Sites and Tissues

Allografts to certain sites ordinarily are not immunorejected. For example, the avascularity of corneas apparently makes the foreign antigens of the graft inaccessible to the immune response system. Tissue typing is not advantageous unless a second graft is required because of vascularization of the first graft. Grafts that become vascularized often are treatable with topical steroids to provide localized immunosuppression. Brain, because it lacks lymphatic drainage, and testicular antigens, because they are sequestered, are referred to as privileged sites or tissues.

The Fetus as an Allograft

The fetus is like an allograft because of paternally determined MHC antigens. Why then is the fetus not immunorejected? The reasons for this paradox still are baffling despite about 20 years of research. There are two main hypotheses, each supported by some evidence. One proposes that a barrier masks the paternal antigens on the trophoblast. The trophoblast is the part of the placenta that forms an interface between the fetal and maternal tissues. Maternal antibodies, for example, may be blocking the paternal antigen, or sulfated mucoproteins may be covering the antigens of the trophoblast. The other leading hypothesis is that the maternal immune system is regulated by fetal sources of steroid hormones, interferon, an interleukin-2 blocking substance, and other factors that suppress maternal antigraft responses.

CANCER AND THE IMMUNE SYSTEM

The central questions in tumor immunology are whether tumor antigens exist on the surface of tumor cells and whether they are recognizable and destroyable by the immune system. Such antigens are demonstrable in many mouse tumor models but this is less easily done with human tumor cells. There are two broad categories of tumor immunotherapy, active and passive.

1. Active tumor immunotherapy. Attempts are made to induce the patient's immune system to augment its production of immune products against the tumor antigens. Attempts along these lines are being made:
   a. Stimulating the immune system to expand its responses. A variety of synthetic chemicals and certain microorganisms or their derivatives are used as immunostimulants. Two of the microorganisms used for this purpose are *Corynebacterium parvum* and mycobacteria that are in the BCG vaccine used for active immunization against tuberculosis.
   b. Modifying the tumor cell surface to increase antigenicity. The tumor cell surface is altered by treatment with synthetic chemicals, or sialic acid residues that "cover" the antigens are stripped off with neuraminidase.
   c. Formation of tumor hybrids. Tumor cells from one species are fused with normal cells from another species, thereby making the hybrid cell more immunogenic because of the foreign antigens.
   d. Use of cytokines. Interferons (IFNs) and interleukin-2 (IL-2) have antitumor effects in murine and human models. Both are now available in quantity through recombinant DNA techniques. The postulated antitumor activities of IFNs: they directly prevent tumor cells from proliferating; they induce an increase of activated effector lymphocytes; they induce tumor cell membrane antigens allowing for better recognition by the immune system. IL-2 fosters lymphocyte activation and proliferation, and the release of other lymphokines and hormones.

2. Passive tumor immunotherapy. Immunologically reactive antitumor reagents are introduced into the patient.
   a. Monoclonal antibodies (Chapter 13) currently are receiving much attention for this purpose. Over the years, before the factors and reactions involved in an immune response were understood, there were many empirical attempts to produce antitumor antibodies in other animals. Patients' tumor cells were injected into animals, the serum was harvested after an appropriate induction period, and the antiserum was injected into the patient. The results were disappointing. Monoclonal antibodies offer the advantage that they can be produced in quantity and they are precisely specific for, say, a tumor antigen. Production of human-source monoclonal antibodies has not been very successful in contrast to the readily available mouse antibodies. Recently, recombinant technology has been used to couple mouse genes that are coding for the Fab portion of a monoclonal antitumor antibody with human genes that code for the Fc portion of the immunoglobulin molecule. The objective of the hybridization is to prevent an immune response to the mouse antigens and the subsequent elimination of the tumor specific monoclonal antibodies. Another promising and highly important application of monoclonal antibodies is as a tumor-seeking device. Radioactive labels are conjugated to tumor-specific monoclonal antibodies and tumor deposits/metastases localized through use of appropriate radioactivity-sensing devices. Other tumor-destroying modalities can then be directed at the metastases.
   b. Experimental gene therapy was approved late in 1990 (see Boxed Essay, page 353) for treatment of patients with advanced malignant melanomas. Genetic manipulation is

used to amplify the natural cancer-killing power of tumor-infiltrating lymphocytes (TIL). TIL cells obtained from cancer patients are cultured to yield billions of cells. A gene is inserted into the TIL cells that commands the cells to produce a protein called *tumor necrosis factor* (TNF). The genetically engineered TIL cells when reintroduced into the patient are expected to localize in the tumor itself and produce the tumor-killing protein. Experiments in mice, according to National Institutes of Health researcher Stephen A. Rosenberg, showed that TIL-TNF altered cells are very powerful against cancer cells.

SUMMARY

1. The immune system does not always provide protection, even though that is its primary function. The immune response may be deficient because of developmental or acquired defects, or the response may be outside the normal range, as in allergies.

2. Hereditary or developmental defects are referred to as primary immunodeficiencies. They are usually manifested in neonates and children.

3. Acquired defects result from malignancy, infections, drugs, and aging and are referred to as secondary immunodeficiencies.

4. Some hypersensitivities are categorized as immediate or delayed, depending on how soon a sensitized individual reacts when skin-tested with the appropriate antigen. Those of the immediate type are antibody (IgE) mediated, the delayed type are cell mediated.

5. There are four types of hypersensitivities on the basis of the mechanism of allergic injury. Type I are the IgE-mediated, hereditarily predisposed local (atopic) and systemic anaphylactic type. IgE antibodies that are attached to mast cells from prior sensitization, when bridged by more of the same antigen, activate mast cells to release pharmacologically active substances. The substances affect blood vessels, smooth muscles, and exocrine glands. The effects of these responses range from localized allergic manifestations (atopic allergies) to the systemic and sometimes fatal reactions of anaphylactic shock.

6. In Type II hypersensitivities host cells or transfused cells are damaged or destroyed when antigens that are part of the host cell surface or that become attached to host cells react with IgG or IgM antibody and complement. Red blood cells and platelets often are the cell types destroyed.

7. In Type III hypersensitivities, the immune complex type, host tissues are damaged because of the vascular effects and intense inflammatory reactions that are initiated by complexes formed by soluble antigen and antibody of classes IgG or IgM, and activated complement.

8. In Type IV hypersensitivities, the delayed or CMI type, tissue damage results from the activation of T cells, which through lymphokines attract and activate tissue-damaging macrophages.

9. Immunopathologists frequently include descriptions of graft rejection, cancer surveillance by the immune system, and the immunology of the fetal-maternal relationship with Type IV hypersensitivities because of the involvement of CMI in these clinical entities.

QUESTIONS FOR STUDY

Select the best response or responses for each of the following:

1. Anaphylactic-type hypersensitivity reactions primarily involve the release of
   A. IgM class antibodies by plasma cells
   B. Pharmacological mediators by mast cells
   C. Prostaglandins by macrophage cells
   D. Lymphokines by effector T cells
   E. Hydrolytic enzymes by neutrophils

2. Alteration of a self antigen so it is recognized as foreign, exposure of sequestered (hidden) self antigen, and infection with a microorganism that carries cross-reactive antigen are possible factors that lead to the development of
   A. An atopic allergy
   B. Systemic anaphylactic reaction
   C. A primary immunodefect
   D. Allergic contact dermatis
   E. Autoimmune disease

3. A kidney transplanted from brother to sister (the siblings are not twins) is an example of a(n)
   A. Allograft
   B. Autograft
   C. Isograft
   D. Xenograft

4. The hypersensitivity reaction to tuberculin observed in skin tests for tuberculosis is a consequence of
   A. Pharmacological mediators released by mast cells
   B. Hydrolytic enzymes released by neutrophils
   C. Destructive effects of activated complement
   D. Lymphokines secreted by T_{DTH}
   E. Natural killer cell activity

5. Systemic anaphylactic type hypersensitivity reactions:
   A. Are violent reactions to allergens occurring even in unsensitized individuals
   B. Are readily treated with antihistamines
   C. Are frequently associated with the intravenous or intramuscular injection of drugs such as penicillin to priorly sensitized individuals
   D. Occur 24 to 48 hours after a sensitized individual contacts the allergen
   E. Usually occur following inhalation of the allergen

6. Transplantation patients receiving immunosuppressive drugs exhibit an increased incidence of infection. This is an example of
   A. Hyposensitization
   B. An acquired immunodeficiency
   C. Immunological tolerance
   D. The emergence and selection of drug-resistant mutants
   E. A primary immunodeficiency disease

7. The consequences of DiGeorge syndrome may be attributed to
   A. The failure of PMNs to respond to chemotactic factors
   B. A poorly developed thymus
   C. The selective inability to synthesize antibodies of the IgM class
   D. Increasing age or malnutrition
   E. The uncontrolled activation of complement

8. Immune complex–type hypersensitivity reactions (Type III) usually involve
   A. The kidneys, blood vessels, and joints as the primary sites of antigen–antibody deposition
   B. IgA and antigen in slight excess
   C. Ingestion of antigen and subsequent formation of immune complexes in the lower GI tract
   D. T killer cell–mediated cytolysis of tissue cells

E. Hydrolytic enzymes released by macrophage cells

9. Which one of the following situations would most likely result in a cytotoxic type (Type II) hypersensitivity reaction?
   A. Inhalation of pollen
   B. Adsorption of certain drugs to the surface of a patient's red blood cells
   C. Repeated skin contact with specific cosmetics or chemicals
   D. Chronic infections by microorganisms not readily eliminated by an immune response

10. In an individual suffering from a severe combined immunodeficiency disease, "combined" refers to a combination of
    A. Primary and secondary immunodeficiency diseases
    B. Defects in both cell-mediated and antibody-mediated immune responses
    C. Defects in both acquired immunity and nonspecific host resistance
    D. Defects in both active and passive immunity
    E. Defects in both antibody-mediated and humoral-mediated immunity

11. Epinephrine is administered in an ongoing systemic anaphylactic reaction for the purpose of
    A. Preventing more antigen from combining with antibody
    B. Directly neutralizing histamine
    C. Limiting the discharge of histamine from mast cells
    D. Counteracting the physiological effects of histamine
    E. Preventing the union of antigen with sensitized lymphocytes

12. Of necessity, most tissue and organ grafts among humans are grafts between individuals who are
    A. Autogeneic   C. Allogeneic
    B. Isogeneic   D. Xenogeneic

True or false:

13. A T-cell immunodefect usually is more serious than a B-cell defect because many of the antigens that B cells respond to are T-dependent antigens.
    A. True   B. False

14. Hydrolytic enzymes released by neutrophils are a major factor in the tissue destruction associated with cytotoxic-type hypersensitivity reactions.
    A. True   B. False

ADDITIONAL READINGS

American Cancer Society. Immunology and cancer. CA 38:66, 1988.

Bach, F. H., and Sachs, D. H. Transplantation immunology. *N. Engl. J. Med.* 317:489, 1987.

Bagshawe, K. D. Towards generating cytotoxic agents at cancer sites. *Br. J. Cancer* 60:372, 1989.

Buckley, R. Immunodeficiency diseases. *J.A.M.A.* 258(20):2841, 1987.

Burnett, J. W., Reisman, R. E., and Yunginger, J. W.

Taking the sting out of hymenoptera. *Patient Care.* p. 93, June 15, 1988.

Condemi, J. The autoimmune diseases. *J.A.M.A.* 258(20):1920, 1987.

Erffmeyer, J. E., and Blaiss, M. S. Proving penicillin allergy. *Postgrad. Med.* 87(2):33, 1990.

Johnson, K. J., Chensue, S. W., Kunkel, S. L., and Ward, P. A. Chapter 4, "Immunopathology," in E.

Rubin and J. L. Farber, *Essential Pathology*. Philadelphia: Lippincott, 1990.

Lieberman, P. Rhinitis: Allergic and nonallergic. *Hosp. Pract.* 23:117,1988.

Rodger, J. C., and Drake, B. L. The enigma of the fetal graft. *Am. Sci.* 75:51,1987.

Salvin, R. G., and Ducomb, D. F. Allergic contact dermatitis. *Hosp. Pract.* 24:39,1989.

Serafin, W. E., and Austen, K. F. Mediators of immediate hypersensitivity reactions. *N. Engl. J. Med.* 317:30,1987.

Walker, E. C. Food allergy. *Amer. Family Physician* 38:207,1988.

Weisdorf, D. J. Bone marrow transplantation. *Postgrad. Med.* 87(1):91,1990.

Yunginger, J. W., Sweeney, K. G., Sturner, W. Q., et al. Fatal food-induced anaphylaxis. J.A.M.A. 260:1450, 1988.

V. BACTERIA THAT CAUSE INFECTIOUS DISEASE

15. INTRODUCTION TO THE BACTERIAL DISEASES

OBJECTIVES

To summarize how bacterial diseases and the
bacteria that cause them are explained in a
taxonomically organized medical microbiology
textbook

To explain what information is gathered and how it
is used to control bacterial diseases
To provide and suggest study aids for the student

This textbook uses a *taxonomic approach* to the discussion of infectious diseases; that is, the properties of a microbial genus or family are described. Each chapter on a given genus or family of bacteria usually includes the topics given in the outline of this chapter. A generalized discussion of what the reader can expect to find under each heading follows.

GENERAL CHARACTERISTICS OF THE TAXONOMIC GROUP

The chapters begin with a generalized description and enumeration of characteristics of the family or genus and the various species within the taxonomic group. Much of the information presented here is in the nature of a preview or summary of what will be spelled out in greater detail in the remainder of the chapter. Included is such information as Gram-stain reaction, morphology, oxygen requirements, spore formation, encapsulation, cultural characteristics, noteworthy diseases caused by members of the taxonomic

group, and major properties that are relevant to the group.

DISEASES CAUSED BY MEMBERS OF THE FAMILY OR GENUS

SIGNS AND SYMPTOMS

Many of the signs and symptoms (disease manifestations) that are evoked by infectious agents are common to many infectious diseases—headache, malaise, nausea, fever, pain, enlarged lymph nodes, and so on. There may be differences, however, in the combination, degree, sequence, and location of these, depending on the particular infectious agent. There are also diseases in which the signs are very distinctive. This is especially so with the readily observable rashes and lesions of the skin and of the mucosa that occur in some diseases.

The impression sometimes exists that each infectious agent causes only one clinical condition. That is the case with a few microorganisms.

Many bacteria, however, are able to cause a number of clinical conditions. The gram-positive cocci are especially noted for the variety of clinical entities in which they may be involved. *Staphylococcus aureus*, for example, in addition to causing infections commonly associated with it, such as skin lesions (boils, bullous impetigo), bone inflammation (osteomyelitis), and food poisoning, can cause infections that involve the lung (pneumonia), central nervous system (meningitis), urinary bladder (cystitis), heart (endocarditis), blood (septicemia), and other disorders. Conversely, bacterial pneumonia may be due to a *Staphylococcus, Streptococcus, Hemophilus, Klebsiella*, or other bacterial agent.

The reader should note that Appendix A contains Tables of Infectious Agents Based on Site of Infection and Appendix B, Table of Normal Microbial Flora of the Human Body.

PATHOGENESIS AND PATHOLOGY

There usually is an account of how the infectious disease develops. It includes the progression of *changes in the functioning and architecture of the affected tissues* and the microbial factors that are responsible for those changes.

BACTERIAL VIRULENCE FACTORS AND OTHER IMPORTANT FACTORS

Research has produced voluminous information about the differing toxins, enzymes, antigens, and other products and factors of each bacterial species. Textbooks emphasize the factors that have a role in the pathogenesis, identification, epidemiology, and control of a disease.

It is helpful to understand the development and the usage of the terminology that is applied to microbial factors. On discovery, a microbial factor usually is named according to its activity (fibrinolysin; spreading factor; hemolysin) or after the discoverer (Duran-Reynals factor; Panton-Valentine leukocidin). Often the chemical nature

eventually is determined. The streptococcal product that was originally called spreading factor, or Duran-Reynals factor, for example, is now known as the enzyme hyaluronidase.

It sometimes happens that one substance produced by a species of bacteria is responsible for several biological activities and the substance remains known under several names. Thus the alpha staphylolysin, the dermonecrotic toxin, and the lethal factor that are produced by *S. aureus* are, insofar as is presently known, all the same substance.

Certain substances are associated mainly with one genus or species of bacteria. Mention oxidase-positive bacteria and the clinical microbiologist thinks first of members of the genus *Neisseria*. Similarly, coagulase is associated with *S. aureus* and lecithinase with *Clostridium perfringens*. These substances often contribute to the virulence of the respective bacteria, and they are often useful in laboratory identification. The association of such substances with a certain bacterial species does not always mean that some other species do not also produce the same substance.

LABORATORY IDENTIFICATION

A good portion of the time of the clinical laboratory microbiologist is expended in identifying infectious agents in the laboratory.

OVERVIEW OF THE IDENTIFICATION PROCESS

The clinical disease serves as the starting point for the laboratory investigation. The attending physician has a mental list of the microorganisms most likely to cause a given condition. Judgments are based on such considerations as the patient's age, signs and symptoms, contacts, geographical and dietary history, predisposing conditions, and what is currently "going around." The type of specimen to be obtained, the culture media to be used, the conditions of incubation, and the tests to be conducted are guided by those clinical judgments.

The first steps in identification usually seek to identify the genus of the isolated bacterium. Next, since most genera contain a number of species with different properties, it becomes necessary to identify the species and possibly strains within the species.

IMPORTANCE OF IDENTIFYING STRAINS

Mutation and selection give rise to many strains within the same species. Strains can differ from the *type species* (the one that typifies the characteristics of the species and against which strains are compared) in a number of important ways: virulence, susceptibility to chemotherapeutic agents, physiological/biochemical activities, antigenic composition, presence or absence of structures (capsules, for example), temperature sensitivity, and susceptibility to bacterial viruses. These differences confer properties that are important for identification, assessing pathogenicity and drug susceptibility, epidemiologic tracing, and immunization. The strains or variants are usually placed into groups or types that are variously designated as *serogroups, serotypes, biotypes, phage groups and types*, and so on. The groups or types are symbolized by various lettering (capitalized, lowercase, Greek alphabet) and numbering (Roman numerals, Arabic numbers) systems. Encapsulated strains of *Hemophilus influenzae*, for example, are placed into types a, b, c, d, e, and f on the basis of antigenic differences in capsular composition; *Staphylococcus aureus* strains are placed into phage groups I to IV on the basis of susceptibility to lysis by different strains of viruses (staphylophages) that specifically infect *S. aureus* (see Fig. 10-4 and text, page 253).

IDENTIFICATION OF NONPATHOGENS

Most of the genera of bacteria studied in medical microbiology contain both pathogenic and nonpathogenic species. Learning the characteristics of the nonpathogens may seem an unproductive pursuit, yet in many instances it is necessary to be able to differentiate the pathogens from the nonpathogens, particularly the nonpathogens that constitute the normal microflora. Furthermore, a number of the nonpathogens may opportunistically cause infections in a debilitated individual or under other predisposing conditions.

LABORATORY IDENTIFICATION PROCEDURES

Seldom does a single laboratory finding conclusively identify the microorganism. Identification involves combinations of the five general laboratory approaches: microscopical study, cultural examination, biochemical techniques, serological techniques, and animal identification procedures.

As a basic step in traditional laboratory identification a pure culture must almost always be obtained. Pure cultures are obtained by such means as the streak plate, the pour plate, and the use of selective and sometimes differential media.

Microscopical Characteristics

Gram-straining is routinely performed in the identification of bacteria. It is a process that eliminates from the investigation those bacteria that differ in morphology and staining reaction from the bacterium under scrutiny. Thus if it is determined that the bacterium under study is a gram-negative bacillus, then gram-positive cocci and bacilli and gram-negative cocci are eliminated. Nevertheless there remain hundreds of gram-negative bacilli to consider.

There are situations when the result of the Gram-staining of clinical material, together with a knowledge of the patient's history and symptoms, is enough information to make a presumptive diagnosis as to the causal agent of the disease. The physician with this information may be able to initiate specific chemotherapy immediately while waiting for definitive laboratory test results. When clinical material is stained, it is important also to note the type of host cells on the slide. For example, the presence of large numbers of neutrophils indicates an acute bacterial infection. Clinical materials that routinely are Gram-stained because the findings may lead to a presumptive diagnosis include: sputum and transtracheal exudates for the causal agents of pneumonia, sputum for pulmonary TB, urine accompanied by pus for bladder and urethral infections, urethral exudate for gonorrhea, cerebrospinal fluid for the causal agents of meningitis, and brain abscesses.

Staining may also be used to identify specific structures on or in the bacterial cell that may be of value in the identification process: capsules, pili, spores, metachromatic granules, or flagella.

Cultural Characteristics

Colonial characteristics such as size, shape, pigmentation, elevation, consistency when touched with a bacteriological loop, and types of indentation of the colony edge are helpful to the laboratorian in deciding which identification avenues to pursue. A large, flat, irregularly shaped colony, for example, is more likely to be formed by a member of the genus *Bacillus* than is a smaller, round, convex colony, which is more typical of different genera of cocci and small bacilli.

Blood agar plate hemolysis. Certain bacterial species characteristically produce hemolysins. When the bacteria are cultured on blood agar plates their hemolysins affect the red blood cells (RBCs) in the zone surrounding the hemolytic colony. Blood agar plate hemolytic activity is of the following types.

1. *Alpha hemolysis*. There is partial destruction of RBCs with a loss of some hemoglobin resulting in a greenish-brownish discoloration of the medium. RBC membranes are visible when examined with a lens.
2. *Beta hemolysis*. RBC membranes disappear and a clear, colorless zone surrounds the colony.
3. *No hemolysis*. When there is no apparent hemolytic activity the bacteria are said to be *nonhemolytic* or *anhemolytic*.

The readily observed presence of hemolysis and the type of hemolysis supply valuable information because the trained observer knows which species produce blood agar plate hemolysis.

Biochemical Characteristics

Biochemical testing most often leads to the specific identification. The clinical impression and the information obtained from microscopical and cultural observations for the most part merely guide the reasoning as to which of the multitude of biochemical tests to use for the specific identification. Bacteria produce nearly a thousand different enzymes. Species differentiation based on biochemical testing is feasible because bacterial species differ as to which enzymes they possess; that is, each species has its own characteristic enzyme "fingerprint."

Most of the tests are conducted in specially designed culture media that contain defined compounds. A set of differing media is inoculated from a pure culture, incubated, and examined for evidence of metabolism. Results are directly evident in some test media because of observable changes, such as changes in the color of a pH indicator. In other tests specific reagents need to be added to produce an observable change. Products that typically are formed are: organic acids such as lactic, acetic, formic, and pyruvic; gases such as carbon dioxide, methane, and hydrogen sulfide; and waste products such as indole, nitrite, and acetylmethylcarbinol.

Following is a sampling of biochemical tests.

1. Fermentation. Fermentation tests are the most frequently used of all the biochemical tests. The broth test type contains a minimal broth, a single carbohydrate, a pH indicator, and an inverted vial that serves as a gas trap. A change in the color of the pH indicator indicates acid formation and the appearance of a bubble in the inverted vial indicates gas formation. An organism that ferments the carbohydrate may be acid positive, or acid and gas positive.

2. Catalase production. The transfer of hydrogen to oxygen in the respiration of some microorganisms results in the production of hydrogen peroxide (H_2O_2). Most aerobic organisms produce an enzyme, catalase, that is capable of oxidizing H_2O_2 to water and oxygen. When colonies on an agar surface are flooded with H_2O_2, bubbles of oxygen will appear if the cells in the colony produce catalase.

3. Hydrogen sulfide production. Some microorganisms are capable of reducing sulfur to hydrogen sulfide (H_2S). A medium containing high concentrations of the amino acid cysteine and iron salts is inoculated with the test organisms. After suitable incubation, a black or brown precipitate will appear if the organisms remove sulfur from cysteine and reduce it to H_2S. The precipitate is ferrous sulfide (FeS), formed according to the following reaction:

$$FeSO_4 + H_2S \longrightarrow FeS + H_2SO_4$$

4. Indole production. Breakdown of the amino acid tryptophan by bacteria leads to the accumulation of indole. Indole can be detected in the broth culture by addition of a color reagent called Kovac's solution. A positive test result is the appearance of a red ring in the broth.

5. Nitrate reduction. The enzyme nitratase can be produced by a wide variety of microorganisms. It is responsible for the catalytic reduction of nitrate (NO_3) to nitrite (NO_2). Nitrite accumulates in the broth culture and can be detected by addition of a special color reagent that reacts with the nitrite to produce a red ring. Some bacteria will further reduce NO_2 to nitrogen gas (N_2) or ammonia (NH_3), and if this occurs the nitrite test is apparently negative. The negative tube should be checked for the appearance of unreduced nitrate by the addition of zinc dust besides the nitrite color reagents. The development of a red color confirms the absence of nitrate reduction.

Many other biochemical tests are used in the laboratory. They will be discussed as they apply to specific groups of microorganisms.

Serological Characteristics

Antigen–antibody interaction can be used for the purposes of laboratory identification in two ways:

1. Known microorganisms are injected into animal hosts. Immune sera or antisera specific for each injected microorganism are prepared and refrigerated (they can also be obtained commercially). If at some time an organism is isolated from a patient, the unknown microorganism can be tested against one of the known antisera.

2. Known antigen suspensions of whole cells, capsules, flagella, or other structures are prepared in the laboratory. Unknown antisera from infected hosts can be tested against known antigen preparations. A positive reaction with one of the known antigens indicates which microorganisms have infected the host and caused the production of the antibodies. Some of the serological tests used in the clinical laboratory were discussed in the chapters on immunology; others will be discussed in the chapters on specific infectious agents such as the viruses.

The Use of Animals for Identification

Animals are not routinely used in microbial identification procedures. Some bacteria, however, do not grow in culture media. A specimen suspected to contain the leprosy bacillus, for example, might be injected into the footpad of a mouse. Syphilis bacteria are injected into rabbit testicles to obtain enough live spirochetes to conduct the Treponema Pallidum Immobilization (TPI) Test. Sometimes animals are used by microbiologists to determine whether a microorganism is virulent or not, to follow functional and tissue changes as a disease progresses (pathogenesis), to obtain specific antisera that are used for serological testing, and to determine the in vivo effectiveness of chemotherapeutic agents.

Rapid Identification Techniques

Beginning in the 1970s, methods of identification were developed that departed from the traditional methods that had been used since the time of Koch. One of the new methods is in the form of kits, which are referred to by such terms as *rapid identification* kits, *multitest,* and *miniaturized* kits. It was found that the use of a good-sized inoculum with small amounts of culture media and reagents could produce rapid, accurate biochemical test results. The number of tests conducted simultaneously usually is a battery or panel of about 8 to 24 tests. The number is governed by the type of organism being tested—enterics, staphylococci, streptococci, and so on— and by the manufacturer's design. Some kits have compartments with different, already prepared agars in each compartment; pH indicators and reagents appropriate to each test are incorporated right into the media. Some kits have cupules or wells that contain dehydrated powdered media or discs of culture media that dissolve when saline or broth suspensions of the test organism are added. Some kits are so designed that certain of the compartments are incubated under anaerobic conditions, or so designed that the test reagents can be added later. Interpretation of results is done through the use of manuals, codes, and computer discs supplied by the manufacturer.

The advantages are many. The inoculum for each culture medium is uniform. The kits require minimum storage and incubation space, they have a long shelf-life, and they are disposable.

Time-consuming preparation of conventional culture media is avoided. Many culture media are inoculated at one time, often with a single manual application. Cost per isolate usually is lower than with the conventional methods. There is no problem maintaining quality control.

The first kits available were for *biochemical testing.* Test systems are now available that *detect antigens, preformed enzymes,* and *antibiotic susceptibility.* Semi-automated and automated equipment has become available in the last decade (Fig. 15-1). The user merely adds inoculum to a disposable tray or cassette. Incubation, test reading, and reporting are done by machine.

More sensitive technologies are being added to the expanding list of improved methods of microbial identification. Two that are already being used are nucleic acid probes and monoclonal antibody techniques (Chapter 13). Increasing numbers of applications are expected as more nucleic acid probes and monoclonal antibodies become available and as the techniques and instrumentation are refined for routine usage.

EPIDEMIOLOGY

Epidemiologic information, which may include such considerations as incidence, age, race, sex, nutritional status, life-style, travels, and geographical location, has a bearing on the clinician's level of suspicion as to the causal agent of the patient's disease and indicates the preventive measures that may have to be undertaken for family, contacts, or the public at large. This information also indicates the effectiveness of, or the necessity for, immunization and community control measures, and it is a reflection of the disease-causing opportunities and capabilities of a given infectious agent.

A variety of laboratory procedures are available for determining the source of infectious agents. They include biotyping, serotyping, phage typing, antibiograms, and molecular techniques described in Chapter 10.

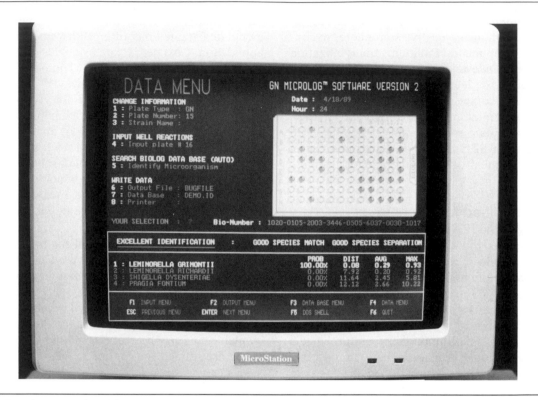

Fig. 15-1. Automated multitest system. The 96-well MicroPlate (upper right) before inoculation contains a dried film of nutrients and reagents. Addition of a bacterial cell suspension activates the identification process. If the cells oxidize the carbon source, a purple-colored dye product forms after 4 to 24 hours of incubation; 95 reactions from the MicroPlate can be read directly from the MicroStation Reader into the MicroStation Computer yielding an identification in seconds from a database of over 300 species/groups of gram-negative aerobes. (From Barry Buchner, Biolog Inc., Hayward, CA.)

TREATMENT AND PREVENTION

CHEMOTHERAPY

Research, experience, and susceptibility testing provide guidelines as to which chemotherapeutic agents are effective against which species and strains of bacteria. It is customary to cite the chemotherapeutic agents of choice and also the alternative agents that may be prescribed if the identified bacterium is resistant to the first-choice chemotherapeutic agent, or if the patient has a hypersensitivity or toxic reaction to the first-choice agent.

ACTIVE IMMUNIZATION

Some infectious diseases are completely preventable through active immunization. The type of immunizing material that is available for the disease is given—toxoid, an attenuated strain, a killed suspension, or whatever (Chapter 12). The description includes the immunogenic component (subunit) of the bacterial cell, when it is known (e.g., capsule, cell wall fraction, and so on), that elicits the protective immune response.

PASSIVE IMMUNOTHERAPY

An account of the available passive immunotherapy or immunoprophylaxis is included. Thus the administration of antiserum (serotherapy) for diseases such as diphtheria or botulism, or the administration of gamma globulin for diseases such as hepatitis A or tetanus, may be advised.

OTHER FORMS OF TREATMENT

Other examples of forms of treatment that may be recommended include *surgical intervention*—for example, *surgical debridement* in gas gangrene; *enzymatic debridement* to speed up removal of pus, fibrin, or edema fluid; and exposure to high concentrations of oxygen (*hyperbaric oxygen therapy*) for patients who are suffering from certain kinds of anaerobic infections.

STERILIZATION AND DISINFECTION MEASURES

Sometimes it is necessary to point out the sterilization and disinfection measures that are to be employed against the disease agent when these measures differ from those that are routinely used against other bacteria.

STUDY AIDS

REGULARLY CITED BACTERIAL PROPERTIES

The following generalizations make it easier to remember some of the regularly cited properties of bacteria. The description of most bacterial species includes their morphology, grouping and Gram's stain reaction, oxygen requirements, whether they are spore formers, and whether they are motile.

1. Gram's stain reaction and shape. The Gram's stain reaction and the shape of one genus member almost always apply as well to all members of the genus. *Hemophilus influenzae* is a gram-negative bacillus; therefore, any *Hemophilus* species will also be a gram-negative bacillus. The student is likely to be expected to know the Gram's stain reaction of the major pathogenic bacteria. The sequence in which the bacterial genera are presented in most textbooks is customarily based on their Gram's stain reaction and their shape: gram-positive cocci, gram-negative cocci, gram-positive bacilli, and gram-negative bacilli. The mycobacteria and the spirochetes usually are not categorized in those terms. The principal genera of medically important bacteria and their Gram's stain reaction and morphology are as follows:

Gram-positive cocci
 Staphylococcus
 Streptococcus
Gram-negative cocci
 Neisseria
Gram-positive bacilli
 Corynebacterium
 Bacillus
 Clostridium
Gram-negative bacilli
 Hemophilus
 Bordetella
 Brucella
 Pasteurella
 Escherichia
 Salmonella
 Shigella
 Bacteroides
 Rickettsia

2. Endospore formation. The only genera of medical importance in which spore formers are found are *Clostridium* and *Bacillus*.

3. Oxygen requirements. Most bacteria en-

countered in an infectious disease are facultatively anaerobic, that is, they are capable of metabolizing under either aerobic or anaerobic conditions. A few genera and species of bacteria are strict or obligate anaerobes. Especially noted for this trait among the bacteria of medical importance are the members of the genera *Clostridium* and *Bacteroides*.

4. Motility. Among the bacteria that are considered in medical microbiology, none of the cocci are motile, all the spiral-shaped forms are motile, and among the rod-shaped bacteria there is no general rule in respect to motility—some are motile, others are not.

ORGANIZATIONAL AID

As a memory and organizational aid, the student might well maintain a running table that summarizes the leading information or features of the major bacteria of medical importance. Table 15-1 shows the headings such a table might include (using *Staphylococcus* as an example).

TERMINOLOGY

Infectious disease is a pathological condition, and a number of terms and concepts from pathology are used to describe it. An understanding of the following terms will improve the student's comprehension of the discussion of infectious dis-

eases. It is advisable to review the events of inflammation and the cell types that participate in inflammation, antibody formation, cell-mediated immunity, phagocytosis, and allergic reactions that are described in Part IV, Immunology.

ABSCESS   a circumscribed accumulation of pus

DIFFERENTIAL BLOOD COUNT   an enumeration of white blood cell (WBC) types with the purpose of detecting changes from the normal WBC range (changes in WBC proportions and numbers are brought about by many infectious agents)

EDEMA   the accumulation of fluid portions of the blood in tissues; accounts for or contributes to the swelling, blockage, pain, induration, and blanching of the affected site

EMBOLUS   a pathological space-occupying aggregate that moves in the vascular system with the constant threat of blocking important vascular channels or spaces (examples: gas bubbles, lipids, pyogenic masses, and, most important, clots [thrombi])

EXUDATE   blood components, both fluid and formed (e.g., cells) elements, which accumulate in tissues, spaces, and surfaces (mucosa) as one manifestation of an inflammatory response

ICTERUS   jaundice

ISCHEMIA   lack or diminution of blood in a tissue; may be due to blockage, vascular collapse or interruption, pressure, or hemorrhage

Table 15-1. Format of Suggested Study Guide

Gram's stain, shape	Genus and species	Culture media	Lab tests	Diseases	Other characteristics
+ c	*Staphylococcus aureus*	Mannitol salt agar	Coagulase CHO utilization Superoxol	Boils Impetigo Osteomyelitis Food poisoning Scalded skin syndrome Toxic shock syndrome	Enterotoxin Hospital-acquired infections Penicillinase Exfoliatin Staphylolysins Protein A

+ c = gram-positive coccus

LEUKOCYTOSIS temporary increase in white blood cells, which may occur in response to injury or disease; may be more specifically termed, depending on which WBC type shows an increase—for example, lymphocytosis, an increase in lymphocytes

LEUKOPENIA temporary pathological diminution of white blood cells; may be more specifically termed, depending on cell type involved

MUCOSA internal epithelial surface lubricated by enzyme-carrying mucus

PATHOGENESIS the in vivo progression or sequence of events leading to the disease state; the development of the pathological condition

PATHOGNOMONIC pertaining to a clinical or laboratory finding that is so distinctive as to be self-identifying (e.g., the inclusion body elicited in neurons by rabies is so characteristic in appearance that the trained observer recognizes that this cell was infected by the rabies virus and not some other agent)

PURULENT pus-containing

PYOGENIC pus-inducing, pus-eliciting, pus-generating

PYROGENIC fever-inducing, fever-eliciting, fever-generating

SIGNS disease manifestations that are detectable by an observer; objective indications such as a rash, swelling, and vomiting

SYMPTOMS disease indications felt by the patient; subjective experiences such as headache, malaise

THROMBUS an in vivo blood clot attached in the cardiovascular system (a thrombus or portion thereof may break away to become an embolus [thromboembolus])

ULCER a circumscribed, necrotic, denuded surface area of the skin or mucosa

VESICLE a blister; a small, circumscribed, elevated area of the skin or mucosa that contains clear fluid

Several combining terms (prefixes and suffixes are used repeatedly, and an understanding of these helps to interpret the meaning of many words):

PREFIXES

a(n)- negative, lack of, deficient, against, reverse of

adeno- pertaining to the glands

arthro- pertaining to the joints

ecto- external

endo- internal

entero- pertaining to the intestines

hema-, hemato- pertaining to the blood

hyper- above, increased, more than the normal; equivalent to *super-*

hypo- below, decreased, less than the normal; equivalent to *sub-*

inter- between

intra- within

myo- pertaining to muscle

oligo- few

peri- around

poly- many

stomato- pertaining to the mouth

SUFFIXES

-algia pain

-dynia pain

-ectomy surgical excision

-emia a condition of the blood

-genic causing, eliciting, generating

-itis inflammation

-lytic dissolving, causing to flow

-oma tumor

-ostomy surgical opening

-rrhea flowing, discharge

-trophic nourishing

-tropic turning toward or attaching to

-uria a condition of the urine

SUMMARY

1. There are a great number and variety of infectious diseases and infectious disease agents. Health care personnel are expected to know the

characteristics of the diseases and of the infectious disease agents.

2. Customarily textbook descriptions include the signs and symptoms of the disease, the microbial (virulence) and host factors involved in the development of the disease (pathogenesis), the mode of transmission of the disease, the extent of the population affected in the past (morbidity and mortality statistics), the laboratory tests and procedures that are used to identify the infecting microorganism, and the treatment.

3. Identification requires knowledge of the cultural conditions and of the components, products, and antigens that are peculiar to a given species.

4. This information is pertinent to deciding the chemotherapy and immunotherapy that is to be applied and to judging the severity of the illness, the prognosis, the expected signs and symptoms in the patient, and the time course of the illness.

5. The availability of vaccines and immunotherapy that protect individuals and populations is also relevant, as are aseptic and sanitary measures that prevent transmission of the disease agents.

6. As a mnemonic aid, the chapter includes a condensed version of some of the routinely required basic information about bacteria: Gram's stain reactions, oxygen requirements, spore formation, and motility.

QUESTIONS FOR STUDY

Select the best response or responses for each of the following:

1. The clear zone surrounding certain colonies on blood agar plates is called
   A. Zone of equivalence
   B. Zone of inhibition of growth
   C. Beta hemolysis
   D. Alpha hemolysis
   E. Twilight zone

2. The culture medium for the indole test must contain
   A. Glucose
   B. Kovac's reagent
   C. Catalase
   D. Nitrates
   E. Tryptophan

3. In the diagnostic laboratory identification of bacteria to the species level is usually accomplished via
   A. Examination of cultural (usually colonial) characteristics
   B. Observation of the microscopical characteristics

C. Biochemical activities testing
D. Serological testing
E. Animal inoculation

True or False:

4. The inverted tube that is placed in fermentation tubes is placed there to ensure anaerobic conditions for obligate anaerobes.
   A. True   B. False

5. One reason rapid, multi-test, miniaturized identification kits/systems are cost-effective, especially in low-volume laboratories, is that the time-consuming preparation of small amounts of numerous conventional media is avoided.
   A. True   B. False

6. In a fermentation test one is usually seeking to detect the name of the specific acid that is a product of the fermentation.
   A. True   B. False

ADDITIONAL READINGS

Baron, E. J., and Finegold, S. M. *Bailey and Scott's Diagnostic Microbiology* (8th ed.). St. Louis: Mosby, 1990.

D'Amato, R. F., McLaughlin, J. C., and Ferraro, J. J. 6. Rapid and Mechanized/Automated Systems in Microbiology. In E. H. Lennette et al., *Manual of Clinical Microbiology* (4th ed.). Washington, DC: American Society for Microbiology, 1985.

Kleger, B., et al. *Rapid Methods in Clinical Microbiology*. New York: Plenum, 1989.

Koneman, E. W., et al. *Color Atlas and Textbook of Diagnostic Microbiology* (3rd ed.). Philadelphia: Lippincott, 1988.

Lambert, H. P., Farrar, W. E., and Swartz, M. N. *Infectious Diseases Illustrated*. Philadelphia: Saunders, 1982.

Mackowiak, P. A. The normal microbial flora. *N. Engl. J. Med.* 307:83,1982.

16. THE GRAM-POSITIVE COCCI

OBJECTIVES

To describe the infectious diseases caused by staphylococci

To list the various factors associated with the virulence of *Staphylococcus aureus* and the streptococci

To describe those laboratory tests that differentiate *S. aureus* from *S. epidermidis*

To briefly describe the techniques for laboratory diagnosis, treatment, and control of staphylococcal and streptococcal infections

To comment on the increasing importance of coagulase-negative staphylococci as causative agents of disease

To describe the laboratory tests used to identify group A streptococci

To list those diseases associated primarily with group B, group C, and group D streptococci and enterococci

To describe *Streptococcus pneumoniae* in terms of virulence factors, disease associations, and laboratory identification

Cocci of medical importance are members of the genera *Staphylococcus*, *Streptococcus*, *Enterococcus*, and *Neisseria*. Staphylococci, streptococci, enterococci, and micrococci are gram-positive; neisseriae are gram-negative. The pathogens can cause infection in virtually any tissue, organ, tract, or system of the body. Since the majority of the infections are acute, the pathogenic cocci are often referred to as the *pyogenic*—pus-eliciting or pus-generating—cocci.

THE STAPHYLOCOCCI

GENERAL CHARACTERISTICS

Members of the genera *Staphylococcus* and *Micrococcus* belong to the family Micrococcaceae. There are 23 recognized species of staphylococci,

12 of which are part of the normal or occasional microflora of humans. Only three are recognized as being clinically important, namely, *S. aureus*, *S. epidermidis*, and *S. saprophyticus*. *S. aureus* is a pathogen. The other two are regarded as opportunistic or nosocomial pathogens. *S. aureus* is the only coagulase-positive (see under Laboratory Identification) human species, so all other human species collectively are referred to as *the coagulase-negative staphylococci* (*CONS* or *CNS*). *S. hominis*, *S. haemolyticus*, and *S. simulans* and other species to an even lesser extent account for a small percentage of infections.

Staphylococci characteristically aggregate in irregular groups like clusters of grapes (Figs. 16-1 and 16-2). They grow regularly on routinely used laboratory media. Staphylococci are aerobic to facultatively anaerobic, nonmotile, and non-spore-forming. They are strongly *catalase positive* (that is, if one adds hydrogen peroxide to colonial growth, immediate evolution of bubbles of oxygen will be visible).

Staphylococci, with *S. epidermidis* and *S.*

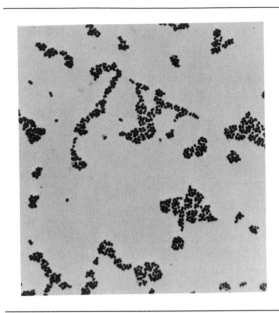

Fig. 16-2. Light micrograph of a smear of *Staphylococcus aureus* taken from a broth culture. (From A. S. Klainer and I. Geis, *Agents of Bacterial Disease*. New York: Harper & Row, 1973.)

Fig. 16-1. Scanning electron micrograph of microcolonies of *Staphylococcus aureus*. (× 14,000.) (Courtesy Z. Yoshii.)

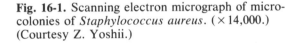

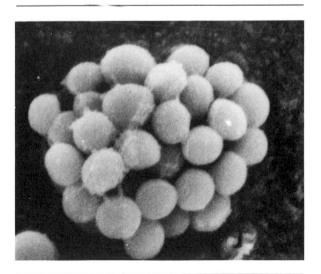

hominis as the most prevalent and persistent, are among the major natural inhabitants of the skin. Large populations are present in the axillae (armpits), anterior nares, and perineum. Staphylococci may also be found in the throat, mouth, vagina, intestinal tract, and mammary glands, but in smaller numbers than on the skin.

STAPHYLOCOCCUS AUREUS

PATHOGENESIS

S. aureus causes a broad range of serious infections throughout the body. The infections and diseases specifically or primarily associated with *S. aureus* are boils, carbuncles, bullous impetigo, scalded skin syndrome, staphylococcal food poisoning, staphylococcal enterocolitis, staphylococcal osteomyelitis, and toxic shock syndrome.

Infections of the Skin

Pyoderma: Abscesses, Furuncles, Sties, Carbuncles, Impetigo. *S. aureus* causes various types of purulent skin infections (pyoderma) and subcutaneous infections. The infection of hair follicles—*folliculitis*—leads to the formation of furuncles (boils) in the skin or sties in the eyelids. *Carbuncles* represent a deeper, more serious condition, which results from tunneling, coalescing abscesses (Fig. 16-3). Either *S. aureus* or *Streptococcus pyogenes* alone or the two agents as coinfectors cause *impetigo* (Fig. 16-4), a skin infection found primarily in children. Impetigo often begins in the nasal area and spreads from there over the face. Impetigo is characterized by fragile blisters, which when broken leave erosions covered by honey-colored crusts.

Scalded Skin Syndrome. Scalded skin syndrome (SSS) is an exfoliative dermatitis that encompasses several clinical conditions. It is most often observed in infants and young children. The syndrome usually begins as erythema around the

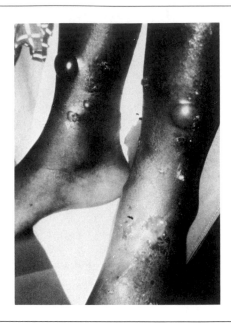

Fig. 16-4. Bullous impetigo caused by *Staphylococcus aureus*. (Courtesy H. Dillon.)

Fig. 16-3. Carbuncle caused by *Staphylococcus aureus* in a diabetic patient. (From F. H. Top, Sr., and P. F. Wehrle [eds.], *Communicable and Infectious Diseases* [8th ed.]. St. Louis: Mosby, 1976.)

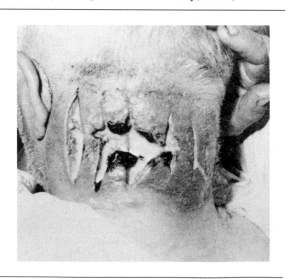

mouth and nose and spreads rapidly to affect the skin of the neck, the trunk, and sometimes the extremities. The epidermal necrolysis, mediated by the toxin *exfoliatin*, results in *extensive areas of denuded skin* as sheets of the overlying epidermis loosen. Transudates and exudates are not copious and fatalities are infrequent because the condition is limited largely to the superficial layer of the skin.

Gastrointestinal Tract Staphylococcal Disease

Staphylococcal Enterocolitis. *Staphylococcal enterocolitis may follow intensive antibiotic therapy or gastrointestinal surgery.* Antibiotics taken orally may reduce the normal intestinal microflora, thereby creating conditions for an antibiotic-resistant, endogenous staphylococcus to multiply and produce what is known as a *super-*

infection. Clinical manifestations include diarrhea, fever, abdominal cramping, electrolyte imbalance, and loss of fluids. Most cases of enterocolitis associated with bacterial overgrowth, however, are due to *Clostridium difficile* (Chapter 18) following antibiotic treatment.

Staphylococcal Food Poisoning. Certain strains of *S. aureus* excrete into foods the heat-stable exotoxin called *staphylococcal enterotoxin*. When ingested with the food, the enterotoxin causes a type of food poisoning that is accompanied by vehement vomiting (projectile vomiting), cramps, diarrhea, and prostration 2 to 8 hours after ingestion. Enterotoxin food poisoning is rarely fatal. The patient is fully recovered in 24 to 48 hours. Many foods support the growth of staphylococci, particularly those that contain a high amount of protein—ham, poultry, and potato and egg salads, for example. Outbreaks occur when a contaminated food is held at inappropriate temperatures long enough to allow the bacteria to elaborate toxin. Food preparers and handlers who have staphylococcal lesions of the skin, especially of the hands, and nasopharyngeal carriers are the most likely to contaminate food. Absence of lesions is no guarantee of safety.

Deeper Infections

Extensive and deeper infections may be primary infections or may stem from an infection that has metastasized from a cutaneous infection or from a carrier site. Serious staphylococcal infections are not likely to occur in healthy individuals but rather in those who have a precondition such as extensive surgery, burns, diabetes, cystic fibrosis, lower respiratory tract viral infection, or decubitus ulcers, and in those who are immunosuppressed or immunodefective, especially in some aspect of their phagocytic system (see Immunodeficiencies in Phagocytes, Chapter 14). *S. aureus* can cause infections in many tissues and organs: endocarditis, meningitis, pneumonia, cystitis, septicemia, infection of postoperative wounds, vascular and valvular infections, and others.

Osteomyelitis. Most cases of osteomyelitis (inflammation of bone) are due to *S. aureus*. The bacteria arrive at the site of infection via hematogenous (blood) spread from a focus of infection such as a furuncle or they enter because of surgery or deep penetrating trauma. In the latter instance the bones are likely to be those that require surgical pinning after a compound fracture. Symptoms of acute osteomyelitis include fever, chills, pain over the bone, and muscle spasms in the affected bone area.

Toxic Shock Syndrome. Toxic shock syndrome (TSS) is a multisystem, febrile illness with abrupt onset and with hypotension (shock). Vomiting, diarrhea, a diffuse macular erythematous rash with subsequent palmar and plantar desquamation (peeling of the skin on the palms of the hands and soles of the feet), and hyperemia of mucous membranes regularly occur. Disseminated intravascular clotting is an occasional complication. Death may be caused by profound shock, respiratory failure, and disseminated intravascular coagulopathy. The abrupt onset of TSS in the absence of a clinical prodrome suggests that a toxin is involved. The toxin responsible for the illness is called *toxic shock syndrome toxin-1* (*TSST-1*).

TSS was first described as a syndrome in 1978. A high percentage of cases occurred in young menstruating females who used tampons. High-absorbency tampons were promptly identified as a high-risk factor. The number of TSS tampon-associated cases decreased substantially starting in 1981 when manufacturers lowered the absorbency of tampons. Nonmenstrual high-risk groups are postpartum women, patients with focal staphylococcal and surgical wound infections, and infections associated with nasal surgery and packing. The highest risk is in children and young adults but cases occur in any age group. Approximately two to five percent of patients with TSS may die. TSS requires fluid replacement, drainage of any foci of infection, and chemotherapy.

VIRULENCE FACTORS RELATED TO S. AUREUS INFECTIONS

S. aureus strains may produce as many as 25 to 30 proteins, some of which are associated with pathogenesis. The factors that are either specifically or primarily related to *S. aureus* are coagulase, staphylolysins, dermonecrotic toxin, lethal factor, Panton-Valentine leukocidin, staphylococcal enterotoxin, toxic shock syndrome toxin-1, and protein A.

Coagulase

Coagulase, a plasma-clotting protein, although produced by some other bacteria, is almost exclusively associated with *S. aureus*. A role for coagulase in causing disease has not been discovered, although it is suggested that the coating of the staphylococci with fibrin inhibits their being phagocytosed. The laboratory tests for coagulase production are described under Laboratory Identification.

Staphylolysins

Staphylolysins are hemolysins that are categorized among the staphylococcal exotoxins. They also are cytotoxic for cells other than red blood cells such as macrophages, platelets, and neutrophils. They can disrupt lysosomes, causing phagocytes to degranulate. They are of several types: alpha, beta, gamma, and delta. They differ in the species of red cells that they are able to lyse, in the cations that are required for their activation, in the cell membrane substrates on which they act, in toxic activities, and in antigenic composition. The alpha lysin lyses rabbit, sheep, and calf red blood cells; the delta lysin lyses human, sheep, rabbit, horse, mouse, rat, and guinea pig red blood cells. More than 90 percent of the staphylococcal strains that are pathogenic for humans produce a combination of the alpha and delta lysins. Alpha and delta staphylolysins also serve as the dermonecrotic toxin and

the lethal factor of *S. aureus*. The toxins cause necrosis when injected into the skin, and death when injected intravenously into laboratory animals.

Panton-Valentine Leukocidin

Many *S. aureus* strains produce a leukocidin different in action and composition from the leukotoxic staphylolysins. Leukocidin increases the permeability of leukocytes to cations and so leads to the swelling and rounding up of the cells. The membranes of cytoplasmic granules fuse with the cytoplasmic membrane of the cell, causing release of the cytoplasmic granules and cell disruption.

Staphylococcal Enterotoxins

There are six (A, B, C1, C2, D, and E) chemically and immunologically related staphylococcal enterotoxins. Under suitable conditions of incubation, approximately one-third of *S. aureus* strains shed staphylococcal enterotoxins into food. The toxin can withstand 30 minutes of boiling (it is *thermostable*) and is not inactivated by the digestive enzymes.

Toxic Shock Syndrome Toxin-1

This toxin is thought to stimulate the production of interleukin-1 (IL-1) by macrophages. IL-1 has numerous biologic effects, among which are fever induction and the release of acute-phase proteins from the liver. About 90 percent of healthy individuals have protective antibodies against TSST-1.

Exfoliatin or Exfoliative Toxin

There are two exfoliatins, A and B. One is heat labile and its production is coded for by a plasmid; the other is heat stable and is chromosomally mediated. These exfoliatins are responsible for *scalded skin syndrome*.

Protein A

Protein A is a surface component of most *S. aureus* strains. It is linked to the peptidoglycan layer of the cell wall, but some of it is released extracellularly. Protein A has the unusual property that the Fc portion of IgG nonspecifically binds to it.* Note that we usually find a protein such as protein A serving as an antigen, and if so it is the other end of the Ig molecule, the Fab portion, that we normally expect to bind to the protein, not the Fc portion as here. (Protein A can serve as an antigen, however, and as such does interact with the Fab portion of specific antibody.) Protein A, because of this property of binding immunoglobulin, is believed to be antiphagocytic by competing with neutrophils for the Fc portion of specific opsonins. Protein A has other biologic effects: it elicits hypersensitivity and inflammation, it injures platelets, and it prevents the absorption of bacterial viruses (bacteriophages) that are specific for *S. aureus* (these viruses are called staphylophages).

Other Substances

Staphylococci produce other substances that may contribute to their virulence and antigen composition: hyaluronidase, staphylokinase, lipase, proteinase, thermostable nucleases (DNase and RNase), and a capsule or a microcapsule in some strains.

LABORATORY IDENTIFICATION

The routine clinical laboratory identification of staphylococci poses one of the less difficult bac-

* *Coagglutination test:* A cleverly designed serological test, the coagglutination test is based on the unusual property of protein A to bind nonspecifically to the Fc portion of IgG. Antibodies that are specific for other bacteria such as streptococci, salmonellae, neisseriae, and Hemophilus are allowed to couple via the Fc portion of the antibody molecule to protein A that is bound to killed staphylococci. This leaves the antigen-specific end of the molecule, the Fab end, free to attach to the bacteria for which the Fab is specific. When bacteria for which the Fab is specific are added, a lattice is formed that is visible as a coagglutinate (clumps of the staphylococci and the test bacteria).

terial identification problems. It may be necessary first to differentiate among the gram-positive cocci, namely staphylococci, streptococci, and micrococci. Differentiation from the streptococci is done by means of the catalase test, colony characteristics, type of blood agar plate hemolysis, and microscopical characteristics. Differentiation from micrococci is described at the end of this chapter under The Micrococci.

Once it is established that the isolate is a *Staphylococcus*, some clinical laboratories go no further than to differentiate *S. aureus* and *S. epidermidis*. However, there are more and more instances in which coagulase-negative staphylococci are the agents of nosocomial infections and should therefore be identified to the species level. The other important clinical laboratory procedure is the testing of the isolate for antimicrobial susceptibility.

When contamination by other organisms is likely to be minimal (for example, in a specimen from a boil), blood agar containing sheep red blood cells is the recommended medium. A selective medium is employed when contamination by other organisms is expected to be heavy, as in a fecal specimen from a patient with a suspected staphylococcal enteritis. Staphylococci tolerate high concentrations of salt (7.5 to 10 percent) and they are relatively resistant to polymyxin, phenylethyl alcohol, and tellurite, and so selective media that contain these substances are employed in the isolation of staphylococci.

One of the better-known selective media used for staphylococcal isolation and identification is mannitol salt agar (MSA). It contains a high concentration of NaCl, 7.5 percent (about 0.5 percent is the usual concentration in other culture media), which is extremely inhibitory to most other bacteria. In addition to being a selective medium, MSA is a differential medium. The carbohydrate mannitol and a pH indicator, phenol red, serve as its differential components. The medium surrounding a mannitol-positive colony turns from the typical red color of the indicator to a yellow color when acid is produced from the fermentation of mannitol. Mannitol fermentation under anaerobic conditions helps in differentiating *S. aureus* from *S. epidermidis*.

Differentiation Between *S. Aureus* and *S. Epidermidis*

Coagulase positiveness is considered by most laboratories as the definitive identifying characteristic of *S. aureus*, which differentiates it from all other staphylococci associated with humans. *S. epidermidis*, in contrast to *S. aureus*, is coagulase, DNAse, thermostable nuclease, and mannitol negative, and it is usually nonhemolytic.

Coagulase Test

Two types of coagulase tests are used, the tube test and the slide test. The slide test is performed by making a heavy suspension of bacteria in distilled water, adding a drop of plasma, and observing for clumping within 10 seconds. False-negatives occur about 17 percent of the time and must be confirmed by the tube test. The tube test is the more definitive test. The test bacteria are suspended in citrated or oxalated plasma (rabbit plasma is the preferred animal plasma) and the inoculated plasma is incubated. Clotting usually occurs within a range of a few minutes to several hours, but the test is observed for 24 hours before it is declared negative. An alternative to the coagulase test is a commercially available rapid test in which immunoglobulin bound to latex beads reacts with protein A of the *S. aureus* cell wall.

Serological tests are of limited usefulness and are not part of routine laboratory diagnosis of *S. aureus*. The detection of antibodies to cell wall teichoic acids of *S. aureus* correlates with the presence of staphylococcal infective endocarditis or deep tissue infection.

EPIDEMIOLOGY

Staphylococci are found on the skin and mucous membranes of humans and so are readily deposited on items that can serve as fomites (e.g., towels, sinks, drawer pulls). There is a comparatively high carrier rate of *S. aureus*—about 30 percent in the general population, and considerably higher in certain segments of the population, notably among hospital personnel. The principal carriage site from which staphylococci are disseminated is the anterior nares. The perineum and intertriginous areas are other common carriage sites. With so high a carrier rate, the source of infection may well be an individual's own microflora.

Particularly susceptible to serious staphylococcal infections are the newborn and those in a debilitated condition: the aged, the chronically ill, persons with metabolic disorders (classically, diabetics), and persons with traumatic or surgical wounds. Aside from urinary tract infections caused by gram-negative bacteria, *S. aureus* is the most frequently isolated pathogenic bacterium in the hospital laboratories of the United States and Europe.

Phage typing (Chapter 10) at one time was very important for tracing and controlling hospital-acquired (nosocomial) staphylococcal infections. It is used much less now because it is cumbersome and somewhat difficult technically, and because methicillin-resistant strains that now are prevalent in nosocomial infections cannot be typed by staphylophages.

TREATMENT AND PREVENTION

Superficial infections in an otherwise healthy person require no chemotherapy; treatment consists of drainage, application of moist heat, and immobilization. Deep-seated infections require intensive prolonged chemotherapy, often with a multidrug regimen.

S. aureus is very adaptable in its consistent ability to develop resistance to many antimicrobials. The corollary to that is that any isolated *S. aureus* (and coagulase-negative staphylococci) should be promptly assayed for susceptibility or resistance to antimicrobials. The majority of *S.*

aureus strains were sensitive to penicillin when penicillin was first introduced in 1940. Now, however, many of the strains, through the plasmid-mediated production of penicillinase (a beta-lactamase), have become resistant to penicillin. The introduction of methicillin in 1959 and 1960 as the first penicillinase-resistant penicillin appeared to solve the penicillin resistance problem. Methicillin-resistant strains, however, became apparent almost immediately. Numerous outbreaks of nosocomial infections caused by methicillin-resistant *S. aureus* have been reported since the 1960s. Methicillin-resistant strains are also reported outside hospital settings, notably among intravenous drug users. Many penicillin-resistant isolates furthermore exhibit multiple drug resistance to such drugs as cephalosporins, aminoglycosides, macrolides (erythromycin, oleandomycin), and lincosamides (lincomycin, clindamycin).

When antibiotic susceptibility information is not available, a beta-lactamase-resistant synthetic penicillin (nafcillin, methicillin,* or oxacillin) is usually chosen. Patients allergic to penicillin are given cephalosporins, clindamycin, or vancomycin. Once the antibiotic susceptibility of the isolated organism is known, selection of antibiotics is based on those results.

The control of staphylococcal infections includes measures to interrupt transmission and to suppress the carrier state by the administration of topical antibiotics. The antigens responsible for inducing immunity to *S. aureus* have not been identified, so routine immunization is not available.

---

* Most strains of methicillin-resistant staphylococci contain both relatively susceptible cells and highly resistant cells. The pattern of resistance exhibited by a strain may be affected by the growth conditions. Subculturing of the strain in beta-lactam antibiotics, the addition of NaCl or sucrose to the culture medium, or incubation at 30°C enhances the expression of resistance. Growth at pH 5.2 or lower or incubation at 43°C suppresses resistance. Antibiotic passage eliminates the methicillin-susceptible cells and selects out the highly resistant subpopulation. Vancomycin is the first-choice drug for treatment of methicillin-resistant *S. aureus* and *S. epidermidis* infections. Rifampin or gentamicin or both should be added if it appears that vancomycin treatment is failing.

In hospitals persons with lesions should not be allowed to come in contact with susceptible patients. Carriers among hospital personnel should be identified when hospital outbreaks occur. Since nursery and surgery patients are especially vulnerable to staphylococcal infections, personnel in these sections must be particularly diligent about aseptic practices.

It has not been possible or practical to eliminate permanently the principal reservoir of staphylococci, the nasal carrier. Topical applications of neomycin, bacitracin, and gentamicin ointments have been attempted for protracted periods of time, especially for those who repeatedly experience staphylococcal infections, to reduce the numbers of cultivable organisms.

COAGULASE-NEGATIVE STAPHYLOCOCCI

There is an increasing interest in coagulase-negative staphylococci (CONS) because of the number of reports that document them as causal agents in bacteremia and infections of prosthetic devices, indwelling catheters, vascular grafts, and wounds. Infections by CONS seldom occur in patients free of predisposing factors such as immunosuppression, surgery, and indwelling devices. The CONS bind to the surface of indwelling devices and some produce a slime layer (biofilm) that acts as a barrier to antibiotic penetration. Slime also stimulates neutrophil degranulation, thus reducing uptake and killing of bacteria.

It has become important to identify the individual species of CONS involved in an infection because of the clinical, economic, and therapeutic implications. Conventional laboratory tests and observations used to differentiate among the CONS include novobiocin resistance, colonial pigmentation, hemolysis, nitrate reduction, alkaline phosphatase and urease production, arginine utilization, and fermentation of selected carbohydrates. Identification of CONS species should no longer be a major problem because of the availability of commercially available, rapid, and miniaturized CONS identification systems. Six such systems are currently available. Because the antimicrobial susceptibility of CONS is extremely variable, susceptibility testing is required.

Staphylococcus epidermidis

S. epidermidis is the organism most frequently associated with CONS endocarditis, colonization of prostheses, bacteremia, wound infections, and urinary tract infections in elderly hospitalized men.

Staphylococcus saprophyticus

S. saprophyticus has a predilection for the urinary tract, especially in young women. *S. saprophyticus* is novobiocin-resistant—a major and reliable characteristic in differentiating *S. saprophyticus* from *S. epidermidis*.

THE MICROCOCCI

Members of the genus *Micrococcus* bear certain resemblances to staphylococci: micrococci are gram-positive cocci, the colonies are similar to staphylococcal colonies, and micrococci may be transients on the skin and mucous membranes. Micrococci are widely distributed in soil and fresh water and are commonly recovered from environmental samples. Species include *M. luteus*, *M. roseus*, and *M. varians*. In rare instances they cause endocarditis. They may appear in specimens as contaminants and must therefore be differentiated from other gram-positive cocci. Micrococci are distinguished from staphylococci by the former group's lack of susceptibility to lysis by lysostaphin, by their failure to ferment glucose anaerobically, and by their failure to produce acid from glycerol when they are grown in the presence of erythromycin. Three commercially available, easily performed disc tests also differentiate micrococci and staphylococci: the

furazolidone susceptibility test (micrococci are resistant); the bacitracin susceptibility test (micrococci are susceptible); and the modified oxidase test (micrococci are modified oxidase positive).

THE STREPTOCOCCI

The streptococci are gram-positive spherical microorganisms that appear in chains or clusters (Fig. 16-5). Most species are facultative anaerobes, although species of *Peptococcus* and *Peptostreptococcus* that inhabit the intestinal tract and female genital tract are strict anaerobes. The genus *Streptococcus* is homofermentative; that is, the end product of glucose fermentation is primarily lactic acid. Streptococci do not produce cytochrome oxidase, and this characteristic, along with the Gram stain and cellular morphol-

Fig. 16-5. Scanning electron micrograph ($\times 6800$) of *Streptococcus mutans*. (Courtesy of S. Hamada.)

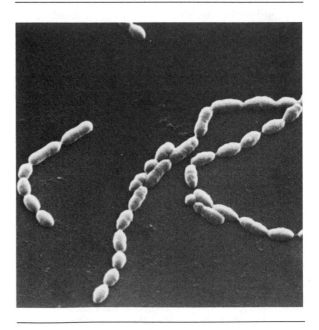

ogy, help distinguish them from *Neisseria* species.

Streptococcal disease in humans includes pharyngitis, scarlet fever, impetigo, rheumatic fever, pneumonia, meningitis, and other pathological conditions. Streptococci also cause mastitis in cows and can therefore be found in milk used for human consumption. This again indicates the importance of pasteurization to prevent human disease.

CLASSIFICATION

Hemolytic activity (see page 384) has been used as a preliminary criterion for differentiating various species of *Streptococcus*. Most of the alpha-hemolytic species are members of a group referred to as the viridans group. The beta-hemolytic streptococci are the most important group because they contain the major human pathogens. Some beta-hemolytic streptococci are, however, not pathogenic. The gamma-hemolytic or nonhemolytic streptococci are a heterogeneous group and are not considered primary pathogens. Many are found as commensals in humans and animals. Although hemolytic activity is a good presumptive criterion for differentiation, it is not suitable for determining pathogenicity, and immunological differences must be used. Rebecca Lancefield and her co-workers developed a technique for differentiation of the streptococci. They placed them into serological groups A through O on the basis of the antigenic characteristics of a cell wall carbohydrate called the *C substance*. The main pathogenic groups for humans are A, B, C, D, and G, and each group is given a species name. Some groups have but a single species. More than 90 percent of streptococcal disease in humans is caused by group A beta-hemolytic streptococci. This group has been given the species name *Streptococcus pyogenes*. Group B streptococci are named *S. agalactiae*; groups C and D are composed of several species to be discussed later. Each group can be further separated into serological types according to the

antigenic characteristic of certain cell wall proteins: the M, R, and T proteins.

GROUP A STREPTOCOCCI (STREPTOCOCCUS PYOGENES)

Streptococcal Antigens and/or Virulence Factors

The antigenic components of the streptococcal cell wall are shown in Figure 16-6. Their importance in pathogenesis and classification will now be described.

Hyaluronic Acid Capsule. Hyaluronic acid is a capsular material produced primarily by streptococcal species in groups A and C. Hyaluronic acid is not immunogenic, which appears to be related to the fact that it is also a prominent component of mammalian connective tissue. The hyaluronic acid capsule is an antiphagocytic substance that disappears during the later stages of the streptococcal growth cycle.

Cell Wall Proteins (M, R, and T). The *M protein* of the streptococcal cell wall is the major virulence factor of group A beta-hemolytic streptococci (Fig. 16-7). It enables the bacterial cell to inhibit phagocytosis. Cells from which the M protein has been removed lose their antiphagocytic ability. On the basis of differences in their M pro-

Fig. 16-6. Relative position of the molecular components lying outside the streptococcal cytoplasmic membrane. Not all capsules are antigenic.

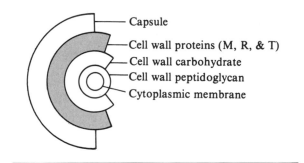

- Capsule
- Cell wall proteins (M, R, & T)
- Cell wall carbohydrate
- Cell wall peptidoglycan
- Cytoplasmic membrane

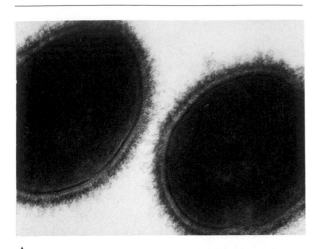

A

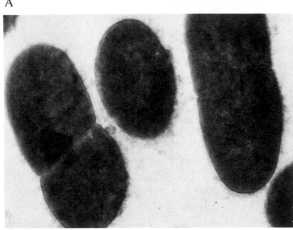

B

Fig. 16-7. Electron micrograph (× 84,000 before 33% reduction) of cross-sections of *Streptococcus pyogenes* with M protein (A) and without M protein (B). M protein appears as pilus-like appendages on the bacterial surface. (From E. H. Beachey and G. H. Stollerman. In D. C. Dumonde [ed.]. *Infection and Immunology in the Rheumatic Diseases*. Oxford, England: Blackwell, 1976.)

tein the members of group A streptococci have been separated into more than 70 different types. Theoretically, one could expect 70 different *S. pyogenes* infections in one's lifetime before becoming completely immune to *S. pyogenes*. An-

tibodies produced in a patient to a type-specific M protein have been shown to confer long-lasting immunity against infection from the same streptococcal strain.

The T protein provides a system of serotyping strains that cannot be typed by means of their M protein. T protein is often used for identification of streptococcal strains isolated from patients with impetigo.

The R protein has no clinical or pathogenic importance.

Cell Wall Carbohydrate. The cell wall carbohydrate, or C substance of group A streptococci, is related chemically to the carbohydrate found in the heart valves of humans. Patients with rheumatic fever, a complication following streptococcal infection, have high levels of serum antibodies to the group A carbohydrate. These serum antibodies may contribute to the heart valve damage associated with rheumatic fever.

Cell Wall Peptidoglycan. Peptidoglycan has been shown to be antigenic and is capable of producing fever, dermal necrosis, carditis, and lysis of red blood cells in rabbits and other animals. Its toxicity is similar to that of the endotoxins of gram-negative bacteria.

Cytoplasmic Membrane. Antigenic components in the cell membrane cross-react with heart, kidney, and connective tissue. It has been suggested that these streptococcal components can interact with host tissue and cause severe damage. As with many other streptococcal antigens, no direct relationship has ever been established between the membrane antigen and the disease condition.

Extracellular Streptococcal Products

The streptococci elaborate extracellular products in vivo and in vitro. Many of these products are believed to be important in the pathogenesis of streptococcal infections. They are used in diagnosing such infections.

Erythrogenic Toxin. In some upper respiratory infections the infecting streptococcal strain produces an extracellular toxin called *erythrogenic toxin.* Erythrogenic strains are phage infected and the toxin determinant is carried in the phage genome. The toxin is responsible for the rash associated with scarlet fever. Injection of antiserum (antitoxin) intradermally causes the rash to disappear. This technique is the basis of the Schultz-Charlton reaction, which is used in the diagnosis of scarlet fever.

Erythrogenic toxin has been shown to be composed of three potent exotoxins, A, B, and C, of which type A is the most potent. Exotoxin A-producing strains are believed by some to be responsible for septic shock, a condition of scarlet fever that was common in the early part of this century. There has been a reemergence of exotoxin A-producing strains and with it increasing episodes of septic shock. (Muppet creator Jim Henson, for example, died suddenly in 1990 from infection by a particularly virulent strain of group A streptococcus.)

Cardiohepatic Toxin and Nephrotoxin. A low molecular weight compound excreted by virulent strains of streptococci is capable of producing lesions in the heart and liver tissue when injected into susceptible laboratory animals. The exact nature or function of this cardiohepatic exotoxin in human infection is not clear. It is believed that by damaging tissue the toxin prepares the way for streptococcal colonization.

Hemolysins. The hemolytic activity of many streptococcal strains is due to the production of two distinct extracellular hemolysins, called *streptolysin O (SLO)* and *streptolysin S (SLS).* SLO is oxygen labile, and its activity is dependent on reducing conditions. It is immunogenic, and detection of anti-streptolysin O antibodies is extensively used in the diagnosis of streptococcal infections. When SLO is injected into susceptible laboratory animals, it can lyse red blood cells and leukocytes and is especially toxic to cardiac tissue. SLO has been implicated as a factor in the pathogenesis of rheumatic fever.

SLS is oxygen stable and is responsible for the zone of beta hemolysis seen around surface colonies of streptococci on blood agar plates. Like SLO, SLS is capable of lysing mammalian red blood cells and leukocytes. Unlike SLO, SLS is nonimmunogenic. The role of SLS in pathogenesis is not known.

Spreading Factors. In primary streptococcal infections the infecting strain is often capable of spreading to surrounding tissue. This capability is probably due to the formation of extracellular products that can dissolve the matrix of connective tissue and clotted material accumulated as a result of host inflammatory responses. The spreading factors include the following:

1. Hyaluronidase. Hyaluronic acid, the substrate for the enzyme hyaluronidase, is a component of intercellular substance. Depolymerization could therefore enhance the spread of streptococci in the tissue.
2. Proteinase. A proteolytic enzyme released by many group A streptococci can digest some peptides and proteins. The purified proteinase when injected into susceptible animals has been shown to cause extensive lesions in the connective tissue of the heart.
3. Streptokinase. Streptokinase is produced by most group A streptococci. It can interact with the proenzyme plasminogen of human serum, converting it to plasmin. Plasmin can digest fibrin and other serum factors important in the formation of blood clots.
4. Nucleases. At the site of infection the host's inflammatory response results in the accumulation of nuclear exudate from dead or injured white blood cells. Virulent streptococci can produce nucleases such as ribonuclease and deoxyribonuclease that will digest the DNA or RNA of the exudate, thus facilitating the spread of trapped streptococci. The released purine and pyrimidine bases can also be used nutritionally by the streptococci.

Pathogenesis and Epidemiology

As stated previously, more than 90 percent of streptococcal diseases are caused by the group A streptococcus, *Streptococcus pyogenes*. Transmission from person to person is usually by contact with an asymptomatic carrier who harbors the organism in the upper respiratory tract, skin, or rectum. Occasionally food contaminated by a carrier may be a source of infection.

Streptococcal disease is divided into two categories: the suppurative, or primary, infections, and the nonsuppurative, or those regarded as complications following primary streptococcal infections.

Suppurative Diseases. Suppurative diseases are those in which pus is formed. One group of suppurative streptococcal diseases often begins as acute pharyngitis, which can be complicated by meningitis, otitis media, and pneumonia. The other group includes puerperal fever, as well as such skin infections as impetigo, cellulitis, and erysipelas. In about 25 percent of the patients a carrier state will develop despite appropriate therapy.

Impetigo is a highly contagious skin disease found primarily in children. The infection begins as small blisters that can spread to adjacent areas. The sores become covered with crusts. If the infecting strain is nephritogenic, a streptococcal complication called acute glomerulonephritis (AGN) can result (see later).

Cellulitis is an inflammatory condition associated with streptococcal invasion of connective tissue. This type of disease can occasionally result in gangrene with subsequent invasion of the bloodstream. *Puerperal fever* is a uterine infection that frequently accompanies childbirth when aseptic techniques are not followed. *Erysipelas* is an infection of the skin or mucous membrane and is characterized by a spreading inflammation (Plate 7). It is frequently seen on the face.

In suppurative infections the virulence of the streptococcus is directly related to the presence of M protein, the antiphagocytic factor. In the majority of primary streptococcal infections the microorganisms are destroyed by the host's immune system. In some instances, however, because of either the particular streptococcal strain involved or the host's immunological state, nonsuppurative complications develop.

Nonsuppurative Diseases. The principal nonsuppurative complications that follow primary streptococcal infections are *scarlet fever, rheumatic fever, acute glomerulonephritis*, and *erythema nodosum*. Their exact cause is still in doubt. One theory holds that a toxin or toxic factor directly affects the tissue; another maintains that it is the host's response to the microbe or its products that damages the tissue.

Scarlet fever is associated with the formation of erythrogenic toxin by group A streptococci and has already been discussed.

Rheumatic fever is a condition that follows about five weeks after pharyngeal infection by any number of group A streptococcal types. It is characterized by heart muscle damage and is often accompanied by tissue destruction of heart valves as well as inflammation of the joints. The highest incidence of rheumatic fever is among those aged 5 to 19 years, especially among the urban poor of all races and ethnic groups. Rheumatic fever is rarely seen in the United States, but recent outbreaks of the disease have been observed in some military facilities, and in some large cities.

Many authorities consider rheumatic fever an autoimmune disease. This theory is related to the finding that many antigenic components of the streptococcal cell wall can cross-react with cardiac tissue. For example, there is a cross reactivity between the group A polysaccharide of the cell wall and heart valve glycoprotein. In rheumatic fever, if there is heart valve damage, group A polysaccharide antibodies are at a high level. If the damaged valves are manipulated during surgery, the level of antibodies increases. If the damaged valves are removed, the antibody level decreases. In addition, antigens are present in the cytoplasmic membrane of the group A streptococcus that are related to antigens in the heart muscle. There is a sustained rise in the titer of antibodies to streptococcal membrane that cross-react with cardiac tissue preceding an attack of rheumatic fever. This suggests, but does not prove, that antibodies may play a role in the pathogenesis of rheumatic fever.

None of the antibodies described above has been found to be toxic to heart tissue and thus the pathogenesis of rheumatic fever may be caused by factors other than or in addition to immunologic factors. Studies in animals indicate that streptococcal extracellular toxins or cellular components may be directly toxic to heart tissue. Streptolysin S or O, for example, has been shown to be toxic to cellular membranes. Streptococcal cell wall components have been shown to persist in tissues such as skin, heart, and liver for long periods of time. The length of time in the tissue correlates with the duration of the disease. These cell wall components are presumably present in the lesion because of the poor hydrolytic activity of phagocytic enzymes on the streptococcal cell wall. When streptococcal fragments containing the C substance are injected into mice, they bring about heart lesions similar to those seen in rheumatic fever. Injections of whole cells, however, have no effect unless the heart tissue has already been damaged.

Acute glomerulonephritis (AGN) is a nonsuppurative complication that follows throat or skin infections by a relatively few serological types of group A streptococci. Clinical symptoms, which appear 1 to 4 weeks after the primary infection, include proteinuria, hematuria, and oliguria, but no bacteria can be recovered. The pathogenesis of AGN is believed to be due to an immune complex reaction. Antigens from the cytoplasmic membrane of the bacterial cell are believed to cross-react with the basement membrane of the glomerulus of the kidney, precipitating the immune complex reaction. Antibiotics are of no use in the treatment of AGN; only bed rest and administration of salicylates are of therapeutic value.

Erythema nodosum is a skin condition in which small red nodules appear under the surface of the skin. It exists in a variety of other diseases such as tuberculosis and coccidioidomycosis. Many authorities believe that erythema nodosum is the result of hypersensitivity to the peptidoglycan portion of the streptococcal cell wall.

Bacteremia by group A beta-hemolytic streptococci can affect all age groups but occurs primarily in the elderly, especially those with an underlying disease. In addition, trauma, surgery, or other disruptions to the skin may predispose an individual to bacteremia. Despite appropriate therapy, disease can progress to shock, disseminated intravascular coagulation, and death. Mortality rates may vary from 5 to 47 percent.

A *streptococcal toxic shock–like syndrome* has also been reported recently. The condition, which produces fever, shock, renal failure, severe tissue injury, and respiratory distress is associated with an exotoxin-producing strain (see page 405).

Laboratory Diagnosis

The clinical symptoms of many streptococcal infections are shared by other bacterial and viral diseases. The clinical symptoms of acute pharyngitis, for example, are similar to those of numerous respiratory virus infections. In a certain percentage of patients with streptococcal disease the "typical" symptoms or host immunological responses do not appear. Accurate diagnosis of most streptococcal infections requires, therefore, both clinical and bacteriological support. The most accurate identification of groups A, B, and G beta-hemolytic streptococci is made by serological procedures while physiological tests are used in identification of other groups such as group D streptococci. Presumptive identification in the clinical laboratory can be made by using a series of tests outlined in Table 16-1. Presumptive diagnosis of group A streptococcal infection can be made on throat cultures if the throat swab contains sufficient numbers of microorganisms. The swab can be treated with nitrous acid to produce an extract containing streptococcal antigens. An aliquot of the extracted antigen is added to a

Table 16-1. Tests Used in the Presumptive Identification of Streptococci

Test	Group A	Group B	Group D	Viridans	Pneumococcus
Susceptibility to bacitracin	+	−	−	+[a]	+
Susceptibility to sulfamethoxazole and trimethoprim	−	−	−[b]	+	?
Hippurate hydrolysis	−	+	−[a]	−[a]	−
PYR hydrolysis	+	−	+	−	−
Growth in 6.5% NaCl	−	+[a]	+[c]	−	−
Optochin susceptibility and bile solubility	−	−	−	−	+
CAMP reaction[d]	−	+	−	−	−

+ = positive or susceptible reaction; − = negative or resistant reaction; PYR = L-pyrrolidonyl-β-naphthylamide.
[a] Occasional exceptions.
[b] Some group D non-enterococci are susceptible.
[c] Group D non-enterococci will not grow in 6.5% NaCl.
[d] A discussion of CAMP test is presented under Group B.

coagglutination group A antibody reagent (for example, the Phadebact system). A positive test is represented by an agglutination reaction. The test can yield results in 30 minutes after taking the swab. Several commercial kits are now available for testing swab as well as blood cultures. The kits contain material for extracting streptococcal antigen by enzymatic or nonenzymatic means. The antigen detection system may be a group of agglutination reagents or an enzyme-linked immunoabsorbent assay.

Two antibody determinations that are useful in evaluating patients with recent streptococcal disease are the anti-streptolysin O (ASO) test and the anti-DNase B(ADN-B) test. The ADN-B test is believed to be the superior test because it is more reliable in confirming streptococcal infection when rheumatic fever or acute glomerulonephritis is suspected. For example, the ASO titer in about 15 to 20 percent of rheumatic fever patients is not significantly elevated.

Treatment and Prevention

To date, all strains of group A beta-hemolytic streptococci have been shown to be susceptible to penicillin. Penicillin is therefore the drug of choice in infections caused by this group. Penicillin G benzathine is usually prescribed because

of its prolonged action. Follow-up cultures should be taken after discontinuation of therapy to determine whether all streptococci have been eliminated. The prevention of streptococcal infections also prevents rheumatic fever. Penicillin treatment does not alter the course of rheumatic fever. To minimize the risk of streptococcal infections in rheumatic fever patients, an injection of penicillin G benzathine is usually prescribed each month. This regimen is considered necessary for at least 5 years after the rheumatic attack. For individuals sensitive to penicillin, erythromycin is a suitable alternative. Vaccines prepared from streptococcal type–specific M protein have been used successfully as immunizing agents against group A infections. Because of the many different streptococcal types, a vaccine utilizing all the type–specific M proteins has proved impractical.

GROUP B STREPTOCOCCI

S. agalactiae is the species designation for members of group B streptococci (GBS). Group B streptococci are commensals found in the oral cavity, intestinal tract, and vagina. For the past two decades GBS streptococci have been important pathogens in neonates, young infants, and postpartum women. In the United States GBS are the most frequent cause of life-threatening disease in newborns. The incidence of GBS infection in the United States is 1.1 to 3.7 per 1000 live births. Factors conducive to GBS infection are premature labor, prolonged rupture of placental membranes, and birth weight less than 3 pounds.

There are two forms of GBS disease in neonates; *early onset* and *late onset*. Early onset disease results from the vertical transmission of GBS from mother to infant in utero or during passage through the birth canal. Early onset disease occurs within a few days of delivery and has a high mortality rate as the result of sepsis or pneumonia. GBS in late onset disease may be acquired from mothers, hospital personnel, or contacts outside the hospital. Most late onset disease in infants is believed to occur by contact with the contaminated hands of hospital personnel. Meningitis is the most frequent complication of late onset disease.

Group B infection in adults is seen in those compromised by chemotherapy, diabetes, or pregnancy. Adult diseases include endocarditis, meningitis, pneumonia, and postpartum infection.

Group B streptococci can be divided into five distinct serotypes. One of these, type III, is the most common cause of neonatal infection. Experimental studies with type III have demonstrated that a capsular polysaccharide component, sialic acid, appears to be an important virulence determinant. Sialic acid has been shown to inhibit the alternative complement pathway; thus resistance to disease requires specific antibodies.

Group B streptococcal infections can be treated with penicillin; however, GBS are not so susceptible to penicillin as are group A streptococci. Ampicillin or ampicillin plus gentamicin has been shown to be effective in treatment. Prevention of disease has been approached in two ways. Intravenous intrapartum therapy with ampicillin has been shown to prevent neonatal colonization with GBS. A second technique is to treat the neonate with penicillin less than 2 hours after birth. Prophylaxis is recommended when the factors conducive to group B streptococcal infection (listed earlier) are encountered.

Group B strains are easily distinguished from other streptococci by their ability to hydrolyze hippurate and their resistance to the antibiotic bacitracin. The CAMP test is also used as a presumptive test for GBS identification. The CAMP test, named from the initials of the investigators who perfected it, is based on the production of a "CAMP factor"—a protein elaborated by group B streptococci. The test is performed by making a single streak of a streptococcal strain perpendicular to but not touching a disk containing betalysin on a sheep blood agar plate. If the streptococcal strain produces the CAMP factor, a crescent-shaped clearing appears at the juncture of the betalysin-containing disk and the streptococci. The CAMP factor thus enlarges the zone of lysis produced by betalysin.

Tests such as latex particle agglutination are now being evaluated for testing the presence of GBS in human amniotic fluid. If these tests are found to be successful and are approved, they will allow early identification and treatment of infants at risk of serious GBS disease.

A chemiluminescent DNA probe assay has recently been developed for identification of group B streptococci. The probe is a DNA oligomer having a sequence complementary to a segment of *S. agalactiae* ribosomal RNA. The probe is labeled with an acridinium ester. Results can be obtained in 40 minutes.

GROUP C STREPTOCOCCI

Group C streptococci are a frequent cause of infection in many animal species but are a rare cause of infection in humans. This group of streptococci is composed of four species: *S. equi*, *S. dysgalactiae*, *S. equisimilis*, and *S. zooepidemicus*. Only the latter two species are more commonly associated with human infection. *S. equisimilis* is primarily associated with human illness in the United States. Human illnesses include endocarditis, pneumonia, meningitis, epiglottitis, and wound infections. Outbreaks of disease have been associated with unpasteurized milk or cheese made from unpasteurized milk. *S. zooepidemicus*, a group C streptococcus, has been associated with outbreaks of pharyngitis and nephritis in Europe and recently with illness in the United States.

VIRIDANS STREPTOCOCCI

The viridans streptococci are for the most part alpha-hemolytic but some are also nonhemolytic. Viridans streptococci do not react with Lancefield grouping sera. In addition, they are commensals and a major component of the oral flora of humans.

Newer methods, which have elucidated the natural genetic relationship of bacteria, have also created some confusion, particularly in naming the viridans streptococci. There are six species, which in the past have been given a variety of other names. These six species are *S. angiosus*, *S. bovis* variants, *S. mitis*, *S. mutans*, *S. salivarius*, and *S. sanguis*. In 1988 a seventh species was isolated from the oral cavity and was named *S. vestibularis*. These species are not primary pathogens but act as opportunistic challengers to the host. *S. mutans*, for example, is the causative agent of tooth decay.

The major disease associated with some viridans streptococci is subacute bacterial endocarditis (SBE). SBE, a suppurative disease, is generally preceded by dental extraction or some type of oral surgery that displaces the alpha-hemolytic species from the oral cavity into the bloodstream. The disease occurs most frequently in patients with rheumatic fever or congenital heart disease. The dislodged streptococci are capable of localizing on the affected heart tissue and can bring about further heart valve damage. Left untreated, SBE can lead to heart failure, but the disease can be treated with antibiotics. The antibiotic regimen includes penicillin plus an aminoglycoside.

Treatment failures have been noted, particularly when the endocarditis is caused by *nutritionally deficient streptococci*. These variant streptococci, which were first described in 1961, have a requirement for pyridoxal. The taxonomy of the nutritionally deficient streptococci is unsettled. They are, however, a cause of 5 to 6 percent of the cases due to viridans streptococci. Their poor response to antibiotics appears to be due to their slow rate of metabolism. Measures can be taken to prevent endocarditis among compromised patients. The American Heart Association has recommended the following prophylactic regimen:

1. For those with congenital heart disease or rheumatic fever, penicillin G plus penicillin G procaine is given intramuscularly 30 minutes to 1 hour before oral surgery (some physicians prefer erythromycin to penicillin because rheumatic fever patients already use penicillin to prevent recurrences of the disease). Penicillin V (phenoxymethyl penicillin) is taken orally every 6 hours for 48 hours after surgery. Vancomycin may be substituted if the patient is allergic to penicillin.
2. For those with prosthetic valves, regimen 1 may be used, or penicillin G plus penicillin G procaine plus streptomycin is administered intramuscularly 30 minutes to 1 hour before oral surgery. Penicillin V is taken orally every 6 hours for 48 hours after oral surgery.

GROUP D STREPTOCOCCI AND ENTEROCOCCUS

Group D streptococci are commensals in the intestinal tract. They had been previously divided into two groups: enterococcal and nonenterococcal. Enterococcal members, such as *S. faecalis*, *S. faecium*, and *S. durans*, have now been assigned the genus name *Enterococcus* (*E. faecalis*, *E. faecium*, etc.). Most species of *Enterococcus* possess these characteristics: ability to grow in 6.5% NaCl and pH 9.6, to grow at 10 and usually 45°C, and, for the most part, to survive at 60°C for 30 minutes. Nonenterococcal group D streptococci are *S. bovis* and *S. equinus*.

Enterococci are found in the feces of most healthy adults. The two most commonly encountered species are *E. faecalis* and *E. faecium*. From 80 to 90 percent of all clinical isolates have been *E. faecalis* with *E. faecium* representing most of the remainder of isolates. These organisms cause an estimated 5 to 15 percent of bacterial endocarditis. Enterococci are also a frequent cause of urinary tract infections, particularly in hospitalized patients. Studies by the Centers for Disease Control indicate that enterococci cause 10 to 15 percent of all hospital-associated urinary tract infections. Enterococci are also recognized as an important cause of neonatal infections such as meningitis.

The enterococci show an intrinsic resistance to many beta-lactam antibiotics and quickly develop resistance to other antimicrobials. Treatment of endocarditis can be accomplished through the use of penicillin plus streptomycin; however, high doses of ampicillin have also been shown to be effective. Susceptibility testing should be routinely performed on clinical specimens.

GROUP F STREPTOCOCCI AND OTHER STREPTOCOCCI

Group F streptococci are commensals in the oropharyngeal and bowel area of humans. They are not frequent causes of human infection. Group F streptococci have a tendency to cause cutaneous abscesses following trauma. Abscesses can also occur in the cervicofacial and intraabdominal areas. Group F streptococci are susceptible to penicillin.

Group G streptococci are known to be associated with clinically symptomatic pharyngitis. Approximately 20 to 25 percent of humans carry group G streptococci in the pharynx. Epidemic pharyngitis caused by this group of organisms is usually associated with food contamination but

contaminated respiratory secretions may also be a source of infection.

Human infections by other groups of streptococci (E, L, M, etc.) are rare but they are important in veterinary medicine.

ANAEROBIC STREPTOCOCCI

The anaerobic streptococci are classifed in the genera *Peptococcus* and *Peptostreptococcus*. Most are nonhemolytic. Anaerobic streptococci are found in the oral cavity, intestinal tract, and vagina. They have been incriminated in such infections as puerperal sepsis, subacute bacterial endocarditis, and deep wound abscesses. Many strains are resistant to penicillin but sensitive to bacitracin and chloramphenicol. Teichoplanin, a new glycoprotein antibiotic, is active against anaerobic streptococci.

STREPTOCOCCUS PNEUMONIAE (PNEUMOCOCCI)

General Characteristics

The pneumococci are inhabitants of the upper respiratory tract and, depending on seasonal variations, can be found in 30 to 70 percent of the population. They are gram-positive cocci that occur singly, in pairs (diplococci) (Plate 8), or in chains. The typical paired or short-chain forms appearing primarily in clinical specimens are often lancet shaped and surrounded by a capsule (Fig. 16-8). Only encapsulated (smooth form) strains are virulent. On repeated subculture in the laboratory the capsule is lost (rough form). There are approximately 83 pneumococcal serotypes, differing in the composition of their capsular polysaccharide.

The pneumococci are facultative anaerobes that are very fastidious in their cultural requirements. Some strains need an elevated level of CO_2 for initial isolation. Meat extracts supplemented with defibrinated blood are one of the best cultural media for isolation of pneumococci.

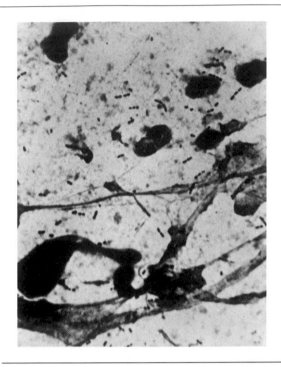

Fig. 16-8. Sputum sample taken from patient with pneumococcal pneumonia. The pneumococci appear lancet-shaped in pairs or short chains. (From A. S. Klainer and I. Geis, *Agents of Bacterial Disease.* New York: Harper & Row, 1973.)

The addition of blood to culture media supplies the enzyme catalase, which is not produced by the pneumococci. Under aerobic conditions the pneumococci produce hydrogen peroxide, which can be toxic to the pneumococci. The enzyme catalase acts to remove the accumulated hydrogen peroxide. On blood agar pneumococcal colonies exhibit alpha hemolysis and closely resemble colonies of alpha-hemolytic streptococci.

Pathogenesis

Streptococcus pneumoniae is the primary cause of community-associated pneumonia. It is also the most frequent cause of otitis media (inflammation of the middle ear) and bacteremia in in-

fants and children. In compromised patients *S. pneumoniae* is often the cause of meningitis.

The primary virulence factor of the pneumococci is the capsular polysaccharide. The capsule prevents binding of antibody to the cell wall of the pneumococcus and thus inhibits phagocytosis. Pneumococci also produce a hemolysin (pneumolysin) and neuraminidase. Their role in pathogenicity is not known.

As much as 70 percent of the population at any one time may carry pathogenic pneumococci in the upper respiratory tract. Pneumonia and related pneumococcal infections are acquired endogenously through lowered host resistance rather than exogenously by direct contact. Age, underlying illness, and viral infections of the upper respiratory tract are important predisposing factors to pneumococcal infections. In the healthy individual numerous barriers prevent establishment of infection in the lungs and bronchioles. Mucus-laden pneumococci can be expelled naturally by the combined action of ciliated epithelium and the cough reflex or through the phagocytic action of macrophages lining the alveoli of the lungs. If the physical and immunological barriers of the host are impaired—as, for example, in the debilitated person or chronic alcoholic—the pneumococci can infect the respiratory tree. The encapsulated pneumococci become trapped in the bronchioles, where they proliferate and eventually infect the alveoli. The inflammatory response of the host leads to the accumulation of an alveolar exudate consisting of large numbers of neutrophils and red blood cells. During this stage the patient's sputum also resembles the alveolar exudate and will appear bloody. During the recovery stage the pneumococci are phagocytized, the alveolar exudate is resorbed, and the lung tissue appears as healthy as before infection. When immediate recovery does not take place, the alveoli can become fibrous and inelastic because of deposition of fibroblasts, and breathing becomes difficult.

In the inflammatory stage of pneumonia, as well as with other diseases in which there is an inflammatory process, a special protein called the *C-reactive protein* is found in the blood (see Chapter 11). It precipitates a polysaccharide component of the pneumococcal cell wall called the C substance (discussed earlier in this chapter).

Laboratory Diagnosis

Presumptive identification of pneumococci can be made by Gram-staining sputum cultures. This procedure is complicated by the fact that, microscopically, pneumococci resemble alpha-hemolytic streptococci, which are often found as contaminating species in clinical specimens. A more rapid and accurate identification procedure involves applying an anticapsular serum to the sputum samples and observing capsular swelling (called the *quellung* reaction). If sputum samples cannot be obtained for examination, swabs of the laryngeal area or material aspirated from involved areas of the lung should be examined. Transtracheal aspiration is also widely used for obtaining samples for direct examination.

Latex agglutination and coagglutination tests can be used to detect pneumococcal antigen in respiratory samples. Both tests provide the most reliable diagnostic methods of the evidence of pneumococcal etiology when later confirmed by other methods. The only reliable technique for detecting antigen in urine specimens involves the use of CIE with pneumococcal omniserum as a source of antibodies.

A definitive diagnosis of pneumococcal pneumonia can be made only if the microorganisms are isolated directly from the blood or from other clinical specimens by plating onto blood agar and incubating overnight. A useful adjunct to direct isolation is identification of specific pneumococcal antibodies by counterimmunoelectrophoresis of body fluids—pleural fluid, blood, urine. Once cultured, the pneumococci can be differentiated from alpha-hemolytic streptococci by the following procedures:

1. Quellung reaction. Provided antiserum is available, the quellung reaction is the most accurate and specific test for identification of the pneumococci (Fig. 16-9). Emulsified sputum or exudative material is spread on a slide and mixed with antiserum against type–specific

Fig. 16-9. Quellung reaction. A. Control (absence of antiserum). B. Capsular swelling of bacteria after application of antiserum. A capsular halo can be observed around the diplococci. (Courtesy R. Austrian.)

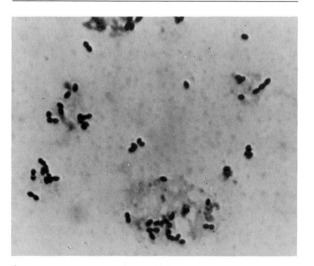

A

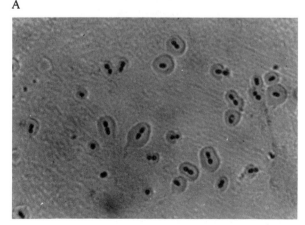

B

polysaccharide or the polyvalent antiserum, which contains antibodies to 33 of the most prevalent types in the United States or all 83 pneumococcal types.

2. Optochin susceptibility test. Optochin is an antimicrobial drug derived from quinine. When disks containing the drug are placed on blood agar previously seeded with pneumococci, zones of inhibition can be observed around the optochin. Alpha-hemolytic streptococci are resistant to optochin (see Table 16-3).

3. Bile solubility test. The pneumococci produce an enzyme (amidase) that cleaves specific covalent bonds in the peptidoglycan layer. This enzyme is activated by bile or bile salts such as sodium deoxycholate. When a few drops of 10% sodium deoxycholate solution are added to a broth culture of pneumococci, the cells are rapidly lysed. Alpha-hemolytic streptococci are not lysed by bile (see Table 16-3).

4. Mouse virulence test. Most pneumococcal strains, when injected intraperitoneally into mice, can induce death of the animals within 24 to 48 hours. Alpha-hemolytic streptococci, used under the same procedures, are not lethal to mice.

Treatment and Prevention

Penicillin is the drug of choice in the treatment of pneumococcal infections. Very few strains become resistant to penicillin. In patients harboring penicillin-resistant strains or those who are sensitive to the drug, erythromycin or tetracycline is an effective substitute. Multiantibiotic-resistant strains of *S. pneumoniae* are relatively few. One or two clusters of such isolates have been found in the United States, Africa, and Czechoslovakia. They are resistant to penicillin and other drugs such as ampicillin, erythromycin, tetracycline, chloramphenicol, and streptomycin.

Although there are 83 different pneumococcal types, only 23 are usually associated with disease. In 1983 a vaccine containing polysaccharide antigens from these 23 types was approved for use in the United States. Each polysaccharide is extracted separately and combined into a final product (polyvalent vaccine). The vaccine is used for high-risk groups: the aged, those compromised by underlying illnesses, and persons in epidemic-prone areas such as military bases. The polyvalent vaccine causes a twofold or greater increase in type–specific antibody within 2 to 3 weeks after vaccination. The vaccine is less antigenic for children under 2 years of age. The vaccine is recommended for children over 2 years of age with chronic illness specifically associated with increased risk for pneumococcal disease. The adverse reactions from vaccination are usually very mild but can be severe if the vaccine is given more than once. Arthus reactions and systemic reactions have been reported when "booster doses" of vaccine were administered.

SUMMARY

1. The staphylococci are gram-positive spherical cells arranged in grape-like clusters. They are aerobic to facultatively anaerobic. Staphylococci can be found as commensals in various areas of the body, particularly the skin and nares.

2. The staphylococci produce a wide range of infections throughout the body, with *S. aureus* the most common culprit. *S. epidermidis* is primarily an opportunistic pathogen. Table 16-2 describes the various types of infections caused by staphylococci.

3. Laboratory identification of staphylococci may first require differentiation from micrococci and streptococci. Mannitol salt agar is used as a selective medium for isolation and identification of staphylococci. The coagulase test is considered the most important test for differentiating *S. aureus* (coagulase positive) from *S. epidermidis* (coagulase negative).

4. The staphylococci are frequently resistant to a host of antimicrobials, particularly penicillin and its derivatives. This resistance is usually due

Table 16-2. Characteristics of Gram-Positive *Staphylococci*

Genus/species	Site of commensalism or source of infection	Major disease association	Treatment*
Staphylococcus aureus (coagulase positive)	Commensal on skin	Abscess, carbuncle, impetigo, sties	None usually required
		Scalded skin syndrome (SSS). Exfoliative toxin produced	None usually required
	Intestinal commensal	Enterocolitis often occurs following intensive chemotherapy for other illness	Discontinuation of chemotherapy
	Skin, particularly hands, and nasopharynx	Food poisoning due to heat-stable exotoxin released in high-protein foods	None usually required
	S. aureus skin infection seeding bloodstream	Osteomyelitis	Synthetic penicillin such as methicillin, vancomycin
	Commensal on skin; genitourinary tract	Toxic shock syndrome, associated primarily with highly absorbent tampons but various types of surgeries also important	Fluid replacement, drainage of foci of infection, antimicrobial therapy
S. epidermidis (coagulase negative)	Commensal in nares and on skin, especially axillae, head, legs, and arms	Endocarditis, colonization of prostheses, bacteremia from indwelling venous catheters	Removal of foreign body or prosthesis, drainage of infection site, antimicrobial therapy such as nafcillin, oxacillin, cephalothin
S. saprophyticus (coagulase negative)	Occasionally isolated from skin; but has predilection for urinary tract	Major cause of acute, recurrent cystitis in young women	Antimicrobial therapy. Organism is susceptible to most common antimicrobials

* Prevention of most *Staphylococcus* infections can be accomplished by frequent handwashing by health-care personnel, maintaining aseptic technique in surgery, and proper insertion and management of intravenous and arterial catheters.

to the formation of enzymes called beta-lactamases.

5. The streptococci are gram-positive, spherical cells that occur in chains of varying length. Most are facultative anaerobes but a few are obligate anaerobes. They are classified primarily by hemolytic behavior and antigenic characteristics associated with a cell wall carbohydrate called the C substance.

6. Beta-hemolytic group A streptococci (*S. py-*

ogenes) are the most important human pathogens. The major antigen associated with pathogenesis is the M protein, which inhibits phagocytosis. Other antigens associated with pathogenesis include various toxins, hemolysins, and spreading factors. The primary virulence factor for *S. pneumoniae* is the capsular polysaccharide that inhibits phagocytosis. The major

streptococcal groups and the diseases with which they are associated are outlined in Table 16-3.

7. Serological detection of group-specific antigens of beta-hemolytic streptococci provides the most accurate method of identification but presumptive identification can be made (see Table 16-1). Various kits are available for detecting group A beta-hemolytic streptococcal an-

Table 16-3. Characteristics of the Pathogenic Streptococci

Species and/or group	Site of commensalism	Major disease associations	Treatment/prevention
Group A beta-hemolytic (*S. pyogenes*)	Nasopharynx, skin, vagina, rectum	*Suppurative*: Impetigo, cellulitis, puerperal fever, erysipelas. *Nonsuppurative*: Rheumatic fever, acute glomerulonephritis, erythema nodosum, scarlet fever	Penicillin
Group B (*S. agalactiae*)	Oral cavity, intestinal tract, vagina	Neonatal disease: Early onset (pneumonia, sepsis). Late onset (meningitis). Adult disease (pneumonia, meningitis, endocarditis) in compromised patients	Penicillin
Group C (*S. equisimilis* et al.)	Not a commensal in humans but associated with infected animals	Endocarditis, meningitis, pneumonia, pharyngitis	Penicillin
Group D (*S. faecalis* et al.)*	Intestinal tract	Wound infections, bacteremia, urinary tract infections, endocarditis	Penicillin plus streptomycin
Group F	Oropharynx and bowel	Abscess formation following trauma	Penicillin
Viridans (*S. mitis* et al.)	Oral cavity	Caries (*S. mutans*) and endocarditis	Penicillin plus aminoglycoside (endocarditis)
Anaerobic streptococci	Intestinal tract and vagina	Subacute bacterial endocarditis and wound abscesses	Bacitracin, chloramphenicol
S. pneumoniae	Upper respiratory tract	Otitis media and bacteremia in children; pneumonia and meningitis in all populations	Penicillin; polyvalent vaccine for compromised adults

* Now referred to as *Enterococcus*.

tigens from throat cultures. The anti-streptolysin O (ASO) titer is the principal diagnostic test for post-streptococcal disease such as rheumatic fever. The quellung reaction is the most definitive test for *S. pneumoniae*. Cultured pneumococci can be differentiated from alpha-hemolytic streptococci by various tests such as optochin susceptibility, bile solubility, and quellung reaction.

8. Nearly all streptococci are susceptible to penicillin (see Table 16-3). A polyvalent vaccine is available for adults who have been compromised by some underlying disease or illness. The vaccine is not suitable for children under 2 years of age.

QUESTIONS FOR STUDY

Select the best response or responses for each of the following:

1. All of the following are disease manifestations of infection with *Staphylococcus aureus* EXCEPT
   A. Folliculitis
   B. Impetigo
   C. Toxic shock syndrome
   D. Scalded skin syndrome
   E. Scarlet fever

2. Staphylococcal enterocolitis:
   A. Is associated with poor nutrition and overcrowded living conditions
   B. Follows contact with infected wild rodents
   C. May follow use of broad-spectrum antibiotics
   D. May follow acute viral infection
   E. Precedes acute glomerulonephritis

3. In which group would you expect to find a very high number of *Staphylococcus aureus* carriers?
   A. Farmers
   B. Pregnant women
   C. Hospital staff
   D. Newborn infants
   E. Veterinarians

4. Which of the following are factors in the development of staphylococcal food poisoning? (1) reduction in host resistance; (2) use of broad-spectrum antibiotics; (3) a food handler who is a carrier of an enterotoxin-producing strain; (4) a protein-rich food such as meat; or (5) inadequate refrigeration.
   A. 1,2,3
   B. 1,3,4
   C. 2,3,4
   D. 2,4,5
   E. 3,4,5

5. Following dental extraction, subacute bacterial endocarditis in compromised patients would most probably be caused by
   A. *S. pneumoniae*
   B. Group D streptococci
   C. Viridans streptococci
   D. Group B streptococci

6. The streptococcus most frequently associated with severe neonatal disease is
   A. *S. pyogenes*
   B. *S. agalactiae*
   C. *S. faecalis*
   D. *S. pneumoniae*

7. Which of the following is not a presumptive test in the identification of streptococci?
   A. Susceptibility to bacitracin
   B. CAMP reaction
   C. Hippurate hydroylsis
   D. Quellung reaction

Fill in the blank:

8. The major virulence factor of *S. pneumoniae* is the _____ while the major virulence factor of *S. pyogenes* is the _____.

9. Rheumatic fever and acute glomerulonephritis are sequelae to infection by _____.

10. The antibiotic to which most streptococci are susceptible is _____.

Match the disease, activity, or characteristic on the left with the appropriate microorganism on the right. A microorganism may be used more than once.

11. Subacute bacterial endocarditis

12. Acute bacterial endocarditis

13. Produces an enterotoxin

14. Toxic shock syndrome

15. Normal microflora of the skin

16. Opportunistic infections following bowel surgery

17. Lancefield Group A

18. Antibiotic resistance is a major problem

19. Rheumatic fever

A. *Streptococcus pyogenes*
B. *Staphylococcus aureus*
C. *Streptococcus faecalis*
D. *Streptococcus sanguis*
E. *Staphylococcus epidermidis*

ADDITIONAL READINGS

Baker, C. J., and Kasper, D. L. Group B streptococcal vaccines. *Rev. Infect. Dis.* 7:458, 1985.

Bisno, A. L., and Waldvogel, F. A. *Infections Associated with Indwelling Medical Devices.* Washington: American Society for Microbiology, 1990.

Dillon, H. C., Jr., Khare, S., and Gray, B. M. Group B streptococcal carriage and disease: A 6 year perspective study. *J. Pediatr.* 110:31, 1987.

Gillum, R. F. Trends in acute rheumatic fever and chronic rheumatic heart disease: A national perspective. *Am. Heart J.* 111:430, 1986.

Gray, B. M., and Dillon, H. C., Jr. Clinical and epidemiologic studies of pneumococcal infections in children. *Pediatr. Infect. Dis.* 5:201, 1986.

Kloos, W. E. Natural populations of the genus *Staphylococcus. Ann. Rev. Microbiol.* 34:559, 1980.

Mufson, M. A. Pneumococcal infections. *J.A.M.A.* 246:1942, 1981.

Musher, D. M. The gram-positive cocci: II and III staphylococci. *Hosp. Pract.* 23:179, 1988.

Murray, B. E. The life and times of the *Enterococcus. Clin. Microbiol. Revs.* 3(1):46, 1990.

Pfaller, M. A., and Herwaldt, L. A. Laboratory, clinical, and epidemiological aspects of coagulase-negative staphylococci. *Clin. Microbiol. Revs.* 1:281, 1988.

Todd, J. K. Toxic shock syndrome. *Clin. Microbiol. Revs.* 1:432, 1988.

Wickboldt, L. G., and Fenske, N. A. Streptococcal and staphylococcal infections of the skin. *Hosp. Pract.* 21:41, 1986.

17. THE GRAM-NEGATIVE DIPLOCOCCI: THE *NEISSERIA* AND RELATED GENERA

OBJECTIVES

To describe the properties of the *Neisseria* that distinguish them from other genera of bacteria

To describe the properties that are used to differentiate the species within the genus *Neisseria* and the properties that differentiate the pathogens from the nonpathogens

To describe *Neisseria meningitidis* in terms of the diseases it causes, epidemiology, antigens,

laboratory diagnostic procedures, chemotherapy, and active immunization

To describe the prominent clinical aspects of genital and extragenital gonorrheal infections and the laboratory diagnostic procedures, chemotherapy, virulence factors, and prospects for a vaccine

To name other members of the Neisseriaceae family that are opportunistically pathogenic

The medically important members of the genus *Neisseria* are *N. meningitidis* (*the meningococcus*) and *N. gonorrhoeae* (*the gonococcus*). The other members included in Table 17-1 are non-pathogens that colonize the oral cavity and the upper respiratory tract.

GENERAL CHARACTERISTICS OF *NEISSERIA*

1. All species are *gram-negative diplococci*. Where the members of the paired bacteria abut, they are flat sided, so that each member of the pair presents a bean-shaped configuration (Fig. 17-1).
2. All species *parasitize the mucous membranes of humans*.
3. All species are aerobic or facultatively anaerobic. *The pathogens grow better in 5 percent to 10 percent CO_2.*
4. *All species produce the enzyme cytochrome oxidase.* Members of the genus are said to be oxidase positive as determined by the oxidase test.

The major species of the genus *Neisseria* and some of their differentiating properties are listed in Table 17-1. Nonpathogenic *Neisseria* microorganisms are almost always present in specimens obtained from the oro- and nasopharynx. There is an appreciable carrier rate of the meningococcus in the nasopharynx, and not infrequently the meningococcus is found in the genital tract and rectum of male homosexuals. The gonococcus does cause infections of the oral cavity and of the pharynx, infections that are usually relatable to oral-genital contact.

NEISSERIA MENINGITIDIS— THE MENINGOCOCCUS

PATHOGENESIS

It is convenient to divide meningococcal disease into three clinical entities: nasopharyngitis, meningococcal septicemia, and meningococcal meningitis. The latter two are the major invasive disease entities. Other forms of invasive menin-

Table 17-1. Differentiative Properties of *Neisseria*

Species	Acid produced from					Pro- duction of IgA protease	Pro- duction of pig- ment	Growth on			Reduction of	
	Glu- cose	Mal- tose	Su- crose	Fruc- tose	Lac- tose			Nutrient agar at 35°C	Chocolate blood agar at 22°C	MTM, ML, or NYC medium	NO$_3$	NO$_2$
*N. gonorrhoeae**	+	−	−	−	−	+	−	−	−	+	−	−
N. meningitidis	+	+	−	−	−	+	−	−	−	+	−	d
N. lactamica	+	+	−	−	+		−	−	−	+	−	d
N. cinerea	−	−	−	−	−		−	−	−	−	−	+
N. polysaccharea	+	+	−	−	−		−	+	−	+	−	d
N. flavescens	−	−	−	−	−	−	+	−	−	+	−	−
N. sicca	+	+	+	+	−	−	d	+	+	−		
N. subflava	+	+	d	d	−	−	+	+	+	−	−	+
N. mucosa	+	+	+	+	−		+	+	+	−	+	+

d = some strains positive, some negative
* Superoxol test: Only *N. gonorrhoeae* and *N. kochii* (not listed here) are superoxol positive. They give a strong reaction (bubbles of oxygen) when 30% hydrogen peroxide is applied to colonies.

Fig. 17-1. Electron micrograph of *Neisseria* (×27,000). (From A. S. Dajani, *Infect. Immun.* 14:776, 1976.)

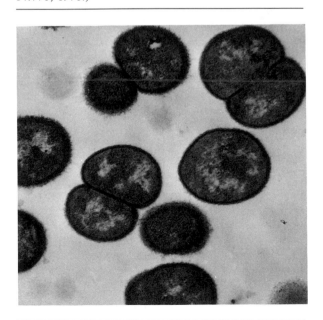

gococcal disease include septic arthritis, endocarditis, osteomyelitis, and pneumonia. Infections usually are acute. Chronic infections are rare and are characterized by recurrent episodes of fever, rashes, and arthritis.

Nasopharyngitis
Infection of the nasopharynx is usually short-lived and frequently symptomless; in fact, it is not regarded as a genuine clinical entity by some. Meningococci that colonize the nasopharynx can spread from that site into the bloodstream to cause meningococcal septicemia, or they can spread to adjacent sites and into the bloodstream to cause meningococcal meningitis.

Meningococcal Septicemia
Infection of the blood can be accompanied by high fever, arthritis, blockages of small vessels, and a rash that starts as *pinpoint hemorrhages (petechiae)* of the skin and mucous membranes.

In severe infections the skin lesions become more extensive. Irregularly shaped, *dusky red blotches (purpura)*, hemorrhage, and necrosis occur (see Plate 9 for massive cutaneous hemorrhage). A serious development is a *fulminating sepsis*, which produces *hemorrhagic necrosis* in the cortex of both adrenal glands (adrenal apoplexy). The profound physiological effects of adrenal insufficiency and the vascular effects lead to rapid collapse and death. Probably no other acute bacterial infection is so swiftly fatal as meningococcal septicemia. The complex of changes accompanying the bilateral adrenal cortical hemorrhage is termed the *Waterhouse-Friderichsen syndrome*, a syndrome that is most frequently associated with the meningococcus.

Meningococcal Meningitis

Meningitis can be caused by a variety of microorganisms and by noninfectious conditions such as cancer, systemic lupus erythematosus, and injected chemicals. Eighty-four percent of reported cases of bacterial (septic) meningitis in patients over one month old are caused by *Neisseria meningitidis, Streptococcus pneumoniae*, and *Hemophilus influenzae*, all three of which normally colonize the nasopharynx. Because the meningococcus is the only microorganism to cause septic meningitis in epidemic form, it is designated the causal agent of epidemic meningitis. *Spinal meningitis* and *cerebrospinal meningitis* are terms used to indicate central nervous system infections caused by the meningococcus.

Meningococcal meningitis usually begins suddenly with high fever, severe headache, and pain and stiffness of the neck, back, and shoulders. Nausea and vomiting occur frequently. Petechial or purpuric lesions occur in about 50 percent of meningococcal meningitis patients. Survivors may suffer major *residual effects (sequelae)* such as deafness, mental retardation, and behavioral defects.

Virulence factors that enable the meningococcus to initiate an infection include: *pili*, which mediate the attachment of the bacterium to mucus-secreting cells; *a mechanism by which the meningococcus is transported within host cell vesicles to the submucosa; surface polysaccharides* (capsules) that are anti-phagocytic; *protease that cleaves IGA₁* antibodies; a unique *mechanism for obtaining essential iron from host transferrin molecules*. It is difficult to pinpoint how the meningococcus, once established, can cause such devastating disease manifestations. Meningococcal endotoxins appear to have an enhanced potency over the endotoxins of some other gram-negative bacteria. Why this is so is open to speculation. Meningococcus strains that do not have the oligosaccharide side chain of the endotoxin molecule ("rough" strains) cause more severe endotoxic reactions in experimental animals than do strains with intact endotoxins. Loss of the side chain exposes the lipid A toxic moiety, which theoretically then can home in on and destroy the cell membranes of the host's defensive cells. The meningococcal endotoxins are noted for inducing disseminated intravascular clotting and vessel damage because of intense inflammation abetted by complement factors. Other virulence mechanisms that may be involved in meningococcal disease are: vessel-damaging immune complex formation (Chapter 14—Type III hypersensitivity); the release of host-cell thromboxane, a potent vasoconstrictor, which may be a factor leading to shock; suppression of leucotriene B4 (LTB4) synthesis, which would depress the release of potent pharmacological mediators and chemotactic factors from leukocytes.

LABORATORY DIAGNOSIS

The organism can be isolated from blood, the nasopharynx, skin lesions, cerebrospinal fluid (CSF), and other sites, such as the urethra, the endocervix, and the anal canal of homosexuals. Specimens should be cultured as soon as possible because the *Neisseria* pathogens *autolyze readily* and are somewhat temperature sensitive. Specimens are cultured on supplemented chocolate agar or *Thayer-Martin, Martin-Lewis*, or *New*

York City medium. The latter three media are made selective by the addition of combinations of six different antimicrobials. The antimicrobials prevent the growth of the nonpathogenic *Neisseria,* as well as yeasts, gram-negative bacilli, and other forms. Growth is augmented by incubation in an *elevated CO_2 environment.*

The examination of clinical materials, especially of cerebrospinal fluid (CSF), yields important information for diagnosis. The cornerstone of diagnosis of all acute bacterial (septic) meningitis, not only of meningococcal meningitis, is a lumbar puncture to obtain CSF. The CSF in acute bacterial (septic) meningitis, as opposed to acute aseptic meningitis, is under increased pressure and cloudy, the white blood cell count is increased, protein is elevated, and glucose is reduced. Some of the CSF is Gram-stained for a presumptive diagnosis. In acute infections the meningococcus (and the gonococcus) characteristically appear in their distinctive morphology and grouping within the cytoplasm of neutrophils (Fig. 17-2).

Colony characteristics and Gram-stained smears prepared from colonies are examined and the *cytochrome oxidase test* (simply referred to as the "*oxidase test*") is performed to identify the isolate as a member of the genus *Neisseria.* The oxidase test is performed by dropping oxidase reagent directly onto colonies or by transferring some of the growth from a colony onto a filter strip moistened with the reagent. In a positive test the colony or the filter strip progressively changes color from pink to maroon or black. Carbohydrate utilization tests are used to differentiate *N. meningitidis* from the other *Neisseria* species, along with other selected differential tests (Table 17-1).

Rapid Test Methods

Rapid test methods (see Chapter 15) available for the identification of *Neisseria* include tests to detect acid production from carbohydrates, tests to detect specific enzymes, serologic tests, and DNA probe tests (Chapter 13, Avidin-Biotin Technique).

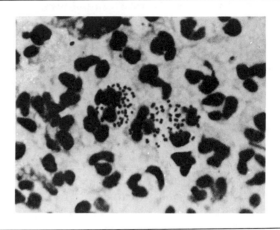

Fig. 17-2. Smear of urethral pus containing gonorrhea organisms. In acute infections the paired, bean-shaped *Neisseria* appear mostly within the cytoplasm of neutrophils (*center*). The large, dark structures are the lobed nuclei of the neutrophils. The circular grouping of the gonococci is due to their confinement within the indistinct cytoplasmic membrane of the neutrophils. (From R. W. Thatcher and T. H. Pettit. Reprinted from the *Journal of the American Medical Association,* March 1, 1971, Volume 215, Copyright © 1971, American Medical Association.)

Serological Tests

Knowledge of the surface antigens of the meningococcus is important to understand serological testing, epidemiology, and active immunization. There are three ways in which the antigens of serologically and chemically different strains of meningococci are organized: serogroups, serotypes, and subtypes. Serogrouping is based on chemical and structural characteristics of the meningococcal capsular polysaccharides. Serotyping and subtyping are based on outer membrane proteins of the cell wall. At present, meningococci are referred to primarily on the basis of their serogroup antigens. *The classical serogroups are A, B, C, D, X, Y, Z, 29E, and W135.*

The serological tests that may be performed directly on CSF include the fluorescent antibody staining procedure and counterimmunoelectrophoresis (CIE). Traditional agglutination tests can also be performed on fresh cultures. Latex agglutination tests (using anti-meningococcal antibodies attached to latex particles) and coagglutination tests (Chapter 16—*Staphylococccus aureus*, Protein A) for detecting meningococcal antigens in body fluids are commercially available. Monoclonal antibodies against serogroup B are available, and they can be used to detect the bacterium in CSF, blood, and urine.

EPIDEMIOLOGY

Humans are the only natural host for *N. meningitidis*. *Spread is via respiratory droplets.* Rates of endemic disease in the United States are 1 to 3/100,000; in parts of the developing world the rates are 10 to 25/100,000. In epidemic periods the rates may be as high as 500/100,000.

Approximately 90 percent of illness is caused by serogroups A, B, and C. When epidemics occur Group A meningococci most often are involved. Epidemics occur primarily in the developing countries, where the conditions for epidemic spread are more likely to exist: presence of virulent strains, low socioeconomic conditions, and appropriate climatic conditions. Outbreaks in sub-Saharan Africa (the "meningitis belt") tend to appear at 8- to 12-year intervals in the dry season, apparently related to constant irritation of the respiratory mucosa during that season. The condition of the pharyngeal mucosa and respiratory epithelium seems to be an important factor in protection from invasive disease. Concurrent viral upper respiratory tract illness appears to be a predisposing factor, as is poor general health.

Occurrence of disease is highest in children aged three months to one year and decreases with age. Peak attack rates are in infants six to nine months old when maternal antibodies have disappeared. Close contacts of persons with meningococcal disease are several hundred-fold more likely to develop disease than the general population. Persons at highest risk are household contacts, day care center contacts, and persons who have had oral contact or who have shared food and beverages with infected persons. Nearly one-third of the contacts who develop meningococcal disease do so within four days after the index (source) patient is hospitalized.

The *asymptomatic nasopharyngeal carrier* is an important link in the transmission of meningococci. Meningococci have also been isolated from uro- and anogenital sites. The carriage rate varies with age, socioeconomic status, and the presence of an ongoing outbreak. The carriage rates are highest among school-age children and young adults. The overall carriage rate in the United States appears to be between 0.6 to 5.7 percent. The rate increases markedly in community epidemic situations, in close contacts with patients, and in closed populations such as occurred formerly in military installations that processed recruits.

TREATMENT AND PREVENTION

The seriousness of meningococcal disease makes it imperative to initiate treatment promptly; the use of antimicrobial drugs should not await the completion of laboratory studies. At one time the sulfa drugs were the drugs of choice, but because there are now so many sulfonamide-resistant strains these drugs should not be used unless susceptibility is established by susceptibility tests. Penicillin is now the drug of choice, with chloramphenicol an alternative choice when there is sulfa drug resistance or penicillin hypersensitivity. A combination of ampicillin and moxalactam is highly active against the major meningeal bacterial agents including the meningococcus.

There are *four licensed vaccines* available in the United States for serogroups or combinations of serogroups: A, C, AC, and ACYW135. The antigens are highly purified, chemically defined polysaccharides. The antibodies formed in response to the antigens activate the complement system. The membrane attack complex (MAC—Chapter 12) of the complement system lyses the meningococci. Infants respond poorly to the polysaccharide antigens, and so the vaccines are least efficacious for the group at highest risk. Antibody level, furthermore, declines rapidly in young children and there is no secondary immune response of note. Experimental conjugate vaccines of meningococcal polysaccharides covalently attached to proteins such as tetanus toxoid and bovine serum albumin are highly immunogenic in mice. A similar polysaccharide-protein conjugate vaccine for *Hemophilus influenzae* type b (Chapter 23) has been shown to be safe and much more immunogenic in young children than the polysaccharide alone.

Group B meningococci account for about 50 percent of meningococcal illness in the United States. There is only a weak response to the B polysaccharide in humans and so no vaccine is available. Current experimental approaches to Group B vaccines include conjugate vaccines and preparations of fragments of outer membrane proteins from which lipopolysaccharides (endotoxins) have been removed.

Currently, routine immunization in the industrialized nations is not recommended. The risk of infection is low, vaccines are not very efficacious in infants—the group at highest risk—and there is no vaccine available against Group B.

Early use of rifampin is recommended for close contacts of persons with meningococcal disease. An adjunct to chemoprophylaxis is active immunization. Over 50 percent of the high-risk close contacts who get a meningococcal infection develop the infection more than five days after contact with the primary case—sufficient time for the active immunization potentially to yield some benefit against disease serogroups A, C, Y, and W135.

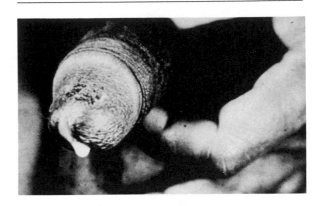

Fig. 17-3. Purulent discharge typical of gonorrhea in men. Often it is only a drop of pus noticed on arising, but in severe cases the discharge is continuous and heavy. (From B. N. Morton, *VD: A Guide for Nurses and Counselors*. Boston: Little, Brown, 1976.)

sations of discomfort and pain. The inflammatory response initially triggers a mucoid discharge followed by a purulent exudate, usually in 2 to 5 days (Fig. 17-3). The infection can progress from the anterior urethra to the posterior urethra in 10 to 14 days, with increasing *dysuria (difficult urination), polyuria (frequent urination),* and occasionally general symptoms including headache and fever. The glands, ducts, and vesicles of the male genitourinary tract may become sites of local complications. Chronic infections of the prostate, seminal vesicles, and epididymides may ensue. *Urethral strictures* may occur.

At one time it was believed that asymptomatic infections did not occur in men, but asymptomatic infections are now known to occur in as high as 40 percent of the infected male population.

NEISSERIA GONORRHOEAE— THE GONOCOCCUS

PATHOGENESIS

Genitourinary Tract Infections in the Male

Infection in men usually takes the form of acute urethritis. Among the early symptoms are sen-

Genitourinary Tract Infections in the Female

In females acute gonorrhea may involve the urethra, Skene's and Bartholin's glands, and the endocervix (Fig. 17-4). The *endocervical glands* are the traditional site of infection, but the rectum is

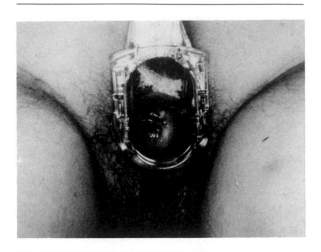

Fig. 17-4. The discharge caused by gonorrhea in women is noticeable on the cervix rather than on the vaginal walls. The test sample is taken from the cervical os, the small opening at the center of the cervix. (From B. N. Morton, *VD: A Guide for Nurses and Counselors*. Boston: Little, Brown, 1976.)

also a common site. Exudate from the endocervix probably contaminates the perineum, and the microorganisms spread to the rectal mucosa. There is no gonococcal vaginitis in the postpubertal female. Symptoms of acute infection of the lower tract are seldom severe. The most prevalent symptoms of acute infection are abdominal or pelvic pain, vaginal discharge (which originates in the endocervix), and dysuria. Chronic infections may be indicated by tenderness of the lower abdomen, backaches, low-grade inflammations of the urethra and genitourinary tract-associated structures, and profuse menstrual flow. Asymptomatic carriers present a major obstacle in controlling the spread of gonorrhea.

Pelvic Inflammatory Disease. There may be an ascending spread of gonococci from the endocervical glands along the endometrium (the inner mucous membrane of the uterus) to the fallopian tubes (where it causes salpingitis) and from there to adjacent structures. The ascending infection is termed *upper tract disease* or *pelvic inflammatory disease (PID)*. PID also is caused by other agents, such as *C. trachomatis*, anaerobic bacteria (*Bacteroides* and gram-positive cocci), *Actinomyces israelii*, and *Mycoplasma hominis*. It is estimated that 30 to 80 percent of the cases of PID are gonococcal, but polymicrobial PID is quite usual. PID most often occurs within 7 days of the previous menstrual period. Signs and symptoms typical of acute upper tract disease include chills, fever to 102°, severe bilateral lower abdominal pain, and rebound tenderness (pain on the release of manual pressure). Those who experience recurrences are at increasing risk of infertility and ectopic pregnancies with each succeeding infection.

Extragenital Infections

Local Infections. Local infections occur in various areas of the body, determined usually by the mode of contact: *pharyngitis, conjunctivitis*, and *proctitis* are examples. *Blindness in the newborn (ophthalmia neonatorum)* can develop from infection of the eyes as the child passes through the birth canal of an infected mother.

Disseminated Gonococcal Infection (DGI). Gonococci from primary sites of infection (endocervix, rectum, pharynx, male urethra) can spread via the bloodstream (hematogenous route) to cause, most commonly, an *arthritis-dermatitis syndrome* and, occasionally, meningitis, endocarditis, and other conditions. One to 3 percent of individuals with genital infections develop disseminated gonococcal infection (DGI). Those who develop DGI are usually asymptomatic in regard to the primary site of infection. Fever, chills, myalgia, and malaise are nonspecific symptoms of the bacteremic phase of DGI. Between 50 and 70 percent of patients with DGI have dermatitis and more than 90 percent have arthropathy. Active skin lesions are usually found in those who have joint involvement (Fig. 17-5). An average of 5 to 30 lesions appear, mostly on the extremities, and they progress from

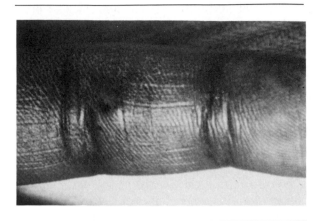

Fig. 17-5. Example of a skin lesion caused by gonococcemia. Metastatic gonorrhea may cause arthritic symptoms accompanied by red papules, vesicles, or pustules typical of those shown. (Courtesy N. J. Fiumara, Massachusetts Department of Public Health, Division of Communicable and Venereal Diseases.)

red papular lesions to pustular, hemorrhagic, or necrotic lesions. The presence of such lesions in various stages of development in sexually active individuals should lead the physician to suspect and rule out DGI. The arthritis is usually felt in several joints, with the knees, ankles, and wrists being the most frequently involved. Joint destruction can occur if the infection is left untreated.

Just as with the meningococcus, the *pathogenic mechanisms of the gonococcus* are not well understood. *Piliated gonococci* are regarded as virulent because they produce infection in volunteers. Pili apparently represent only one type of adhesion involved in pathogenicity (see Chapter 9 for further discussion of epithelial adherence and penetration by the gonococcus). Strain-specific secretory IgA is found in genital secretions. Secretory IgA functioning as topical antibody blocks attachment of microorganisms to host cells. *N. gonorrhoeae* elaborates an *IgA protease* that cleaves and inactivates the secretory IgA subclass IgA1. Nonpathogenic Neisseria species do not produce IgA protease. The persistence of

the gonococcus in the carrier state may be due to *epithelial endocytosis*. Gonococci have been found in epithelial cells obtained from the cervix of carriers. The gonococci attach to the epithelial cells of the cervix, are endocytosed, multiply within the cell, and are protected there from the phagocytic activities of leukocytes. Gonococcal lipopolysaccharide (LPS) is not so apparent a virulence factor as are the endotoxins of some of the other gram-negative bacteria when the gonococcal infection is a mucosal one. Gonococcal endotoxin, however, is probably responsible for some of the pathophysiological effects observed in DGI

LABORATORY DIAGNOSIS

The laboratory characteristics that were cited for the meningococcus apply as well to the gonococcus: the fragility of the bacterium, types of culture media employed for isolation, requirement for elevated CO_2 environment for growth (more important for gonococci), typical gram-negative diplococci appearing in the cytoplasm of pus cells, and the availability of like rapid identification methods.

The finding of intracellular gram-negative diplococci in *smears of urethral pus* is viewed as presumptive evidence of gonorrheal infection in men (Fig. 17-2). Smears of specimens from the female genital tract are much less reliable for diagnostic purposes; acute infections are not nearly so apparent as in the male, and other gram-negative diplococci and other organisms that resemble the gonococcus may appear in such specimens. Smears from the pharynx or rectum have little reliable diagnostic value.

In order to diagnose a gonorrheal infection reliably, it is necessary to culture out the organisms to establish its identity. It is important to give careful attention to the collection of appropriate specimens and to the processing of the specimens. Oropharyngeal and anorectal specimens should also be obtained along with the regularly collected urethral and endocervical specimens when there is reason to believe that oral or anal contact has occurred. Colonial and microscopic characteristics, the oxidase test, and carbohydrate (CHO) utilization tests are the principal observations and tests that are routinely conducted on the isolated organisms. Additional tests are indicated in Table 17-1.

N. gonorrhoeae displays four colony types. Colony types T1 and T2 are small, sticky, and dark (when obliquely lighted); they develop in primary culture from clinical material. T1 and T2 colonies are correlated with virulence.

The *Superoxol test*, which is like the conventional catalase test except that the concentration of hydrogen peroxide (H_2O_2) is 30% rather than 3%, is an inexpensive, rapid screening test for organisms growing on selective media. Any organism that grows on these media and that is Superoxol positive (bubbles of oxygen appear when the reagent is applied to colonies) is likely to be *N. gonorrhoeae*.

There are two generally accepted serological tests used in the identification of *N. gonorrhoeae*: the direct fluorescent antibody technique and the staphylococcal coagglutination technique. The latter technique employs a strain of protein A–containing staphylococci that are coated with antigonococcal antibodies (see under Protein A in Chapter 16).

EPIDEMIOLOGY

Except for vulvovaginitis in prepubertal (usually institutionalized) girls and conjunctivitis in the newborn, gonococcal infections are usually spread by sexual contact. As of 1989 the number of cases of gonorrhea reported to the Centers for Disease Control (CDC) has averaged about 800,000 per year for the past several years. This figure exemplifies the extent of infection in the population and the enormity of the control problem.

Among the factors that predispose to the epidemic proportions of gonorrhea are the high degree of transmissibility; short incubation period; high rate of asymptomatic carriers; lack of protective immunity; increasing resistance to antibiotics; and, conceivably, changes in sex mores and practices.

TREATMENT AND PREVENTION

Several observations and reports affect the treatment recommendations. There is a high frequency—as high as 45 percent in some studies—of *co-transmitted and coexisting gonococcal and chlamydial infections*. Concern is growing about the serious complications that accompany these infections. In a surveillance of gonococcal susceptibilities to antibiotics conducted in 1988 and 1989 by the CDC, more than 20 percent of the gonococcal strains were resistant to penicillin and tetracycline, the drugs that have been used for some years for gonorrheal infections. Resistance to an alternative drug, spectinomycin, has also been reported. Susceptibilities to antibiotics vary in parts of the country. State and local health departments are encouraged to determine antimicrobial susceptibilities of isolates from selected patients to detect emerging resistance, which may necessitate revisions of therapy recommendations for their area.

In view of the possibility of co-transmitted chlamydial infection and the increasing number of resistant strains, the generally recommended regimen for uncomplicated urethral, endocervical, or rectal infections is *ceftriaxone* 250 mg intramuscularly (IM) once plus *doxycycline* 100 mg orally twice per day for 7 days. For patients who cannot take ceftriaxone, the preferred alternative is spectinomycin 2 grams IM in a single dose followed by doxycycline. Ceftriaxone is also recommended for virtually all other types of gonococcal infections: pharyngitis, meningitis, endocarditis, adult ophthalmia, disseminated gonococcal infection, infections in pregnancy, and infections in infants and children. The regimens for these other types vary in respect to dosage, number and spacing of doses, and additional or alternative drugs.

PLASMID-MEDIATED ANTIMICROBIAL RESISTANCE IN NEISSERIA GONORRHOEAE, UNITED STATES, 1988 AND 1989

Because the prevalence of antimicrobial resistance in *Neisseria gonorrhoeae* increased during the early 1980s, in 1986 CDC implemented the Gonococcal Isolate Surveillance Project (GISP) to monitor antimicrobial susceptibilities at 21 collaborating sexually transmitted disease clinics in 21 cities. Although national gonorrhea rates changed little from 1988 (302 per 100,000 persons) to 1989 (298 per 100,000), important increases occurred in the percentage of isolates with plasmid-mediated resistance.

PPNG (penicillinase-producing *Neisseria gonorrhoeae*) was first isolated in the United States in 1976. From 1976 through 1981, the prevalence of PPNG infections increased slowly; foci of infections were identified in Los Angeles, Miami, and New York City. From 1981 through 1986, the prevalence of PPNG infections increased more than fivefold. This increasing prevalence prompted the recommendation that penicillins be virtually abandoned as single-dose, primary therapy for gonorrhea. From 1988 through 1989, PPNG was isolated at all clinics participating in GISP. The percentage of PPNG infections in the clinics participating at GISP indicates that PPNG has spread beyond its initial geographic foci and now represents a public health problem in all regions of the United States.

TRNG (tetracycline-resistant *N. gonorrhoeae*) was first described in 1986. Infections with TRNG appear to be most common in the eastern United States; in 1989, however, of the four clinics reporting substantial increases in the percentage of TRNG, one was in the midwest (St. Louis), and one in the west (Denver). These data suggest that further spread of TRNG from eastern to western cities is likely. In 1985, based on previously described resistance caused by chromosomal mutations, CDC recommended that tetracycline not be used as sole therapy for gonorrhea; the subsequent emergence of TRNG has further emphasized the importance of this recommendation. TRNG is important for two reasons: first, because it has high-level resistance to tetracycline, and second, because experimentally its plasmid may transfer both itself and β-lactamase plasmids to *Neisseria* and related species.

The conjugative ability of the TRNG plasmid may have resulted in the emergence of strains that are both penicillinase-producing and tetracycline-resistant (PPNG/TRNG). PPNG/TRNG accounted for a small proportion of all isolates examined in 1988 and 1989. However, because these isolates accounted for 9.7% of all *N. gonorrhoeae* isolates from the Philadelphia clinic in 1989, and because the frequency of

PPNG/TRNG isolates identified from other clinics increased almost threefold between 1988 and 1989, infections caused by these strains will further challenge the selection of gonorrhea therapies.

Despite the increase in the frequency of strains with plasmid-mediated resistance to penicillins and tetracycline, all isolates examined were susceptible to ceftriaxone, and fewer than 1% were resistant to spectinomycin (CDC, unpublished data). Initial therapy for gonococcal infection with ceftriaxone (250 mg intramuscularly), or an antimicrobial agent with proven equivalency, remains an integral component of the strategy for gonorrhea control.

Excerpted from *M.M.W.R.* 39(17):284, May 4, 1990.

A well-standardized laboratory method to monitor the susceptibilities of gonococcal isolates to penicillin, tetracycline, spectinomycin, and ceftriaxone has been recommended by the National Committee for Clinical Laboratory Standards.

Most states have a law that requires the instillation of a prophylactic agent into the eyes of newborn infants *immediately postpartum to prevent gonococcal ophthalmia neonatorum*. Silver nitrate solution 1% (Credé's method) is effective for gonococcal ophthalmia neonatorum but is not effective against chlamydial conjunctivitis. Either erythromycin (0.5%) ophthalmic ointment or tetracycline (1.0%) ointment is effective against both agents.

Long-lasting immunity does not appear to develop as a result of natural infections with *N. gonorrhoeae*. Repeated infections occur in an individual, and an acute infection may be superimposed on a chronic one. Antigonococcal secretory IgA is found, however, in genital secretions. Bactericidal serum antibodies can be demonstrated.

Extensive efforts have been made to develop a vaccine against gonorrhea. The best antibody response is to pili, outer membrane protein II, and lipooligosaccharide (LOS—a small form of bacterial endotoxin). One thing that occurs that probably affects protection is that the *antigens shift from one antigenic form to another*. The shifting is of such frequency that each gonococcus possibly is antigenically distinct from other gonococci. A number of other candidate antigens besides pili, protein II, and LOS have been tried, but with little success. Investigations have been initiated to determine whether a cell-mediated immune response might provide protection. Despite these many efforts, a vaccine for gonococcal infection remains elusive.

OTHER MEMBERS OF THE FAMILY NEISSERIACEAE

NONPATHOGENIC NEISSERIA SPECIES

Members of the genus *Neisseria* (see Table 17-2) other than *N. gonorrhoeae* and *N. meningitidis* are not frequently involved in overt disease. Their importance lies in the following facts: (1) they are the second most prevalent aerobic microorganisms in the oral cavity and upper respiratory tract, and some are occasionally recovered from genital sites; (2) it is usually nec-

Table 17-2. Characteristics of the Pathogenic *Neisseria*

	Disease association	Morphological and physiological characteristics	Virulence factors	Mode of transmission	Treatment and prevention
N. meningitidis	Septicemia: high fever, disseminated intravascular clotting, vascular damage, shock Septic meningitis: high fever, severe headache, nausea, disorientation, sequelae	Gram-negative diplococci, intracellular habitat in smears of pus, Thayer-Martin medium and elevated CO_2 for laboratory growth, cytochrome-oxidase positive	Pili, capsules, IgA_1 protease, ability to remove iron from host transferrin, mechanism to traverse mucosa; endotoxins	Respiratory droplets	Penicillin; chloramphenicol; rifampin prophylactically for close contacts
N. gonorrhoeae	Males: acute urethritis; chronic infection of other GU tract sites; asymptomatic carrier state Females: infection of endocervix, rectum, periurethral glands; pelvic inflammatory disease; asymptomatic carrier state Extragenital infections: local—governed by mode of contact, pharyngitis; proctitis, conjunctivitis; systemic—arthritis-dermatitis, endocarditis, meningitis	Same as above	Pili, IgA, protease, epithelial endocytosis; endotoxins	Venereal	Ceftriaxone; use of penicillin, tetracycline, spectinomycin determined by patient hypersensitivity or regional occurrence of resistant strains; 1% silver nitrate or erythromycin or tetracycline into eyes of newborn

essary to differentiate them from the pathogens; (3) occasionally they are found as causal agents of infections such as meningitis, endocarditis, pneumonia, osteomyelitis, and septicemia.

ACINETOBACTER

Acinetobacter is a genus with many species of gram-negative diplococci or coccobacilli. Its members are widely distributed in nature and often are part of the normal human flora, especially that of the skin. There is one recognized species, *Acinetobacter calcoaceticus* (which includes the former *Herellea vaginicola* and *Mima polymorpha*), that is being reported with increasing frequency as an opportunistic pathogen that causes a variety of infections, especially hospital-associated infections: pneumonia, bacteremia, nongonococcal urethritis, meningitis, and wound infections.

BRANHAMELLA

Branhamella catarrhalis is a gram-negative diplococcus, formerly known as *Neisseria catarrhalis*. This species recently has come to be recognized as a significant cause of maxillary sinusitis and otitis media in children. The organism is an infrequent but significant cause of pneumonia, bronchitis, endocarditis, meningitis, conjunctivitis, and septicemia, especially in individuals with a compromised health status. Characteristics that help differentiate *B. catarrhalis* from other *Neisseria:* it does not produce acids from the dissimilation of carbohydrates, it reduces nitrates, colonies are non-pigmented or gray, growth is variable on selective media (MTM, ML, NYC), it produces deoxyribonucleases, and it is Superoxol negative.

KINGELLA

Members of *Kingella* (three recognized species) are gram-negative cocobacilli that occur in pairs and short chains. Members of the genus are opportunistically pathogenic and have been associated with cases of endocarditis, septic arthritis, septicemia, and other lesions.

MORAXELLA

Members of *Moraxella* (six recognized species) are plump, gram-negative bacilli. *Moraxella lacunata* occasionally causes conjunctivitis in humans.

SUMMARY

1. The *Neisseria* are gram-negative diplococci that colonize, and sometimes infect and cause disease in, the mucous membranes of humans. Members of the genus are cytochrome-oxidase positive and that, coupled with their gram-negative diplococcal features, differentiates *Neisseria* from other genera.

2. Differentiation of species within the genus is based primarily on carbohydrate utilization.

3. The two pathogens, *N. meningitidis* (meningococcus) and *N. gonorrhoeae* (gonococcus), are delicate, culturally fastidious microorganisms. Special culture media such as supplemented chocolate agar or Thayer-Martin medium and CO_2 elevation are used for successful cultivation. The pathogens typically appear in the cytoplasm of neutrophils in acute infections.

4. The two best-known meningococcal infections are septic meningitis, which can occur in epidemic form, and fulminant meningococcemia, which is rapidly fatal.

5. There are nine classical meningococcal serogroups: A, B, C, D, X, Y, Z, 29E, and W135. Vaccines against A, C, Y, and W135 are available.

6. Penicillin, with choramphenicol as an alter-

native, is used when there is sulfa drug insusceptibility.

7. Gonorrhea is a major sexually transmitted disease (STD). In men, acute genital infections are usually manifested as an urethral exudate. In women, the primary site of genital infection is the endocervical glands. The development of pelvic inflammatory disease (PID) is not uncommon.

8. Asymptomatic infections are a problem in controlling infections.

9. The site of localized extragenital infections (pharyngitis, proctitis, conjunctivitis) usually is determined by mode of contact. Disseminated gonococcal infections (DGI) are spread via the hematogenous route and mostly take the form of an arthritis-dermatitis syndrome.

10. Imputed gonococcal virulence factors are pili, IgA protease, intraendothelial cell habitat, and endotoxins.

11. Chemotherapy is somewhat varied and is based, for one thing, on whether the infection is uncomplicated or complicated (e.g., by pregnancy or youth). Ceftriaxone and several forms of penicillin and tetracycline are the principal chemotherapeutic agents. One percent $AgNO_3$ or erythromycin or tetracycline ointments are used prophylactically in neonates to prevent blindness.

QUESTIONS FOR STUDY

Select the best response or responses for each of the following:

1. Members of the genus *Neisseria* have an affinity for
   A. Nerve cells
   B. Muscle fibers
   C. Endocrine glands
   D. Mucous membranes
   E. Renal parenchymal tissue

2. The gonococcal arthritis-dermatitis syndrome is the most common manifestation of disseminated gonococcal disease. This syndrome occurs only when the patient has
   A. A gonococcal bacteremia
   B. Had oral-genital contact
   C. Gonococcal endocarditis
   D. A positive Credé test
   E. An infection with non-piliated strains of gonococci

3. The principal method for differentiating the various species within the genus of *Neisseria* is
   A. The oxidase test
   B. Colonial morphology
   C. Carbohydrate utilization reactions
   D. Carbon dioxide requirements
   E. Bacteriophage typing

4. A spinal tap specimen (i.e., cerebrospinal fluid) from a young adult who was experiencing a severe headache, vomiting, and a stiff neck, when streaked on a Thayer-Martin medium, yielded virtually a pure culture of oxidase-positive colonies when incubated under an elevated CO_2 environment. A stained smear of the spinal tap material was most likely to contain
   A. Gram-positive cocci in pairs
   B. Clue cells
   C. Gram-negative coccobacillary forms
   D. Intracytoplasmic gram-negative bean-shaped diplococci
   E. Pleomorphic forms

5. A throat culture was obtained from a patient and a variety of colony types representing different bacterial genera appeared on the agar surface after a suitable period of incubation. What would be a good way to detect

potential colonies of *Neisseria* species in that mixture of colonies?

A. Apply drops of safranin to different colonies
B. Look for colonies that are emitting CO_2
C. Look for colonies that are beta hemolytic
D. Look for colonies that appear in pairs
E. Apply drops of oxidase reagent to different colonies

6. Certain enzymes are prominently associated with certain bacterial species because the enzymes are important in such roles as the virulence, the resistance, and the identification of the species. Enzymes of *Neisseria gonorrhoeae* that are accorded such important roles are (1) cytochrome oxidase; (2) lecithinase; (3) sIgA protease; (4) beta lactamase (in plasmid-producing strains, i.e., PPNG); or (5) collagenase.

A. 1,2,4
B. 1,3,4
C. 1,3,5
D. 2,3,4
E. 2,5

True or false:

7. The most common clinical form of DGI (disseminated gonococcal infection) is proctitis in male homosexuals.
   A. True   B. False

8. In order to prevent serious ocular infections in the newborn a 1% silver nitrate solution is introduced into the vagina of the mother just prior to giving birth.
   A. True   B. False

9. The combination of drugs that is currently recommended for the treatment of uncomplicated gonococcal infections is ceftriaxone and doxycycline.
   A. True   B. False

10. Chlamydial infections frequently are co-transmitted or coexist with gonococcal infections.
    A. True   B. False

Fill in the blank:

11. In females the ascending spread of gonococcal infection from the endocervical glands along the endometrium to the fallopian tubes and from there to adjacent structures or areas is called _____ .

12. In meningococcal infections the dusky red rash that resembles small bruises is called _____ .

ADDITIONAL READINGS

Centers for Disease Control. Disk diffusion antimicrobial susceptibility testing of Neisseria gonorrhoeae. *M.M.W.R.* 39(10):167, 1990.

Centers for Disease Control. Sexually transmitted diseases treatment guidelines. *M.M.W.R.* 38(S-8), 1989.

DeVoe, I. W. The meningococcus and mechanisms of pathogenicity. *Microbiol. Rev.* 46:162, 1982.

Frasch, C. E. Vaccines for prevention of meningococcal disease. *Clin. Microbiol. Rev.* 2(Suppl.): S134, 1989.

Handsfield, H. H. Sexually transmitted diseases. *Hosp. Pract.* 17(1):99, 1982.

Heerema, M. S. Diagnosis: Meningitis. *Hosp. Med.* 18:13, 1982.

Knapp, J. S. Historic perspectives and identification of Neisseria and related species. *Clin. Microbiol. Rev.* 1:415, 1988.

PID: Often subtle, always dangerous. *Patient Care* 22:220, 1988.

Tramont, E. C. Gonococcal vaccines. *Clin. Microbiol. Rev.* 2(Suppl.):S74, 1989.

18. THE GRAM-POSITIVE SPOREFORMERS: THE BACILLI AND CLOSTRIDIA

OBJECTIVES

To describe the types of disease caused by the genus *Bacillus* and the virulence factors associated with them

To discuss the techniques used to treat and control disease caused by *Bacillus* species

To list the major species of *Clostridium* and the diseases they cause in humans

To explain the various laboratory techniques used to differentiate species of *Clostridium*

To explain the mechanism of action of the clostridial toxins

To describe the methods used to treat and prevent the various clostridial infections

The gram-positive sporeformers comprise two major genera of bacteria: *Bacillus* and *Clostridium*. In culture they appear as long rods varying in length between 3 and 8 μm. In the spore state they are relatively resistant to heat and many chemicals. Autoclaving for 15 minutes at 120°C and 15 pounds per square inch pressure is the most effective way to destroy them. Most species exist as saprophytes in soil, water, and vegetation although some are harbored in the intestinal tract of animals and humans. Only a few species are pathogenic to humans. They are, however, among the most virulent.

BACILLUS

The two major pathogens in the genus *Bacillus* are *B. anthracis*, the etiological agent of *anthrax*, and *B. cereus*, the agent causing a form of food poisoning.

BACILLUS ANTHRACIS

General Characteristics

The anthrax bacillus is a nonmotile, facultative anaerobe that is 3 to 5 μm in length and 1.0 to 1.5 μm in width. The spore, located in the center of the cell (endospore), is produced only when the cells are cultivated outside animal host tissue. Colonies on blood agar or other laboratory media have a rough texture (ground-glass appearance) and a serrated edge. As the colonies age, the edge gives the appearance of undulating bands and is referred to as "medusa head." When *B. anthracis* is cultivated in the presence of elevated concentrations of CO_2 the colonies become mucoid from capsule formation. The capsule is a polypeptide (polyglutamic acid) and its formation in the presence of CO_2 is characteristic of virulent *B. anthracis*. This trait is not characteristic of any other *Bacillus* species.

The vegetative cells of *B. anthracis* in clinical

specimens occur as nonsporeforming cells in short chains (Fig. 18-1). In culture long chains of endospore-forming rods are observed and resemble a jointed rod. Vegetative cells are easily stained with ordinary laboratory dyes. The M'Fadyean stain is used to detect the capsule but the latter can be detected by fluorescent antibody as well.

Antigens and/or Virulence Factors

To be fully virulent, *B. anthracis* must produce a capsule and a protein exotoxin. The polypeptide capsular material enables the microorganism to evade phagocytosis. The capsular material, however, does not stimulate the formation of protective antibodies. The protein exotoxin, whose genetic determinants are carried on a single plasmid, is a complex of three protein factors: *edema factor (EF), protective antigen (PA)*, and *lethal factor (LF)*. Separately the toxins are nontoxic but act in combinations of two to produce two distinct toxic responses: edema in skin and lethality. Edema factor has been found to be an inactive form of *adenylate cyclase*, whose function is to convert adenosine triphosphate to cyclic adenosine monophosphate (see page 231). Apparently PA binds to the cytoplasmic membrane of host cells and then interacts with EF, causing the latter to be transported into the cytoplasm of the host cell (Fig. 18-2). In the cytoplasm EF interacts with a cellular molecule called calmodulin to become an active adenyl cyclase. The production of cyclic AMP causes mammalian cells to oversecrete (edema).

PATHOGENESIS AND EPIDEMIOLOGY

Anthrax is primarily a disease of herbivorous animals—sheep, horses, and cattle—that can be acquired by humans. The spores, which are found in the soil and on vegetation, are ingested or inhaled and gain entrance to the subcutaneous tissue through abraded skin or mucosa. After the spores germinate in the tissue, the vegetative cells produce an exotoxin that, in combination with the capsule, inhibits phagocytosis. If the bacilli reach the lymph and bloodstream, fatal septicemia may develop. The pathophysiology of toxin and infection is not completely understood. Some observers believe the primary site of action is the capillaries, whose altered permeability by toxin results in severe loss of vascular fluid. Others believe the central nervous system to be the primary site of action, with death resulting from respiratory failure.

In humans the disease is considered an occupational hazard for those working in areas where livestock is handled or where animal hides and hair are processed, and in microbiology laboratories. Inhalation of anthrax spores can result in a condition referred to as *woolsorters' disease*. The inhaled spores settle in the respiratory tract, producing local hemorrhaging and edema. Sep-

Fig. 18-1. Appearance of anthrax bacillus as observed in tissue. (Courtesy Armed Forces Institute of Pathology, AFIP 28-59.)

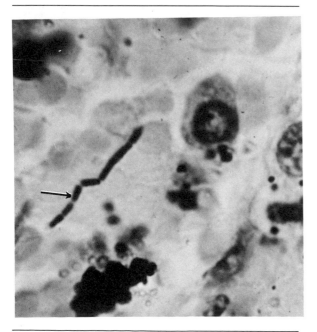

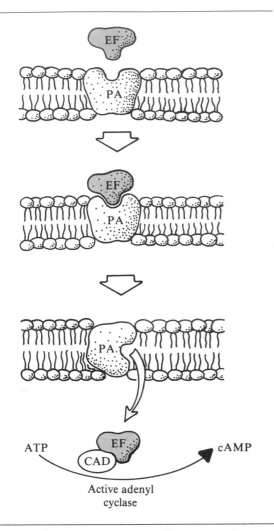

Fig. 18-2. Mechanism for internalization of edema factor and its activation. Edema factor binds to protective antigen (PA) factor, which is inserted into cytoplasmic membrane of host cell. Protective antigen facilitates transfer of edema factor into cytoplasm, where it interacts with calmodulin to become an active adenyl cyclase.

ticemia sometimes occurs, leading to meningitis. The most common form of the disease in humans, however, is called *cutaneous anthrax*. The organisms gain entrance to the body by contact with an abraded portion of the skin (Fig. 18-3). Flies and mosquitoes have been implicated as vectors

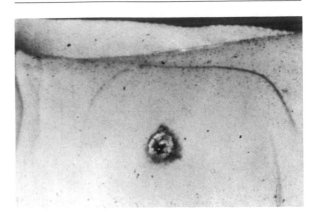

Fig. 18-3. Cutaneous anthrax. Lesion containing a central dark area (eschar) is observed on the forearm. (Courtesy P. Brachman.)

in transmission from animals to humans in large outbreaks of anthrax in African communities. The vectors feed on bacteremic animals and then bite humans to produce cutaneous anthrax (see Boxed Essay). The fully developed lesion appears as a dark necrotic area surrounded by a rim of edema. In severe cases the regional lymph nodes may enlarge, and once the blood is invaded the disease may prove fatal. Another form of the disease called *gastrointestinal anthrax* is uncommon in the United States but occurs more frequently in underdeveloped countries where contaminated meats are sold. The toxin produced in the intestinal tract forms a necrotic lesion in the ileum or cecum. Case fatality rates for this condition are very high.

IMMUNITY

Recovery from infection by *B. anthracis* brings permanent immunity for humans and animals. Protective antibodies are produced as a result of the host's response to the exotoxin complex. At present the only vaccine safe enough for human use is a toxoid prepared from a fraction of the exotoxin.

HUMAN CUTANEOUS ANTHRAX—*NORTH CAROLINA, 1987*

On July 10, 1987, a 42-year-old male maintenance worker at a North Carolina textile mill noticed a small, red, pruritic, papular lesion on his right forearm. Over the next week, the lesion became vesiculated and then developed a depressed black eschar with surrounding edema. Cutaneous anthrax was diagnosed. After the patient was treated with intravenous ampicillin and cephalosporins, his condition improved, and he was discharged on a regimen of oral cephalosporin.

The textile mill has been in operation for 25 years and employs about 210 workers. No known cases of anthrax have occurred among the workers before, and there has never been a vaccination program. The mill produces yarn from domestic wool and wool imported from Australia and New Zealand; cashmere goat hair from China, Afghanistan, and Iran; and camel hair from China and Mongolia.

To assess the degree of *Bacillus anthracis* contamination in the mill, investigators collected samples of raw and processed materials and environmental debris from the plant. *B. anthracis* was grown from 8 (14 percent) of the 59 samples tested. Five samples of West Asian cashmere were positive for *B. anthracis*, as was one sample of Australian wool and two samples of surface debris from the storage area. All cashmere used in the mill is first washed in a plant in Texas. Eight of 12 cashmere samples in the Texas plant were shown to be positive for *B. anthracis*. The West Asian cashmere was probably the contaminant at the mill. Western Asia is an endemic area for anthrax.

This is the first case of human anthrax to occur in the United States since 1984. Only 9 cases have occurred in this country in the past decade. The practice of vaccinating workers involved in the industrial processing of imported animal products and the decline in using fibers of animal origin are the primary factors in the current low incidence of human anthrax in this country.

From *M.M.W.R.* 37:413,1988

LABORATORY DIAGNOSIS

The anthrax bacillus can be cultured from the soil, cutaneous lesions, the respiratory tract, or blood (Fig. 18-1). The appearance of other sporeforming bacilli from some of these sites occasionally makes identification difficult. A motility test is a reliable technique for the screening of *Bacillus* isolates for *B. anthracis*. Any *Bacillus* isolate showing motility is assumed to be a species other than *B. anthracis*. Some of the recommended procedures for identification of *B. anthracis* include the following:

1. Culture the specimen on sheep blood agar or a selective medium when highly contaminated specimens are encountered.
2. Isolates of #1 above should be cultured in a bicarbonate- and serum-containing medium in presence of 5 percent CO_2. Determine the presence of a capsule.
3. Determine the presence of toxin by using antitoxin. Positive reaction confirms *B. anthracis*.
4. Determine susceptibility to penicillin. *B. anthracis* is susceptible to penicillin; other bacilli are resistant.
5. Determine susceptibility to gamma phage. *B. anthracis* is sensitive to gamma phage while all other *Bacillus* species (except *B. mycoides*) are invariably sensitive to gamma phage.

TREATMENT AND PREVENTION

Penicillin is often the drug of choice, but streptomycin, tetracycline, and erythromycin are also effective against the anthrax bacillus. Treatment before the appearance of bacteremia is important because the antibiotics are not effective against the toxin.

Anthrax is endemic in many areas of the world, especially the underdeveloped ones. Epizootic outbreaks still occur in the United States when unusual climatic conditions such as prolonged and heavy rains prevail. The most effective control program is vaccination of cattle, cremation or burial with quicklime of infected animals, and restricted movement of livestock.

Cutaneous anthrax is infrequently observed in the United States. Many of the cases recorded result from contact with goat hair or with animal hides that have not been decontaminated. Overseas travelers buying articles made of animal products must be made aware of these potential sources of infection.

Control of the disease in humans, whose occupation may be a predisposing factor, is provided by immunization with the toxoid.

Animals can be immunized with live spore vaccine; the Sterne strain vaccine is prepared from avirulent anthrax spores.

BACILLUS CEREUS AND OTHER BACILLI

B. cereus produces two enterotoxins that are responsible for two clinical entities: one that is a typical gastroenteritis, characterized by diarrhea and abdominal pain, and the other in which vomiting (emetic type), not diarrhea, takes place. Gastroenteritis occurs 8 to 16 hours after ingestion of contaminated food, while the emetic type occurs 1 to 5 hours after ingestion of contaminated food, particularly rice dishes. Both conditions are self-limiting and require no special treatment.

B. cereus is also being recognized as a major cause of ocular disease following trauma from nonsurgical penetrating objects. The organism infects the vitreous humor of the eye and can cause retinal damage with loss of vision. Therapy for infection includes clindamycin plus an aminoglycoside.

In the compromised patient other species of *Bacillus* such as *B. circulans*, *B. macerans*, *B. brevis*, and *B. coagulans* are occasionally associated with a variety of infections.

Because of ease in cultivation and heat resistance the spores of some bacilli are routinely used in the laboratory for experimental and testing procedures. *B. subtilis* is employed as a test organism to measure the effectiveness of ethylene oxide sterilization. Spores of *B. stearothermophilus*, because of their unusually high resistance to heat, are employed to test the efficiency of autoclaving. Finally, spores of *B. pumilus* are used to test the efficiency of sterilization by radiation.

CLOSTRIDIUM

The genus *Clostridium* includes many species that inhabit water, soil, and vegetation and play a major role in animal and plant putrefaction. Some species are commensals in the mammalian intestinal tract. A few species from these habitats are pathogenic and are the causative agents of botulism, tetanus, gas gangrene, and other clinical entities.

GENERAL CHARACTERISTICS

All clostridia are gram-positive spore-forming rods varying in length from 3 to 8 μm and in width from 0.4 to 1.2 μm. In most species the sporangia (vegetative cells with the enclosed spores) appear swollen (Fig. 18-4). Most clostridia are obligate anaerobes and some are aerotolerant. Most species of *Clostridium* are motile by peritrichous flagella with the notable exception being *C. perfringens* which is nonmotile. With few exceptions the spores of this genus do not germinate unless suitable reducing conditions are available and oxygen is absent. The spores are unusually resistant to heat and can withstand temperatures of 120°C for as long as 10 to 15 minutes.

The clostridia are easily cultivated in the laboratory when anaerobic conditions prevail. The most commonly used method for isolation of anaerobes is streaking blood agar and egg yolk agar plates and incubating anaerobically for 48 to 72 hours. After incubation the blood agar colonies should be examined for hemolysis, colony structure, and swarming of motile cells. Egg yolk agar

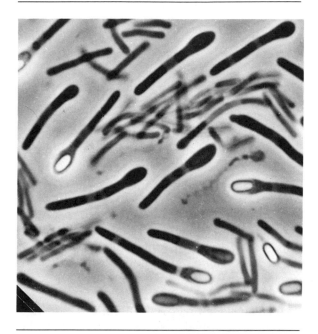

Fig. 18-4. Phase-contrast micrograph (×3600) of the endospores of a species of *Clostridium*. Note the refractile spore body and the swollen appearance of the vegetative cell. (Courtesy P. C. Fitz-James.)

should be examined for evidence of lecithinase and lipase activity. Lecithinase activity is indicated by an opaque, whitish precipitate within the agar while lipase activity is indicated by an iridescent sheen on the surface growth. Many specimens suspected of containing clostridia are often contaminated with gram-negative species, and primary isolation on plates incubated anaerobically is difficult. Some alternatives to primary isolation are as follows: (1) The specimen is heated to 80°C for 10 to 15 minutes to destroy any vegetative bacteria and then incubated at 37°C before being subcultured on laboratory media. This spore selection technique can also be accomplished by treating the specimen with ethyl alcohol. (2) The specimen (except for some strains of *C. tetani*) is placed in tubes of thioglycolate broth containing glucose, incubated for 24 to 48 hours, and subcultured. In the thioglycolate broth the clostridial species ferment glucose, and the acids produced inhibit the growth of gram-negative organisms. (3) The specimen is transferred to chopped meat medium and sealed with petrolatum. The latter procedure is routinely used in isolation of anaerobic bacteria, especially when they appear to be in small numbers in the specimen. After suitable incubation at 37°C a subculture is made on other media.

The fermentation of various sugars is an important characteristic used in separating species of clostridia. Table 18-1 illustrates some fermentative and biochemical properties of the major species. In addition, some clostridia produce a considerable amount of gas during growth, a property that may be used in identifying *C. perfringens*. When milk is inoculated with this organism, the clotted milk is torn apart by the accumulated gas ("stormy fermentation").

An unusually large number of enzymes and toxins have been recovered from the filtrates of cultured clostridial species. They include hemolysins, collagenase, lipase, deoxyribonuclease, hyaluronidase, and the two potent exotoxins that cause tetanus and botulism. Many of these products are helpful in the identification or separation of species within the genus. For example, toxin tests are occasionally necessary for the identification of a few species. Sometimes only a toxin neutralization test will distinguish *C. botulinum* from *C. sporogenes* and *C. novyi*.

DISEASES CAUSED BY THE CLOSTRIDIA

C. botulinum, C. perfringens, and *C. tetani* produce potent toxins responsible for potentially fatal diseases: botulism, gas gangrene, and tetanus, respectively. However, the majority of clinical clostridia diseases are caused by other species.

Food Poisoning (Botulism)

Botulism is a noninfectious disease that results from the ingestion of preformed toxin in foods. About 25 percent of the incidences of clostridial food poisoning can be directly attributed to the species *C. botulinum*. *C. perfringens*, the primary causal agent of gas gangrene, is involved in the remainder of clostridial food poisonings. Food botulism is rarely seen in the United States (24 cases in 1989), but when outbreaks occur they are associated primarily with home canning procedures and not with commercial preparations. Most outbreaks are due to improper cooking of low acid vegetables or to fermentation procedures. Eskimos, for example, now ferment foods in plastic containers, which provide an anaerobic environment for clostridial growth.

Clostridium botulinum *Toxin*. *C. botulinum* produces eight immunologically distinct neurotoxins

Table 18-1. Characteristics Distinguishing Some of the Important Species of *Clostridium*

Species	Motility	Gelatin hydrolysis	Milk digestion	Fermentation Glucose	Maltose	Lactose	Sucrose	Mannitol	Indole formation	Spores
C. botulinum[a]	Yes	+	+[b]	+	+	−	−	−	−	OS
C. tetani	Yes	+	−	−	−	−	−	−	V	RT
C. perfringens	No	+	+	+	+	+	+	−	−	OS
C. ramosum	Yes	−	−	+	+	+	+	V	−	R/OT
C. innocuum	Yes	−	−	+	−	−	V	+	−	OT
C. difficile	Yes	V	−	+	−	−	−	+	−	OS
C. butyricum	Yes	−	−	+	+	+	+	−	−	OS

+ = positive reaction; − = negative reaction; V = variable reaction; / = either/or; O = oval; R = round; S = subterminal; T = terminal.
[a] Toxin neutralization test required for identification.
[b] Only group I species are positive.

(A, B, C_1, C_2, D, E, F, and G), permitting its separation into types. Types A, B, E, and F are responsible for human food poisonings (see Boxed Essay, p. 446). The toxins of some non-proteolytic strains are not completely active unless activated by proteolytic enzymes such as trypsin. Proteolytic strains produce their own enzymes to activate the toxin.

Type A toxin, which is responsible for most outbreaks of food poisoning associated with *C. botulinum*, is a complex consisting of the neurotoxin and a hemagglutinin. Since at least 1000 times more neurotoxin than neurotoxin-hemagglutinin complex is required to cause food poisoning in animals, it is believed that the hemagglutinin protects the neurotoxin from stomach acids and enzymes. Neurotoxin alone is rapidly inactivated by gastric enzymes and lowered pH. The complete toxin is sensitive to heat. To give some idea of the toxicity of *C. botulinum* toxin, less than 1×10^{-9} gm of toxin can kill a mouse. Its toxicity is similar to that of the neurotoxin produced by *C. tetani*. For comparison, the lethal concentration of diphtheria toxin is 1.5×10^{-6} gm; for *C. perfringens* toxin, 3.6×10^{-6} gm.

Pathogenesis. Botulism resulting from the ingestion of toxin-contaminated food is considered an *intoxication* rather than an infection. Once the active toxin is released in the intestine, it is absorbed and transported into the lymph and then the bloodstream. Clinical symptoms usually appear between 24 and 72 hours after the toxin has been absorbed from the intestinal tract. The toxin acts specifically on the peripheral nervous system, particularly the cranial nerves, and not the central nervous system. It prevents the release of acetylcholine at the neural synapses. Thus, muscle response to a nerve impulse is blocked because no neurotransmitter (acetylcholine) is released to excite the muscle. Symptoms of intoxication include double vision (diplopia) and dizziness, often followed by difficulty in swallowing and breathing. Nausea and vomiting may also be present during these manifestations. Death is usually due to respiratory failure from paralysis of the diaphragm. Fatality rates are high for type A poisoning (75 percent), lower for the other types (20 percent). The severity of type A intoxication may be related to the greater affinity of type A neurotoxin for nerve fibers.

Botulism may also be caused by the production of toxin by *C. botulinum* in wounds. *Wound botulism* has been recognized as a clinical entity since 1976, but only four or five cases per year are reported. The symptoms are the same as those in food poisoning caused by *C. botulinum*. Type A is usually implicated, with a case fatality rate of 25 percent. Although microorganisms are present in the wound, chemotherapy with antibiotics has not proved efficacious, probably on account of lack of blood supply in necrotic areas.

Infant botulism is the most frequently reported form of botulism, with approximately 60 cases being reported each year in the United States. Infant botulism is an infection resulting from ingestion of spores that germinate in the intestine and release toxin. Ingestion of honey contaminated with botulinal spores has been implicated in several cases of the disease. The CDC recommends that honey not be fed to infants less than one year old.

Most of the infants affected by infant botulism are less than 6 months old. The first signs of infection are constipation, followed by weakened sucking and swallowing and diminished gag reflex. Later there is a loss of head control. The most important aspect in the treatment of infant botulism is supportive care because of the possibility of respiratory insufficiency. The effect of antibiotics and antitoxin has not been established. Infant botulism is currently being investigated as one of the causes of sudden infant death syndrome.

Laboratory Diagnosis. Initial diagnosis depends on the identification of the toxin in the serum or stools of the affected individual. (In infant botulism only stools will consistently reveal the presence of toxin.) This is often followed by intraperitoneal injections of extracts of the patient's serum or liquefied stool samples into lab-

INTERNATIONAL OUTBREAK OF TYPE E BOTULISM ASSOCIATED WITH UNGUTTED SALTED WHITEFISH

On November 2, 1987, a 39-year-old Russian immigrant and his 9-year-old son were admitted to a suburban New York hospital with symptoms indicative of botulism. The father had 10 days earlier purchased a whole, ungutted, salted, air-dried whitefish known as either ribyetz or kapchunka from a delicatessen in Queens, New York City. He and his son had eaten the fish on October 30 and 31. On November 3, 1987, CDC received a report from the Ministry of Health, Jerusalem, Israel, of five additional cases suspected to be botulism; one case was fatal. The patients had eaten ribyetz purchased in a grocery in New York City on October 17 and taken to Israel. The fish as well as a serum sample from one surviving patient subsequently yielded type E botulinum toxin.

The company distributing the whitefish was identified and the New York City Department of Health issued an embargo on the sale and distribution of ribyetz or kapchunka and removed the implicated product from the shelves of stores selling it.

Ribyetz or kapchunka is an ethnic food consumed in this country primarily by Russian immigrants. It has been implicated as a vehicle for botulism twice in recent years and two Russian immigrants died after eating the fish. The mechanism of contamination of the ribyetz has not been established. However, *Clostridium botulinum* spores can be found in the intestinal contents of fish, and the fact that the fish were uneviscerated may have been important.

In addition to halting the distribution of the fish, officials in New York City and New York State are developing regulations that would in effect prohibit the production and sale of such uneviscerated whitefish.

From *M.M.W.R.* 36:812,1987

oratory mice. The mice will succumb in 1 to 4 days if *C. botulinum* toxin is present in the specimens. If the suspect food is available, it too can be checked for the presence of toxin or anaerobic sporeformers (Fig. 18-5).

Treatment and Prevention. The earlier botulism is detected, the better the prognosis. Case fatality rates in the 1950s were near 60 percent but have since declined to less than 15 percent because of advances in acute respiratory intensive care. Even before a bacteriological diagnosis is made, trivalent antitoxin, prepared against the toxins of types A, B, and E, is given intravenously to patients with foodborne or wound botulism but not to patients with infant botulism. Because the antitoxin is prepared from horse serum, the patient is generally tested for sensitivity before injection. If the patient has neurological symptoms, he or she should be placed in an intensive care unit, where cardiac and respiratory function may be

Fig. 18-5. Sporulating cells of *Clostridium botulinum* type A. Spores are subterminal. (Courtesy P. D. Walker.)

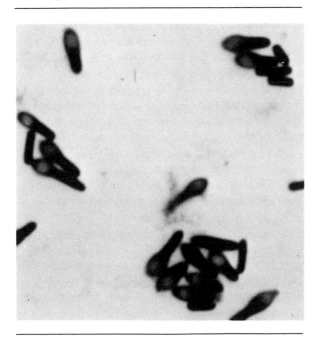

monitored. Guainidine hydrochloride is sometimes used during treatment to enhance the release of acetylcholine in the nerve junctions to prevent respiratory failure.

Prevention of botulism is best accomplished in the home by using sterilized containers and pressure cookers. Since the *C. botulinum* toxin is heat-labile, it is suggested that whenever possible home-canned fruits and vegetables be heated to 100°C for 10 minutes before ingestion.

Medicinal Uses of Botulinal Toxin. Type A botulinal toxin has recently (January, 1990) been approved for treating eye disorders. Some eye disorders, such as cross-eye and blepharospasm, in which muscle spasms cause the eyes either to wander or close involuntarily, can be controlled by the toxin. The toxin is injected directly into specific sites where it blocks muscular response to the nerve impulses responsible for the disorder. The toxin interferes with the release of the neurotransmitter acetylcholine. The drug has not yet been approved for use in children under 12 years of age.

Gas Gangrene

Gas gangrene is a disease in which there is severe muscle necrosis and invasion of the bloodstream by clostridial species, particularly *C. perfringens*. Other species that may act in concert with *C. perfringens* are *C. novyi*, *C. septicum*, and *C. histolyticum*. *C. perfringens* is a non-motile aerotolerant organism that does not produce spores in ordinary culture media. All the *Clostridium* species associated with gas gangrene can be found as commensals in the intestinal tract of humans and animals. All of them produce potent toxins.

Clostridium perfringens *Toxins.* Of the 11 toxins produced by *C. perfringens*, four are used to separate the species into five toxigenic groups (A, B, C, D, and E). Only types A and C produce disease in humans. All five types produce various proportions of four toxins (alpha, beta, epsilon, and iota), but the most important is the *alpha toxin*, also called *phospholipase C*. Alpha toxin acts as a lecithinase and hydrolyzes lecithin, a component of eukaryotic membranes, and during infection destroys red blood cells and leukocytes. Other toxins released during infection that may take part in pathogenesis are collagenase, hemolysin, proteinase, and deoxyribonuclease. The toxin demonstrating collagenase activity is believed to attack healthy connective tissue in the skin and the connective tissue supporting muscle fibers. It is the probable cause of the extensive muscle destruction observed in gas gangrene. Hemolysin lyses the red blood cells of most mammalian species. Proteinase is thought to be important in degrading necrotic tissue, while deoxyribonuclease may destroy leukocytes by its ability to depolymerize DNA.

Pathogenesis. Gas gangrene is an infection that requires a site for germination of spores and replication of vegetative cells. Such a site is available when tissue has been traumatized by foreign bodies (for example, puncture wounds) and is devitalized, thereby offering an anaerobic environment. Clostridial wound infection may be divided into two major clinical conditions: *anaerobic cellulitis* and *anaerobic myositis* (true gas gangrene). Anaerobic cellulitis involves necrotic tissue, but the organism does not invade healthy muscle. Anaerobic cellulitis is the less severe infection. There is seldom toxemia or shock. True gas gangrene is often a mixed infection involving several *Clostridium* species. Most cases of the disease appear during war or after automobile accidents or surgical procedures such as those involving the uterus. Deep wounds and areas of dead tissue favor germination. Toxins are liberated by vegetative cells, and during the course of infection gases such as hydrogen and carbon dioxide may be released by metabolizing bacteria. The first symptoms of gas gangrene are usually observed 72 hours after traumatization of tissue. Severe local pain is felt in the area of the wound. A few hours later there is swelling of the wound, giving it a stretched and reddened appearance. Still later the skin ruptures, revealing a necrotic, foul-smelling wound. The most important symptoms of gas gangrene are the delirium, apathy, and disorientation exhibited by the patient in the early stages of the disease. Death is believed to be due to severe toxemia and to the effect of toxin on vital organs.

Laboratory Diagnosis. A tentative diagnosis of gas gangrene is often made by examination of the wound for gram-positive spore formers. This is usually difficult because *C. perfringens* does not often sporulate in tissue. In addition, the wound may contain a wide variety of other microorganisms including nonpathogenic clostridia. Presumptive identification of *C. perfringens* can be made by first inoculating a blood (rabbit, sheep, or human) agar plate with the specimen and incubating it anaerobically. Gram-stained cells show a typical "boxcar" shape as opposed to the rounded ends of other clostridial species (Fig. 18-6). Colonies of *C. perfringens* appear surrounded by an inner zone of complete hemolysis and an outer zone of incomplete hemolysis. The isolated colonies may also be subcultured to egg yolk agar plates to demonstrate the production of alpha toxin (lecithinase).

Treatment and Prevention. Successful treatment of gas gangrene consists in the immediate debridement of the wound to remove all dead tissue, application of antiserum that has been prepared from filtrates of the major clostridial species that produce gas gangrene, and antibiotic therapy. Penicillin and tetracyclines have been the antibiotic drugs of choice.

Treatment of gas gangrene patients with high concentrations of oxygen at elevated pressures is receiving a great deal of attention today. This procedure, called *hyperbaric oxygen therapy*, at one time was used almost exclusively for persons suffering from carbon monoxide poisoning and decompression sickness. The patient inhales 100

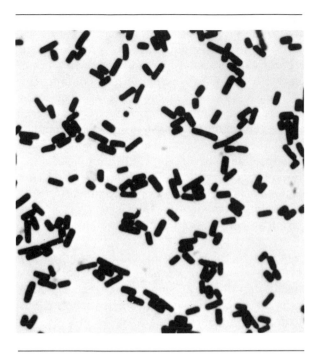

Fig. 18-6. Photomicrograph of *Clostridium perfringens*. Note the boxcar shape of the cells. (Courtesy P. D. Walker.)

percent oxygen through an aviator's mask in a chamber initially pressurized to approximately 3 atmospheres of air for a period of 1 hour. Then follows a 30-minute period of 100 percent oxygen at 2 atmospheres of pressure, and finally comes a 30-minute period of 100 percent oxygen at 1 atmosphere of pressure. The treatment is repeated every 8 hours, the total number of treatments seldom exceeding eight. The principle behind this treatment is that anaerobes in the presence of oxygen produce a strong oxidizing agent, hydrogen peroxide, which can be lethal to the organisms. Oxygen has no effect on the circulating toxin, which must be detoxified in the body. Hyperbaric oxygen treatment is potentially very dangerous and must be administered by qualified personnel.

Gas gangrene is always a possible hazard when surgery is being performed on areas of the body that are easily contaminated by one's intestinal microflora—the lower limbs, thighs, and buttocks. Infections have been greatly reduced when the area to be operated on and surrounding tissue are first swabbed with compresses of iodophors. Best results are obtained when the area is swabbed just 15 minutes before surgery.

Food Poisoning
(*Clostridium perfringens*)

C. perfringens is a common cause of a mild form of food poisoning in humans. The condition is the result of ingestion of a large number of viable vegetative cells. Foodborne disease in the United States is due to type A *C. perfringens* and is most frequently associated with a meat product. The organism survives cooking by sporulation and then germinates when the food is cooled. If the food is not reheated, many vegetative cells are produced. Ingestion of approximately 10^8 cells will cause food poisoning. The ingested bacteria sporulate in the intestine and produce an enterotoxin that is part of the spore coat. The enterotoxin causes secretion of fluid and electrolytes (sodium and chloride ions).

Foodborne disease caused by *C. perfringens* type C is associated with a high mortality. The illness is referred to as *enteritis necroticans* and is characterized by hemorrhaging and gangrene of the intestine. The severity of the disease is believed to be due to a beta toxin that is normally inactivated by proteolytic enzymes. The disease is observed primarily in areas outside the United States. Large outbreaks of disease have been observed in New Guinea. Infection is associated with feasts where contaminated and improperly cooked pork is ingested. The disease is called "pig-bel."

C. perfringens type A food poisoning ranks high in terms of number of cases per year in the United states (see Table 10-5, p. 246). The vehicles implicated in disease, in order of importance, are beef, Mexican food, turkey, ham, and chicken. Improper storage or holding temperature and inadequate cooking of food are the principal causes of disease. The major symptoms are abdominal pain, diarrhea, nausea, and vomiting. The incubation period is 24 to 30 hours and rarely are fatalities encountered.

Confirmation of foodborne illness can be determined by (A) count of more than 10^5 C. perfringens per gram of suspected food, (B) median spore count of greater than 10^6 C. perfringens per gram of stool, or (C) isolation of same serotype of C. perfringens from food and stool. Serological tests for enterotoxin detection in feces are now available and include reversed passive latex agglutination test.

Treatment of C. perfringens food poisoning does not require antibiotics since the disease is mild and self-limiting. It is important that body fluids and electrolytes be replenished. This type of food poisoning can be prevented by properly cooking food and, if food is to be reheated, by ensuring that the internal temperature of the food is greater than 75°C so that vegetative cells are destroyed.

Enterotoxin-Associated Diarrhea

There is accumulating evidence that enterotoxin-induced diarrhea can occur in the absence of a food vehicle. The diarrhea is associated with antibiotic treatment and occurs almost exclusively in the hospitalized elderly patient. The patients were observed to have stools in which C. perfringens numbered 5×10^7 to 4×10^9 per gram of stool. The diarrhea lasted at least 7 days and this is to be compared to the 24 hours seen in foodborne diarrhea.

Tetanus

Tetanus, like gas gangrene, is an infection often stemming from a complication of traumatized tissue. The causative agent, C. tetani, is found primarily in cultivated soil but also appears in the intestinal tract of about 25 percent of humans. In underdeveloped countries tetanus is a common cause of neonatal death. In the United States, 53 cases of tetanus were recorded in 1989.

Tetanus Toxins. The complications of tetanus are due to the release of a potent neurotoxin called *tetanospasmin.* Tetanospasmin is a heat-labile protein with a toxicity similar to that of C. botulinum toxin. Every milligram of toxin-nitrogen is lethal for 2×10^8 laboratory mice. The toxin that is released on lysis of the vegetative cell acts on the central nervous system. Unlike botulinum toxin, which blocks transmission of nerve impulses, tetanus toxin causes the continued excitation of motor neurons in the spinal cord. This occurs because tetanus toxin prevents the release of inhibitory mediators. The effect of tetanus toxin can be observed as a spastic paralysis.

Pathogenesis. C. tetani gains entrance to the body through wounds or abrasions. The spores germinate only in the absence of oxygen, and such a condition is encountered when the wound is deep or contains considerable necrotic tissue. Piercing of the ears, circumcisions, and abortions are also predisposing factors that can lead to tetanus when hygienic precautions are not taken. *Tetanus neonatorum,* for example, is a frequent cause of death in developing countries. This type of tetanus is the direct result of cutting the umbilical cord with unsterilized instruments or packing the umbilical stump with mud. Once the organism germinates in the tissue, the toxin acts directly on the motor neurons of the central nervous system. The toxin causes the continued contraction of various voluntary muscles, which is referred to as *tetany.* The symptoms of the disease appear in 4 to 6 days as a rule; however, up to 6 weeks is not unusual. This wide range in incubation time seems to depend on two factors: the time for anaerobic conditions to develop at the site of infection and the time required for any toxin to reach the central nervous system. The predominant symptoms of tetanus are primarily muscle rigidity and muscle spasm. Rigidity affects the muscles of the jaw (masseter muscles), abdomen, and spine. Muscle spasm is seen most often in the mouth but may occur in any part of the body. The convulsive contraction of the voluntary muscles of the jaw is referred to as *lockjaw* (*trismus*). Death is often the result of some type of respiratory failure—pneumonia, pulmonary edema, or asphyxia.

Laboratory Diagnosis. Diagnosis can be made on clinical grounds. Patients usually have a wound, exhibit trismus, and have a history of no immunization. Stained smears of the material from a wound are very unreliable for the identification of *C. tetani* because of the presence of other clostridia. Material from the wound can be cultured directly on blood agar or transferred to cooked meat medium heated to 80°C for 10 to 15 minutes to destroy nonsporeformers. After 24 hours' incubation on blood agar, the plate should be examined for swarming (motility). A spore stain reveals characteristic terminal spores shaped like tennis rackets (Fig. 18-7). Definitive proof that the isolated species is *C. tetani* is obtained by determining neurotoxin production. This is measured by injecting the filtrate from a pure culture of *C. tetani* into the leg of a mouse; a second mouse receives an injection of the filtrate plus the tetanus antitoxin. After a few hours the unprotected mouse displays stiffness and muscular spasms in the injected leg that extend to the tail and then to the opposite leg. The protected mouse shows no adverse effects from the toxin.

Treatment. Suspected cases of tetanus, even before isolation of *C. tetani*, are first treated by administration of tetanus antitoxin to neutralize any toxin in the blood. The antitoxin will not neutralize toxin already fixed to nerve cells. Antibiotics such as penicillin are usually given to destroy any clostridial cells and prevent further toxin production. Where there is a foul contaminated wound, it is important to remove surgically the necrotic tissue or debris that is creating the anaerobic environment. Even if all these measures are performed, once the toxin is attached to the nerve cells they will not alter the course of the disease. The basic treatment is symptomatic; that is, the convulsions and spasms must

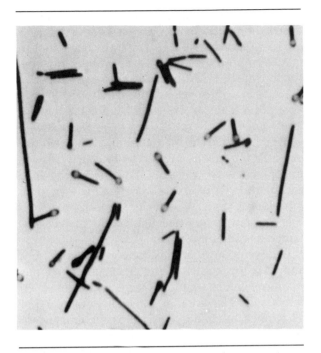

Fig. 18-7. Photomicrograph of *Clostridium tetani* demonstrating the characteristic tennis racket–shaped terminal spores. (Courtesy P. D. Walker.)

be controlled by drugs. Barbiturates are therefore routinely employed to sedate the patient and to control the spasm.

A great deal of controversy had been centered around the use of antitoxin prepared from horse serum (tetanus immune globulin, or TIG). Some physicians will not administer such antitoxin because many individuals are sensitive to the horse serum proteins. It is also believed that the body's immune system eliminates the injected antitoxin too rapidly, and thus it provides inadequate protection. For these reasons some hospitals and private practitioners use only antitoxin prepared from the gamma globulin fraction of humans.

Prevention. The only effective way to control tetanus is through the prophylactic use of the tetanus toxoid. The toxoid, which incorporates an adjuvant (aluminum salts) to increase its immunizing potency, is given routinely with diphtheria toxoid and pertussis vaccine (DTP). An initial dose is normally administered a few months after birth, a second dose 4 to 6 months later, and finally a reinforcing dose 6 to 12 months after the second injection. A final booster is given between the ages of 4 and 6 years. For many years booster doses of tetanus toxoid were administered every 3 to 5 years; that practice has been discontinued since it has been shown that a single booster dose can afford protection for 10 to 20 years. Serious hypersensitivity reactions have occurred when too many doses of toxoid were administered over a period of years. Booster doses today are generally given only when an individual has sustained a wound infection.

In developing countries, where health services and delivery teams are limited, neonatal tetanus is a problem that requires special strategies. Continuous immunization of pregnant women and of all women of childbearing age is recommended. In addition, the training of midwives has caused a precipitous drop in neonatal tetanus. These strategies are used in addition to the primary immunization in early childhood and at schools.

Other Clostridial Conditions

Antibiotic-Associated Clostridial Disease. The microflora of the gut serves as a barrier against colonization by pathogens. Oral antibiotics used to treat infection disturb the gut microflora and make the host susceptible to colonization by pathogens and to overgrowth by commensal species. An important disease associated with antibiotic therapy, particularly in compromised elderly patients, is called *pseudomembraneous colitis*. This disease is characterized by an inflammation of the colonic mucosa and the formation of a pseudomembrane composed of fibrin, mucus, necrotic epithelial cells, and leukocytes. Symptoms of disease include diarrhea, fever, and nausea, which may progress to dehydration, septicemia, shock, and death. The organism responsible for this condition is *Clostridium difficile. C. difficile* is found as a commensal in the gut of only a small percentage of healthy adults but is highly visible in the hospital environment. Patients with pseudomembranous colitis have diarrhea and the organism can be released into the environment. In addition, infants carry high levels of *C. difficile* in the intestine but are refractory to the disease. Hospital personnel are often responsible for transmitting the microorganisms to patients. *C. difficile* can persist in the environment for months because of its ability to produce spores.

C. difficile produces two toxins, A and B. Toxin A is primarily an enterotoxin while toxin B is a cytotoxin. Toxin A is more responsible for leakage of fluids while toxin B directly affects the structure of mucosal cells.

Treatment of pseudomembranous colitis can often be achieved by discontinuation of the offending antibiotic. The most common method, however, is to use an antibiotic such as vancomycin, which is bactericidal for *C. difficile*. In Europe metronidazole is an effective and less costly antimicrobial in treatment of the disease.

Necrotizing Enterocolitis. Necrotizing enterocolitis is a fulminating, sometimes lethal condition of sick premature babies. Symptoms include abdominal distention, blood in stools, shock, and gas in the bowel wall. Breast-fed babies are protected against this disease. It is hypothesized that immunoglobulins or other factors in the mother's milk protect the baby from the overgrowth of clostridial species in the intestinal tract.

Neutropenic Enterocolitis. Neutropenic enterocolitis is an infection associated with congenital neutropenia, or neutropenia associated with cancer chemotherapy, leukemia, and cancer of the colon. The most commonly associated pathogen is *C. septicum*, but other indigenous *Clostridium* species may also be involved. Infection results in edema, hemorrhage, and necrosis of cecum and colon. The case-fatality rate is 50 to 100 percent. Surgical intervention is required to prevent fatal outcomes.

There are a wide variety of toxins produced by species of *Clostridium* and keeping track of them is difficult. We have outlined some but not all of the clostridial toxins and their known activities in human disease in Table 18-2.

Table 18-2 Some of the Important Species of *Clostridium* and Their Toxins That Are Associated With Human Disease

Species	Toxin	Activity/disease
C. botulinum	Neurotoxin	Prevents release of acetylcholine from nerve ending/botulism
C. tetani	Neurotoxin	Prevents release of inhibitory mediators of spinal cord motor neurons/tetanus
C. perfringens	Major	
	Alpha	Phospholipase C/gas gangrene (myonecrosis)
	Beta (B and C strains)	Necrotic enteritis(pig-bel)/enterotoxemia
	Epsilon (B and D strains)	Increases permeability of intestine/ enterotoxemia
	Iota	ADP-ribosylation/enterotoxemia
	Other	
	Enterotoxin	Altered membrane permeability/foodborne diarrhea
	Delta (B and C strains)	Hemolysin/gas gangrene
	Kappa	Collagenase/gas gangrene
	Lambda (B, D, E strains)	Protease (digests gelatin, hemoglobin)/gas gangrene
	Mu	Hyaluronidase/gas gangrene
	Nu	DNase/gas gangrene
	Neuraminidase	Hydrolysis of neuraminic acid/gas gangrene
C. difficile	Toxin A	Enterotoxin-altered membrane permeability/ antibiotic-associated pseudomembranous colitis
	Toxin B	Cytotoxin/antibiotic-associated pseudomembranous colitis
C. sordelii (*C. bifermentans*)	Alpha	Phospholipase C/acute edematous wound infections
	Beta	Contains lethal and hemorrhagic components that are equivalent to toxins A and B, respectively, of *C. difficile*/acute edematous wound infections
C. novyi	Alpha	Lethal/gas gangrene
	Beta and Gamma	Phospholipase C
C. chauvoei (*C. septicum*)	Alpha	Lethal, necrotizing/gas gangrene, neutropenic enterocolitis
	Beta	DNase
	Gamma	Hyaluronidase
C. histolyticum	Alpha	Lethal, necrotizing/toxemia of gas gangrene
	Beta	Collagenase/gas gangrene

Table 18-3. Characteristics of the Major Species of *Bacillus* and *Clostridium*

Genus and species	Important morphological, physiological, and staining traits	Disease association	Mechanism of transmission	Virulence factors	Treatment and prevention
Bacillus	Gram-positive aerobic spore-formers				
B. anthracis	Capsule produced in culture	Anthrax—cutaneous, respiratory, and gastrointestinal	Contact with contaminated animals or hides	Capsule; protein exotoxin composed of three fractions	Penicillin; vaccination of cattle; toxoid for humans to prevent occupation-associated infections
B. cereus		Food poisoning, ocular disease	Ingestion of contaminated food; ocular disease from penetrating wounds	Two enterotoxins for gastrointestinal disease	None required for food poisoning; clindamycin plus aminoglycoside for ocular disease
Clostridium	Gram-positive anaerobic spore-formers				
C. botulinum	Motile	Food poisoning, wound botulism, infant botulism	Ingestion of contaminated food; soil contamination of wound; ingestion of spore-contaminated foods by infants	Neurotoxin	Trivalent antitoxin for food-borne and wound botulism; supportive care for infant botulism
C. perfringens	Non-motile	Gas gangrene	Soil contamination of deep wounds	Alpha toxin (lecithinase)	Wound debridement, application of antiserum, and penicillin therapy; hyperbaric oxygen for extreme cases
		Food poisoning	Ingestion of contaminated food	Enterotoxin	Replenishment of body fluids
C. tetani	Motile, terminal spores	Tetanus	Soil contamination of deep wounds	Neurotoxin	Tetanus antitoxin plus penicillin; toxoid as part of DTP immunization
C. difficile		Antibiotic-associated pseudomembranous colitis	Contact with infected hospital personnel or contaminated environment	Enterotoxin and cytotoxin	Vancomycin for treatment and discontinuation of original antibiotic therapy

SUMMARY

A summary of the characteristics of *Bacillus* and *Clostridium* species is presented in Table 18-3.

QUESTIONS FOR STUDY

Select the best response or responses for each of the following:

1. Which of the following is *not* characteristic of *Bacillus anthracis*?
   A. Produces a polysaccharide capsule.
   B. Produces a complex exotoxin one of whose activities is called edema factor.
   C. Is susceptible to penicillin.
   D. Produces disease primarily in animals.

2. The organism responsible for causing foodborne disease associated with rice dishes is:
   A. *Bacillus circulans*
   B. *Bacillus subtilis*
   C. *Bacillus cereus*
   D. *Clostridium botulinum*

3. Egg yolk agar is frequently used to identify clostridia that produce
   A. Proteinases
   B. Hyaluronidase
   C. Neurotoxin
   D. Lecithinase

4. Antibiotic-associated pseudomembranous colitis:

   A. Is caused by the overgrowth of *C. perfringens* in the intestine.
   B. Is due to toxins released by *C. botulinum*.
   C. Is caused by *C. difficile*.
   D. Is caused by the toxicity of certain antibiotics such as clindamycin.

5. The two most frequent causes of foodborne disease outbreaks in the United States, in order of importance, are
   A. *C. botulinum* and *Staphylococcus aureus*
   B. *S. aureus* and *Bacillus cereus*
   C. *C. perfringens* and *S. aureus*
   D. *S. aureus* and *C. perfringens*

6. Infant botulism may be caused by
   A. Toxin released in honey-containing formula
   B. Overgrowth of *C. difficile* in the intestine
   C. Toxin released by spores germinating in the intestinal tract
   D. Overgrowth of *C. botulinum* in the intestine

Fill in the blank:

7. In Third World countries contamination of the umbilical cord at birth frequently leads to infection by *Clostridium* _____ .

8. Hyperbaric oxygen treatment is used as a last resort in the treatment of an infectious disease called _____ .

9. The only clostridial species that is nonmotile is _____ .

10. The spores of *Bacillus* _____ are routinely used to test the efficiency of autoclaving.

11. The edema associated with *B. anthracis* infection is believed to be caused by the enzyme _____ .

ADDITIONAL READINGS

Finegold, S. M., George, W. L., and Mulligen, M. E. Anaerobic infections. Part I. *Disease of the Month* 31:50,1985.

Lyerly, D. M., Krivan, H. C., and Wilkins, T. *Clostridium difficile:* Its diseases and toxins. *Clin. Microbiol. Rev.* 1(1):1,1988.

Peterson, D. R., Eklund, M. W., and Chinn, N. M. The sudden infant death syndrome and infant botulism. *Rev. Infect. Dis.* 1:639,1979.

Smith, L. D. S. *The Pathogenic Anaerobic Bacteria.* Springfield, IL: Thomas, 1975.

van Heyningen, S. Tetanus Toxin, in F. Dorner and J. Drew (eds.). *International Encyclopedia of Pharmacology and Therapeutics.* Section 119, page 549. Oxford, England: Pergamon Press, 1986.

Hatheway, C. L. Toxigenic clostridia. *Clin. Microbiol. Rev.* 3(1):66,1990.

19. CORYNEBACTERIUM DIPHTHERIAE

OBJECTIVES

To describe the symptoms associated with diphtheria

To describe the mechanism of action of diphtheria toxin

To describe the in vivo test for determining the toxigenicity of *C. diphtheriae*

To describe those methods used to treat and prevent diphtheria

To outline the schedule for immunization against diphtheria

To explain the importance of diphtheroids, *Listeria*, and *Erysipelothrix rhusiopathiae* as agents of disease

Corynebacterium is a genus belonging to a group of bacteria called *coryneforms*. Coryneforms include several genera that are plant and animal pathogens. The most important human pathogen, *Corynebaceterium diphtheriae*, is the etiological agent of the disease diphtheria. Diphtheria is rarely seen in developed countries because of mass immunization programs but it is still an im-portant disease in developing countries. The effect that the immunization program has had on the incidence and mortality of the disease in the United States is illustrated in Figure 19-1.

We will first discuss the characteristics of *C. diphtheriae* and then examine related groups of organisms.

Fig. 19-1. Diphtheria annual incidence and mortality ratios and case fatality ratios in the United States, 1920–1988. (From Centers for Disease Control, Atlanta, GA.)

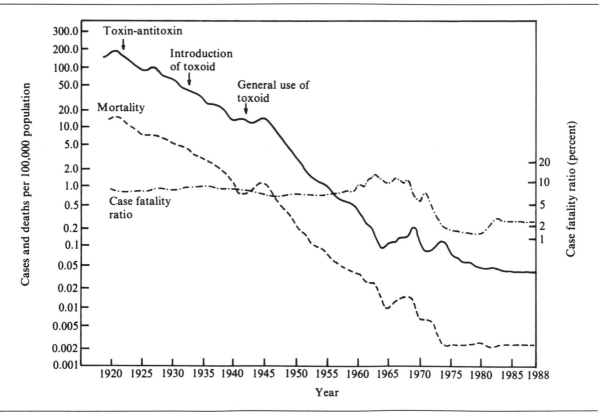

GENERAL CHARACTERISTICS

Corynebacterium diphtheriae is an obligate aerobe found in the upper respiratory tract of humans. It is a nonmotile, gram-positive pleomorphic bacillus averaging between 2 and 6 μm in length and 0.5 and 1.0 μm in diameter. In older cultures the bacilli appear club shaped. The bacilli are capable of concentrating phosphate in the form of polymerized metaphosphate granules. When the cell is stained with methylene blue, the metaphosphate granules become apparent and give the bacillus a beaded appearance (Fig. 19-2). These granules are called *metachromatic granules*. Because of their unusual arrangement after cell division the bacilli appear in palisades (parallel rows) and resemble Chinese letters. *Corynebacterium* and other coryneforms have a close relationship with the mycobacteria and nocardiae (see Chapters 24 and 28) because of their cell walls. The cell walls of these groups possess arabinose, galactose, meso-diaminopimelic acid, and mycolic acids.

There are three characteristic biotypes of *C. diphtheriae*: *gravis*, *intermedius*, and *mitis*. Their

Fig. 19-2. Stained smear of diphtheria bacilli. The darkly stained areas are polyphosphate or metachromatic granules. (From R. R. Gillies and T. C. Dodds, *Bacteriology Illustrated*. London: Churchill Livingstone, 1976.)

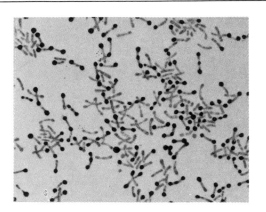

names purportedly correspond to the severity of the disease; however, this is not always the case. The toxigenicity of these strains is directly related to the presence of a temperate (does not lyse the cell) bacteriophage that carries information for toxin production (tox gene). If "cured" of its temperate virus, the bacterium is no longer toxigenic. Many normally nontoxigenic strains of corynebacteria can be converted to toxigenic strains by infecting them with the appropriate temperate bacteriophage.

PATHOGENESIS

Humans are the only natural host of *C. diphtheriae*. The organism is found in the upper respiratory tract but skin lesions may also be a source of the organisms (cutaneous diphtheria). Contact with respiratory or cutaneous discharges is the means of transmission from person to person.

Diphtheria may be divided into two types, respiratory and cutaneous. The incubation period for respiratory diphtheria is 2 to 6 days. Symptoms initially include sore throat, slight fever, and malaise. The bacilli are harbored in the mucous membranes of the passageways of the oral cavity. The toxin elaborated by the bacilli causes necrosis of the mucosal cells, which aids in bacterial multiplication. The bacilli do not invade any underlying tissue, nor do they enter the bloodstream. The inflammatory response of the infected tissue causes the accumulation of a grayish white exudate that clots and attaches to various passageways, forming a pseudomembrane. The pseudomembrane consists of neutrophils, corynebacteria, and desquamated epithelial cells enmeshed in a dense fibrinous network. The membrane can be found over the mucosa of the mouth, pharynx, larynx, or trachea. If the inflammatory response involves the laryngeal or tracheal areas, respiratory obstruction can occur.

If not remedied by tracheostomy or intubation, this condition can cause suffocation. Death in most instances, however, results from heart failure owing to the effects of the toxin on heart tissue. Nontoxigenic strains of gravis, intermedius, and mitis have been isolated from patients with clinical symptoms similar to those of diphtheria. In these patients a sufficient level of antitoxin was still present in the serum for protection against toxigenic strains. It has been suggested that other bacteria or viruses may cooperate with the nontoxigenic strains to produce a diphtheria-like illness. In the majority of such infections the clinical symptoms are less severe than those produced by toxigenic biotypes.

A great deal of research in the past 10 to 15 years has been directed at the genesis, chemistry, and physiological effects of diphtheria toxin. Expression of the tox gene is controlled by the level of iron in the cell. Maximum levels of toxin are produced only when iron becomes the growth-limiting nutrient. Studies with phage mutants have indicated that a bacterial factor is also involved in control of toxin production. It is currently believed that *C. diphtheriae* synthesizes an inactive molecule that in the presence of iron becomes activated and represses the synthesis of toxin. Toxin is released by the bacterial cell as a single inactive polypeptide but is later cleaved into two fragments, A and B. Toxin is believed to enter eukaryotic cells and inhibit protein synthesis in the following way:

1. The hydrophilic (carboxyl) end of the toxin is positively charged and interacts with specific receptors on the cytoplasmic membrane of the eukaryotic cell.
2. A cellular protease nicks the polypeptide, causing the release of the carboxyl tail (Fig. 19-3), and also affects the amino end of the polypeptide.
3. Release of the carboxyl tail allows the hydrophobic portion of the molecule (fragment B) to enter the lipid bilayer of the cell. Fragment B forms a channel in the lipid bilayer and facilitates the transport of fragment A into the cytoplasm.
4. Both fragment A and fragment B are required to halt protein synthesis in living cells, but only fragment A is enzymatically active in inhibiting eukaryotic peptide chain elongation. The toxin accomplishes this by catalyzing the transfer of the ADP-ribose component from NAD^+ to a single amino acid residue of elongation factor, which is thus inactivated.

Once the toxin has entered the cell, antitoxin has no effect on its activity. If the toxin is only ab-

Fig. 19-3. Proposed action of cellular protease on the polypeptide toxin of *Corynebacterium diphtheriae*.

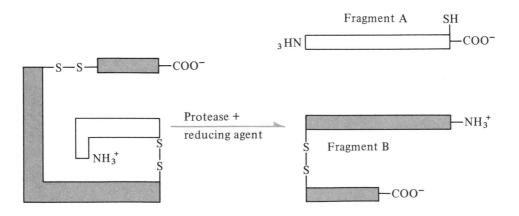

sorbed to the cell surface, antitoxin can neutralize it.

Cutaneous diphtheria can be manifested as an impetigo-like lesion occurring on the face, or the lesions may appear on the legs. Both toxigenic and nontoxigenic strains can be found in the lesions. The intensity of the infection is unaffected by a strain's toxigenic potential. Infections are often the result of insect bites or other skin trauma as well as poor personal hygiene. Cutaneous diphtheria is more common in tropical areas. In the United States most cases occur in the southern states. Some studies have demonstrated that the strain carried in the cutaneous lesion is also carried in the respiratory tract in more than 50 percent of the cases. It has been suggested, but not proved, that the cutaneous carrier, particularly in crowded living conditions, is a source of respiratory diphtheria.

IMMUNITY

Because diphtheria is much less severe in the fully immunized individual, all members of the community should have access to prophylactic immunization with the diphtheria toxoid. Many people who have an artificially acquired or a natural immunity are hypersensitive to the toxoid and should not be given injections of such a preparation. The *Schick test* is a screening device used to separate immune from susceptible individuals. In the test a small amount of dilute toxin is injected intracutaneously in the forearm. A positive test, which indicates that there is little or no antitoxin in the serum, is characterized by a localized erythema 24 to 48 hours after injection. A negative test or no erythema at the site of injection indicates that there is sufficient antitoxin in the serum to protect the individual. False-positives often arise among older children and adults despite high levels of antitoxin in their serum. For this reason a control test is performed on the opposite arm by using toxin detoxified by heating. An allergic response, however, to the detoxified protein can still occur. If the tissue response at the control site parallels that at the test site in size and duration, the Schick test is considered negative.

LABORATORY DIAGNOSIS

The symptoms suggestive of diphtheria are fever, chills, sore throat, serosanguineous nasal discharge, and enlarged cervical nodes. Fluorescent antibody provides a rapid presumptive test but should be used in conjunction with other laboratory tests. Swab cultures should be taken from the nares, pharynx, nasopharynx, or cutaneous sites and plated on Loeffler (coagulated serum) medium. The overnight culture can be stained with methylene blue for presumptive diagnosis (metachromatic granules) and observed for typical morphology. Growth from the overnight culture should be subcultured to a blood agar and cysteine-tellurite medium. On cysteine-tellurite medium corynebacterium reduces tellurite and the colonies appear black or gun-metal gray. Each colony type should be gram stained. Coryneforms on the cysteine-tellurite plates should be subcultured for biochemical and toxin testing (see Table 19-1 for important biochemical tests). The blood agar plate is used to screen beta-hemolytic streptococci and *Staphylococcus aureus* and any corynebacteria not growing on cysteine-tellurite.

All *C. diphtheriae* isolates are sent to a reference laboratory for toxin testing. The toxin tests used may be of the in vitro or in vivo types. In the in vivo test a small area of the abdomen of two guinea pigs is shaved. One animal is administered diphtheria antitoxin intraperitoneally. After 2 to 4 hours both animals are injected intradermally with a dilution of the unknown suspension of bacilli. If toxigenic bacilli were

Table 19-1. Characteristics of Some Important Species of *Corynebacterium* That Cause Disease in Humans

Species	Normal habitat	Disease	Important biochemical properties
C. diphtheriae	Normal flora of upper respiratory tract of humans	Respiratory (diphtheria), cutaneous	Ferments glucose and maltose, produces catalase; most strains reduce nitrate; acid without gas is produced from glucose and maltose
C. equi (Rhodococcus equi formerly)	Found in soil near livestock	Pulmonary infection in patients with neoplastic disease	Cannot ferment carbohydrates
C. xerosis	Normal flora of skin and nasopharynx of humans	Endocarditis in patients with prosthetic cardiac valves	Can reduce nitrate, ferments several carbohydrates
C. pseudodiphtheriticum (C. hofmannii)	Normal flora of pharynx of humans	Endocarditis	Cannot ferment carbohydrates, produces urease, can reduce nitrate
C. jeikeium (formerly called CDC Group JK)	Indigenous to skin	Blood, tissue, and wound infections in those with indwelling catheters	Cannot produce urease, cannot reduce nitrate, cannot ferment carbohydrates
C. ulcerans	Pharynx of humans	Diphtheria-like illness	Produces urease, does not reduce nitrate
C. pseudotuberculosis (C. ovis)	Respiratory tract of domestic animals	Lymphadenitis, pneumonia	Produces phospholipase D and urease
Arcanobacterium (Corynebacterium haemolyticum)	Occasionally isolated from throat	Pharyngitis, skin lesions	Demonstrates beta hemolysis and is catalase-negative
C. urealyticum (CDC coryneform group D-2)	May be found on healthy skin in 35% of hospitalized patients	Urinary tract infections	Produces urease

present in the unknown suspension, only the animal unprotected by antitoxin will sustain any ill effects. The animal protected by antitoxin will show no adverse effects. In the in vitro test (*Elek method*) a sterile strip of filter paper impregnanted with diphtheria antitoxin is pushed below the surface of a molten enriched agar medium. After the agar hardens, an inoculum of the unknown culture is streaked at right angles to the filter strip. If the unknown bacilli are toxigenic, a precipitate, indicating specific antigen–antibody interaction, will be formed (see Fig. 19-4).

EPIDEMIOLOGY

Eradication of the diphtheria microorganism in carriers and maintenance of immunization levels in children have removed diphtheria from the list of major infectious diseases in the United States. Epidemics do occur periodically, but they are limited to very small geographical areas. Most vulnerable to diphtheria are people of low socioeconomic status with limited access to health care facilities. More than 80 percent of the

physician should therefore determine the patient's sensitivity to the serum before administration of the antitoxin. Antibiotics, although not a substitute for the antitoxin, will destroy the toxin-producing bacilli. Penicillin and erythromycin are effective in destroying the bacilli. Erythromycin is especially valuable in the eradication of the carrier state.

For cutaneous diphtheria, compresses soaked in penicillin can be applied to the lesions.

Mass immunization has been a major factor in the control of diphtheria. It is generally recommended that the diphtheria toxoid be mixed with tetanus toxoid and pertussis vaccine (DTP) and administered as early as 3 months after birth, followed by second and third injections at 6- to 8-week intervals. A booster dose is recommended before entry into school. Immunity persists for nearly 10 years after full immunization. For unimmunized persons 7 years and older a series of three doses of tetanus and diphtheria toxoid (*Td*) is administered. Pertussis vaccine is not administered because pertussis is infrequent and less severe in this age group. Diphtheria prophylaxis is recommended for household contacts of patients with respiratory diphtheria—especially those previously unimmunized or inadequately immunized. The contacts should receive diphtheria toxoid as well as an intramuscular injection of penicillin G benzathine. The major problem in diphtheria control is elimination of the carrier state. Present control efforts include (1) isolation and treatment of clinical cases, (2) use of erythromycin and penicillin in treatment of household and other contacts shown to be carriers of *C. diphtheriae*, and (3) full immunization of all preschool children with diphtheria toxoid and maintenance of diphtheria antitoxin serum levels by booster injections.

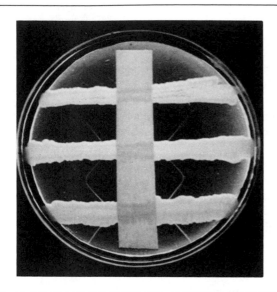

Fig. 19-4. Gel diffusion plate for demonstrating the toxigenicity of strains of *Corynebacterium diphtheriae* (Elek method). A filter strip soaked in diphtheria antitoxin is placed in the center and just below the surface of the agar. The plate is inoculated on each side of the strip and incubated for 24 to 48 hours. In the figure, three test strains have been inoculated. A positive test (toxigenic strain) is evidenced by the formation of one or more white lines of toxin-antitoxin precipitate. The two lower test cultures are positive. (From R. J. Olds, *Color Atlas of Microbiology*. London: Wolfe, 1975.)

recorded cases of diphtheria occur in the 1- to 19-year-old age group, with the highest incidence among those between 10 and 14 years of age. Disease is also frequent in older adults because of low immunization status. Complications after infection are severe in older adults.

TREATMENT AND PREVENTION

In any suspected cases of diphtheria the antitoxin should be administered to neutralize preformed toxin. The antitoxin is still prepared from horse serum, and approximately 10 percent of persons receiving therapy develop allergic reactions. The

OTHER CORYNEBACTERIA, *LISTERIA*, AND *ERYSIPELOTHRIX RHUSIOPATHIAE*

Many species of *Corynebacterium* are found in humans and animals. Some have been implicated

ACNE AND PROPIONIBACTERIUM ACNES

Propionibacterium acnes is a microorganism found in high numbers on or in the skin. This commensal is usually harmless, but it has been associated with a skin condition called *acne vulgaris*. Acne vulgaris is a consequence of oversecretion of sebum, a fluid secreted by sebaceous glands. Stimulation of sebaceous glands is controlled by hormones such as testosterone, as well as adrenal and ovarian hormones. *Propionibacterium acnes* produces enzymes that partially degrade the sebum and release products that cause inflammation. Severe inflammatory lesions (pimples, blackheads, etc.) occur in some individuals and treatment may be necessary. *Propionibacterium acnes* is sensitive to tetracycline, which is used in treatment. Tetracyclines themselves are sensitive to light; therefore, affected skin areas should be covered and protected from the sun.

in human infection, while others are considered nonpathogens. The nonpathogenic corynebacteria, which are collectively called *diphtheroids*, reside on the skin and in the mouth, vagina, and urethra. The anaerobic corynebacteria have now been reclassified in the genus *Propionibacterium*. For example, *C. acnes* is now *P. acnes* (see Boxed Essay, p. 464). The diphtheroids exhibit the same morphology and biochemical characteristics as other coryneforms.

Although not primary pathogens, the diphtheroids are opportunistic. They are known to be the cause of endocarditis in cases in which the patient has been compromised by cardiac surgery or valvular prostheses. Diphtheroids have also been implicated in meningitis and osteomyelitis. Since diphtheroids do not elaborate exotoxin, the toxigenicity test is critical in determining the presence of *C. diphtheriae*.

Bacteriological diagnosis of diphtheroid infections is difficult because of the confusion with strains of *Streptococcus*, which under certain growth conditions appear rod shaped, and with *Listeria monocytogenes*, a motile, gram-positive diphtheroid bacillus that is also catalase positive. Isolation of diphtheroids can be achieved by using a selective medium containing a base of trypticase soy and yeast extract supplemented with polysorbate 80 (Tween 80) to support the growth of lipophilic strains, oil red to distinguish lipophilic from nonlipophilic, and Furoxone to inhibit growth of gram-negative bacilli and gram-positive cocci. Differentiation of *Corynebacterium* species is routinely performed through biochemical reactions. Characteristics of some of these species are listed in Table 19-1.

The genus *Listeria* was previously classified in the family *Corynebacteriaceae* but now is included with another genus, *Erysipelothrix*, as "genera of uncertain affiliation" in *Bergey's Manual of Determinative Bacteriology* (ninth edition). *Listeria monocytogenes*, the primary human pathogen, is found in soil, water, and vegetation. It is an important veterinary pathogen, causing abortions and encephalitis in sheep and cattle. Listeria disease in humans (*listeriosis*) oc-

curs primarily in compromised patients, pregnant women, neonates, alcoholics, diabetics, and the elderly. Meningitis is the most commonly reported form of listeriosis in humans and in some areas of the United States is second only to group B streptococci as a cause of neonatal meningitis. The source of infection has not been clearly determined, but contaminated foods (cheeses, milk, etc.) have been implicated in several outbreaks (Boxed essay, p. 466). Infection by *L. monocytogenes* begins as a bacteremia with the organism capable of infecting any organ; however, nervous tissue is the primary site of disease. *L. monocytogenes* causes approximately 1,700 cases of meningitis and sepsis in the United States each year, with a case-fatality rate of 25 percent.

Certain cultural characteristics of *L. monocytogenes* provide a means of identification as well as differentiation from diphtheroids:

1. Clinical specimens from blood or cerebrospinal fluid can be inoculated onto sheep blood agar plates. Colonies of *L. monocytogenes* are surrounded by a narrow zone of beta hemolysis. If isolated on tryptose agar, the colonies appear green when observed with light reflected obliquely through them.
2. Isolates of *L. monocytogenes* can be inoculated into two tubes of semisolid motility medium, one at room temperature (20–25°C) and the other at 35°C, for 2 to 5 days. At room temperature the microorganism produces an "umbrella" growth below the surface of the medium. Most other diphtheroids are nonmotile and do not grow below the surface of the motility medium. Motility at 35°C is minimal.
3. Pathogenic strains of *L. monocytogenes* may be differentiated from nonpathogenic strains by an ocular test. A drop from an overnight culture is introduced into the conjunctival sac of a rabbit. Purulent conjunctivitis develops in a few days and then heals.

Treatment of listeriosis includes administration of antibiotics such as ampicillin and tetracycline.

LISTERIOSIS AND PASTEURIZED MILK

Listeria monocytogenes can be cultured from approximately 5 percent of raw unpasteurized milk samples and case reports have shown that disease in humans can be caused by consumption of unpasteurized contaminated milk. *L. monocytogenes* can cause serious infections in compromised patients in whom meningitis is a frequent cause of death. Other reports suggesting that *L. monocytogenes* is relatively resistant to heat have raised concern about the effectiveness of pasteurization for eliminating this organism from milk. In an outbreak of listeriosis that occurred in Massachusetts in 1983, pasteurized whole or 2 percent milk was implicated as the source of infection. An inspection of the milk-producing plant detected no apparent breach in the pasteurization process, thereby prompting further interest in the effectiveness of pasteurization.

In a pasteurization study designed to simulate the natural situation more closely, milk from cows that had been purposefully infected with *L. monocytogenes* was used along with several different *L. monocytogenes* isolation procedures. Proper pasteurization was found to inactivate *L. monocytogenes* in milk contaminated through natural as well as in artificially inoculated milk.

Improperly performed pasteurization and the occurrence of contamination after pasteurization are the most likely explanations for the presence of *L. monocytogenes* in pasteurized milk. Two percent of pasteurized milk samples from more than 700 United States milk-producing plants were culture-positive for *Listeria* species, primarily *L. monocytogenes*, in a survey conducted during 1987 and 1988 as part of the Food and Drug Administration's Dairy Product Safety Initiatives. Efforts to ensure that milk is safe from *L. monocytogenes* contamination should focus on promoting proper methods of pasteurization and on identifying and eliminating of postpasteurization contamination.

From *M.M.W.R.* 37:764,1988

Table 19-2. Tests Used in Differentiation of *Erysipelothrix rhusiopathiae* from *Corynebacterium* Species, *Lactobacillus** Species, and *Listeria monocytogenes*

Characteristic	E. rhusiopathiae	Corynebacterium	Lactobacillus	Listeria monocytogenes
Hemolysis on blood agar	Beta hemolysis	Variable	None	Beta hemolysis
Motility	−	−	−	+
Catalase reaction	−	+/−	−	+
H₂S formation in triple sugar iron agar	−	+	−	−

+ = positive reaction or characteristic; − = negative reaction or characteristic.
* Lactobacilli are gram-positive, non-sporeforming anaerobic bacilli found as commensals in the oropharynx, intestinal tract, and vagina.

Erysipelothrix rhusiopathiae is a gram-positive facultative anaerobic, non-sporeforming, rod-shaped bacterium. It is found everywhere in nature where nitrogenous materials decompose. The organism has been isolated from a variety of animals and also fish, shellfish, and birds. It is believed that excretion of the organism by infected and colonized animals leads to contamination of the environment and to acquisition of infection by humans.

E. rhusiopathiae infection in humans is primarily an occupational disease. Infections occur primarily among those who are in contact with contaminated organic matter or infected animals. There are three types of human infection: (1) a mild cutaneous form, usually found on the hands, which is known as *erysipeloid*, "whale finger," or "seal finger," (2) a rare but severe cutaneous form, and (3) a septic form associated with endocarditis. Penicillin is the drug of choice in treatment of all forms of the disease.

Blood culture media are used to culture the microorganism from specimens. After preliminary identification as a gram-positive rod, the organism can be differentiated from *L. monocytogenes*, lactobacilli, and corynebacters (Table 19-2).

SUMMARY

1. The corynebacteria and related bacteria are gram-positive, aerobic, pleomorphic bacilli that concentrate phosphate into stainable granules. *C. diphtheriae* is the etiological agent of diphtheria. Its virulence is due to a toxin whose genetic determinant is carried on a bacteriophage.

2. Diphtheria toxin is composed of two fragments; one attaches to the host cell cytoplasmic membrane and affects the transport of the other fragment into the cytoplasm of the cell. Diphtheria toxin acts on respiratory tissue and results in the formation of a pseudomembrane. The toxin penetrates to the bloodstream and affects protein synthesis in all tissue, especially the heart.

3. Diphtheria may also be of the cutaneous type, which is found in tropical and semitropical climates. Cutaneous diphtheria is not a fatal disease but it may be a source of microorganisms for respiratory diphtheria. Penicillin can be used in the treatment of both cutaneous and respiratory diphtheria.

4. Diphtheria is practically nonexistent in developed countries because of mass immunization programs with diphtheria toxoid. The toxoid is part of the complex (DTP) containing pertussis vaccine and tetanus toxoid.

5. *C. diphtheriae* can be detected in the laboratory by cultivation of specimens on appropriate media, staining to observe metachromatic granules and cellular morphology, and observation of colony appearance. All isolates are tested for toxin production by in vivo (guinea pig) and in vitro (gel diffusion) tests.

6. *Corynebacterium* species other than *C. diphtheriae* are found in the soil or as part of the

normal flora of animals and humans. These species are pathogenic primarily in the compromised host and are not considered major pathogens.

7. Two groups of bacteria that may be confused with *Corynebacterium* are *Listeria* and *Erysipelothrix*. *L. monocytogenes* is found in nature and is a cause of disease primarily in compromised patients such as pregnant women, neonates, alcoholics, etc. It has a predilection for nervous tissue, and for this reason meningitis is the major pathological consequence of infection.

8. *Erysipelothrix rhusiopathiae* is found in nature where nitrogen material decomposes. It causes occupation-associated diseases, particularly for those in contact with infected animals or organic matter. Cutaneous infections and endocarditis are the principal forms of disease caused by this organism. Penicillin is the drug of choice in treatment.

QUESTIONS FOR STUDY

Select the best response or responses for each of the following:

1. The source of organisms responsible for diphtheria is (are)
   A. The upper respiratory tract
   B. Cutaneous lesions
   C. The intestinal tract
   D. The lower respiratory tract

2. DTP vaccine is composed of
   A. Diphtheria toxin, tetanus toxoid, heat-killed *Bordetella pertussis*
   B. Diphtheria toxoid, tetanus toxoid, *B. pertussus* toxoid
   C. Diphtheria toxoid, tetanus toxoid, heat-killed *B. pertussis*
   D. Diphtheria toxoid, tetanus toxoid, heat-killed *Pseudomonas aeruginosa*

3. Diphtheria toxin affects host cells by
   A. Inhibiting sterol synthesis, thus affecting membrane permeability
   B. Inhibiting polypeptide chain elongation
   C. Inhibiting mRNA synthesis
   D. Inhibiting protein synthesis by binding to the 50S subunit of the ribosome

4. *Listeria monocytogenes* is an opportunistic pathogen that is an important cause of which of the following conditions?
   A. Endocarditis
   B. Gastroenteritis
   C. Nephritis
   D. Meningitis

Fill in the blanks:

5. Erysipeloid is a cutaneous infection caused by _____ .

6. The Elek method is used to detect toxigenic strains of *C. diphtheriae* by streaking specimens at right angles to a filter strip containing diphtheria _____ .

7. Methylene blue staining of *C. diphtheriae* is a presumptive test that permits observation of _____ granules.

8. Both *Streptococcus pyogenes* and *C. diphtheriae* produce toxins because of the presence of _____ .

ADDITIONAL READINGS

Gorby, G. L., and Peacock, J. R., Jr. *Erysipelothrix rhusiopathiae* endocarditis: Microbiologic, epidemiologic, and clinical features of an occupational disease. *Rev. Infect. Dis.* 10(2)317,1988.

Lipsky, B. A., et al. Infections caused by non-diphtheria corynebacteria. *Rev. Infect. Dis.* 4:1220,1982.

Samara, Y., Hertz, M., and Altmann, G. Adult listeriosis—a review of 18 cases. *Postgrad. Med. J.* 60:267,1984.

Stephen, J., and Pietrowski, R. A. *Bacterial Toxins (2nd ed.).* Aspects of Microbiology 2. Washington, DC: American Society for Microbiology, 1986.

20. GRAM-NEGATIVE ENTERIC BACILLI

OBJECTIVES

To list the important traits that are common to the
majority of Enterobacteriaceae

To briefly outline in a flowchart the laboratory
procedures used to isolate and differentiate
members of the Enterobacteriaceae

To describe the intestinal and extraintestinal
diseases caused by *Escherichia coli*

To describe the virulence factors associated with
infections caused by *E. coli*, *Salmonella* species,
Shigella species, and *Yersinia* species

To explain the methods of treatment for intestinal
and extraintestinal disease caused by the
Enterobacteriaceae

To describe the different disease states associated
with salmonella infections

To describe the epidemiology of plague

To list the opportunistic Enterobacteriaceae and the
types of infections with which they are associated

Many gram-negative non-sporeforming bacilli are commensals in the intestinal tract of humans and animals. These enteric bacilli for the most part belong to the family Enterobacteriaceae (Table 20-1). Other gram-negative bacilli that are either found as intestinal pathogens or are recovered from infections associated with enteric bacilli belong to the families Vibrionaceae and Pseudomonadaceae. They will be discussed in subsequent chapters.

The term *coliform* has sometimes been used to denote all the enteric bacilli. It is used more often, however, to describe gram-negative, fermentative inhabitants of the intestinal tract: *Escherichia coli, Klebsiella pneumoniae*, and *Enterobacter aerogenes*.

In the past 20 years the overuse of antibiotics has caused a dramatic increase in the number of hospital-associated (nosocomial) diseases caused by enteric bacilli. As a group the enteric bacilli have replaced the gram-positive microorganisms, such as the staphylococci and streptococci, as the major cause of disease in the hospital. Enterobacteriaceae may account for approximately 50 percent of all clinically significant isolates. They are the major cause of septicemia, urinary tract infections, and intestinal infections in the hospital.

CHARACTERISTICS OF THE ENTEROBACTERIACEAE

No single morphological or biochemical characteristic can be used to differentiate all the Enterobacteriaceae. However, some generalizations can be made about the majority of them.

1. All members of the family Enterobacteriaceae are gram-negative aerobic or facultatively anaerobic rods varying in length from

Table 20-1. Current Classification of Enterobacteriaceae Based on *Bergey's Manual of Determinative Bacteriology* (9th ed.)*

FAMILY: Enterobacteriaceae
  GENUS: *Escherichia*
    SPECIES: *E. coli*
  GENUS: *Shigella*
    SPECIES: *S. dysenteriae*
          S. flexneri
          S. boydii
          S. sonnei
  GENUS: *Edwardsiella*
    SPECIES: *E. tarda*
  GENUS: *Citrobacter*
    SPECIES: *C. freundii*
          C. diversus
  GENUS: *Salmonella*
    SPECIES: *S. choleraesuis*
          S. typhi
          S. paratyphi A
          S. typhimurium
          S. enteritidis
          S. arizonae
  GENUS: *Klebsiella*
    SPECIES: *K. pneumoniae* subsp. *pneumoniae*
          K. pneumoniae subsp. *ozaenae*
          K. pneumoniae subsp. *rhinoscleromatis*
          K. oxytoca
  GENUS: *Enterobacter*
    SPECIES: *E. cloacae*
          E. aerogenes
          E. agglomerans
  GENUS: *Hafnia*
    SPECIES: *H. alvei*
  GENUS: *Serratia*
    SPECIES: *S. marcescens*
          S. liquifaciens
  GENUS: *Proteus*
    SPECIES: *P. vulgaris*
          P. mirabilis
  GENUS: *Providencia*
    SPECIES: *P. alcalifaciens*
          P. rettgeri
  GENUS: *Yersinia*
    SPECIES: *Y. pestis*
          Y. pseudotuberculosis
          Y. enterocolitica

* Not all the genera or species are indicated, only those that are major human pathogens.

1 to 8 μm. They ferment glucose, do not produce oxidase, and reduce nitrates to nitrites.

2. Most can be cultivated on ordinary laboratory media and stained with aniline dyes.

3. Most species are active fermenters of glucose and other carbohydrates. Many of the pathogens can be separated from the nonpathogens on the basis of the former's inability to ferment lactose.

4. Motile as well as nonmotile species are found in the group. Those that are motile are peritrichous (have flagella over their entire surface).

5. Pili are found on the cell surface of members of the Enterobacteriaceae (Fig. 20-1). The sex pili are important in the conjugation process, particularly for the transfer of antibiotic resistance factors (R factors) between the same or different family members. The more numerous adhesive pili found on the surface of the organisms are responsible for the adherence of some species to epithelial surfaces. These antigens are protein and are also called K antigens, but they are to be distinguished from the capsular K antigens, which are polysaccharide.

6. Because of the ability of members of the Enterobacteriaceae to transfer antibiotic resistance plasmids, antibiotic susceptibility testing must be routinely performed on clinical isolates before an antibiotic regimen can be instituted. Some clinical isolates have shown resistance to one to ten different major therapeutic agents.

7. The lipopolysaccharides of the cell wall of the enteric bacilli are toxic and are called *endotoxins*. As yet no direct relationship has been established between pathogenicity and the endotoxin of the enteric microorganisms. The biological properties of the endotoxins are discussed in Chapter 9.

8. Many enteric species are capable of producing bacteriocins that are bactericidal to related species of bacteria but not themselves (see page 254).

9. Many of the Enterobacteriaceae are classi-

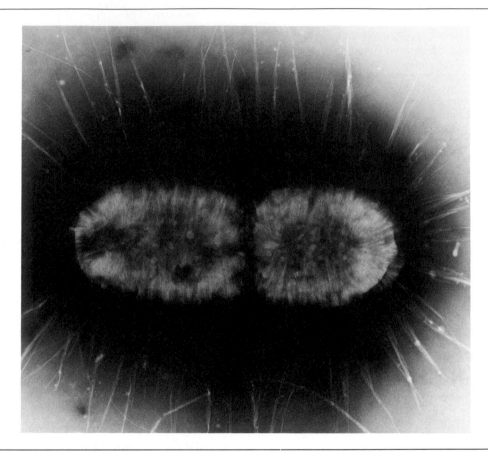

Fig. 20-1. Electron micrograph (×60,000) of *E. coli*, demonstrating pili used in attachment to epithelial surfaces. (From C. F. Deneke, G. M. Thorne, and S. L. Gorbach, *Infect. Immun.* 26:362, 1979.)

fied by their cell envelope–associated antigens, that is, the O, K, and H antigens (Fig. 20-2). The *O* or *somatic antigen* is the O-specific polysaccharide of the lipopolysaccharide (LPS) component of the cell wall (see Fig. 9-9, page 227). The O polysaccharide is responsible for the O antigen specificity of the Enterobacteriaceae. There are 164 known somatic O antigens. The O-specific polysaccharide protects the cell against host resistance factors. Certain O antigens seem to be associated with certain diseases.

Lipid A is the toxic component of the LPS complex. It is similar in all of the different Enterobacteriaceae.

The capsular polysaccharide of the Enterobacteriaceae is referred to as the *K antigen*. Among the *E. coli* strains there are 100 different K antigens. Not all species in the family possess K antigens, but those that do are usually more pathogenic. The K capsular polysaccharide provides a barrier to phagocytosis because of its ability to resist activation of the alternate complement pathway.

Flagellar protein antigens are referred to as *H antigens*. They are responsible for motility.

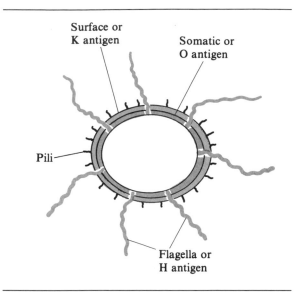

Fig. 20-2. The antigenic components found on the surface of members of the Enterobacteriaceae.

Their identification often represents the last step in the procedure of serotyping various strains within a genus of bacteria. (Serotypes are divisions based on antigenic relatedness—for example, similarity of O antigens. Biotypes are strains of the same serotype that differ in a biochemical characteristic—for example, sugar fermentation.)

10. Because of the ease of cultivating them, many Enterobacteriaceae have been used in research efforts, especially in the elucidation of metabolic pathways, protein synthesis, and genetic mechanisms. *E. coli*, for example, is the most studied of all bacteria and it is used as a vehicle in recombinant DNA technology (see Chapter 6).

ISOLATION OF THE ENTEROBACTERIACEAE

The enteric laboratory represents the largest division in the clinical microbiology section of a hospital. For this reason we will provide more detailed descriptions of laboratory isolation and identification techniques than will appear with microorganisms in other chapters. Enteric bacilli are involved in numerous hospital-associated diseases. They can be isolated from feces, urine, blood, and cerebrospinal fluid. The kind of medium to use for isolation depends on the source of the specimen. If it is from a nonintestinal source such as the blood or urine, the organisms may be a practically pure culture because human blood and urine are usually sterile. Hence the specimen may be plated on blood agar and a differential medium. If the specimen is from an intestinal source, the infecting pathogen will be greatly outnumbered by commensal species and will initially require a selective enrichment medium. A variety of selective, differential, and enrichment media are available to resolve these problems.

SELECTIVE ENRICHMENT MEDIA

If the infecting pathogen (for example, *Salmonella* or *Shigella* species) is from an intestinal source, a selective medium is often needed. Selective media such as tetrathionate, Hajna GN broth, and selenite broth inhibit gram-positive bacteria and coliforms, permitting the rapid multiplication of *Salmonella* and *Shigella* species. Once the pathogen has been grown to sufficient numbers, it can be inoculated into various selective or differential media.

PRIMARY ISOLATION MEDIA

Primary isolation media include eosin–methylene blue (EMB) and MacConkey agar. These media contain chemicals that inhibit gram-positive organisms. They also contain lactose, a disaccharide that permits a presumptive differentiation of lactose fermenters from non-lactose fermenters. Lactose fermenters such as *E. coli* and *Enterobacter aerogenes* produce colored colonies, while the non-lactose fermenters such as *Salmonella* and *Shigella* exhibit colorless colonies because they do not ferment lactose.

DIFFERENTIAL SELECTIVE MEDIA

Differential selective media such as *Salmonella-Shigella* (SS), deoxycholate-citrate, bismuth sulfite, and brilliant green agars are used primarily for the isolation of *Salmonella* and *Shigella* species. These media are selective against gram-positive organisms as well as most coliforms.

SCREENING AND IDENTIFICATION OF THE ENTEROBACTERIACEAE

Many biochemical tests can be used to identify a member of the *Enterobacteriaceae*. A spot test for oxidase, performed immediately on isolates, will separate oxidase-negative *Enterobacteriaceae* from oxidase-positive gram-negative organisms such as *Pasteurella*. A battery of 28 biochemical tests will differentiate all of the pathogenic *Enterobacteriaceae*. A battery of 14 primary tests, however, is sufficient to differentiate most isolates to the genus and some to the species level. The primary tests are outlined in Table 20-2. The secondary tests are primarily fermentation tests. Several of the primary tests can be determined in a single medium. For example, triple sugar iron agar provides results for gas and hydrogen sulfide production and glucose fermentation. Phenylalanine-urease broth provides testing for phenylalanine deaminase and urease while motility-indole-ornithine medium provides results for motility, indole production, and ornithine decarboxylase production. Since triple sugar iron (TSI) agar is so important, we will briefly describe the test.

An isolated colony from the selective or differential media is first stabbed into the butt of a TSI agar slant, then streaked onto the surface of the slant. The TSI agar tube contains glucose (0.1%), sucrose (1%), and lactose (1%), plus phenol red to indicate fermentation and ferrous sulfate to detect hydrogen sulfide production. The small amount of glucose in the TSI agar slant, as compared to the other carbohydrates, enables one to detect the fermentation of this sugar. If glucose is the only carbohydrate fermented, the small amount of acid produced on the slant is oxidized, and the slant remains alkaline (red). Acid produced in the butt is not oxidized, and the butt remains yellow. All inoculated TSI tubes are read after 18 to 24 hours (Table 20-3).

Rapid identification methods for enteric bacilli have recently been developed. These are microsystems often consisting of a set of plastic strips or tubes each containing one of 15 or more different media used in enteric identification. Once a species of bacteria is isolated, a small inoculum is added to each of the media, incubated, and read in 5 hours or after overnight incubation. Up to 95 percent correlation has been found between results obtained with the microsystems and those produced by the conventional methods.

ESCHERICHIA COLI

PATHOGENESIS

E. coli is an abundant commensal found in the intestinal tract of humans and animals. One gram of feces may contain from 1×10^7 to 1×10^8 *E. coli*.* Despite being a commensal, some strains of *E. coli* are pathogenic and cause diarrheal disease and extraintestinal infections. Classification

---

* Species of *Bacteroides*, an anaerobe, are the most abundant group of bacteria in the intestinal tract. Some species are also found in the oral cavity and vagina. *Bacteroides* is implicated in diseases such as brain abscesses, respiratory tract disease, diseases of the female genital tract, such as pelvic inflammatory disease (PID), and bacteremia.

Table 20-2. Primary Biochemical Tests (14) Used to Identify Some of the Major Species in the Enterobacteriaceae

Test or substrate	E. coli	Salmonella typhi	Shigella dysenteriae	Klebsiella pneumoniae	Enterobacter sakazii	Serratia marcescens	Proteus mirabilis	Yersinia pestis
D-adonitol	∓	–	–	±	–	V	–	–
Voges-Proskauer	–	–	–	±	+	±	∓	–
Citrate utilization	–	–	–	±	+	±	±	–
Arginine dihydrolase	∓	∓	∓	–	+	–	–	–
Motility	±	±	+	–	±	±	±	–
Indole production	+	–	V	–	∓	∓	∓	–
H₂S (on TSI agar)	–	±	–	–	–	–	±	–
Urease production	–	–	–	±	–	∓	±	∓
Phenylalanine deaminase	–	–	–	–	V	–	±	–
Ornithine decarboxylase	V	–	–	–	±	+	+	–
Lysine decarboxylase	±	±	–	±	–	+	–	–
Sucrose	V	–	–	+	+	+	∓	–
DNase	–	–	–	–	–	±	–	–
Gas from glucose	+	–	–	±	±	V	±	–

∓ = over 90 percent of isolates are negative; ± = over 90 percent of isolates are positive; V = variable, that is, as many positive as negative isolates; TSI = triple sugar iron agar.

of pathogenic *E. coli* isolates according to serotypes has been difficult since there are over 160 O-antigens, 100 K-antigens, and 55 H-antigens. Some of these surface antigens are important adhesins that enable *E. coli* to attach to epithelial cells. The majority of pathogenic as well as nonpathogenic *E. coli* strains possess a common type of pilus called *type 1*.

Extraintestinal Disease

Extraintestinal disease caused by *E. coli* is usually the result of person-to-person contact. The organism may also travel from the intestine to the urinary tract. In the community outside the hospital *E. coli* is the most common cause of urinary tract infection, probably on account of the close association between the organisms' normal habitat and the urinary tract (especially in women), as well as special properties possessed by the *E. coli* strain. Hospital-associated infections represent another group of extraintestinal infections caused by *E. coli*. Again, the most frequent site of infection is the urinary tract. *E. coli* is implicated in approximately 20 percent of all urinary tract infections in the hospital.

The severity of urinary tract infections appears to be associated with adhesins called *P pili* (some *E. coli* strains can make both type 1 or P pili). The presence of P pili enables *E. coli* to avoid

Table 20-3. Key to Identification of the Enterobacteriaceae on Triple Sugar Iron Agar

Reaction	Biochemical interpretation	Organisms most likely to be involved
Acid slant, acid-gas butt, no H$_2$S produced	Glucose fermented and lactose or sucrose fermented with acid and gas produced	*Escherichia coli, Enterobacter, Klebsiella*, and *Proteus* species
Acid slant, acid-gas butt, H$_2$S produced	Glucose fermented and lactose or sucrose fermented with acid and gas produced	*Citrobacter* species
Alkaline slant, acid butt, no H$_2$S produced	Glucose fermented with acid and no gas produced	*Proteus, Shigella*, and *Serratia* species
Alkaline slant, acid-gas butt, no H$_2$S produced	Glucose fermented with acid and gas produced	*Proteus, Citrobacter, Salmonella, Providencia*, and *Hafnia* species
Alkaline slant, acid-gas butt, H$_2$S produced	Glucose fermented with acid and gas produced	*Proteus, Arizona, Salmonella*, and *Edwardsiella* species
Alkaline slant, acid butt, H$_2$S produced	Glucose fermented with acid and no gas produced	*Salmonella* species
No reaction, but green pigment produced	Peptone only source of carbon and energy	*Pseudomonas* species

phagocytic cells. *E. coli* strains that cause acute *pyelonephritis* (inflammation of the kidney usually arising from ascending infection from the ureter) have virulence factors not found in the usual fecal *E. coli* strains. These virulence factors include (1) P pili, (2) presence of hemolysin, (3) presence of aerobactin, an iron scavenging molecule, and (4) capsular K antigen.

E. coli can also cause life-threatening infections, such as septicemia, meningitis, and pneumonia, in compromised hosts. For example, *E. coli* is a common cause of neonatal meningitis in which the mortality rate is between 40 and 75 percent. Eighty percent of all *E. coli* strains involved in neonatal meningitis produce the K1 capsular polysaccharide.

Intestinal Disease

There are five groups of *E. coli* strains that are associated with diarrhea and gastrointestinal illness, but only four have been well defined and they are: (1) *enterotoxigenic E. coli*, (2) *enteroinvasive E. coli*, (3) *enteropathogenic E. coli*, and (4) *enterohemorrhagic E. coli*. All these

groups are distinct but they do have some common underlying characteristics:

1. Important virulence traits are encoded on plasmids.
2. They interact with the intestinal mucosa (Fig. 20-3).
3. They produce enterotoxins or cytotoxins.
4. Within each category the strains fall within certain O:H serotypes.

Table 20-4 characterizes the four major groups of diarrheagenic *E. coli*.

Laboratory Diagnosis

E. coli is a lactose fermenter and is readily separated from other enteric species by its characteristic colonial appearance on EMB agar and biochemical reactions outlined in Table 20-2. Since the biochemical activities of the pathogenic species of *E. coli* are identical to those of the nonpathogenic species of the gut, other tests are needed to detect specific groups of diarrheagenic *E. coli*. These tests may include enterotoxin test-

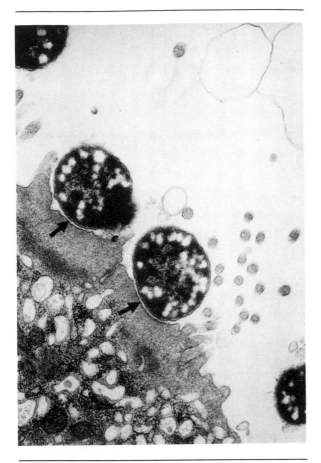

Fig. 20-3. Transmission electron micrograph of *E. coli* adhering to epithelial cells of colon. Arrows point to apical membrane of epithelial cells, which form a pedestal when microorganisms become adherent. From M. K. Wolf et al., *Infect. Immun.* 56(8):1846, 1988.

ing and serotyping. Serotyping has been used in identifying enteropathogenic *E. coli* but this is not a routine procedure applicable to most clinical laboratories. DNA probes are now being developed to identify toxigenic strains of *E. coli* in the clinical laboratory.

Treatment and Prevention
In gastrointestinal infections antibiotics are not recommended. Successful treatment depends on the replacement of water and electrolytes. Chloramphenicol, tetracyclines, and nalidixic acid are used to treat urinary tract infections. Many enteric bacilli are notoriously resistant to a wide variety of antibiotics. It is advised that isolated species be subjected to in vitro antibiotic susceptibility tests if antibiotic therapy is undertaken.

Prophylactic drugs are recommended for prevention of travelers' diarrhea. The drugs are for (1) persons visiting high-risk areas (Mexico, for example) for short periods (2–5 days) and (2) persons with underlying disease that might increase susceptibility to diarrhea during travel in high-risk areas. Chemoprophylaxis is to be avoided if visits to high-risk areas last more than two weeks. Trimethoprim-sulfamethoxazole is an effective chemoprophylactic drug. Bismuth subsalicylate has also been shown to be effective in preventing traveler's diarrhea.

SALMONELLA *SPECIES*

Members of the genus *Salmonella* are rod-shaped cells that with few exceptions are actively motile. They are capable of causing disease in both animals and humans. Salmonellae are hardy microorganisms that can survive in moist environments and in the frozen state for several months. All *Salmonella* diseases are the result of ingestion of the bacilli from contaminated water, food, or fomites.

The three recognized species of *Salmonella* are *S. typhi*, *S. choleraesuis*, and *S. enteritidis*. *S. enteritidis* includes all the *Salmonella* organisms except those of *S. typhi* and *S. choleraesuis*. Although there are more than 1500 serotypes of *S. enteritidis*, about 70 percent of human *Salmonella* infections in the United States are caused by 10 serotypes, the most common of which is *S. enteritidis* serotype typhimurium. (Many investigators still prefer to use the serotypes of *S. enteritidis* as species names; for example, *S. enteritidis* serotype typhimurium is called *S. typhimurium*. We will follow this practice.) The genus

Table 20-4. Characteristics of the Major Groups of Diarrheagenic *Escherichia coli*

E. coli group	Epidemiology and disease symptoms	Mechanism of transmission and site of action	Virulence factors
Enterotoxigenic	Major cause of infant diarrhea in less developed countries and travelers' diarrhea. Diarrhea in the United States rarely caused by this agent. Watery diarrhea, abdominal cramps, low-grade fever	Ingestion of contaminated food (raw vegetables, fish, meat) or water. Colonizes proximal small intestine	Heat-labile (LT) or heat-stable (ST) enterotoxin. LT resembles cholera toxin in chemistry and action. Fimbrial adhesin called colonization factor (CFA)
Enteropathogenic	Not well defined. In some countries it is the most important cause of infant diarrhea. Fever, vomiting, diarrhea with large amounts of mucus. Distinctive lesions in which microvilli are destroyed	Ingestion of contaminated food or water. Proximal intestine	Cytotoxin similar to Shiga toxin produced by *Shigella dysenteriae* type 1
Enteroinvasive	Diarrhea in adults and infants. Resembles shigella in pathogenicity, i.e., causes epithelial cell death. Fever, severe abdominal cramps, watery diarrhea followed by gross dysentery with bloody stools and mucus	Ingestion of contaminated food or water. Predilection for mucosa of the colon	Several outer membrane proteins, similar to shigella, involved in invasiveness. Shiga-like toxin produced
Enterohemorrhagic	Sporadic and epidemic cases of gastrointestinal illness in United States, Canada, and Great Britain since 1982. Affects both adults and children. Severe abdominal cramps and copious bloody diarrhea. No fever or fecal leukocytes—which distinguishes it from dysentery due to shigella. A hemolytic uremic syndrome may also appear to be characterized by hemolytic anemia and renal failure. Farm animals may serve as reservoirs of infectious agent	Ingestion of contaminated food or water. Person to person transmission, as in nursing homes, during epidemic disease. Proximal intestine	Potent toxins called Verotoxin or Shiga-like toxins that are related to Shiga toxin of *Shigella dysenteriae* type 1

Arizona is so similar to strains of *Salmonella* that it is now considered a *Salmonella* serotype.

Pathogenesis

The manifestations of disease caused by the salmonellae may include gastroenteritis, enteric fever, and bacteremia, and each may be associated with the carrier state. Most infections in the United States are of the gastrointestinal variety and result from the ingestion of contaminated food or water. Enteric fevers (for example, typhoid fever) are seldom observed in the United States, although they are quite common in developing countries.

The factors that determine the severity of infection by salmonellae are size of the inoculum, the serotype, and the state of health of the host. The number of viable salmonellae that are required to cause infection after ingestion of contaminated water or food depends on the serotype and host factors. The calculated doses involved in *Salmonella* outbreaks have been determined in recent studies in which the vehicle was obtained. They have demonstrated that as few as 17 or as many as 1×10^9 microorganisms may be required to cause disease.

Gastroenteritis. When contaminated material has been ingested, the bacilli multiply in the intestinal tract. Later they penetrate the epithelial mucosal cells of the ileum and cause an inflammatory response in the lamina propria of the intestinal villi. Lymphatic barriers prevent the less virulent serotypes from invading the bloodstream, and the infection remains intestinal. Symptoms appear 4 or 5 days after ingestion of the bacilli and include diarrhea, which is not dependent on the production of an enterotoxin. The mechanism of diarrhea production is believed to be similar to that caused by *Vibrio cholerae* and pathogenic *E. coli*; that is, adenyl cyclase is induced with the formation of adenosine 3′5′-cyclic phosphate (cyclic AMP), resulting in the hypersecretion of fluid. The diarrhea lasts 3 to 5 days and is accompanied by fever and abdominal pain. During acute gastroenteritis 10^6 to 10^9 salmonellae per gram of feces may be present.

Enteric Fever (Typhoid, Paratyphoid, and Nontyphoidal Fevers). The ingested bacilli that cause enteric fever are more invasive than those that cause only gastroenteritis. They are capable of resisting host defenses and can multiply in the macrophage (Plate 10). The primary step in pathogenesis is penetration of the intestinal mucosa. Presumably there is alteration of the mucosal surface that permits the pathogen to gain access to the epithelial cell. Once contact has been made with the epithelial surface there is localized degeneration of the brush border of the epithelial cell. The microorganism is then surrounded by the cytoplasmic membrane of the epithelial cell and is subsequently observed in a vacuole within the cytoplasm. Salmonellae are transported through the epithelial cells within these vacuoles. The salmonellae eventually enter the lamina propria and can enter lymph nodes, where they colonize the macrophage. Organisms that have infected the lymph system can enter the circulation, from whence they can infect any tissue of the body including the intestine. The reinfection of lymph tissue in the intestine provides an avenue for shedding in the stool. The bacilli routinely infect the gallbladder, where they multiply and provide a focal point for shedding of bacilli into the intestinal tract.

The major species or serotypes that cause enteric fevers are *S. typhi* (typhoid fever), *S. paratyphi A* and *S. paratyphi B* (paratyphoid fever), and *S. schottmülleri* (nontyphoidal enteric fever). The incubation period for enteric fever is approximately 1 to 2 weeks. During the first week there is a gradual increase in fever accompanied by anorexia and general aches and pains. A continual headache is the principal symptom, and more than 60 percent of patients demonstrate a nonproductive cough. During the second week the fever remains as high as 104°F, and there are symptoms of diarrhea and abdominal discomfort and general weakness. During this period, which corresponds to the chronic bacteremic stage, rose-colored spots may appear on the abdomen. If no complications occur, the disease begins to terminate during the third week. Complications include abscess formation, intestinal perforation (Fig. 20-4), pneumonia, and thrombophlebitis. The death rate for typhoid fever varies from 2 to 10 percent. Paratyphoid fever is similar to typhoid fever but of shorter duration and milder.

The virulence factors of *S. typhi* are still a subject of controversy. One of the surface antigens is a K antigen called *Vi antigen*. The Vi antigen is believed to be important in the pathogenesis of and immunity to typhoid fever. The Vi antigen does not appear to be needed as an invasive factor, but as a protective factor, for the O antigen, against phagocytosis and the bactericidal action of serum. The invasiveness of *S. typhi* appears to be directly associated with motility. Nonmotile mutants of *S. typhi* are unable to invade epithelial cells.

The manifestations of typhoid fever are believed to be a result of molecules released from infected macrophages. These molecules include arachidonic acid metabolite and free oxygen radicals. The endotoxin of *S. typhi* appears to contribute to the pathogenesis of typhoid fever by enhancing local inflammatory responses at the tissue site of *S. typhi* multiplication.

Bacteremia

Salmonellae may be transiently present in the bloodstream or may persist for long periods of time. The more invasive species such as *S. typhimurium* and *S. choleraesuis* are usually involved in sustained bacteremia. The most serious consequence of bacteremia is metastatic infection, which may involve the bones and joints, the cardiovascular system, and the meninges. Fever and chills are the symptoms associated with bacteremia.

Carrier State

It has been suggested that the asymptomatic carrier state is a more frequent consequence of *Sal-*

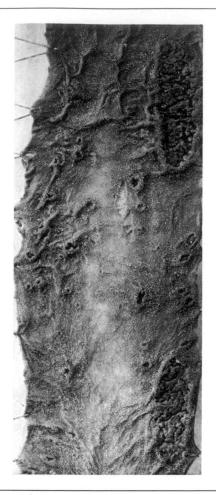

Fig. 20-4. Typhoid ulceration of ileum. Ulcerations appear as small craters. (Courtesy Air Force Institute of Pathology, AFIP 2803.)

monella infection than is gastroenteritis. Shedding of salmonellae normally occurs 5 to 6 months after the development of an acute infection. Carriers, however, are classified as those who shed bacilli for one year after infection. The factors that appear to determine whether the carrier state will develop are (1) the species or serotype involved (*S. typhi*, *S. paratyphi A*, and *S. paratyphi B* are frequently associated with the carrier state), (2) the dose of salmonellae (doses too small to cause overt disease may induce the

TYPHOID MARY

Mary Mallon was a cook in a family for 3 years, and in 1901 she developed typhoid fever. About the same time a visitor to the family had the disease. One month later the laundress in this family was taken ill.

In 1902, Mary obtained a new job, and 2 weeks after her arrival the laundress was taken ill with typhoid fever. In a week, a second case developed, and soon seven members of the household were sick.

In 1904, Mary went to a home on Long Island. There were four in the family, besides seven servants. Within 3 weeks after her arrival, four servants were attacked.

In 1906, Mary went to another family, and 6 of the 11 members of this family were attacked with typhoid between August 27 and September 3. At this time, the cook was first suspected. She entered another family on September 21, and on October 5 the laundress developed typhoid fever.

In 1907, she entered a home in New York City and 2 months after her arrival 2 cases developed, one of which proved fatal. During these 5 years, "Typhoid Mary" is known to have been the cause of 26 cases of typhoid fever.

She was virtually imprisoned by the New York Department of Health in a hospital from March 19, 1907. Cultures taken every few days showed bacilli now and then for 3 years. Sometimes the stools contained enormous numbers of typhoid bacilli and again for days none could be found.

Typhoid Mary then escaped from observation until 1914. In October of that year, she was engaged as cook in the Sloane Hospital for Women in New York. In January and February of 1915, an outbreak of typhoid occurred, principally among the doctors, nurses, and help of the institution, involving 25 cases. The cook was suspected but she left the premises on a few hours' leave, and did not return or leave her address. She was, however, located by the health department under an assumed name, and an investigation established her identity as the famous Typhoid Mary.

A subsequent study of her career showed that she had infected still other individuals beyond those already mentioned, and that she may have given rise to the well-known waterborne outbreak of typhoid in Ithaca, New York, in 1903, involving over 1300 cases. The fact is that a person by the name of Mary Mallon had been employed as a cook in the vicinity of the place where the first case appeared, and from which contamination of the water supply occurred.

From M. J. Rosenau, *Preventive Medicine and Hygiene* (6th ed.). New York: Appleton, 1935.

carrier state), and (3) disorders of the biliary tract (diseases of the biliary tract are asymptomatic and serve as a source for the shedding of bacilli). Chronic carriers are most often elderly people (see Boxed Essay, p. 483).

EPIDEMIOLOGY

Approximately 40,000 cases of salmonellosis are reported each year to the CDC and fewer than 500 are typhoid fever. Salmonellosis is an underreported infection and the actual yearly incidence of infection is believed to be one million. The estimated incidence of typhoid fever throughout the world, excluding China, is 12.5 million cases per year. The highest incidence of disease occurs among young children and the elderly. The greatest number of cases occurs in children less than 1 year old, and it is in this age group that mortality is highest. The increased susceptibility of this age group may be related to several factors. One of these factors may be the hydrochloric acid in the stomach. The stomach is a barrier to many microorganisms, including the salmonellae. Children less than 2 months of age produce little hydrochloric acid. Patients with gastrectomies or who are taking antacids are also more susceptible to infection by ingested salmonellae.

S. typhi, *S. paratyphi A*, and *S. paratyphi B*, unlike most other *Salmonella* species, are harbored by humans and not animals. Transmission of these species is from person to person via fecally contaminated food or water. Contamination of food occurs only by secondary contamination during the processing or handling of meat and animal products by human carriers. Often asymptomatic carriers of *S. typhi* have caused large epidemics. The death rate for typhoid fever in the United States is less than 1 percent, but in developing countries both the number of cases and the death rate are high.

Nontyphoidal *Salmonella* species can be found in a wide variety of animal species, which serve as a common source of infection to humans. The main sources are turkeys, chickens, eggs and egg products, swine, and other domestic animals. Since 1979 most of the outbreaks caused by *S. enteritidis* were associated with Grade A shell eggs. (See Boxed Essay, p. 485). Because of the mass processing of meats and other animal-related products used for human consumption, the number of cases of salmonellosis is rising. *S. typhimurium* is the most frequently reported serotype, followed by *S. enteritidis* (Fig. 20-5). Nontyphoidal *Salmonella* infections are spread from animal to animal and then to humans either directly or indirectly via animal-processing procedures. Person-to-person transfer seems to be less important than contaminated foodstuffs. The majority of cases of salmonellosis occur when large groups of people are served dishes that were prepared 24 to 48 hours before and were perhaps left standing for several hours at room temperature.

Salmonella infections are commonly associated with enclosed environments such as hospitals, homes for the mentally retarded, and nursing homes. These institutions also have the highest mortality. Most epidemics begin by ingestion of contaminated foodstuffs or medical products of

Fig. 20-5. Salmonella isolation rates by total, and serotypes *S. typhimurium* and *S. enteritidis* and year, United States, 1970–1986. (From Centers for Disease Control.)

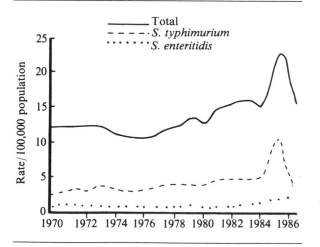

SALMONELLA ENTERITIDIS *INFECTIONS AND GRADE A EGGS*

Between 1976 and 1985 New England and the Middle Atlantic regions experienced a fivefold increase in the reported isolation rate of *Salmonella enteritidis*. Investigations of these outbreaks and related studies suggested that most of the infections were associated with eggs.

In many of the outbreaks the vehicles of transmission were either eggs or foods which contained raw or undercooked eggs (homemade eggnog prepared with store-bought eggs, Monte Cristo sandwiches made of sliced cooked meat and cheese or bread dipped in raw egg and grilled, and Caesar salad dressing made with raw eggs). The outbreak-associated eggs were all USDA grade A shell eggs.

Large outbreaks of salmonellosis before 1970 led to the passage of the Egg Product Inspection Act in 1970. This law required pasteurization of all bulk egg products and federally supervised inspection of shell eggs for cracks. Outbreaks of salmonellosis associated with bulk eggs have not been reported since 1970 but frequent outbreaks of salmonellosis from shell eggs still occur. Eggs can be contaminated by organisms entering through hairline cracks in the shell. In addition if there is an ovarian infection in the hen, an egg yolk may become infected by *Salmonella* species before the shell is formed. Most outbreaks of salmonellosis associated with eggs occur during the summer months. Warm temperature may provide opportunities for *Salamonella enteritidis* to multiply and survive in eggs during production, transport, storage, or use. *S. enteritidis* infections can occur even when acceptable food preparation techniques have been used. Proper handling and cooking of eggs can minimize the risk of salmonellosis; thorough cooking kills Salmonella.

From *M.M.W.R.* 36:204, 1987; *M.M.W.R.* 37:490, 1988.

animal origin—pancreatin, vitamins, gelatin. From these initial cases of infection the organisms may be spread by contact between persons. Person-to-person spread is particularly important in mental institutions, where personal hygiene is at a minimum. Nursery epidemics are often related to the presence of an infant "shedder" of the salmonellae.

LABORATORY DIAGNOSIS

Diagnosis of *Salmonella* infections rests on isolation and identification of the suspected species from feces, urine, blood, or contaminated food.

In typhoid fever the organism can generally be isolated from the blood during the first week of illness. Later it may be isolated from the urine or stools. The suspected samples are first plated on the various media, as indicated under Isolation of the Enterobacteriaceae earlier in this chapter. The isolated species is then subjected to biochemical tests (see Table 20-2), followed by serological tests of the O, H, or Vi antigens.

The O (somatic) antigen has been assigned arabic numbers from 1 to 64. For convenience the salmonellae have been placed in serogroups A through Z, each group containing specific O antigens. For example, one serotype in group A might contain O antigens 1, 4, 12, and 27 while another serotype in group B might contain O antigens 1, 6, 14, and 25. For identification of the most important salmonellae a commercial grouping serum is available. Nearly 95 percent of the serotypes isolated from humans and animals can be found in groups A through O. Some groups contain common antigens, and single-factor antiserum is available for more specific identification. The *Vi* antigen surrounds *S. typhi* and can prevent agglutination of O antigens. When negative reactions occur with O grouping sera, the Vi antiserum should be applied.

Serotype identification is based on the characteristics of the H or flagellar antigen. Most salmonellae have two different H antigens. The H antigens are designated by a lowercase letter: a, b, c, and so on. The two different H antigens occur in phases, which are genetically controlled and can be influenced by the age and composition of the culture medium. Speciation of salmonellae requires identification of both phases. Serotyping is provided only by special reference laboratories.

In gastroenteritis, specimens of feces, vomit, or foodstuffs are analyzed in the laboratory. The same procedures that are used for the enteric fever group can be applied. Salmonella isolates should be identified to the genus and serogroup level. Phage typing is used epidemiologically to match patient isolate with contaminated food.

Blood samples are also used to isolate *Salmonella* species involved in septicemia.

Diagnosis of enteric fever in endemic areas, where physicians do not have access to facilities for bacteriologic examination, can be accomplished by confirmation of any of the eight following events:

1. Positive Widal test at a screening dilution of 1:40 (this is an agglutination test to detect H or O agglutinins in patient's serum)
2. Peak temperature of more than 39°C
3. Previous antibiotic treatment
4. A white blood cell count greater than 9×10^9/liter
5. A PMN cell count of more than 3.5×10^6/liter
6. Splenomegaly
7. Hepatomegaly
8. Fever duration of more than seven days

TREATMENT

Salmonella infection responds to four drugs: chloramphenicol, ampicillin, amoxicillin, and trimethoprim-sulfamethoxazole. For gastroenteritis, antibiotics are contraindicated unless chronic bacteremia is also present. Replenishment of lost fluids and electrolytes is the most important aspect of gastroenteritis management, particularly for young children.

For enteric fevers and bacteremia, chloramphenicol is one choice for antimicrobial therapy. Ampicillin and trimethoprim-sulfamethoxazole are used if the species is resistant to chloramphenicol. Surgery may be required if there has been perforation of the ileum.

PREVENTION AND CONTROL

Salmonella infections can be controlled or at least reduced by (1) proper sanitation with special emphasis on sewage disposal and maintenance of unpolluted water supplies; (2) supervision of the preparation of products by the food industries; (3) proper refrigeration of foods, particularly poultry and related products; and (4) detection of asymptomatic carriers and their removal from occupations involved in the handling of food or care of the hospitalized until the carriers are adequately treated.

S. *typhi* vaccines are seldom administered in the United States; however, they are employed for military personnel and those traveling to areas where typhoid fever is endemic. The vaccine used is an acetone-killed suspension of S. *typhi* that has been shown to give a high degree of protection.

The vaccines used in most parts of the world where typhoid fever is endemic are administered parenterally. These vaccines frequently cause adverse reactions such as inflammation, fever, and headache and need to be readministered periodically. Currently two vaccines are being tested in several Third World countries. One of them is an oral attenuated vaccine, which has been recently licensed in the United States. The other is an injectable vaccine made from the capsular polysaccharide or Vi antigen.

SHIGELLA SPECIES

Shigella species are the cause of a gastrointestinal disease called *bacillary dysentery*. There are four species of *Shigella*: S. *dysenteriae*, S. *flexneri*, S. *boydii*, and S. *sonnei*. With few exceptions the shigellae are harbored by humans and transferred by the fecal-oral route. Shigellae are also important historically because they were the first recognized microorganisms isolated from humans that carried multiple antibiotic resistance markers on plasmids.

PATHOGENESIS

Like the salmonellae, the shigellae are transferred from person to person by contaminated food, water, or fomites. The incubation period for shigellosis is 36 to 72 hours. As few as 200 ingested *Shigella* organisms are enough to initiate infection. The shigellae invade the intestinal epithelium like the invasive *Salmonella* species. Shigellae, however, unlike the salmonellae, are found free in the cytoplasm of the epithelial cell. It appears that when engulfed by the cytoplasmic membrane of the epithelial cell the shigellae digest the membrane of the phagocytic vacuole. Shigellae then spread laterally to invade adjacent epithelial cells. Epithelial invasion is not sufficient to cause disease; the organism must also replicate and be capable of persisting in the mucosa. A transient inflammation may result from penetration of the epithelium, but the mucosal ulceration associated with disease occurs only after microbial multiplication. Up to 10^{10} organisms can be found per gram of stool during disease. Abdominal cramps, fever, and watery diarrhea occur early in the disease. Dysentery occurs during the ulceration process with high concentrations of neutrophils in the stools.

The symptoms of shigellosis are mild or severe depending on the species causing infection. The severest forms of shigellosis are caused by S. *dysenteriae* type 1, also called the *Shiga bacillus*. *Shigella dysenteriae* produces a toxin called the *Shiga toxin*, which may contribute to the necrotic lesions of the colon (cytotoxic activity) and probably the diarrhea associated with disease (enterotoxic activity). Shiga toxin belongs to the group of toxins (cholera, diphtheria, and pertussis, for example) that possess A and B subunits. In other words, the B subunit is responsible for binding to the mammalian cell while the A subunit is the toxic fraction. The Shiga toxin, released by *Shigella* during infection, is taken up by mammalian cells (intestinal microvilli, for example) and this leads to cell death. The primary site of Shiga toxin action is the ribosomal binding site for aminoacyl tRNA, that is, the 60 S ribosomal subunit. *Shigella* species other than *S. dysenteriae* produce a toxin referred to as *Shiga-like*, which is similar in chemistry and action to toxins produced by *E. coli*, *Campylobacter*, and others. Shiga-like toxins are not produced in sufficient quantities to cause disease so severe as that caused by *S. dysenteriae*.

EPIDEMIOLOGY

The number of cases of shigellosis reported in the United States in 1989 was 25,010. *S. sonnei* accounts for nearly 80 percent of all *Shigella* isolates while *S. dysenteriae* accounts for approximately 1 percent. The highest rates of shigellosis are in the western states and among children from 1 to 5 years of age (Fig. 20-6).

Epidemics of shigellosis occur in crowded communities where reservoirs are human carriers of *Shigella*. *Shigella* can be spread by flies, fingers, food, or feces. Many cases of shigellosis are associated with day care centers, prisons, and institutions for the mentally retarded. Military field groups and travelers to countries with unsanitary conditions are also likely victims.

LABORATORY DIAGNOSIS

As a presumptive test for shigellosis some clinicians examine fecal specimens for the presence of sheets of neutrophils. Confirmatory tests are carried out by plating the specimen on various selective or differential media. Isolated species are then subjected to specific biochemical tests. Species that are nonmotile, do not ferment lactose, produce no gas from carbohydrate fermen-

Fig. 20-6. Rate of reported isolates of *Shigella* by age. (From Centers for Disease Control.)

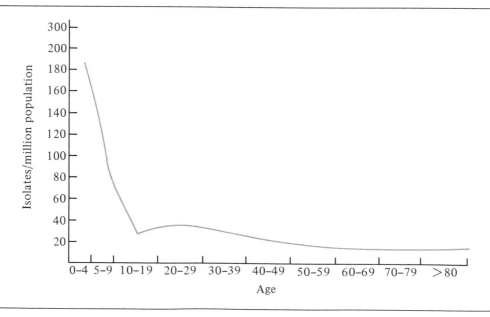

tation, and fail to produce hydrogen sulfide are possibly *Shigella*. Three biochemical tests are helpful in separating species of *Shigella* (Table 20-5), but serological testing is needed for confirmation. There are four serogroups corresponding to the four species of *Shigella*: Group A (*S. dysenteriae*), Group B (*S. flexneri*), Group C (*S. boydii*), and Group D (*S. sonnei*). Agglutination of isolated colonies in one of the four antisera, plus the biochemical reactions, provides species identification.

Colicin typing of strains of *S. sonnei* is performed in some laboratories. The colicin determinants appear to be relatively stable in the various serotypes. Colicin typing is based on ability to produce colicins and not on susceptibility to colicins.

TREATMENT

Although most cases of shigellosis are mild and do not require antibiotics, the latter can shorten the duration of diarrhea and eliminate the bacillus from the stool, preventing possible spread to others in the community.

The World Health Organization (WHO) suggests that in shigellosis only *S. dysenteriae* warrants antibiotic administration. Trials in several countries have shown that norfloxacin, a new fluoroquinolone derivative, provides clinical and microbiological cure. If other antibiotics are to be used, there is really no drug of choice because susceptibility patterns differ from one region to another. Many *Shigella* species show multiple drug resistance. Patients who experience dehydration should have oral fluid and electrolyte replacement. Oral rehydration, however, is ineffective in changing the course of the disease.

PREVENTION AND CONTROL

Improving sanitation and hygienic practices is the most important factor in the control of shigellosis. Because of overcrowding and sometimes poor hygienic practices or procedures, custodial institutions are a major reservoir of disease. Control measures in institutions should include isolation of the infected patient, restriction of infected personnel from handling food or working with patients, and in-service training for all personnel. An oral attenuated *Shigella* vaccine has been very successful in reducing epidemics in custodial institutions. The vaccine consists of streptomycin-dependent *Shigella* strains that cannot multiply in the intestine but are capable of stimulating antibodies.

Table 20-5. Biochemical Tests Used to Differentiate Species of *Shigella*

Test	Response of			
	S. dysenteriae	*S. flexneri*	*S. boydii*	*S. sonnei*
Mannitol fermentation	−	+	+	+
ONPG	V	−	V	+
Ornithine decarboxylase	−	−	−	+

− = ≤9 percent of strains are positive; V = 10 to 89 percent of strains are positive; + = ≥ 90 percent of strains are positive; ONPG = ortho-nitrophenyl-beta-D-galactopyranoside.

YERSINIA SPECIES

The genus *Yersinia* (formerly *Pasteurella*) has three important pathogenic species: *Y. pestis*, *Y. pseudotuberculosis*, and *Y. enterocolitica*. *Y. pestis* is the causative agent of *bubonic plague* (black death) in humans. *Y. pseudotuberculosis* causes epizootic disease in animals and is a minor gastrointestinal pathogen. *Y. enterocolitica* is now being recognized as an important agent of gastrointestinal illness in humans.

YERSINIA PESTIS

In the fourteenth century bubonic plague was responsible for the deaths of more than 25 percent of the population of Europe. The most recent pandemic occurred in Asia in 1904, when more than a million people succumbed. Today the disease, which is harbored by rodents and transmitted to humans by insect vectors, is a rarity, partly because of the widespread use of insecticides and other measures that have controlled the insect vectors responsible for its transmission.

The plague bacillus, *Yersinia pestis*, is a gram-negative, nonmotile, facultative anaerobe that possesses bipolar granules. It produces a capsule in animal tissue. It grows optimally on blood agar or media supplemented with blood at temperatures ranging from 27 to 30°C.

Pathogenesis

Plague is a disease found naturally in rats and other rodents. The primary vector in transmission of *Y. pestis* is the rat flea, which picks up the plague bacillus by biting an infected rodent. The plague bacillus readily adapts to conditions in the alimentary tract of the flea, where it multiplies and accumulates. The bacilli are then transmitted to humans through the bite of the infected flea. During the incubation period, which may last from 1 to 5 days, the patient is subject to vomiting and high fever. From the site of the fleabite the bacilli migrate to regional lymph nodes, such as axillary and inguinal nodes, causing their enlargement. The enlarged nodes are called *buboes*; hence the term *bubonic plague*. The bacilli proliferate in the mononuclear phagocytes and there develop antiphagocytic factors: a capsule and two antigens called the *V* and *W* factors. The enlarged lymph nodes contain numerous bacilli and bacterial products, which have free access to lymphatic tissue. If the plague bacilli enter the circulation (*septicemic plague*), they can infect a number of different organs. On rare occasions the plague bacilli infect the lungs (*pneumonic plague*), producing massive hemor-

rhages. From the infected lungs the plague bacilli can enter the bloodstream. All forms of plague can be fatal, but the pneumonic type is invariably the most lethal if left untreated, on account of the toxemia caused by the lipopolysaccharide endotoxin of *Y. pestis*.

Yersinia Virulence Determinants

All the pathogenic *Yersinia* share a marked tropism, or affinity, for lymphoid tissue. As yet there are no conclusive answers to the mechanisms of virulence but several factors are believed to be involved. From their site of invasion (lung or intestinal tract) *Yersinia* adhere to the cytoplasmic membrane of host cells and then are ingested by endocytosis with vacuole formation. The vacuolar membrane dissolves, allowing the bacteria to migrate in the cytoplasm of host cells. The invasion process appears to be associated with determinants encoded on the chromosome. All the other potential virulence determinants appear to be associated with a plasmid called *pYV*, which codes for 16 different proteins, some of which are outer membrane proteins. *Yersinia* resistance to phagocytosis by macrophages is also associated with the pYV plasmid. *Y. pestis* produces a capsule that resists phagocytosis, but other *Yersinia* appear to rely on outer membrane proteins or on the V antigen to prevent phagocytosis. The virulence determinants on the pYV plasmid appear to be controlled by the *calcium concentration*. Calcium dependence is viewed as a transition between free growth and protection against the immune system. Within the macrophage, for example, the concentration of calcium induces *Yersinia* to produce outer membrane proteins that prevent digestion of the bacteria.

Epidemiology

Plague, primarily a disease of rodents, is transmitted from animal to animal or animal to human by infected fleas (Fig. 20-7). In bubonic plague, rats are the primary reservoir of *Y. pestis*. Most cases are found in Southeast Asia. In the United

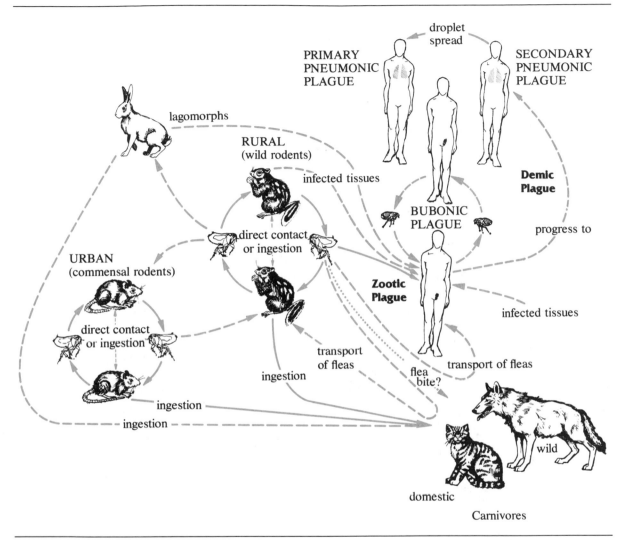

Fig. 20-7. Epidemiology of infection by *Yersinia pestis*. Solid lines = usual pathway; dashed lines = occasional pathway; dotted lines = rare or theoretical pathway. (From J. Poland. In P. Hoeprich [ed.], *Infectious Diseases*. Hagerstown, MD: Harper & Row, 1977.)

States most cases of plague (approximately 15–20 per year) are seen in New Mexico and Arizona. Most cases are seen among Indians in the Navajo tribe. The infectious agent is harbored primarily by rodents such as the rock squirrel and prairie dog and infrequently by coyotes, dogs, cats, and rabbits. Rodents, which have a high mortality in epizootics of plague, carry a large

number of fleas during the summer months. Human disease may result from direct exposure to infected rodents, rabbits, or carnivores as well as the bite of an infected flea. Plague among wild rodents is referred to as wild or *sylvatic plague*. Plague transmitted from person to person is called *demic plague*. (See Boxed Essay, p. 492).

Pneumonic plague, in which quantities of ba-

PLAGUE—SOUTH CAROLINA

On August 5, 1983, plague was diagnosed in a 13-year-old girl in South Carolina. She became ill while en route to Maryland from her previous residence in Santa Fe, New Mexico, and subsequently died. The area in which she had lived had been recognized as a locality where sylvatic plague was enzootic.

On July 25, the girl, a horsewoman who spent considerable time outdoors, handled and then released a wild chipmunk.On July 27, she flew to Atlanta, Georgia, and spent the night with friends; the following day she was driven to Seneca, South Carolina. That evening, she complained of a sore throat and tenderness in her right groin and reportedly had a temperature of 40.0°C (104°F). On July 29, she saw a physician, who noted an oral temperature of 38.3°C (101°F), pharyngeal erythema, tender cervical lymph nodes and a 1-×-2-cm tender right inguinal lymph node. Laboratory tests, including complete blood count, urinalysis, and throat culture, and tests for mononucleosis were done, and oral penicillin was prescribed. Three days later she was seen again, still febrile and with expanding right inguinal nodes. Because of her history of residence in a plague-enzootic state, a diagnosis of plague was considered. She was hospitalized and given parenteral therapy, including streptomycin. By the following morning, she was tachypneic, with productive bloody sputum, and appeared moribund. Despite intensive supportive care and therapy with intravenous chloramphenicol, she developed overwhelming sepsis and died on August 2. A chest radiograph taken before death revealed extensive pulmonary infiltrates.

Based on the clinical picture and the positive fluorescent antibody results from sputum, it appears that pneumonic plague and the potential for human-to-human transmission existed terminally. Local health care providers had placed her in complete isolation before this development. Hospital staff directly in contact with her at this point were given prophylactic tetracycline and followed up for evidence of illness. No secondary cases appeared during the expected incubation period.

Primary pneumonic plague in the United States has been described as rare, with only three cases between 1926 and 1977—all in laboratory workers. Recent investigations suggest that plague pneumonia (i.e., secondary to bubonic plague) is more common.Thus far in 1983, 24 cases of human plague have originated in New Mexico, and three (13 percent) of them have had pneumonic involvement. No transmission to contacts of patients with pneumonic plague has been documented in the United States since 1925.

From *MMWR* 32:417, 1983

cilli are found in the sputum, can be transmitted to others by respiratory droplets. Pneumonic plague is seen infrequently today but when it does occur it is usually an extension of septicemia and is seldom due to inhalation of the pathogen. Primary pneumonic plague is occasionally the result of contact with household pets that have plague pneumonia.

Only 4 cases of plague were reported in 1989 in the United States.

Laboratory Diagnosis

Depending on the nature of the plague, blood cultures, sputum samples, or aspirates of buboes should be examined for typical bacilli. The isolated bacilli can be identified by (1) staining with Wayson's technique (methylene blue plus basic fuchsin) to demonstrate bipolar staining of the granules (Fig. 20-8), (2) fluorescent antibody technique using *Y. pestis* antiserum, and (3) phage typing.

Treatment

Because of the severity of the disease, rapid treatment is required, even before final laboratory diagnosis. Successful treatment can be secured with streptomycin, chloramphenicol, tetracycline, or the combination of trimethoprim and sulfamethoxazole. A permanent immunity is obtained after recovery from infection.

Prevention and Control

It is neither possible nor desirable to eliminate the rodent population. The major avenue of control is directed at eliminating or reducing the flea population. Fumigation of ships traveling to and from various ports has proved effective in controlling the transmission of plague. In the United States, when epidemics occur among the wild rodent population, bait stations are set up in certain tracts of land, particularly wooded areas. These stations contain rodent attractants as well as in-

Fig. 20-8. Smear prepared from lymph gland for demonstration of *Yersinia pestis*. Note bipolar staining. (From R. R. Gillies and T. C. Dodds, *Bacteriology Illustrated*. London: Churchill Livingstone, 1976.)

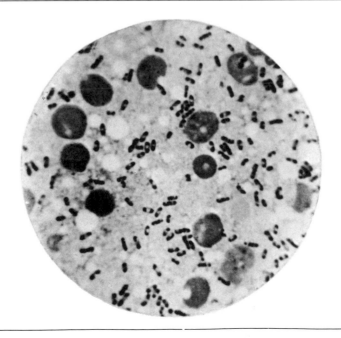

secticides such as permethrin, which is lethal to the flea.

Vaccines have had limited success. Dead, whole-organism plague vaccines are still believed to be the most useful for human vaccination. A formalin-killed vaccine is currently being used for people working in areas where plague is endemic. Vaccination is recommended for laboratory personnel who are working with *Y. pestis* organisms resistant to antimicrobials, persons engaged in aerosol experiments with *Y. pestis*, and persons working in areas with enzootic plague. Vaccination should also be considered for laboratory personnel working with plague-infected rodents and those whose occupation or residence brings them into continual contact with wild rodents or rabbits in enzootic areas.

YERSINIA ENTEROCOLITICA AND *Y. PSEUDOTUBERCULOSIS*

Diseases caused by *Yersinia* species other than *Y. pestis* are called *yersinoses*. Two species are associated with yersinosis, *Y. enterocolitica* and *Y. pseudotuberculosis*. Both species are found in many domestic animals, and thus yersinoses are zoonotic diseases in which humans become accidentally infected. Human carriers are rare. Disease in humans is caused primarily by ingestion of fecally contaminated food, water, milk, or milk products, but some diseases result from animal-to-human transmission. *Y. enterocolitica* is the most frequent isolate from yersinosis cases in the United States. Gastroenteritis is the chief manifestation of disease in all age groups. Diseases occur more frequently in the colder months. In infants the most common manifestation is enterocolitis, in which there is severe diarrhea and fever. The stool often contains blood and mucus. The disease resembles gastroenteritis caused by species of *Salmonella*, *Shigella*, and *E. coli*. In infants the diarrhea is usually self-limiting. In older children and adults, there is invasion of the mesenteric lymph with or without diarrhea. Ar-

thritis involving ankles, fingers, and knees and erythema nodosum with subcutaneous nodules on the legs are common complications following infection by *Y. enterocolitica* in Scandinavia. Septicemia is not usually encountered unless the patient has some underlying illness. The fatality rate in this septicemia is higher than 50 percent because, like other gram-negative septicemias, it is difficult to diagnose.

Laboratory diagnosis of *Y. enterocolitica* and *Y. pseudotuberculosis* is complicated by the fact that these organisms are not usually sought in the laboratory. There are some biochemical tests that can aid in separating the three major *Yersinia* species (Table 20-6).

Antibiotics are not required for gastroenteritis but rather only replacement of lost fluids. Chloramphenicol, gentamicin, tobramycin, and the combination trimethoprim-sulfamethoxazole are all effective in the treatment of systemic disease.

Table 20-6. Biochemical Tests Used in Differentiating Pathogenic *Yersinia* Species

Test	Response of		
	Y. pestis	*Y. enterocolitica*	*Y. pseudotuberculosis*
Melibiose fermentation	V	–	V
Ornithine decarboxylase	–	+	–
Raffinose fermentation	–	–	V
Rhamnose fermentation	–	–	V
Sucrose fermentation	–	+	–
Urease formation	–	V	+

– = ≤9 percent of strains are positive; V = 10 to 89 percent of strains are positive; + = ≥90 percent of strains are positive.
Tests are performed at 37°C and may vary if performed at 25°C.

OPPORTUNISTIC ENTERIC BACILLI

Several genera of enteric bacilli are seldom encountered in community-associated infections. Instead, these bacilli are causes of a variety of infections in the compromised host, especially those who have been hospitalized. Table 20-7 outlines the characteristics of these opportunistic bacteria.

SUMMARY

1. The Enterobacteriaceae are facultative, gram-negative rods that ferment glucose, are oxidase negative, and reduce nitrates to nitrite.

They may be motile by peritrichous flagella or nonmotile.

2. Enterobacteriaceae are widely distributed on plants, in the soil, and in the intestines of humans and animals. They are associated with many types of infections, some of which are community-associated while others are opportunistic and associated with compromised patients. The lipopolysaccharide of the outer membrane of the Enterobacteriaceae is probably responsible for the devastating effects of shock and death in patients with septicemia.

3. The characteristics of the major pathogenic genera of the family Enterobacteriaceae are outlined in Table 20-8. The characteristics of opportunistic species were described in Table 20-7.

4. The pathogenic genera of Enterobacteriaceae can be identified in the laboratory by bio-

Table 20-7. Characteristics of Some Genera of Opportunistic Enteric Bacilli That Occasionally Cause Opportunistic Infections in Humans*

Genus	Clinically important species	Primary site of infection or disease	Treatment
Enterobacter	*E. aerogenes,* *E. cloacae,* *E. agglomerans*	Extraintestinal (pulmonary, bloodstream, central nervous system, etc.)	Aminoglycosides, chloramphenicol, tetracyclines
Providencia	*P. alcalifaciens,* *P. rettgeri,* *P. stuartii*	Urinary tract infections, burn wound infections	Resistant to many antimicrobials in vivo. Antimicrobial susceptibility testing critical
Klebsiella	*K. pneumoniae,* *K. ozaenae,* *K. rhinoscleromatis,* *K. oxytoca*	*K. pneumoniae* important cause of septicemia in pediatric wards. Pneumonia and other respiratory tract infections in compromised patients *K. ozaenae* may cause middle ear and soft tissue infections	Some aminoglycosides, tetracyclines
Proteus	*P. mirabilis,* *P. penneri,* *P. vulgaris*	Urinary tract infections	Ampicillin, cephalothin, aminoglycosides
Serratia	*S. marcescens*	Extraintestinal (urinary tract, septicemia, central nervous system)	Gentamicin, carbenicillin, kanamycin

* Not all enteric bacilli are represented in this table.

Table 20-8. Characteristics of the Major Pathogenic Species in the Family Enterobacteriaceae

Genera	Major pathogenic species	Disease	Virulence factor	Mechanism of transmission	Treatment and prevention
Escherichia	*E. coli*	Extraintestinal: urinary tract in compromised host. Neonatal meningitis. Intestinal: see Table 20-4	Pili; K1 polysaccharide See Table 20-4	Person to person (extraintestinal). Ingestion of contaminated food or water (intestinal)	Chloramphenicol, tetracycline in extraintestinal. Replacement of fluids and electrolytes in intestinal infections
Salmonella	*S. typhi, S. paratyphi A, S. paratyphi B*	Enteric fever: gastrointestinal illness followed by bacteremia. Complications may occur (e.g., perforated intestine)	Vi antigen to prevent phagocytosis. Endotoxin for inflammation (*S. typhi*)	Person to person via fecally contaminated food or water	Chloramphenicol, ampicillin, trimethoprim-sulfamethoxazole. Surgery for perforated intestine. Killed vaccine for travelers to areas endemic for typhoid
	Many serotypes other than those causing enteric fevers	Gastroenteritis: diarrhea	Enterotoxin similar to cholera toxin	Ingestion of food products contaminated by salmonella indigenous to animals	Replenishment of fluids and electrolytes
Shigella	*S. dysenteriae* type 1, *S. sonnei, S. flexneri, S. sonnei*	Bacillary dysentery: *S. dysenteriae* type 1 produces most severe symptoms	Shiga toxin (*S. dysenteriae*). Shiga-like toxin for other species	Ingestion of fecally contaminated food or water	Replenishment of fluids and electrolytes. Ampicillin, trimethoprim-sulfamethoxazole to prevent spread
Yersinia	*Y. pestis*	Bubonic plague: infection of lymph tissue. Pneumonic plague: infection of lung	pYV plasmid encodes several virulence factors: capsule, V antigen, and outer membrane proteins	Bite of infected flea (bubonic plague). Contact with respiratory secretions or via bacteremia (pneumonic plague)	Streptomycin, chloramphenicol, trimethoprim-sulfamethoxazole. Killed vaccine in areas endemic for disease
	Y. enterocolitica, Y. pseudotuberculosis	Gastroenteritis: diarrhea. Sometimes complicated by arthritis and erythema nodosum	Probably same as *Y. pestis*	Ingestion of contaminated food or water	Replenishment of fluids and electrolytes. Chloramphenicol, gentamicin, trimethoprim-sulfamethoxazole for systemic infection

chemical testing but genera such as *Escherichia*, *Shigella*, and *Salmonella* are also identified by O antigens and sometimes by H and K antigens.

5. Enterobacteriaceae are frequently resistant to many antimicrobials and susceptibility testing is required. Most species are susceptible to some type of aminoglycoside, a tetracycline, or trimethoprim-sulfamethoxazole.

QUESTIONS FOR STUDY

Select the best response or responses for each of the following:

1. All of the following are characteristics of the Enterobacteriaceae *except*
   A. Most species ferment glucose and reduce nitrates to nitrites.
   B. Pili are the principal adhesins.
   C. Antimicrobial resistance can be transferred between different species.
   D. Most have complex nutritional requirements.

2. Which of the following Enterobacteriaceae demonstrate the least metabolic activity when identified in the clinical laboratory?
   A. *E. coli*
   B. *Yersinia pestis*
   C. *Salmonella typhi*
   D. *Proteus mirabilis*

3. If glucose is the only sugar fermented in a triple sugar iron agar slant
   A. The slant will retain its original red color.
   B. The entire tube will be yellow including the slant.
   C. The slant will appear yellow but the remainder of the tube will be red.
   D. The entire tube will be red including the slant.

4. The most abundant group of bacteria found in the intestinal tract is
   A. *E. coli*
   B. *Bacteroides* species
   C. *Salmonella* species
   D. *Proteus* species

5. The main virulence determinant that is found in most *E. coli* strains causing neonatal meningitis is
   A. Pili
   B. Enterotoxin
   C. K1 capsular polysaccharide
   D. Cytotoxins

6. The major cause of bacterial infant diarrhea in developing countries is
   A. Enterotoxigenic *E. coli*
   B. *Salmonella* species
   C. Enteropathogenic *E. coli*
   D. *Shigella* species

7. Which of the following enteric pathogens would be most likely to survive as an intracellular parasite, for example, in the macrophage?
   A. Enterotoxigenic *E. coli*
   B. *Salmonella typhi*
   C. *Shigella dysenteriae*
   D. Enteropathogenic *E. coli*

8. Gastroenteritis in several individuals attending a party for which the lunch meat was catered would most likely be caused by
   A. *E. coli*
   B. *Shigella dysenteriae*
   C. *Clostridium perfringens*
   D. *Salmonella enteritidis*

Fill in the blank:

9. Replacement of water and electrolytes is the primary treatment regimen for most infections in which _____ is the primary symptom.

10. Plague is a disease that is naturally found in _____.

11. _____ species are opportunistic enteric bacilli that are an important cause of pneumonia in compromised patients.

12. In addition to biochemical testing genera such as *Escherichia*, *Shigella*, and *Salmonella* can be identified by their _____ antigens.

13. Enlarged lymph nodes caused by *Yersinia pestis* infection are called _____.

ADDITIONAL READINGS

Chalker, R. B., and Blaser, M. J. A review of human salmonellosis. III. Magnitude of salmonella infection in the United States. *Rev. Infect. Dis.* 10(1): 111,1988.

Cornelis, G., Laroche, Y., Balligand, G., and Sory, M. P. *Yersinia enterocolitica*, a primary model of invasiveness. *Rev. Infect. Dis.* 9(1):64,1987.

Hale, T. L. Virulence mechanisms of enteric pathogens. *Curr. Opin. Infect. Dis.* 2(6):781,1989.

Hornick, R. B. Selective primary health care. Strategy for control of disease in the developing world. XX. Typhoid fever. *Rev. Infect. Dis.* 7(4):536,1985.

Law, D. Virulence factors of enteropathogenic *Escherichia coli*. *J. Med. Microbiol.* 26:1,1988.

Levine, M. M. *Escherichia coli* that cause diarrhea. Enterotoxigenic, enteropathogenic, enteroinvasive, enterohemorrhagic, and enteroadherent. *J. Infect. Dis.* 155(3):377,1987.

National Institutes of Health Consensus Development Conference. Traveler's diarrhea. *Rev. Infect. Dis.* 8(Suppl. 2):1986.

O'Brien, A. D., and Holmes, R. K. Shiga and shiga-like toxins. *Microbiol. Rev.* 51(2):206,1987.

21. *PSEUDOMONAS* AND RELATED ORGANISMS

OBJECTIVES

To describe those virulence factors associated with
  Pseudomonas infections
To explain the techniques used to identify strains of
  Pseudomonas aeruginosa
To list the drugs most effective in treatment of *P.*

aeruginosa infections and to explain why the
  organism is so resistant to most antimicrobials
To list some *Pseudomonas* species other than *P.
  aeruginosa* that are associated with human
  infection

The genus *Pseudomonas* belongs to a group of bacteria that are characterized as gram-negative, nonfermentative, aerobic bacilli. Pseudomonads are opportunistic pathogens and like other members of the group—*Alcaligenes, Achromobacter, Acinetobacter, Moraxella, Flavobacterium, Eikenella,* and *Agrobacterium*—are associated with disease in the hospital setting. Pseudomonads are known for their ability to catabolize a wide variety of carbon sources. For this reason they can be found in soil and water and related habitats. The most important species in terms of causing disease is *Pseudomonas aeruginosa*.

PSEUDOMONAS AERUGINOSA

GENERAL CHARACTERISTICS

P. aeruginosa rods are from 2 to 4 μm in length, and most are motile. *Pseudomonas* produces a slime layer at all times, but in certain instances an exopolysaccharide is produced by mucoid strains, for example, those strains found in the lungs of cystic fibrosis patients. The success of *P. aeruginosa* in colonizing and multiplying in a wide variety of environments is due to its biphasic growth patterns. Sometimes the organism exists as a highly motile cell capable of swimming from site to site; at other times it produces a slimy layer that enables it to multiply in the form of an adherent microcolony. Another distinguishing characteristic of most *P. aeruginosa* mucoid strains is their ability to produce yellowish water-soluble fluorescent pigments called *pyoverdins*. Only *P. aeruginosa* produces the nonfluorescent water-soluble pigment called *pyocyanin*. Strains of P. aeruginosa, which produce pyocyanin and pyoverdin, frequently impart a greenish color to culture media. Cultures of *P. aeruginosa* or wounds infected by this organism give off a distinctive grape-like odor due to one of their pigments, *2-aminoacetophenone*.

PATHOGENESIS AND EPIDEMIOLOGY

P. aeruginosa is a ubiquitous organism, and most persons have antibodies to the species. Most *Pseudomonas* diseases are associated with those who are severely compromised. For example, *P. aeruginosa* has become the predominant organism isolated from patients with cystic fibrosis and severe lung diseases. The organism is also one of the leading causes of gram-negative infections of the urinary tract, surgical wounds, and burn wounds (Fig. 21-1). It is second only to *E. coli* as the major cause of hospital-associated disease. The increasing number of hot tubs and whirlpools in private residences has also resulted in increasing numbers of *Pseudomonas* infections. These infections are of the cutaneous type (folliculitis). When recreational water is maintained at pH 7.2 to 7.8 with residual chlorine, outbreaks of cutaneous infections do not occur.

The ubiquitous nature of *P. aeruginosa*, particularly in water, has created concern in the area of ophthalmology. This organism is one of the most common pathogens associated with bacte-

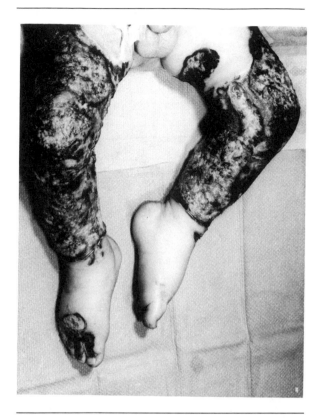

Fig. 21-1. Generalized invasive *Pseudomonas* burn wound sepsis in a child. (From B. A. Pruitt, et al., *Rev. Infect. Dis.* 5 [Suppl. 5]:889. © 1983 University of Chicago.)

Table 21-1. Possible Virulence Determinants of *Pseudomonas aeruginosa*

Determinant	Biological activity
CELLULAR FACTORS	
Pili	Adherence to epithelial cells
Slime polysaccharide	Neutrophil toxicity
Mucoid exopolysaccharide	Antiphagocytic; decreased pulmonary clearance
Lipid A	Endotoxic effects; induces protective antibodies
EXTRACELLULAR FACTORS	
Proteases (e.g., elastase, alkaline protease)	Tissue adherence, tissue invasion and damage
Exotoxin A	Cytotoxicity, macrophage toxicity; induces protective antibodies
Phospholipase	Degradation of cytoplasmic membrane components

rial corneal ulcers. Corneal injury is a major predisposing factor to infection. Recently, keratitis due to *P. aeruginosa* has also been observed in the wearers of extended-wear contact lenses.

Pseudomonas is well suited to habitation in mammalian hosts because it possesses components and elaborates products that are believed to be associated with virulence. We will discuss some of the more important virulence determinants. Some of the others are outlined in Table 21-1.

Pili

Pili appear to be the adhesins involved in binding of nonmucoid strains of *P. aeruginosa* to the mu-

cins covering the tracheobronchial tree and receptors on tracheal cells.

Proteases

P. aeruginosa releases proteases that have been shown to be virulence factors. Alkaline proteases and elastase, for example, have been shown to cause proteolytic cleavage of receptors on neutrophils that are involved in binding to target *P. aeruginosa* cells. Thus, proteases interfere with normal neutrophil function.

The ability of *P. aeruginosa* to cause tissue necrosis and invade epithelial surfaces appears to be due also to the action of alkaline proteases and elastase. Elastase, for example, acts as an endopeptidase (cleaves proteins internally) and is capable of digesting human proteins, including elastin, collagen, fibrin, immunoglobulin G (IgG), and IgA.

Exopolysaccharide

Mucoid strains of *P. aeruginosa* isolated from the respiratory tract of patients with cystic fibrosis produce an exopolysaccharide. The exopolysaccharide is an alginate composed of mannuronic-glucuronic acids. This polysaccharide is different in chemical composition from the polysaccharide slime produced by nonmucoid cells. The exopolysaccharide alginate allows the organism to form microcolonies. (see Boxed Essay, p. 503) When artificially produced microcolonies are introduced into the lungs of normal rats, disease can be induced. The microcolony withstands clearance mechanisms in the host's respiratory tract and also inhibits phagocytosis. Host cells are killed by the microcolony, and the pathogens multiply and spread to form other microcolonies.

Exotoxin A

Exotoxin A is an extracellular enzyme produced by most clinical strains of *P. aeruginosa*. The exotoxin is a protein composed of two polypeptide chains, A and B. Fragment B is the receptor-binding portion of the exotoxin A molecule and is believed to initiate the transport of fragment A, the enzymatic fragment. The intact polypeptide is probably transported across the cytoplasmic membrane by an endocytic mechanism (Fig. 21-2). Once inside the cytoplasm, fragment A is separated from fragment B and becomes activated. Exotoxin A, like diphtheria toxin, is a proenzyme consisting of an enzymatically active NH_2 terminal portion (fragment A) and the COOH terminal binding portion (fragment B). Exotoxin A enzymatically catalyzes the transfer of the adenosine diphosphate ribosyl (ADPR) moiety from nicotinamide-adenine dinucleotide (NAD) to a covalent linkage with elongation factor 2 (EF2), which is involved in protein synthesis:

$$NAD + EF2 \xrightarrow{\text{exotoxin A}} ADPR\text{-}EF2 + \text{nicotinamide} + H^+$$

Thus ribosomal translocation along the messenger RNA (mRNA) is stopped, and protein synthesis is inhibited.

After injection of exotoxin A into animals there is necrosis of liver cells followed by a decrease in cardiac output and systemic arterial blood pressure. Death results from respiratory failure. The exotoxin may also be immunogenic and affect human macrophages. The toxin is one-tenth as toxic as diphtheria toxin. Since many other products are released by *P. aeruginosa* it is difficult to assess the complete role of exotoxin in the disease process.

Phospholipase

Phospholipase is an extracellular product that liberates phosphorylcholine from lecithin, the component of eukaryotic membranes. Phospholipase is capable of causing pulmonary necrosis in laboratory animals.

LABORATORY DIAGNOSIS

Clinical specimens from blood, burns, and other sources can be cultured on ordinary peptone agar media. Specimens contaminated with nonpseudomonads can be cultured on media that selects pseudomonads (cetrimide agar is one example of a selective agar). Isolated colonies can be examined for odor and pigmentation. Isolates from colonies should be gram-stained and observed for morphology and motility. Suspected *Pseudomonas* isolates should be transferred to triple sugar iron agar. *Pseudomonas* species are primarily nonfermenters and on TSI agar they do not produce an acid butt or slant and H_2S is not formed. *Pseudomonas* isolates should be inoculated into oxidative fermentative media. Other tests that are employed and offer a presumptive identification of *P. aeruginosa* are outlined in Table 21-2.

Phage typing, serotyping, and pyocin typing are three methods of identifying and establishing relationships among strains of *P. aeruginosa*. Phage typing is not always effective because many strains are resistant to lytic phage. Serotyping is of limited value because most strains fall into relatively few serotypes. *Pyocin* (a bac-

EXOPOLYSACCHARIDE AND HOSPITAL-ASSOCIATED INFECTIONS

The exopolysaccharide of *P. aeruginosa* is an important virulence factor in patients with cystic fibrosis but this material appears to be also indirectly involved in hospital-associated infections.

There have been 3 instances since 1981 of clusters of *P. aeruginosa* and *P. cepacia* infections in hospitalized patients. In each case it was suspected that povidone-iodine disinfectant solutions had been contaminated by these microorganisms. In one instance the disinfectant had been used to disinfect the tops of blood-culture bottles before inoculation while in another instance the disinfectant was used as a peritoneal catheter disinfectant. Investigators now believe that *Pseudomonas* species, which are commonly found in water, colonize water distribution pipes or filters in plants that manufacture iodine solutions. The exopolysaccharides enable *Pseudomonas* species to adhere to the surface of polyvinylchloride distribution pipes and pipes of other composition. The development of microcolonies with a slime layer could enable individual bacteria to be protected from the bactericidal action of the iodophor solution.

From *M.M.W.R.* 38 (No. 8):133,1989

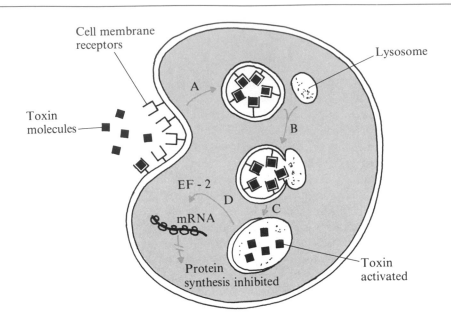

Fig. 21-2. Mechanism of exotoxin A transport and activation in the cell. A. Toxin binds to cell receptors and is transported into the cytoplasm within a vesicle. B. Lysosome fuses with the toxin-containing vesicle, and lysosomal activity activates the toxin. C. Activated toxin is released into the cytoplasm where it inhibits cellular protein synthesis by interfering with elongation factor (*EF2*).

Table 21-2. Minimal Characteristics for Identification of *Pseudomonas aeruginosa* Strains

Characteristic	Sign
Gram-negative rod	+
Motility (polar monotrichous)	+
Oxidative-fermentative glucose medium, open, acid	+
Oxidative-fermentative maltose medium, acid	−
Indophenol oxidase	+
L-lysine decarboxylase	−
L-arginine dihydrolase	+
Black butt (hydrogen sulfide) in triple sugar iron agar	−
Growth at 42°C	+

teriocin) typing is effective in determining the source of hospital-acquired infections. In this procedure the liquid pyocin in the broth culture is added to lawns of indicator strains, and growth inhibition is measured (see Chapter 10).

TREATMENT AND PREVENTION

P. aeruginosa is resistant to most antibiotics. The various mechanisms of antimicrobial resistance have been found to be combined in *P. aeruginosa*. This organism can produce beta-lactamase (plasmid-associated), has cell wall channels (porins) that are too small to allow transport of many antimicrobials, and contains altered penicillin-binding proteins. In vitro antibiotic sensitivity tests should be done before antibiotic therapy is begun. Most strains are susceptible to polymyxin B, colistin, and gentamicin, but these are very toxic and must be used sparingly. Severe infections are usually treated with carbenicillin, carbenicillin plus gentamicin, or tobramycin plus azlocillin.

Ciprofloxacin, a new quinolone, has been shown to be effective in the treatment of many multi-resistant strains of *P. aeruginosa*. Antibiotics rarely eradicate *P. aeruginosa* from the lungs of cystic fibrosis patients but early treatment improves lung function and long-time patient survival.

For patients with severe burns antibiotic therapy, combined with IV infusions of human immunoglobulin (IgG) containing antibodies to lipopolysaccharide antigens of *P. aeruginosa*, significantly lowers mortality better than when antibiotics are used alone.

Two *P. aeruginosa* vaccines have been eval-

Table 21-3. Characteristics of *Pseudomonas* Species Other than *P. aeruginosa* and Related Bacilli

Species	Disease association	Other characteristics
Pseudomonas fluorescens	Respiratory and urinary tract, wounds, bacteremia	Produces pyoverdins but not pyocyanin, no growth at 42°C, produces lecithinase
P. putida	Same as *P. fluorescens*	Does not produce pyocyanin or lecithinase, no growth at 42°C
P. cepacia	Endocarditis, septicemia, wound infections	No growth at 42°C
P. stutzeri	Same as *P. fluorescens*	No growth at 42°C
P. maltophila	Found normally in oral cavity; urinary tract infections; except for *P. aeruginosa* most frequently isolated *Pseudomonas* species	Growth at 42°C, lavender-green color on blood agar, only oxidase-negative *Pseudomonas* species
P. mallei	Cause of glanders, a disease of horses occasionally transmitted to humans	Nonmotile, no growth at 42°C
P. pseudomallei	Cause of melioidosis, a pneumonia that may progress to fatal septicemia, in humans. Septicemic melioidosis is a major cause of morbidity and mortality in northeast Thailand but is rare elsewhere in the world.	Pyocyanin and pyoverdins not produced, growth at 42°C
Acinetobacter species	Part of indigenous flora of humans; respiratory and urinary tract infections, bacteremia	Coccobacillary, confused with *Neisseria* (see Chapter 17)
Alcaligenes species	Recovered from urinary tract and blood	Oxidase positive, asaccharolytic
Achromobacter species	Isolated from blood, spinal fluid, urine, and respiratory tract	Saccharolytic, oxidase positive
Moraxella species	Isolated from blood, respiratory tract, and urine	Oxidase positive, asaccharolytic
Flavobacterium species	Rarely pathogenic but occasionally cause neonatal meningitis	Nonmotile, proteolytic, prefer cool environment
Eikenella corrodens	Isolated from wounds, respiratory tract, blood, and bone	Nonmotile, asaccharolytic, produces craters in agar
Agrobacterium species	Plant pathogens, but one species, *A. radiobacter*, isolated from wounds and spinal fluid in humans	Motile, oxidase positive

uated clinically on burn patients. A polyvalent vaccine containing a crude whole-cell extract has demonstrated protective capacity with only minor adverse reactions. A new vaccine containing *P. aeruginosa* lipopolysaccharide conjugated to exotoxin A is currently being evaluated.

OTHER *PSEUDOMONAS* SPECIES AND RELATED BACILLI

A number of other *Pseudomonas* species as well as related bacilli occasionally cause disease in humans. These species, which play a role in hospital-acquired infections, are outlined in Table 21-3.

SUMMARY

1. *Pseudomonas* is the most important member of a group of bacteria that are gram-negative, non-fermentative, aerobic, and facultatively anaerobic bacilli. The most important pathogen is *Pseudomonas aeruginosa,* which causes infections primarily in compromised patients such as burn patients, cystic fibrosis patients, and other hospitalized individuals.

2. The reason *P. aeruginosa* is observed so frequently in hospitalized patients is related to several factors, which include (1) ability to survive in moist environments, (2) ability to catabolize many varieties of carbon compounds, and (3) resistance to many antimicrobials.

3. The virulence-associated factors of *P. aeruginosa* include (1) pili for adherence, (2) proteases to destroy neutrophil receptors and prevent capture, (3) slime production, which inhibits neutrophil function, (4) exopolysaccharide, which is antiphagocytic and helps in establishing microcolonies in the host, (5) exotoxin A, which inhibits protein synthesis in host tissue, and (6) phospholipase, which attacks cellular membrane components.

4. *P. aeruginosa* produces various pigments, some of which give colonies a distinctive odor. Laboratory identification of this organism includes this feature as well as others outlined in Table 21-2. Pyocin typing is a useful epidemiologic tool.

5. Because there are many multi-resistant strains of *P. aeruginosa*, antibiotic susceptibility tests should be performed on clinical isolates before treatment is initiated. An aminoglycoside plus a penicillin derivative is a frequent treatment regimen. Antibiotic therapy can be combined with administration of human immunoglobulin in burn patients. A polyvalent vaccine is also available for burn patients.

6. Several genera of pseudomonas-related non-fermentative bacilli are important in hospital-associated infections and these are outlined in Table 21-3.

QUESTIONS FOR STUDY

Select the best response or responses for each of the following:

1. All of the following are characteristics of *Pseudomonas aeruginosa except*
   A. Produces a slime layer
   B. Is a gram-negative motile rod
   C. Produces water-soluble fluorescent pigments called pyoverdins
   D. Excretes an exotoxin that has an affinity for nervous tissue

2. All of the following are virulence factors for *P. aeruginosa* except
   A. Exotoxin A
   B. Phospholipase
   C. Lipid A
   D. Enterotoxin

3. The activity of exotoxin A is similar to that of toxin produced by
   A. *Streptococcus pyogenes*
   B. *Corynebacterium diphtheriae*
   C. *Clostridium perfringens*
   D. *Clostridium botulinum*

4. Which of the following characteristics is distinctive of *Pseudomonas* species?
   A. Are nonfermenters
   B. Cannot be cultivated on ordinary media
   C. Produce H_2S on triple sugar iron agar
   D. Are nonmotile

Fill in the blank

1. _____ typing is the most effective typing technique for determining the source of *P. aeruginosa*.

2. _____ is the nonfluorescent water-soluble pigment produced by *P. aeruginosa*.

3. IV infusions of human IgG, used for burn patients, contain antibodies to _____ antigens of *P. aeruginosa*.

4. Except for *P. aeruginosa*, *Pseudomonas* ____ is the most frequently isolated *Pseudomonas* species.

ADDITIONAL READINGS

Bodey, G. P., et al. Infections caused by *Pseudomonas aeruginosa*. *Rev. Infect. Dis.* 5:279,1983.

Pseudomonas aeruginosa—Biology, immunology, and therapy: A cefsulodin symposium. *Rev. Infect. Dis.* 6(Suppl. 3):1984.

Rubin, S. J., Granato, P. A., and Wasilauskas, B. L. Glucose-Nonfermenting Gram-Negative Bacteria, in E. H. Lennette (ed.), *Manual of Clinical Microbiology* (4th ed.). Washington, DC: American Society for Microbiology, 1985.

Sabath, L. D. (ed.). *Pseudomonas Aeruginosa*. Bern, Switzerland: Hans Huber Publishers, 1980. Symposia on *Pseudomonas aeruginosa* infections. *Rev. Infect. Dis.* 5(Suppl.5),1983.

22. VIBRIONACEAE

GENUS *VIBRIO*

Vibrios are straight or curved rods that belong to the family Vibrionaceae. Four genera are included in this family: *Vibrio, Aeromonas, Plesiomonas,* and *Photobacterium. Photobacterium* is not a human pathogen, while *Vibrio* is the major human pathogen. Vibrios are gram-negative facultative anaerobes that are motile by means of a polar flagellum (flagella). They demonstrate both respiration and fermentation and, like the Enterobacteriaceae, do not have exacting nutritional requirements. They are found in marine and fresh waters and some are common causes of intestinal and extraintestinal disease in humans.

There are several species of Vibrio, the most important of which is *V. cholerae,* the etiological agent of cholera. Other species include *V. parahaemolyticus, V. vulnificus,* and *V. alginolyticus.* Each will be discussed separately.

VIBRIO CHOLERAE

V. cholerae (serotype 01, biotype *cholerae*) is the cause of classical Asiatic cholera that devastated populations for several centuries (Fig. 22-1). In 1961 the biotype (biotypes differ in biochemical characteristics) of *V. cholerae,* called *el tor*, emerged as an important cause of cholera pandemics. Cholera is still a major cause of gastrointestinal illness in developing countries but is seldom observed in the United States (no cases reported in 1989). Worldwide, 48,403 cases of cholera were reported to WHO in 1989. In the United States *V. cholerae* non-01 (those strains that are not agglutinated by 01 antiserum) cause more gastroenteritis than *V. cholerae* 01.

Pathogenesis of *V. cholerae* 01

Cholera caused by *V. cholerae* 01 is spread from person to person by ingestion of contaminated water or uncooked foods, especially fish. *V. cholerae* is very susceptible to gastric secretions, and ingestion of approximately 10^9 vibrios in food or

Fig. 22-1. Scanning electron micrograph ($\times$ 12,000) of *Vibrio cholerae* adhering to intestinal epithelium. (From J. Teppema et al., *Infect. Immun.* 55:2093, 1987.)

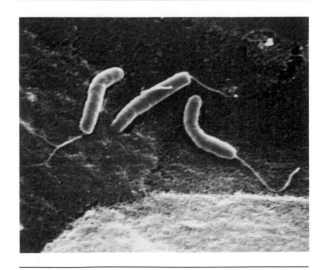

water is required to initiate disease (compare this to previously given numbers of gram-negative bacteria required to cause disease). If the individual's gastric contents have been neutralized by bicarbonate or other antacids, 10^6 vibrios may cause disease. The incubation period is approximately 2 to 3 days and is followed by a period of vomiting and diarrhea. Ten to twenty-five liters of fluid may be lost during the course of infection. Rapid dehydration is accompanied by a loss of electrolytes such as potassium and bicarbonate. The loss of electrolytes during diarrhea is due to an enterotoxin. Prostration can occur at any time and is directly related to the amount of fluids lost. Most fatalities occur when electrolytes have not been replenished. The major causes of death are shock, metabolic acidosis, and renal failure. *V. cholerae* 01 rarely causes extraintestinal infections. There is apparently no complete immunity to reinfection by *V. cholerae* since reinfection does occur in areas where the disease is endemic.

The mechanism by which cholera vibrios attach to the intestinal epithelium has not been fully elucidated. The mucous gel covering the intestinal epithelial surface is believed to be a normal barrier to invasion by many microorganisms. Vibrios penetrate the mucous gel because of their motility. Once the mucous gel has been penetrated, it is believed that a surface component of the vibrio that has protease and hemagglutinin activity enables the organism to attach to the microvilli of host epithelial cells. Once attached, the microorganism can multiply and produce enterotoxin. *Cholera enterotoxin,* which is responsible for the watery diarrhea (*rice water stool*) associated with disease*, is a protein composed of one A subunit and five B subunits. After cholera toxin binds to the cell surface the A subunit passes into the host cell membrane. The A subunit, which is activated by a cellular protease, affects the enzyme adenyl cyclase (see Boxed

* Mutants of *V. cholerae* that cannot produce toxin have been known to elicit diarrhea in one-half of orally challenged volunteers. Apparently, attachment to intestinal mucosa is a factor that can also promote diarrhea.

Essay, p. 231). The A subunit is actually an *adenosine 5'-diphosphate (ADP)-ribosyltransferase* that catalyzes the transfer of the ADP-ribose moiety of nicotinamide adenine dinucleotide (NAD) to a membrane protein. It is the ADP-ribosylated membrane protein that activates adenyl cyclase and causes the conversion of ATP to cyclic AMP (cAMP). The increase in cAMP alters the ion transport mechanisms associated with the cytoplasmic membrane. Changes in cell membrane permeability to ions, such as sodium (Na^+) and chlorine (Cl^-), cause an efflux of water from the mucosal surface and hence causes diarrhea.

Pathogenesis of *V. cholerae* non-01

Non-01 *V. cholerae* are those strains that are not agglutinated by 01 antiserum. Non-01 are found in sewage, estuarine waters (both polluted and unpolluted), seafoods, and animals. Those strains found in estuarine waters appear to be indigenous free-living forms. They are found in greater numbers during the summer months than during other seasons, but their role in pathogencity is not known.

Non-01 *V. cholerae* has been isolated in outbreaks involving gastrointestinal disease but, unlike *V. cholerae* 01, it has also been associated with extraintestinal disease. Non-01 organisms have been isolated from blood and wound infections, primarily in patients already compromised by some underlying disease. Non-01 organisms produce a cholera-like toxin that is believed to be associated with the diarrhea of gastrointestinal disease. Most cases are sporadic and not associated with pandemics, as classical cholera is. The symptoms of non-01 disease are similar to those of classical cholera but are less severe. Many outbreaks result from ingestion of mollusks, especially raw oysters. Most disease in the United States occurs in southern coastal waters. The first reported case of non-01 *V. cholerae* from New England waters was recorded in 1981 and resulted from ingestion of raw clams. The reservoir of non-01 strains of *V. cholerae* that cause human disease is not known. Humans may be the reservoir, and occasional carriers have been identified.

Epidemiology

Over 35,000 cases of cholera are reported each year and most of these are seen in Asia and Africa. Less than 1 percent of these cases result in patient death. Fewer than 20 cases of cholera are reported each year in the United States. Because of the milder symptoms associated with non-01 *V. cholerae* infection, many infections are probably not reported. Nearly all cases of cholera in the United States are associated with coastal waters, particularly in areas such as Louisiana and Texas.

Humans are the primary host of *V. cholerae* and thus the principal source of new cases of cholera. Cholera organisms are harbored by convalescent as well as chronic carriers and are shed into the environment in large numbers. Ingestion of fecally contaminated food or water can lead to disease.

Laboratory Diagnosis

Separation of *Vibrio* species from other clinically important bacteria with which they may be confused can be carried out by using the following tests:

1. The indophenol oxidase test differentiates Enterobacteriaceae (oxidase negative) from *Vibrio* (oxidase positive).
2. The oxidative-fermentative test differentiates oxidase-positive *Pseudomonas* (oxidative) from *Vibrio* (fermentative).
3. The NaCl requirement for growth differentiates *Vibrio* (requires NaCl) from *Aeromonas* and *Plesiomonas* (do not require NaCl).
4. Susceptibility to compound 0/129 differentiates *Vibrio* (susceptible) from *Aeromonas* (resistant) and *Plesiomonas* (variable).

When vibrios are suspected in a gastrointestinal illness their isolation from fecal material is fairly easy to carry out because they are able to tolerate alkaline pH and are motile. It has been recommended that one enrichment medium, and at least one plating medium, be used in the isolation and identification procedures. The enrichment medium is alkaline peptone broth (pH 8.4), which suppresses the growth of other intestinal microorganisms. The most frequently used plating medium is thiosulfate citrate bile salts sucrose (TCBS) agar, which is a selective medium. *V. cholerae* produces yellow colonies on TCBS agar. Typical colonies are then streaked on appropriate media or tested with *V. cholerae* polyvalent 01 antiserum. Final identification rests on certain biochemical tests that differentiate the species of *Vibrio* and other related species. The *el tor* biotype is distinguished from the *cholerae* biotype by the former's resistance to polymyxin B, resistance to phage group IV, ability to hemolyze sheep red blood cells, and a positive Voges-Proskauer test at 22°C.

Prevention and Treatment

Cholera can be prevented by adhering to certain sanitary procedures. There must be adequate sewage treatment and purification of water supplies. Travelers to foreign countries, especially Asia and Africa, are advised against eating raw seafood and uncooked vegetables. Thorough cooking of potentially contaminated food and careful storage of food will prevent food-borne cholera and related gastrointestinal disease. *V. cholerae* 01 can survive in crabs boiled for 8 minutes but not in crabs boiled for 10 minutes. Storage of food should be at temperatures too low (less than 4°C) or too high (greater than 60°C) to permit microbial multiplication. Extraintestinal infections can be prevented by avoiding contact with potentially contaminated water. This is especially true for those with skin abrasions or underlying illnesses.

Currently two oral cholera vaccines are under investigation. These vaccines consist of killed *V. cholerae* 01 whole cells of the different biotypes and serotypes, either with or without addition of the B subunit of cholera toxin. Preliminary results indicate that the vaccines can induce high levels of protective antibodies with little side effects. Vaccines have proved ineffective in reducing the incidence of clinical illness. Vaccination is not required for travelers to areas endemic for cholera unless the country demands it.

Cholera is self-limiting within a few days, if water and electrolytes are replaced. A replacement fluid consisting of 5 gm NaCl, 4 gm NaHCO$_3$, and 1 gm KCl per liter of sterile water given intravenously has met with great success. Electrolyte solution may also be given orally, but it must contain glucose to enhance absorption. It is used in milder cases of cholera. Antibiotics, although not required, will lessen the duration and volume of diarrhea and will reduce the vibrio population in the intestinal tract and prevent shedding. Most vibrios are susceptible to tetracyclines, chloramphenicol, and aminoglycosides, which are required to treat bacteremia and other potentially life-threatening infections in compromised patients.

OTHER PATHOGENIC VIBRIOS

Several species of *Vibrio* are infrequently pathogenic for humans, but we will discuss only three of them: *V. parahaemolyticus*, *V. vulnificus*, and *V. alginolyticus*.

Vibrio parahaemolyticus

V. parahaemolyticus is part of the normal flora of estuarine and other coastal waters throughout the world. Most of the organisms are associated with zooplankton. During winter months these microorganisms remain in the sediment, but as the waters warm the vibrios are released and become attached to minute crustaceans, where they proliferate. Most infections result from ingestion of improperly cooked crabs.

V. parahaemolyticus is associated with two types of clinical gastrointestinal syndromes. The most common manifestation of disease is watery diarrhea, accompanied by abdominal cramps, nausea, and vomiting. The disease is self-limiting. A more severe syndrome may be manifested by dehydration, dysentery, and acidosis. This syndrome too is usually self-limiting, but occasionally hospitalization is required. No deaths have been recorded in the United States, but some have been recorded in other countries. The microorganism may also cause extraintestinal disease and has been isolated from wounds and blood. Extraintestinal infections may require antimicrobial therapy (chloramphenicol, tetracyclines, aminoglycosides, etc.).

Few cases of *V. parahaemolyticus* disease have been recorded in the United States. Most are reported from Asia, where the disease is usually transmitted by raw or uncooked seafood. Raw food if left at refrigeration temperatures sustains the growth of vibrios. *V. parahaemolyticus* has a maximum generation time of 9 minutes and grows well at temperatures between 25 and 44°C. Even at less than ideal conditions, large numbers of vibrios can be obtained in only a few minutes. The principal reservoir of these vibrios is seafoods and seawater. Carriers do not appear to be important in disease transmission.

Pathogenic strains of *V. parahaemolyticus* can be differentiated from nonpathogenic strains by the Kanagawa test. This test is based on the detection of a heat-stable hemolysin in a special medium (Wagatsum agar) that contains human erythrocytes. Pathogenic strains hemolyze the erythrocytes while nonpathogenic strains do not.

Vibrio vulnificus

V. vulnificus is believed to be part of the normal flora of seawater. Disease caused by this microorganism has been reported in the United States as well as Japan and Belgium. Many cases of the disease are extraintestinal and are associated with wounds. Such diseases are the result of patient contact with seawater or with saltwater crustaceans. Septicemia is believed to result from ingestion of raw seafood. Most infections are incurred by those with some underlying disease or condition.

Patients with wound infections develop rapid swelling around the wound. Infection may also involve surrounding tissue. Large vesicles or bullae with necrosis are common. Patients with septicemia complain of fever and chills, and most have cutaneous lesions after the incubation period. These lesions are believed to result from hematogenous seeding of the microorganism. Surgical procedures—debridement, incision, and drainage of wounds—are often required in those with septicemia. Fatality rates are frequently high (45–60 percent) among those with septicemia because most of these patients have an underlying disease or condition and septicemia is recognized too late. *V. vulnificus* infections can be treated with antimicrobials such as ampicillin, chloramphenicol, tetracyclines, and aminoglycosides.

Vibrio alginolyticus

V. alginolyticus is a normal inhabitant of seawater and has a worldwide distribution. The organism is associated with extraintestinal infections such as wounds or ear infections. Most of these infections occur after swimming or activities at the seashore. Most lesions require debridement or drainage, but no serious complications occur and most patients respond to antibiotic (chloramphenicol, gentamicin, or nalidixic acid) therapy.

GENUS *AEROMONAS*

The genus *Aeromonas* has been recognized for years as a pathogen in reptiles, amphibia, and fish, but infections occur infrequently in humans. The habitat of *Aeromonas* species is various bodies of water, sewage, marine life, and foods. The species pathogenic for humans is *A. hydrophila*.

Most infections involve the intestinal tract, resulting in diarrhea that may last up to 7 days. Ingestion of contaminated water is the mechanism of transmission of *Aeromonas*-associated gastroenteritis. The second most prevalent form of disease caused by *Aeromonas* is wound infections, in which there is inflammation of connective tissue (cellulitis). This condition often follows accidents in fresh or salt water, alligator bites, or puncture wounds sustained from crabs, fishbone, aquarium, boats, and broken glass. Septicemia is the most invasive form of *Aeromonas* infection and may be community- as well as hospital-associated. *Aeromonas* cells are believed to enter the bloodstream following gastrointestinal or wound infections. *Aeromonas* septicemia in patients already compromised by underlying disease or conditions has a high mortality rate (25–75 percent). Very rare *Aeromonas* infections may involve the respiratory tract, eyes, and bone.

Aeromonas hydrophila is susceptible to several antibiotics, including chloramphenicol, gentamicin, kanamycin, nitrofurantoin, tetracyclines, and trimethoprim-sulfamethoxazole.

GENUS *PLESIOMONAS*

The type species for the genus *Plesiomonas* is *P. shigelloides*. It is found primarily in freshwater or estuarine environments and disease may follow ingestion of, or contact with, contaminated water or consumption of raw shellfish. Gastroenteritis is the most common form of the disease believed to be associated with *Plesiomonas* infection. Symptoms include fever, abdominal pain, vomiting, headache, and dehydration. Diarrhea may be prolonged and can last up to 3 weeks with numerous bowel movements (up to 30) per day. Over 60 percent of the cases of gastroenteritis require hospitalization and/or antimicrobial therapy. Most patients with plesiomonas-as-

Table 22-1 Characteristics of *Vibrio*, *Aeromonas*, and *Plesiomonas* Species

Species	Primary disease associations	Virulence factor	Mechanism of transmission	Treatment/prevention
Vibrio cholerae 01	Cholera—a severe gastroenteritis	Cholera enterotoxin affects adenyl cyclase activity	Ingesting contaminated water or foods (fish)	Replenishment of fluids and electrolytes; oral killed vaccine under trial
V. cholerae non-01	Cholera-like gastroenteritis less severe than 01; extraintestinal infections involving blood and wounds	Cholera-like toxin	Ingestion of mollusks (e.g., raw oysters) or contact with contaminated water	Replenishment of fluids
V. parahaemolyticus	Gastroenteritis—one type severe with dehydration and dysentery, the other a less severe diarrhea; extraintestinal infections involving blood and wounds	None firmly established as cause of disease	Ingestion of raw seafood; contact of wound with water or object contaminated by water	Gastroenteritis (a self-limiting disease); antimicrobials for extraintestinal disease (chloramphenicol, tetracyclines)
V. vulnificus	Wound infections and septicemia	None firmly established as cause of disease	Contact with contaminated water	Surgical debridement, antimicrobials (ampicillin, chloramphenicol, gentamicin)
V. alginolyticus	Wounds, ear infections	None firmly established as cause of disease	Contact with contaminated water (e.g., after swimming)	Debridement or drainage, antibiotics such as tetracyclines, erythromycin
Aeromonas hydrophila	Gastroenteritis, wounds, septicemia	None firmly established as cause of disease	Ingestion of contaminated water; contact of lacerated skin with contaminated water	None usually required for gastroenteritis; septicemia requires antibiotics (chloramphenicol, aminoglycosides)
Plesiomonas shigelloides	Gastroenteritis	None firmly established as cause of disease	Ingestion of or contact with contaminated water	Antimicrobial therapy (chloramphenicol, tetracyclines, aminoglycosides) required in over 60% of cases

sociated diarrhea have an underlying illness (for example, cancer) or risk factor such as consumption of raw seafood. Extraintestinal infections by *Plesiomonas* are severe but rare and include, in order of importance, meningitis, sepsis, cellulitis, and arthritis. The portal of entry for these infections has not been determined. *Plesiomonas* is susceptible to several antibiotics, including chloramphenicol, tetracycline, trimethoprim-sulfamethoxazole, and the aminoglycosides.

Plesiomonas can be differentiated from *Aeromonas* by several biochemical tests. For example, *Plesiomonas*, in contrast to aeromonas, ferments inositol and does not ferment mannitol or sucrose.

SUMMARY

Vibrio, Aeromonas, and *Plesiomonas* are straight or curved, gram-negative, motile rods that are aerobic to facultatively anaerobic. They are found in fresh, marine, or estuarine waters. The major characteristics of these genera and species are outlined in Table 22-1.

QUESTIONS FOR STUDY

Select the best response or responses for each of the following:

1. All of the following are characteristics of *Vibrio* species *except*
   A. They all possess polar flagella.
   B. They are easily cultivated in the laboratory.
   C. They have a requirement for NaCl.
   D. They can be found only in marine waters.

2. Cholera enterotoxin:
   A. Is an enzyme called adenyl cyclase
   B. Causes an increase in cyclic AMP in the intestinal tract
   C. Causes an influx of water and electrolytes into the intestinal mucosa
   D. Exhibits cytotoxic activity

3. Which of the following procedures is an enrichment technique for isolating *Vibrio* species in the laboratory?
   A. Adding thiosulfate to the medium
   B. Adding tetrathionate to the medium
   C. Incubating the culture at 47.4°C
   D. Increasing the pH of the medium to 8.5

4. *Vibrio alginolyticus* and *V. vulnificus* are pathogens associated primarily with
   A. Infections of the intestinal tract
   B. Infections of the respiratory tract
   C. Cutaneous infections
   D. Infections of the central nervous system

5. Gastroenteritis caused by which of the following most often requires hospitalization?
   A. *Aeromonas hydrophila*
   B. *V. parahaemolyticus*
   C. *Plesiomonas shigelloides*
   D. *V. cholerae* non-01

Fill in the blank:

1. The _____ test is used to differentiate pathogenic strains of *V. parahaemolyticus* from nonpathogenic strains.

2. The _____ test differentiates *Vibrio* species from Enterobacteriaceae.

3. Gastroenteritis caused by *V. parahaemolyticus* is usually due to eating _____.

4. In epidemic cholera the source of infectious microorganisms is _____.

ADDITIONAL READINGS

Brenden, R. A., Miller, M. A., and Janda, J. M. Clinical disease spectrum and pathogenic factors associated with *Plesiomonas shigelloides* infection in humans. *Rev. Infect. Dis.* 10(2):303,1988.

Janda, J. M., and Duffey, P. S. Mesophilic aeromonads in human disease: Current taxonomy, laboratory identification, and infectious disease spectrum. *Rev. Infect. Dis.* 10(5):980,1988.

Janda, J. M., Powers, C., Bryant, R. G., and Abbott, S. L. Current perspectives on the epidemiology and pathogenesis of clinically significant *Vibrio* species. *Clin. Microbiol. Rev.* 1(3):245,1988.

Khardori, N., and Fainstein, V. Aeromonas and Plesiomonas as etiological agents. *Annu. Rev. Microbiol.* 42:395,1988.

Morris, J. G., Jr., and Black, R. E. Cholera and other vibrios in the United States. *N. Engl. J. Med.* 312:343,1985.

Safranin, S., et al. Non-0:1 *Vibrio cholerae* bacteremia: Case report and review. *Rev. Infect. Dis.* 10(5):1012,1988.

23. GRAM-NEGATIVE COCCOBACILLARY AEROBIC BACTERIA

OBJECTIVES

To understand the types of infections associated with *Hemophilus influenzae* type b

To describe the various stages in whooping cough and the microbial factors believed to be associated with their appearance

To understand the importance and risks of vaccination against whooping cough

To explain the various ways in which the agents of brucellosis and tularemia may be transmitted to humans

To outline the methods used to treat and prevent *H. influenzae* type b infections, brucellosis, whooping cough, and tularemia

The genera *Hemophilus*, *Bordetella*, *Brucella*, and *Francisella* belong to a group referred to as gram-negative coccobacillary bacteria. They are the causative agents of meningitis, whooping cough (pertussis), brucellosis (undulant fever), and tularemia, respectively. All are nonmotile and are aerobic or microaerophilic. Their growth on laboratory media is favored by the addition of blood or serum or elevated concentrations of CO_2. Except for species of *Hemophilus*, most are resistant to penicillin.

HEMOPHILUS

GENERAL CHARACTERISTICS

Hemophilus influenzae is the predominant pathogenic species of the genus. This small bacillus is found exclusively in the upper respiratory tract of humans. Other species of *Hemophilus* inhabiting the upper respiratory tract are *H. hemolyticus*, *H. parainfluenzae*, *H. parahemolyticus*, *H. aphrophilus*, and *H. paraphrophilus*. Strains of *H. influenzae* can be divided into two groups: nonencapsulated and encapsulated.

H. influenzae is fastidious in its growth requirements. It grows best on chocolate agar or enriched media supplemented with two nutritional factors called *X* (hemin) and *V* (nicotinamide-adenine dinucleotide[NAD]). Incubation under CO_2 enhances the growth of most species. Colonies of *H. influenzae* increase in size if they are cultivated in the vicinity of other bacterial colonies—staphylococci, for example. This cooperative effect is called the *satellite phenomenon* and is due to the production of NAD by the staphylococcal colonies (see Plate 11).

PATHOGENESIS

Encapsulated *Hemophilus influenzae*

Encapsulated strains of *H. influenzae* are primary pathogens, and the most invasive is type b, the main cause of bacterial meningitis and acquired mental retardation in children under 4 years of age (Table 23-1). The major virulence factor of *H. influenzae* type b is the polysaccharide capsule surrounding the organism. The capsule inhibits phagocytosis. During the first 6 months of life *H. influenzae* type b is found in the upper respiratory tract of less than 1 percent of children, but this increases to at least 5 percent

Table 23-1. Causative Agents of Meningitis and the Frequency with Which They Are Associated with Disease

Agent	Frequency[a] (percent)
Hemophilus influenzae[b]	40–50
Neisseria meningitidis	20–25
Streptococcus pneumoniae	20–25
Escherichia coli	4–5
Other species	3–5

[a] The values are approximate and vary from year to year as well as from one community to another.
[b] In children under 4 years of age *H. influenzae* accounts for over 65 percent of the cases of meningitis.

for the remainder of childhood. Those individuals colonized by the organism develop resistance to disease by 5 years of age, because of antibody. Infection with *H. influenzae* occurs following inhalation of respiratory droplets from patients or carriers. In infants there is no detectable level of antibody so disease leads to serious consequences. Meningitis in this group, even after chemotherapy, leads to serious sequelae such as mental retardation. *H. influenzae* type b infections may also lead to conditions such as pneumonia, bronchitis, otitis media, and epiglottitis. Several studies have revealed that *H. influenzae* type b is one of the major causes of otitis media in children. What is particularly alarming about this statistic is that many of the strains are resistant to ampicillin, the drug most widely prescribed for infection.

H. influenzae type b infections in adults are rare. Adult infections occur more frequently when the patient is compromised by respiratory problems, diabetes, or alcoholism. Infection is manifested as pneumonia and may be caused by encapsulated as well as nonencapsulated strains.

Resistance to type b infections is believed to be associated with the production of antibodies to capsule as well as outer membrane proteins. The capsule is a polyribitol phosphate that was developed as a vaccine in 1985.

Nonencapsulated *Hemophilus influenzae*

Nonencapsulated *H. influenzae* is present in the pharynx of the majority of healthy children but with increasing age becomes less frequent as a commensal. These organisms cause disease in both children and adults. They are a frequent cause of otitis media, particularly in children between 6 and 24 months of age. Neonatal infections from nonencapsulated strains are severe and are believed to arise by transmission from mother to newborn. Meningitis in adults and children usually occurs as a result of secondary infection following primary infection of the paranasal sinuses. Nonencapsulated strains are an important cause of pneumonia, particularly in the elderly and in patients with chronic bronchitis.

EPIDEMIOLOGY

Approximately 12,000 cases of *H. influenzae* type b meningitis are reported each year in the United States. The mortality rate is less than 10 percent but 10 to 15 percent of the survivors are left with neurologic complications. Several studies indicate that children at day-care centers are at an increased risk of infection. *H. influenzae* meningitis has a seasonal distribution, with major incidences of the disease in the fall and spring. Higher rates of the disease occur in blacks, American Indians, and Eskimos.

LABORATORY DIAGNOSIS

Specimens (usually blood or cerebrospinal fluid for type b organisms) can be gram-stained for identification of coccobacilli. The capsule can be demonstrated by a capsular swelling reaction (quellung; see page 413) after using type b antiserum. Immunofluorescent technique using fluorescein-conjugated anti-type b serum is another way to identify the organism in clinical specimens. Isolation of *H. influenzae* is achieved by culturing specimens on chocolate agar (heated blood agar) or richer media such as Levinthal's medium. Both media contain X and V factor. Colonial isolates can be identified by serological tests discussed above plus others such as counter-immunoelectrophoresis, latex agglutination, and coagglutination using antisera.

All *Hemophilus* species except *H. aphrophilus* and *H. ducreyi* require V-factor (see Table 23-2). Paper disks containing V-factor can be placed on blood agar medium (devoid of V factor) to identify V-factor-requiring species. X-factor requirements for further differentiation of *Hemophilus* species can be obtained on the basis of the ability of species to utilize γ-aminolevulinic acid, a precursor in the biosynthesis of heme. Species requiring the X factor do not possess the enzymes to metabolize γ-aminolevulinic acid. Further differentiation of *Hemophilus* species is also based on growth response to CO_2, fermentation, hemolysis, and catalase production.

TREATMENT AND PREVENTION

Ampicillin and chloramphenicol were once considered the most effective drugs in treating infections caused by *H. influenzae*, but drug-resistant strains have now become prevalent. In some areas of the world as many as 50 percent of the clinical isolates of *H. influenzae* are resistant to both drugs. Sensitivity tests should be used on clinical isolates before an antimicrobial regimen is begun. Ampicillin resistance is caused primarily by beta-lactamase production and one treatment-regimen includes the combination of a beta-lactamase inhibitor (sulbactam, for example) plus ampicillin. Other drugs that show promise include the newer cephalosporins (ceftriaxone, ceftizoxime, etc.) and trimethoprim-sulfamethoxazole.

Although early treatment of *H. influenzae* infections with antimicrobials is almost 100 percent effective, a few patients who recover have residual central nervous system injury. A vaccine containing capsular polysaccharide of *H. influenzae* type b was licensed in the United States in 1985. The vaccine was not effective in children younger than 18 months of age and sometimes failed to prevent disease even in older children. Some studies suggest that genetic differences in humans may account for some unresponsiveness to polysaccharide vaccines. In late 1987 a conjugate vaccine was licensed to provide a more effective

Table 23-2. Characteristics of Species of *Hemophilus* Occasionally Associated with Disease

Species	Disease association	Other characteristics
H. aegyptius	Communicable form of conjunctivitis (pinkeye)*	Requires X and V factors; serologically related to *H. influenzae*
H. hemolyticus	Sinusitis, otitis media, and lower respiratory disease	Found normally in upper respiratory tract; beta hemolytic; requires X and V factors
H. parainfluenzae	Respiratory tract infection and endocarditis	Found normally in respiratory tract; requires V factor
H. ducreyi	Sexually transmitted disease (chancroid)	Fastidious growth requirements; difficult to isolate from lesions; requires X factor
H. paraphrophilus	Infrequent cause of disease but disease is usually severe—endocarditis, septicemia, and meningitis	Does not require V or X factor

* Bacteremia following recovery from conjunctivitis can lead to a frequently fatal illness (called Brazilian purpuric fever) in young children. This disease has been seen almost exclusively in Brazil.

response in infants and younger children. Three conjugate vaccines of *H. influenzae* type b polysaccharide are now available. One conjugate includes meningococcal protein, while the other two are diphtheria proteins. The conjugated vaccines are now recommended for children over the age of 2 months. Three doses are to be given over 2-month intervals, and a booster dose at the age of 15 months.

There is an increased risk of disease in children who come in contact with a person with *H. influenzae* type b meningitis because the organism is transmitted by respiratory droplets. The attack rate is highest in those under 2 years of age. The Immunization Practices Advisory Committee (ACIP) recommends that the drug rifampin be considered for all classroom contacts of a child with invasive *H. influenzae* type b disease if any exposed classroom contact is under 2 years of age. Rifampin should not be used for pregnant women because of the drug's teratogenic (capable of causing congenital malformation) potential.

PATHOGENIC SPECIES OTHER THAN H. INFLUENZAE

Several species of *Hemophilus* are occasionally associated with disease (Table 23-2). One of the more important of these is *H. ducreyi*, the causal agent of the sexually transmitted disease *chancroid*. *Chancroid* refers to the soft, painful ulcers seen in the genital area. The base of the chancroid ulcer, in contrast to the smooth base of the syphilis ulcer, is irregular and is granular in appearance. Little inflammation surrounds the ulcer. In males the distal prepuce is the most common site of involvement while in females most of these lesions are at the entrance of the vagina. Painful, tender inguinal lymphadenopathy is a characteristic feature in up to 50 percent of the patients. Involved lymph nodes (buboes) may spontaneously rupture (Plate 12).

Chancroid is prevalent in developing countries but uncommon in the United States. Just over 5100 cases were reported to the CDC in 1987. The disease is probably underreported. Whether asymptomatic carriers play a role in disease transmission is uncertain at this time.

Definitive diagnosis of chancroid requires the isolation and identification of *H. ducreyi*; however, isolation of the organism is difficult and the presently available media will not support the growth of all strains. Chocolate agar containing hemoglobin, fetal bovine serum, and vancomycin (to inhibit gram-positive species) appears to be the most effective isolation medium.

Chancroid can be effectively treated with erythromycin, ceftriaxone, amoxicillin, or the combination sulfamethoxazole-trimethoprim.

BORDETELLA

GENERAL CHARACTERISTICS

Species of *Bordetella* are common inhabitants of the human upper respiratory tract. *B. pertussis* is the causative agent of *whooping cough (pertussis)* and is morphologically indistinguishable from other coccobacillary forms. *B. pertussis* is a strict aerobe and is among the most fastidious pathogenic bacteria. Two other species that share antigens with *B. pertussis* are *B. parapertussis* and *B. bronchiseptica*. *B. parapertussis* can also cause whooping cough while *B. bronchiseptica* may cause respiratory or wound infections. These two species are less fastidious than *B. pertussis* and can be differentiated from the latter in tests outlined in Table 23-3.

EPIDEMIOLOGY AND PATHOGENESIS

B. pertussis is a pathogen only in humans. Pertussis is worldwide in distribution and most in-

Table 23-3. Characteristics Differentiating Species of *Bordetella*

Test	*B. pertussis*	*B. parapertussis*	*B. bronchiseptica*
Pigment production	−	+	−
Urease production	−	+	+
Oxidase production	+	−	+
Nitrate reduction	−	−	+
Motility	−	−	+
Citrate utilization	−	+	+

stances of disease occur in the very young, particularly in those less than 6 months of age. Pertussis is highly communicable and is spread by exposure of susceptible individuals to aerosols generated by infected persons.

Pertussis is divided into three symptomatic stages: *catarrhal, paroxysmal,* and *convalescent.* Following exposure to the infectious agent, symptoms of infection may appear from 6 to 20 days later. In the catarrhal stage the symptoms are similar to those of a cold: conjunctivitis, watery eyes, mild cough, and low-grade fever. The catarrhal stage may last from one to two weeks or more with episodes of severe coughing.

The paroxysmal (sudden attacks occurring periodically) stage is characterized by severe coughing, first at night and then during the day as well. As many as 15 to 25 coughing episodes may occur within a 24-hour period. The coughing leads to mucus expulsion and this is followed by inspiration of air into the lungs, causing the classic "whooping" associated with the disease (whooping is not usually observed in adult pertussis). The paroxysmal stage is the most contagious phase of the disease, and the bacilli can be seen attached to the epithelium of the bronchi or trachea (Fig. 23-1). As the disease progresses and more respiratory tissue is involved, blockage of the bronchial passages may take place, leading to lung infection from pyogenic cocci, convulsions, and sometimes death. The bacteria never invade the bloodstream. The paroxysmal stage may last from one to four weeks, followed by fewer and less severe symptoms of the disease (the convalescent stage). During convalescence

mild to severe coughing may occur periodically for up to six months after infection.

B. pertussis produces several potential virulence factors. *Filamentous hemagglutinin (FHA)* is a surface protein, similiar to pili, that is believed to be important for colonization of the upper respiratory tract. *Pertussus toxin (PT)* is a protein exotoxin of the A-B subunit type (see page 226) in which the B subunit enables the enzymatic or toxic A subunit to reach its site of action in the cell. The A subunit possesses ADP-ribosyltransferase activity; that is, it catalyzes the transfer of the ADP-ribose moiety from NAD to a cell membrane protein. This cell membrane protein is usually involved in controlling cyclic AMP (cAMP). Thus, the pertussis toxin directly affects the cAMP content of the host cell, a characteristic similar to cholera toxin (see Boxed Essay, p. 231). Pertussis toxin has a variety of biological effects, such as histamine sensitization, which may be responsible for the cough, and impaired monocyte migration to the site of infection. The latter may be responsible for maintaining the infection as well as contributing to secondary infections. *Adenylate cyclase* is an enzyme found on the surface of *B. pertussis* cells. This enzyme is believed to inhibit phagocytic activity. The enzyme apparently enters phagocytic cells, where it is activated by a mammalian protein called calmodulin (see also *B. anthracis* pathogenesis, page 439). Activation of adenylate cyclase induces high levels of intracellular cAMP, which impairs the bactericidal activity of PMNs and macrophages. Suppression of phagocytic activity could permit establishment and mainte-

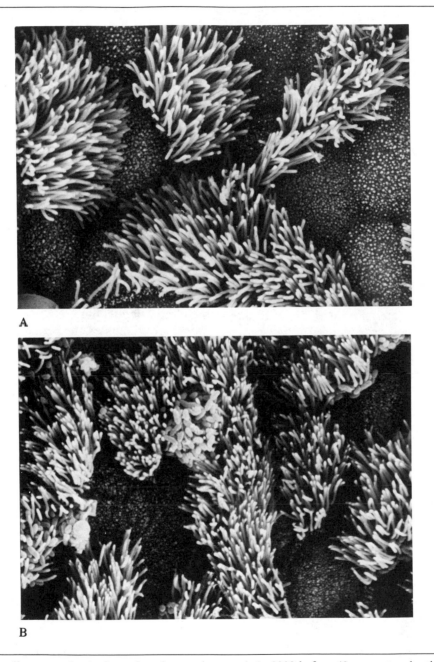

Fig. 23-1. *Bordetella pertussis*. A. Scanning electromicrograph (×3000 before 40 percent reduction) of mouse tracheal epithelium incubated in sterile medium. B. Scanning electron micrograph of mouse tracheal epithelium infected with *B. pertussis*. (From L. B. Opremcak and M. S. Rheins, *Can. J. Microbiol.* 29:415, 1983.)

nance of infection. Other potential virulence factors include a hemolysin, fimbriae, tracheal cytotoxin, lipopolysaccharide, and heat-labile dermonecrotic factor. The last three probably are involved in the damage associated with the ciliated epithelium of the respiratory tract but studies so far are not conclusive.

LABORATORY DIAGNOSIS

No single laboratory or clinical diagnostic test has been shown to be optimally sensitive and specific for *B. pertussis*. Culture of *B. pertussis* from nasopharyngeal secretions, although specific as a diagnostic test, shows low sensitivity. The tip of a Nichrome wire is covered with cotton, and the wire is passed through the nose and allowed to touch the nasopharyngeal wall. The wire is removed and the material on it is streaked on a charcoal-horse blood agar plate. The plates are incubated and examined daily since colonies may not appear before three days. Typical colonies are tiny and glistening and resemble bisected pearls. Colonies should be gram-stained. If small, gram-negative rods, or coccobacilli, are observed, fluorescent antibody tests can be used for serological confirmation. Direct fluorescent antibody testing, however, has been shown in some studies to lack sensitivity. Laboratory tests combined with clinical criteria (cough, for example) are suggested for diagnosis of pertussis. Biochemical tests can be used to differentiate *Bordetella* species (see Table 23-3).

TREATMENT AND PREVENTION

Although whooping cough is often self-limiting, antibiotics such as erythromycin, tetracycline, and chloramphenicol are important in lessening its communicability. These antibiotics are also helpful in reducing the possibility of secondary pneumonia infections. Treatment administered after infection has been established has little effect on the course of the illness. Penicillin may be given, however, to reduce secondary infections by pyogenic cocci.

Since the first vaccine for pertussis was administered, the number of cases of whooping cough has decreased from a high of 120,000 per year in 1950 to 4,157 cases in 1989. Active immunization of all children 2 to 3 months old is highly recommended. The initial vaccination is generally followed by two injections at monthly intervals and booster doses at ages 1 and 5. The vaccine contains killed *B. pertussis* cells and is usually combined with diphtheria and tetanus toxoids (collectively called the DTP).

The pertussis vaccine when administered to infants does not confer as long-lasting immunity as do other vaccines. Probably the reason is the inability of the vaccine to stimulate sufficient concentrations of IgA, which is important in circumventing the attachment of *B. pertussis* to ciliated respiratory epithelium. Natural infection with *B. pertussis* stimulates the formation of high levels of IgG and IgA.

More than 80 percent of children exposed to pertussis who have received three doses of DTP vaccine will be protected. The number of cases of pertussis in those younger than 6 months of age is reduced indirectly because of vaccination of older children. Killed whole cells, however, can cause severe side effects such as shock and encephalopathy, which can terminate in death. In the United States between 1984 and 1985, 5865 cases of vaccine-associated pertussis were reported with 19 deaths. Results like these frighten many parents to the point that they refuse to have their children vaccinated. Vaccination apathy in Japan and England in the 1970s, for example, resulted in large epidemics of pertussis and many pertussis-associated deaths. These results demonstrate the importance of vaccination. A noncellular vaccine was developed in Japan and has been used in that country since 1982. The Japanese vaccine is composed of two cellular proteins that exhibit hemagglutinin activity. It appears to be protective without inducing serious side effects. A noncellular vaccine is being considered for use in the United States.

BRUCELLA

GENERAL CHARACTERISTICS

Members of the genus *Brucella* are facultative intracellular parasites that cause chronic disease in animals and humans. There are three major pathogenic species of *Brucella*: *B. abortus*, which infects cattle; *B. melitensis*, which infects goats and sheep; and *B. suis*, which infects swine. Human infection caused by brucellae is referred to as *brucellosis* or *undulant fever*.

The *Brucella* are gram-negative, nonmotile, and coccobacillary in shape. Capsules if present are small. Brucellae are strict aerobes that require complex media for cultivation.

EPIDEMIOLOGY AND PATHOGENESIS

Brucellosis is primarily a zoonosis and is transmitted to humans through consumption of raw milk or its products, through contact with products of conception, or sometimes through ingestion of meat from infected animals. *B. abortus* infection in cattle is responsible for bovine abortions. The pathogen exhibits an affinity for placental tissue by virtue of its requirement for the sugar erythrose, which is abundant in bovine placenta. Brucellosis is worldwide in distribution, and travelers to areas where the disease is endemic in animals are at increased risk. In the United States fewer than 125 cases are reported each year but in areas of Africa the annual incidence of brucellosis per 100,000 population is as high as 128. Outbreaks in the United States are frequently associated with ingestion of cheese from unpasteurized goats' milk. Sporadic cases of disease in the United States may occur among farmers, veterinary surgeons, and slaughterhouse personnel who come in contact with infected animals. Hunters slaughtering infected animals such as moose, elk, bison, etc. can also acquire the disease. Domestic swine are the major source of infection in the United States, and *B. suis* the most frequently isolated species.

Brucella organisms gain entrance to the body through abraded skin or mucous membranes of the intestinal or respiratory tract. They do not persist long at the site of entry and are ingested by neutrophils and then quickly settle in regional lymph nodes. In the intracellular environment of the neutrophil the bacilli reproduce and subsequently lyse the cell. The released bacteria at this stage may be destroyed by phagocytes, or they may overcome the host defenses and be transported within macrophages via the blood to many areas of the body. The bacilli localize in tissue (liver, bone, spleen), where granulomas similar to those found in tuberculosis are produced. Viable bacilli may persist for several months in the granulomas, giving rise to acute or chronic symptoms. For this reason the incubation period in brucellosis may be very long. The acute stage, which usually appears approximately 1–2 weeks after infection, is characterized by fever and enlargement of the lymph nodes, spleen, and liver. Patients' temperature during the acute phase ranges between 101 and 104°C and may continue for several weeks with intermittent remissions (undulant fever). About 80 percent of the patients recover spontaneously during the acute stage. The chronic stage is generally associated with a hypersensitivity in which there is swelling of the joints and persistence of a low-grade fever. Inflammation of spinal vertebrae (spondylitis) resulting in severe back pain is a common complication of brucellosis, particularly in older men.

LABORATORY DIAGNOSIS

Diagnosis of brucellosis is difficult because the disease is generally chronic and is accompanied by fever and few symptoms. The microorganisms are best recovered from the blood during the fever stage. Blood cultures often become negative after the first few weeks of infection because of the presence of patient antibodies.

Culture and isolation of *Brucella* can be made

from blood, abscesses, and tissues. Clinical specimens are cultured on tryptose agar or brucella agar in an atmosphere of 2 to 10 percent CO_2. Plates should be incubated for 10 days at 35 to 37°C. Colony isolates should be gram-stained. Nonhemolytic colonies that are gram-negative coccobacilli, do not ferment lactose or glucose, are obligate aerobes, and are oxidase positive are tested for agglutination in *Brucella* antiserum. These tests define the genus *Brucella*. Other tests are used to differentiate species and biotypes of *Brucella* (see Table 23-4).

The tube agglutination test (TAT) is the standard method for serodiagnosis of brucellosis. Standarized *Brucella* antigen can be obtained commercially to determine the immune response to brucellosis. Definitive results are obtained when multiple blood cultures have been procured: acute-phase serum followed by convalescent serum from 14 to 21 days after onset of disease.

Several screening tests are available for conducting serological surveys in support of epidemiologic investigations. Two important screening tests are the card agglutination and microagglutination tests.

TREATMENT AND PREVENTION

Mass testing, slaughter of infected cattle, and vaccination of heifers have reduced the infection rate of cattle in the United States to less than 5 percent. Infection in swine, however, remains at a very high level, and the disease is highest among personnel at slaughterhouses.

A satisfactory vaccine for humans has not yet been produced.

Because of the presence of brucella within host cells, effective treatment is often difficult. Brucellae are susceptible to ampicillin, streptomycin, and tetracycline. Tetracyclines are the first choice in treatment. Successful treatment is best obtained during the acute stage of the disease. During chronic infections antibiotics are unsatisfactory and relapses are common.

FRANCISELLA

GENERAL CHARACTERISTICS

The most important species in the genus *Francisella* is *F. tularensis*, the causative agent of *tularemia*. The genus name honors Dr. Francis, while the species name indicates Tulare County in the state of California, where the disease was first described. Tularemia is a disease of rodents, particularly rabbits, and is transmissible to humans.

F. tularensis is a gram-negative, nonmotile bacillus that can produce a capsule in vivo. Like the *Brucella*, *Francisella* species are facultative

Table 23-4. Characteristics Used in Differentiating the Three Major Species of *Brucella*

| Species | H$_2$S production | Growth in presence of | | | Urease activity | Reaction to monospecific/serum of | |
		Basic fuchsin (1:25,000)	Thionin (1:25,000)	CO$_2$ requirement		B. abortus	B. melitensis
B. abortus	±	±	−	±	+	+	−
B. melitensis	−	+	+	−	V	−	+
B. suis	∓	V	±	−	+	+	−

± = most biotypes are positive; ∓ = most biotypes are negative; V = variable; as many positive biotypes as negative biotypes.

intracellular parasites. The organism is highly pleomorphic in culture and can resemble filamentous, coccal, or bacillary forms. It is fastidious in its cultural requirements. Reducing agents such as cystine or thioglycolate must be supplied in the medium if it is to achieve maximum growth.

EPIDEMIOLOGY AND PATHOGENESIS

Humans acquire tularemia by direct contact with infected animals, by handling or ingesting contaminated meat, by the bite of infected insect vectors such as ticks or deerflies, or by inhalation of contaminated aerosols. From 200 to 250 cases of tularemia are reported each year in the United States. Rodents or rabbits are the major reservoirs of infection but wild and domestic animals including fox, deer, opossum, dogs, and sheep can become infected. Most cases of tularemia result from contact with infected animal tissue, for example, skinning rabbits (so-called *rabbit fever*), or eating infected meat. One-third of the cases of tularemia in the United States are the consequence of bites of infected ticks or deerflies. Laboratory personnel caring for animals can contract tularemia through contaminated aerosols generated by sneezing animals.

Two types of *F. tularensis*, each with different characteristics, have been described. Type A strains are more virulent than type B strains. They cause 5 to 7 percent mortality in untreated cases and are usually associated with rabbits and tick vectors. Type B strains are less virulent, rarely cause death in untreated cases, and are associated primarily with rodents, such as muskrats. Type A strains are found only in North America, where they cause 80 to 90 percent of the reported cases.

The incubation period in tularemia is from 2 to 10 days and is coupled with fever and headache. From the original site of infection the bacilli migrate to regional lymph nodes, causing their enlargement. Like the brucellae, *F. tularensis* can persist within the phagocyte. No explanation has been given for the microorganism's ability to sur-

vive phagocytosis. During their intracellular travels the bacilli can enter the bloodstream and infect a number of organs, including the spleen, liver, and lungs, where they produce granulomas.

The manifestations of tularemia often depend on how the microorganism was acquired. The most common type is the *ulceroglandular* variety, which usually results from contact of abraded skin with infected animal tissue (skinning infected rabbits, for example). The primary lesion, usually found on the hands and arms, becomes ulcerated in 6 to 8 days (Fig. 23-2). During this period there will be fever and involvement of local lymph nodes. The lesions may take four to seven weeks to heal.

Accidental contamination of the eye can result in *ocularglandular* tularemia, in which there is ulceration of the conjunctiva.

The most severe form of tularemia is the pneumonic variety, usually contracted through contaminated aerosols. If left untreated, this clinical type of tularemia can be fatal to 30 percent of the persons infected.

Recovery from all three forms of tularemia confers permanent immunity.

Fig. 23-2. Typical cutaneous lesion of tularemia. (Courtesy Armed Forces Institute of Pathology, AFIP 83587-2.)

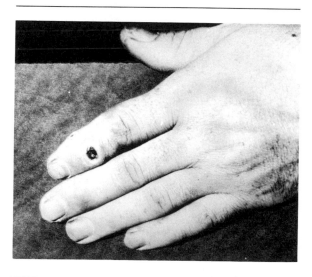

Table 23-5. Characteristics of the Gram-Negative Coccobacillary Bacteria

Genus	Major pathogenic species	Disease	Virulence factors	Mechanism of transmission	Treatment and prevention
Hemophilus	*H. influenzae* type b	Meningitis in children under 4 years; otitis media in children	Capsule (polyribitol phosphate)	Inhalation of respiratory droplets from active cases or carriers	Ampicillin, chloramphenicol, or ampicillin plus a beta-lactamase inhibitor
	H. influenzae nonencapsulated	Otitis media in children; neonatal infections; pneumonia in elderly	Unknown	Inhalation of respiratory droplets; mother to newborn	Same as for *H. influenzae*
Bordetella	*B. pertussis* *B. parapertussis*	Pertussis (whooping cough)	Filamentous hemagglutinin, pertussis toxin, adenylate cyclase	Inhalation of aerosols generated by infected individuals	Erythromycin, tetracycline, chloramphenicol; killed vaccine as part of DTP
Brucella	*B. abortus* (cattle) *B. melitensis* (goats, sheep) *B. suis* (swine)	Brucellosis (undulant fever)	Unknown	A zoonosis transmitted to humans by consumption of raw milk or its products; contact with products of conception; or ingestion of meat from infected animals	Ampicillin, streptomycin, tetracycline; mass testing, slaughter of infected cattle, and vaccination of heifers
Francisella	*F. tularensis*	Tularemia (rabbit fever)	Unknown	Direct contact with infected animals by handling or ingesting contaminated meat; bite of insect vectors; or inhalation of contaminated aerosols generated by infected animals	Streptomycin; attenuated vaccine for laboratory personnel

LABORATORY DIAGNOSIS

The risk to laboratory personnel of infection by *F. tularensis* is so high that tularemia is diagnosed on the basis of clinical findings and the patient's history of recent animal or tick exposure. In addition, it is very difficult to isolate this very fastidious organism. *F. tularensis* specimens from local lesions, regional lymph nodes, sputum, or conjunctival scrapings must be cultured on media rich in cystine or other reducing agents. The most popular medium is blood-cystine-dextrose agar. The colonies appear about 3–5 days after incubation of the specimen and are minute and transparent. Biochemical characterization is not necessary or recommended for identification. Direct or indirect fluorescent antibody techniques are considered the best tools for rapid and specific identification of *F. tularensis* in exudates, tissue sections, etc. Serodiagnosis can be accomplished by using an agglutination test on the patient's serum. The test becomes positive about 10 to 14 days after infection. The titer rises significantly at three weeks after infection.

TREATMENT AND PREVENTION

Streptomycin is the most effective drug in the treatment of tularemia, although chloramphenicol and tetracycline are sometimes employed. Relapses are more common when tetracycline or chloramphenicol are used because they fail to penetrate the phagocyte, where the bacilli may be located. If precautions are taken laboratory personnel are at minimal risk of incurring infection. An attenuated vaccine is available for use by laboratory personnel who are continually in contact with potentially infected animals.

SUMMARY

The gram-negative coccobacillary bacteria include *Hemophilus*, *Bordetella*, *Brucella*, and *Francisella*. They are nonmotile and aerobic to microaerophilic, and their growth on laboratory media is favored by the addition of blood, serum, or elevated concentrations of CO_2. The clinical importance of these groups is outlined in Table 23-5.

QUESTIONS FOR STUDY

Select the best response or responses for each of the following:

1. Which of the following is the cause of conjunctivitis?
   A. *Hemophilus hemolyticus*
   B. *H. ducreyi*
   C. *H. aegyptius*
   D. *H. influenzae*

2. A patient exhibits a high fever and lymph node enlargement. You discover that he has recently returned from Greece, where his diet consisted largely of milk products including many cheeses. Which of the following microbial agents might be suspected of causing infection?

   A. *Brucella* species
   B. *H. influenzae*
   C. *Francisella tularensis*
   D. *Bordetella pertussis*

3. Tularemia:
   A. Is caused by a nonmotile bacillus that produces a capsule in vivo
   B. Is caused by the ingestion of contaminated milk products
   C. Is most often characterized by ulcerated lesions and enlarged lymph nodes
   D. Can be caused by inhalation of contaminated aerosols

4. *Hemophilus influenzae*:
   A. Is the cause of influenza
   B. Type b strains are an important cause of meningitis in infants
   C. Has a requirement for NAD that can be supplied when it is cultivated in close proximity to *Streptococcus pyogenes* on blood agar
   D. Consists of capsulated and nonencapsulated strains that are present in the upper respiratory tract of healthy children

Fill in the blank:

5. Chancroid is a sexually transmitted disease caused by _____ .

6. The pertussis toxin is similar in its activity to the toxin produced by _____ .

7. Colonies of _____ on charcoal-blood agar resemble bisected pearls.

8. Antimicrobial therapy for *H. influenzae* type b infections has become more difficult because of the increased resistance of strains of the organism to _____ .

9. The drug _____ is recommended for all classroom contacts of a child with invasive *H. influenzae* type b disease.

ADDITIONAL READINGS

Friedman, R. L. Pertussis: The disease and new diagnostic methods. *Clin. Microbiol. Rev.* 1(4): 365,1988.

Morse, S. A. Chancroid and *Haemophilus ducreyi*. *Clin. Microbiol. Revs*. 2(2):137,1989.

Mousa, A. R.M., Elhag, K. M., Khogali, M., and Marafie, A. A. The nature of human brucellosis in Kuwait: Study of 379 cases. *Rev. Infect. Dis.* 10(1):211,1988.

Murphy, T. F., and Apicella, M. A. Nontypable *Haemophilus influenzae*: A review of clinical aspects, surface antigens, and the human immune response to infection. *Rev. Infect. Dis.* 9(1):1,1987.

Needham, C. A. *Haemophilus influenzae*: Antibiotic susceptibility. *Clin. Microbiol. Rev.* 1(2):218,1988.

Weiss, A. A., and Hewlett, E. L. Virulence factors of *Bordetella pertussis*. *Annu. Rev. Microbiol.* 40:661,1986.

Winter, A. J. Brucella and brucellosis: An update. *Ann. Inst. Pasteur Immunol.* 138:135,1987.

24. MYCOBACTERIA

OBJECTIVES

To describe the stages from inhalation of the tubercle bacillus to the formation of a tubercle

To outline the drugs used in the treatment and prevention of tuberculosis

To understand the immune response associated with tuberculosis and its relationship to vaccination and resistance to infection

To briefly describe the techniques used to identify mycobacteria in the laboratory

To briefly outline the features of nontuberculous mycobacterioses that distinguish them from *M. tuberculosis* disease

To describe the clinical features of indeterminate, tuberculous, and tuberculoid leprosy

The mycobacteria are ubiquitous microorganisms that can be readily found in animals and humans. Two diseases of medical importance, tuberculosis (TB) and leprosy, are caused by *Mycobacterium* species. Diseases caused by the mycobacteria are called *mycobacterioses*. The causative agents of tuberculosis in humans are *M. tuberculosis*, the human strain, and *M. bovis*, the strain found in cattle. Tuberculosis is particularly injurious to lung tissue and is widespread throughout the world. Although control measures have reduced the mortality in the United States and other developed countries, as many as 4 to 5 million people each year die of TB. Leprosy, a disease that produces lesions of the skin and nerves, is caused by *M. leprae*. This disfiguring ailment is found in Asia, islands of the South Pacific, and other tropical areas. There are approximately 5 million lepers in the world; few deaths, however, are directly related to the disease.

MYCOBACTERIUM TUBERCULOSIS

GENERAL CHARACTERISTICS

There are several characteristics that distinguish *M. tuberculosis*, as well as other mycobacteria, from most gram-positive and gram-negative bacteria. Most of these differences are due to the nature of the cell wall.

1. Mycobacteria possess a peptidoglycan layer but the usual gram-staining reagents cannot penetrate it. The reason is that layers of lipid surround the mycobacterial peptidoglycan. The majority of these lipids are called *mycolic acids*. The lipid content of the mycobacteria may be as high as 60 percent of the cell weight (5–20 percent lipid in most gram-negative bacteria).

2. Mycobacteria resist the acid-alcohol decolorization step and thus are referred to as *acid-fast bacilli*. Acid-fast stains such as the Ziehl-Nielsen procedure are used to literally force, by means of heat, stains into the cell (see Chapter 3).

3. Some mycolic acids are called the *cord factor* because they are responsible for the serpentine cords that mycobacteria produce when cultured on certain media (Fig. 24-1).

4. Mycobacterial cells divide every 18 to 24 hours (every 30 minutes for *E. coli*). This lengthy doubling time is reflected in the time it takes for visible colonies to develop on laboratory media (from 2 to 10 weeks, depending on the species) and in the time for symptoms to develop in disease (several weeks to months).

5. Mycobacteria produce pigments that are constitutive (produced under any environmental conditions) and are called *scotochromogens*. Some mycobacteria produce pigments that are produced only in the presence of light and are called *photochromogens*.

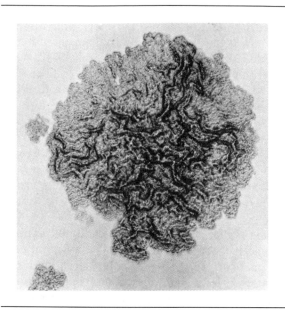

Fig. 24-1. Serpentine cord colony of *Mycobacterium tuberculosis*. (From E. H. Runyon, A. G. Karlson, G. P. Kubica, and L. G. Wayne. In F. H. Lennette, A. Balows, W. J. Hausler, Jr., and J. P. Truant [eds.], *Manual of Clinical Microbiology* [3rd ed.]. Washington, DC: American Society for Microbiology, 1980.)

PATHOGENESIS

Tuberculosis, like syphilis, is an infectious granulomatous disease that may last the lifetime of the patient; that is, it is a chronic disease. The TB bacillus can infect any organ of the body but is usually associated with the lungs. Because of current control measures on dairy cattle, *M. bovis* is not a major factor in the disease in the developed countries of the world, but *M. tuberculosis* is still an important pathogen even in developed countries such as the United Sates. Infection occurs mostly by direct contact with the infecting bacilli via droplet nuclei, ingestion of contaminated milk, or inhalation of contaminated dust particles. The extent of the disease is not related to the virulence of the infecting bacilli but to such factors as the *immunity of the host, the hypersensitivity of the host*, and the *infecting dose of bacilli*.

First infections are more prevalent in children than in adults. After inhalation of the bacilli, a lesion develops in the alveoli of one lung. This is followed by an inflammatory response in which there is an accumulation of neutrophils and macrophages. The bacilli are often carried to regional lymph nodes. Bacilli in the lung and lymph tissue lesions are ingested by macrophages and continue to multiply. The primary lesion may heal, with resorption of the exudate and destruction of the bacilli, but many bacilli survive. Surviving bacilli may reach the thoracic duct and bloodstream, eventually finding their way to other parts of the body.

At 3 to 12 weeks after the initial infection an immunological response can be detected. T cells and B cells appear at the lesion and respond to the appearance of the mycobacteria. The lesions, whether in the lung or other organs and tissues, are walled off in up to 85 to 95 percent of those infected. These sites of infection, however, still retain viable bacilli, which can later be reactivated. These individuals show no symptoms of disease although they do exhibit a delayed hypersensitivity. The remaining 5 to 15 percent show foci of infection that result in a specific pathological response, and bacilli proliferate; that is, the patient exhibits evidence of tuberculosis that may be respiratory or involve other organs or tissues. These manifestations of disease are referred to as *primary tuberculosis*. Microorganisms that persist and multiply at the site of infection are joined by mononuclear cells, tissue macrophages, and other cells. Dense connective tissue surrounds this site of cellular accumulation, which is referred to as a *tubercle* (Fig. 24-2). The tubercle observed microscopically appears as a granular nodule (granuloma) and represents the individual's hypersensitive response to the invading bacilli.

If large numbers of bacilli are produced in the tubercle, the number of neutrophils at the lesion will also increase. The release of lysosomal en-

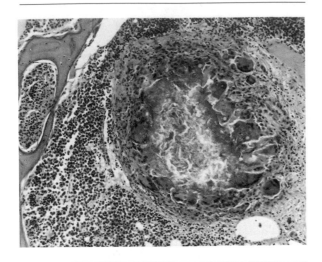

Fig. 24-2. Histology of a tubercle (×160 before 35 percent reduction). Tubercle is in the bone marrow of wild turkey. Central necrosis can be observed with multinucleated giant cells surrounding it. A well-defined capsule delineates the tubercle. (From C. O. Thoen, A. G. Karlson, and E. M. Himes, *Rev. Infect. Dis.* 3:960. © 1981 University of Chicago.)

zymes destroys not only the bacilli but the tubercle as well, and so functional host tissue is destroyed. A coagulated mass of host cells and bacilli referred to as *caseation necrosis* thus appears. The caseous lesion may heal by calcification with bacilli remaining viable within it for years. The calcification of the lesion permits its radiographic visualization. If the caseous lesion ruptures, viable bacilli can be disseminated by a systemic or pulmonary vessel to other organs of the body to form tubercles. This type of disseminated tuberculosis is called *miliary tuberculosis* (Fig. 24-3). If the caseous lesion ruptures, viable bacilli are carried to a bronchus, where they can infect healthy lung tissue. Bacilli can be aspirated into the lower portions of both lungs (Fig. 24-3). The bacilli may also be aspirated in the sputum. In some individuals the tuberculous cavity becomes encapsulated by fibrous walls of connective tissue and persists for years, constantly draining bacilli into the bronchi.

Even when the disease has apparently terminated, reinfection may occur by (1) activation of the bacilli that survived the primary infection or (2) inhalation or ingestion of new bacilli from the environment. This manifestation of disease is called *reactivation tuberculosis* and occurs primarily in the elderly. Malnutrition, diabetes mellitus, prolonged corticosteroid therapy, and chronic alcoholism are factors that predispose the patient to reactivation of tuberculosis. A strong tuberculin skin sensitivity is an indicator that an infected individual has a greater probability of developing active disease (see Immunity).

The ability of *M. tuberculosis* to inhibit phagosome-lysosome fusion is one of the principal mechanisms for escaping host defense mechanisms. Initially bacteria and macrophage live in apparent harmony but later when some bacteria die an immune response occurs. This immune response results in hypersensitivity, and macrophages, bacilli, and host tissue become destroyed by microbial products or toxic components released by dead macrophages. What components of *M. tuberculosis* are associated with virulence is not known, but the cord factor (Fig. 24-4) may be an important one. Cord factor inhibits the migration of leukocytes, and organisms lacking it have reduced virulence. Cord factor injected into mice causes the formation of pulmonary granulomas indistinguishable from those elicited by injection of *M. bovis* into healthy mice.

IMMUNITY

Infection by the tubercle bacillus results in delayed hypersensitivity by the host. The magnitude of the hypersensitivity, however, cannot be correlated with the degree of acquired resistance. The intensity of the hypersensitivity response is directly proportional to the amount of mycobacterial antigen present in the infected host. Large numbers of tubercle bacilli in tissue are associated with a highly destructive lesion because of the sensitivity to mycobacterial antigens (tuber-

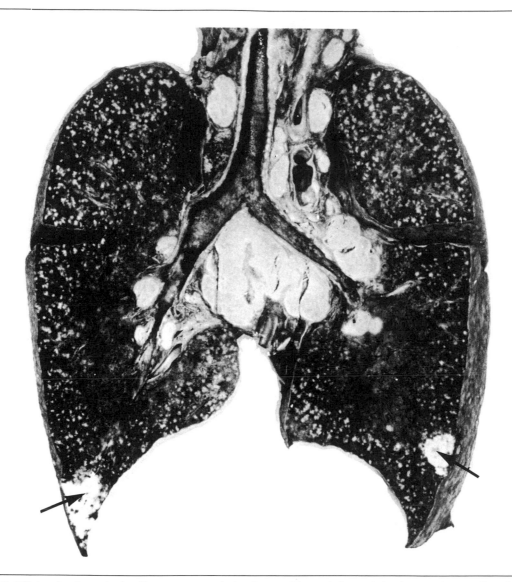

Fig. 24-3. Bilateral tuberculosis. Caseous necrosis is observed in each lower lobe (*arrows*) as well as in hilar and tracheobronchial nodes. Advanced miliary dissemination can be seen (as white speckled areas) throughout both lungs. (From W. Giese. In E. Kaufmann and M. Staemmler [eds.], *Lehrbuch der speziellen pathologischen Anatomie*, Vol. 2, Berlin: Walter De Gruyter, 1959–1960.)

culin). This hypersensitivity does not prevent the bacilli from multiplying in tissue.

Resistance to tuberculosis is related to the ability of macrophages to kill the bacilli or to prevent them from multiplying. The immune cells that

carry out the killing or inhibition of microbiol growth are primarily activated macrophages. Activation is brought about by lymphokines released by sensitized T cells. Activated macrophages are rich in lysosomes and the enzymes

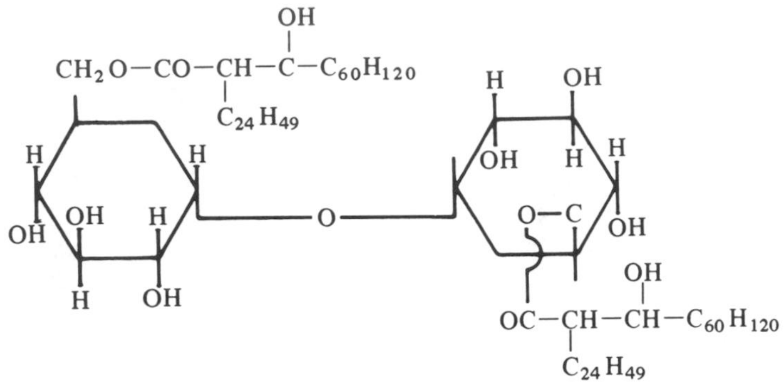

$$CH_2O-CO-CH-\overset{\overset{\displaystyle OH}{|}}{C}-C_{60}H_{120}$$
$$\underset{C_{24}H_{49}}{|}$$

Fig. 24-4. Structure of the cord factor.

they contain as well as oxygen-derived substances such as hydrogen peroxide, superoxide ion, and hydroxyl radical. An individual can remain infected for many years without demonstrating overt disease if macrophages can prevent the bacilli from multiplying.

T-cell sensitivity to *M. tuberculosis* does not apparently provide life-long immunity. Studies in nursing homes indicate that immunocompetent elderly persons who were at one time tuberculin positive may become nonreactive to *M. tuberculosis*. Such nonreactive persons are at risk of contracting an entirely new or primary infection.

Tuberculin Tests

Purified tuberculin protein derivative (PPD) is used in skin sensitivity tests. When injected intracutaneously (*Mantoux test*) into hypersensitive individuals, tuberculin evokes an intense inflammatory reaction (delayed hypersensitivity) at the site of injection. The activity of PPD is standardized into tuberculin units from 1 to 100. The standard dose in testing procedures is 5 tuberculin units. The degree of induration at the site of injection is an indication of the individual's present or past association with the TB bacillus. An induration of 1 to 5 mm after 48 to 72 hours is considered a negative response. The test is usu-

ally repeated, with a greater dose strength of PPD, for confirmation. If both tests are negative, the individual has presumably not had contact with the TB bacillus. An induration of 5 to 9 mm is called a *doubtful reaction*, and the test is usually repeated. An induration of 10 to 33 mm reflects a hypersensitivity resulting from either previous or present infection with the TB bacillus. Depending on their clinical presentation appropriate treatment may be necessary for these individuals. The skin test does not turn positive during the first 3 to 7 weeks after infection.

LABORATORY DIAGNOSIS

The techniques used for detecting tuberculosis and determining possible communicability to others are the tuberculin skin test, chest x-ray, and examination of sputum smears and cultures for *M. tuberculosis*. Because tuberculosis is primarily a disease of the lungs the major source of infecting bacilli for laboratory diagnosis is the sputum or lung secretions. When sputum samples cannot be obtained, gastric contents can be collected and examined. Tuberculosis may affect other areas of the body, and clinical material can be obtained from the cerebrospinal fluid, urine, bone, joints, or feces. Confirmation of *M. tuber-*

culosis infection is established by identification of the bacilli in a stained smear of clinical material (smears are not performed on urine or gastric aspirations), by cultivation of the microorganisms from clinical material on suitable laboratory media, and by biochemical and other tests.

Presumptive identification of *M. tuberculosis* can be made by demonstration of acid-fast bacteria in sputum samples or other clinical material (Plate 5). When 10^5 bacilli per milliliter are present, the smear is considered positive. An alternative to the acid-fast staining procedure, which is used in many laboratories, is fluorescent microscopy. Fixed smears are stained with auramine-rhodamine dye and then observed with a fluorescent microscope. By staining with fluorochrome dyes, such as auramine-rhodamine mixture, one can readily detect the bacilli in clinical material as bright yellow-green microorganisms (Plate 2). Although direct microscopical examination is the least sensitive of all tests, it does indicate—especially if the clinical material is sputum—that the patient may be highly infectious.

Accurate identification of the mycobacteria is obtained by cultural methods. Sputum samples, because of their viscosity and the presence of contaminating microbial species, are digested with a mucolytic agent containing N-acetyl-L-cysteine or sodium hydroxide. The sample is centrifuged and the neutralized sediment cultured on selective Löwenstein-Jensen medium as well as selective 7H11 media and examined weekly for 4 to 8 weeks for the appearance of characteristic colonies. Plated on clear 7H10-OADC media, pathogenic species of mycobacteria produce typical corded colonies. A niacin test is usually performed to identify the isolate as *M. tuberculosis*. *M. tuberculosis* is a strong producer of niacin. Recently, however, a species of *Mycobacterium* not pathogenic for humans has been found to be niacin positive. It is therefore recommended that combinations of various tests be used to identify and differentiate tubercle bacilli from other mycobacteria. Although tuberculosis by definition

is a disease caused by tubercle bacilli (*M. tuberculosis* and *M. bovis*), other species of *Mycobacteria* can cause disease in humans (see Nontuberculous Mycobacteria). It is therefore necessary to differentiate the tubercle bacilli from the other mycobacteria. Differentiation is based largely on the following characteristics and procedures:

1. Colonies may be examined for pigmentation, a characteristic not found in *M. tuberculosis* or *M. bovis* but common to many other species, especially those in group II (see Table 24-1).
2. Species plated on clear media such as 7H10-OADC produce corded, serpentine colonies characteristic of pathogenic species of mycobacteria.
3. Biochemical tests can be used to differentiate pathogenic from nonpathogenic species (except *M. microti*).
   a. Niacin production. Niacin production is characteristic of human tubercle bacilli and not of other species (except *M. microti*).
   b. Nitrate reduction. Most pathogenic species can reduce nitrate, while nonpathogens do not.
   c. Catalase production. Cultures of *M. tuberculosis* heated to 68°C for 20 minutes cannot produce catalase. The nonpathogens are not affected by temperature and continue to produce catalase. It has been observed that pathogenic species of *Mycobacteria* unable to produce catalase are also resistant to isoniazid.
   d. Polysorbate 80 (Tween 80) hydrolysis. Polysorbate 80, a derivative of sorbitan monooleate, is hydrolyzed by pathogenic species in 10 to 20 days, while nonpathogenic species hydrolyze polysorbate 80 in 5 days or less.

Many other tests can differentiate various pathogenic and nonpathogenic species. Those just mentioned, however, are the most important.

Table 24-1. Characteristics of the Most Frequently Isolated Nontuberculous *Mycobacterium* Species

Runyon group	Species	Source	Most common clinical manifestation	Basis of grouping	Treatment
I	*M. kansasii*	Milk, water; natural reservoir unknown	Pulmonary disease similar to tuberculosis	Pigment produced when exposed to light (photochromogen)	Two or more antituberculosis drugs, one of which is rifampin
	M. marinum	Water; found in fish	Cutaneous and disseminated disease		Lesions may resolve spontaneously but drainage or excision of lesion may be required. Antituberculosis drugs for disseminated disease (e.g., rifampin, ethambutol)
	M. simiae	Water; found in monkeys	Chronic pulmonary disease, osteomyelitis		No recommended therapeutic approach, but antituberculosis drugs stabilize disease
II	*M. scrofulaceum*	Water, soil, milk and dairy products	Cervical adenitis in children	Pigment produced in dark (scotochromogens)	Resistance to many antimicrobials. Rifampin usually suggested
	M. szulgaii	Soil, water; natural reservoir unknown	Pulmonary disease, cervical adenitis		Sensitive to antituberculosis drugs
	M. xenopi	Soil, water; birds may be reservoir	Pulmonary disease, bone and lymph node involvement		Sensitive to antituberculosis drugs (e.g., rifampin, ethambutol, isoniazid)
III	*M. avium-intracellulare* complex (MAC)	Soil, water	Pulmonary disease similar to tuberculosis, but disseminated infection in AIDS patients	Nonpigmented	Antituberculosis drugs; but surgical excision may be required
	M. malmoense	Natural reservoir unknown	Chronic pulmonary disease		Sensitive to antituberculosis drugs; but treatment usually unsatisfactory
	M. haemophilum	Natural reservoir unknown	Cutaneous lesions		Rifampin, isoniazid, and ethambutol plus surgical debridement
IV	*M. fortuitum-chelonae* complex	Water, soil	Pulmonary, cutaneous, abscesses; postoperative wound infections	Rapid growth (3–5 days)	Resistance to many antimicrobials; amikacin plus cefoxitin in combination

EPIDEMIOLOGY

Tuberculosis is treatable and curable, yet many die each year from this disease. The fatality rate in 1900 in the United States, before the introduction of antimicrobials, was approximately 200 per 100,000 population. The current rate is approximately 1.5 per 100,000 (Fig. 24-5). Tuberculosis is still a major problem in the United States, where approximately 24,000 new cases are recognized each year. In some of the larger cities death rates as high as 6 per 100,000 are still

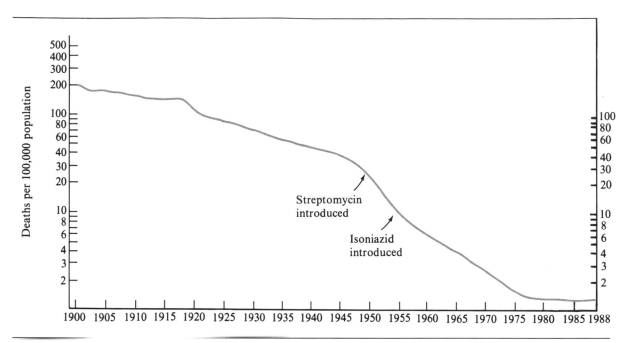

Fig. 24-5. Tuberculosis death rate in the United States, 1900–1988. (From Centers for Disease Control.)

observed. It is estimated that more than 10 million people in the United States are infected with tubercle bacilli. There has been an obvious apathy toward the disease, since nearly 50 percent of those currently dying from tuberculosis in the United States were undiagnosed during their lifetime. The treatment of infected individuals with antimicrobials for as little as 2 months can reduce the risk of disease by as much as 90 percent. A major increase in tuberculosis has resulted from the emigration of foreign persons into the United States. In addition, persons infected with the human immunodeficiency virus (HIV), the cause of AIDS, are extremely susceptible to tuberculosis. HIV-infected patients are 300 to 500 times more likely to acquire tuberculosis than those who are not infected by the virus.

Susceptibility to tuberculosis is influenced by age. The very young (younger than 5 years of age) are extremely susceptible, and in this group the disease is often fatal. Susceptibility decreases up to the early teens, then increases again, reaching a peak in old age. The variation in age suscep-

tibility is associated with the effectiveness of the cell-mediated response; that is, the cell-mediated response is greatly reduced in those at either end of the age spectrum. Such factors as poor nutrition and overcrowded living conditions also play an important role in susceptibility to infection.

TREATMENT AND PREVENTION

Several drugs have been used successfully in the treatment of TB. The chronic nature of the disease requires that therapy be continued for long periods of time, thus providing the opportunity for drug-resistant bacterial strains to emerge. To prevent the emergence of resistant forms of the bacilli, drugs are used in combination. At present, a 6-month drug regimen is used for treatment of tuberculosis. Isoniazid, rifampin, and pyrazinamide are administered for 2 months, and rifampin plus isoniazid for 4 months. If resistance to isoniazid is probable, a fourth drug, either ethambutol or streptomycin, is added and the treatment is prolonged for 12 months. Antimicrobial susceptibility testing usually is not required for newly diagnosed patients with tuberculosis. Antimicrobial susceptibility testing should be performed on a patient who has previously received antituberculosis drugs, or who has not responded to therapy after 3 to 4 months.

Modern treatment of tuberculosis can take place in the home, and most patients do not require hospitalization. Hospitalization may be required only if the patient has an additional severe disease or if a diagnostic procedure such as lung biopsy is required. Once the patient is undergoing treatment, any tubercle bacilli that might have been transmitted by the sputum are destroyed and thus transmission to healthy persons is no longer considered a factor in prevention of the disease.

A person with active tuberculosis can prevent the spread of bacilli by covering the mouth and nose when coughing or sneezing. A cough may produce up to 10^5 droplet nuclei, and each nucleus may contain one or more bacilli. More than half of the droplet nuclei remain suspended in the air for at least 30 minutes. Adequate ventilation and use of UV lights help to prevent dissemination of the bacilli. Areas in which these procedures are most important are sites of potential transmission, such as mycobacterial laboratories, chest clinic waiting areas, and shelters for the homeless. Chemotherapy is the best method of control. Isoniazid can be used in preventive therapy as well as for treating infectious cases of tuberculosis. It is recommended for individuals who have an induration greater than 5 mm in the tuberculin skin test. Included among positive reactors who should receive chemoprophylaxis are persons with progressive tuberculosis, those who have recently converted from a negative to a positive tuberculin test, and members of households with patients with recently diagnosed tuberculosis. Isoniazid prophylaxis is usually carried out for 6 months to 1 year. Patients should be carefully monitored because prolonged use of isoniazid has been known to cause liver damage. Isoniazid should be discontinued, of course, when

such toxic effects can be demonstrated. Poor patient compliance with the 6- to 12-month preventive therapy has prompted investigations into the use of other drugs for shorter periods. Among those being considered are rifampin and pyrazinamide, rifampin alone, and aconiazide, a compound related to isoniazid.

In the past patients cured by chemotherapy were advised to have follow-up examinations and x-ray tests. Today persons who have responded to treatment and are considered cured are no longer advised to return for examination. If the discharged patient develops tubercular symptoms, such as persistent fever and cough and loss of weight, a follow-up examination and x-ray should be initiated.

The bacillus of Calmette and Guérin (BCG), isolated from a strain of *M. bovis*, has been used since 1921 in a live vaccine for the prevention of TB. The vaccine has been used more frequently in other countries than in the United States. The vaccine is not recommended in the United States because it results in the recipient's having a positive tuberculin test; hence a valuable diagnostic aid is lost. BCG vaccination is recommended for infants and children with negative tuberculin tests who are exposed for long periods to (1) patients who are untreated or ineffectively treated or (2) patients who have bacilli resistant to isoniazid and rifampin. BCG is also recommended for tuberculin-negative infants and children in groups in which the rate of new infection exceeds 1 percent per year—for example, in groups to whom health care is not regularly accessible.

Those receiving the BCG vaccine should have a repeat tuberculin test 3 months later. If the skin test is negative, the vaccination should be repeated. For newborns, the dose of vaccine is one-half that used for adults. If revaccination is necessary, a full dose of vaccine is administered. The vaccine should not be given to anyone who is tuberculin positive or to individuals with impaired immune responses. It has been known to cause death in children with immunological disorders. In the United States isoniazid chemoprophylaxis rather than BCG vaccine is recommended for prevention. In developed countries, where the level of resistance to tuberculosis is relatively high, it is much cheaper to treat the disease with drugs than to use preventive methods on a large segment of the population.

NONTUBERCULOUS MYCOBACTERIOSES

Mycobacteria other than *M. tuberculosis* (MOTT), differ from *M. tuberculosis* in several ways. First, person-to-person transmission seldom occurs. Second, MOTT are ubiquitous in nature and can be found as saprophytes in the environment. Third, MOTT may colonize an individual without causing disease. Infections caused by MOTT are not invasive unless the patient has some predisposing condition. To distinguish MOTT from *M. tuberculosis* and *M. bovis*, Runyon in 1959 proposed a classification scheme in which there were four groups, each group containing several species (Table 24-1). These groups were differentiated on the basis of colony pigmentation and growth rate.

PATHOGENESIS

Because the human pathogenic nontuberculous mycobacteria are not infectious for animals, much concerning the transmission and host response to infection remains unknown. *M. kansasii* is the most frequently isolated species from human infections. *M. kansasii*, *M. avium*, and *M. intracellulare* produce pulmonary infection that is indistinguishable from that produced by *M. tuberculosis* or *M. bovis*. Infection is more common in patients compromised by chronic pulmonary conditions such as emphysema and bronchitis. In all nontuberculous mycobacterioses, dissemination from the initial site of infection is rare except in some immunologically compromised patients.

A more careful examination of natural waters and community water supplies has revealed the presence of nontuberculous mycobacteria. They have often gone unrecognized because of their slow growth on laboratory media but are now recognized as common contaminants of water. They are especially troublesome in the hospital because of their resistance to disinfectants such as chlorine and glutaraldehyde, and they have been incriminated in infections following such hospital procedures as dialysis, open-heart surgery, and insertion of implant devices (for example, porcine heart valves).

Isolates of *M. avium* and *M. intracellulare* (collectively referred to as members of the *M. avium* complex [MAC]) have been frequently isolated from AIDS patients. Up to 50 percent of AIDS patients develop a mycobacterial infection at some stage in their disease. Two-thirds of the isolates are MAC serotypes. MAC infection may involve the liver, lung, bone marrow, kidney, spleen, central nervous system, and intestinal tract. Approximately 5 percent of AIDS patients develop disseminated mycobacterioses, which are directly responsible for the death of the patient. The prognosis for MAC-infected AIDS patients is very poor due to the resistance of these microorganisms to antimicrobials.

LABORATORY DIAGNOSIS, TREATMENT, AND PREVENTION

Clinical characteristics may suggest nontuberculous mycobacteriosis, but repeated isolation of the organism from specimens such as sputum is required. Identification of the mycobacterial species is required if optimal therapy is to be obtained. Nontuberculous mycobacteria do not always respond to the usual antituberculosis drugs (see Table 24-1). Besides pigment production and growth rate, several biochemical and cultural tests are used in the identification of nontuberculous mycobacteria (see *Manual of Clinical Microbiology* (4th ed.), pages 218 and 219). No vaccines are available for immunization.

MYCOBACTERIUM LEPRAE

The causal agent of leprosy (Hansen's disease), *M. leprae* has the potential for causing disfigurement. Infected individuals who show maximum resistance to the bacilli demonstrate a disease affecting the superficial nerve endings and related skin areas. In persons with minimal resistance the bacilli may be disseminated throughout the body.

GENERAL CHARACTERISTICS

M. leprae is an intracellular parasite that can be cultivated only in vivo and not on laboratory media. The bacillus can be cultured on mouse foot pads or armadillos. Like most other mycobacteria, *M. leprae* exhibits slow growth and has a generation time of 12 days (when cultivated in armadillo or mouse foot pad).

EPIDEMIOLOGY AND PATHOGENESIS

Leprosy is a disease found primarily in Asia and Africa. The total number of leprosy patients in the world is estimated at 10.6 million. In 1989, 163 cases in the United States were reported to the CDC. These cases were clustered in states such as Hawaii, California, and Texas.

Transmission of the leprosy bacillus is believed to occur through (1) inhalation of bacilli onto nasal mucosa, (2) intact skin, or (3) penetrating wounds such as by thorns. Inhalation of aerosols generated by infected patients is believed to be the most common method of transmission. Leprosy is a natural infection of wild armadillos, but whether these animals are a source of infection to humans is not clear since most leprosy cases occur where armadillos are absent.

Most people in areas endemic for leprosy become infected without any overt symptoms being manifested. Disease symptoms appear from 2–4 years after infection. In one form of the disease, called *indeterminate leprosy* (*IL*), a few hypo-

pigmented areas of the skin plus a dermatitis may be the first clinical manifestations of disease. Most (75 percent) of these individuals will recover spontaneously but the remainder will progress to one of the established forms of the disease, called *lepromatous leprosy* (*LL*) or *tuberculoid leprosy* (*TL*). Lepromatous leprosy is the most disfiguring form of the disease because of the host's lack of immunity to the bacillus (Plate 13). Skin lesions range from diffuse to nodular (the nodules are called *lepromas*). The skin lesions appear in the cooler parts of the body (nasal mucosa, anterior one-third of the eye, and peripheral nerve trunks at specific sites, as elbow, wrist, and ankle). The patient in lepromatous leprosy has few symptoms other than those caused by the nodular masses. In advanced cases there is sensory loss due to involvement of nerve fibers. The lesions are filled with macrophages, which contain large numbers of bacilli.

Tuberculoid leprosy (Plate 14) represents a localized form of the disease, in which there are a few well-circumscribed skin lesions. The lesions appear flat, are blanched, and contain few bacilli. The clinical picture of tuberculoid leprosy is due to bacterial proliferation followed by a relatively efficient immune response of the host to the bacilli.

In most leprosy patients there is some degree of irreversible peripheral nerve damage. In advanced cases, widespread destruction of nerve trunks can result in loss of feeling and permanent paralysis involving face, hands, and feet. The lack of pain sensations allows the patient to suffer self-damage and self-deformation through continued use of an extremity.

The pathogenic mechanisms of *Mycobacterium leprae* have never been clearly defined, but recent studies have incriminated a few chemical substances. *M. leprae* is able to live intracellularly because it is a poor stimulator of the respiratory burst in human monocytes. *M. leprae* possesses a phenolic glycolipid that is released extracellularly. This compound can be released in macrophages, where it acts as an antioxidant and scavenges various oxygen-derived metabolites that are believed to be important in microbial killing. A surface compound of *M. leprae*, called *lipoarabinomannan*, inhibits the proliferation of T cells. These two chemical compounds may represent mechanisms for preventing effective responses by the host during infection.

LABORATORY DIAGNOSIS, TREATMENT, AND PREVENTION

Scrapings from skin, nasal secretions, or lymph fluids removed from punctured skin nodules are stained for the presence of acid-fast bacilli, which often appear in parallel rows. Infection of the mouse foot pad is sometimes used to confirm the diagnosis of leprosy. The appearance of characteristic lesions is a confirmation of the leprosy bacillus.

At present, four drugs are used to control proliferation of the leprosy bacillus: dapsone, rifampin, clofazimine, and either ethionamide or prothionamide. In some areas dapsone is used alone; however, the World Health Organization (WHO) recommends a multidrug regimen. Current United States recommendations for tuberculoid leprosy is 6 months of rifampin plus dapsone daily and then dapsone alone for 3 years. Lepromatous leprosy patients are treated with rifampin plus dapsone daily for at least three years and dapsone is given alone for the remainder of the patient's life. Management of leprosy patients also includes minimizing permanent disability by controlling peripheral nerve damage and irreversible eye damage. These goals can be accomplished by using topical corticosteroids plus high doses of antibacterial drugs such as clofazimine. Prophylaxis is considered for family members of leprosy patients.

SUMMARY

1. The major human pathogenic species of *Mycobacterium* are *M. tuberculosis* and *M. bovis*, the causative agents of tuberculosis, and *M. leprae*, the cause of leprosy. Nontuberculous mycobacteria found in the environment (soil and water) are causes of respiratory and extrarespiratory disease, primarily in compromised hosts (see Table 24-1). Some nontuberculous species are associated with compromised hosts, such as in AIDS patients.

2. *Mycobacterium* differs from other bacteria in certain respects: (1) mycobacteria have a high lipid content; (2) they are acid-fast bacilli; (3) they produce serpentine colonies on specific agar; (4) they divide every 18 to 24 hours; and (5) they produce pigments that may be induced or they may be constitutive.

3. Tuberculosis is primarily a respiratory disease, but any organ can be infected. TB bacilli are ingested by macrophages but apparently only activated macrophages can kill them. In the lung, infected macrophages can persist and multiplying bacilli cause an inflammatory response and formation of dense areas of connective tissue and debris called a tubercle. Tubercles can become liquefied to produce areas of cascation necrosis.

4. Caseous lesions may heal and retain active bacilli for years or bacilli may spill out into the bloodstream to infect any organ. Some caseous lesions can rupture, allowing bacilli to be carried to healthy lung tissue. Bacilli in healed lesions can be reactivated years later to cause active disease.

5. The virulence of *M. tuberculosis* is associated with its ability to prevent phagosome-lysosome fusion in the macrophage. The cord factor may be the virulence factor.

6. Tuberculosis is a disease that is manifested as a hypersensitivity to antigens of the TB bacillus. Once infected by the bacillus, the host is sensitive to antigens such as purified tuberculin protein. This is the basis of the tuberculin test, which determines one's present or past contact with the TB bacillus.

7. Laboratory diagnosis of tuberculosis relies on detecting bacilli in sputum or other secretions via acid-fast stain or fluorescent antibody. The TB bacillus can be cultured on special media and

then subjected to biochemical and colonial identification tests.

8. Anyone is susceptible to tuberculosis, which is spread by contact with infected respiratory secretions. The very young and older adults are the most susceptible to infection. Approximately 24,000 cases are reported each year in the United States but as many as 10 million people may be infected.

9. Treatment of tuberculosis requires a multidrug regimen in which combinations such as isoniazid plus rifampin or ethambutol plus pyrazinamide are used over a period of 6 to 9 months. Izoniazid is used prophylactically. A vaccine, BCG, is used in Europe but is not ordinarily recommended in the United States. Isoniazid treatment is the preferred method of prevention in the United States.

10. The leprosy bacillus cannot be cultivated in vitro but can be cultured in the armadillo and the mouse foot pad. Leprosy is seen primarily in Asia and Africa, but a few cases (15–20 per year) are reported in the United States.

11. Leprosy is believed to be acquired primarily by inhalation of contaminated aerosols generated by infected patients. Most individuals have a natural resistance to the leprosy bacillus and when infected do not demonstrate overt symptoms. Those individuals who do respond to the leprosy bacillus usually demonstrate one of three forms of the disease: indeterminate leprosy (IL), tuberculoid leprosy (TL), or lepromatous leprosy (LL).

12. Indeterminate leprosy is manifested as only a few hypopigmented areas on the skin plus dermatitis, and most of the patients will recover spontaneously. The remainder, however, progress into TL or LL. In tuberculoid leprosy the patient has some immunity and the disease is localized. In lepromatous leprosy immunity is lacking; and this is the most disfiguring form of the disease, in which large nodules may form on areas of the body.

13. Diagnosis of leprosy is usually based on the appearance of lesions but acid-fast bacilli can be identified in scrapings from skin, nasal secretions, etc. Four drugs, including dapsone and rifampin, are the principal drugs in treatment of leprosy and these are used in combination. Some form of treatment may be required for the life of the patient, as in lepromatous leprosy.

QUESTIONS FOR STUDY

Select the best response or responses for each of the following:

1. Tuberculosis resembles brucellosis in that
   A. Both are caused by intracellular parasites.
   B. Both can be acquired by ingestion of contaminated milk.
   C. Both are characterized by granulomas in organs and tissue such as bone, spleen, and liver.
   D. Both are caused by organisms whose cell walls have a high concentration of mycolic acids.

2. Which of the following could be considered valid candidates for BCG immunization in the United States?
   A. Tuberculin-negative infants in metropolitan areas
   B. Tuberculin-negative adults
   C. Tuberculin-positive individuals who are not responding to chemotherapy
   D. Tuberculin-negative infants or children who are exposed for long periods to patients who have bacilli resistant to isoniazid and rifampin

3. The drug used in tuberculosis treatment as well as prophylaxis is
   A. Rifampin
   B. Isoniazid
   C. Streptomycin
   D. Ethambutol

4. The component or product of *M. tuberculosis* that is believed to be the major virulence factor is
   A. The capsule
   B. An exotoxin
   C. Mycolic acids
   D. Peptidoglycan

5. The most frequently isolated nontuberculous *Mycobacterium* species are found primarily
   A. As commensals in the respiratory tract of mammals
   B. In water
   C. As commensals in the intestinal tract of mammals
   D. In birds

Fill in the blank:

6. Only pigments produced by mycobacteria in the presence of light are called _____ .

7. The nontuberculous *Mycobacterium* species that causes a pulmonary disease similar to tuberculosis is _____ .

8. The coagulated mass of host cells and bacilli that results from destruction of the tubercle is called _____ .

9. The localized form of leprosy is called _____ .

10. Leprosy is a natural infection found in wild _____ .

ADDITIONAL READINGS

ACIP. Use of BCG vaccines in the control of tuberculosis. *M.M.W.R.* 37(43):663,1988.

American Thoracic Society, C.D.C. Treatment of tuberculosis and tuberculous infection in adults and children. *Am. Rev. Resp. Dis.* 134:355,1986.

Dannenberg, A. M., Jr. Immune mechanisms in the pathogenesis of pulmonary tuberculosis. *Rev. Infect. Dis.* 11(Suppl. 2):369,1989.

Hastings, R. C., et al. Leprosy. *Clin. Microbiol. Rev.* 1(3):330,1988.

Hastings, R. C. (ed.). *Leprosy.* Edinburgh: Churchill Livingstone, Ltd., 1985.

Sunderam, G., et al. Tuberculosis as a manifestation of the acquired immune deficiency syndrome (AIDS). *J.A.M.A.* 256:362,1986.

Woods, G. L., and Washington, J. A. II. Mycobacteria other than *Mycobacterium tuberculosis*: Review of microbiologic and clinical aspects. *Rev. Infect. Dis.* 9(2):275,1987.

25. SPIROCHETES AND SPIRAL AND CURVED RODS

OBJECTIVES

To outline the various symptoms associated with the stages of syphilis

To outline the types of treatment for the different groups of individuals who have syphilis

To briefly describe the most important laboratory tests used to identify the syphilis organism

To list the causative agent, method of transmission, site of infection, and method of treatment for leptospirosis, relapsing fever, Lyme disease, rat bite fever, and *Campylobacter* infection

A number of helical and curved bacteria are indigenous to soil and water, and some can be found as commensals in animals. Only a few, however, are human pathogens. The *spirochetes* are a group with a distinct morphology and method of movement that distinguishes them from the *spiral and curved rods*. There are three important genera of human pathogenic spirochetes: *Treponema*, *Borrelia*, and *Leptospira*. The spiral and curved rods include two important genera: *Spirillum* and *Campylobacter*.

THE SPIROCHETES

The spirochetes are long, slender, helically shaped cells that are actively motile by means of flagella-like filaments called *axial filaments*. The axial filaments, which originate at each pole of the cell, are located between an outer envelope or sheath and an inner protoplasmic cylinder. The number of axial filaments varies depending on the genus.

Spirochetes are gram-negative (but the Gram procedure is rarely used to identify them). They are from 3 to 500 μm in length and from 0.2 to 0.75 μm in diameter. Human pathogens, however, are seldom more than 40 μm in length. They all divide by transverse fission and may be aerobic, facultatively anaerobic, or anaerobic. Routine staining procedures are not ordinarily employed for most genera because the width of many spirochetes is at or just below the resolving power of the light microscope. Spirochetes are best recognized by dark-field microscopy. The only reliable method for differentiation among the pathogenic spirochetes is based on the size, number, and spacing of the helical coils (Fig. 25-1).

GENUS TREPONEMA (TREPONEMA PALLIDUM)

Treponemal species can be found as commensals in the oral cavity, gastrointestinal tract, and urogenital tract of animals. The pathogenic treponemes are *T. pallidum*, the causative agent of ve-

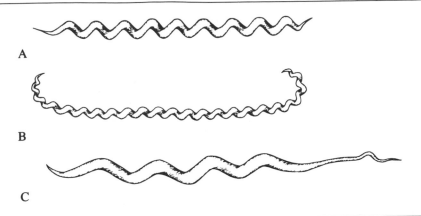

Fig. 25-1. Relative size and shape of the spirochetes. A. Genus *Treponema*. B. Genus *Leptospira*. C. Genus *Borrelia*.

nereal syphilis; *T. pertenue*, the agent of *yaws*, which is a tropical disease; and *T. carateum*, the agent of a chronic skin disease found in Central and South America called *pinta*. Diseases caused by species of *Treponema* are called *treponematoses*.

General Characteristics of *Treponema pallidum*

T. pallidum, the agent of venereal syphilis, is 6 to 14 μm in length with a width of 0.1 to 0.2 μm. The organism cannot be stained easily by ordinary dyes and is best observed by dark-field microscopy. When observed microscopically, the coils are seen to be evenly spaced 1 μm from each other (Fig. 25-2).

Pathogenic treponemes are not cultivable with any consistency in artificial laboratory media. They are ordinarily cultivated in rabbit testicular tissue, which provides a source of substantial numbers of treponemes. *T. pallidum*, originally considered to be an anaerobe, has been shown to be microaerophilic. The organism is sensitive to environmental influences and is easily inactivated by heat (temperatures above 42°C), cold, dessication, osmotic changes, and heavy metals. Heavy metals such as arsenic, antimony, and bismuth were used to treat syphilis before the discovery of antibiotics.

Fig. 25-2. Electron micrograph of *Treponema pallidum* attached to rabbit testes. (From T. J. Fitzgerald, *J. Bacteriol.* 130:1333, 1977.)

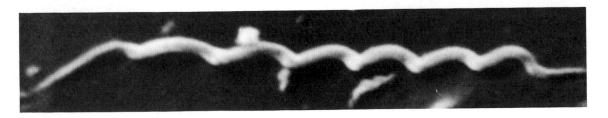

PATHOGENESIS

Syphilis is almost always contracted by direct transmission. Direct contact takes place by sexual means or by accidental contact with infectious lesions such as those that occur in the mouth. Congenital transfer between mother and fetus may also occur. Almost 90 percent of the cases of syphilis are caused by sexual contact.

Untreated, syphilis either progresses through a number of stages to debilitation and death or terminates spontaneously with no apparent detrimental effects. The symptoms in each stage, if present, are varied and often unpredictable.

Primary Syphilis

In more than 90 percent of the cases a single lesion appears on the cervix of the female or the penis of the male. The primary lesion may also be evident on any cutaneous or mucous membrane surface, as on the scrotum, labia, nipples, rectum, eyelids, fingers, or mouth. At the initial site of infection, a papule, the base of which is hard but painless, develops into an ulcerated sore (Fig. 25-3). This lesion is called a *hard chancre.* The time required for appearance of the chancre varies between 10 and 90 days, the average being about 3 weeks. In women a lesion on the cervix may go unnoticed. If treated immediately with antibiotics, the chancre will disappear within a week. Untreated, it may disappear spontaneously within 4 to 12 weeks. Accompanying the primary chancre is the development of enlarged lymph nodes near the initial lesion. Once into the lymph, the organism is capable of reaching the bloodstream and infecting other tissues.

As many as 25 percent of patients with primary syphilis have a negative serological test. At this stage the only absolute diagnostic test is darkfield microscopic examination of material from the lesions. Material from the lesions is highly infectious.

Studies in Europe during the early 1900s of untreated syphilis patients revealed that 75 percent of cases did not progress beyond the primary

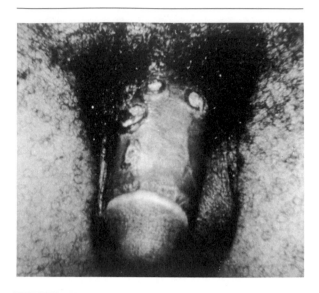

Fig. 25-3. Primary stage of syphilis. Chancres on the penis. (Courtesy Centers for Disease Control.)

stage. This implies that a certain degree of immunity results from primary infection.

Secondary Syphilis

The chancre produced in the primary stage may still be present during the secondary stage. Symptoms of the secondary stage, which is the result of systemic dispersal of the organism, may appear from six weeks to several months after infection. They are manifested by the development of cutaneous as well as mucous membrane lesions.

In more than 80 percent of persons infected, a macular skin rash appears on the trunk or limbs but seldom on the face. The macular lesions are round and flat and fade within a few weeks. A papular rash may occur in which the lesion is raised and indurated (Fig. 25-4). The papules usually develop on the trunk and limbs as well as the palms of the hands and soles of the feet. They also appear on the face. The papular lesion may break down, resulting in ulceration. Lesions on the scalp can cause temporary loss of hair (alopecia).

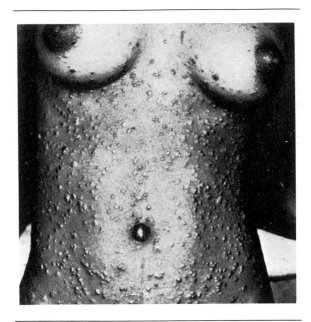

Fig. 25-4. Secondary cutaneous syphilis. (From A. H. Rudolph. In P. F. Wehrle and F. H. Top, Sr. [eds.], *Communicable and Infectious Diseases* [8th ed.]. St. Louis: Mosby, 1976.)

Mucous membrane lesions can occur at the mucocutaneous junctions. Sometimes these lesions coalesce to form large masses called *condylomata lata* (Plate 15). They are more prevalent around the anus and labia. Lesions of the mucous membrane are also common in the mouth and on tongue and tonsils. Such a lesion is known as a *mucous patch* and is raised and covered with a gray-white membrane.

The spirochete can be demonstrated in any of the cutaneous or mucous membrane lesions by dark-field microscopy. Serological examination of patients during this stage reveals high antibody titers that remain relatively high for up to two years after infection—after that the serological tests are often negative. Patients in the primary and secondary stages are highly infectious. The infectious stage usually ends when the lesions of the secondary stage have healed and the treponemes are no longer demonstrable in them. Some treponemes, however, remain viable after the

disappearance of the secondary symptoms and give rise to a quiescent period called *latent syphilis*.

Latent Syphilis

In latent syphilis a relatively high serological titer is evident, but clinical symptoms are lacking. This stage is subdivided into early and late latent periods. Early latent syphilis is a latent infection of two years or less. During this period the patient may suffer relapses in which secondary lesions reappear and render the patient potentially infectious. The late latent period, considered a noninfectious stage, is a latent infection of more than two years. This stage may last the lifetime of the patient or until certain clinical symptoms are manifested that occur in the tertiary stage of syphilis.

Tertiary or Late Syphilis

Lesions of the tertiary stage may occur any time after the appearance of the primary and secondary stages, or they may never arise. In this noninfectious stage the lesions may or may not be debilitating. *Gummas* are the most typical tertiary lesions. Gummas contain no treponemes but rather are due to a hypersensitivity on the part of the host. They are granulomatous lesions of the skin, subcutaneous tissue, mucous membrane, bone, or viscera. Gummas of the skin (Fig. 25-5) are painless, firm, indurated nodules and may show scaling. Gummas of the subcutaneous tissue result in ulceration, with the lesion giving the appearance of being punched out. They may be found on the leg, hand, scalp, or face. Gummas of mucous membranes can eventually destroy deeper tissue such as bone and cartilage. Gummas of the mouth can lead to perforation of the hard palate as well as deformities of the soft palate and uvula. Glossitis, a superficial inflammation of the tongue, causes an initial swelling that may later result in the formation of deep fissures.

Syphilis of the bone may result in periostitis,

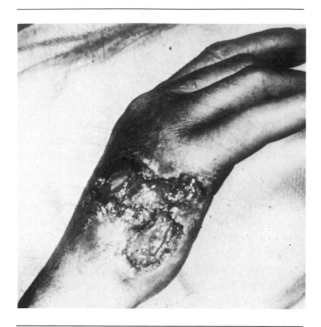

Fig. 25-5. Gumma of the hand, characteristic of tertiary syphilis. (Courtesy Centers for Disease Control.)

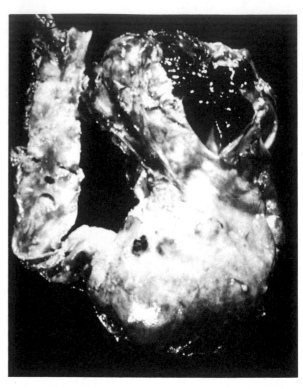

Fig. 25-6. Syphilitic aneurysm of the thoracic aorta. (Courtesy Armed Forces Institute of Pathology, AFIP 82-6064.)

in which there is proliferation of the bone under the periosteum, or osteitis, in which destructive lesions are produced. Periostitis of the tibia causes a bowing of the front of the bone and is called *saber shin syndrome*. In osteitis, flat bones, particularly those of the skull, as well as the nasal bones and the palate may be severely affected and become deformed. Gummas of the viscera are manifested most frequently in lesions in the liver.

The most destructive and debilitating lesions involve the cardiovascular and central nervous systems. The prognosis for cardiovascular syphilis is death, often as a result of aneurysms in the vessels of the heart a few months after the appearance of the symptoms (Fig. 25-6). Organisms that infect the central nervous system give rise to the following conditions: (1) In *tabes dorsalis* the spinal cord is affected, resulting in loss of control of the lower extremities; in such cases death is often the result of some other compli-

cation. (2) In *paresis*, also called *general paralysis of the insane*, there is first a personality change and then the patient becomes demented and bedridden.

Dark-field examination of tertiary lesions for spirochetes is usually negative because of the relatively few treponemes present. Serological tests can disclose the presence of antibodies in more than 70 percent of the cases. In other cases antibodies cannot be detected.

Studies on mechanisms of pathogenesis for *T. pallidum* have been difficult because of problems in cultivation in the laboratory. Currently these problems are being circumvented by utilization of recombinant DNA technology. Some important aspects of pathogenesis have come to light in recent years. Attachment to host cells is an important step in initiating disease.One type of receptor appears to be the glycoproteins, called *fibronectins*, which are present on eukaryotic cell surfaces. Projections on the tips of treponemes are the organelles believed to promote attachment to fibronectins, but other treponeme–cell interactions may be involved. The lesions associated with the secondary stage are believed to represent an immune complex disorder; however, we still are not sure if the immune complexes are merely by-products of the infection. To date no *T. pallidum* antigen has been shown conclusively to be a virulence factor.

Congenital Syphilis

A mother with untreated primary or secondary syphilis is a potential threat to the fetus. After the sixteenth week of pregnancy the fetus is vulnerable to infections by *T. pallidum*. Treatment of the mother before the sixteenth week almost always prevents infection in the newborn. Treatment after the sixteenth week brings about an in utero cure but may not be in time to prevent bone or joint involvement, deafness, or interstitial keratitis. If infected fetuses are left untreated, 20 to 25 percent will die as stillbirths or spontaneous abortions, another 20 to 25 percent will die soon after birth, and 50 percent of the survivors will have severe infection. Although many infected infants appear healthy at birth, after 2 weeks symptoms begin to manifest themselves. The syphilitic is often born with or develops a rash similar to that incurred in secondary syphilis. The rash is papular and may cover the entire body but is particularly evident on the palms, soles, and areas about the mouth. Mucous patches may also appear. In the nose these patches give rise to a nasal discharge called *snuffles*. Snuffles often progresses to inflammation of the bone (osteitis), causing a deformity referred to as a *saddle nose*. The liver is often enlarged, causing a distended abdomen. The bones can also be affected, resulting in periostitis of the long bones, a very painful condition.

After the second year of life noninfectious manifestations of congenital syphilis occur. Gummas can destroy the nasal septum and perforate the soft and hard palates. Periostitis of the tibia leads to the bowing of the leg known as saber shin (Fig. 25-7). The most common lesion is interstitial keratitis, which can involve both eyes. Each attack leaves some scarring on the cornea, which eventually impairs vision. Hutchinson's teeth, a condition in which the central incisors of the permanent teeth are notched and translucent, is also a common late congenital symptom. Failure of the maxilla to develop makes the jaw look prominent, producing a bulldog appearance.

EPIDEMIOLOGY

In 1989, 44,540 cases of primary and secondary syphilis were reported in the United States. This represents a substantial increase over the 1987 total of 34,550 cases and the 1986 total of 27,883 cases. The greatest increases were seen in large metropolitan areas of the states of Florida, New York, and California. These increases in 1989 and 1988 reverse the downward trend observed between 1983–1987 (Fig. 25-8). The greatest relative increase in syphilis was among females and heterosexual males of all racial and ethnic backgrounds. Several factors may be involved in the dramatic increases in syphilis in recent years, including: (1) nonintravenous drugs (such as crack cocaine) being exchanged for sex; (2) routine use of spectinomycin (which does not cure syphilis) in areas where a number of gonorrhea infections are caused by beta-lactamase-producing organisms; and (3) decreased resources available for syphilis control programs. Infectious syphilis, however, has decreased among homosexual and bisexual men. This decrease is apparently due to changes in sexual behavior in response to AIDS infections in these groups. There were 859 cases of congenital syphilis in 1989 in the United States. Most cases were observed among minority women, who are less likely to receive adequate prenatal care.

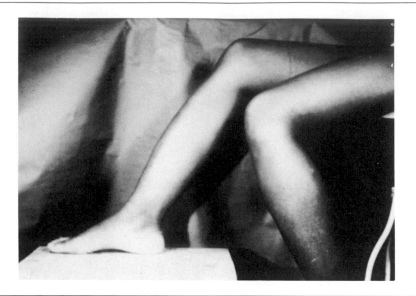

Fig. 25-7. Saber shin, characteristic of congenital syphilis. (Courtesy Centers for Disease Control.)

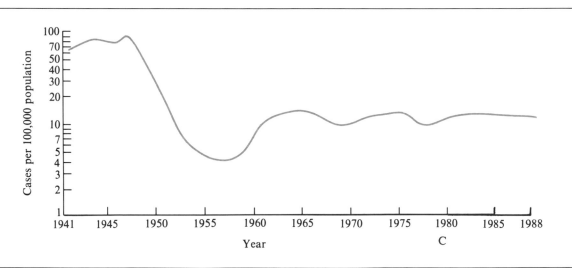

Fig. 25-8. Reported civilian case rates by year of primary and secondary syphilis in United States, 1941–1988. (From Centers for Disease Control.)

The increases in syphilis can be reversed by (1) removing financial barriers that prevent access to quality care, (2) screening for sexually transmitted diseases in high-risk populations, (3) utilizing interviews for locating and treating sexual partners, and (4) providing the necessary information to educate all age groups about the disease and how it can be avoided.

LABORATORY DIAGNOSIS

Dark-field Examination

Examination of exudate from syphilitic lesions or rashes by dark-field microscopy is the only absolute diagnostic test for *T. pallidum* (Plate 1). Such examination cannot be used in all stages of syphilis because suspected lesions may not exist or may be inaccessible. The suspected lesions may also reveal no spirochetes if they are from the tertiary stage of syphilis or if the patient has received antibiotic treatment before examination.

Immunofluorescence

The exudate from tissue can be fixed to a slide and stained with a fluorescein-labeled antitreponeme serum. Identification is made by fluorescence microscopy.

Serological Tests

Two types of antibodies are produced in response to treponemal infections: *reagin*, a nonspecific nontreponemal antibody, and a specific antitreponemal antibody. Several tests can be used to detect each. None of the tests, however, is absolute because biological false-positives can occur in any of them.

Reagin is a nonspecific antibody produced by all syphilitics, but it is not a protective antibody. It is a mixture of IgG and IgM antibodies produced in a number of other conditions and diseases besides syphilis. Reagin reacts with a cardiolipin extracted from beef heart. The most common tests used to detect the reagin-cardiolipin complex are the agglutination tests.

The *Venereal Disease Research Laboratories (VDRL)* test is an agglutination test. A positive reaction is the appearance of discrete clumps when the cardiolipin antigen is added to the patient's serum. The VDRL is employed primarily as a screening test in the laboratory. The rapid plasma reagin (RPR) card test is a modification of the VDRL test. It also detects reagin but uses charcoal particles so the test can be read macroscopically. A positive reaction is the clumping of the charcoal particles. The RPR test is used mainly in the field in surveying large groups such as migrant workers. The VDRL and RPR tests are very sensitive in the late primary and secondary stages. They are least sensitive in early primary and late latent syphilis.

Nontreponemal tests are not ideal because they cannot distinguish between IgG and IgM without previous separation of serum. Detection of IgM is important for the diagnosis of congenital syphilis because IgM does not cross the placenta and IgM in newborns indicates active syphilis. A VDRL ELISA has been developed for large-scale testing and detection of IgG and IgM antibodies.

Antitreponemal antibody tests are more specific than the nontreponemal antibody tests and are used mostly to resolve problems that arise from the initial screening procedures. Antitreponemal tests include the following:

1. The *fluorescent treponemal antibody (FTA) test* is sensitive in all stages of syphilis. The most widely used variant of this test is the FTA absorption (FTA-ABS) test, in which nonspecific treponemal antibodies are removed from the test serum by absorption with an extract of Reiter protein (which is prepared from a nonpathogenic treponemal strain called the Reiter strain). The test is performed as follows:
   a. Killed *T. pallidum* is fixed to the slide.
   b. The patient's serum is applied to the slide and incubated for 30 minutes. If antibodies

to *T. pallidum* are present in the serum, they will bind to the spirochete.

c. Goat or rabbit anti-human globulin previously tagged with fluorescein is added to the slide. If the test is positive, a fluorescein-antibody-spirochete complex will be formed. The immunoglobulin to which the fluorescein dye is conjugated is IgG. For the detection of congenital syphilis IgG human immunoglobulin has been replaced by IgM in some laboratories. It has been found to be more specific than any of the STS tests generally used for congenital syphilis because total IgM is elevated in the umbilical cord or blood during syphilis infection.

2. *T. pallidum* hemagglutination (TPHA) tests have become popular in recent years. Red blood cells from certain animal species plus Reiter treponeme components are used. The test detects, by hemagglutination, the presence of treponemal antibodies. This test is very inexpensive and easy to perform. It compares favorably with the FTA-ABS test except in primary syphilis.

3. An alternative to the FTA-ABS test is called the BIO-ENZ Bead test. The test is a modification of the ELISA and uses ferrous metal beads and a solid-phase carrier for antigen prepared from *T. pallidum*. The presence of treponemal antibody in a test serum sample is indicated by enzyme-substrate color intensity, which may be read visually or spectrophotometrically. The advantages of the test are: (1) there is no need for expensive microscopy equipment, (2) tests can be performed quickly, and (3) little training is needed by the serologist.

Biological False-Positives

In some individuals, serological tests for syphilis are positive when in fact the patient does not have and never had syphilis. Such tests are called *biological false-positives* (BFP). Any serological test for syphilis may give a false-positive. Reagin, which is what the VDRL test detects, can be produced in a number of conditions other than syphilis, including immunization, drug addiction, lupus erythematosus, connective tissue diseases, and hepatitis. Pregnant women, diabetics, and persons with immune disorders also sometimes produce reagin. BFP in the FTA-ABS test may result from the appearance of abnormal immunoglobulins in the patient's serum arising from any number of immune disorders. Most studies have shown that 1 in 4000 nonsyphilitic patients will give a BFP. Chronic BFPs may be a clue to certain underlying diseases or may represent latent or asymptomatic treponemal disease.

Antitreponemal antibodies persist for years after successful antibiotic therapy, while reagin declines more rapidly. A positive test for antitreponemal antibodies could also be considered a false-positive since antibodies may be present in the absence of infection.

TREATMENT

Penicillin is the drug of choice in the treatment of all stages of syphilis. Because the generation time of *T. pallidum* is 30 to 33 hours, it is important to maintain a level of antibiotic to cover a sufficient number of divisions. The following are the Venereal Disease Control Advisory Committee's recommendations for the treatment of syphilis:

1. Primary, secondary, and latent syphilis of less than one year's duration: Penicillin G benzathine, aqueous penicillin G procaine, or penicillin G procaine in oil may be administered intramuscularly. If the patient is allergic to penicillin, tetracycline or erythromycin may be administered orally.

2. Syphilis of more than one year's duration (including latent syphilis, cardiovascular syphilis, and neurosyphilis): Penicillin G benzathine or aqueous penicillin procaine may be injected intramuscularly. Tetracycline or erythromycin can be used for those allergic to penicillin.

3. Syphilis in pregnancy: Penicillin is given in dosage schedules appropriate for the stage of

syphilis as recommended for the treatment of nonpregnant patients. Tetracyclines are not recommended because of their toxic effect on both patient and fetus.

4. Congenital syphilis: Aqueous penicillin G, aqueous penicillin G procaine, or penicillin G benzathine may be administered, depending on the extent of infection and condition of the cerebrospinal fluid.

5. Neurosyphilis: A total dose of 6.0 to 9.0 million units of penicillin G over a three- to four-week period is satisfactory for over 90 percent of the cases.

6. Syphilis in HIV-infected patients: Penicillin regimens should be used whenever possible for all stages of syphilis.

7. Follow-up and retreatment: All patients with early syphilis and congenital syphilis are encouraged to repeat quantitative nontreponemal tests 3, 6, and 12 months after treatment. Patients with syphilis of more than one year's duration should also have a repeat serological test 24 months after treatment. Retreatment should be considered when
   a. Clinical signs or symptoms of syphilis persist or recur.
   b. There is a fourfold increase in titer of a nontreponemal test.
   c. An initially high-titer nontreponemal test fails to show a fourfold decrease within a year.

In many cases of syphilis a local or generalized reaction follows the administration of penicillin. Called the *Jarisch-Herxheimer reaction*, it is characterized by headache, fever, and joint pains followed by an intensification of the syphilitic symptoms, particularly those of the secondary stage. Steroid hormones can prevent or diminish the reaction. Herxheimer-like reactions have also been detected in other diseases including borreliosis, brucellosis, and trypanosomiasis. The reasons for these reactions are not known.

Prophylactic use of penicillin before intercourse is not recommended because of the danger of masking the usual symptoms of syphilis.

PREVENTION AND CONTROL

To date no active immunizing agent has been produced as a prophylaxis to syphilis infection. Although sexual abstinence would certainly be the ultimate weapon against this disease, that proposal would not be met with a great deal of enthusiasm. Control of the disease is difficult because of the high rate of travel, mildness of symptoms, infectiousness in early stages, and ignorance about the transmission, diagnosis, and treatment of syphilis. Prevention should be the ultimate goal, and this can be accomplished by

1. Education. The transmission, diagnosis, and treatment of syphilis among all age groups, especially the young, must be understood.

2. Routine serological testing programs. Many infected individuals unaware of their condition have been detected by these programs, which include testing before issuance of marriage licenses, testing of patients admitted to the hospital, and preemployment examination.

3. Investigation—as rapid as possible—concerning the treated syphilitic so that his or her contacts can be found, tested, and if necessary treated for possible infection.

NONVENEREAL SYPHILIS

Yaws, bejel, and pinta are three diseases that resemble syphilis. They are endemic, nonvenereal, and transmitted primarily by contact with eating and drinking utensils in areas lacking adequate hygiene. Yaws is caused by *T. pertenue*, which is morphologically and serologically indistinguishable from *T. pallidum*. Yaws is endemic in Africa, India, and parts of South America. The primary lesion, called a "mother yaw," heals and later develops into a secondary lesion (Fig. 25-9). Tertiary lesions may involve the skin and occasionally the bones. Penicillin is effective in treatment.

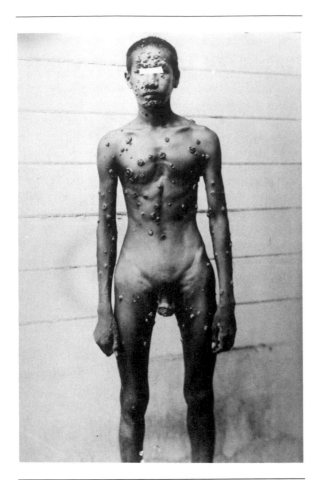

Fig. 25-9. Characteristic yaws lesions. (Courtesy Air Force Institute of Pathology, AFIP 39201.)

Pinta, a disease found in Central and South America, is caused by *T. carateum*. This organism, like *T. pertenue*, is morphologically and serologically indistinguishable from *T. pallidum*. Primary lesions develop that do not become necrotic but do become hyperpigmented. As the lesions heal the affected skin area becomes depigmented. Penicillin is effective in treatment.

Bejel is an endemic syphilis occurring primarily in the Middle East. The disease is usually contracted during childhood and is treatable with penicillin.

GENUS *BORRELLIA*

GENERAL CHARACTERISTICS

The borrelias are the largest of the pathogenic spirochetes, ranging in size from 10 to 30 μm in length and 0.3 to 0.7 μm in width (Fig. 25-10). They are actively motile, exhibiting a lashing, twisting movement. They have irregularly spaced

Fig. 25-10. *Borrelia* species (×1000) in rodent blood. (From W. Burgdorfer. In E. H. Lennette et al. [eds.], *Manual of Clinical Microbiology* [3rd ed.]. Washington, DC: American Society for Microbiology, 1980.)

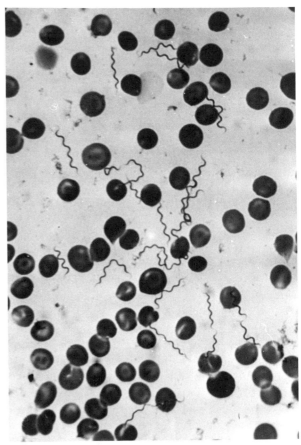

coils that may range in number from 4 to 30. Borrelia are distinguished from the other spirochetes in that they can be stained by ordinary dyes such as crystal violet or carbolfuchsin. When artificial media are supplemented with serum or blood, these organisms can be cultivated in the laboratory.

EPIDEMIOLOGY AND PATHOGENESIS

All borrelia are transmitted to their hosts by arthropod vectors. The hosts infected by borrelia include rodents, domestic animals and birds, as well as humans. There are two important human diseases caused by borrelia: *relapsing fever*, which is transmitted by body lice or soft-shelled ticks, and *Lyme disease*, which is transmitted by ixodid ticks.

Relapsing Fever

Louse-borne relapsing fever is caused by *B. recurrentis* while tick-borne disease in North America is caused by *B. hermsii*, *B. turicatae*, and *B. parkeri*. In louse-borne disease humans acquire infection by crushing the arthropod and rubbing its infected parts into the bite wound. Humans are the only reservoir. In tick-borne disease the infectious microorganisms are transferred via tick saliva or body fluids while the tick is feeding on its host. Rodents are the reservoir of tick-borne disease.

About 3 to 4 days after infection there is an onset of chills and fever caused by excessive numbers of borrelia in the bloodstream. The organs containing high levels of borrelia are the spleen, liver, kidney, and eye, as well as the brain. Tenderness of the liver and spleen, jaundice, and a macular rash are characteristic symptoms during the first episode of fever. The initial attack, which may last 3 to 7 days, is followed by an asymptomatic period and then a relapse with symptoms resembling the first attack. Four or more relapses may occur, with each slightly shorter than the previous one and each with less severe symptoms.

The recurrent fever is coincidental with the immune response of the host. Relapses are related to the antigenic variation of the microorganism. Experimental infections in animals have revealed that as many as four major serotypes can be recovered. Microorganisms disappear from the blood after the initial symptoms of disease and this coincides with high level of antibodies to the infecting serotype. Those microorganisms that undergo antigenic variation are resistant to the antibody present and begin to multiply. The multiplication cycle results in the return of clinical symptoms. Once the immune system has responded to the new serotype, the clinical manifestations of disease disappear.

Louse-borne relapsing fever is seen predominantly in Africa while tick-borne disease occurs sporadically throughout the world. In the United States approximately 10 to 15 cases of tick-borne disease are reported each year. Most of the cases occur in western states such as California, Oregon, Colorado, and Texas.

Lyme Disease

Lyme disease is a systemic tick-borne illness in humans caused by *B. burgdorferi*. There is evidence that Lyme disease may also affect dogs and other domestic animals. Lyme disease has been the most frequently reported tick-borne disease in the United States since it was first reported in 1977. In 1988, for example, 4,572 cases of Lyme disease were reported to the CDC. A history of tick bites, outdoor activities, or pets carrying ticks is associated with most cases of Lyme disease.

The North American distribution of Lyme disease parallels known bird migration routes. Birds are therefore believed to be important local reservoirs and long-distance dispersal agents for *B. burgdorferi*-infected ticks.

Lyme disease, which was first reported in North America in Lyme, Connecticut, is an infection that may be brief and inconsequential or chronic and disabling. It is transmitted to humans by ixodid ticks. The first stage of infection is characterized by an expanding skin lesion called erythema chronicum migrans (ECM). ECM develops at the site of tick bite sustained 3 to 14 days previously. The patient often complains of headache, low fever, stiff neck, and arthralgia. Skin lesions may also appear at sites distant from the original lesion.

The second stage of Lyme disease appears from a few weeks to a few months after the primary stage. The secondary stage is characterized by arthritis and pain in tendons, bursa, and muscle. Arthritis usually involves a knee or other large joint. Untreated arthritis may become destructive and involve erosion of cartilage and bone. Lyme arthritis that continues for years is considered part of the third stage of disease. Neurologic disorders may also appear during the second stage and there is evidence of aseptic meningitis. Patients with chronic meningitis complain of altered mental states and persistent fatigue. In the second and third stages of Lyme disease there may also be cardiac involvement or myocarditis but this is usually self-limiting.

LABORATORY DIAGNOSIS

The borrelias of relapsing fever are easily observed in stained blood smears, provided the blood is sampled during the fever period and antibiotics have not been used previously. The microorganisms can also be detected in unstained preparations by phase-contrast microscopy. When spirochetes cannot be detected in blood smears, a blood sample or other tissue specimen from the infected patient can be injected intraperitoneally into white mice. After 48 hours borrelia can be perceived in the tail blood of the infected mouse.

Lyme disease borrelias can be detected in blood but often they are not present there and skin biopsies are required. When fluorescein-labeled antibodies are used to detect *B. burgdorferi* large or small blebs can be detected on the cells.

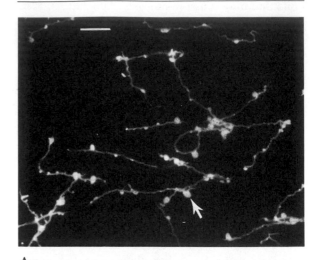

A

B

Fig. 25-11. Lyme disease spirochetes. A. Indirect fluorescence of fixed spirochetes isolated from *Ixodes* ticks and incubated with monoclonal antibodies. Arrow points to outer membrane bleb. Bar = 5 μm. B. Phase-contrast micrograph after illumination with epifluorescence and low-intensity transmitted light. Bar = 5 μm. (From A. G. Barbour, S. Tessier, and W. Todd, *J. Infect. Immun.* 41:795, 1983.)

These blebs are antibodies binding to the outer membranes that become disrupted during drying and fixation (Fig. 25-11). Determination of serum antibodies is often helpful in the diagnosis of Lyme disease because, unlike relapsing fever, the Lyme disease spirochetes have stable surface antigens. Established tests include indirect fluorescent antibody and ELISA; however, cross-reactivity with other spirochetes may occur. A commercial test utilizing the technique, polymerase chain reaction, is being developed. This test (see Chap. 10) is so sensitive that it can detect *B. burgdorferi* DNA in a sample containing as few as five spirochetes.

TREATMENT AND PREVENTION

Tetracyclines and chloramphenicol are drugs of choice in the treatment of relapsing fever. If drugs do not cause an immediate cure, they do reduce the rate of relapses. Tetracycline treatment does incite a Jarisch-Herxheimer-like reaction, but the reaction is not severe.

Lyme disease patients with first-stage disease are treated with oral antibiotics such as phenoxymethyl penicillin or tetracycline. Patients with neurologic disease or arthritis are given penicillin G, chloramphenicol, or ceftriaxone intravenously. Antibiotic failures increase the longer the patient has chronic symptoms.

No prepared vaccine has proved effective in relapsing fever and none has been developed for Lyme disease. Prevention is centered on control of insect vectors. In building sites where ticks may be present, sprays containing 1 percent aldrin or 0.5 percent malathion can be applied. Persons going into areas that are potential tick habitats should cover as much of their bodies as possible and check their skin periodically for the presence of ticks.

GENUS LEPTOSPIRA

The genus *Leptospira* contains a large number of species that are saprophytes and are harmless to humans or animals. Several species, however, are parasitic and cause infections (*leptospiroses*) characterized by their effect on the liver, kidney, lungs, and meninges. The pathogenic leptospires are classified under the species name *L. interrogans*, with serogroups such as *canicola*, *pomona*, and *iceterohaemorrhagiae*. Each subgroup can be divided into serologically distinct types called serovars.

GENERAL CHARACTERISTICS

Leptospires are thin and spiral-shaped, range in length from 6 to 20 μ, and are 0.1 μm in width. The spirals have numerous coils and hooked ends (Fig. 25-12). The coils can be observed when a living culture is examined by dark-field microscopy. The leptospires are not readily stained by ordinary dyes but can be perceived in stained preparations by means of silver impregnation methods. Most species can be cultivated on ordinary media supplemented with animal serum fractions. The leptospira are obligate aerobes.

Fig. 25-12. Scanning electron micrograph of a leptospire. Note the compactness of the coils. (Courtesy Z. Yoshii.)

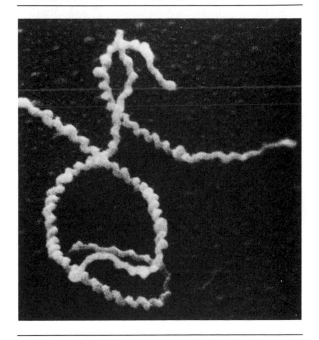

EPIDEMIOLOGY AND PATHOGENESIS

The pathogenic leptospires are harbored by wild rodents and domestic animals. It has been estimated that as many as 10 to 30 percent of the wild rat population are hosts to them. *L. icterohaemorrhagiae* is the most pathogenic serogroup, although most of the other serogroups produce some disease symptoms. In wild rodents, in which the infection is almost never fatal, the organisms localize in the kidneys and are shed in the urine. Up to 1 million leptospires per milliliter can be excreted by infected rodents. Transmission from animals to humans is usually indirect. Animal urination in soil or water, for example, is a frequent mode of transmission. Swimming or other recreational activity that brings individuals, especially teenagers, young adults, and household pets in contact with contaminated water is responsible for outbreaks of disease. In 1989 in the United States, 93 cases of human leptospirosis were reported to the CDC.

The microorganism multiplies in the blood and can infect other areas of the body such as the liver, kidney, lung, and meninges. The incubation period of 8 to 12 days is followed by chills, fever, headache, and severe muscular pain. The most serious form of leptospirosis, called *infectious jaundice*, is often characterized by jaundice and hemorrhage in the skin and subcutaneous tissue (hence the name *L. icterohaemorrhagiae*). The disease is frequently diagnosed improperly because jaundice appears in only 50 percent of infected individuals. Since there is no vaccine against the organism, prevention is achieved by avoiding contact with contaminated water.

LABORATORY DIAGNOSIS AND TREATMENT

During the first week of disease, blood and urine samples can be collected and introduced into suitable media for cultivation of leptospires. Leptospires can also be detected in the blood by dark-field microscopy. Antibodies can be detected by the microscopic agglutination test; however, the test is very laborious. The counterimmunoelectrophoresis (CIE) technique is more suited for the smaller laboratory because of its ease in operation.

If diagnosis of leptospirosis is made during the early stages of infection, penicillin, streptomycin, or tetracycline is an effective chemotherapeutic agent. Once the disease has progressed beyond the fever stage, antibiotic therapy is usually ineffective.

SPIRAL AND CURVED RODS

The motility of spiral and curved rods arises from the presence of polar flagella and not axial filaments, as in the spirochetes. Two important genera are *Spirillum* and *Campylobacter*.

GENUS SPIRILLUM

Spirillum minor is the only human pathogen in the genus and is the cause of a form of *rat-bite fever*. The organism has not been cultivated in the laboratory. Identification was originally derived from the experimental inoculation of humans with blood containing the microorganisms.

Rat-bite fever is a disease of rats that is transmissible to humans by the bite of an infected animal (for example, rats or cats). The incubation period lasts 6 to 14 days, followed by the swelling of the wound site and formation of an ulcer. There is fever and swelling of local lymph nodes. The fever is undulating and may continue for several weeks. During the fever period a maculopapular rash appears on the arms, legs, and trunk but subsides with a drop in the patient's temperature. The disease is self-limiting unless a secondary infection arises at the site of the bite, thereby requiring antibiotic therapy. Penicillin is the drug of choice when complications do arise.

Diagnosis of disease can be made by microscopic examination of blood or material from the bite. The organisms can be stained by the Giemsa or Wright technique. If this is not possible animals must be inoculated and their blood examined for the organisms.

GENUS CAMPYLOBACTER

Campylobacter are gram-negative, slender, spirally curved rods from 0.2 to 0.5 μm wide and 0.5 to 5.0 μm in length. They are motile by a single polar flagellum (Fig. 25-13). The campylobacter were recognized for years as important pathogens in animals. They are important causes of infertility and abortion in cattle, sheep, and swine but only in the past 10 years have they been shown to be important causes of disease in humans. Some species are believed to play a role in the diarrhea associated with homosexual men. We will discuss those species known to cause diarrhea in humans that is *C. jejuni* and others. In addition, we will discuss a recently discovered species, *Helicobacter pylori* (formerly *Campylobacter pylori*) that is believed to play a role in human gastritis and pyloric ulcers.

CAMPYLOBACTER JEJUNI

Four species that are causes of diarrhea in humans are *C. fetus* (subsp. *fetus*), *C. coli*, *C. laridis*, and *C. jejuni*. Over 90 percent of the campylobacter isolates in the United States are *C. jejuni* and our discussion will center on this organism.

C. jejuni is widely distributed in nature and the most common source of infection for humans is unpasteurized milk, raw or partially cooked poultry, and contaminated water (Table 25-1). The principal source of sporadic outbreaks of disease is poultry.

The dose of organisms required to cause disease depends on the vehicle (milk, water, etc.) and the susceptibility of the host. As few as 500

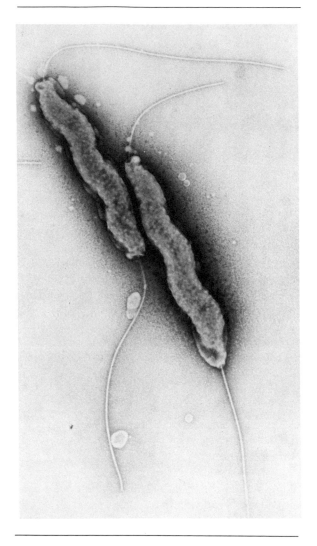

Fig. 25-13. Electron micrograph of *Campylobacter fetus* subspecies *jejuni* (×33,740 before 37 percent reduction). Note curved shape of organisms and polar flagella. (From P. J. Pead, *J. Med. Microbiol.* 12:383, 1979.)

organisms or as high as 10^6 organisms may be required to initiate disease. The mechanism of adherence to intestinal epithelium and penetration of mucus gel is not known but the flagellum may play an important role. The incubation period is 1 to 7 days and enteritis is usually observed

Table 25-1. Reported Outbreaks of *Campylobacter* Infections, by Vehicle of Transmission, United States, 1978–1986.

Vehicle	No. of outbreaks	No. of ill persons
All foodborne	45	1308
Raw milk	26	829
Poultry	3	27
Egg	1	26
Other	6	87
Unknown	9	339
All waterborne	11	4983
Community water supply	7	4930
Other	4	53
Travel-associated	1	150
Total	57	6441

Source: *CDC Surveillance Summaries*, Vol. 37. No. SS-2, June 1988.

Table 25-2. Some Tests That Aid in the Differentiation of the Four Major Species of *Campylobacter* Causing Diarrhea in Humans

Organism	Growth at 25°C	Hippurate hydrolysis	Nalidixic acid*	Cephalothin*	C-19-0 fatty acid
C. jejuni	–	+	S	R	+
C. coli	–	–	S	R	d
C. laridis	–	–	R	R	–
C. fetus subs. fetus	+	–	R	S	–

d = 11 to 89 percent of the strains are positive; S = sensitive; R = resistant.
* 30-μg disk.

as a mild diarrhea that is self-limiting, but a dysentery-like syndrome may also appear. There is evidence that *C. jejuni* produces an enterotoxin similar in activity to cholera toxin; that is, it exhibits adenylate cyclase activity (see page 231). *C. jejuni* does not appear to be very invasive since bacteremia is seldom reported. Several studies suggest that repeated exposure to *C. jejuni*, for example, in raw milk, leads to acquisition of immunity.

Plating on solid selective media is the standard technique used for isolation of *C. jejuni* from human stools. *C. jejuni* is a thermotolerant species and 42°C is the temperature of incubation. In addition, the atmosphere for incubation should be oxygen (5 percent), carbon dioxide (10 per-

cent), and nitrogen (85 percent). Disposable gas-generating systems such as polybags are sometimes used for incubating the plates. Following a 48-hour incubation period, presumptive identification of colonies can be made by three tests: dark-field microscopy (motility and morphology), oxidase reaction, and gram reaction. Identification of isolates requires several tests including growth temperatures, catalase activity, nitrate reduction, hippurate test, etc. Table 25-2 lists some of the tests that differentiate the four major species of *Campylobacter* that cause diarrhea in humans.

Whether antibiotics should be administered in disease is a matter of controversy. Erythromycin is suggested for prolonged illnesses.

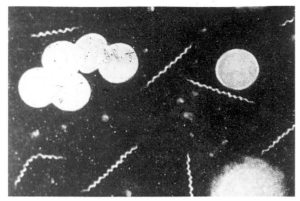

Plate 1. Dark-field microscopy of spirochetes (spiral-shaped organisms). (Courtesy Centers for Disease Control, Atlanta, Georgia.)

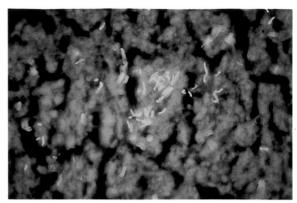

Plate 2. Yellow fluorescing *Mycobacterium tuberculosis*. (From H. M. Sommers. In E. H. Lennette [Ed.], *Manual of Clinical Microbiology* (4th ed.). Washington, D.C.: American Society for Microbiology, 1985.)

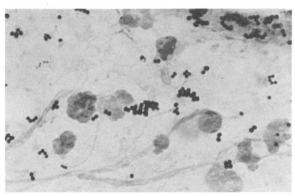

Plate 3. Gram-stain of gram-positive staphylococci (purple, clustered spherical cells). (From J. H. Stein [Ed.], *Internal Medicine* [3rd ed.]. Boston: Little, Brown, 1990.)

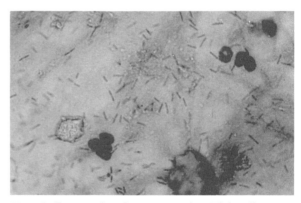

Plate 4. Gram-stain of gram-negative *Klebsiella pneumoniae*. The red-stained bacterial cells are short, thin rods in the photomicrograph. (From J. H. Stein [Ed.], *Internal Medicine* [3rd ed.]. Boston: Little, Brown, 1990.)

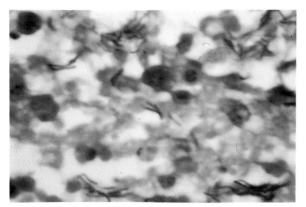

Plate 5. Ziehl-Neelsen acid-fast stain of *Mycobacteria*. (From H. M. Sommers. In E. H. Lennette [Ed.], *Manual of Clinical Microbiology* [4th ed.]. Washington, D.C.: American Society for Microbiology, 1985.)

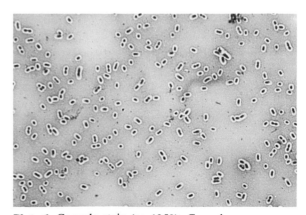

Plate 6. Capsule stain (× 1250). Capsule appears as white halo in a blue background that has been stained by a dye. Bacterial cells were counterstained with a red dye. (From R. E. Corstvet et al., *J. Clin. Microbiol.* 16:1123, 1982.)

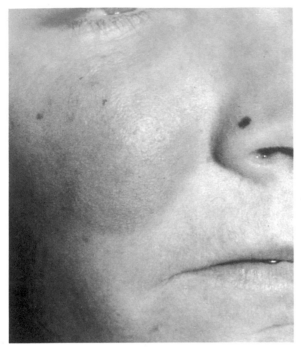

Plate 7. Erysipelas. (From J. H. Stein [Ed.], *Internal Medicine* [3rd ed.]. Boston: Little, Brown, 1990.)

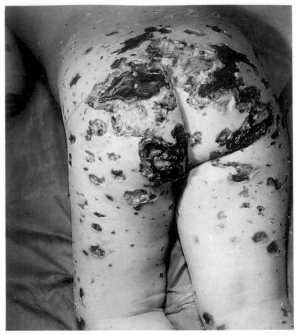

Plate 9. Massive cutaneous hemorrhage from meningococcal disease. (From H. Peltola and I. Simula, *Rev. Infect. Dis.* 5:71, 1983.)

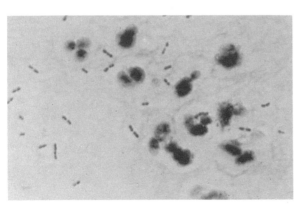

Plate 8. Gram-positive diplococci (*Streptococcus pneumoniae*) as seen in high power (× 1000). (From J. H. Stein [Ed.], *Internal Medicine* [3rd ed.]. Boston: Little, Brown, 1990.)

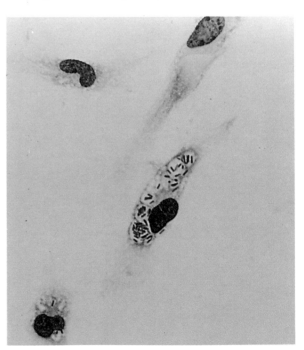

Plate 10. Peritoneal macrophage (× 2000) with intracellular *Salmonella typhimurium* bacilli. (From J. V. DeSiderio and S. Campbell, *J. Infect. Dis.* 148:563, 1983.)

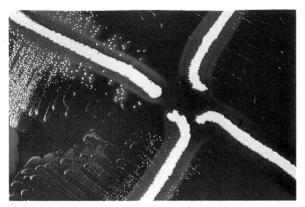

Plate 11. Satellite phenomenon. Small colonies of *Hemophilus influenzae* are observed in the vicinity of large streaks of *Staphylococcus aureus*.

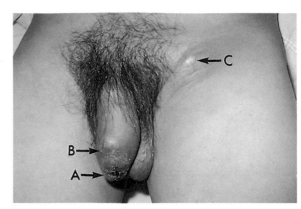

Plate 12. Chancroid. A. Ulceration of prepuce. B. Lymphadenopathy. C. Inguinal buboe about to rupture. (From G. W. Hammond, *Rev. Infect. Dis.* 2:867, 1980.)

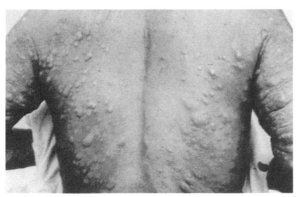

Plate 13. Lepromatous leprosy. (From J. H. Stein [Ed.], *Internal Medicine* [3rd ed.]. Boston: Little, Brown, 1990.)

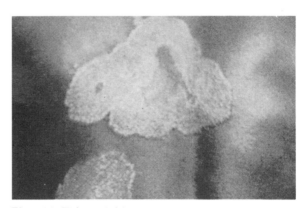

Plate 14. Tuberculoid leprosy. (From J. H. Stein [Ed.], *Internal Medicine* [3rd ed.]. Boston: Little, Brown, 1990.)

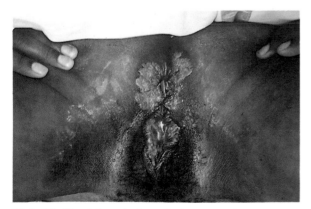

Plate 15. Condylomata lata during secondary stage of syphilis. (From P. S. Friedman, *Br. J. Vener. Dis.* 53:276, 1977.)

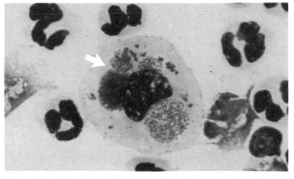

Plate 16. Giemsa stain of conjunctiva scraping showing typical cytoplasmic inclusion of *Chlamydia trachomatis*. (From J. H. Stein [Ed.], *Internal Medicine* [3rd ed.]. Boston: Little, Brown, 1990.)

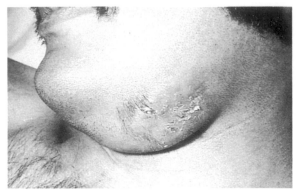

Plate 17. Actinomycosis. (From J. H. Stein [Ed.], *Internal Medicine* [3rd ed.]. Boston: Little, Brown, 1990.)

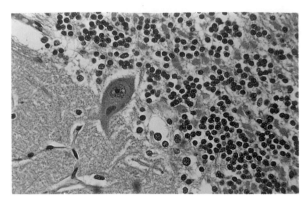

Plate 18. Negri body in human rabies. In the center is a well-defined cell with nucleus and Negri body. (Courtesy F. A. Murphy.)

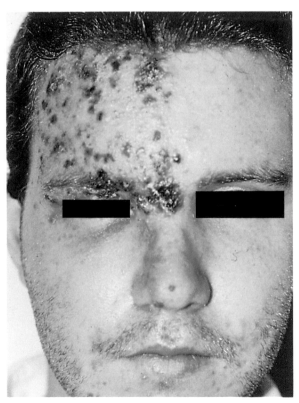

Plate 19. Herpes zoster of the face. (Courtesy H. E. Kaufman, M.D.)

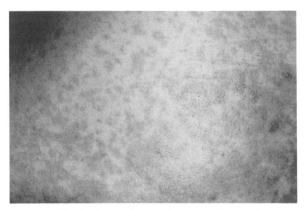

Plate 20. Typical maculopapular rash of measles. (From J. H. Stein [Ed.], *Internal Medicine* [3rd ed.]. Boston: Little, Brown, 1990.)

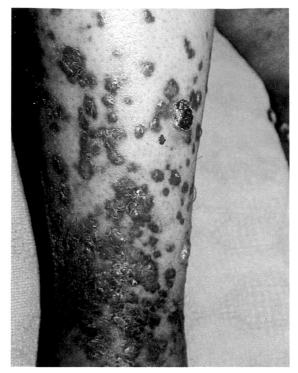

Plate 21. Kaposi's sarcoma. (From J. H. Stein [Ed.], *Internal Medicine* [3rd ed.]. Boston: Little, Brown, 1990.)

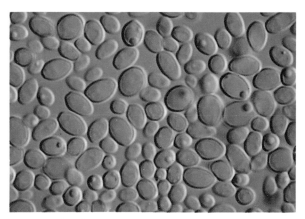

Plate 22. Oval yeast cells as seen by Nomarsky interference microscopy (× 1000). (From M. Ogawa et al., *Appl. Environ. Microbiol.* 46:912, 1983.)

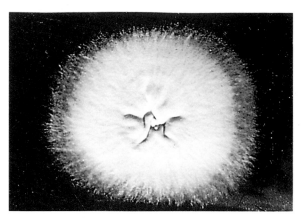

Plate 23. Typical "mold" colony showing cottony appearance.

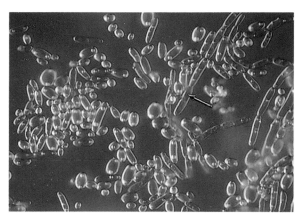

Plate 24. Pseudohyphae (arrow) formation in *Candida* as seen by Nomarsky interference microscopy (× 400). (From M. Ogawa et al., *Appl. Environ. Microbiol.* 46:912, 1983.)

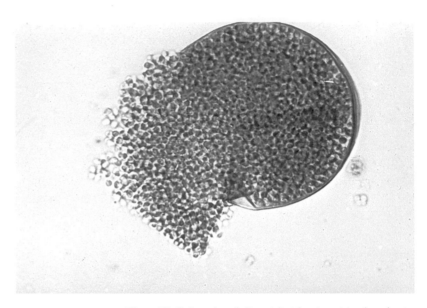

Plate 25. Spherule of *Coccidioides immitis* showing endospores. (From S. M. Finegold and E. J. Baron. In *Bailey and Scott's Diagnostic Microbiology* [7th ed.]. St. Louis: C. V. Mosby, 1987.)

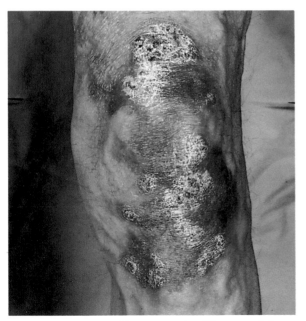

Plate 26. Cutaneous blastomycosis. (Courtesy John Utz, M.D.)

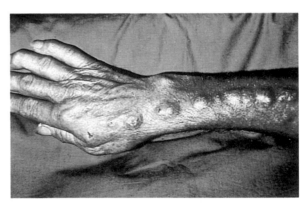

Plate 27. Sporotrichosis. (From J. H. Stein [Ed.], *Internal Medicine* [3rd ed.]. Boston: Little, Brown, 1990.)

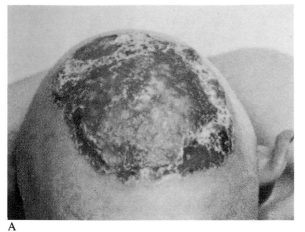

A

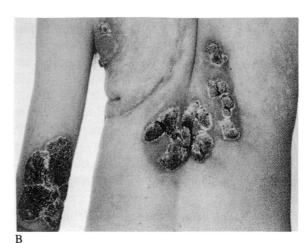

B

Plate 28. Chronic mucocutaneous candidiasis involving head (A) and back (B). (From P. Phillips et al., *Rev. Infect. Dis.* 9[Suppl. I]:87, 1987.)

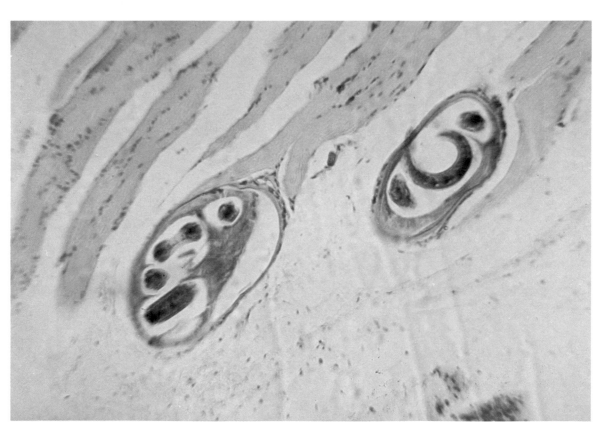

Plate 29. *Trichinella* larvae encysted in muscle. (From S. M. Finegold and E. J. Baron. In *Bailey and Scott's Diagnostic Microbiology* [7th ed.]. St. Louis: C. V. Mosby, 1987.)

HELICOBACTER PYLORI (FORMERLY CAMPYLOBACTER PYLORI)

H. pylori was first isolated from human gastric mucosa in 1983. Gastritis had been believed to be a normal condition that accompanied aging, but it is now believed that this condition may also have a bacterial etiology. In addition, as many as 70 percent of the patients with stomach ulcers and as many as 90 percent of those with duodenal ulcers have large concentrations of spiral bacteria in biopsied tissue, but not in healthy tissue. *H. pylori* colonizes only gastric-type epithelium, and surface pili are believed to be the adhesions associated with this process (Fig. 25-14). At high levels the microorganism produces the enzyme, urease, which is also believed to be associated with pathogenicity. Ammonia, which is one of the

Fig. 25-14. Scanning electron micrograph (×3441) of *Helicobacter pylori* adhering to gastric cells. (From V. Neman-Simha and F. Mégraud, *Infect. Immun.* 56[12]:3329, 1988.)

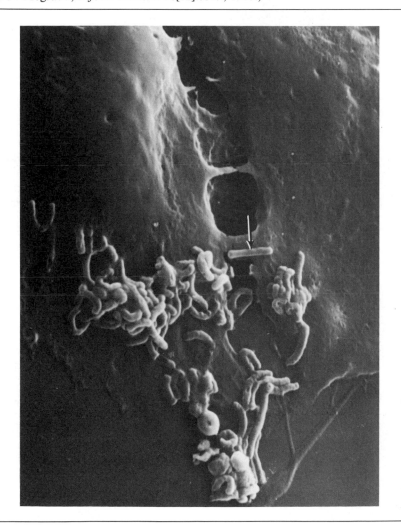

Table 25-3. Characteristics of the Diseases Caused by Spirochetes and Spiral and Curved Rods

Group and species	Disease	Mechanism of transmission	Treatment and prevention
Spirochetes			
Treponema pallidum	*Syphilis:* Primary stage: chancre. Secondary stage: rash and mucous membrane lesions. Tertiary stage: lesions called gummas. Congenital: stillbirth, abortion, or secondary syphilis	Sexual contact, accidental contact with lesions Congenital transfer	Penicillin, tetracycline or erythromycin. Treatment of contacts to prevent spread
T. pertenue	*Yaws:* Primary and secondary skin lesions	Contact with eating and drinking utensils	Penicillin. Improve hygiene
T. carateum	*Pinta:* Skin lesions, hyperpigmented	Same as for *T. pertenue*	Penicillin. Improve hygiene
Borrelia recurrentis *B. hermsii* *B. turicatae* *B. parkeri*	*Relapsing fever:* Bloodstream infected—followed by invasion of kidney, liver, eye, brain. Episodes of fever caused by antigenic variation of borrelia	Louse-borne relapsing fever (*B. recurrentis*); tick-borne relapsing fever caused by remaining borrelia	Tetracyclines, chloramphenicol. Avoid tick-infested areas
B. burgdorferi	*Lyme disease:* Skin lesions in first stage. Second and third stages: arthritis; neurologic and cardiac symptoms	Ixodid ticks	Oral phenoxymethyl penicillin or tetracycline for first stage. Penicillin G, chloramphenicol, or ceftriaxone for second stage
Leptospira interrogans, serogroup *icterohaemorrhagiae*	*Infectious jaundice:* Bloodstream invaded—followed by liver, kidney, lung, and meninges	Ingestion of water contaminated by urinating animals	Penicillin, streptomycin, tetracycline
Spiral and curved rods			
Spirillum minor	*Rat-bite fever:* Formation of ulcer at site of bite plus body rash	Bite of infected animal such as cat	Self-limiting; but penicillin treatment if complications occur
Campylobacter jejuni	*Diarrhea* (or dysentery-like syndrome)	Ingestion of contaminated food or water, unpasteurized milk	Self-limiting; but erythromycin used in prolonged illnesses
Helicobacter pylori	*Possible gastritis and stomach or duodenal ulcers*	Unknown	Bismuth subsalicylate with amoxicillin or tinidazole

products of urease activity, probably protects the bacteria from stomach acids. Scientists are still seeking to fulfill Koch's postulates by reproducing the disease in an animal model system. One study in germ-free piglets has shown that many of the features of gastritis in humans can be reproduced by infecting animals with *H. pylori*.

H. pylori may be diagnosed by culture of gastric biopsy specimens, examination of stained biopsies for presence of bacteria, or detection of urease activity in the biopsies. Cultured *H. pylori* can be readily identified on the basis of characteristic colonial and microscopic morphology, positive oxidase and catalase tests, and rapid hydrolysis of urea. Noninvasive methods include serologic techniques and detection of serum antibodies.

Evaluation of treatment regimens indicates that bismuth subsalicylate (Pepto-Bismol) combined with amoxicillin or tinidazole affect a long-time cure.

SUMMARY

1. Spirochetes and curved rods, although exhibiting spiral morphology, differ in certain aspects of motility. Specifically, spirochetes possess flagella that originate at the poles and wrap around the body of the microorganism. The flagella of spirochetes do not come into contact with the environment. Curved rods have polar flagella, either single or multiple, that are in contact with the environment.

2. The characteristics of the diseases caused by spirochetes and curved rods are outlined in Table 25-3.

QUESTIONS FOR STUDY

Select the best response or responses for each of the following:

1. All of the following are characteristic of secondary syphilis *except*
   A. Papular rash
   B. Condylomata lata
   C. Mucous patches
   D. Gummas of the bone, skin, etc.

2. Dark-field examination of which of the following host specimens would probably not reveal treponemes?
   A. Primary chancre
   B. Mucous patch
   C. Blood from a patient with tertiary syphilis
   D. Skin lesion from a patient with tertiary syphilis

3. A patient with syphilis was treated with penicillin. A few days later he developed fever, an intense papular rash, and joint pain. The reason for these symptoms is that

A. The infectious agent was resistant to penicillin and the course of the illness was not diminished.
   B. Penicillin can produce a generalized reaction called Jarisch-Herxheimer.
   C. Penicillin is relatively toxic when used in the treatment of any disease.
   D. Penicillin is known to concentrate in joints.

4. Which of the following would best detect congenital syphilis?
   A. Dark-field examination of the blood
   B. FTA-ABS using immunoglobulin IgG
   C. VDRL
   D. FTA-ABS using immunoglobulin IgM

5. During a summer outing you observed the presence of several cattle upstream from where you and your friends were swimming.

About 8 days later three of your friends develop chills, fever, and headache. Which of the following microbial agents would you suspect as responsible for these infections?
A. *Campylobacter fetus*
B. *Mycobacterium bovis*
C. *Leptospira icterohaemorrhagiae*
D. *Borrelia recurrentis*

6. A patient complains of constant headache, persistent fatigue, stiff neck, and considerable joint pain, particularly in the knee. In addition, there are unusual lesions on the skin. The physician discovers the patient recently spent two months in Connecticut, Maine, and New Jersey, where he was collecting various mosses from wooded areas. The patient indicated he had been bitten by ticks. The physician would suspect which of the following infectious agents?

A. *Borrelia recurrentis*
B. *Helicobacter pylori*
C. *Borrelia burgdorferi*
D. *Lepstospira interrogans*

Fill in the blank:

7. Erythema chronicum migrans refers to a skin lesion associated with _____ disease.

8. Some forms of gastric ulcer are now believed to be caused by a member of the genus ___ .

9. *Campylobacter jejuni* is an animal pathogen that is now regarded as a frequent cause of _____ in humans.

10. Relapsing fever is a disease caused by a spirochete belonging to the genus _____ .

ADDITIONAL READINGS

Barbour, A. G. Laboratory aspects of Lyme borreliosis. *Clin. Microbiol. Rev.* 1(4):399,1988.

Barbour, A. G., and Hayes, S. F. Biology of *Borrelia* species. *Microbiol. Rev.* 50:381,1986.

Buck, G.E. *Campylobacter pylori* and gastroduodenal disease. *Clin. Microbiol. Rev.* 3(1):1,1990.

CDC. *Campylobacter* isolates in the United States, 1982–1986. *CDC Surveillance Summaries*. Vol. 37/No. SS-2, June 1988.

CDC. Guidelines for the prevention and control of congenital syphilis. *M.M.W.R.* 37(Suppl. S-1),1988.

CDC. Syphilis and congenital syphilis—United States, 1985–1988. *M.M.W.R.* 37(32):486,1988.

Engelstein, L. Syphilis, historical and actual: Cultural geography of a disease. *Rev. Infect. Dis.* 8 (6):1036,1986.

Marshall, B. *Campylobacter pyloridis* and gastritis. *J. Infect. Dis.* 153(4):650,1986.

Penner, J. L. The genus *Campylobacter*: A decade of progress. *Clin. Microbiol. Rev.* 1(2):157,1988.

Tramont, E. C. Syphilis in the AIDS era. *N. Engl. J. Med.* 316:1600,1987.

Walker, R. I. Pathophysiology of *Campylobacter* enteritis. *Microbiol. Rev.* 50(1):81,1986.

26. MYCOPLASMAS AND L-FORMS

OBJECTIVES

To describe the differences between mycoplasmas and L-forms

To outline the mechanism of transmission, symptoms, and treatment for *Mycoplasma pneumoniae* infection

To describe the relationship between genital mycoplasmas and the diseases they may cause in males and females

The mycoplasmas are a unique group of bacteria in that they lack a cell wall and yet are free-living. They can be found in animals, humans, soil, and plants. They are so small (0.2 to 0.3 μm) that until the late 1930s many investigators referred to them as small bacteria or even viruses because of their ability to pass through bacterial filters. The mycoplasmas belong to three families: Mycoplasmataceae, Acholeplasmataceae, and Spiroplasmataceae. Only the Mycoplasmataceae contain important human pathogens. The Spiroplasmataceae are plant pathogens. The major mycoplasmas causing disease in humans are: *M. pneumoniae* (atypical pneumonia), *M. hominis* (upper urinary tract disease), and *Ureaplasma urealyticum* (nongonococcal urethritis).

At about the same time that the mycoplasmas were first being described, it was observed that colonies of *Streptobacillus moniliformis** resembled, in appearance and structure, the colonies of *Mycoplasma*. The cells in the *S. moniliformis* colonies lacked cell walls and could not be stained by the usual methods. These cells, now called *L- (Lister) forms*, are variants of the cell wall-containing parent cell. They differ from mycoplasmas in that they are capable of reverting back to the typical parental form. L-forms have now been found in most species of bacteria.

---

* *S. moniliformis* is one of the etiological agents of rat-bite fever. Infections are usually acquired after the bite of a rat, mouse, or cat (see page 607).

GENERAL CHARACTERISTICS OF THE MYCOPLASMAS

Mycoplasmas can assume a variety of morphological forms, such as coccoid, filamentous, or cocci in chains, because they lack a cell wall determinant. The small coccoid units vary in diameter from 0.2 to 0.3 μm in diameter. Some of the different morphological forms are illustrated in Figure 26-1. Although lacking a cell wall, the

Fig. 26-1. Electron micrograph of a species of *Mycoplasma* showing different morphological forms. (Courtesy E. S. Boatman.)

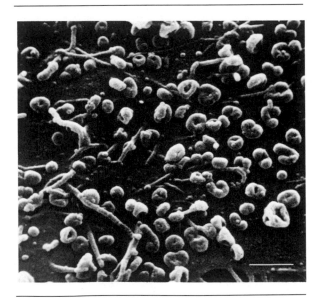

mycoplasmas are stable in ordinary culture media, apparently because of the presence of sterols in the cytoplasmic membrane. These sterols are not found in any other bacterial cells or their L-forms.

Most *Mycoplasma* species are aerobes or facultative anaerobes, although a few species require anaerobic conditions for initial isolation in the laboratory. For laboratory cultivation the mycoplasmas need a basal medium of meat infusion and peptone supplemented with horse serum or ascitic fluid. The serum or ascitic fluid supplies the fatty acids or lipid precursors required by many species. The medium is usually supplemented with penicillin and thallium acetate to inhibit the growth of any bacterial contaminants. Most mycoplasmas exhibit optimal growth at temperatures between 30° and 36°C in media at alkaline pH's. *Ureaplasma* exhibits optimal growth at acid pH's and is capable of hydrolyzing urea, a property useful in distinguishing it from other mycoplasmas.

Cells from broth culture are best visualized by dark-field or phase-contrast microscopy. Mycoplasmas are best recognized by their colony formation on semi-solid media. Colonies that are 10 to 300 μm in diameter give the appearance of "fried eggs" and are visible only with the aid of a microscope (Fig. 26-2).

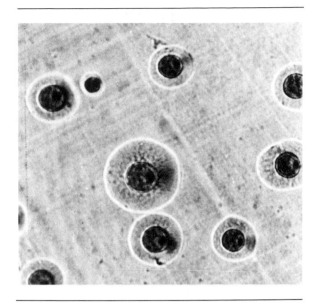

Fig. 26-2. Colony of *Mycoplasma salivarium* showing typical umbonate (button-like) or fried egg shape. Colonies are 0.1 mm in diameter. (From P. F. Smith, *The Biology of the Mycoplasmas.* New York: Academic Press, 1971.)

GENERAL CHARACTERISTICS OF L-FORMS

The L-form is a wall-deficient bacterial variant that may occur spontaneously in a bacterial culture or may be induced by certain agents. Two of the agents used to induce microbial transformation are penicillin and ultraviolet light.

In a population of L-forms some are stable (that is, they fail to revert to the parental type), while others are unstable (they revert to the parental type). In a few instances it has been shown that by proper adaptation a stable L-form may be maintained on isotonic media. Most stable L-forms, however, require high concentrations of an osmotic stabilizer. The fact that L-forms are without walls does not mean they are unable to produce cell wall products. L-forms of various gram-positive and gram-negative bacteria can produce wall biosynthetic intermediates. For example, lipoteichoic acid, which binds cell wall to the cell membrane, is formed by an L-form of *Streptococcus pyogenes*. The endotoxin of such gram-negative species as *Proteus* and *Salmonella* is produced, albeit in reduced quantities, by L-forms of these genera. The inability of the L-forms to form complete cell walls may be due to some conformational change in surface geometry or to a lack of appropriate enzymes. The L-forms are similar to the mycoplasmas but differ in the following ways:

1. L-forms can be cultivated only in a culture medium that has a high concentration of non-metabolizable solute (NaCl, for example). These solutes contribute to the high osmotic pressure required to prevent lysis of L-forms. Mycoplasmas do not require these osmotic forces.
2. L-forms can revert to the stable bacterial parental type. Mycoplasmas do not revert to any other bacterial form.
3. L-forms do not have a high lipid content or sterols in the membrane as do the mycoplasmas.
4. Reproduction of L-forms is inhibited in the presence of penicillin. Penicillin has no effect on the mycoplasmas.
5. The guanine-cytosine content of L-forms is the same as that of the bacterial species they were derived from. Most mycoplasmas have a much lower guanine-cytosine content than do other bacterial species.

PATHOGENESIS

MYCOPLASMA PNEUMONIAE

M. pneumoniae is a noncommensal that produces a human disease called *atypical pneumonia*. This organism infects the upper and lower respiratory tract and usually produces epidemic disease in confined populations such as in military barracks and institutions. The organism is usually transmitted by coughing or sneezing.

Atypical pneumonia (walking pneumonia) is slow to develop, and the incubation period for the disease may be up to 3 weeks. The disease is usually mild and self-limiting with infrequent complications. Symptoms include fever, headache, and a persistent nonproductive cough.

The mechanisms of virulence of *M. pneumoniae* have received considerable attention in the past 15 years, but no absolutely conclusive results have been obtained. Experimental studies

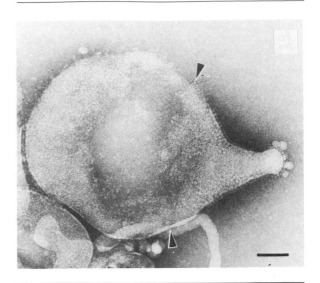

Fig. 26-3. Electron micrograph of *Mycoplasma genitalium*. The terminal structure is the organelle of attachment and is covered with a nap that extends to the areas indicated by arrows. The nap is apparently the protein called P1 that initiates attachment to respiratory epithelium. (From P. C. Hu et al., *Infect. Immun.* 55:1126, 1987.) Bar = 0.1 μm.

with tracheal tissue in organ culture have revealed some interesting details of the pathogenic mechanisms. Mycoplasmas are believed to attach to the ciliated cells of the trachea by means of the microorganisms' *attachment organelle*, which gives the organism the appearance of a flask. The attachment organelle is coated with a protein called P1 that mediates initial binding to respiratory epithelium (Fig. 26-3). The terminal tip structure or attachment organelle is also observed in another pathogenic mycoplasma, *M. genitalium*. The chemical nature of the binding site on the microbial surface has not been determined but is probably a protein. Once mycoplasmas are adsorbed to the cilia, epithelial cell injury, vacuolization, nuclear swelling, and loss of cilia ensue. The mechanism by which epithelial cells are injured is not known.

The level of immunity acquired after infection by *M. pneumoniae* is related to the intensity of the disease. Immunity lasts longer after pneumonia than after less severe infections. Even so, immunity after pneumonia is short-lived and lasts no more than 7 to 8 years. There is a decreasing attack rate after the age of 10, which represents an acquired immunity from early childhood disease. Immunity is probably built up after the age of 10 by repeated subclinical disease.

OTHER MYCOPLASMAS AND L-FORMS

Ureaplasma urealyticum and *M. hominis* are mycoplasmas that may colonize both the male and female genital tracts. Studies have revealed that as many as 60 percent of healthy women carry *U. urealyticum* in the genital tract and 20 percent carry *M. hominis* in the vagina. Both organisms are opportunistic pathogens and can be transmitted by sexual contact. Colonization occurs initially during birth as the infant passes through the birth canal. The rate of isolation of these organisms appears to decline after birth but increases in both sexes after puberty and increased sexual activity. There is an apparent decline in genital mycoplasmas after menopause. The importance of these organisms in disease has been difficult to establish. Both *U. urealyticum* and *M. hominis* are linked to pelvic inflammatory disease (PID)* but their exact roles are not known. Recently a newly isolated species, *M. genitalium*, has been implicated in acute PID. *M. genitalium*, when injected intraurethrally, induces urethritis in male chimpanzees. These *Mycoplasma* species may also contribute to infertility following salpingitis (inflammation of the fallopian tubes). In men *U. urealyticum* may play a role in nonspecific urethritis, but it is not so important as the chlamydiae (see Chapter 27). *M. hominis* does not appear to play any role in male urethritis but ureaplasmas may play a role in chronic prostatitis. *U. urealyticum* and *M. hominis* have recently been linked to perinatal disorders. Women

* Pelvic inflammatory disease is caused primarily by chlamydiae, discussed in Chapter 27.

carrying genital mycoplasma deliver smaller infants than women who do not carry these microorganisms. The presence of genital mycoplasma in blood sampled shortly after delivery is significantly associated with stillbirth and prematurity. An association has also been demonstrated between the carriage of ureaplasmas and the presence of chorioamnionitis. *M. hominis* can also be involved in nongenitourinary infections such as bacteremia, wound infections, and joint infections. The source of *M. hominis* for these infections is the genitourinary tract.

One researcher has isolated *Mycoplasma* from AIDS patients with Kaposi's sarcoma. It is speculated that *Mycoplasma* and the virus-causing AIDS (human immunodeficiency virus [HIV]) may actually act in concert to lyse infected cells. The isolated *Mycoplasma* can also cause death on their own when injected into silverleaf monkeys. These studies are undergoing close scrutiny by the scientific community to determine if this speculation is correct. There is only one recorded instance in which an L-form was considered the causal agent of disease. Most information on the pathogenicity of L-forms is circumstantial. It has been suggested that the L-form is a survival mechanism for the bacterial cell. For example, under adverse environmental conditions such as the presence of an antibiotic that inhibits cell wall synthesis, the cell could maintain its viability by remaining as an L-form until environmental conditions improved. In the L-form state some pathogenic mechanisms could still be in operation. Studies have shown that L-form gram-negative species produce endotoxin; L-forms of *S. pyogenes* produce a lipoteichoic acid that mimics the destructive effect of intact microorganism on heart, kidney, and liver tissue; L-forms of *Hemophilus parainfluenzae* cause a pneumonia in pigs that is indistinguishable from that produced by natural infection with *H. parainfluenzae*.

LABORATORY DIAGNOSIS

Isolation of mycoplasmas from clinical material is accomplished by swabbing infected areas and inoculating onto a selective agar medium containing penicillin and thallium acetate to inhibit bacterial growth. Thallium acetate should not be used if *M. genitalium* or *U. urealyticum* is to be isolated. In one week microscopical examination of the colonies can be made by inverting the culture dish and looking for the characteristic fried egg appearance. Identification of specific *Mycoplasma* species may require the following techniques:

1. *M. pneumoniae* is presumptively identified by its typical growth on agar, its ability to ferment glucose (*U. urealyticum* and *M. hominis* do not ferment glucose), and hemolysis testing. The hemolysis test is carried out by flooding guinea pig erythrocytes over suspected *M. pneumoniae* colonies. After overnight incubation at 37°C a zone of hemolysis will be seen around

M. pneumoniae colonies. Absolute identification is by the *growth inhibition test* on solid media. Paper disks are impregnated with specific antiserum and are placed on the agar after the agar has been streaked with the test organism. Zones of inhibition can be identified and measured after 4 to 7 days' incubation.

2. *U. urealyticum* can be differentiated from all other mycoplasmas because of its ability to hydrolyze urea. *U. urealyticum* colonies turn brown when reagent containing urease is added, while *M. hominis* colonies are unaffected by the reagent.

Culturing as a means of identification of mycoplasmas is time-consuming; it may take 2–3 weeks. Serological tests such as the complement fixation test are recommended for rapid presumptive diagnosis of infection by *M. pneumon-*

Table 26-1. Pathogenic Characteristics of the Mycoplasmas

Species	Site of infection and pathogenesis	Mechanism of transmission	Treatment and prevention
Mycoplasma pneumoniae	Respiratory tract; self-limiting pneumonia with infrequent complications	Sneezing, coughing in confined areas	Erythromycin, tetracycline; vaccine under investigation
M. hominis	Urogenital tract; several possibilities: pelvic inflammatory disease, infertility following salpingitis, perinatal disorders, stillbirth, prematurity, chorioamnionitis	Opportunistic but may be transmitted sexually or congenitally	Erythromycin, tetracycline
M. genitalium	Urogenital tract; possibly associated with acute pelvic inflammatory disease	Opportunistic pathogen; may be transmitted sexually	Erythromycin, tetracycline
Ureaplasma urealyticum	Urogenital tract; several possibilities: pelvic inflammatory disease, infertility following salpingitis, nonspecific urethritis in men, chronic prostatitis, perinatal disorders as with *M. hominis* infection	Opportunistic pathogen	Erythromycin, tetracycline

iae but these tests are laborious and not very sensitive. Most serological tests so far have not proved reliable because of variability and nonspecificity. In addition, it appears that *M. pneumoniae* shares antigenic determinants with *M. genitalium*. Rapid diagnosis may require the development of DNA probes specific for the organism in question.

The isolation and identification of L-forms has never been part of the usual regimen in the clinical laboratory and is more suited to the research laboratory. If L-forms are found to be responsible for certain infections, the clinical laboratory may require, in addition to the usual media for isolation of the natural agent, special hypertonic media. Some studies have shown that when both types of media are used a greater percentage of positive cultures is obtained. Thus some so-called negative specimens may actually be positive because of the presence of L-forms. The implications could be important if the individual is a carrier of a very contagious agent such as *Neisseria gonorrhoeae*.

TREATMENT AND PREVENTION

Erythromycin as well as several tetracyclines are effective in the treatment of mycoplasmal pneumonia. Erythromycin is preferred in the treatment of children because of the risk of staining immature teeth when tetracyclines are used over prolonged periods of time.

Formalin-killed vaccines of *M. pneumoniae* have been used with some success in the military. Live vaccines are currently being evaluated.

Nongonococcal urethritis caused by *Ureaplasma urealyticum* or *M. hominis* infection responds to treatment with tetracycline. Patients allergic to tetracyclines may take erythromycin. Female sexual partners of men with nongonococcal urethritis should also be treated with tetracycline.

SUMMARY

1. Bacteria without cell walls belong to two groups: the mycoplasmas, a group containing several species of bacteria, and L-forms, which are variants of any cell wall–containing species.

2. Mycoplasmas are aerobic to facultative anaerobes that are pleomorphic and about the size of large viruses. Unlike wall-containing bacteria, mycoplasmas have sterols in their cytoplasmic membranes that provide cellular stability. L-forms, unlike mycoplasmas, can revert to the parental wall-containing types and can be isolated only on media that have a high osmotic pressure.

3. The pathogenic characteristics of mycoplasmas are outlined in Table 26-1.

QUESTIONS FOR STUDY

Select the best response or responses for each of the following:

1. Mycoplasmas are able to survive despite their lack of a cell wall because
   A. They are found only as commensals in humans.
   B. Their cell membrane is enforced with sterols.
   C. They are so small that the environment has no effect on them.
   D. They are obligate intracellular parasites.

2. The following are characteristics of L-forms *except*
   A. They can be cultivated on ordinary lab-

oratory media as long as the media contain a fermentable sugar.
B. They can revert back to the parental form by producing cell wall.
C. Reproduction of L-forms is inhibited by penicillin.
D. They can be obtained from nearly all bacterial species.

3. Which of the following statements is not characteristic of *Ureaplasma urealyticum*?
A. Its ability to hydrolyze urea is an important differentiating test.

B. As many as 60 percent of healthy women carry it in the respiratory tract.
C. It may be associated with chronic prostatitis in men and pelvic inflammatory disease in women.
D. It is found in the genitourinary tract.

4. Which of the following would never be considered in the treatment of atypical pneumonia caused by *Mycoplasma pneumoniae*?
A. Bacitracin
B. Erythromycin
C. Cephalosporins
D. Tetracyclines

Fill in the blank:

5. Inflammation of the fallopian tubes is called _____ .

6. Mycoplasmas produce distinctive colonies on agar that resemble _____ .

7. The *Mycoplasma* species that may be associated with sexually transmitted disease is *M.* _____ or *M.* _____ .

ADDITIONAL READINGS

Cassell, G. H., and Cole, B. C. Mycoplasmas as agents of disease. *N. Engl. J. Med.* 304:80,1981.
Hu, P. C., et al. *Mycoplasma pneumoniae* infection: Role of a surface protein in the attachment organelle. *Science* 216:313,1982.

Lin, J. L. Human mycoplasmal infections: Serologic observations. *Rev. Infect. Dis.* 7(2):216,1985.
Madoff, S., and Hooper, D. C. Nongenitourinary infections caused by *Mycoplasma hominis* in adults. *Rev. Infect. Dis.* 10(3):602,1988.

27. RICKETTSIAE AND CHLAMYDIAE

OBJECTIVES

To outline the differences and similarities between the rickettsiae and chlamydiae

To list the causative agent, method of transmission, pathogenesis, symptoms, and treatment for Rocky Mountain spotted fever, epidemic typhus, Q fever, trench fever, and ehrlichiosis

To describe the types of disease and groups affected by infection with *Chlamydia trachomatis* and by *C. psittaci*

To list the methods of treatment and prevention for chlamydial disease

The rickettsiae and chlamydiae are both intracellular parasites (*Rochalimaea quintana* is the only species that can be cultivated on ordinary laboratory media) that are found in invertebrates and vertebrate hosts, including humans. Although originally believed to be viruses because of their size and difficulty in cultivation, they are now recognized as bacteria. There are many similarities between the rickettsiae and chlamydiae. The chlamydiae, however, are easily distinguished from the rickettsiae because of their unique cell cycle. In addition, none of the chlamydiae is transmitted by an insect vector.

THE RICKETTSIAE

GENERAL CHARACTERISTICS

The rickettsial family of obligate intracellular parasites includes three genera: *Rickettsia*, *Coxiella*, and *Ehrlichia*. *Rochalimaea* also belongs to the rickettsial family but it is not an intracellular parasite and lives extracellularly. The typical rickettsial species is approximately 0.3 to 0.7 μm in diameter and 2.0 μm in length. Rickettsial species are pleomorphic but usually appear as rods. They possess a cell wall that is structurally and biochemically similar to the gram-negative cell wall (Fig. 27-1).

Rickettsial species, except for *Coxiella*, possess no glycolytic activity and their major metabolic pathway is the Krebs cycle. The biosynthetic potential of these intracellular parasites is limited primarily to synthesis of those molecules that cannot be obtained from the host cytoplasm. Species of *Rickettsia* use the high-energy phosphates of the cell but if necessary they can generate their own ATP by oxidative phosphorylation. Rickettsiae can be cultivated in the yolk sac of embryonated eggs, in laboratory animals, in certain arthropods, and in some tissue cultures.

Members of the rickettsial family are very similar in many ways but there are some major differences. One of these differences relates to their intracellular environment and how they cope with it. When these bacteria are taken up by host cells they enter the cytoplasm as part of a vacuole (phagosome) that displays different host–parasite

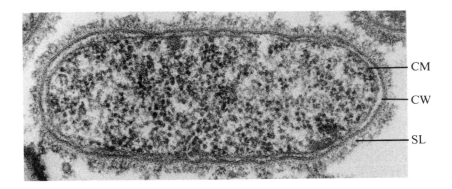

Fig. 27-1. Electron micrograph (×69,500) of *Rickettsia rickettsii*. The cell wall is typical of gram-negative bacteria. CM = cytoplasmic membrane; CW = cell wall; SL = slime layer. (From D. J. Silverman and C. L. Wisseman, Jr., *Infect. Immun.* 21:1020, 1978.)

relationships depending on the microbial species (Fig. 27-2). When phagosome-containing *Coxiella* enter the cytoplasm the phagosome fuses with the lysosome to form a phagolysosome. *Coxiella*, unlike other bacteria, are naturally resistant to the acid hydrolases of the phagolysosome. In fact, the acidification that occurs in the phagolysosome stimulates replication of *Coxiella*. The genus *Rickettsia* escapes from the phagosome before it fuses with the lysosome by producing a phospholipase that breaks down cytoplasmic membrane lipids. The genus *Rickettsia*, therefore, lives directly in the cytoplasm of the host cell. *Ehrlichia* apparently replicates within the phagosome and somehow prevents fusion with the lysosome. *Rickettsia* species differ from *Coxiella* in other respects, such as:

1. *Coxiella* metabolism is activated by acid pH while other rickettsiae are inactivated by acid pH.
2. *Coxiella* is resistant to dessication and can survive in water and milk for up to three years. *Coxiella* is also resistant to disinfectants at concentrations that would kill most other bacteria, including other rickettsiae. *Rickettsia* species are very sensitive to environmental conditions.

3. *Coxiella* possess a special developmental cycle that is not present in other rickettsiae.

EPIDEMIOLOGY AND PATHOGENESIS

With the exception of *Coxiella burnetii*, the rickettsiae are transmitted to humans exclusively by insect vectors: ticks, mites, lice, and fleas. The rickettsiae multiply in the salivary glands of ticks and mice and can be transmitted to the host by biting, but in fleas and lice the rickettsiae multiply in the gut and are excreted in the feces. Transfer of rickettsiae from fleas and lice to a human host occurs by crushing of the arthropod or by arthropod defecation at the site of the bite.

In general, the pathological features of all rickettsial diseases except Q fever differ only in the severity of the clinical symptoms. Once the rickettsiae have penetrated the skin, they quickly reach the bloodstream. In the vascular system they have an affinity for the endothelial cells of small blood vessels. The rickettsiae replicate in the infected endothelial cells and become detached from the blood vessels. In the bloodstream infected endothelial cells can bring about vascular obstruction that eventually leads to tis-

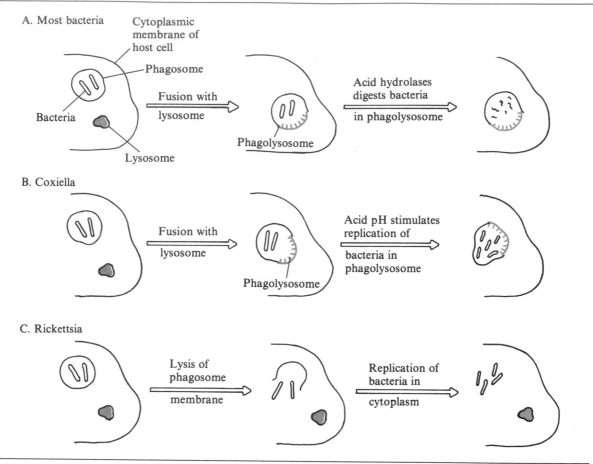

Fig. 27-2. Host-parasite response to phagocytosis by most bacteria (A), by *Coxiella* (B), and by *Rickettsia* (C). See text for details.

sue necrosis. Many of the symptoms of rickettsial infection—rash, myocarditis, and neurological changes—are due to rickettsiae in the vascular tissue of such organs as the skin, heart, and brain, respectively. At the site of the arthropod bite, an encrusted ulcer (*eschar*) may appear. Later during the disease, the ulcer develops a black necrotic center. The eschar is not found in all rickettsial diseases, but when it is it provides a diagnostic clue.

The rickettsial diseases of humans can be classified into five major groups: the *typhus group*, the *spotted fever group*, *scrub typhus*, *Q fever*,

and *trench fever* (Table 27-1). *Ehrlichiosis* is a rare rickettsial disease of humans that will be discussed separately.

Typhus Group

Epidemic or Louse-borne Typhus. Louse-borne typhus is caused by *Rickettsia prowazekii* and is transferred to humans by the body louse. The organisms are passed in the louse feces during biting and enter the wound around the bite. Before the discovery and use of DDT and other insecticides, severe epidemics of louse-borne ty-

Table 27-1. Human Rickettsial Diseases

Group	Causative agent	Common name	Mode of transmission	Reservoir of Rickettsiae	Geographic distribution
Typhus	*Rickettsia prowazekii*	Epidemic typhus*	Louse feces rubbed in skin	Humans, flying squirrels	Worldwide
	R. typhi (R. mooseri)	Murine typhus	Flea feces rubbed in skin	Rodents	Worldwide
Spotted fever	*R. rickettsii*	Rocky Mountain spotted fever	Ixodid tick bite	Rodents	Western hemisphere
	R. sibirica	Siberian tick typhus	Ixodid tick bite	Rodents	Central Asia, Siberia, Mongolia, Central Europe
	R. conorii	Boutonneuse fever	Ixodid tick bite	Rodents, dogs	Mediterranean, Black Sea, Middle East, India, Africa
	R. australis	Queensland tick typhus	Tick bite	Marsupials, mice	Australia
	R. akari	Rickettsialpox	Mite bite	House mice	North America, USSR, South Africa, Korea
Scrub typhus	*R. tsutsugamushi*	Scrub typhus	Mite bite	Rodents	Asia, Australia, Pacific Islands
Q fever	*Coxiella burnetii*	Q fever	Inhalation of contaminated aerosol, tick bite	Cattle, sheep, goats, rodents	Worldwide
Trench fever	*Rochalimaea quintana*	Trench fever	Infected louse feces rubbed into skin	Humans	Europe, Africa, North America

* Epidemic typhus infections may become latent and the infected carrier develops disease in the future (called *Brill-Zinsser disease*).

phus were common during times of war and famine. The disease today is no longer a major public health problem and appears to be confined to certain areas of Africa and Asia, where it is still an important cause of illness. The fatality rate of epidemics can run as high as 30 percent. In areas where socioeconomic standards are low and body lice are prevalent, epidemics remain a constant threat to the population.

Thirty cases of illness caused by *R. prowazekii* were documented in the United States from 1976 to 1983. These cases were unusual in that they were sporadic. In several cases flying squirrels or nests of flying squirrels were found in the homes of the patients. Flying squirrels often nest in attics during the winter months, and 75 percent

of the cases of disease occurred during the winter months. *R. prowazekii* appears to be enzootic in flying squirrels from Virginia to Florida in the eastern United States. The disease is sometimes referred as *sylvatic typhus*. The mechanism of transmission of the rickettsial agent is not known.

The incubation period of louse-borne typhus lasts 10 to 14 days and is characterized by a high fever, which tends to remain during the course of the illness. On the fourth or fifth day a rash appears on the trunk and spreads to the extremities. The rash is seldom seen on the face, palms, or soles. Death is the result of myocardial or neurological involvement.

In some individuals who have recovered from an initial attack of epidemic typhus, surviving rickettsial microorganisms may enter a latent stage. The infected carrier can develop disease in the future but will not have the characteristic rash. The carrier state has been referred to as *Brill-Zinsser disease*.

Endemic Typhus. Endemic or murine typhus is a mild form of typhus transmitted to humans by the rat flea. The causative agent is *Rickettsia typhi* (*R. mooseri*). The symptoms of endemic typhus are similar to those of epidemic typhus but are much milder. Immunity to infection by epidemic typhus also confers immunity to endemic typhus.

As many as 5000 cases of murine typhus were reported in the United States in the 1940s. Today fewer than 100 cases are reported annually to the Centers for Disease Control, with most of these reported from Texas.

Spotted Fever Group

Rocky Mountain Spotted Fever. Of reported rickettsial diseases in the United States, 90 percent are Rocky Mountain spotted fever (RMSF). RMSF is primarily a disease of children and young adults. More than 60 percent of all cases occur in persons younger than 20 years old. Since 1960 there has been a 200 percent increase in the number of reported cases (Fig. 27-3). The causative agent is *Rickettsia rickettsii*. Most cases are found east of the Mississippi, particularly in Virginia, North Carolina, and Tennessee. In the

Fig. 27-3. Rocky Mountain spotted fever, reported cases by county, United States, 1987. (From Centers for Disease Control.)

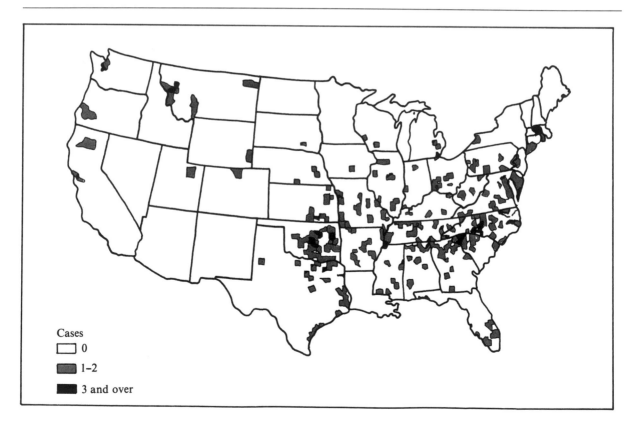

Cases
☐ 0
▨ 1–2
■ 3 and over

eastern United States the American dog tick, the primary vector in transmission of the rickettsiae to humans, is harbored by the rabbit, raccoon, fox, woodchuck, and deer. The wood tick is responsible for the transmission of RMSF in the western United States.

Clinical symptoms, which appear on the average 2 to 5 days after the tick bite, include fever, headache, lymphadenopathy, and rash. Only 3 percent of patients with RMSF have the classic fever, rash, and history of tick bite during the first 3 days of illness. The rash generally starts on the wrists and then spreads to the trunk, face, and extremities. In contrast with other rickettsial infections, an eschar seldom develops at the site of the tick bite. The symptoms are often misdiagnosed as those of measles, encephalitis, meningococcemia, or rubella, and consequently the case fatality rate may reach as high as 15:1. Death usually occurs 10 days after the appearance of the first symptoms and is due to development of progressive hypotension culminating in convulsions or cardiac arrest. In some instances death results from intravascular coagulation. The case fatality rate is higher for persons 30 years of age or older than for younger individuals.

Boutonneuse Fever. The agent of *boutonneuse fever Rickettsia conorii* is carried by ticks. The clinical symptoms are similar to those of RMSF except that an eschar develops at the site of the tick bite. The disease is seldom fatal.

Siberian Tick Typhus. Siberian tick typhus, like boutonneuse fever, occurs rarely, and the clinical symptoms are mild. The causative agent is *Rickettsia sibirica.*

Rickettsialpox and Queensland Tick Typhus. Rickettsialpox and Queensland tick typhus are the mildest of all rickettsial diseases. They are caused by *R. akari* and *R. australis*, respectively. Rickettsialpox is found in North America, the USSR, South Africa, and Korea, while Queensland tick typhus is found in Australia. The vector for transmission is the tick.

Scrub Typhus

Scrub typhus was first recognized during the sixteenth century in China. It is caused by *Rickettsia tsutsugamushi* and is transmitted to humans by mites carried on rodents. Today the disease is more prevalent in eastern Asia and the islands of the South Pacific. Clinical symptoms include a maculopapular rash that covers most of the body and an eschar at the site of the mite bite. Enlargement of the spleen occurs in more than 50 percent of the cases. Treatment with antibiotics brings complete recovery; untreated, the disease progresses until there are serious respiratory, neurological, and cardiovascular complications, often leading to death.

Q Fever

Q fever is caused by *Coxiella burnetii*, a microbial agent that differs from other rickettsiae in ways discussed under General Characteristics. The designation *Q* was used to indicate fever of unknown origin, or "query" fever. Q fever has a worldwide distribution but is rarely observed in Scandanavian countries or New Zealand. The primary reservoirs of *C. burnetii* are sheep, goats, and ticks but other arthropods as well as birds, fish, rodents, camels, and livestock are known to be infected. Q fever in animals is a subclinical disease with rickettsiae being excreted in large numbers in the milk, urine, or feces. In the pregnant ewe, for example, Q fever rickettsiae are found in large numbers in the amniotic fluid. Q fever rickettsiae released in the afterbirth, milk, or urine of animals can survive in the inanimate environment for long periods. This survival characteristic is associated with a developmental cycle in which there is believed to be a vegetative and spore-forming state. The spore resembles an endospore and is the resistant form of the organism (Fig. 27-4).

Humans acquire Q fever by inhalation of aerosols that have been generated from the dried parturition products of farm animals. *C. burnetii* is highly infectious and a single inhaled organism is believed to be sufficient to cause disease. The

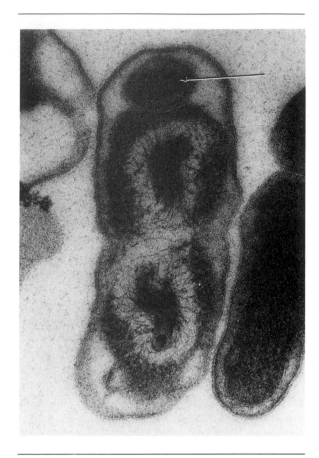

Fig. 27-4. Electron micrograph of *Coxiella burnetii*, demonstrating the endospore-like component (arrow). (From T. F. McCaul and J. C. Williams, *J. Bacteriol.* 147:1963, 1981.)

incubation period is from 14 to 39 days. The fever is intermittent, with spikes of fever to 104 to 105°F and is accompanied by headache, persistent cough, myalgia, and chest pain. Pneumonia is one manifestation of illness, but its incidence may vary from 0 to 90 percent, depending on the particular outbreak of disease. Q fever may also be manifested by liver involvement (hepatitis). Complications from acute disease are rare and are usually self-limiting. A rare but severe and often fatal complication of Q fever is endocarditis (endocarditis is seldom seen in North America).

Q fever is primarily an occupational disease that is rarely reported in the United States. Persons working with goats or sheep or other infected animals in the field, in research facilities, or in abattoirs are at risk of infection by *C. burnetii*.

Trench Fever

R. quintana is the causative agent of trench fever. Human beings are the reservoir of infection, and the body louse is the only known vector. Trench fever was an important clinical entity during the two world wars. Because the symptoms are mild, trench fever is not considered a public health problem.

Ehrlichioses

Ehrlichioses are diseases caused by species of *Ehrlichia*. *Ehrlichia* have been known for years to cause disease in animals but only two species to date have been implicated in human infection: *E. sennetsu* and *E. canis*. *E. sennetsu* (*sennetsu* from the Japanese, meaning glandular fever) is the cause of glandular fever in humans and is observed only in western Japan and Malaysia. So far it is not known how the infectious agent is transmitted to humans, but presumably an insect vector is involved. The incubation period for glandular fever is about 14 days. The symptoms of disease resemble those of infectious mononucleosis. There is remittent fever with daily fluctuations accompanied by headache, chills, joint pain, sore throat, and sleeplessness. About 5 days after these initial symptoms there is lymph node enlargement about the face and neck. Hepatosplenomegaly is observed in about one-third of the patients. *E. sennetsu* is sensitive to tetracyclines; they should be administered for about 7 days to eliminate organisms from the lymph nodes.

E. canis, which before 1986 was associated with canine ehrlichiosis, has been associated with human infection in the United States. It is not known how the disease is transmitted in humans but in dogs it is transmitted by the brown dog tick. The symptoms of disease are similar to those of Rocky Mountain spotted fever except that the rash is seen less often in ehrlichiosis. Tetracyclines are effective in treatment.

LABORATORY DIAGNOSIS

Rickettsiae are difficult and dangerous to work with in the laboratory. The single most important diagnostic aid in identification of rickettsial disease is the demonstration of a rise in serum antibody during the course of illness. The complement fixation test is the most widely used test for serological diagnosis of rickettsial disease. A number of agglutination tests have been used diagnostically, particularly for epidemic typhus and Q fever. Because of the excessive amounts of rickettsial antigen required for the tests and the difficulty in preparing such quantities, a microagglutination technique has been devised. The agglutination tests are much more sensitive than the complement fixation tests and can distinguish between epidemic and endemic typhus.

The *Weil-Felix test* is a test used in the serological diagnosis of all rickettsial diseases except Q fever, trench fever, and rickettsialpox. It is based on the antigenic relationship between strains of the bacterium *Proteus* (OX-19, OX-2, and OX-K) and rickettsiae. *Proteus* strains can be agglutinated by antibodies induced by various rickettsiae. The test is not valuable in establishing a presumptive diagnosis of rickettsial disease since nonspecific reactions can frequently occur. Only 50 to 70 percent of patients with scrub typhus show a rise in OX-K agglutinins. In murine and louse-borne typhus most patients are positive for OX-19 agglutinins. For Rocky Mountain spotted fever, Weil-Felix agglutinins are seldom constant and false-positive and false-negative reactions are common.

Many of the serological techniques do not yield rapid results because of the time required for production of a sufficient antibody titer in the infected host. Immunofluorescence is a useful serologic method, which can identify rickettsiae in infected tissue as well as detect rickettsial antibodies in serum. The direct method, relatively inexpensive and simple, uses specific antiserum conjugated with fluorescein isothiocyanate (FITC) to discover rickettsiae in tissue. In the indirect method, which is employed to detect antibody, specific antibody is fixed to rickettsial antigen. The latter complex is allowed to combine with FITC-conjugated antibody against specific antiserum. In recent years the indirect fluorescent antibody test has replaced the direct method in the diagnosis of RMSF. Latex agglutination is an alternative to indirect fluorescent antibody in RMSF diagnosis.

C. burnetii is a very contagious agent and can be easily acquired by laboratory personnel if certain precautions are not taken during culturing techniques. For this reason it is much safer to use serological tests such as the complement fixation test. Recently, an ELISA for diagnosis of Q fever has been described.

TREATMENT, PREVENTION, AND CONTROL

Treatment of rickettsial disease with tetracycline or chloramphenicol often results in complete recovery. Because of the toxic effects of chloramphenicol, tetracycline is the preferred drug. In some rickettsial diseases, such as RMSF, early treatment is absolutely necessary. Antibiotic treatment should therefore be initiated on the basis of clinical symptoms and not serological diagnosis since antibodies do not always develop in the early stages of the disease. Many of the fatalities from rickettsial infections have occurred because of misdiagnosis and administration of antibiotics such as penicillin and ampicillin that have no effect on the infecting microorganisms. Early therapy, particularly in scrub typhus, does not allow enough time for immunity to develop, and relapses are possible unless treatment is extended for several weeks.

Since many rickettsial diseases are self-limiting and occur infrequently, vaccination programs

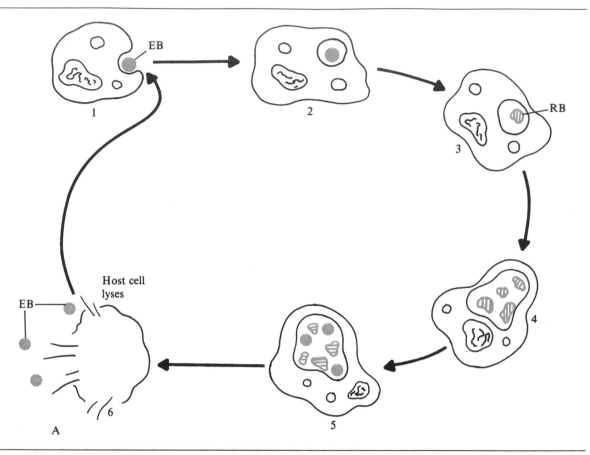

Fig. 27-5. Developmental cycle of chlamydiae. A. Diagrammatic illustration: 1, infectious elementary body (EB) is internalized by host cell; 2, EB within phagosome; 3, EB reorganizes into reticulate body (RB); 4, RB multiplies and phagosome occupies most of internal contents of cell; 5, some RBs become EBs; 6, infected host cell dies and releases infectious EB, which infects adjacent cells. B. Electron micrograph of EB and phagosome formation: one EB (arrow) is internalized, while in cytoplasm four vesicles (phagosomes) can be observed to contain 2 to 3 EBs. (From P. Wyrick, *Infect. Immun.* 56[6]:1456, 1988.) (Fig. 27-5 continued on next page)

have met with little success. A vaccine for Q fever has been developed to prevent shedding of *C. burnetii* in cows. A Q fever vaccine has been available since 1967 for use by laboratory personnel and others who are in contact with the organism. This vaccine is prepared from what we would now call phase II organisms. There has been no vaccine for national distribution. Since 1979 there have been four large-scale outbreaks of Q fever at major teaching universities. A commercial vaccine for RMSF, prepared from yolk sacs of embryonated eggs, was thought to provide protection but was removed from the market in 1978. Since that time no RMSF vaccine has been available in the United States. A new formalin-inactivated vaccine was developed in 1983 and is currently under evaluation.

Chemical control with insecticides can be easily applied against fleas and lice since they are closely associated with humans and rats. Control of woodland ticks and mites is more difficult because of the variety of mammals that harbor the

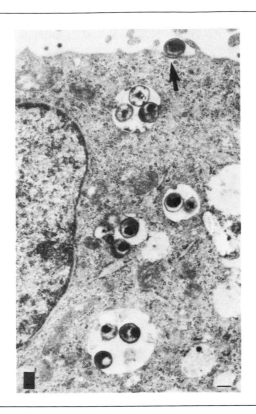

Fig. 27-5. (continued)

arthropod vectors. The most practical protection is the use of repellents and personal cleanliness.

THE CHLAMYDIAE

The chlamydiae, like the rickettsiae, are intracellular parasites. They are found throughout the animal kingdom and are recognized as important animal pathogens. Only a few species of *Chlamydia* cause infections in humans but one of them, *C. trachomatis*, is the leading cause of sexually transmitted disease in the United States, affecting up to 5 million persons. The group at greatest risk are females of child-bearing age, in whom infection can lead to infertility or ectopic pregnancies.

GENERAL CHARACTERISTICS

Chlamydiae range in size from 0.2 to 1.0 μm. They have no peptidoglycan layer in the cell wall and this distinguishes them from rickettsiae. The chlamydial cell wall does contain an outer membrane of the gram-negative cell wall type. Chlamydiae can make their own DNA, RNA, and protein but are unable to produce their own energy sources such as ATP.

Three species of *Chlamydia** are recognized: *C. trachomatis*, *C. pneumoniae* (formerly called *Chlamydia* sp. strain TWAR), and *C. psittaci. C. trachomatis* is divided into three biovars (biological varieties), two of which cause human disease: *lymphogranuloma venereum*, the agent of the sexually transmitted disease of the same name (LGV), and *trachoma*, the agent of oculogenital diseases other than LGV.

Chlamydiae have an unusual developmental cycle, in which two forms of the microorganism exist: the *elementary body*, which is the extracellular and infectious form, and the *reticulate body*, which is the intracellular, noninfectious form of the organism. The developmental cycle can be broken down into the following stages (Fig. 27-5):

1. The infectious elementary body (EB) is internalized by host cells and in the process forms a phagosome.
2. Chlamydiae, once internalized, remain within the phagosome and in some as yet unknown way prevent phagosome-lysosome fusion.
3. Elementary bodies undergo a reorganization into another form, the reticulate body (RB).
4. The reticulate bodies multiply by binary fission. During this multiplication process the phagosome enlarges and is referred to as an *inclusion body* (Plate 16).
5. Some of the reticulate bodies, instead of multiplying, undergo reorganization and become elementary bodies.

* A strain of *C. psittaci*, called TWAR, discovered in 1986 as a potential pathogen, has been assigned the species name *C. pneumoniae*. It is associated with respiratory disease.

Table 27-2. Properties of Chlamydial Particles

Property	Elementary body	Reticulate body
Size	0.2–0.4 μm	0.6–1.0 μm
Rigid cell wall	Yes	No
Extracellular stability	Yes	No
Infective	Yes	No
Induces phagocytosis	Yes	No
Inhibits phagosome fusion with lysosome	Yes	No
Toxic	Yes	No
Metabolic activity	No	Yes
Replication	No	Yes

Source: J. Schachter and H. D. Caldwell, Chlamydiae. *Annu. Rev. Microbiol.* 34:285, 1980.

6. Elementary bodies are released from the inclusion body and the host cell. These EBs are ready to infect adjacent host cells. The properties of EBs and RBs are outlined in Table 27-2.

EPIDEMIOLOGY AND PATHOGENESIS

Chlamydia trachomatis

Ocular Disease. *Trachoma* is an ocular disease that is worldwide in distribution but is endemic in certain areas such as the Punjab region of India, isolated regions of Africa, and a few south-central states in the United States. Worldwide trachoma affects nearly 500 million people. The microorganism is spread by (1) contaminated fingers, (2) items such as facecloths and clothing, (3) infective discharges on bed linen, pillows, etc., and (4) direct contact between parents and children. In communities where trachoma is endemic, clinically active disease is found primarily in the very young and less so in older adults. Apparently, repeated infections among family members lead to chronic disease and blindness. Trachoma begins as a chronic conjunctivitis in which there is an accumulation and coalescence of lymphocytes and macrophages that form discrete red or yellow follicles on the conjunctiva. The follicles eventually enlarge and involve greater areas of the conjunctiva. Necrosis of the follicles may result in conjunctival scarring. Over a period of years these scars contract and turn in the upper eyelid, resulting in abrasions of the cornea by eyelashes. Blindness may result from mechanical scarring and secondary bacterial infections by species of *Hemophilus* and *Moraxella*, for example. The incidence of trachoma can be reduced significantly when there is (1) water available for washing the body (especially the face), clothes, and linen, (2) adequate living space, and (3) elevated, separated, and ventilated living space. Thus, any cultural practice that reduces intrafamilial transmission reduces the incidence as well as the severity of the disease.

Inclusion conjunctivitis is a general term referring to ocular chlamydial infection in adults and infants that does not usually result in blindness. Infants become infected during passage through the birth canal of infected mothers. This type of infection, called *ophthalmia neonatorum*, can also be caused by *Neisseria gonorrhoeae* (see Chapter 17). In the United States about 5 percent of the women having vaginal deliveries are infected with *C. trachomatis*. Of those infants exposed to infected mothers, about 20 percent will develop inclusion conjunctivitis and another 15 percent will develop pneumonia. *Neonatal pneumonia* is a frequent complication after inclusion conjunctivitis but it can also occur in the absence of eye infections. Inclusion conjunctivitis in adults occurs primarily by contact with microorganisms derived from the genital tract. Many cases of adult ocular disease can be traced to swimming in pools contaminated with the microorganisms. Inclusion conjunctivitis in infants and adults is usually a self-limiting disease; however, scarring has been noted in infants in whom treatment was delayed.

Male Genital Tract Disease. *C. trachomatis* is the primary agent of a sexually transmitted disease in men called *nongonococcal urethritis (NGU)*. NGU is less frequently caused by *Ureaplasma urealyticum* plus other microbial agents. NGU keeps increasing each year despite well-developed medical systems for control of sexually transmitted diseases in developed countries. Part of the problem stems from the fact that many men with NGU also have gonococcal urethritis. Treatment regimens for gonococcal urethritis (penicillin, for example), are not effective against *C. trachomatis*.

The highest rate of *C. trachomatis* among men is found in those who are sexually promiscuous or who have recently changed sex partners. Most of the female sex partners of men with chlamydial infection also carry *C. trachomatis* on the cervix. *C. trachomatis* is seldom isolated from the female sex partner of men without NGU. NGU is considered self-limiting, although a small proportion of men incur epididymitis. It takes 2–3 weeks for the manifestation of NGU—that is, a white urethral discharge—to occur (the incubation period for gonorrhea is 2 to 7 days).

Female Genital Tract Disease. Chlamydial infection in the genital tract of women usually involves the cervix. The infected cervix may be the source of infection for neonates (that is, inclusion conjunctivitis and pneumonia). From 2 to 18 percent of women may be infected by *C. trachomatis* and infection may develop into more serious consequences. Chlamydial genital tract infection in women is initially asymptomatic but frequently leads to symptomatic *pelvic inflammatory disease (PID)*. PID is often manifested as salpingitis, in which there is first inflammation followed by necrosis and obstruction of the fallopian tubes. Acute PID is a leading cause of infertility and ectopic pregnancies. Over 1 million cases of acute salpingitis are reported each year in the United States. PID in the United States causes more morbidity among women aged 15 to 25 than all other serious infections combined. Several microbial agents may cause PID (*N. gonorrhoeae*,

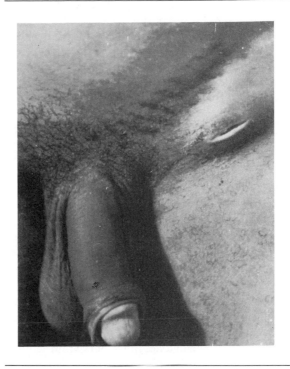

Fig. 27-6. Lymphogranuloma venereum. Acute buboe, which has been surgically incised. (From E. V. Hamm. In W. A. D. Anderson and J. M. Kissane [eds], *Pathology* [7th ed.]. St. Louis: Mosby, 1977.)

Mycoplasma hominis, Chlamydia trachomatis, and *Ureaplasma urealyticum*) but *C. trachomatis* is more frequently associated with the complication of infertility. Women with tubal infertility begin sexual activity sooner, have more sex partners, and more often have a history of sexually transmitted disease.

Lymphogranuloma Venereum. Lymphogranuloma venereum (LGV) is a sexually transmitted disease caused by *C. trachomatis*. Fewer than 400 cases are reported each year in the United States, and the majority of these are from the southern states. A lesion develops at the site of inoculation after an incubation period of 1 to 4 weeks (Fig. 27-6). This is followed by lymphatic involvement and enlarged inguinal lymph nodes. As the disease progresses more lymph nodes become involved and exhibit a purplish cast. Lymph nodes may become necrotic, but they eventually heal. The most severe complications of this disease are associated with perianal abscesses and fistulas that may develop 1 to 10 years after infection.

Chlamydia psittaci

C. psittaci is the causal agent of *psittacosis*. *C. psittaci* infections occur in avian and mammalian populations, but only the avian strains are known to cause disease in humans. Psittacosis is primarily an occupational disease of those working in poultry-processing plants. Pet birds and occasionally wild birds transmit the infectious agent to humans. Infected birds usually show no clinical signs of disease.

Psittacosis in humans is usually asymptomatic, but an atypical pneumonia may develop. The incubation period of 1 to 3 weeks is followed by chills, fever, headache, and persistent cough. The symptoms subside in less than 2 weeks.

A strain of *C. psittaci* now called the TWAR (Taiwan-Acute-Respiratory) agent was first isolated in 1965. A variety of lower respiratory diseases have been ascribed to the TWAR agents and human exposure is prevalent. The exact route of transmission is unclear but is believed to be via human-to-human respiratory contact. Recent studies indicate the TWAR agent differs from other chlamydiae in its mode of attachment and internalization by host cells. The species name *C. pneumoniae* has been proposed for this agent.

Chlamydia pneumoniae

C. pneumoniae (formerly called *Chlamydia* sp. strain *TWAR* or Taiwan-Acute-Respiratory) was first isolated in 1965. Infection with this organism appears to be very prevalent, with 40–60 percent of all adult populations showing serological evidence of current or past infection. *C. pneumoniae* has the same developmental cycle as other *Chlamydiae*, however, its mode of attachment and internalization differ from other *Chlamydiae*.

A variety of lower respiratory tract diseases have been ascribed to this microorganism. In young adults, for example, 4 percent of bronchitis has been shown to be associated with *C. pneumoniae*. Pharyngitis is frequently associated with *C. pneumoniae* infection. About 5 percent of primary sinusitis in young adults has also been associated with *C. pneumoniae*.

C. pneumoniae infection is transmitted from person to person. However, the mode and place of transmission, incubation period, and infectiousness of this organism are, as yet, unknown.

LABORATORY DIAGNOSIS

Growth of chlamydiae in cell culture has been the established way to identify chlamydial infection. However, the demand for identification exceeds the availability of laboratory services because tissue culture is complicated and time-consuming. Most laboratories cannot provide these services and other methods of identification have been sought. Tests that have received considerable attention involve the detection of antigens through the use of monoclonal antibodies. Specimens for these tests are obtained by swabs and transferred to transport media. The specimens can then be shipped to central laboratories and identified on slides by direct immunofluorescence or by ELISA. These rapid testing procedures are still less sensitive than culture techniques.

Cell culture systems are commercially available and identification is based on observation of intracytoplasmic inclusions. Intracytoplasmic inclusions can be identified by staining (Giemsa or iodine). Staining techniques do not differentiate *C. trachomatis* from *C. psittaci*. Chlamydial inclusions can be detected by staining by immunofluorescence with monoclonal antibodies. This technique is more sensitive, more rapid, and yields higher isolation rates than conventional staining procedures.

Physicians who wish to determine if a first-visit

patient requires treatment for nongonococcal urethritis can perform the simple leukocyte esterase test on voided urine specimens. This test is a more accurate indicator of urethritis than the Gram stain and is an excellent screening device for identifying sexually active individuals who should then be cultured for *N. gonorrhoeae* and *C. trachomatis*.

The complement fixation test is the most widely used serological test for diagnosing chlamydial disease, particularly neonatal pneumonia. It is useful for diagnosing psittacosis and LGV but less useful in diagnosing oculogenital infections and nearly useless in diagnosing trachoma. A more sensitive serological test is the microimmunofluorescence (MIF) test, which is useful in diagnosing oculogenital infections and trachoma. A commercial antigen, however, is not available for the MIF test, and each laboratory must prepare the antigen by growing *Chlamydia* in yolk sacs. Diagnosis of *C. pneumoniae* infection is based on isolation of organisms and serological testing. When *C. pneumoniae* elementary body antigen is used, MIF is specific for *C. pneumoniae* and distinguishes between antibodies in the IgM and IgG serum fractions. A complement fixation test recognizes lipopolysaccharides of the genus.

Table 27-3. Characteristics That Distinguish Rickettsiae from Chlamydiae

Characteristic	Group	
	Rickettsiae	Chlamydiae
Size	2.0 μm in length	0.2 to 1.0 μm in length
Cell wall composition	Contain peptidoglycan	Do not contain peptidoglycan
Developmental cycle	Simple binary fission except for *Coxiella burnetii*, which exists in endospore and vegetative state	Two forms of the agent: the infectious or elementary particle and the noninfectious reticulate body
Energy source	Can produce their own	Cannot produce their own
Method of evasion of phagocytes	Break down membrane of phagosome and survive in cytoplasm; *Coxiella* resistant to acid hydrolases of phagolysosome	Developmental cycle occurs in phagosome and somehow prevents fusion with lysosome
Transmission to humans	Insect vectors (tick, mite, flea, louse); *C. burnetii* transmitted via inhalation of aerosols from dried parturition products	Direct sexual contact (nongonococcal urethritis, neonatal inclusion conjunctivitis, neonatal pneumonia, salpingitis, lymphogranuloma venereum); indirect contact (trachoma, psittacosis)
Disease characteristics	Affinity for vascular tissue eventually causes obstruction; rash often characteristic of infection; Q fever (*C. burnetii*) associated with lung tissue and no rash is involved	Affinity for tissue of eye (trachoma, inclusion conjunctivitis) and genital tract (nongonococcal urethritis, salpingitis, lymphogranuloma venereum); affinity for respiratory tissue (psittacosis)
Laboratory diagnosis	Serological tests (complement fixation) performed during course of illness	Cell culture or detection of antigens in specimens by immunofluorescence or ELISA
Antibiotic sensitivity	Sensitive to tetracyclines but *not* sensitive to penicillins	Sensitive to tetracyclines, erythromycin, and penicillins

TREATMENT AND PREVENTION

Individuals who have acquired and recovered from chlamydial infection remain susceptible to reinfection. Reinfection occurs despite development of antibody in both serum and secretions such as genital secretions.

Doxycycline and tetracycline are the drugs of choice in the treatment of most chlamydial disease; erythromycin is sometimes an alternative, particularly in pregnancy. If erythromycin is not tolerated, sulfisoxazole is an alternative. Amoxicillin is an alternative to erythromycin if the latter drug cannot be tolerated. In pelvic inflammatory disease, the antimicrobial regimen may include cefoxitin or other cephalosporins plus doxycycline as well as clindamycin to also inhibit anaerobes. Sulfisoxazole is a useful alternative to tetracycline in the treatment of those who are pregnant. Erythromycin syrup administered orally is used in the treatment of established inclusion conjunctivitis in the newborn as well as for infant pneumonia.

Vaccines have been used on a trial basis for preventing trachoma, but they have so far demonstrated little success. Prevention of psittacosis is dependent on preventing avian infection by chemoprophylaxis. Imported birds are supposed to be treated at quarantine stations; however, these measures are oftentimes ignored or improperly carried out.

Silver nitrate drops, which were originally used on newborns to prevent gonococcal infection of the eye, have been replaced by antibiotics such as erythromycin or tetracycline. These agents can prevent chlamydial conjunctivitis.

SUMMARY

Both rickettsiae and chlamydiae are gram-negative intracellular parasites that cannot be cultivated on ordinary laboratory media. There are differences that distinguish most rickettsiae from chlamydiae and these are outlined in Table 27-3.

QUESTIONS FOR STUDY

Select the best response or responses for each of the following:

1. Rickettsia are able to resist destruction in the phagocyte by
   A. Releasing enzymes that lyse the phago-lysosome membrane
   B. Producing a capsular polysaccharide
   C. Producing an enzyme that digests the phagosome membrane
   D. Remaining as extracellular parasites

2. A number of farmhands developed intermittent fever, accompanied by headache and a persistent cough. Three weeks previously the farmhands were involved in lambing. Which of the following agents would be the prime suspect for causing such infections?
   A. *Rickettsia rickettsii*
   B. *Ehrlichia sennetsu*
   C. *Brucella abortus*
   D. *Coxiella burnetii*

3. A child from a rural area in Virginia has fever, headache, lymphadenopathy, and a rash that appears on the wrist. The physician suspects a bacterial infection and prescribes

ampicillin. The child does not improve and the rash now covers her body. The physician prescribes tetracyclines and the child recovers. Which of the following microorganisms might have been involved?

A. *Coxiella burnetii*
B. *Chlamydia psittaci*
C. *Chlamydia trachomatis*
D. *Rickettsia rickettsii*

4. All of the following statements about *Chlamydia trachomatis* are true *except*:

A. It causes several conditions including trachoma, inclusion conjunctivitis, and nongonococcal urethritis.

B. It can cause neonatal pneumonia following vaginal deliveries.
C. It is the leading cause of pelvic inflammatory disease.
D. Some strains can be transmitted by arthropods.

5. If you were examining patients who had been in concentration camps during wartime, which of the following microbial agents might you recover from the majority of them?

A. *Coxiella burnetii*
B. *Rickettsia australis*
C. *Chlamydia psittaci*
D. *Rickettsia prowazekii*

Fill in the blank:

6. The infectious forms of chlamydia are referred to as _____.

7. An encrusted black ulcer at the site of an arthropod bite would be referred to as a(an) _____.

8. The chlamydial cell wall differs from the rick-

ettsial cell wall in that the former contains _____.

9. Chlamydiae and rickettsia are uniformly sensitive to the drug _____.

10. The chlamydial disease acquired by contact with birds is called _____.

ADDITIONAL READINGS

Baca, O. G., and Paretsky, D. Q fever and *Coxiella burnetii*: A model for host parasite interactions. *Microbiol. Rev.* 47:127,1983.

Brunham, R. C., et al. Etiology and outcome of acute pelvic inflammatory disease. *J. Infect. Dis.* 158(3):510,1988.

Burnakis, T. G., and Hildebrandt, N. B. Pelvic inflammatory disease. A review with emphasis on antimicrobial therapy. *Rev. Infect. Dis.* 8(1):86,1986.

CDC. Human ehrlichiosis—United States. *M.M.W.R.* 37(17):270,1988.

Heggie, A. D., et al. *Chlamydia trachomatis* infection in mothers and infants: A perspective study. *Am. J. Dis. Child.* 135:507,1981.

Infectious causes of blindness. *Rev. Infect. Dis.* 7(6):711,1985.

McCutchan, J. A. Epidemiology of venereal urethritis: Comparison of gonorrhoea and nongonococcal urethritis. *Rev. Infect. Dis.* 6(5):669,1984.

McDade, J. E., and Newhouse, V. F. Natural history of *Rickettsia rickettsii*. *Annu. Rev. Microbiol.* 40:287,1986.

Sawyer, L. A., Fishbein, D. B., and McDade, J. E. Q fever: Current concepts. *Rev. Infect. Dis.* 9(5):935,1987.

Schachter, J., et al. Perspective study of perinatal transmission of *Chlamydia trachomatis*. *J.A.M.A.* 255:3374,1986.

Schachter, J., and Grossman, M. Chlamydial infections. *Annu. Rev. Med.* 32:45,1981.

Weiss, E. The biology of rickettsiae. *Annu. Rev. Microbiol.* 36:345,1982.

28. ACTINOMYCETES

OBJECTIVES

To list the most important species of *Actinomyces* and the types of infections with which they are associated

To briefly describe the association between *Actinomyces* species and caries and periodontal disease

To outline the similarities and differences between *Nocardia* and *Actinomyces*

To describe the types of infections associated with *Nocardia*

To describe the types of treatment required for actinomycoses and nocardioses

Actinomycetes are a large group of bacteria that have characteristics of bacteria and fungi. Most of the species in this group have the ability to form branches or filaments, referred to as *hyphae*—a fungal characteristic (Fig. 28-1). In addition, the diseases that actinomycetes cause resemble fungal diseases. The cell walls and other structural components of the actinomycetes are, however, prokaryotic in composition and function. Moreover, the growth of actinomycetes is inhibited by penicillin—a characteristic of bacteria but not fungi. The classification of the ac-

tinomycetes and related bacteria has not been uniformly agreed on. Some artificial schemes include genera that form hyphae, which fragment into coccoid- or rod-like elements, while other genera are characterized by the formation of spores. Many species, particularly species of *Streptomyces* (Fig. 28-2), which are found in the soil, are widely known because of their use in the production of antibiotics and other commercial products. Actinomycetes also include genera such as *Corynebacterium* and *Mycobacterium*, which are widely known because of their pathogenic potential. There are other actinomycetes that are less widely known as human pathogens and these are the major focus of this chapter. We will discuss three types of infections caused by actinomycetes: actinomycosis, nocardiosis, and actinomycetoma.

Fig. 28-1. Scanning electron micrograph of *Actinomyces israelii* microcolony. Note the branching filaments. (From J. M. Slack and M. A. Gerencser, *Actinomyces, Filamentous Bacteria: Biology and Pathogenecity*. Minneapolis: Burgess, 1975.)

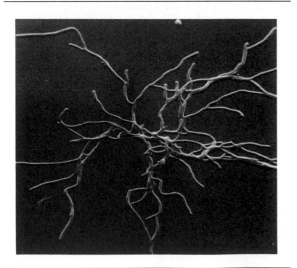

ACTINOMYCOSIS

Actinomycosis may be caused by several actinomycete species belonging to several genera (*Actinomyces, Rothia, Arachnia, Bifidobacterium, Corynebacterium*, et al.), but the most important are species of the genus *Actinomyces*. *Actinomyces* are facultative anaerobes that make up the microbial flora of the oral cavity, intestinal tract, and pelvic area. *Actinomyces* produce branching filaments during growth but do not produce aerial filaments. The most frequently re-

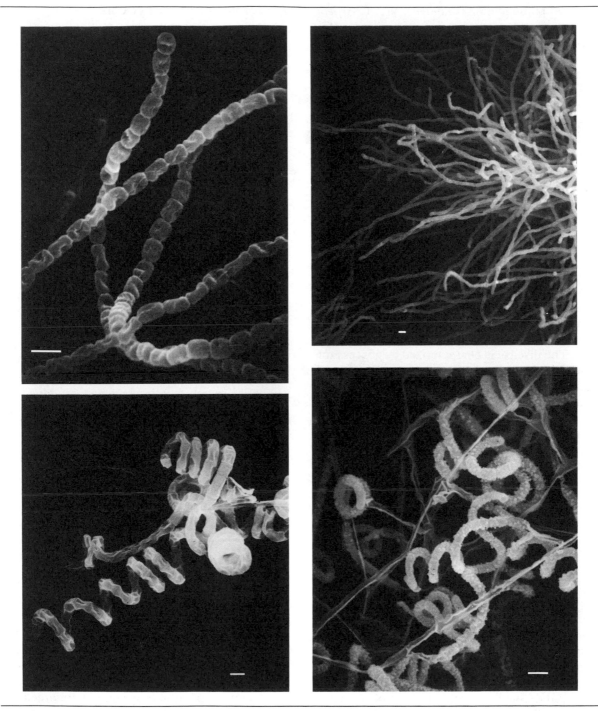

Fig. 28-2. Types of *Streptomyces* species found in the soil. Bar = 1 μm. (From S. Omura, *Microbiol. Revs.* 50[3]:259, 1986.)

covered pathogenic *Actinomyces* are *A. israelii*, *A. naeslundii*, and *Arachnia propionica* (formerly *Actinomyces propionicus*).

Actinomycosis is a chronic, suppurative infection characterized by abscess formation and draining sinuses. The draining sinuses contain white or yellow granules (called *sulfur granules*) composed of microcolonies of the branching actinomycete. The major forms of the disease involve the cervicofacial, abdominal, thoracic, and genital regions.

PATHOGENESIS

Cervicofacial Actinomycosis

Cervicofacial actinomycosis is the most common type of actinomycosis and is usually associated with the lower jaw. Individuals predisposed by conditions such as tooth decay, jaw fracture, or tooth extraction are most susceptible to infection. The disease is characterized by abscess formation and development of sinus tracts (Plate 17) that eventually reach the skin, producing nodules that can break and form fistulas. The tissue around the fistulas often shrinks, leaving an area of depression. In advanced cases the infection may penetrate the orbital cavity, causing blindness.

Thoracic Actinomycosis

Thoracic actinomycosis can result from the aspiration of microorganisms from the oral cavity, by extension from cervicofacial actinomycosis, or by hematogenous spreading. Lesions occur in the lung and may involve both lobes. The infection extends to the pleura and eventually penetrates the thoracic wall through multiple draining sinuses. Fistulas and the characteristic depression on the chest are also evident. During the course of the disease there may be chest pain, fever, and cough resembling those of other respiratory diseases, such as tuberculosis.

Abdominal Actinomycosis

Abdominal actinomycosis results most frequently from trauma of the intestinal tract or abdominal wall. Many cases of the disease are a consequence of appendectomies that fail to heal or of perforated appendixes. Sinus tracts may develop and penetrate the abdominal wall.

Genital Actinomycosis

Genital actinomycosis is a relatively new clinical syndrome, resulting from the wearing of intrauterine devices. Uterine actinomycosis may be superficial or invasive and fatal. Metastatic spread of infection to the brain has been reported following pelvic abscesses.

LABORATORY DIAGNOSIS

Pus from fistulas and sputum can be examined for the appearance of yellow or white granules; however, they are not always present. When granules are not present in the fistulas, the wound should be covered with gauze and examined the next day. Gram-staining the granules permits the identification of gram-positive filamentous or diphtheroid bacilli. Clinical specimens or granules should be inoculated into thioglycolate broth or brain-heart infusion agar and incubated anaerobically for 2 to 5 days. When colonies develop, the growth should be checked for the appearance of gram-positive bacilli. Species of *Actinomyces* can be identified directly in clinical specimens by immunofluorescent techniques.

TREATMENT

Surgical debridement of damaged tissue is the prerequisite to antibiotic therapy. Penicillin G administered over a period of 3 to 4 weeks remains the drug regimen. Recent evidence indicates that combinations of trimethoprim and sulfamethoxazole have resulted in more rapid cures, particularly in cervicofacial and abdominal infections. It has been recommended that asymptomatic women found to have pelvic infection due to *Actinomyces* be treated only by removal of the IUD, but that patients with pelvic symptoms should receive a full course of antibiotic therapy to prevent systemic dissemination of the infection.

NOCARDIOSIS AND ACTINOMYCETOMA

Nocardioses are infections caused by species of *Nocardia* (Fig. 28-3) that are indigenous to soil and water. *Nocardia* also differ from *Actinomyces* in that they are aerobic and produce aerial filaments that can undergo fragmentation. The most important human pathogens are *N. asteroides*, *N. brasiliensis*, and *N. caviae*.

PATHOGENESIS

Nocardioses are usually found in compromised patients, for example, those being treated with immunosuppressive drugs for neoplastic disease and transplantation or those with underlying chronic pulmonary disease. There have been reports that up to 15 percent of transplant patients and 53 percent of those receiving immunosuppressive therapy for other conditions develop nocardiosis. Corticosteroids have been shown to adversely affect tissue macrophage activity at sites such as liver, spleen, and lung. *Nocardia* is more resistant than most other microorganisms to oxidative killing by macrophages. Steroid administration, therefore, makes some patients more susceptible to infection by *Nocardia*.

Most *Nocardia* infections result from the inhalation of the organism (usually *N. asteroides*) but direct inoculation into traumatized tissue (usually *N. brasiliensis* and *N. caviae*) can also occur. In lung infections nodular abscesses can

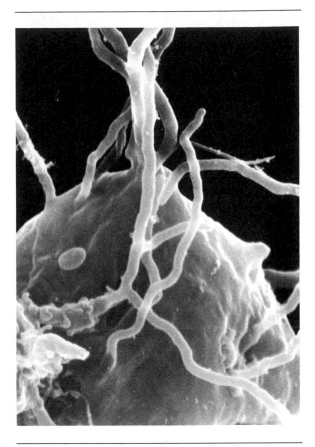

Fig. 28-3. Scanning electron micrograph of rabbit alveolar macrophage infected with filamentous *Nocardia*. (From B. L. Beaman, *Infect. Immun.* 15:925, 1977.)

be observed. Fever and dry cough are symptoms sometimes observed, but many times no symptoms are evident. If not diagnosed and treated early, the infection may become metastatic and involve the central nervous system and kidneys. Fatality rates approach 80 percent in undiagnosed disseminated disease. *Nocardia* can also cause infections in the skin and subcutaneous tissue, usually in a lower extremity following trauma. Infection is localized and chronic and is characterized by draining sinuses and the presence of granules. As the infection becomes more chronic, the sinus tracts extend more deeply into the body and involve both muscle and bone. These types of infections, called *actinomycetoma* (Fig. 28-4), may also be caused by other microorganisms, including *Actinomadura madurae*, *A. pelletieri*, *Streptomyces somaliensis*, and *S. paraguayensis*.

LABORATORY DIAGNOSIS

Diseases caused by *Nocardia* and *Actinomyces* are very similar. Differentiation of these genera is important because successful treatment requires different therapeutics. Exudative material from lesions should be examined microscopically for microcolonies of granules. Sputum, spinal fluid, urine, and exudative material can be examined microscopically for the typically thin, highly branched filaments. Acid-fast staining techniques have revealed that young colonies are strongly acid-fast, while older cultures are variable. Specimens should be planted on Sabouraud dextrose agar (without antibiotics) and streaked on beef heart infusion agar plates and incubated

Fig. 28-4. Mycetoma of the foot caused by *Actinomadura madurae.* (Courtesy V. V. Pankaja Lakshmi.)

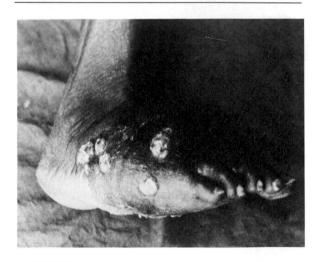

aerobically at 25 to 30°C. Cultures are examined at 48-hour intervals for 2 weeks or more. Colonies on both media initially appear yellow but on further incubation they turn a dark orange. Aerial filaments can be discerned microscopically. Filaments have a tendency to break up into bacillary forms. A variety of biochemical tests can be used to differentiate *Nocardia* from other actinomyces. Rapid diagnosis of nocardiosis may become a reality since a specific protein of *N. asteroides* has recently been identified and isolated. An enzyme immunoassay is currently under investigation to evaluate patients with possible nocardiosis.

TREATMENT

As in actinomycosis, surgical debridement of damaged tissue should be performed whenever possible before chemotherapy is initiated. *N. asteroides* responds quickly to treatment. Early diagnosis is important since recovery rates after systemic infection are very low. Sulfonamides are the drug of choice in treatment. Trimethoprim-sulfamethoxazole is highly effective, but whether it is better than sulfonamides is not yet known.

CARIES, PERIODONTAL DISEASE, AND ACTINOMYCETES

A variety of nonbiological and biological factors are associated with diseases of the teeth (*caries*, or tooth decay) and tissues surrounding the teeth (periodontal disease). Microorganisms form only one link in the chain of events that lead to tooth decay and periodontal disease. Actinomycetes represent but one group of bacteria that play a role in these diseases, and that role is in the formation of *plaque*. Plaque is a structureless accumulation of bacteria, microbial polysaccha-

Table 28-1. Characteristics of *Actinomyces* and *Nocardia*

Characteristics	Actinomyces	Nocardia
Oxygen requirements	Facultative anaerobes	Aerobes
Environmental source of human pathogens	Oral cavity, intestinal tract, and pelvic region	Soil and water
Morphology	Do not produce aerial filaments	Do produce aerial filaments
Disease characteristics in humans	Chronic, suppurative, infections with sinus tracts that may cause dissemination	Same as *Actinomyces*
Site of disease in humans	Cervicofacial, thoracic, abdomen, and genital tract	Lung; subcutaneous tissue, especially of extremities
Mechanism of transmission of infectious agent	Opportunistic because of underlying condition (cervicofacial), aspiration (thoracic), trauma (abdominal), wearing intrauterine devices (genital)	Most infections from inhalation of organisms but some infections from trauma to skin, particularly in extremities
Treatment of infection	Surgical debridement followed by penicillin G therapy	Surgical debridement followed by sulfonamide therapy

rides, and host proteins that is attached to the enamel surrounding the tooth's surface. Plaque formation is invariably a prerequisite to caries and periodontal disease. Two actinomycetes that appear to be important in the formation of plaque are *Actinomyces viscosus* and *A. naeslundii*. Both species produce fimbriae and extracellular polysaccharides. Bacterial polysaccharides are sticky enough to enable various bacterial species to aggregate and to attach to the tooth's surface. Plaque represents a thin sticky environment that becomes a structured ecosystem where various bacterial species reside and thrive. When we eat foods high in sucrose, this sugar is metabolized by plaque bacteria such as actinomycetes and others, and acids are produced that cause demineralization of tooth enamel. In other words, a cavity or tooth decay has taken place. If plaque is not removed it thickens and the bacteria and the products they release cause inflammation of the gums (gingivitis). This inflammatory condition leads to destruction of the bone supporting the teeth and *periodontitis* is the result.

SUMMARY

Actinomycetes are bacteria having the characteristics of bacteria and fungi. They produce hyphae and the diseases they cause resemble fungal diseases, with fungal characteristics. The cell wall and other structural components of actinomycetes are bacterial in composition and function. Table 28-1 outlines the characteristics of the two major pathogenic actinomyces: *Actinomyces* and *Nocardia*.

QUESTIONS FOR STUDY

Select the best response or responses for each of the following:

1. Actinomycetes resemble fungi in which of the following ways?
   A. Their cell wall composition is similar.
   B. Both are inhibited by penicillin.
   C. Both can exist in filamentous forms.
   D. Both contain species that produce antibiotics.

2. The term *sulfur granule* refers to
   A. Lesions caused by actinomycetes that concentrate sulfur
   B. The characteristic color of actinomycete colonies on certain media
   C. The accumulation of yellow or white filaments of actinomycetes in a lesion
   D. The color of actinomycete colonies in the soil

3. Each of the following is a predisposing condition that can lead to actinomycosis *except*
   A. Various intrauterine devices
   B. Broken jaw
   C. Sexual promiscuity
   D. Aspiration of saliva during anesthesia

4. The following statements about *Nocardia* and the diseases they cause are true *except*
   A. *Nocardia* are aerobic organisms.
   B. Nocardioses are found primarily in compromised patients.
   C. Most nocardioses resolve on their own.
   D. *Nocardia* colonies appear yellow to orange on laboratory media.

Fill in the blank:

5. The single most important treatment regimen for actinomycosis and nocardiosis prior to antibiotic administration is _____ .

6. The structureless accumulation of bacteria and host material attached to the surface of the tooth is called _____ .

7. *Actinomyces* _____ and *A.* _____ are believed to be somehow involved in periodontal disease.

8. The term _____ is used to describe sinus tracts produced by actinomycetes that extend deeply into muscle and bone.

ADDITIONAL READINGS

Reiner, S., et al. Primary actinomycosis of an extremity. A case report and review. *Rev. Infect. Dis.* 9(3):581, 1987.

Schaffner, A., and Schaffner, T. Glucocorticoid-induced impairment of macrophage antimicrobial activity: Mechanisms and dependence on the state of activation. *Rev. Infect. Dis.* 9 (Suppl. 5):620, 1987.

Smego, R. A., Jr. Actinomycosis of the central nervous system. *Rev. Infect. Dis.* 9(5):855, 1987.

Tight, R. R., and Bartlett, M. S. Actinomycetoma in the United States. *Rev. Infect. Dis.* 3:1139, 1981.

29. MISCELLANEOUS PATHOGENS

OBJECTIVES

To describe the method of transmission, sources of disease, site of infection, and treatment for Legionnaires' disease.

To list the type of infection associated with *Capnocytophaga* species, *Actinobacillus, Calymmatobacterium, Streptobacillus, Chromobacterium, Eikenella,* and *Gardnerella*

Legionella is a recently discovered (1976) human pathogen that, like several other bacteria, is an infrequent cause of disease. The classification of many of these bacteria is not complete and in *Bergey's Manual* they are referred to as Other Genera in the various groups that are classified. The list of infrequent pathogens discussed in this chapter is not complete but represents those for which some clinical information is available. Most of our attention will be given to the genus *Legionella*, while the remaining genera are outlined in Table 29-1.

LEGIONELLA

More than 200 persons were stricken with a respiratory disease of unknown origin at the American Legion Convention in Philadelphia in 1976 and 34 died. The causal agent of the disease at first resisted isolation, but researchers at the Centers for Disease Control in Atlanta identified the previously unknown bacterium and called it the *Legionnaires' disease bacterium* (LDB), now classified as *Legionella pneumophila*. The genus *Legionella* belongs to the family Legionellaceae. Currently there are 24 described species comprising 39 serogroups. For example, there are 12 serogroups in the species *L. pneumophila*. Some of the most frequently isolated species of *Legionella* are outlined in Table 29-2.

GENERAL CHARACTERISTICS

The causal agent of Legionnaires' disease is a gram-negative aerobic bacillus that is 0.3 to 0.4 μm in diameter and 2.0 to 3.0 μm in length (Fig. 29-1). Occasionally the organism appears filamentous, reaching up to 20 μm in length. The organism does not grow on the usual bacteriologic media. Clinical specimens from lung tissue taken at autopsy were originally cultivated in the yolk sac of embryonated eggs. Supplemented laboratory media have now been used to cultivate the bacillus (see Laboratory Diagnosis).

EPIDEMIOLOGY

L. pneumophila is an organism found primarily in water. It has been found in thermal effluent water, creek water, mud, water from cooling towers, and water from freshwater lakes. *L. pneumophila* is not thermophilic but it can survive in water at temperatures from 6 to 67°C. Outbreaks of disease have been associated with heat-exchange apparatus, shower water, tap water, and potable water after chlorination. The most important mechanism of transmission of the organism to humans is by aerosols.

The incidence of *Legionella* pneumonia in the United States is believed to be somewhere between 25,000 and 30,000 cases per year. (Only 1100 were reported to the CDC in 1989.) *L. pneumophilia* may be acquired in the community or in the hospital. In about 70 percent of the cases the patient has some underlying condition or ill-

Table 29-1. Characteristics of Miscellaneous Bacterial Species Pathogenic to Humans

Species	Characteristics of disease	Characteristics of organism	Treatment
Calymmatobacterium granulomatis	*Granuloma inguinale*, an infrequent sexually transmitted disease: lesions in pubic area that may lead to elephantiasis; occasionally found in southern United States	Pleomorphic facultative anaerobe, gram-negative, nonmotile rod that is heavily encapsulated	Streptomycin, tetracycline, or trimethoprim/sulfamethoxazole
Streptobacillus moniliformis	One type of *rat-bite fever* acquired by bite of rat or ingestion of contaminated food; fever, rash, and polyarthritis are major symptoms	Pleomorphic, facultatively anaerobic gram-negative rod; normal inhabitant of rat throat and nasopharynx	Penicillin or streptomycin; penicillin induces L-forms
Actinobacillus actinomycetemcomitans	Primarily endocarditis	Nonmotile, gram-negative, facultatively anaerobic coccobacillus; part of human oral flora	Tetracyclines, chloramphenicol, trimethoprim-sulfamethoxazole
Capnocytophaga species	Juvenile periodontosis and bacteremia in immunosuppressed	Gram-negative gliding bacterium; normal inhabitant of human oral cavity; *C. ochracea* most important pathogen	Penicillin
Cardiobacterium hominis	Recovered in cases of endocarditis	Pleomorphic, gram-negative, nonmotile rod; normal inhabitant of respiratory and intestinal tract of humans	Penicillin, tetracyclines, aminoglycosides
Chromobacterium violaceum	Abscess formation and bacteremia; human infections often fatal; septicemia invariably fatal; most cases in Southeast Asia and southeastern United States	Motile, gram-negative, slightly curved rod; found in soil and water; produces violet pigment in broth and on agar	Aminoglycosides, chloramphenicol, tetracyclines
Eikenella corrodens	Often in mixed infections involving mucous membranes of oral cavity, intestinal tract, and genitourinary tract; infections from trauma such as fist fights or human bites	Inhabitant of oral cavity and upper respiratory tract; gram-negative facultative anaerobic bacillus; pits agar surface	Ampicillin
Gardnerella vaginalis (See Boxed Essay, p. 608)	One of a complex of organisms associated with nonspecific vaginitis (*bacterial vaginosis*); originally classified as *Hemophilus vaginalis*	Gram-negative facultatively anaerobic bacillus; increases in vagina with decrease in lactobacilli and increase in anaerobes; difficult to cultivate	Metronidazole, if condition does not resolve on its own

BACTERIAL VAGINOSIS

Microbial infections of the vagina are rather common and involve bacterial as well as fungal and protozoal agents. The infectious agent may in some instances be transmitted to a sex partner or the fetus. The fungal agent associated with vaginitis is *Candida albicans* (see p. 779), while the protozoal agent is *Trichomonas vaginalis* (see p. 815). The etiology of bacterial vaginosis is still controversial and no single organism is associated exclusively with this clinical condition.

The organisms most frequently associated with bacterial vaginosis are the facultative anaerobes *Gardnerella vaginalis* and *Mycoplasma hominis*, and anaerobes such as *Bacteroides* species, *Fusobacterium* species, and *Mobiluncus* species. *G. vaginalis* is the organism most often suggested as playing a role in bacterial vaginosis. However, as many as 55 percent of the women in whom the organism can be isolated are asymptomatic. *G. vaginalis* does not appear to be sexually transmitted.

The diagnosis of bacterial vaginosis is made when three of the following criteria have been established:

1. Homogenous vaginal discharge
2. pH of vaginal discharge less than 4.7
3. Release of an aminelike odor when the vaginal discharge is mixed with potassium hydroxide
4. Clue cells representing more than 20 percent of the vaginal epithelial cells

Clue cells are vaginal epithelial cells covered by adherent gram-negative rods present in vaginal smears of women with bacterial vaginosis but not in clinically normal women. *G. vaginalis* occurs in higher counts on clue cells than in any other bacterial species. The finding of clue cells is vital to the diagnosis of bacterial vaginosis.

The treatment options for bacterial vaginosis are (1) no treatment, since many cases resolve on their own, (2) local treatment with chlorhexidine, and (3) oral therapy with metronidazole or medicated sponges containing metronidazole.

Table 29-2. Some of the Isolated Species of *Legionella*

Species	Original source of isolation
L. pneumophila	Human respiratory tissue
L. bozemanii	Human respiratory tissue
L. dumoffii	Human respiratory tissue
L. micdadei	Enzootic in pigs
L. gormanii	Creek bank
L. jordanis	Water and sewage
L. longbeachae	Human respiratory tissue

ness that predisposes him or her to disease by *Legionella*. Predisposing factors contributing to disease are diabetes, cancer, immunosuppressive therapy, cigarette smoking, renal dialysis, transplantation, advancing age, and alcohol abuse. Surveys of several healthy populations have demonstrated a high titer of antibody to *L. pneumophila*. This may indicate that the organism is abundant in the environment and is responsible for asymptomatic infection in the general population.

PATHOGENESIS

Legionella species behave as facultative intracellular parasites that multiply within the mononuclear phagocyte but not in neutrophils or lymphocytes. Within the monocyte the bacteria are surrounded by a membrane (phagosome) that is studded with ribosome-like particles. *Legionella* can be phagocytosed by neutrophils and monocytes but only in the presence of complement and antibody. The immune cells do not destroy all the bacilli and surviving bacilli are capable of multiplication in the monocyte. Fusion of lysosome with phagosome and phagosome acidification is inhibited by virulent *Legionella*.

Disease caused by *L. pneumophila* is respiratory and may be mild, requiring no hospitalization, or it may be a severe pneumonia requiring hospitalization. The incubation period is 2 to 10 days. The onset of disease is usually gradual except in severely compromised patients such as those who are immunosuppressed. The first symptoms are fever, headache, and weakness,

Fig. 29-1. Photomicrograph of *Legionella pneumophila*. Bacterial cells are observed as plump rods (*arrow*). (Courtesy Centers for Disease Control.)

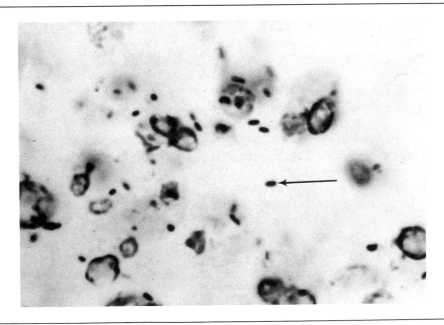

followed by sore throat and rhinitis. Diarrhea may appear before or after respiratory symptoms. The fever is unremitting, and in about one-third of the cases there are lethargy, confusion, disorientation, and other central nervous system symptoms. The major pathological findings are confined to respiratory tissue. Severe bronchopneumonia with inflammation in the alveoli and respiratory bronchioles is common. Extrapulmonary manifestations include central nervous system symptoms such as tremors of the extremities and hyperactive reflexes. Most extrapulmonary manifestations are found in immunosuppressed patients.

What factors are responsible for the damage to lung tissue are not yet known. Several bacterial products are suspected, including a protease and a toxin. It appears that the cellular immune system is critical to recovery but the role of the humoral immune system is not clear. It is also unclear whether humans who have had Legionnaires' disease are immune to reinfection.

LABORATORY DIAGNOSIS

Legionella infections can be diagnosed by demonstrating a serological response to the bacteria, by recognition of bacterial antigen or nucleic acid in clinical specimens, and by recovery of the pathogen in culture.

The most widely used serological technique is the indirect immunofluorescent method for detecting changes in serum antibody titers during the course of infection. An increase in titer levels from less than 1:32 to more than 1:128 is considered confirmatory. Only 75 percent of patients with clinical disease develop a fourfold or greater rise in titer early in the disease process.

Direct immunofluorescence has been used to detect bacterial antigen in clinical specimens. Polyclonal antibody reagents and a monoclonal antibody directed against all serotypes of *Legionella* are used. Cross-reactions with other bacteria, however, have been reported. A DNA probe is commercially available to identify all strains of

Legionella species; however, the current radio-labeled probe has a short half-life.

Recovery of *Legionella* in culture is the mainstay of diagnosis. The organism can be recovered on BYCE-a (buffered charcoal yeast extract supplemented with alpha-ketoglutaric acid) containing selective agents such as cefamandole or polymyxin B. At least two days are needed for colonies to be recognized. Colonial appearance is characteristic and is described as resembling cut glass (Fig. 29-2). A Gram stain should be performed on suspected *Legionella* colonies with basic fuchsin rather than safranin as the coun-

Fig. 29-2. Colonies of *Legionella pneumophila* on buffered charcoal yeast extract agar. Colonies resemble cut glass. (From W. C. Winn, Jr., *Clin. Microbiol. Revs.* 1[1]:60, 1988.)

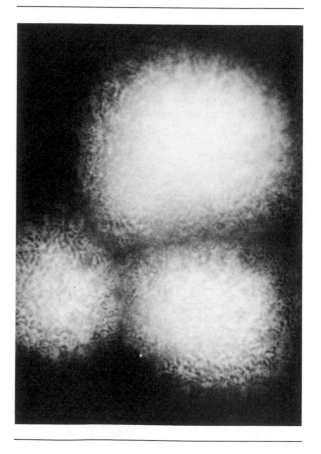

terstain. Subcultures should be made to a BYCE-a medium containing L-cysteine and to tryptic soy agar. If there is growth on the medium containing L-cysteine, the isolate is probably not *Legionella*. If there is growth on tryptic soy agar, the isolate is not *Legionella*. Presumptive identification can be made by direct fluorescent antibody. Identification to the species level is not important other than for epidemiologic purposes.

TREATMENT

Oral administration of erythromycin results in rapid effects in 12 to 36 hours. Studies have demonstrated that erythromycin reduces the case–fatality ratio about fourfold compared to those who do not receive antibiotic therapy. In immunosuppressed patients without therapy the disease is invariably fatal. One of the more promising groups of antimicrobial agents are the quinolone derivatives. They have demonstrated effectiveness equal to or greater than that of erythromycin.

SUMMARY

1. *Legionella* is a recently discovered respiratory pathogen. It is a gram-negative aerobic bacillus that is easily recovered from aqueous environments. There are currently 24 species comprising 39 serogroups.

2. The most important mechanism of transmission of *Legionella* to humans is via aerosols. The compromised patient is most susceptible to infection.

3. *Legionella* is an intracellular parasite that can survive in the monocyte by preventing fusion of the phagosome with lysosomes.

4. *Legionella* are able to damage respiratory tissue, but what factors are involved are not known. Infections resemble bronchopneumonia and can be fatal if not treated. Extrapulmonary disease is seen primarily in immunosuppressed patients.

5. Laboratory diagnosis of *Legionella* is best accomplished by recovery of the pathogen in culture. *Legionella* does not grow on ordinary media and special media such as BYCE-a with supplements and selective agents are required for recovery of the organism. Use of indirect immunofluorescence is the most used serological technique for identifying changes in serum antibody during infection. Direct immunofluorescence or DNA probes can be used to detect bacterial antigen or nucleic acid, respectively, in clinical specimens.

6. Erythromycin is the drug of choice in treatment of *Legionella* pneumonia.

7. Several miscellaneous pathogens that cause disease in humans are outlined in Table 29-1.

QUESTIONS FOR STUDY

Select the best response or responses for each of the following:

1. Which of the following characterizes *Legionella pneumophila*?
   A. It can be transmitted by aerosols.
   B. It is an aerobic bacillus.
   C. It produces respiratory illness.
   D. It is sensitive to erythromycin.

2. The following laboratory characteristics of *L. pneumophila* are true *except*
   A. It is fastidious in its growth requirements.
   B. It is gram-negative.
   C. Colonies resemble cut glass.
   D. Colonies appear within 24 hours following incubation.

3. The species that is an inhabitant of the oral cavity and pits agar is
   A. *Streptobacillus moniliformis*
   B. *Gardnerella vaginalis*
   C. *Eikenella corrodens*
   D. *Chromobacterium hominis*

4. The organism that is the cause of an infrequently described sexually transmitted disease is
   A. *Calymmatobacterium granulomatis*

   B. *Gardnerella vaginalis*
   C. *Cardiobacterium hominis*
   D. *Streptobacillus moniliformis*

5. The organism that is transmitted by the bite of a rat is
   A. *Actinobacillus actinomycetemcomitans*
   B. *Streptobacillus moniliformis*
   C. *Eikenella corrodens*
   D. *Capnocytophaga* species

ADDITIONAL READINGS

Fraser, D. W. Potable water as a source of legionellosis. *Environ. Health Perspect.* 62:337, 1985.

Grace, C. J., Levitz, R. E., Katz-Pollak, H., and Brettman, L. R. *Actinobacillus actinomycetomitans* prosthetic valve endocarditis. *Rev. Infect. Dis.* 10(5)L922, 1988.

Kaufman, R. H. The origin and diagnosis of "nonspecific vaginitis." *N. Engl. J. Med.* 303:637, 1980.

Parenti, D. M., and Snydam, D. R. *Capnocytophaga* species: Infection in nonimmunocompromised and immunocompromised hosts. *J. Infect. Dis.* 151-(1):140, 1985.

Reingold, A. L., et al. Legionella pneumonia in the United States: The distribution of serogroups and species causing human illness. *J. Infect. Dis.* 149:819, 1984.

Stoloff, A. L., and Gillies, M. L. Infections with *Eikenella corrodens* in a general hospital: A report of 33 cases. *Rev. Infect. Dis.* 8(1):50, 1986.

Winn, W. C., Jr. Legionnaires' disease: Historical perspective. *Clin. Microbiol. Rev.* 11(1):60, 1988.

VI. VIROLOGY

30. VIRUSES

OBJECTIVES

To outline the steps and mechanisms involved in the infection of a host cell by animal and bacterial viruses

To list the cytopathic effects on host cells following viral infection

To explain the mechanisms by which viruses transform mammalian cells

To outline the effects of viral transformation on mammalian cells

To explain which DNA and RNA viruses are thought to cause cancer in humans

To outline the techniques used in the cultivation and/or identification of animal viruses

To list the principal viral chemotherapeutic agents and the diseases for which they are prescribed

To describe the component parts of the T4 bacterial virus and their function in the infectious process

To compare and contrast the infection process by temperate and lytic bacterial viruses

To compare and contrast the processes of restricted and generalized transduction carried out by bacterial viruses

Until the latter half of the nineteenth century, it was believed that certain mammalian infectious agents, capable of passing through porcelain bacterial filters and microscopically unobservable, were merely small forms of bacteria. The fact that these so-called bacteria could not be cultivated on any laboratory medium only implied that they were fastidious in their requirements and that their nutritional needs had not been discovered. After the turn of the century some scientists proposed that these submicroscopic agents were a subcellular form of life and called them *viruses*. About 1915 it was discovered that even bacteria were subject to disease and that the infectious agent resembled in many ways the mammalian viruses. The bacterial invaders were called *bacteriophages* or simply *phages*. Not until the advent of the electron microscope and other technological advances were many of the hypotheses concerning these viruses either substantiated or discarded. In the past 40 years a mass of information concerning viral structure and physiology has been forthcoming. A virus is now defined as a *subcellular agent, consisting of a core of nucleic acid surrounded by a protein coat that must use the metabolic machinery of a living host to replicate and produce more viral particles.*

We will begin our discussion of animal viruses

and then conclude with a brief discussion of bacterial viruses.

ANIMAL VIRUSES

STRUCTURE AND COMPOSITION

Morphology

Animal virus morphology can be divided into two important types on the basis of how the nucleic acid is packaged: *rod-like*, or *helical*, and *spherical*, or *isometric*. The nucleic acid of the virus is surrounded by a specific geometric array of protein molecules that form a coat called the *capsid*. The capsid itself is made up of identical subunits called *capsomeres*. When the protein subunits bind in a periodic way along the nucleic acid, a helical shape is produced. The helical shape is frequently observed as a rod containing flexible coils. The tobacco mosaic virus is a plant virus having a helical or rod shape similar to helical animal viruses (Fig. 30-1). In spherical viruses the nucleic acid, which is condensed within the virus, is independent of the organization of protein subunits surrounding it. The capsid surrounding the nucleic acid of spherical viruses has icosahedral (20-sided object) symmetry. Most animal viruses, such as the adenoviruses (Fig. 30-2) exhibit icosahedral symmetry. When electron micrographs of spherical viruses are observed the capsomeres are readily visible. The capsid together with the nucleic acid form what is called the *nucleocapsid*. As you will soon discover, many nucleocapsids with helical symmetry are surrounded by other structures that protect them. The poxviruses exhibit a combination of both helical and spherical symmetry and are referred to as *complex*. Complex symmetry is more characteristic of bacterial viruses.

Animal viruses range in size from 25 to 30 nm for smaller viruses, such as the poliovirus, to 225 to 300 nm for the poxviruses.

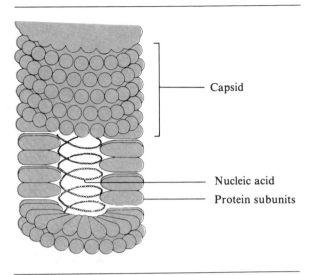

Fig. 30-1. Tobacco mosaic virus, a helical virus that infects plants.

Nucleic Acids

The nucleic acid of the animal virus is either DNA or RNA and may be single- or double-stranded. Most viral nucleic acids are linear molecules, but the papovavirus DNA is an exception to this rule and is circular. The molecular weight of animal virus nucleic acids ranges from 1.5 to 3 $\times 10^6$ for picornaviruses to 1 to 2 $\times 10^8$ for the largest viruses, the poxviruses. Some viruses also have segmented genomes. The reoviruses and rotaviruses consist of 10 and 11 segments, respectively. The genomes of the influenza viruses, bunyaviruses, and arenaviruses are also segmented. One of the consequences of this segmentation is that genetic recombination can occur more efficiently than in unsegmented viral genomes. Thus, strains of these viruses may demonstrate considerable antigenic variability (see page 695).

Lipids

Many nucleocapsids are surrounded by an *envelope* of lipid that mimics the composition of the cytoplasmic membrane of the infected host (Fig. 30-3). The lipid envelope is a bilayered structure

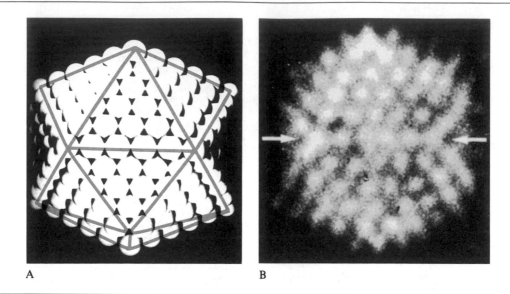

A   B

Fig. 30-2. Icosahedral symmetry. A. Model of capsid exhibiting icosahedral symmetry. Colored line outlines the various facets of the icosahedron. B. Negatively stained adenovirus particle showing the arrangement of capsomeres. (From R. W. Horne and P. Wildy, *Br. Med. Bull.* 18:199, 1962.)

that acts as a protective device for the nucleo-capsid. If the envelope is removed, the virus loses its infectivity. Various proteins may be associated with the lipid envelope and these are discussed in the next section. The envelope viruses are outlined in Tables 30-4 and 30-5 at the end of the animal virus section.

Proteins

In addition to the structural proteins that make up the capsid there are other proteins that have enzymatic as well as structural functions. Some enveloped viruses have nucleocapsids that are tightly enclosed within an assembly of proteins called a *viral core* (Fig. 30-3). The nucleocapsid or core in enveloped viruses is surrounded by a layer of protein called a *protein shell* (Fig. 30-3). The proteins that surround the core or nucleo-capsid are protective structures. Complex proteins, such as glycoproteins, are found on the surface of viral envelopes and are in the form of projections or *spikes* (also called *peplomers*).

Glycoprotein spikes are important as antigenic determinants, and some are involved in binding of virus to host tissue. One type of glycoprotein spike found on viruses, such as the influenza viruses, has the ability to agglutinate red blood cells and is called a *hemagluttinin spike*.

Enzymatic proteins are also found in or on viruses. Some viruses, such as the poxviruses, contain a DNA-dependent RNA polymerase, while RNA tumor viruses possess an RNA-dependent DNA polymerase. These enzymes and others are found in the core of the virus and they become active once the virus has invaded the cell and the capsid has been partially degraded. The influenza virus also possesses a surface spike, embedded in its lipid envelope, that has enzymatic activity. This surface spike exhibits *neuraminidase* activity. The neuraminidase spike is used by the virus to dissolve neuraminic acid, a component of the cytoplasmic membrane of mammalian cells. Neuraminidase activity enables the virus to spread in host tissue.

A completely assembled and infective virus is

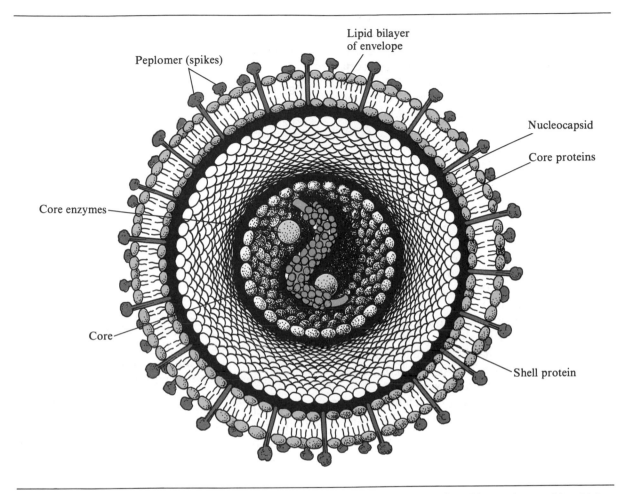

Fig. 30-3. Idealized structure of an enveloped helical virus as seen in cross-section. The nucleocapsid, which is helical, is itself encased in a core of structural protein molecules. The core may also contain enzymes that are used by the virus to replicate in the infected mammalian cell. The core may in turn be surrounded by an outer shell of structural proteins. Adjacent to the shell is an envelope, or lipid bilayer, within which are embedded glycoprotein spikes called peplomers.

called a *virion*. Defective or incompletely assembled viruses are usually noninfective; for example, enveloped viruses without their envelope are noninfective. If you do not know whether a virus is infective it is referred to as a *viral particle*.

EPIDEMIOLOGY AND PHYSIOLOGY OF ANIMAL VIRUS INFECTION

Viruses enter the mammalian host primarily via the respiratory tract, gastrointestinal tract, direct inoculation by arthropods into the bloodstream, or breaks in the skin.* These routes of viral transfer from one individual to another are called routes of *horizontal transmission*. Viruses can also be transferred from parent to offspring—for example, from the blood of an infected mother through the placenta. This type of transfer is

* Tables outlining the viral diseases affecting specific tissues and organs are found in Appendix A.

called *vertical transmission*. Viruses have specific target cells (tissue tropisms) in which they will replicate; however, not all viruses are created equal. Viruses have an affinity for certain cells and this seems to be based on the chemical composition of the viral surface and the cytoplasmic membrane of the host cell. Some viruses are very selective in the type of host they will infect. For example, the poliovirus and measles virus infect only humans. Viruses such as the rabies virus are relatively nonspecific and can infect several different animal species, including humans. Even the rabies virus will not infect all animals. Occasionally viral strains that are specific for one host may undergo mutation and expand their host range. For example, outbreaks of human influenza have been associated with individuals working with influenza-infected swine. The swine-associated virus apparently underwent a mutation that altered a surface protein, thereby making it capable of infecting human cells. Once the host has been invaded, the infection process can be broken down into five stages: *adsorption, penetration and uncoating, genome expression, maturation and assembly,* and *release*.

Adsorption

The host cell invaded by virus possesses many *receptors* which are dispersed over its surface. The number of receptors may be from 10^4 to 10^5 per cell and are probably major determinants in susceptibility to infection. Most cell receptors appear to be glycoproteins whose composition varies from one cell type to another. The influenza virus, for example, uses its neuraminidase-containing glycoprotein spikes to adhere to the neuraminic acid–containing glycoprotein receptors on the cell membrane. Sometimes the binding process alters the virus. When some viruses bind to cell receptors there is apparently a rearrangement of capsid proteins and this is believed to enable viral nucleic acid to be released from the capsid. Once virus has adsorbed to the cell membrane, its infectivity is lost. This period of loss

of infectivity is called the *eclipse* and is due to partial or total uncoating of the virus, as discussed in the next section.

Penetration and Uncoating

We are not sure how most virions enter the cell. There are believed to be three major mechanisms of viral entry and a single virus may use more than one mechanism:

1. Endocytosis. Virus binds to specific receptors on the cell membrane surface. Virus-receptor complexes are concentrated in pits, which invaginate to form vesicles (Fig. 30-4A). As these vesicles move deeper into the cytoplasm they fuse with lysosomes to produce a *lysosomal vesicle*. Lysosomal enzymes digest away the viral layers and release the nucleocapsid into the cytoplasm.
2. Fusion. Some enveloped viruses gain access to the cytoplasm of the cell by fusing with the cytoplasmic membrane. Fusion produces an opening through which the nucleocapsid may pass directly into the cytoplasm (Fig. 30-4B).
3. Direct penetration. Some nonenveloped viruses may be so small that they are able to pass directly through the cytoplasmic membrane and enter the cytoplasm (Fig. 30-4C). It is possible that the attachment process disrupts the capsid so that uncoating takes place.

Depending on the site of viral multiplication, viral nucleocapsids may be uncoated in the cytoplasm or enter the nucleus to be uncoated. For example, the nucleocapsid of the adenovirus is uncoated near the nuclear pores, with viral DNA penetrating into the nucleus, but for other viruses uncoating appears to occur in the nucleus. Most viral uncoating occurs in the cytoplasm. Once uncoating occurs, the viral nucleic acid is released and ready to be expressed.

Genome Expression

Viral genomes are so diverse—that is, they may be single-stranded, they may contain RNA or

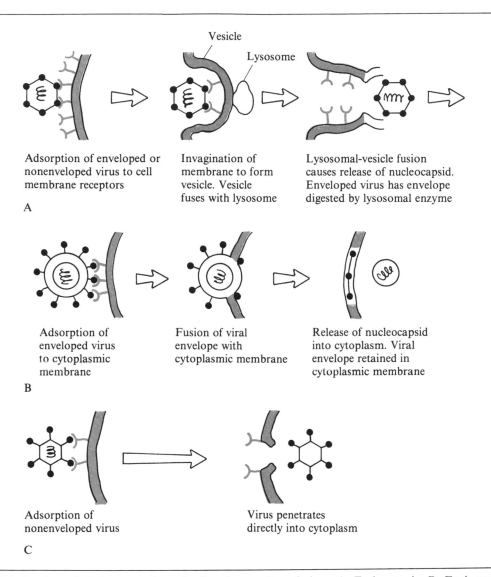

Fig. 30-4. Mechanism of viral penetration of cell and uncoating of virus. A. Endocytosis. B. Fusion with cytoplasmic membrane. C. Direct penetration.

DNA, or they may be segmented or nonsegmented—that describing the various mechanisms for transcribing them can be confusing. The pattern of animal virus expression can be divided into six classes (Fig. 30-5). For each class keep in mind that two functions must be fulfilled. First, a strand of the genome will be utilized in the formation of messenger RNA (expressed as having plus [+] polarity) that will be translated into specific viral proteins. Many of these proteins will be used as enzymes in the replication of viral nucleic acid while others will be used for assembly

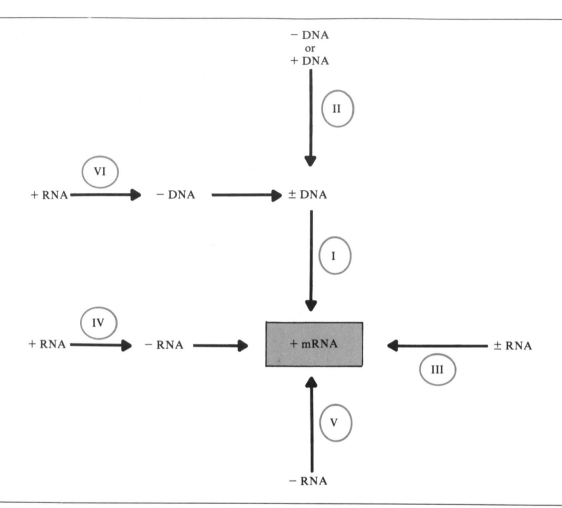

Fig. 30-5. Virus classes depicting the expression of various virus genomes. Regardless of the polarity of the viral genome a process is utilized to produce viral mRNA that has plus (+) polarity. The template for (+) mRNA synthesis in each case is a minus (−) strand of nucleic acid. (From D. Baltimore, *Bacteriol. Rev.* 35:235, 1971.)

of new virus. Second, to replicate the viral nucleic acid so that each viral particle produced in the infected cell will contain a genome.

Expression of DNA Genomes. Except for the poxviruses, replication of DNA viruses occurs in the nucleus. Most DNA viruses contain a double-stranded molecule (*Class I*) in which a minus strand is transcribed into mRNA by the enzyme RNA polymerase. Both DNA strands are repli-

cated to produce plus (+) and minus (−) strands that form double-stranded molecules as genomes for new viral particles (Fig. 30-5).

Single-stranded DNA viruses (family Parvoviridae) belong to *Class II*. The viral genome is converted to a double-stranded replicative form, from which mRNA can be produced as well as DNA replicas for use as viral genomes.

Expression of RNA Genomes. Double-stranded

(±) RNA viruses (*Class III*) include the reovirus and rotavirus, both of which possess segmented genomes. Each of the double-stranded segments is transcribed into single-stranded mRNA. The mRNAs are translated into protein. Each of the double-stranded segments is also replicated to produce progeny RNA (Fig. 30-6A).

Plus (+)-stranded RNA viruses (*Class IV*) include the families Picornaviridae and Togaviridae. Since the viral genome has the same polarity as mRNA, the naked RNA can by itself initiate infection in the host. The viral genome is translated into proteins, some of which aid in the transcription of the genome into a *minus-strand replicative complex*, from which positive strands can be produced (Fig. 30-6B). The newly synthesized plus strands become the genomes of new viral particles.

Minus (−)-stranded RNA viruses (*Class V*) include Orthomyxoviridae, Paramyxoviridae, and Rhabdoviridae. The viral genome is used as a template for transcription into mRNA (Fig. 30-6C). The mRNA is translated into protein and is also used to produce minus-strand replicas, which will become the genomes of new viral particles.

Some RNA viruses have a DNA intermediate (*Class VI*) and this is characteristic of the family Retroviridae or those viruses that cause tumors (Fig. 30-6D). Retroviruses possess an RNA genome containing two identical positive strands. A minus strand of DNA is produced with the aid of an unusual enzyme called *reverse transcriptase* (an RNA-dependent DNA polymerase). In other words, the reaction (RNA → DNA) is the reverse to the usual flow of information in the cell (DNA → RNA). The minus DNA strand binds to a plus RNA strand to produce an RNA-DNA hybrid. The RNA in the hybrid is later degraded and the DNA acts as a template for formation of double-stranded DNA. The DNA can be transcribed into mRNA and is also replicated to form plus (+) RNA strands, which will provide the genetic material for a new generation of virus (see page 634, Oncogenic Viruses, for a more detailed discussion of these viruses).

Maturation and Assembly

The maturation of viruses can be viewed as a growth cycle (even though viruses do not grow like other infectious agents) during which viral nucleic acids and proteins are produced. As stated previously, after adsorption there is a period, called *eclipse*, during which no new viral particles can be detected (Fig. 30-7). During this period of growth *early proteins* are synthesized. Some proteins are used to inhibit host function, with the degree of inhibition depending on the virus and host cell involved. Many proteins, such as DNA and RNA polymerase, are synthesized in the early period that is used to produce viral genomes. The very small viruses do not possess enough genetic information to synthesize nucleic acid polymerases and must use the enzymes of the host cell. The synthesis of viral nucleic acids may occur in the cytoplasm or nucleus depending on the final site of viral assembly. Even during the period of early protein synthesis proteins to be used late in the maturation process are also produced. These *late proteins* are primarily structural and are used in the construction of the capsid.

As the concentration of structural proteins increases capsid assembly begins and there is formation of nucleocapsids. Nucleocapsids of most DNA viruses are assembled in the nucleus while most RNA-containing nucleocapsids are assembled in the cytoplasm. Despite the site of nucleocapsid assembly the viral proteins are always synthesized on ribosomes in the cytoplasm.

The assembly of viruses is an autocatalytic process based primarily on interaction of capsid polypeptides. During assembly of virus large quasicrystalline arrays are produced that are microscopically observable in the nucleus or cytoplasm (Fig. 30-8).

Release

Some nonenveloped viruses are released from the cell only after the cell has disintegrated and thus no specific mechanism for release is involved.

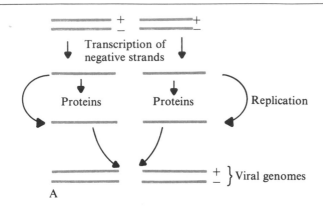

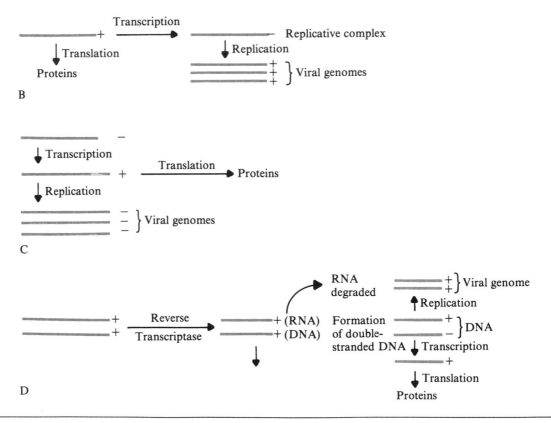

Fig. 30-6. Replication mechanisms for RNA viruses. A. Double-stranded RNA ($\pm$) virus. B. Plus ($+$)-strand RNA virus. C. Minus ($-$)-strand RNA virus. D. Identical positive-strand RNA virus.

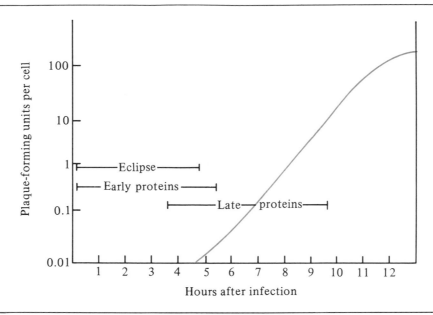

Fig. 30-7. Growth cycle of animal virus. Mature particles do not make their appearance until nearly 5 hours after infection. The maximum number of virus particles appear about 12 hours after infection. The time periods will vary from one virus to another.

The release of enveloped virus is more complex because, in addition to the capsid, an envelope must be acquired. The lipid bilayer of the viral envelope can be acquired from the host's membrane system, that is, the nuclear membrane, if the nucleocapsid is assembled in the nucleus, or cytoplasmic membrane if the nucleocapsid is assembled in the cytoplasm. The viral envelope, however, also possesses glycoprotein spikes that are encoded by the virus. If the cell membrane is to be used as a viral envelope it must undergo reorganization. What happens is that protein of the glycoprotein is synthesized on the endoplasmic reticulum. Sugars are added to the protein in the endoplasmic reticulum and then the glycosylated protein is transported to the Golgi, where it undergoes further modification. The viral glycoprotein is transported to and inserted into the cell membrane. The viral nucleocapsid makes contact with the patch of cell membrane containing viral glycoproteins. This causes the membrane to protrude and it literally encloses the nucleocapsid. The enveloped nucleocapsid then pinches off or *buds* from the cell membrane (Fig. 30-9). The cell membrane beneath the bud reforms and the continuity of the cell membrane is retained.

The multiplication cycle for animal viruses varies from 6 to 8 hours for the poliovirus to 24 to 48 hours for release of the adenovirus from the infected cell.

EFFECTS OF VIRAL INFECTION ON THE HOST CELL

Despite all the research on viral infection over the past 80 years, we still know very little about how viruses damage host cells. It seems logical that if a virus is to survive it must engage in an association with one or more of its hosts in such a way that the host is not killed. Viruses replicate

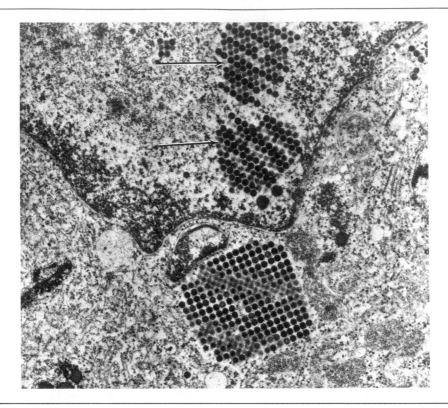

Fig. 30-8. Electron micrograph (×30,000) of quasicrystalline accumulations of adenovirus. Two accumulations of virus appear in nucleus (*arrows*) and one is free in the cytoplasm. (From R. Wigand, H. Gelderbloom, and H. Brandis, *Arch. Virol.* 64:225, 1980.)

only in living cells! Some viruses appear to replicate in cells of the infected host without causing any obvious damage while other viruses bring about a variety of changes, which may be lethal to the cells they infect. These alterations are referred to as *cytopathic effects (CPE)*. Let us examine some of the ways in which viral infection affects host cells.

Direct and Indirect Damage

Some viruses are able to shut down host macromolecule synthesis and thus directly damage host cells. The damaged cells lyse and this cytopathic effect can be detected in the laboratory by the formation of lesions on cultured cells (see Cultivation of Viruses). Lysis of infected cells in vivo may result in temporary or permanent loss of function. For example, during poliovirus infection motor neuron involvement can cause loss of function of the corresponding muscles. As yet no viral toxin has been discovered for any viruses but the accumulation of capsid proteins may be sufficient to produce cytopathic effects.

Some virus infections indirectly affect the function of tissues or organs in the host. This effect is illustrated during influenza virus infection. The influenza virus damages the respiratory epithelium and ciliary activity is severely affected. This results in the accumulation of bacteria that normally would be eliminated by ciliary action. Bacteria, such as staphylococci, streptococci, and hemophili, adhere to respiratory tissue, multiply, and cause disease. Thus, death

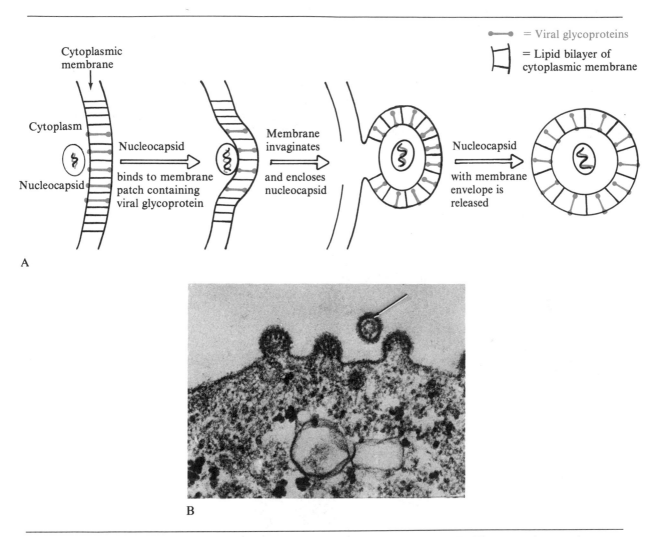

Fig. 30-9. Budding process for enveloped viruses. A. Diagrammatic illustration. B. Electron micrograph (×86,000) showing a budded virus (*arrow*) and three viruses in various stages of budding. (From E. Norby, H. Marusky, and L. Orvell, *J. Virol.* 6:237, 1979.)

from influenza is often due to pneumonia caused by *Staphylococcus aureus*, *Streptococcus pneumoniae*, or *Hemophilus* species. Another example of the indirect effect of viral infection is the AIDS virus, which affects immune cells. The virus brings about immunological changes that result in the patient's dying from infections caused by other infectious agents (see page 717 for a discussion of AIDS).

Inclusion Body Formation

The replication of virus in the cytoplasm or nucleus of infected cells often results in the accumulation of viral as well as cellular products. These accumulations, which may be nucleic acids, proteins, etc., can be stained and are referred to as *inclusion bodies*. For example, the quasicrystalline arrays of virus observed in Figure 30-8 are inclusion bodies. Some inclusion bodies are so distinctive that their presence is diagnostic (referred to as *pathognomonic effect*). Rabies virus inclusions, called Negri bodies, for example, are of diagnostic value (Plate 18).

Cell Fusion (Syncytia Formation)

Enveloped viruses, such as the herpesvirus, paramyxoviruses, and the AIDS virus release specific proteins that become incorporated into the cytoplasmic membrane of the infected cell. These proteins act like magnets on the infected cell and attract uninfected cells to their surface. This results in infection of the originally uninfected cell and this process is repeated until a large collection of infected cells is formed. Eventually the cells fuse, producing a giant multinucleated cell or *syncytium* (Fig. 30-10).

Changes in Surface Antigens

During viral infection there are changes in the antigenic character of the surface of the infected cell. One change, discussed previously, that is always found during infection by enveloped viruses is due to incorporation of virus-specified glycoproteins into the cytoplasmic membrane. Nonenveloped viruses also code for proteins that are associated with the cell surface. These viral-specified proteins induce both humoral and cell-mediated immunity in the host. Some of these virus-specified proteins will be discussed later.

Interferon Production

In cell cultures and whole animals, soon after infection, some cells produce a protein that has the ability to prevent the infection of healthy cells by the same virus. This protein, called *interferon*, is an important host defense mechanism, and was discussed in Chapter 11.

Persistent Viral Infection

Up to now we have discussed the effects of acute viral disease, that is, virus replication accom-

Fig. 30-10. Syncytium of giant multinucleated cell caused by viral infection. Several cells can be seen to be enclosed by a single membrane producing a giant cell. Arrow points to an inclusion body. (Courtesy H. M. Yamashiroya, Department of Pathology, University of Illinois Medical Center, Chicago.)

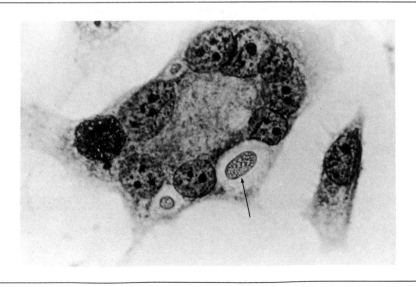

panied by cell damage. The intracellular location of viruses permits them to remain as cellular occupants for prolonged periods of time. This phenomenon, which is referred to as *persistence*, allows virus to remain undetected and safe from immune forces that exist outside the cell. The mechanisms for viral persistence follow.

1. *Virus-produced defective-interfering particles*. During viral infection some viral particles are produced that are defective. The defective particles have the ability to prevent multiplication of complete virus. For example, the disease subacute sclerosing panencephalitis (SSPE) is a late sequela of measles virus infection. The virus appears to be defective in its ability to bud from infected cells.

2. *Integration of the viral genome into the host genome*. DNA viruses can insert their genome into host DNA. As a consequence, the virus replicates only when the cell divides. For RNA viruses, integration of the viral genome requires the formation of a DNA intermediate (Class VI RNA virus, see page 623). Integration of the viral genome is the ultimate mechanism of escape from immune forces. The integrated virus can persist for months or several years until it becomes reactivated by release from the host genome. This reactivation can result in active viral production accompanied by disease symptoms. Several viruses that integrate into the host genome can cause the malignant state, a process called *transformation*, which is discussed at length on page 630.

3. *Thwarting immune responses*. Some viruses escape immune defenses by interfering with immune responses or by not inducing an effective immune response. The cytomegalovirus elicits a late antibody response in the infected host, thereby allowing persistence to be maintained. Viruses such as the rabies virus infect neural cells that are not accessible to antibody. Viruses such as the AIDS virus undergo mutation in the host, thereby changing their antigenic characteristics. Viruses such as the hepatitis B virus release antigens that inactivate immune cells. Viruses such

as the herpes simplex virus invade lymphoid tissue and this can lead to suppression of the immune system.

Persistent infections can be divided into three types: *latent, chronic,* and *slow*. Latent infections are those in which the virus persists in a nonreplicating state or at an undetectable, possibly intermittent, level of replication. Clinical symptoms may or may not be evident during latent infection. Herpesviruses, such as the cytomegalovirus and the herpes simplex virus, are noted for causing latent infections. Herpes simplex virus, for example, causes a latent infection that is expressed in the form of intermittent cold sores. Chronic infections are those in which the virus causes cytolysis, but symptoms are subclinical and do not impair organ function. Hepatitis caused by hepatitis B virus and rubella caused by rubella virus are examples of chronic infections. Slow persistent infections are those in which there is a long incubation period (years) and the virus continues to multiply, albeit slowly, causing a protracted and continued destruction of tissue. An example of a slow virus disease in humans is kuru (*see Slow Virus Diseases in Chapter 31*). Major groups of viruses that cause persistent infections are presented in Table 30-1.

VIRUSES AND CANCER

Cancer can be defined as a malignant growth or tumor resulting from the transformation of cells that demonstrate unrestricted growth. Since cancer has never been shown to be contagious, it is hard to see how this disease could be due to an infectious agent. Cancer in humans is usually caused by chemical or physical agents. Early in the twentieth century, investigators Shope, Rous, and Bittner, among others, demonstrated that in animals viral agents are responsible for some neoplasms (abnormal growth of tissue). There was no reason to believe, however, that viruses might be involved in human cancer until 1951, when Gross discovered that a mouse leu-

Table 30-1. Viruses Causing Persistent Infections in Humans

Viral agent	Disease	Effect on host cell
Rubella virus	Fetal anomalies and panencephalitis	Inhibition of cell division
Measles virus	Subacute sclerosing panencephalitis	Cytolysis
Human papillomavirus	Warts	Transformation
Hepatitis B virus	Hepatitis	Immunopathology
Herpes simplex virus types 1 and 2	Herpes	Cytolysis
Varicella-zoster virus	Zoster (shingles)	Cytolysis
Cytomegalovirus	Mononucleosis	Cytolysis
Epstein-Barr virus	Mononucleosis, Burkitt's lymphoma	Transformation
Kuru virus	Kuru (encephalopathy)	Cytolysis
Creutzfeldt-Jakob virus*	Creutzfeldt-Jakob disease (encephalopathy)	Cytolysis
JC virus	Leukoencephalopathy	Transformation
BK virus	?	None
Adenovirus	?	None

* Creutzfeldt-Jakob disease has recently been demonstrated to be caused by an infectious agent (prion) that does not possess a nucleic acid (see Slow Virus Diseases, Chapter 31).
Source: Adapted from N. Nathanson, D. Schlessinger (eds.), *Microbiology—1977*. Washington, D.C.: American Society for Microbiology, 1977.

kemia induced by an animal virus was very similar to the leukemia that afflicts humans. Since Gross's discovery, scientists the world over have been actively attempting to determine the association between viruses and human cancer. We now know that the human T-lymphotrophic viruses (HTLVs) are causes of certain leukemias and lymphomas in humans. One of the members of HTLV is the cause of acquired immune deficiency syndrome (AIDS), a disease that predisposes its patients to cancers (see page 717).

Viruses classified as tumor viruses may be able to induce tumors, when injected into experimental animals, or to transform cells maintained in culture. Tumor-initiating viruses are called *oncogenic viruses*. Some of these viruses can cause cancer in native animal species under natural circumstances while others must be manipulated in the laboratory to produce the desired effect. Before we discuss the various types of tumor viruses, let us first examine what happens to cells to make them malignant—that is, the properties of transformed cells.

Properties of Transformed Cells

Both DNA and RNA viruses are able to induce tumors in experimental animals. In each instance the tumor cell is transformed and acquires properties that make it distinct from uninfected cells, or infected cells in which tumors are not produced. Depending on the virus and the cell type involved, these transformation properties are quite variable. Some important properties of transformed cells are:

1. The viral nucleic acid becomes integrated into or closely associated with the genome of the cell, and the cell does not lyse.
2. The transformed cells are rounder than normal cells and show irregular patterns of orientation in cell culture (Fig. 30-11).
3. Transformed cells lose the property of contact inhibition (density-dependent growth) and show a loss of growth-inhibiting ability. Changes in the growth patterns of certain transformed cells cause them to form colonies in soft agar. This is a property that permits the

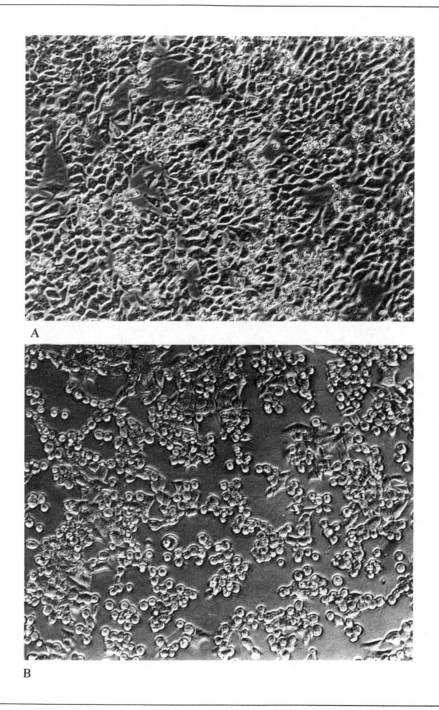

A

B

Fig. 30-11. Transformation of a cell culture by cytomegalovirus. A. Uninfected control. B. Infected culture. (From J. F. Baskar, S. C. Stanat, and E. Huang, *Infect. Immun.* 40:726, 1983.)

investigator to select transformed from untransformed cells.

4. Some transformed cells can produce tumors when injected into susceptible animals. Whether the tumors are benign or malignant is dependent on the transformed cell used and the type of host being challenged.

5. After transformation, a virus-specific antigen appears on the surface of many tumor cells. It is called the *tumor-specific transplantation antigen (TSTA)*. Other antigens may also appear on the surface of the cell that make it recognizable by the host's immune system. These surface antigens may be host- or virus-specified.

6. Chromosomal abnormalities, including breakage of some chromosomes and duplication of others, appear after cellular transformation.

7. Several changes occur in the cytoplasmic membrane of transformed cells. One of the earliest changes involves the permeability mechanism. Transformed cells are more permeable to metabolites, such as sugars, than are normal cells. Chemical changes in the membrane involving lipid, carbohydrate, and glycoprotein composition may occur. These changes are not uniform but vary depending on the composition of the growth medium and the growth rate of the cells.

8. The agglutinability of cells by certain glycoproteins called *lectins* or *agglutinins* is altered in transformed cells. The sources of lectins include plant seeds (wheat germ, jack bean), snails, and crabs. Transformed cells are agglutinated more readily by lectins because of alteration of the lectin-binding sites.

Oncogenic DNA Viruses

There are five families of oncogenic DNA viruses: polyomaviruses, papillomaviruses, adenoviruses, herpesviruses, and hepatitis B virus (HBV). A general scheme of the events that occur when a cell is transformed by a DNA virus is illustrated in Figure 30-12. It should be pointed out that it is not necessary for the viral genome to integrate into the host genome to cause transformation. Many transforming DNA genomes remain outside the host chromosome as episomes and in some instances only the transforming genes appear to be integrated into the host genome.

The HBV, a herpesvirus, and some strains of papilloma virus are considered as likely causes of cancer. It should be noted that none of the DNA viruses can cause cancer by themselves and other factors, in conjunction with presence of virus, are involved.

Hepatitis B Virus (HBV). As many as 300 million people, most of them in Asia, are carriers of HBV. The carrier's risk of acquiring liver cancer is 100 times greater than that of a noncarrrier. Unlike other oncoviruses, HBV does not appear to carry transforming genes. It is believed that the HBV inserts its DNA into the DNA of liver cells and establishes a persistent infection in the host. An immune attack on virus-infected cells causes liver damage. Liver cells divide to regenerate damaged tissue. The repeated cycles of liver cell regeneration may increase the opportunity for carcinogenic mutations to occur. These mutations may lead to abnormal liver cell growth by affecting the cell's normal growth-inhibiting functions.

Herpesviruses. The Epstein-Barr virus is the only herpesvirus that is currently believed to be associated with certain neoplasms. The EBV has an affinity for lymphocytes and is capable of transforming them from end stage to immortal cells with unlimited life spans. The virus was first identified by Epstein and Barr in the early 1960s in cultured lymphoid cells from patients afflicted with Burkitt's lymphoma (this rare disease, endemic in certain areas of Africa, is a cancer of the lymphoid system and affects primarily children).

Early prospective studies of children in Uganda showed elevated titers of antibody to the EBV even before the onset of overt disease.

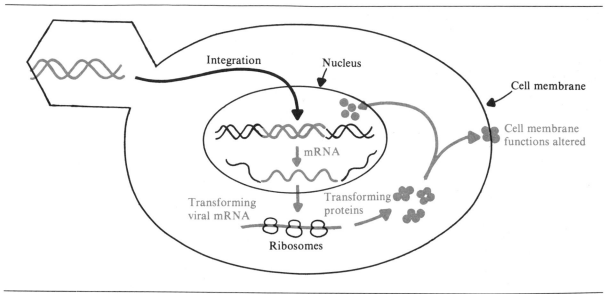

Fig. 30-12. Events that lead to transformation of animal cells by oncogenic DNA virus. Virus infects cell and viral DNA is integrated into host genome. Viral DNA is transcribed into mRNA, a small portion of which contains transforming genes. Transforming genes code for proteins that affect cell membrane and genome function.

Thus, a possible association between EBV and Burkitt's lymphoma was established. There are basically three steps in the pathogenesis of Burkitt's lymphoma:

1. EBV infection induces nonmalignant polyclonal B-cell proliferation.
2. There is T-cell immunodeficiency with B-cell proliferation.
3. Translocations occur in the chromosomes of proliferating B-cells, which affect B-cell differentiation. The genetically altered B-cell outgrows normal cells as the result of enhanced growth and resistance to T-cell surveillance.

EBV is also linked to a rare nasopharyngeal cancer that occurs among adults, primarily in southern China. The evidence that has linked EBV to Burkitt's lymphoma and nasopharyngeal cancer are:

1. In both malignancies EBV-specific membrane antigens have been demonstrated. The protein product encoded by EBV has been detected in the nuclei of infected cells. The nuclear protein of EBV has not been found in cells from other cancers or related malignancies.
2. EBV DNA is always found in malignant tissue from patients with Burkitt's lymphoma and nasopharyngeal cancer. Multiple copies of the EBV genome appear in some of the cells.
3. Cancers have been induced in laboratory animals with EBV-containing materials. The cancer produced is almost identical to that occurring in humans and further implicates EBV as a tumorigenic agent.

In the United States approximately 80 percent of the population have acquired antibody against the EBV with no apparent symptoms from infection. EBV infection seems to produce no symptoms in infants, but in some adolescents and young adults it may lead to infectious mononucleosis (see page 677). Infection is therefore accompanied by the presence of high antibody titers throughout life.

Human Papillomaviruses (HPV). Human papillomaviruses consist of 16 distinct types, which cause a variety of lesions including warts involving the hands and other body sites and warts and papillomas involving the genitalia. The HPV are strong candidates as etiological agents of cancer since they are the only viruses proven to induce tumors (warts and papillomas) in humans. In addition, some papillomas are known to convert to carcinomas.

There appears to be a strong association of HPV with cervical tumors. In some studies the DNA of HPV types 16 and 18 have been found in over 60 percent of the cervical tumors examined. The incidence of genital warts, the incidence of cervical cancer, and the mortality from cervical cancers have increased markedly over the past 20 years. The increase in sexual promiscuity that has occurred during this period provides some circumstantial evidence that there may indeed be a direct link between HPV and some cervical cancers.

Oncogenic RNA Viruses

General Characteristics of Oncogenic RNA Viruses. The oncogenic RNA viruses belong to a group of viruses called *retroviruses* (Table 30-2). Retroviruses are infectious for many mammalian hosts and birds. As briefly described on page 623, retroviruses are a class VI group of viruses in terms of their mode of replication. They produce a double-stranded DNA intermediate with the aid of the enzyme reverse transcriptase. It is the DNA intermediate that is integrated into the host genome as a *provirus*. Once the provirus is integrated into the cellular genome, several pathways are possible:

1. Protected within the genome of the host cell, the provirus may duplicate when the cell DNA duplicates. If the infected cell is a germ cell, the progeny of the host will also carry the provirus; thus vertical transmission may occur.
2. Under certain circumstances, the provirus may become activated and excised from the host genome. In this event new virus particles can be produced that may infect adjacent cells and tissue; that is, horizontal transmission occurs.
3. Under other circumstances the provirus may also carry information that is oncogenic. If the oncogenic information is translated into specific products it may convert the cell into a tumor cell.

Oncogenic retroviruses, unlike other viruses, carry genes that are closely related to cellular genes. These genes are not important for viral replication but they enable the virus to bring about the transformation of the cells they infect.

Table 30-2. Classification of Human Retroviruses

Retrovirus	Classification	Associated pathology	Endemic area
Human T lymphotropic virus type 1 (HTLV-1)	Oncovirus	Adult T cell leukemia/lymphoma	Southeastern United States
HTLV-11	Oncovirus	T-cell hairy leukemia	England, New York (IV drug users)
Human immunodeficiency virus type 1 (HIV-1)	Lentivirus	Acquired immune deficiency syndrome (AIDS); AIDS-related complex (ARC)	Central Africa, Europe, United States
HIV-2	Lentivirus	AIDS	West Africa, Cape Verde
HTLV-V	Not yet classified	Sézary syndrome	Southern Italy

Table 30-3. A List of Some of the Known Oncogenes, Their Sources, and Their Function

Name of Oncogene	Source of retrovirus	Function of protein coded by oncogene
src	Chicken sarcoma	Protein kinase
abl	Mouse and human leukemia	Protein kinase
sis	Monkey sarcoma	Growth factor
Ha-ras	Rat and human sarcoma	Guanosine triphosphate binding
Ki-ras	Rat and human sarcoma	Guanosine triphosphate binding
myc	Chicken and human leukemia	DNA binding

The viral transforming genes are called *onco-genes*, or *v-onc*, while their cellular counterparts are called *c-onc*, or *proto-oncogenes*. Each onc gene is given a trivial three-letter name, for example, *src, ras, mos, fes,* etc. Over 20 v-onc genes have been identified and DNA sequences homologous to them have been identified in normal uninfected cells, including those of humans (Table 30-3).

Oncogenes and Transformation. Two of the most widely studied viral oncogenes are *v-src*, in which the source of the retrovirus is chicken sarcoma, and *v-ras*, in which the source is rat and human sarcoma. Viral oncogenes are nearly identical to their cellular counterparts and they perform equivalent functions in the cell. To better understand the relationship between viruses and cancer we need to answer two basic questions: (1) How do retroviruses obtain cellular information? And: (2) If the cellular proto-oncogenes perform normal functions in the cell, how is transformation induced?

During the infection process retroviruses integrate into the DNA of the cell and several copies of viral DNA may be integrated. It is believed that during the integration process a cellular gene becomes incorporated into the proviral genome (Fig. 30-13). When viral DNA replicates and new virus particles are produced each viral nucleic acid will possess a cellular gene, now called a viral onc-gene. Retroviruses carrying the v-onc gene can infect other cells and several copies of the oncogene can be inserted into the host genome at a site distant from the normal cellular gene site. How oncogenes transform cells is still very much a subject of speculation. The oncogenes that have been identified have also been analyzed in terms of the products they code for. Several of them code for amino acid kinases, some code for growth factors, and others code for DNA-binding proteins. The biological function of these products is still a mystery. Mutations apparently cause changes in the mechanisms of gene expression or changes in product structure that affect cell growth and cause tumor forma-

Fig. 30-13. Postulated mechanism for acquisition of cellular oncogene by retrovirus. A. Retrovirus integrated into cellular DNA (—) near cellular oncogene (c-onc). B. Recombinational event between cellular oncogene and proviral DNA results in copy of oncogene being inserted into proviral DNA. C. Proviral DNA deintegrated from cellular genome now carries viral version of oncogene, v-onc.

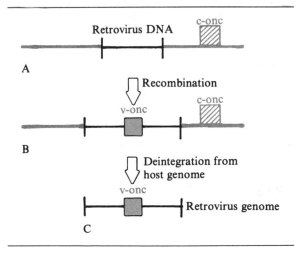

tion. For example, expression of the oncogene may be affected in such a way that its coded product gives the cell a selective growth advantage over other cells. If the c-onc gene has a mutation, the gene product could be altered so that growth is also affected. The altered product could be a regulatory molecule whose function is to turn on synthesis of a growth protein or turn off synthesis of a growth inhibitor. Activated oncogenes have been detected in human tumors. Researchers have shown that about 40 percent of the colon cancers removed from surgery contain active ras oncogenes. The ras protein, which is a mutated version of the normal protein, is produced along with normal protein. The ras proteins, however, are apparently dominant in their activity and bring about transformation.

The only RNA viruses known to cause cancer in humans are the retroviruses called *human T-lymphotropic viruses (HTLV)*. HTLV-I and HTLV-II are linked to human leukemia. The virus causing acquired immune deficiency syndrome (AIDS) is related to these viruses, but the AIDS virus only predisposes its victims to cancer (see Chapter 31).

The previous discussion implied that only mutation was necessary to activate oncogenes, but another mechanism may also be operating. The expression of genes can be affected by relocation, that is, movement of a gene from its normal location to another site on the chromosome. For example, when a c-onc gene is integrated into the virus genome the adjacent regulatory element, such as a promoter, may be different from the promoter adjacent to the proto-oncogene in a normal cell. When the viral DNA is inserted into the chromosome of an infected cell the v-onc gene may be expressed at a different rate from the proto-oncogene at its normal location, and transformation ensues (Fig. 30-14).

DIAGNOSTIC VIROLOGY

Laboratory diagnosis is often unnecessary for viral infections like the usual childhood diseases (for example, mumps, measles, and chickenpox). Diagnosis does become important when (1) it is suspected that the virus is one associated with a high mortality and its spread in the community could be devastating (for example, polio), (2) there is cross-infection in the hospitalized patient resulting in severe illness (for example, influenza A, syncytial virus infections), and (3) a pregnant woman is suspected of carrying viruses that are known to cause abnormalities in the fetus (for example, rubella). At one time even the identification of a virus was of little help because antiviral drugs were unavailable for treatment. More antiviral drugs are now becoming available, and rapid diagnosis of viral agents is becoming more practical.

Many new and exotic techniques for rapid identification of virus are available but the mainstays of diagnostic virology are *viral cultivation* and *serology*.

Cultivation of Virus from Clinical Material

Tissue culture is the most widely used technique for virus isolation. There are three major types of tissue culture: *primary cultures, diploid cell lines,* and *continuous cell lines*. Primary cultures are prepared by removing an organ from a freshly killed animal and then dispersing the cells of the organ by biochemical treatment. The number of cell divisions for primary cultures is relatively small. Diploid cell lines have a finite life span consisting of 50 to 60 passages in vitro. Most of the diploid cell lines used in the laboratory are fibroblasts. Continuous cell lines are derived from normal or malignant tissue and are immortal in that they can grow indefinitely. Examples of continuous cell lines are *Vero cells* from monkey kidney tissue and *HeLa cells* derived from malignant tumor (see Boxed Essay, 638). Which cell line to use depends on its sensitivity to virus.

Cell lines are cultured in glass or plastic vessels containing liquid media. The cells attach to the surface and then begin to divide. Division continues until all the available surface has been cov-

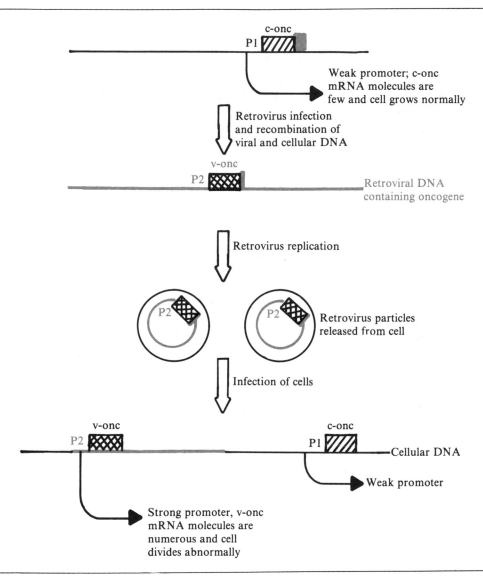

Fig. 30-14. A scheme depicting how relocation of oncogenes can lead to transformation. Host cell with cellular oncogene (c-onc) adjacent to weak promoter (P1) is infected by retrovirus. Retrovirus picks up oncogene and integrates it adjacent to a strong promoter (P2) on the viral DNA. Retrovirus particles are produced and released from infected cell. Infection of new cells by retrovirus results in integration of viral oncogene (v-onc) and its strong promoter into cellular DNA. Transcription of P2 v-onc results in many mRNAs, which are translated into a product that causes abnormal growth response.

THE LEGACY OF HENRIETTA LACKS

The term *HeLa* is derived from a woman named Henrietta Lacks who was born in Virginia in 1920. Henrietta began raising a family in Baltimore, Maryland, and was of normal health. She was relatively free of cares until 1951, when she observed a pink discharge in her underclothes. She went to a women's clinic at Johns Hopkins Hospital, where a gynecologist noted an abnormal growth about the cervix. Biopsy of the tissue revealed that it was malignant and that Henrietta Lacks had cervical cancer. A slice of the tumor was given to George and Margaret Gey, who at the time were pioneers in tissue culture. The Geys' greatest hope was that they would be able to establish a continuous culture of a human tumor that could be studied in the test tube. Every day the Geys would see what operations were being performed in the hospital and then retrieve interesting sources of tissue. They would then race to the lab and try to culture the cells for extended periods of time. But no matter how careful their manipulations and culturing techniques, most human cells would shrivel up and die after a few months.

The malignant tissue taken from Henrietta was code-named with the first two letters of the donor's first and last name (HeLa). Cubes of the malignant tissue were cultivated and fed the usual diet of clotted chicken plasma, chopped beef embryo, and blood from human placentas. Within 48 hours a new band of cells could be seen around each cube of tissue. After 4 days the culture tubes became overrun with new cells and, as Mary Gey described it, "spreading like crabgrass." The tumor cells grew 10 to 20 times faster than normal cervical cells—making them different from any tumor cells previously observed. The tumor within Henrietta Lacks was also different. Most cervical cancers are held in check by radiation, but Henrietta's grew so quickly that it covered the surface of the liver, diaphragm, intestine, appendix, rectum, and heart. In 8 months from the time of discovery of the malignancy Henrietta Lacks was dead; but part of what she had been, escaped and is still surviving.

ered. When the cells reach a state in which their total membrane surface is in contact with adjacent cells, division ceases. This phenomenon, called *contact inhibition*, or *density-dependent growth*, results in the formation of a monolayer of cells in the culture medium. When malignant cells are used to cultivate virus, however, the phenomenon of contact inhibition is lost and the cells pile up.

Sometimes cell cultures are not especially sensitive to virus and other culture systems are required. Two such culture systems are *embryonated eggs* and *suckling mice*. Influenza virus, for example, is cultured in embryonated eggs, while suckling mice are used primarily in the isolation of alphavirus, flaviviruses, and bunyaviruses.

Effects of Virus on Cultured Cells. Regardless of the cell type used for cultivating virus, most viruses will produce a particular cytopathic effect that is measurable. These cytopathic effects include the formation of *plaques, pocks, foci,* and *syncytia* (syncytia were discussed previously).

Some virus-infected cells lyse and progeny virus are released to infect and lyse adjacent cells. After several days a localized area of infection, called a *plaque*, appears (Fig. 30-15). These plaques are similar in appearance to the plaques caused by bacterial viruses on cultured bacteria (see Fig. 30-22, p. 650).

When some viruses are cultivated on the chorioallantoic membrane of embryonated chick eggs, lesions called *pocks* are produced. The membrane can be removed and spread out and the pocks counted. Each pock represents the original site of a single virus infection (Fig. 30-16).

Some viruses that infect cells do not cause visible plaques or pocks. Instead, virus infection stimulates cell proliferation and after a period of time results in the formation of a mass of live cells called a *focus* (Fig. 30-17).

The cytopathic effect produced on host cells offers only a preliminary method of identification of virus. Final identification usually depends on serologic tests.

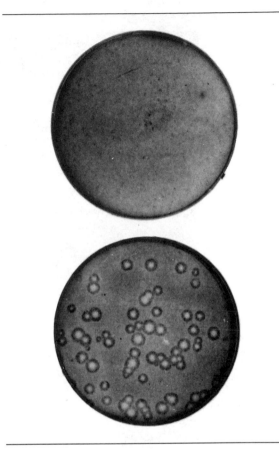

Fig. 30-15. Viral plaques. Influenza virus grown on human amnion cells. A. Uninfected cells. B. Infected cells after 5 days of incubation. (From A. Sugiura and M. Ueda, *Virol.* 7:499, 1977.)

Serologic Methods

Serologic methods are by far the most important in diagnostic virology. They are based on demonstrating a significant increase in the antibody titer to a given virus over the course of the patient's disease—that is, testing acute and convalescent-phase serum. The length of time required for testing is a limitation but serologic methods are more economical than isolation of virus. In order to prevent the hazards associated with handling infectious antigens, the nucleic acid of viruses can be inactivated prior to use by laboratory personnel. A variety of techniques are

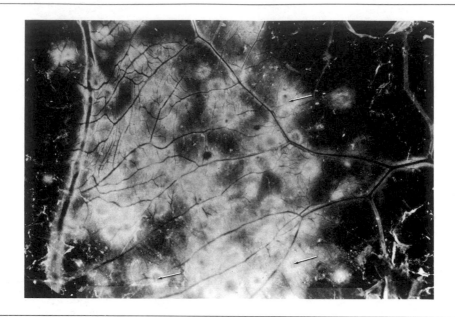

Fig. 30-16. Viral pocks (*arrow*) produced on chorioallantoic membrane of embryonated hen's egg after 5 days' incubation with virus at 35.5°C. (Courtesy Audio Visual Service, Department of Pathology, University of Illinois Medical Center, Chicago.)

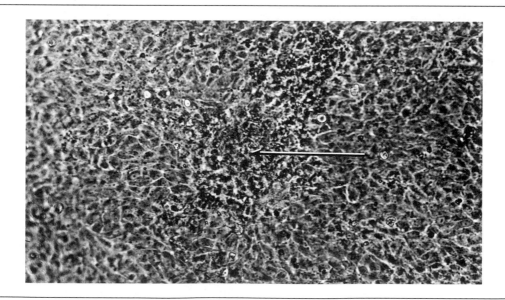

Fig. 30-17. Cell focus (*arrow*) produced by virus-infected cell. (From K. Hamada et al., *J. Virol.* 38:327, 1981.)

now available to detect antibody. Some of these techniques are immunoassays and include the following: radioimmunoassays, enzyme immunoassay, immunofluorescence tests, and avidin-biotin immunoassays. These tests are described in detail in Chapter 13. Other immunological tests that measure antibody include complement fixation, neutralization, hemagglutination, hemagglutination-inhibition, immune-adherence hemagglutination, and single radial diffusion; these are also described in Chapter 13.

Rapid Methods in Diagnostic Virology

The most ideal method for diagnosis of viral infection is to directly detect and identify the infectious agent in clinical material. This can be accomplished by examining clinical material directly by electron microscopy or by using immunological or other techniques on the clinical specimen.

Electron Microscopy. Under most circumstances examination of clinical material by electron microscopy is not feasible or practical. Not all laboratories have an electron microscope. The concentration of virus in a sample is often very small and there is considerable tissue debris that hinders identification. In addition, some viruses are so small that their morphology is not discernible enough to permit identification. Skin lesions may contain high concentrations of virus but techniques other than microscopy are more practical for identification. Electron microscopy can be used for diagnosis if the viral agent, such as the rotavirus, cannot be cultivated by standard procedures. In the case of rotavirus, extracts of infected epithelial cells of the duodenal mucosa contain high concentrations of virus whose morphology is distinctive enough to permit identification (see Fig. 31-24, p. 715).

Electron microscopy can be coupled with serology for rapid detection of virus in a technique called immunoelectron microscopy (IEM). In this procedure antiserum containing antibodies specific for the virus is mixed with a large clinical specimen in which virus concentration may be small. Interaction of antibody with virus produces virus-antibody aggregates that are more easily discernible with electron microscopy. The hepatitis A virus was first identified by this procedure.

Immunologic and Other Methods of Identification. Virus or viral antigens can be detected in clinical specimens either within cells or outside cells (for example, the blood). Reliable identification is dependent on having sufficient virus or viral antigen in the clinical specimen and having highly specific antisera. Lack of highly specific antisera was a problem at one time but the availability of monoclonal antibodies has permitted more precise characterization and identification of viral isolates. For those diseases in which virus is found predominantly in the cell, immunofluorescence or immunoperoxidase is most suitable for identification. Immunofluorescence has been used very successfully to identify influenza viruses, syncytial viruses, mumps virus, and measles virus. In addition, immunofluorescence is the principal technique used to detect the rabies virus in the brains of infected animals.

Assays for detecting virus or viral antigens have been important in the screening of blood. Some of these assays include passive hemagglutination, radioimmunoassays, and enzyme immunoassays. Detection of hepatitis B antigen in blood and rotavirus in fecal specimens offers examples of how these tests have been applied to detecting virus outside cells.

The advent of recombinant DNA technology has permitted investigators to identify virus on the basis of detection of viral genomes. A number of tests are now available for "fingerprinting" viral nucleic acids but most of these are used epidemiologically to distinguish differences or similarities between strains of virus. For example, the changes that occur in the influenza virus from one season to the next can be identified by recombinant DNA techniques. These techniques were discussed in Chapter 10 and some are being evaluated as diagnostic as well as epidemiologic tools. (See Polymerase Chain Reaction in Chap. 10.)

VIRAL CLASSIFICATION

Viral classification has been approached in many ways over the past years. With every major advancement in our understanding of viruses, new classification schemes have evolved, centered on (1) symptoms of the viral disease, (2) method of transmission of the virus, (3) symmetry of the viral capsid, or (4) the tissue or organ affected by the virus. One of the most useful means of separating the viruses is based first and foremost on the type of nucleic acid carried by the virus. Further separation is based on capsid symmetry and on the presence or absence of an envelope. These and other viral properties are summarized in Tables 30-4 and 30-5.

TREATMENT AND CONTROL OF VIRAL INFECTIONS

The most successful approach to the control of viral infection has been the development of vaccines. Unfortunately, vaccines are not available for most viral diseases and in some cases vaccines will never be practical or possible. Chemotherapy, therefore, may be the only effective mechanism for controlling viral infections. We will begin our discussion with chemotherapeutic agents.

CHEMOTHERAPEUTIC AGENTS

Many people find it difficult to understand why viruses cannot be treated with the same drugs that are effective against bacteria. The antibiotics used against bacteria for the most part inhibit some process that is peculiar or specific to the bacteria. For instance, the antibiotics that inhibit bacterial cell wall formation are of obvious value in therapy because mammalian cells have no cell walls and thus are not affected. For antibiotics that do inhibit both bacterial and host metabolism, the concentration of drug required is usually so small that the cells of the body are not adversely affected. The situation with viruses is different because the virus does not have its own metabolic machinery; it relies on the host's metabolic systems and most of the cells' enzymes. Thus, many of the metabolic steps in the cell are common to the steps in virus replication. An antiviral drug that inhibits viral activity will therefore often inhibit cell metabolism. Consequently, development of nontoxic antiviral agents has been difficult. One of the problems in antiviral drug development has been our lack of knowledge about specific mechanisms of viral growth and metabolism. There are some sequences in viral replication that are unique. If we can isolate and identify the specific viral enzymes, nucleic acids, or proteins that are involved in these processes, we may be able to synthesize compounds with antiviral potential. For an antiviral drug to be effective it must either act at the surface of the cell to prevent viral attachment or it must enter the cell and inhibit some step in viral replication. Currently licensed antiviral drugs are outlined in Table 30-6. These licensed drugs and a variety of other antiviral drugs, including interferon, are being screened for their activity in a number of viral diseases. Interferon has been evaluated as a treatment regimen for a number of viral diseases but has been licensed only for the treatment of genital warts, caused by human papilloma viruses, and of hairy cell leukemia. The mechanism of action of interferon was discussed previously on page 275.

VACCINES

The historic epidemics, such as smallpox and yellow fever, that once decimated large populations

Table 30-4. Classification of DNA-containing Viruses of Vertebrates

Capsid symmetry	Cubic					Complex
Virion: naked or enveloped	Naked			Enveloped		Complex
Reaction to ether	Resistant			Sensitive		Resistant
Diameter[a] of virion (nm)	18–26	45–55	70–90	100	130–300	230 × 300
Virus family	Parvoviridae	Papovaviridae	Adenoviridae	Herpesviridae	Iridoviridae	Poxviridae
Important genera	Parvovirus	Papovavirus	Mastadenovirus	Alphaherpesvirinae[b], Betaherpesvirinae[b], Gammaherpesvirinae[b]	—	Orthopoxvirus
Human diseases caused by viral family members	Gastroenteritis	Warts	Respiratory infections	Herpes, chickenpox (varicella), shingles (zoster)	—	Smallpox

Table 30-5. Classification of RNA-containing Viruses of Vertebrates

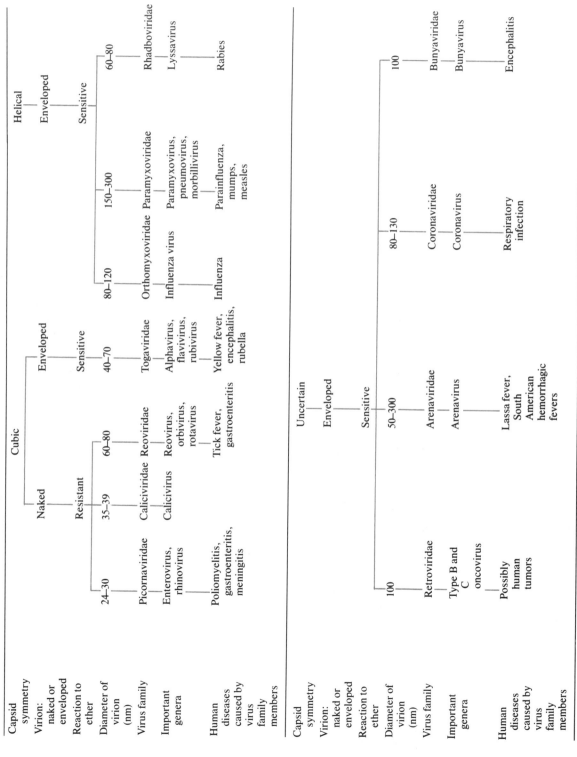

Capsid symmetry	Cubic				Helical	
Virion: naked or enveloped	Naked			Enveloped	Enveloped	
Reaction to ether	Resistant			Sensitive	Sensitive	
Diameter of virion (nm)	24–30	35–39	60–80	40–70	80–120	150–300	60–80
Virus family	Picornaviridae	Caliciviridae	Reoviridae	Togaviridae	Orthomyxoviridae	Paramyxoviridae	Rhabdoviridae
Important genera	Enterovirus, rhinovirus	Calicivirus	Reovirus, orbivirus, rotavirus	Alphavirus, flavivirus, rubivirus	Influenza virus	Paramyxovirus, pneumovirus, morbillivirus	Lyssavirus
Human diseases caused by virus family members	Poliomyelitis, gastroenteritis, meningitis		Tick fever, gastroenteritis	Yellow fever, encephalitis, rubella	Influenza	Parainfluenza, mumps, measles	Rabies

Capsid symmetry	Uncertain		
Virion: naked or enveloped	Enveloped		
Reaction to ether	Sensitive		
Diameter of virion (nm)	100	50–300	100
Virus family	Retroviridae	Arenaviridae	Bunyaviridae
Important genera	Type B and C oncovirus	Arenavirus	Bunyavirus
Human diseases caused by virus family members	Possibly human tumors	Lassa fever, South American hemorrhagic fevers	Encephalitis

Table 30-6. Currently Licensed Antiviral Drugs

Drug	Trade name	Mechanism of action	Diseases recommended for treatment and dosage form
Amantadine	Symmetrel	Inhibits uncoating step in viral replication	Prophylaxis and treatment of influenza A (oral)
Acyclovir	Zovirax	A nucleoside analog that inhibits viral DNA synthesis	Mucocutaneous herpes simplex in compromised patients; primary genital herpes infections (oral and intravenous)
Idoxuridine	Stoxil, Herplex	A nucleoside analog that inhibits viral DNA synthesis	Herpes simplex keratitis (topical)
Trifluridine	Viroptic	A halogenated nucleoside that inhibits viral DNA synthesis	Herpes simplex keratitis (topical)
Vidarabine	Vira-A	A nucleoside analog that inhibits viral DNA synthesis	Herpes simplex encephalitis; neonatal herpes infection of the central nervous system and disseminated infections (intravenous)
Alpha interferon	Intron-A	A cellular glycoprotein now produced by recombinant DNA technology that interferes with protein synthesis	Genital warts from human papillomaviruses (injected directly into lesions)

are no longer a major threat to modern society. In some underdeveloped nations of the world outbreaks still occur, but except in extreme cases they are generally curtailed before they involve large masses of people. One of the primary reasons massive epidemics no longer exist is the development and extensive use of vaccines.

Viral vaccines induce an immune response to virus surface antigens or to viral antigens on the surface of infected cells. Viral suface antigens may be in the form of capsid proteins for icosahedral viruses and in the form of glycoproteins in enveloped viruses. Immunizations are particularly important for children, not only because of the devastating effects of viral infection on this group but because of the ease in communicability of viral disease to other children and adults. Today in the United States child day care centers are arising in an almost exponential fashion. Childhood diseases are quickly transmitted to children and adults in these facilities. Childhood immunization is therefore an important measure

in reducing morbidity and mortality. The recommended viral immunization schedules for children are outlined in Table 30-7.

Viral vaccines may be of the inactivated or live variety and each variety has its advantages and disadvantages, as discussed in Chapter 12. The

Table 30-7. Recommended Immunization (Viral) Schedule for Children

Age	Immunization child should receive
2 months	Trivalent oral poliovirus vaccine (first)
4 months	Trivalent oral poliovirus vaccine (second)
15 months	Measles vaccine ⎫ Mumps vaccine ⎬ May be combined Rubella vaccine ⎭ as single injection
18 months	Trivalent oral poliovirus vaccine (third)
4–6 years	Trivalent oral poliovirus vaccine (fourth)

Table 30-8. Currently Available Viral Vaccines

Vaccine	Vaccine type	Route of administration
Influenza A	Inactivated	Parenteral
Poliomyelitis	Inactivated and live	Parenteral and oral
Rabies	Inactivated	Parenteral
Hepatitis B	Inactivated	Parenteral
Rubella	Live	Parenteral
Yellow fever	Live	Parenteral
Measles	Live	Parenteral
Adenovirus	Live	Oral
Mumps	Live	Parenteral

currently licensed viral vaccines are outlined in Table 30-8.

BACTERIAL VIRUSES

Bacterial viruses or phages have played an important role in the development of molecular biology. Our present knowledge of nucleic acid transcription, replication, mutation, and regulation in higher organisms can be attributed to discoveries acquired from the study of phage genetics. The information obtained from experiments with phages has also been applied to our understanding of the infectious disease process in animal viruses.

COMPOSITION AND STRUCTURE

Most phages possess a protein coat called a *phage head*. The phage head, which exhibits icosahedral symmetry, encloses the nucleic acid of the virus. In most phages the head is attached to a protein tail, which exhibits helical symmetry. Some phages are tailless and still others, which are the least frequently observed, are filamentous (Fig. 30-18). The nucleic acid of phages may be either DNA or RNA and both can be either single- or double-stranded. Most phages possess double-stranded DNA, which has a molecular weight that averages from 1 to 1.5×10^8, while the DNA of their hosts, such as *E. coli*, have molecular weights that average from 1 to 3×10^9.

Much of phage research has been directed at the physiology and structure of a group of double-stranded DNA viruses that infect *E. coli*. This group of viruses is called the *T series*, which includes several strains. *T4 bacteriophage*, for example, possesses a tail, to which is attached a base plate containing spikes, as well as tail fibers (Fig. 30-19). Most of our discussion on phage physiology will describe results obtained from T4 infection of *E. coli*.

PHYSIOLOGY OF VIRUS INFECTION

Three things happen when a phage and a bacterial suspension are incubated together: (1) No infection occurs because the virus is not specific for the bacterial species. (2) Infection proceeds with the production of mature virus and the subsequent lysis of the cell. (3) The virus infects the bacterial cell, but mature virus is not produced because the virus and host enter into a quiescent state, called *lysogeny*, in which the host does not lyse. Our discussion will begin with the physiology of lytic virus infection, followed by a discussion of the process of lysogeny.

Lytic Bacteriophage Infection

Adsorption and Injection. A number of important conditions must be met if the bacterial cell is to be infected by a virus. First, the virus must be specific for the bacterial species. Second, the ratio of virus to bacteria must be correct. A ratio of ten viruses to one bacterium ensures that all the bacteria in a suspension will be infected. If too many viruses are attached to the bacterium, there may be premature lysis without the production of new virus. Third, the bacterial growth

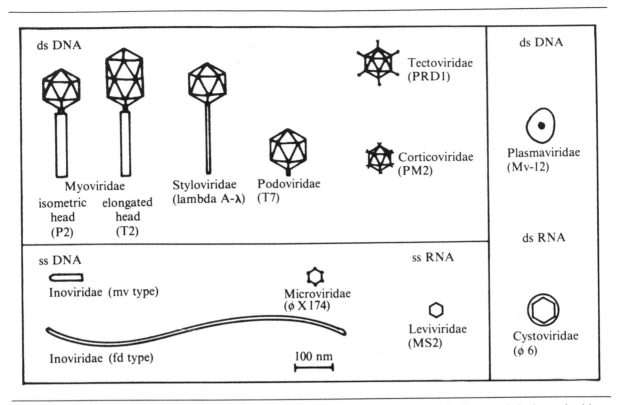

Fig. 30-18. Basic shape of the families of virus that infect bacteria. (Key: ss = single-stranded; ds = double-stranded.)

medium in which the infection process takes place must contain the necessary metabolites to support the synthesis of viral molecules in the bacterial cell.

Virus attaches to the cell wall by means of tail fibers. Attachment of only one fiber to the bacterial cell wall is sufficient to initiate binding of virus (Fig. 30-20). Irreversible binding of virus, however, requires the attachment of other tail fibers to the bacterial surface. The binding of tail fibers brings about the interaction of base plate with bacterial surface. This is followed by contraction of the tail and passage of the tail tube or core through the cell wall and cytoplasmic membrane (Fig. 30-20). DNA is injected into the cytoplasm of the cell when these two bacterial structures have been punctured.

Maturation. Inside the bacterial cell naked viral DNA is protected from bacterial nucleases because of nucleic acid modification. T4 DNA possesses a *glycosylated hydroxymethyl cytosine*, which is not recognized by bacterial nucleases and thus is protected from degradation. Viral transcription and replication require the inhibition of specific host functions and diversion of host metabolic machinery and/or enzymes for viral use. These events, which occur during the "early" period, include the following:

1. Viral genes are transcribed that encode products to be used in repairing the bacterial cell membrane that was damaged during the injection of viral DNA into the cytoplasm.
2. The viral genome encodes a product (or prod-

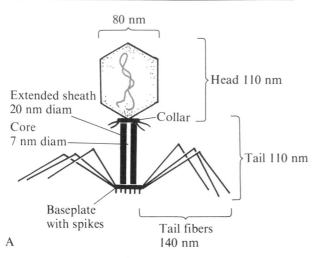

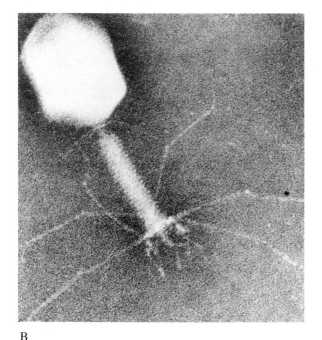

Fig. 30-19. The T4 bacteriophage. A. Diagram. B. Electron micrograph. (From R. C. Williams and H. W. Fisher, *An Electron Micrograph Atlas of Viruses,* 1974. Courtesy of Charles C Thomas, Publisher, Springfield, Illinois.)

ucts) that alter host RNA polymerases so that they can be used to produce only viral and not host mRNA.

3. The viral genome codes for enzymes that degrade host DNA into nucleotides that will be used in the synthesis of viral genomes.

4. The viral genome codes for viral-specific DNA polymerases and other enzymes involved in synthesis of deoxyribonucleoside triphosphates.

After viral DNA synthesis is finished, "late" proteins are synthesized. These proteins are primarily structural (head, tail, tail fibers, etc.) as well as catalytic. Some of the catalytic proteins are used to convert phage DNA into a form suitable for packaging into new viral particles. After the structural proteins are synthesized, assembly of viral particles begins (the period up to the appearance of the first complete viral particle is called *eclipse*—see page 625). The assembly process is divided into three basic pathways: (1) assembly of phage heads and packaging of the viral genome; (2) assembly of tail and base plate and joining to the head; and (3) addition of tail fibers to base plates (Fig. 30-21). Fifty to 1000 phage particles can be assembled in a single bacterial cell.

Release. Release of T4 phage from the bacterial cell is dependent on an enzyme called *lysozyme,* which attacks the peptidoglycan layer of the bacterial cell wall. Lysozyme activity causes the cell to burst and release the virus particles all at once.

Bacteriophage infection can be assayed in the laboratory in the following way. A sample of phages is mixed with a drop of a culture of bacteria plus 1 to 2 ml of soft agar at 44°C. The mixture is shaken slightly and then poured over the surface of hard agar in a Petri dish. The soft agar is allowed to set and the plate is incubated overnight. During the incubation period bacteriophages diffuse through the agar until they find a bacterium to infect. Each infected bacterium produces progeny phage after 30 to 45 minutes, and lysis occurs with release of phage. Several

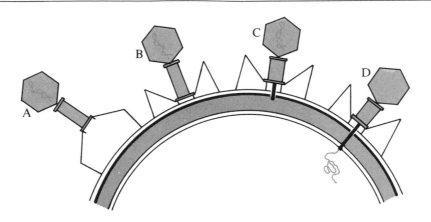

Fig. 30-20. Bacteriophage infection process. A. Attachment of long tail fibers of virus to cell wall. B. Adsorption of viral tail pins to cell wall. C. Contraction of tail sheath and injection of core into cell wall. D. DNA injection through core into cytoplasm of bacterial cell.

Fig. 30-21. Abbreviated scheme showing assembly pathways of bacteriophage. Each pathway leads to the assembly of phage component. The components are then assembled into a mature viral particle.

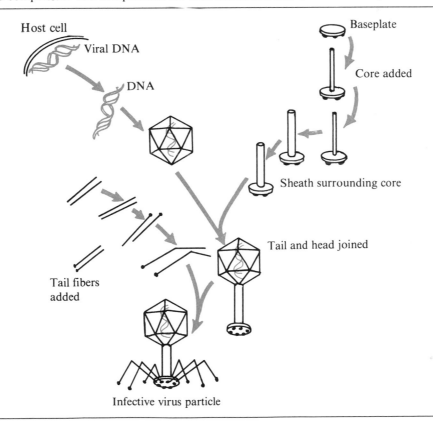

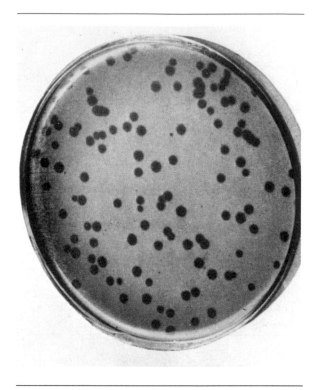

Fig. 30-22. Bacterial plaques. Agar culture medium shows a lawn of *Escherichia coli* growth on which T2 bacteriophages have produced plaques. (From *Molecular Biology of Bacterial Viruses* by Gunther S. Stent. W. H. Freeman and Company. Copyright © 1963.)

hundred phages are released from each bacterium, and they in turn infect adjacent bacteria, causing lysis and release of phages. Uninfected bacteria multiply and produce a lawn over the agar surface except at those sites where phage-infected bacteria have lysed. These areas of lysis appear clear and are called *plaques* (Fig. 30-22). The number of plaques coincides with the number of phages per unit volume that initiated infection in the original sample.

Temperate Bacteriophage Infection (Lysogeny)

Some viruses have evolved mechanisms that control their own replication and allow them to maintain a stable relationship with their host. This stable relationship between virus and host is called *lysogeny*. The cell harboring the virus is called a *lysogen*, and the virus is called a *temperate virus*. Temperate virus DNA may integrate into the host cell (Fig. 30-23C), or it may remain physically independent of the host genome. In either case, replication of the phage genome is coordinated with host genome replication; thus at cell division both bacterial cells receive at least one copy of the viral genome. The expression of the replicative mechanisms of the virus is controlled by a *repressor*, which is coded by a phage gene. In its nonproductive state the genes of the temperate virus (except for the repressor gene) are not expressed because of the binding of repressor to certain sites on the phage genome. The presence of the repressor also makes the lysogenic cell immune to infection by a second phage particle of the same phage species.

If the lysogenic cell is treated with ultraviolet light, x-rays, alkylating agents, or carcinogenic chemicals, the phage genome is released from the effects of the repressor and a productive infection ensues in which mature phage particles are assembled and released from the cell (Fig. 30-23G).

One of the most widely studied temperate viruses is called *lambda* (λ), which can also produce a lytic cycle. During lysogenization lambda becomes inserted into the host genome as a prophage (Fig. 30-23C). Lambda DNA has been used as a vector for molecular cloning (see Chapter 6). Once inserted, phage DNA and its replication mechanisms are regulated by the systems that control replication of the bacterial chromosome. Some prophages are capable of changing the cell's phenotype, a process called *phage conversion*, or *lysogenic conversion*. Some examples in which lysogenic conversion has contributed to the infectious disease process are:

1. *Corynebacterium diphtheriae* is a pathogen whose virulence is related to its ability to produce a toxin. The organism is virulent only when it carries a temperate virus. If the organism is cured of the temperate virus, it is no

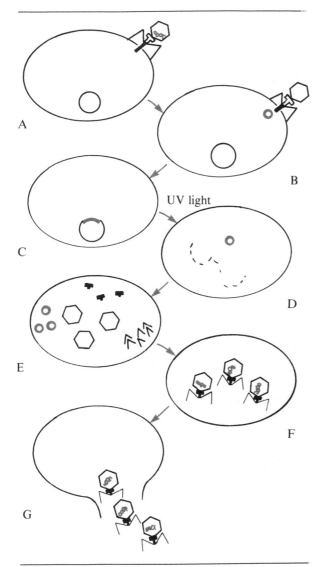

Fig. 30-23. Process of lysogeny and its conversion to the lytic state. A. Virus adsorbs to the cell. B. Viral DNA (*in color*) is injected into the bacterial cell and becomes circular. C. Viral DNA is incorporated into bacterial DNA (prophage state). The bacterial cell is now lysogenized. D. The lysogenized bacterial cell, having been treated with ultraviolet light, releases viral DNA from the bacterial genome. E. Virus behaves as a lytic virus in the bacterial cell; viral components are produced, and bacterial DNA is degraded. F. Mature viral particles are assembled. G. Viral particles are released upon lysis of the bacterial cell.

longer pathogenic. Thus, the gene for toxin production apparently resides in the viral genome and not in the host's genome.

2. Only streptococci carrying a temperate phage can produce the erythrogenic toxin associated with scarlet fever.

3. *Clostridium botulinum* type C in the lysogenic state is nontoxigenic.

4. Some lysogenic bacteria can be distinguished from nonlysogenic ones. Species of *Salmonella*, when infected by a temperate virus, will eventually show changes in their surface component (O antigens). The virus in some way prevents the formation of normal cell surface components. For this reason the antigenic components of the lysogenized cell are different from those of the nonlysogenized cell, and this difference can be detected serologically.

5. The lysogenic state of bacteria is rather similar to the relationship between an animal tumor virus and its host. In both instances the viral DNA is incorporated into the host's genome.

BACTERIOPHAGES AND TRANSDUCTION

Transduction is a mechanism that, like transformation and conjugation, can alter the genotype of the cell. Transduction basically involves the ability of a virus to transfer bacterial genes from one bacterial cell to another. Two types of transduction can be distinguished: *generalized* and *restricted*.

Generalized Transduction

Generalized transduction implies that any bacterial gene can be incorporated into the phage head during the infection process. When a transducing phage infects a bacterial cell, the transduced bacterial DNA is capable of entering into a recombinational event with the DNA of the recipient bacteria (Fig. 30-24), assuming homology

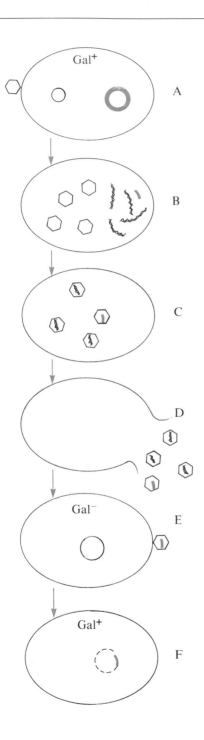

between their genetic determinants. (Generalized transduction was discussed in Chapter 6.)

Restricted Transduction

Restricted (specialized) transduction is based on the ability of phage DNA to integrate into, and to be excised from, the bacterial chromosome. In restricted transduction, as the name implies, only specific bacterial genes can be transduced. Bacterial viruses that exhibit restricted transduction integrate into the bacterial chromosome at specific sites. The bacterial virus lambda, for example, integrates between the galactose gene and the biotin gene on the host genome. When the lysogenic cell is induced to produce lytic virus, lambda prophage is excised from the bacterial genome and in the process the galactose gene is carried with it. These lambda particles are called λ *gal*. Sometimes the excised λ gal lacks certain genes essential for lytic growth. These defective particles are called λ *dgal* (Fig. 30-25). If we use λ dgal particles to infect other bacteria, the transduced galactose gene can enter into a recombinational event with the galactose gene on the bacterial genome.

SUMMARY

1. Viruses are obligate intracellular agents that possess single- or double-stranded DNA or RNA

Fig. 30-24. Generalized transduction. A. Bacterial cell with a functional galactose gene (gal⁺) is infected by a virus. (Bacterial DNA is red; viral DNA is black.) B. Bacterial DNA is degraded. C. Bacterial gal⁺ gene is encased in a viral coat. D. Bacterial cell lyses, releasing virus, one of which carries bacterial gal⁺ gene. E. Another bacterial cell that carries a nonfunctional galactose gene (gal⁻) is infected by the transducing virus. F. The transduced gal⁺ gene engages in recombination with gal⁻ gene of bacterial chromosome, converting the cell to gal⁺. The bacterial cell does not lyse because there was no viral information in the infecting viral particle.

e of
terium

surrounded by a coat of protein. Many animal viruses also possess lipid envelopes but the majority of bacterial viruses, or phages, are free of lipid envelopes.

2. The viral protein coat is called a capsid and is made of protein subunits called capsomeres. The capsid may possess either helical or icosahedral symmetry, depending on how it interacts with the nucleic acid of the virus to produce the nucleocapsid.

3. The lipid bilayer of the viral envelope is derived from the host cell but the glycoproteins that are surface antigens are of viral origin and are referred to as spikes or peplomers. Some peplomers can help the virus bind to the cell but others may possess enzymatic activity that aid in the infectious disease process.

4. The multiplication cycle of animal viruses may range in time from 6 hours to 48 hours and is divided into five stages: adsorption, penetration, genome expression, maturation, and release. Adsorption of virus is dependent on the chemical nature of viral glycoproteins and host receptors. Viruses may penetrate the cell directly, by fusion with the cytoplasmic membrane, or by endocytosis. The viral nucleic acid is released from the nucleocapsid and may remain in the cytoplasm of the cell or it may penetrate the nucleus, depending on site of viral assembly.

5. Expression of viral genomes in mammalian cells can be divided into six classes, depending on polarity (plus or minus), type of nucleic acid, and number of strands of nucleic acid. All classes transcribe the genome into an mRNA molecule and also replicate it to produce many viral genomes.

6. The viral maturation process can be divided into early and late. Early proteins that are synthesized function in the synthesis of viral genomes while late proteins are primarily structural in function. Nucleocapsids of DNA viruses are assembled primarily in the nucleus while most RNA nucleocapsids are assembled in the cytoplasm.

7. Most nonenveloped viruses are released when the cell lyses. Enveloped viruses must ob-

Fig. 30-25. Restricted transduction. Integrated lambda DNA is closely associated with the galactose (*gal*) gene in the bacterial chromosome. Deintegration of the lambda genome causes it to loop out and engage in an incorrect recombination with attachment sites (*in color*) and the gal gene is carried on the viral genome. The defective virus genome (λ dgal) does not carry sufficient viral information for assembly into a lytic phage particle during the next infection cycle. (bio = biotin.)

tain a lipid envelope that may be acquired by release through the nuclear membrane if the nucleocapsid is assembled in the nucleus, or cytoplasmic membrane if the nucleocapsid is assembled in the cytoplasm. The lipid envelope contains glycoprotein spikes that are part of the cell membrane but are virus-encoded. Release of virus through cell membranes is called *budding*.

8. When animal virus is cultured the infected cells show cytopathic effects (CPE). CPE include lysis of cells, inclusion body formation, and syncytia formation. Virus infection also affects the surface antigens of cells, causes the formation of interferon—an antiviral protein—and may also induce persistent infection.

9. Persistent infections can occur in cells if the immune system is somehow evaded by viruses, the virus produces defective-interfering particles, or the viral genome integrates into the genome of the host. Persistent infections are divided into three types: chronic, latent, and slow.

10. Cancers are malignant growths resulting from the transformation of cells. Viruses causing cancers are called oncogenic. Viral transformation causes a number of effects on cells, including: changes in morphology and changes in properties of the cytoplasmic membrane, which include changes in permeability, antigenic characteristics, and agglutinability. In addition, the viral genome becomes integrated or closely associated with the host genome.

11. The oncogenic DNA viruses most closely associated with human cancers are the herpesviruses and human papillomaviruses (HPV). The Epstein-Barr virus is a herpesvirus associated with Burkitt's lymphoma and nasopharyngeal cancer. Strains of HPV that cause genital warts may be precursors of cervical cancer.

12. Oncogenic RNA viruses belong to a group called retroviruses. Retroviruses produce a DNA intermediate via the activity of an enzyme called reverse transcriptase, and insert it into the host genome. Viral transforming genes, or oncogenes, are not associated with viral replication. The only RNA viruses causing cancer in humans are the human T lymphotropic viruses (HTLV).

13. Oncogenes are defective cellular genes called proto-oncogenes that have been picked up by retroviruses during the infection process. There are over 20 known oncogenes that encode proteins with activities affecting cellular growth.

14. A few viral infections can be diagnosed if the symptoms are of obvious clinical significance. The mainstays of diagnostic virology are virus cultivation and serology. Most virus is cultivated in continuous culture, that is, cells from normal or malignant tissue that can be passaged indefinitely. Other culture systems that are infrequently used include embryonated eggs or suckling mice.

15. Infected cultured cells can be observed for cytopathic effects (CPE) such as plaques, pocks, foci, or syncytia. CPE permit only presumptive identification of virus and final identification requires serology. Serologic tests utilize a variety of immunologic techniques to identify antibody to virus and include immunoassays, immunofluorescence, complement fixation, neutralization, hemagglutination, etc.

16. Rapid methods in diagnostic virology rely on identification of virus or viral antigen in the clinical specimen. Electron microscopy is infrequently used, and most rapid tests are of the immunologic variety. Viruses can be detected within cells by using such tests as immunoperoxidase or immunofluorescence and outside cells by hemagglutination, radioimmunoassays, and enzyme immunoassays.

17. Viral classification is based primarily on nucleic acid type, capsid symmetry, and presence or absence of an envelope (see Tables 30-4 and 30-5).

18. The most frequently used antiviral drugs are analogs of nucleosides, which inhibit nucleic acid synthesis. The currently licensed drugs are outlined in Table 30-6.

19. Viral vaccines are still the most effective way of preventing viral diseases. Vaccines can be of the inactivated or live type and the ones available for humans are outlined in Table 30-8.

20. Bacterial viruses, which exhibit primarily icosahedral symmetry, have a capsid head that,

depending on the virus, may have a tail or may be tailless. The most researched viruses belong to the T series, which infect *E. coli*.

21. Phage infection can be lytic or the virus may enter into a state of equilibrium with its host in a process called lysogeny. T4 phage infection is initiated by binding of virus via tail fibers to the bacterial cell wall and injection of DNA into the cytoplasm.

22. Phage maturation can be divided into early and late. Early proteins are used to divert the host's metabolic machinery and to produce viral genomes. Late proteins are used to construct structural proteins. Assembled virus is released when the cell wall is degraded by lysozyme. Viral infection on a lawn of bacteria is observed as cleared areas called plaques.

23. Lysogeny is caused by temperate viruses such as lambda, whose genome may integrate into the host's genome. A viral repressor mole-cule maintains lysogeny but the repressor becomes inactivated if the lysogen is treated with chemical or physical agents. Repressor inactivation induces the lytic state.

24. Temperate viruses can change cells' phenotypes and some of these changes, called *lysogenic conversion*, are associated with virulence.

25. Bacterial viruses can change the genotype of the cell in a process called transduction. There are two types of transduction: generalized and restricted. Generalized transduction involves the transfer of any bacterial gene while restricted transduction involves the transfer of only specific bacterial genes to bacterial cells.

26. Only a few chemotherapeutic agents are available to treat viral disease. Antiviral drugs exhibit a great deal of toxicity to the host because they inhibit processes that are as much a part of host as well as viral replication.

QUESTIONS FOR STUDY

Select the best response or responses for each of the following:

1. Which of the following statements about viruses and virus structure is not true?
   A. Viruses require living cells for their replication.
   B. In spherical viruses the nucleic acid is intimately associated with capsid proteins.
   C. When present, complex proteins, called spikes, are found on the surface of lipid envelopes.
   D. The nucleocapsid or core of enveloped viruses is surrounded by a protective cover called a protein shell.

2. Which of the following enzymes would not be found in the core of the virus?
   A. RNA polymerase
   B. DNA polymerase
   C. Reverse transcriptase
   D. Neuraminidase

3. Which of the following events would not be likely to occur during infection by herpesvirus, a DNA-enveloped virus?
   A. Interaction between cellular receptors and the lipid envelope during adsorption
   B. Fusion of the virus with the plasma membrane during penetration
   C. Assembly of the virus in the nucleus
   D. Final maturation of the virus involving budding from the plasma membrane

4. Which of the following statements concerning nucleic acid replication is untrue?
   A. Minus-stranded RNA viruses use their genome as a template for transcription into mRNA.
   B. Retroviruses, which contain two positive strands, produce a minus strand of RNA

with the aid of the enzyme reverse transcriptase.

C. Double-stranded RNA viruses, which possess segmented genomes, use each segment for transcription into mRNA.

D. Double-stranded DNA viruses use the minus strand for transcription into mRNA.

5. Which of the following statements concerning the effects of virus infection on the host cell is *not* true?
   A. Both enveloped and nonenveloped viruses code for proteins that may become associated with the cell membrane surface.
   B. Integration of the viral genome into the host genome is a mechanism of persistence.
   C. Both enveloped and nonenveloped viruses cause infections in which giant multinucleated cells are formed.
   D. Viral infection can cause the release of interferon from infected cells.

6. Which of the following statements concerning oncogenic viruses is *not* true?
   A. Oncogenic viruses have their genome integrated into or closely associated with the host genome.
   B. Most of the population in the United States at one time or another has been infected by the Epstein-Barr virus, a potentially oncogenic virus.

C. All oncogenic RNA viruses are retroviruses.

D. Viral oncogenes code for enzymes that are unrelated to cellular enzymes.

7. Bacteriophage infection of susceptible bacteria on an agar surface produces areas of clearing called
   A. Foci
   B. Pocks
   C. Plaques
   D. Syncytia

8. Which of the following licensed antiviral agents is *not* used in the treatment of herpesvirus infections?
   A. Acyclovir
   B. Amantadine
   C. Idoxuridine
   D. Vidarabine

9. For which of the following diseases are there both an inactivated and a live vaccine?
   A. Polio
   B. Rubella
   C. Measles
   D. Mumps

10. Henrietta Lacks is best remembered:
    A. For her discovery of the first oncogenic virus
    B. As the first women to succumb to cervical cancer
    C. For her cervical tumor cells, called HeLa cells, which are used in viral research
    D. For her contributions to antiviral chemotherapy

Match the definition or statement on the left with the term or characteristic on the right that best describes it.

11. Protein subunits on the virus coat

12. A complete infective virus

13. Period during virus infection in which mature virus cannot be detected

14. Cytopathic effect that is diagnostic

A. Lysogeny
B. Maturation
C. Epstein-Barr virus
D. Chronic
E. Virus particle
F. Transduction

15. A persistent infection in which there is a long incubation period (years)

16. Believed to be a cause of Burkitt's lymphoma

17. Integrated form of animal virus

18. Cellular counterpart of viral oncogene

19. Virus-associated phenomenon that results in formation of a monolayer of cells

20. Quiescent state following bacteriophage infection

21. Process in which bacteriophage infection causes changes in the bacterium's phenotype

22. The process in which virus transfers bacterial genes to a recipient bacterium

G. Contact inhibition
H. Pathognomonic effect
I. Virion
J. Latent
K. Human papillomavirus
L. Retrovirus
M. Provirus
N. Early period of protein synthesis
O. Eclipse
P. Proto-oncogene
Q. Lysogenic conversion
R. Slow
S. Capsomere

ADDITIONAL READINGS

Bishop, J. M. The molecular genetics of cancer. *Science* 235:305, 1987.

Crowell, R. L., and Lonberg-Holm, K. (eds.). *Virus Attachment and Entry into Cells*. Washington, DC: American Society for Microbiology, 1986.

Dulbecco, R., and Ginsberg, H. S. *Virology* (2nd ed.). Philadelphia: Lippincott, 1988.

Fields, B. N. (ed.). *Virology*. New York: Raven Press, 1985.

Hunter, T. The proteins of oncogenes. *Sci. Amer.* 250:70, 1984.

Lopez, C. (ed.). *Immunobiology and Pathogenesis of Persistent Virus Infections*. Washington, DC: American Society for Microbiology, 1989.

Mims, C. A., and White, D. O. *Viral Pathogenesis and Immunobiology*. London: Blackwell Scientific, 1984.

Notkins, A. L., and Oldstone, M. B. A. (eds.). *Concept of Viral Pathogenesis I and II*. New York: Springer-Verlag, 1984.

Stephnes, E. B., and Compans, R. W. Assembly of animal viruses at cellular membranes. *Annu. Rev. Microbiol.* 42:489, 1988.

Weinberg, R. A. The action of oncogenes in the cytoplasm and nucleus. *Science* 230:770, 1985.

31. VIRAL DISEASES

OBJECTIVES

To group the viruses according to the specific tissue or organ they affect

To outline the various types of herpes viruses and describe the types of infections they cause and what group of individuals are most likely to be affected by infection

To outline those viruses that are likely to have devastating effects on the fetus and/or neonate and how such infections may be recognized and prevented

To briefly describe some of the complications associated with the specific vaccines that are routinely administered in the United States

To list the primary serologic tests that are currently used in the laboratory diagnosis of viral disease

To describe some of the rare sequelae of infection by certain viruses

To understand the concepts of antigenic shift and antigenic drift as they apply to the influenza viruses

To differentiate between the viral agents causing sporadic and epidemic encephalitis

To differentiate among hepatitis B, hepatitis A, and hepatitis C and E as to method of transmission, pathogenesis, laboratory diagnosis, treatment, and prevention

To describe what is meant by slow virus infections and the role of prions

DNA VIRUSES AND ASSOCIATED DISEASES

POXVIRUSES

The poxviruses belong to the family Poxviridae and are divided into subgenera that cause various diseases. The most important genus is called Orthopoxvirus, which contains species called *variola virus, monkeypox virus, vaccinia virus*, and *cowpox virus*. Variola virus is the cause of human smallpox, a disease that was declared eradicated in 1977. Monkeypox, found only in African and Asian monkeys, is poorly transmitted from person to person. Vaccinia virus is a laboratory product that was used to vaccinate humans against smallpox. Cowpox, which is found only in Britain and Western Europe, is a rare disease. The agent of cowpox is isolated from cattle and farmworkers who are in close association with cattle. Rodents, however, may be natural reservoirs for the cowpox virus, which is pathogenic for a wide range of animals, such as camels, cats, gerbils, rats, raccoons, et al.

The poxviruses are the largest of the animal viruses. They range in length from 250 to 300 nm and in width from 200 to 250 nm and are in the shape of a brick (Fig. 31-1). Poxviruses are double-stranded DNA viruses that are assembled in the cytoplasm of the infected cell.

Epidemiology and Pathogenesis

Since smallpox is an eradicated disease, clinical descriptions will not be supplied in any great detail. The student should refer to the readings cited at the end of the chapter in order to know more about this disease. To appreciate the significance of the global vaccine procedures that led to the eradication of the disease, one should be aware of the virulence of smallpox. Smallpox declined in Europe and North America after the introduction of vaccination in 1796 by Edward Jenner (see Chapter 1). Still, in the epidemic years 1930 and 1931, 49,000 cases of smallpox

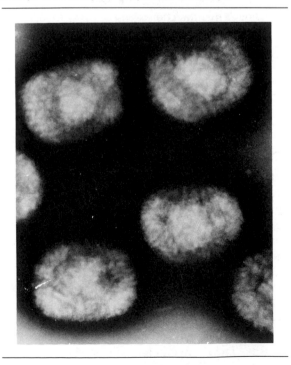

Fig. 31-1. Electron micrograph of smallpox (vaccinia) virus. (Courtesy R. C. Williams, Virus Laboratory, University of California, Berkeley.)

and 173 deaths were recorded in the United States. Fatality rates in developing countries ranged from 15 to 45 percent. In areas endemic for smallpox, such as India, more than one million cases, with 230,849 deaths, were recorded in 1944.

Smallpox is transmitted by inhalation of virus released from lesions in the oropharynx of the infected patient. The incubation period is from 10 to 14 days. The virus spreads rapidly from the oropharynx into the bloodstream, finally lodging in various organs and the skin. Virus lodged in the skin produces a rash about the fourth day of the disease. The rash becomes pustular (Fig. 31-2) and is most profuse about the face. Those who survive infection are scarred for life.

Vaccine

The virus used in vaccines is called the vaccinia virus. There have been many suggestions as to how the virus was derived. Perhaps the most popular theory is that vaccinia virus is a hybrid that arose from inadvertent mixing of the cowpox and smallpox viruses in the laboratory. Vaccination occasionally causes serious complications, especially in those with immunologic deficiencies. Complications may be in the form of (1) encephalitis, which may be fatal in 40 percent of those affected, (2) a spreading necrosis of the inoculated area, and (3) infection of diseased skin in patients with eczema (Fig. 31-3). Vaccination is no longer used in the general population but is still used for:

1. United States and Soviet troops (The reason for vaccination appears to be that each side fears the other might use it in biological warfare.)
2. Laboratory workers who work with the poxviruses
3. Those traveling to certain countries where vaccination is a prerequisite for entry (Some countries in Africa and Asia make this condition.)
4. Those who might be in early contact of someone with a known case of smallpox

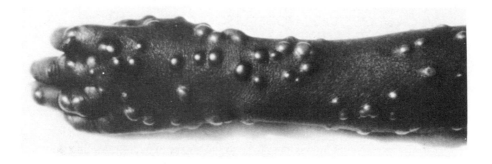

Fig. 31-2. Smallpox pustules on the sixth day of the rash. (Courtesy S. O. Foster.)

Fig. 31-3. Eczema vaccinatum. (Courtesy Department of Pathology, University of Illinois Medical Center, Chicago.)

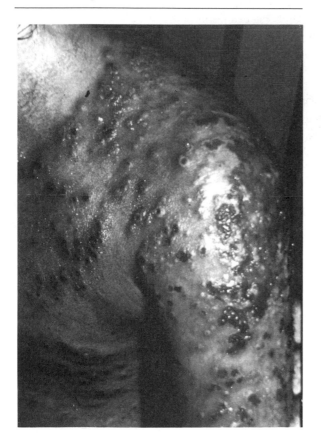

If vaccination in children is required, it should be carried out at ages 1 and 2 years or over to reduce the incidence of complications.

Recombinant vaccinia viruses are currently being used to carry genes for other immunizing antigens. The naked DNA from poxviruses is not infectious and foreign genes with appropriate sequences for expression can be inserted into a nonessential genetic site of a cloned fragment of the vaccinia DNA. Recombinant vaccinia viruses expressing genetic information from influenza, hepatitis B, and herpes simplex have been constructed. Inoculation of these genetically engineered viruses into animals has resulted in production of antibodies directed against the foreign antigen. They may at some time become important human vaccines.

Potential Sources of Infection

Two potential sources of poxvirus infection still remain. The first is accidental infection with laboratory smallpox virus, and the second is infection with animal poxviruses. An example of laboratory-associated smallpox is described in the Boxed Essay (p. 664). Infection with animal poxviruses has been shown to be a distinct possibility. A poxvirus of mammals—namely, monkeypox—has been associated with disease. Monkeys in Africa and Asia are known to harbor the mon-

A CASE OF LABORATORY-ASSOCIATED SMALLPOX: A TRIPLE TRAGEDY

A medical photographer working in a darkroom located above a research laboratory where poxvirus studies were being conducted became a victim of laboratory-associated smallpox in 1978. The photographer had spent most of July 25 telephoning from an office next to her darkroom. The area used for telephoning was close to an ill-fitting inspection panel of the service duct linking the office to the smallpox laboratory one floor below. The smallpox laboratory was due to close at the end of 1978 on the basis of recommendations by the World Health Organization (WHO). The laboratory director and his assistants were working feverishly to complete their studies before the lab was forced to close.

The photographer, who had last been vaccinated for smallpox in 1966, became ill on August 11, 1978, and developed a rash. Her illness was diagnosed by electron microscopy as smallpox by the director of the smallpox laboratory. A few days later a variola strain was isolated from the patient that was identical to the strain being evaluated in the smallpox laboratory. One month later after the onset of symptoms the photographer died of smallpox (renal failure and bacteremia). The director of the laboratory blamed himself for the escape of the virus. He became so depressed that he committed suicide by self-inflicted throat wounds. The father of the photographer also incurred smallpox and was admitted to a hospital. Two days later he died of a heart attack.

Investigations into the cause of this laboratory-associated case of smallpox indicated that the virus had probably escaped from the laboratory to the service duct in the form of an aerosol, which reached the room where the photographer had been phoning. Investigators from other investigation teams, however, dismissed the idea of aerosol transmission, and the mode of transmission to this day has not been satisfactorily explained.

Since 1978 the WHO has attempted to restrict smallpox virus stock to adequate facilities. Presently the CDC in Atlanta, Georgia, and a research institute in Moscow, U.S.S.R., are the containment facilities for storage of smallpox virus.

keypox virus and this virus can be transmitted to humans and produce a disease indistinguishable from smallpox. There is evidence that a person infected with monkeypox virus can transmit the virus to other humans. Human monkeypox, however, is still a rare zoonosis.

There is some fear that animal poxviruses may eventually replace the smallpox virus. Perhaps a mutation could make the animal viruses more easily transmitted to humans. Vigilance by the World Health Organization (WHO) is being exercised to keep track of animal poxvirus infections throughout the world. As a protective measure, the WHO also keeps enough vaccine in stock to inoculate 300 million people.

HERPESVIRUSES

The herpesviruses belong to the family Herpesviridae. They have cubic symmetry, are enveloped (Fig. 31-4), and contain double-stranded DNA as their genetic material. Viral multiplication and assembly take place in the nucleus of the infected cell. The lipid envelope is acquired as the nucleocapsid buds through the nuclear membrane. The important members of this group of viruses are the *cytomegalovirus, varicella-zoster virus, Epstein-Barr virus, herpes simplex viruses*, and *human herpesvirus-6 (HHV-6)*. All herpesviruses are characterized by their ability to persist in their hosts and are therefore associated with recurrent infections.

Cytomegalovirus (CMV)

Pathogenesis. Those groups most susceptible to infection by CMV are infants, renal transplant patients, and those compromised by immunosuppressive drugs or conditions, for example, AIDS patients.

INFECTION IN THE NEWBORN. Pregnant women may acquire CMV by primary infection or by reactivation of a latent infection. Primary infection in the mother results in viremia, and the virus can pass through the placenta and infect the fetus. Nearly every organ of the fetus becomes infected with the virus. Unlike rubella virus infection, which has its worst effects during the first trimester, congenital CMV infection has more deleterious effects on the fetus during the second trimester of pregnancy. It is estimated that approximately 1 percent of all infants (30,000 to 35,000 annually in the United States) are born congenitally infected with CMV. Approximately 90 percent of these have subclinical disease that will remain chronic. From 5 to 10 percent of congenitally infected infants manifest symptoms, which may include intrauterine growth retardation, hepatosplenomegaly, jaundice, and neurological manifestations including deafness and chorioretinitis. A frequent result of symptomatic infection is permanent mental retardation. Childhood retardation from congenital CMV infection is estimated at 2.5 to 10 per 1000 live births (see Boxed Essay, p. 667).

The most common source of perinatal or postnatal infection is reactivation of latent infections in the mother. Virus may be excreted by the mother from the cervix, in breast milk, and in urine and throat secretions. The infant becomes infected during passage through the cervix or acquires the virus from the mother's mouth or breast milk. These infections, which are less severe than congenital infections, because the infants are born with variable levels of maternal antibody, cause mild or marked respiratory disturbances and some liver malfunction. Approximately 2 to 3 percent of all infants are infected perinatally with CMV.

INFECTION IN THE RENAL TRANSPLANT PATIENT. CMV infection is common after renal transplantation (more than 90 percent). The virus may be transmitted via an infected donor kidney, or infection may occur by reactivation of latent virus. Reactivation is sometimes due to immunosuppressive therapy, which is part of the transplantation procedure, or to host-vs.-graft rejection. CMV infection may result in two different syndromes.

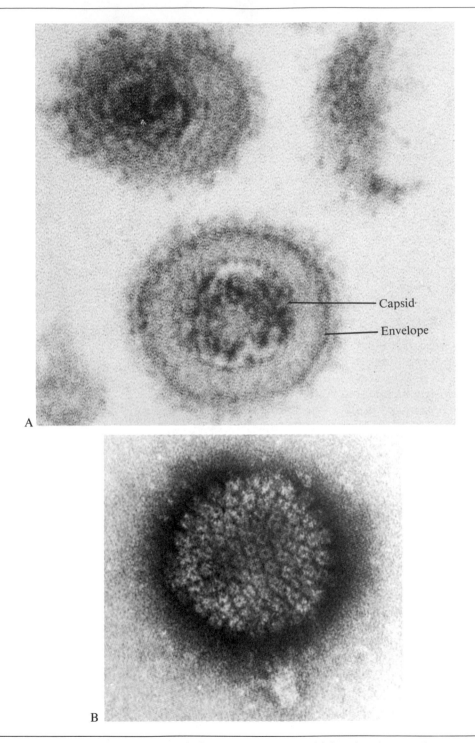

Fig. 31-4. Electron micrographs of herpesvirus. A. Intact herpesvirus particles showing envelope surrounding capsid. (Courtesy B. Roizman.) B. Electron micrograph of the herpesvirus capsid. Note arrangement of the capsomeres. (From R. C. Williams and H. W. Fisher, *An Electron Micrograph Atlas of Viruses*, 1974. Courtesy Charles C Thomas, Publisher, Springfield, Illinois.)

CONGENITAL CYTOMEGALOVIRUS DISEASE: A MAJOR HEALTH PROBLEM

Congenital cytomegalovirus disease is not a reportable disease and the reason given is that infections are not obvious at birth. In addition, many laboratory tests either are too expensive or lack sensitivity. Unfortunately, these reasons do not reflect the seriousness of congenital cytomegalovirus disease. Each year approximately 3000 to 4000 infants are born with symptomatic CMV disease—many of whom die, while the survivors become blind, deaf, or mentally retarded. In addition, each year some of the 30,000 to 40,000 infants who are asymptomatic at birth may also be severely affected by CMV disease. About 15 percent of these infants will either become deaf or suffer a variety of neurological problems. In other words, each year from 7500 to 10,000 infants in the United States will die or require extensive medical care because of CMV disease.

The four avenues of approach to this problem are education, appropriate diagnosis of the disease in infants, treatment of infected infants, and development of a vaccine. Almost all the infants with symptomatic disease are born to mothers who have primary CMV infection during pregnancy. Many young children today are placed in day-care centers to allow mothers the opportunity to work outside the home. It is important that women of childbearing age be aware of their immune status. Relatively inexpensive serological tests are available to determine the immune status of women of childbearing age. The information from these tests would enable women to make informed decisions about pregnancy and its potential risks.

Studies have revealed that women who have a naturally acquired immunity prior to pregnancy may transmit virus to their infants but virtually none of the infants are damaged. A live attenuated vaccine has been tested in renal transplant patients but has not been tested in women of childbearing age. If or when a vaccine is approved it will probably be used for young females.

Lastly, no antiviral agent has yet been approved for treatment of congenital CMV disease. Ganciclovir appears to be a promising drug but has not been approved for use in infants.

1. Six months after transplantation a benign, self-limiting disease may appear, accompanied by fever, leukopenia, and biopsy evidence of rejection. Antibodies to CMV are present in the serum. The deteriorating allograft function improves when immunosuppressive therapy is halted.
2. The same symptoms of fever and leukopenia appear as in the first syndrome but are soon followed by prostration, severe pulmonary and hepatic dysfunction, muscle wasting, central nervous system depression, and death. Antibodies to CMV do not develop, and allograft biopsy shows no evidence of rejection.

Virus shedding occurs in 40 to 80 percent of transplant patients and is more common in those who have antibody to CMV before transplantation. Of those who shed virus, less than one-third have illness. The parent-to-offspring transplant pairing produces more primary infections in recipients than does cadaver-to-recipient pairing.

OTHER CMV INFECTIONS. In patients receiving massive transfusions (for example, during heart surgery), a mononucleosis- or hepatitis-like syndrome may appear. Most *CMV mononucleosis* patients appear well but a few have irregular fever lasting up to three weeks, myalgia, and leukocytosis. Hepatitis is usually mild and liver dysfunction does not become chronic. Primary CMV infection in the immunosuppressed patient can result in severe forms of the disease, especially in younger individuals—the population most susceptible to primary infection. The use of irradiation or drug regimens that suppress the immune system leads to reactivation of virus and disease manifestations such as mononucleosis, pneumonia, and chorioretinitis involving one or both eyes. The overwhelming majority of AIDS patients, especially homosexual men, are positive for CMV and they are more likely to experience reactivation of the disease. Ninety percent of AIDS patients develop active CMV infection and 25 percent of these experience life (encephalitis)- or sight (progressive retinitis)-threatening infections due to this virus. Approximately 10 percent of AIDS patients may also demonstrate CMV-associated gastrointestinal disease, such as colitis, gastritis, or esophagitis.

Epidemiology. The mode of transmission of CMV is not completely understood. The virus is relatively unstable outside the host or body fluids. Few laboratory workers or hospital personnel who are exposed to the virus demonstrate disease. It is therefore believed that CMV is spread by close personal contact, including congenital transfer, direct contact with donor organs or blood transfusions, and contact with body fluids from someone who sheds the virus. By age 50 years about 50 percent of the population in a developed country is seropositive for CMV. Virus excretion persists for years following congenitally, perinatally, or postnatally acquired infections.

Approximately 1 percent of infants excrete CMV at birth and continue to shed it for months to years in the urine or from the throat. Symptomatic congenital infection appears to result from a primary CMV infection during pregnancy. Most infants whose mothers acquire CMV before pregnancy are asymptomatic at birth even though some show a tendency to hearing loss. Fewer than 50 percent of the infants whose mothers acquire primary CMV infections during pregnancy are symptomatic at birth.

The incidence of infection in those who are not congenitally infected increases with age and is correlated with socioeconomic status—the lower the socioeconomic status, the greater the incidence of infection. Most children and adults who acquire infection develop a subclinical form of the disease; fewer than 2 percent of these develop CMV-associated mononucleosis. Excretion of virus by this group may also persist for months or years after symptoms have dissipated.

Laboratory Diagnosis. Diagnosis of CMV infection can be accomplished by several techniques: (1) electron microscopy, (2) detection of typical CMV tissue pathology, (3) isolation of the virus, (4) seroconversion, and (5) detection of CMV antigen or genome in tissue. Electron microscopy is rarely used to identify CMV in the clinical laboratory. Detection of virus in tissue is the hallmark of CMV infection. The infected cell contains a large *intranuclear inclusion*, referred to as "owl's eye" because it is separated from the nuclear membrane by a halo (Fig. 31-5). Cytologic observations are, however, not so sensitive as culture. Virus is most easily isolated from urine or throat washings. Human fibroblasts are used to support the growth of CMV. Incubated samples are observed for CPE from 5 days to 3 to 5 weeks after inoculation of cells. Fluorescent antibody can be used to detect CMV antigen prior to development of CPE. Culture techniques are the preferred diagnostic method in congenital and perinatal infections. Seroconversion, or development of CMV antibody from an initial negative response during the course of infection, is an indication of primary infection. Patients with acute primary infections are usually seronegative and then develop high titers of antibody (IgG or IgM) about 2 weeks later. Antibody is detected by complement fixation. Kits that detect CMV IgG and, especially, IgM are available from a number of commerical sources, but these tests are not rapid. Latex agglutination has become an important method of screening blood and organ donors for CMV antibody. This assay provides results in minutes and is reasonably accurate. Serology, however, does not provide a rapid diagnosis.

Rapid diagnosis is especially important for those in whom CMV infection is life-threatening—for example, AIDS patients. A variety of techniques are now being used to detect CMV antigen in clinical specimens. For example, immunofluorescence using monoclonal antibodies directed against several CMV antigens has been shown to be effective in diagnosis. Experiments are also being conducted on the use of DNA-DNA hybridization to detect CMV in clinical specimens.

Treatment and Prevention. Whenever possible, the blood or organs to be used in transfusion and/or transplantation procedures should be from CMV

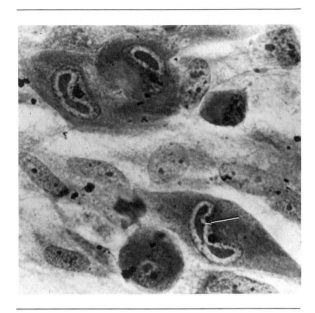

Fig. 31-5. Typical enlarged cytomegalovirus-infected human embryonic fibroblast cells in culture with intranuclear type A inclusions (*arrow*) and cytoplasmic lesion. (Courtesy H. Yamashiroya.)

seronegative donors. In the seronegative, renal transplant recipient and seronegative, bone marrow transplant recipient, the use of CMV-immunoglobulin reduces the risk of CMV disease. In seropositive transplant recipients, acyclovir can be administered orally to reduce the frequency of CMV infection.

Recently two drugs—*foscarnet*, a pyrophosphate analogue, and *ganciclovir*, an analogue of 2' deoxyguanosine—have demonstrated a high degree of potency against CMV. Foscarnet, an inhibitor of DNA polymerase, shows promise in the treatment of AIDS patients with CMV-associated retinitis. Both foscarnet and ganciclovir appear to be effective in the treatment of CMV pneumonitis associated with organ, but not bone marrow, transplantation.

Attenuated vaccines have shown promise in clinical trials. Objection to their use, however, is based on the potential of the virus to become latent and oncogenic.

Varicella-Zoster Virus (Chickenpox and Shingles)

Chickenpox and shingles are different clinical manifestations of infection by the same virus. Chickenpox (*varicella*) is a common benign childhood disease, whereas shingles (*zoster*) is an uncommon disease of later life in which reactivation of the latent varicella infection has occurred.

Pathogenesis. VARICELLA. Varicella infection begins in the upper respiratory tract. The incubation period is between 15 and 18 days. Replication of the virus occurs in the respiratory tract, and viremia ensues. From the blood the virus is taken up by reticuloendothelial cells where it undergoes several replications. The host's immune system becomes overwhelmed and a second viremia develops in which the first symptoms (fever, chills, etc.) of infection are evident. The virus lodges in capillary endothelial cells and then spreads to epithelial cells of the skin producing a rash and this is followed by vesicle formation (Fig. 31-6). The lesions are confined to the thoracic, lumbar, and facial areas. The vesicles of varicella differ from those of smallpox in that all stages of vesicle development may be seen at any one time on the body of the individual infected with varicella. One week after their appearance the vesicles become crusted and fall off, with no visible scarring. The infectious period begins 1–2 days before the rash and lasts up to 1 week after lesions appear. During vesicle development, virus is transported to cranial nerves and dorsal root ganglion cells by centripetal movement along sensory nerve fibers.

Chickenpox is usually regarded as a benign, self-limiting disease. The most common cause of morbidity in normal children is bacterial superinfection. Severe infections caused by either streptococci or staphylococci may occur and may be accompanied by gangrene and deep vein thrombosis. Varicella encephalitis is an infrequent complication. Varicella is more severe in normal adults, and pneumonia has been reported in as many as 16 percent of those infected. In

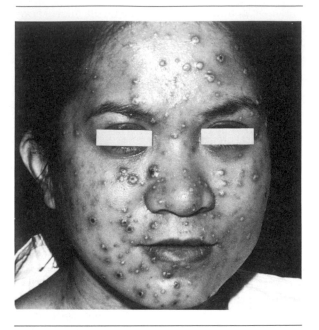

Fig. 31-6. Chickenpox lesions at various stages of development. (Courtesy Department of Pathology, University of Illinois Medical Center, Chicago.)

children and adults who have immunodeficiency disease or who are being treated with immunosuppressive drugs, varicella can become disseminated and is a life-threatening infection. The incidence of disseminated disease in the immunosuppressed is as high as 30 percent, with a mortality as high as 7 percent.

Varicella has teratogenic potential (ability to cause congenital abnormalities) when contracted during the first trimester of pregnancy. If the mother is infected during later stages of pregnancy, the infant develops a rash at birth or shortly thereafter but no congenital anomalies appear. Some of the effects of early fetal infection are low birth weight, bilateral cataracts, an atrophic limb, cortical atrophy, and seizure activity.

ZOSTER. Zoster is attributed to the activation of latent varicella virus that is initially in the cells of the posterior root or cranial sensory nerve ganglia. Its incidence and severity increase with age, and it seldom occurs in the young. Many factors may be responsible for viral reactivation: corticosteroid therapy for nonmalignant diseases, fatigue, sunburn. Once the virus is activated, it moves down the sensory nerves until it reaches the skin, where it replicates and produces localized lesions similar to those of chickenpox. The lesions are confined to the areas affected in varicella—thoracic, lumbar, and facial areas (Plate 19). Before the appearance of the lesions a generalized rash may arise accompanied by fever and intense pain over the involved nerve. In approximately 3 to 5 weeks the lesions heal and the pain subsides.

Postherpetic neuralgia (pain after healing of vesicles) frequently occurs in adults more than 60 years of age and is believed to be due to scarring in the ganglia and afferent portions of the sensory nerve. The symptoms may last as long as 6 months. Facial nerve paralysis is a common complication of zoster. It is not permanent and is resolved within 2 to 3 months after infection.

Zoster may disseminate into various organs, particularly the lungs, in a few patients who have some underlying illness such as Hodgkin's disease or AIDS, or who are being treated with immunosuppressive drugs. AIDS patients, for example, are prone to encephalitis and associated dementia from varicella-zoster–related infection. Untreated disseminated zoster has a high mortality, resulting most frequently from viral pneumonia or secondary bacterial infections.

Epidemiology. Varicella is a very contagious disease found predominately in children, although other age groups may be affected. The disease is believed to be transmitted by the airborne route. Humans are the only known reservoir of infection. The clinical manifestations of chickenpox, as opposed to zoster, are believed to represent the individual's first encounter with the herpes agent. The greatest incidence of the disease is during the spring months and among children 5 to 8 years old. More than 80 percent of the adult population give a history of having had a childhood attack of varicella. In 1988, nearly 193,000 cases of chickenpox were reported in the United States.

Zoster occurs primarily in adults and is neither so seasonal nor so infectious as varicella. Zoster is generally thought to result from the reactivation of virus in those who have had varicella. The frequency and severity of the shingles increase with age, and second attacks are not uncommon. Zoster has been known to give rise to varicella, particularly in nonimmune children who come in contact with zoster patients. Herpes zoster is also infectious, but less so than varicella.

Laboratory Diagnosis. Varicella can ordinarily be diagnosed from the rash or history of recent exposure. The rash can be confused with the smallpox rash. When varicella pneumonia or other complications are evident, a rapid and specific diagnosis is crucial.

A presumptive but rapid test for identification of the varicella-zoster virus involves examination of vesicular material. The degenerated cells at the base of fresh vesicles contain inclusion bodies that can be detected by Giemsa staining. This method serves to distinguish between the poxviruses and the varicella-zoster virus. Presumptive identification can also be made by electron microscopy of vesicular material. Differentiation between varicella-zoster virus and other herpesviruses such as the herpes simplex virus can be accomplished by immunofluorescent staining or gel diffusion tests. In the immunofluorescent staining method, fluorescein-conjugated immunoglobulin from hyperimmune animal serum is used.

The presence of serum antibody to VZV has been shown to correlate with immunity to varicella. Determination of the immune status to varicella is important if hospital-associated infections are to be contained and it is important in deciding whether to administer postexposure prophylaxis with varicella-zoster immune globulin (see Prevention and Treatment). It will also be important in determining the eligibility of some patients for live attenuated vaccine when the vaccine is licensed in the United States. Complement fixation and fluorescent antibody tests are relatively insensitive and time-consuming, respectively. Commercial tests are now available for testing, with rapidity and sensitivity, large numbers of specimens for antibody to VZV. The fluorescent - antibody - to - membrane - antigen (FAMA) test* has been the standard test but because of its cumbersomeness is being replaced by tests such as the indirect fluorescent antibody and ELISA tests.

Immunity. Natural infection or immunization results in the development of varicella-zoster virus–specific IgG and IgM antibodies in the serum. Antibody activity is four to eight times higher after natural infection than after immunization. Antibody that is produced persists for many years, crosses the placenta, and is present before the onset of zoster. Development of serum and nasopharyngeal IgA antibodies occurs with natural infection but not after immunization. Cell-mediated immunity increases immediately after infection and persists for several years. As with other viruses, cell-mediated immunity plays a more important role in recovery from infection than does humoral immunity. The majority of varicella patients develop a permanent immunity.

Prevention and Treatment. Treatment is not necessary in uncomplicated varicella or zoster other than relieving the itching of varicella or the pain of zoster. Vidarabine (adenine arabinoside or ara-A) can be used successfully in complicated cases of varicella, especially varicella pneumonia. The drug should be restricted to immunologically normal patients because it has no therapeutic effect on varicella pneumonia patients compromised by immunodeficiencies. Vidarabine also benefits those with zoster if it is administered within 72 hours after onset of skin eruptions. Acyclovir also benefits the patient and is still effective once disseminated disease has occurred.

Immune globulins have been shown to be ef-

fective in preventing or modifying varicella infection. Two immune globulins are currently available. *Zoster immune globulin (ZIG)* is prepared from the plasma of persons recovering from zoster. *Varicella-zoster immune globulin (VZIG)* is prepared from outdated blood bank plasma from normal persons with high titers of varicella-zoster antibody. Both immune globulins are in short supply and not always available. ZIG and VZIG can prevent varicella in normal children but can only ameliorate the illness of immunosuppressed children. Two groups are eligible to receive ZIG or VZIG: (1) susceptible children with high-risk conditions such as immunodeficiencies or those receiving immunosuppressive drugs who have been exposed to confirmed cases of varicella within the previous 72 hours, and (2) neonates at high risk of having congenital varicella—that is, infants born within 4 days after onset of rash in the mother.

An attenuated varicella-zoster vaccine (OKa strain) has been experimentally evaluated in Japan. It was administered to healthy children, chronically ill children (some of whom were receiving steroid therapy), chronically ill children after the appearance of chickenpox in the ward, and seronegative household contacts within 3 days of exposure. The vaccine proved effective in all cases by preventing infection. Antibody was detectable 2 years after vaccination. Many investigators in the United States believe that further evaluation is needed before licensing the vaccine. Much of their apprehension stems from the possibility that the vaccine itself could cause zoster (and it would take decades to find out), the immunity may not be long lasting, and the result could be a more severe disease later in life. Trials in the United States have shown that the vaccine offers significant protection against severe chickenpox in healthy adults.

Herpes Simplex Virus

Herpes simplex virus (HSV) is the causal agent of several human infections including cold sores, fever blisters, keratitis (inflammation of the cor-

---

* In the FAMA test the membrane antigen of live VZV-infected cells is stained with fluorescent antibody.

nea), encephalitis, and a venereal infection of both men and women. The virus may also be transmitted to the fetus, resulting in a generalized or severe infection. Recurrent herpes simplex infections are common.

There are two serotypes of HSV: types 1 and 2. *Type 1* is associated primarily with lesions in the oral cavity and facial areas. *Type 2* infections are found primarily in the genital area; HSV of either type can cause infection at any site if inoculated at the proper place. A virus called *B virus* is the simian counterpart of HSV (see Boxed Essay, p. 674).

Pathogenesis. HSV infection may be primary (an acute infection that runs its natural course) or recurrent. The cause of recurrent infections is believed to be reactivation of endogenous latent virus. Thus the virus may remain dormant in nervous tissue. Supporting evidence comes from studies in which HSV-1 was isolated from the trigeminal ganglion and HSV-2 from the sacral ganglia of humans. It has been hypothesized that after reactivation the virus in the ganglia travels along the axon of the peripheral nerve to cause a localized infection in the innervated skin. In addition to involvement of the sensory and autonomic nervous systems, HSV is believed to be involved in motor nerves and the central nervous system motor centers. Studies have indicated that HSV can penetrate the neuromuscular junction, travel in a pure motor nerve, and produce a focal encephalitis. The diversity of clinical illness caused by primary HSV infections is outlined in the following paragraphs.

TYPE 1 INFECTIONS

1. *Acute herpetic gingivostomatitis* is a common HSV-1 infection characterized by ulcerative lesions on the mucous membranes of the oral cavity. The disease may be accompanied by fever and cervical lymphadenopathy. The disease is self-limiting and is resolved in 2 to 3 weeks (Fig. 31-7). In immunocompromised patients the infection may extend to the esophageal and laryngeal mucosa.

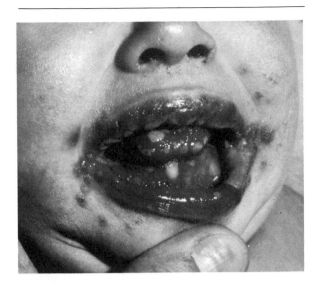

Fig. 31-7. Gingivostomatitis caused by herpesvirus infection. (From J. C. Overall, Jr. In G. J. Galasso, T. C. Merigan, and R. C. Buchanan [eds.], *Antiviral Agents and Viral Diseases in Man.* New York: Raven, 1979.)

2. *Eczema herpeticum* results from accidental inoculation of the virus into the skin lesions associated with eczema. Recurrent attacks are less severe than the initial attack.

3. *Herpetic keratoconjunctivitis* is believed to be the leading cause of loss of vision caused by external eye disease in the United States. Recurrent infections are common and often lead to opacity of the cornea and eventually to impaired vision (Fig. 31-8).

4. *Herpes labialis* is the most prevalent form of herpes type 1 infection. Infections involve the mucocutaneous junction of the lips (fever blisters and cold sores) (Fig. 31-9). Recurrent infections are common and are probably due to activation of latent virus in the sensory cells of the trigeminal nerve ganglion. Many investigators feel that conditions of stress, sunlight, hormones, or menstruation may activate the latent virus. Dental extraction appears also to trigger reactivation of latent HSV in occasional susceptible patients by axonal injury from the local anesthetic injection

B VIRUSES—A SIMIAN COUNTERPART TO HERPES SIMPLEX VIRUS

In 1932 a case of encephalitis caused by B virus in a monkey handler was recorded. The B virus is the simian counterpart of HSV in humans. Only 22 additional cases occurred from 1932 to 1987, but 15 of those patients died of encephalitis. Most cases of human disease are believed to be caused by exposure to contaminated monkey saliva through bites or scratches. Herpesvirus simiae (B virus) is enzootic in rhesus and other Asiatic monkeys. Infection in monkeys is recognized as a gingivostomatitis and, like HSV in humans, remains latent. Viral shedding, in saliva and/or genital secretions is common in infected monkeys.

Of the five cases of B virus infection in 1987, one was apparently caused by person-to-person transmission. Infection has been known to occur following a person's exposure to contaminated cell cultures of simian origin, and one case occurred after the patient had cleaned a monkey skull. B virus infection appears to be treatable with acyclovir (see M.M.W.R. 36 [No. 41]:680, 1987).

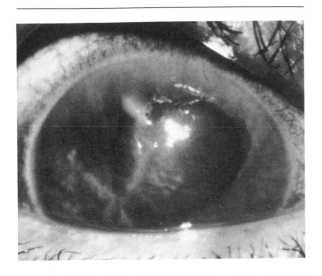

Fig. 31-8. Herpetic keratoconjunctivitis. Dendritic ulcer stained with fluorescein in cornea of patient with recurrent disease. (Courtesy J. Sugar.)

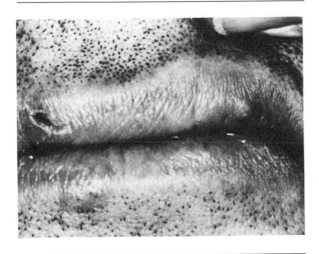

Fig. 31-9. Cutaneous lesions on lips and skin around the mouth of individual with recurrent herpes labialis. (Courtesy L. J. LeBeau.)

or by irritation of the nerve terminals from surgical procedures.

5. *Herpetic encephalitis* acquired after birth is believed to be the most common form of fatal endemic encephalitis in the United States. The virus may enter the host through the nasal cavity and then travel from the olfactory pathway to the base of the brain. Brain infection may also be the result of reactivation of latent virus in the trigeminal ganglion, followed by spread to the brain. The virus tends to localize in the temporal lobes of the brain, where it causes necrosis. Many patients die within 3 weeks of onset of symptoms. Both HSV-1 and HSV-2 are frequently associated with encephalitis. HSV-2-associated encephalitis in children presents with a higher frequency of brain damage and seizures than does HSV-1-associated infections. This finding is the reverse of that seen in adults with HSV encephalitis.

TYPE 2 INFECTIONS. HSV-2 infections include primarily *genital herpes and neonatal herpes*.

1. Genital herpes infection in women generally results in symptoms that do not require medical attention. (In some cases, however, it can be a serious disease causing severe tissue inflammation and pain.) Lesions appear on the vagina, cervix, or vulva and are only mildly discomforting. In men the lesions, which appear primarily on the penis, are painful and are associated with a watery discharge (Fig. 31-10).

2. Neonatal herpes infection may result in three types of disease: (1) disseminated, (2) central nervous system (encephalitis), or (3) skin, eye, and mouth infections. Disseminated infection may involve several organs, such as liver, lung, brain, skin, and/or adrenals. The mortality from disseminated disease is greater than 80 percent. Fewer than 10 percent of the survivors of disseminated or central nervous system disease develop normally. The mortality from central nervous system disease is greater than 50 percent. Babies with skin, eye, or mouth infections do not usually die but about 25 percent of them later develop severe neurological impairment. About 75 percent of the babies with skin, eye, or mouth infections, if left untreated, will progress to either central nervous system or disseminated disease.

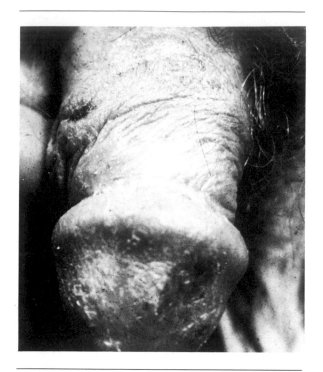

Fig. 31-10. Genital lesions caused by herpes simplex virus infection. (Courtesy L. Solomon, Department of Dermatology, University of Illinois Medical Center, Chicago.)

Neonatal infection is most commonly acquired at the time of delivery by contact of the fetus with infected maternal secretions. Adverse outcomes for the neonate are greater when pregnancies are complicated by a first rather than a recurrent episode of genital herpes.

OTHER MANIFESTATIONS. Lesions on the fingers or hands of physicians, dentists, and medical personnel have been called *herpetic whitlows*. They were originally thought to be caused by type 1 virus acquired through contact with oral lesions of patients. Now it has been discovered that they also occur on the foot and that both types 1 and 2 may be involved. Since type 2 is associated with genital herpes, it is suspected that finger contact with genital lesions is one means of transmission to any part of the body, including the eyes. A

burning or stinging sensation is felt in the lesions. A vesicle is formed, surrounded by a rim of edema and erythema. The vesicles remain unchanged for up to 3 weeks, at which time they begin to heal.

Epidemiology. Herpes simplex infections affect populations throughout the world. It has been difficult to distinguish the true incidence of a primary infection from recurrent disease. Although HSV-1 is associated primarily with oral disease and HSV-2 with genital disease, either strain may be involved with genital or oral disease. For example, pharyngitis due to type 2 has been observed in patients who have engaged in oral sex. It is estimated that 10 percent of genital disease may be caused by type 1 strains. Recurrences of genital herpes are less likely with type 1 strains than type 2 strains. As yet no reasonable explanation for this characteristic has been forthcoming.

The prevalence of genital HSV infection in women during pregnancy and at term, when transmission to the neonate occurs, has not been clearly defined. Most studies indicate that approximately 30 percent of the mothers of neonates have a history of genital herpes. Genital herpes has reached epidemic proportions in the United States. It is estimated that upwards of 30 million people in the United States suffer from genital herpes. Genital herpes is an especially important venereal disease because of its potential effects on the newborn.

Laboratory Diagnosis. The typical herpetic lesion, especially in recurrent infections, can be identified by the physician through patient history and physical examination. This is not true for the lesions in a primary infection, which may resemble lesions caused by a variety of other microbial agents. The diagnosis of HSV infection can be confirmed by serologic diagnosis, but only for primary infections in which the patient has not been previously infected with HSV-1 or HSV-2.

Tissue culture remains the most sensitive method to detect HSV and this is confirmed by observation of cytopathic effects. Although this technique is more sensitive than direct viral antigen or nucleic acid detection in clinical specimens, it requires three days to complete. The importance of early recognition cannot be overemphasized. Several reagents have been manufactured to detect HSV antigens directly in clinical specimens and in cell culture fluid as a means of culture confirmation. These reagents have been used primarily in ELISA assays and direct and indirect fluorescent-antibody assays. The rapid methods detect antigen in less than 24 hours but they are not always reliable because of lack of sensitivity and dependence on the quality of specimen being submitted.

Differentiation of HSV-1 and HSV-2 may be performed by virus isolation and identification of antigen by immunofluorescence. Other techniques such as restricted endonuclease cleaving are also used to type HSV. Differentiation is important because the two HSV types differ in their susceptibility to antiviral agents.

Prevention and Treatment. Effective treatment of herpes simplex infection should be concerned not only with reducing the severity of primary infection but with reducing the severity of recurrent disease, reducing transmission to contacts, and reducing the frequency of recurrences. The drugs currently available for treatment of HSV infections are:

1. Acyclovir. Acyclovir is used for mucocutaneous infections in compromised patients. Acyclovir is also the principal drug for the treatment of primary genital herpes infections. The drug is available in topical or oral form. Continuous oral acyclovir for 6 month periods can suppress recurrent genital herpes.
2. Idoxuridine. This drug is used in topical form for the treatment of keratoconjunctivitis.
3. Trifluridine. This drug is used in topical form for the treatment of keratoconjunctivitis.
4. Vidarabine. Vidarabine is used intravenously for HSV encephalitis and disseminated disease.

There are no vaccines available for preventing HSV infections; however, a subunit glycoprotein vaccine is being used in clinical trials.

Epstein-Barr Virus (EBV)

The Epstein-Barr virus was initially discovered in a Burkitt's lymphoma cell line in 1964 (see Herpesviruses, page 632). Infection by EBV is usually established early in childhood in most parts of the world and remains silent throughout a person's life. EBV is associated with several clinical entities. Its association with Burkitt's lymphoma and nasopharyngeal cancer were discussed previously (Chapter 30). We will discuss three other EBV associations: *infectious mononucleosis, chronic mononucleosis syndrome*, and *EBV-induced disorders in immunodeficient patients*.

When uninfected adolescents and young adults are exposed to EBV about two-thirds of them develop infectious mononucleosis. Symptoms of infection appear about 5 to 10 days after contact with virus. The disease is characterized by sore throat, fever, fatigue, enlarged cervical lymph nodes, and often splenomegaly. The major route of transmission of EBV is through the saliva and very rarely by blood transfusion. In the United States about 15 to 20 percent of young adults are shedders of the virus. Infected individuals who are immunosuppressed (organ transplant patients, for example) are common shedders of virus. EBV inhabits B lymphocytes, where it can remain indefinitely in a latent state. The virus can become activated after recovery from infectious mononucleosis—for example, following immunosuppression. Fortunately, most adults with EBV-infected B lymphocytes do not demonstrate reactivation disease. Infectious mononucleosis generally resolves on its own within one month after infection but occasionally long-lasting fatigue persists. Complications of disease may include hemolytic anemia, aplastic anemia, and agranulocytosis. The sera of patients with infectious mononucleosis contain IgG and IgM antibodies to viral antigens plus IgM heterophile antibodies. Heterophile antibodies are nonspecific and are capable of agglutinating sheep and horse red blood cells.

Chronic mononucleosis syndrome is a protracted illness, usually preceded by infectious mononucleosis, that may last from months to years. Rarely some young children and adults develop life-threatening complications over the course of the disease. The precise mechanism by which EBV causes the syndrome is not known. Some investigators believe that these patients exhibit some immunodeficiency to EBV.

EBV-induced disorders in immunodeficient patients are the result of abnormal proliferation of lymphocytes. AIDS patients, organ transplant recipients, and others with genetically acquired immunodeficiencies may be subject to life-threatening EBV infections. EBV infections may be primary or they may be a result of reactivation of virus. The EBV-associated disorders in AIDS patients, for example, include malignant B-cell lymphoma, colonic lymphoid hyperplasia, and hairy leukoplakia.

Infectious mononucleosis may be presumptively diagnosed on the basis of clinical symptoms plus the finding of elevated lymphocytes. The *Paul-Bunnell-Davidsohn test* detects IgM heterophile antibodies by using sheep or horse erythrocytes as agglutination indicator cells. EBV-induced heterophile antibody can be differentiated from heterophile antibody associated with other diseases by the former's adsorption to beef erythrocytes but not guinea pig kidney.

When cases of infectious mononucleosis are heterophile-antibody negative or when heterophile-antibody–positive patients with atypical manifestations appear, serodiagnostic tests are required for diagnosis of disease. The interpretation of serological tests is based on the profile of antibody titers against four viral antigens: viral capsid, two types of early antigens, and an EBV-determined nuclear antigen. The serologic methods used in diagnosis include immunofluorescence and ELISA.

The diagnosis of lymphoproliferative disorders or malignant lymphoma depends on histologic evaluation of tissue biopsies, but distinguishing between benign and malignant disorders is difficult. Nucleic acid hybridization techniques can be used to detect EBV DNA, which is found only in tissues from patients with active EBV infection having neoplastic or other lymphoproliferative disorders (lymphoma or lymphoproliferative lesions).

Human Herpesvirus-6 (HHV-6)

In 1986 a new herpesvirus was found in the leukocyte cultures of patients with AIDS-associated malignant lymphoma and leukemia. The virus was designated *human lymphotropic virus* or *human herpesvirus-6* (HHV-6).

HHV-6 appears to be distinct from herpes simplex virus types 1 and 2, cytomegalovirus, varicella-zoster virus, and Epstein-Barr virus. The whole virus averages 163 nm in diameter. T cells (CD 4 lymphocytes) appear to be the primary target of the infection by HHV-6. The CD 4 lymphocytes are also the target of the human immunodeficiency virus (HIV), which causes AIDS.

At present it is not known whether HHV-6 causes disease in humans. Like other herpesviruses, it may establish a latent infection after primary infection in the host. Recent serological studies indicate that the virus is acquired early in life and may be the cause of an exanthem (eruption) called *roseola infantum*.

THE ADENOVIRUSES

The adenoviruses belong to the family Adenoviridae. They can be found in many animal species including humans. So far, 41 immunologically distinct adenoviruses of human origin are recognized. The virion is made up of 240 nonvertex hollow capsomeres called *hexons* (surrounded by six capsomeres) in an icosahedral pattern of cubic symmetry (Fig. 31-11). In addition there are 12 vertex capsomeres called *pentons* (surrounded by five capsomeres). Each penton has a fiber attached to it. Some adenovirus

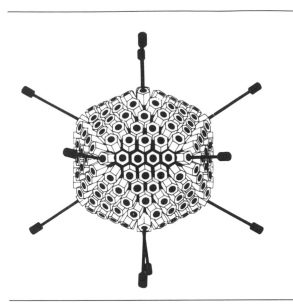

Fig. 31-11. Model of adenovirus showing capsomeres' arrangement as well as placement of the 12 pentons (only 10 are shown in this Figure). Each penton consists of a penton-capsomere, a fiber, and a terminal knob. (From R. W. Horne, I. P. Ronchetti, and J. M. Hobart, *J. Ulstruct. Res.* 51:233, 1975.)

types have a knob attached to the penton fiber, and the complete virion gives the appearance of a laboratory-constructed earth satellite. The penton fibers and the terminal knobs can be seen in electron micrographs. The penton fibers are antigenic and probably serve as organs of attachment. They are responsible for the hemagglutinating activities of the virus (only type 18 fails to hemagglutinate).

Pathogenesis

Adenoviruses have an affinity for mucocutaneous surfaces and are usually associated with respiratory illness, particularly in infants, but gastrointestinal disease is not uncommon. In some instances the association of one viral strain with one clinical syndrome has been demonstrated, but for the most part adenoviruses are associated with a variety of clinical syndromes. Except for pneumonia, most adenovirus infections are not fatal. Occasionally adenoviruses are the cause of meningoencephalitis, acute hemorrhagic cystitis, and neonatal sepsis. Table 31-1 lists the major clinical syndromes in which adenoviruses have been implicated.

The adenoviruses were the first human viruses demonstrated to be oncogenic, but the oncogenicity has been observed only in laboratory rodents. To date there is no proof that the adenoviruses are oncogenic for humans.

Epidemiology

Adenovirus infections are associated with respiratory and ocular disease and occasionally gastrointestinal conditions. Serological surveys indicate that every child in the United States will have had at least one adenovirus infection by the age of 5 years. Respiratory disease is seldom seen in adults except for military recruits. Adenoviruses account for nearly 2 percent of all acute respiratory disease in nonhospitalized children and for 5 to 25 percent in hospitalized children. Of the 41 serological types of adenoviruses only 10 to 12 have been routinely associated with disease. Children under 6 years of age are most susceptible to infection by adenoviruses. The clinical conditions associated with infection in children include pharyngitis, bronchitis, croup, and pneumonia. Types 3, 7, and 21 have been associated with lower respiratory tract disease and "swimming pool" conjunctivitis in children under 6 years of age. Types 4 and 7 are the major cause of epidemic respiratory illness in military recruits. Although type 7 usually produces mild illness it has been associated with respiratory disease of high mortality, particularly in hospitalized children with underlying heart or respiratory illness. Types 8 and 19 are associated with keratoconjunctivitis, a very severe eye disease. Keratoconjunctivitis outbreaks occur frequently in industrial settings and in the offices of ophthalmologists (because of contaminated ophthalmic equipment or solutions). Adenoviruses types 40 and 41 are the second most commonly identified agent after rotavirus in stool samples of patients with infantile gastroenteritis.

Table 31-1. Adenovirus-associated Syndromes and Viral Type Most Frequently Recovered

Syndrome	Adenovirus types	Symptoms and signs
Acute respiratory disease	Types 4 and 7 in military camps; types 3, 14, and 21 in civilian populations	Sore throat, cervical lymphadenopathy, fever
Pharyngoconjunctival fever	Usually types 3 and 7; types 1, 4, and 14 less frequent; worldwide summer epidemics among infants; acute follicular conjunctivitis more frequent in adults	Pharyngitis, conjunctivitis, sore throat, fever, and cervical lymphadenopathy
Pharyngitis	Types 3, 4, 7, 14, and 21	Pharyngitis and intestinal pain often observed in infants
Pneumonia	Types 3 and 7; mortality highest in this syndrome, which occurs primarily in infants	—
Epidemic keratoconjunctivitis	Types 8 and 19 most frequent cause of this syndrome in the United States	A localized infection in which subepithelial opacities occur in the cornea and may remain for up to 2 years.
Gastrointestinal disease	Types 40 and 41	Diarrhea with or without vomiting (second most important cause of infantile gastroenteritis after rotavirus, but milder than rotavirus infections)

Laboratory Diagnosis

Swabs of clinical specimens (except stool samples) are inoculated into primary human embryonic kidney cell cultures and incubated. Cytopathic effects are analyzed after approximately 14 days. For rapid identification of an isolate, fluorescent antibody staining is used. A polyclonal fluorescent antibody reagent is commercially available but monoclonal antibody systems are currently being evaluated. Neutralization with type-specific antiserum is the best method for typing the adenovirus isolate. Typing is an important aspect of identification because a particular set of serotypes is associated with a specific disease.

Types 40 and 41 must be cultivated on special cell lines. Once cultivated, they are typed by viral genome analysis. Direct detection of enteric virus in stool specimens can be obtained by use of a monoclonal antibody-based enzyme immunoassay.

Prevention and Treatment

The frequent outbreaks of respiratory disease caused by type 7 adenovirus in military camps led to the development of a vaccine. Live vaccines of types 4 and 7 have been developed for oral administration. The virus is encased in a capsule, which when released in the intestine causes an asymptomatic response. The virus is nontransmissible. No chemotherapeutic agent has proved effective in treating any adenovirus-associated condition, including conjunctivitis.

THE PAPILLOMAVIRUSES

The papillomaviruses (Fig. 31-12) are structurally similar to the polyomaviruses, such as SV40 and the BK and JC viruses, discussed in Chapter 30, but the former cannot replicate in cultured cells. The papillomaviruses are the cause of warts. Humans are the only hosts for human papillomavi-

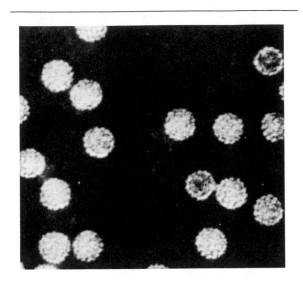

Fig. 31-12. Electron micrograph of human papilloma-virus. (From B. Janis. In P. D. Hoeprich [ed.], *Infectious Diseases* (2nd ed.). New York: Harper & Row, 1977.)

ruses. Warts can be transmitted from person to person. The virus infects cells and stimulates them to divide. Papillomas begin as a proliferation of connective tissue followed by a proliferation of the epidermal cells. It may take 1 to 6 months before the wart becomes evident. Warts are divided into four clinical types: (1) *verruca vulgaris* (common wart), (2) *verruca plana* (flat wart), (3) *verruca plantaris* (plantar wart), and (4) *condyloma acuminata* (venereal warts). Each clinical type is distinct and should be distinguished because therapy for each differs. Each clinical type may be caused by more than one virus type. Most warts regress, but if they persist they can be treated by electrosurgery or cryo-surgery or by topical application of drugs, such as podophyllotoxin or trichloroacetic acid. Podophyllotoxin is contraindicated in pregnancy.

Venereal warts are soft, pink cauliflower-like growths that appear singly or in clusters on the external genitalia and rectum. The disease is one of the most common sexually transmitted diseases in the United States. More than eight mil-lion new and recurrent cases are reported each year in the United States. It is estimated that between 12 and 14 million people in the United States are infected with the papillomavirus. There is a direct association between venereal warts and other sexually transmitted diseases. Nearly 30 percent of women with venereal warts also have gonorrhoea. Most homosexual men with perianal warts also have syphilis or gonor-rhoea. Spontaneous regression of venereal warts occurs, but when they do not regress serious consequences may take place. Large growths may result in transmission to neonates, and such transmission is thought to give rise to childhood laryngeal papillomatosis. There is also some evidence that patients with a history of anogenital warts are predisposed to cervical and perianal neoplasias (see page 634).

Electrocauterization and cryotherapy appear to be the best methods of treatment. Recurrent warts may be removed by surgery. The FDA has recently approved the use of a recombinant version of alpha interferon (Intron-A) to treat genital warts. The drug is injected directly into lesions and it either eliminates or reduces lesions. To date, however, carbon dioxide laser therapy appears to be one of the most satisfactory methods for treating genital warts. Podophyllotoxin can also be used and can be applied by the patient.

The most sensitive method of diagnosing human papillomavirus infection is by DNA hybridization using cloned, type-specific virus probes.

THE PARVOVIRUSES

Parvoviruses belong to the family Parvoviridae. They are nonenveloped single-stranded DNA viruses with icosahedral symmetry. The capsids have a diameter of 20 to 25 nm. Included in this group of viruses pathogenic for humans are the adeno-associated virus (AAV) and parvovirus B19. AAV infection of humans is common but occurs only in association with adenovirus infection. Replication of AAV can occur only with the aid of its helper adenovirus. No unique disease has been associated with AAV.

Parvovirus B19

Parvovirus B19 was first discovered in human blood in 1975. No disease manifestation was associated with the virus, however, until 1981. Individuals with chronic hemolytic anemias—for example, sickle cell anemia and beta-thalassemia—were shown to be susceptible to infection by B19 virus. B19 virus infection in this group produces a condition called *transient aplastic crisis (TAC)*. Patients with TAC have a moderate to severe anemia that may require transfusion and hospitalization if not treated promptly. The serious mainfestations of infection are related to the virus' propensity to infect and lyse erythroid precursor cells and interrupt normal red blood cell proliferation.

Parvovirus B19 infection occurs worldwide and can affect all age groups. The virus is now believed to be associated with other conditions (see Boxed Essay, p. 683).

Norwalk Viruses

The Norwalk virus (identified during an epidemic in Norwalk, Ohio) is a prototype for several viruses that cause a mild epidemic form of gastroenteritis. The virus is a nonenveloped, spherical particle whose nucleic acid content is not known and has not been placed in any family of viruses. Norwalk viruses cannot be cultivated in cell culture by standard techniques. The virus can be identified by immunoelectron microscopy (IEM is a technique in which antibody specific for the virus is added to a specimen containing virus. Specific immune-virus aggregates are formed and are easier to visualize than individual virions).

Norwalk viruses have been associated with disease, primarily in school-age children and adults. The disease is characterized by vomiting, nausea, diarrhea, and abdominal pain. Most epidemics or sporadic cases occur during the winter months, September to March. The mild gastrointestinal disease caused by Norwalk viruses is comparable to infection by two RNA viruses, astroviruses and caliciviruses, which are discussed later in this chapter.

Norwalk virus illness is usually acquired by ingestion of contaminated food or water. Norwalk virus disease is a very mild form of gastroenteritis that resolves on its own. Administration of fluids is suggested to replace the fluids lost through diarrhea. Immunity to reinfection may be short term or long term. Short-term resistance is serotype specific for 6 to 14 weeks after the initial infection. The reasons for long-term immunity are not known, since most individuals who resist viral challenge have little if any antibody to the virus. Studies do indicate that an individual must be exposed to the virus several times before immunity develops.

RNA VIRUSES AND ASSOCIATED DISEASES

MEASLES

Measles as a clinical entity has been recognized for several hundred years. The measles virus was first cultivated in human and monkey kidney cell cultures in 1954. In 1963 an attenuated vaccine was made available to the public, and since that time the number of measles cases in the United States has dropped precipitously. In less well-developed countries, however, the morbidity and mortality in young children from measles infection remain at high levels.

The measles virus is an enveloped, spherical RNA virus measuring approximately 150 nm in diameter. It belongs to the Paramyxoviridae family. The envelope contains hemagglutinin peplomers but does not carry neuraminidase, as many other paramyxoviruses do. The virus is very labile at 37°C but is stable when stored at sub-zero temperatures.

PARVOVIRUS B19: VIRUS IN SEARCH OF A DISEASE

Following the recognition of parvovirus B19 as a cause of hemolytic anemia in sickle cell disease, other diseases of unknown but potential viral etiology were sought in the 1970s. One of the conditions now believed to be parvovirus B19–induced is an infectious exanthem (skin eruption) called *erythema infectiosum (fifth disease)*. Fifth disease derives its name from a nineteenth-century numbering system given to the exanthems during that period (e.g., measles #1, scarlet fever #2, etc.). The disease is common in children 5 to 14 years old and is mildly contagious. The virus is believed to be spread from respiratory secretions and following viremia a rash develops that often resembles rubella (German measles). Sometimes the rash is not present and the disease remains relatively asymptomatic.

Symptoms in children are milder than in adults. There is a three-stage rash in children sometimes preceded by fever. Initially there is an erythematous rash on the face and this is followed by a rash on the extremities 3 to 4 days later. The rash seldom involves the trunk, soles, or palms. During the third stage the rash may remit—to recur with stress, exercise, or sunbathing—and usually disappears within a week or two. In adults infection is more severe and arthralgia or arthritis is commonly observed with or without rash. Adults often complain of fatigue and depression. Numbness and tingling of the fingers often occur in over 50 percent of the patients.

It is now believed that parvovirus B19 may also be associated with many abortions and stillbirths during pregnancy. Like rubella virus, parvovirus B19 is believed to cross the placenta and pose risk to the fetus. In many of the stillbirths and abortions serologic evidence of parvovirus B19 infection has been confirmed but further studies are required.

The epidemic nature of the parvoviruses now makes it seem likely that we should examine other situations in which virus may be spread, such as in the hospital setting, in transplant patients, and in those in whom susceptibility to infection is increased by underlying conditions. (See *Pediatr. Inf. Dis.* 6:711, 1987; *Rev. Inf. Dis.* 10:1005, 1988.)

Pathogenesis

Measles infection is initiated by spread of virus to respiratory tract, mouth, pharynx, and conjunctiva. The incubation period lasts 7 to 10 days, during which time fever, conjunctivitis, sore throat, photophobia, and headache appear. In the incubation period the virus multiplies in the respiratory mucosa and is then disseminated to the entire body via the bloodstream. A rash first appears on the face and then spreads to the extremities. The rash, which is made up of reddish elevated macules that tend to coalesce, lasts for only 3 or 4 days (Plate 20). Throughout the incubation period and up to 2 days after the appearance of the rash the patient is highly contagious. Virus can be shed from the conjunctiva or the respiratory mucosa.

A day or so before the rash is visible, small red macules with a bluish-white center appear on the inside of the cheek in more than 95 percent of persons infected. These lesions are called *Koplik's spots* and are important in measles identification.

Measles is a self-limiting disease; however, secondary infections of the upper respiratory tract such as pneumonia do occur, particularly in patients debilitated by other illnesses. Measles-associated encephalitis occurs in 1 of every 1000 cases. A very small percentage of patients contract a demyelinating encephalitis, which is fatal to one-half of those affected. The remainder of those with encephalitis suffer varying degrees of central nervous system (CNS) injury that may result in loss of mental and motor functions. A rare sequela of measles infection is *subacute sclerosing panencephalitis* (*SSPE*) (see Slow Virus Infections later in this chapter). It is characterized by changes in personality, motor loss, speech difficulty, and mental retardation. Death is the invariable outcome of SSPE.

Severe forms of measles are common in developing countries throughout the world. Overcrowding and intensive exposure are important determinants in the high case–fatality ratio (10–15%) found in developing countries. Thus, when several sick children in a family live under crowded conditions a higher case–fatality ratio is observed than when there are isolated cases.

The measles virus can bridge the placental barrier and infect the fetus, resulting in premature labor and increased rates of spontaneous abortion. First trimester infection may be associated with congenital malformation.

Epidemiology

Measles is one of the most communicable diseases of humans and is seen everywhere in the world. In unimmunized populations almost every child will get measles early in life. Before 1963, when attenuated measles vaccine was first licensed, more than 400,000 cases occurred annually in the United States, with over 400 deaths and 300 cases of encephalitis (Fig. 31-13). In 1989, 18,193 measles cases were reported to the CDC, with complications in approximately 3 percent or 445 cases. Otitis media (5.4%) was reported most frequently and encephalitis least frequently (0.1%). It is estimated that 25 percent of patients with encephalitis caused by measles will be left with residual brain damage manifested by conditions such as mental retardation, seizure disorders, and nerve deafness. Measles is primarily a disease of childhood, but unimmunized adults are just as susceptible as children. Epidemic cycles appear every 2 to 3 years and are related to climate, the season, and the number of unimmunized persons in the community. Since the widespread administration of vaccine in the United States these 2- to 3-year peaks of incidence no longer occur in this country. The administration of vaccine has also resulted in a reduction of the incidence of disease in school-age children. The highest incidence now observed in the United States is in children under 5 years of age (Table 31-2). In unimmunized populations most infections occur in children between 6 months and 2 years of age. Spread of virus is more rapid when younger children are infected because of greater contact with other family members.

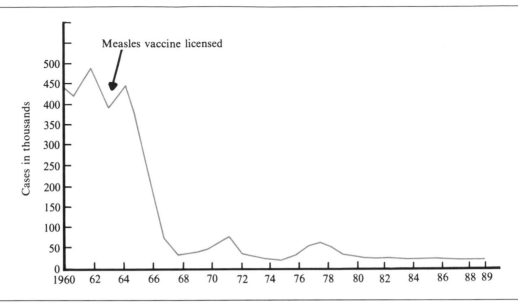

Fig. 31-13. Number of reported cases of measles in the United States, 1960–1988. (From Centers for Disease Control.)

Table 31-2. Age Distribution and Estimated Incidence Rates (per 100,000 Population) of Measles—United States, 1987

Age group (years)	Number of cases	Percent	Rate
0–4	1065	(29.2)	5.9
5–9	337	(9.2)	1.9
10–14	717	(19.6)	4.3
15–19	1047	(28.7)	5.6
20–24	205	(5.6)	1.0
≧25	281	(7.7)	0.2

Source: M.M.W.R. 37 (34):527, 1988.

Laboratory Diagnosis

Measles is diagnosed on the basis of certain clinical features—for example, Koplik's spots and rash. In most measles cases laboratory diagnosis is not needed. In many cases Koplik's spots are not detected and the measles rash may be misdiagnosed. During measles infection the virus causes the formation of multinucleate giant cells 2 to 6 days after the disappearance of the rash. Indirect fluorescent antibody technique can de-

tect these giant cells in nasopharyngeal cells aspirated from the patient. The demonstration of the multinucleate giant cells is a positive test for measles. Complement-fixing, neutralizing, and hemagglutination-inhibiting antibodies develop in the serum at the onset of the rash. The hemagglutination inhibition test is one of the most useful and rapid tests for determining a patient's immunity status. The ELISA, however, is a more sensitive test.

Immunity

Infants are protected for up to 12 months after birth because of maternal antibodies. Following acute disease, lifelong immunity is established. Subclinical infections can occur if virus is circulating in the community.

Prevention and Treatment

The best method for control of measles is vaccination. From 1963 to 1967 an inactivated vaccine was used, and many vaccinations did not take because of nonimmunogenicity of the vaccine or because the vaccine was administered at too early an age, that is, less than 12 months. Probably as a result of this failure, cases of measles among today's 15- to 19-year-olds have increased. An attenuated vaccine, prepared from chick embryo cell culture, has been available since 1968. The vaccine currently used is called the *Moraten vaccine*. The vaccine is available in monovalent form and in combinations: measles-rubella (MR) and measles-mumps-rubella (MMR). Measles vaccines had been routinely administered as a single dose at approximately 15 months of age. Several outbreaks of measles, however, among children less than 15 months of age and among children who had been vaccinated have occurred. These outbreaks have prompted a new strategy for elimination of measles in the United States. A routine two-dose vaccination schedule is now recommended. The first dose is recommended at 15 months of age for children in most areas of the country, but at 12 months of age for children in some areas with recurrent measles transmission. The second dose is recommended when a child enters school at kindergarten or first grade. When outbreaks of measles occur, vaccination is also recommended. For example, if measles is occurring in children less than one year of age, vaccination can be initiated in children as young as 6 months of age. This is followed by revaccination at 15 months of age. If outbreaks occur in day-care centers, K-12th grades, colleges, and other institutions, revaccination is recommended for all students and their siblings and for school personnel born in or after 1957 who do not have documentation of immunity to measles.

Both doses of measles vaccine should be given as combined MMR vaccine when given on or after the first birthday. Measles vaccine should not be given to women who are pregnant or to anyone with a febrile illness.

Immune serum globulin (ISG) provides short-term protection if given less than six days before exposure to the virus. ISG is especially valuable for susceptible household contacts of measles patients, particularly those less than 1 year old. Vaccine should not be given at the time of ISG administration: at least three months should elapse before vaccine is administered. ISG does not prevent infections from occurring at a later date.

MUMPS (EPIDEMIC PAROTITIS)

The mumps virus belongs to the Paramyxoviridae family. The mumps virus is a pleomorphic, roughly spherical, enveloped RNA virus whose size may range from 100 to 600 nm. The RNA genome is single-stranded and nonsegmented. The envelope carries glycoprotein peplomers (hemagglutinins) as well as the enzyme neuraminidase. Neuraminidase can destroy cell receptor sites and thus may interfere with the hemagglutinin reaction. A glycoprotein called *F* (fusion) is also part of the viral envelope. F protein mediates the fusion of the viral envelope with the cytoplasmic membrane of the host cell. (Fig. 31-14). This activity provides the virus with a mechanism for penetration of the nucleocapsid into the host cell.

Pathogenesis

The incubation period of mumps is 16 to 21 days. During this period the virus multiplies in the upper respiratory tract. Later the virus enters the blood and infects other organs and tissues including the CNS. The salivary (parotid) glands are invariably infected, with swelling and sometimes intense pain. (In the view of some researchers, the virus in the oral cavity goes to Stensen's duct and then the parotid gland, where it multiplies and finally causes a general viremia.) Unilateral infection of the testes occurs in approximately 25 percent of men infected. Infections are rare in infants up to 6 months old because of the protective influence of maternal antibody acquired in utero. Early infections of the fetus may cause death or premature onset of labor, but not congenital malformations.

Mumps is a benign disease although complica-

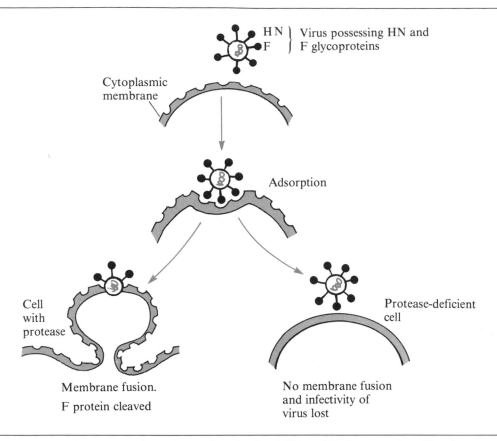

Fig. 31-14. Paramyxovirus penetration of the cell and role of HN and F glycoproteins. HN glycoprotein is required for membrane attachment. Once attachment has taken place, the F protein is cleaved by a protease that promotes membrane fusion and infectivity. Cells deficient in protease do not show membrane fusion, and infectivity is lost.

tions occasionally arise. These include (1) pancreatitis, which may or may not induce diabetes; (2) thrombocytopenia, a disease characterized by bleeding caused by a decrease in the number of blood platelets; (3) aseptic meningitis,* which may occur in up to 10 percent of those infected; (4) meningoencephalitis, a complication of the CNS that may afflict 0.5 to 10 percent of those infected without causing permanent damage; and (5) orchitis (infection of the testes), which may

accompany 20 percent of the clinical cases of mumps in postpubertal males (unilateral infection does not usually result in sterility, but bilateral involvement poses a risk). In females the ovaries may be infected but there is no threat of sterility.

Epidemiology

Mumps is a disease endemic throughout the world. Humans are the only known host of the mumps virus, which is transmitted by respiratory droplets or fomites contaminated with saliva. The peak incidence of the disease is between January and May. Mumps is contagious primarily because

---

* *Aseptic meningitis* refers to viral meningitis, in which spinal fluid is clear. In bacterial meningitis spinal fluid is often purulent (cloudy owing to large numbers of bacteria and leukocytes).

as many as 50 percent of persons infected may be asymptomatic and, in those who develop symptoms, virus is shed from saliva and urine several days before and after symptoms appear. In 1967, the year the vaccine was licensed, 185,691 cases were reported in the United States; in 1989, 5,712 cases were reported. This represents a 98 percent decrease (Fig. 31-15). Most cases used to be found in elementary school children but most outbreaks today occur in high schools and on college campuses. The reason for this trend, which is also characteristic of measles and rubella, is that some individuals do not become vaccinated or have the disease at a younger age.

Mumps is an endemic disease in which about one-third of the infections result in subclinical disease. Immunity to mumps is usually acquired between the ages of 5 and 14 and is long-lived.

Laboratory Diagnosis

Like measles, laboratory diagnosis is not required for mumps. Virus can be isolated from urine, saliva, or CNS specimens within 4 to 5 days after onset of illness. An immunofluorescence test can be used for early diagnosis. It has been reported that virus can be isolated in 80 percent of the cases up to 15 days after onset of the disease. The specimens are inoculated onto monkey kidney or human embryonic kidney cell culture. The virus cultivated in cell culture can be identified by hemagglutination inhibition or fluorescent antibody tests.

Serologic studies are the foundation of laboratory diagnosis of current mumps infection and monitoring effects of vaccination. Complement fixation is used for diagnosis of current infection while ELISA tests are used to monitor vaccination.

Prevention and Treatment

Vaccines appear to produce an immunity equivalent to that obtained in natural infection. An attenuated mumps vaccine prepared in chick embryos is available for children 1 year old or older.

Fig. 31-15. Reported mumps cases per 100,000 population, by year, United States, 1968–1988. (From Centers for Disease Control.)

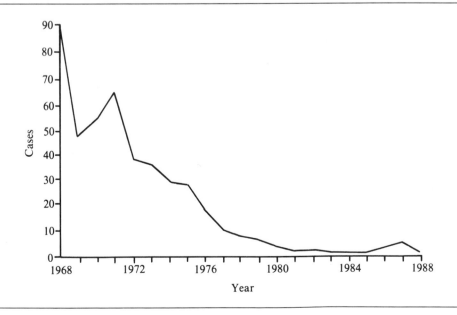

The vaccine is often combined with other vaccines, that is, MMR and rubella-mumps. If used with measles vaccine it should be administered at 15 months of age to ensure maximum seroconversion (antibody production) for measles (maternal antibody can interfere with maximum seroconversion). Mumps vaccine is also recommended for adolescents and adults who have not encountered mumps during childhood. Vaccine should not be administered to persons with febrile illness, congenital immunodeficiencies, leukemia, or lymphoma, or to those receiving immunosuppressive therapy. Because of the theoretical risk of fetal damage, vaccine is also not recommended for pregnant women.

Mumps vaccine is considered one of the safest of the childhood immunizing agents, yet only 31 states require proof of mumps immunity as a condition for entry into school. The incidence of mumps in states without a compulsory school mumps immunization law is twice as high as that in states with such a law.

RUBELLA

Rubella was first described in Germany in the 1800s and was subsequently called German measles. In 1941 Sir Norman Gregg suggested that rubella infection during the first trimester of pregnancy was responsible for crippling effects on the fetus (teratogenic effects), but the virus was not isolated until 1962. The full clinical implications of rubella infection were not realized until the pandemic of 1964, in which more than 30,000 infants were born with congenital abnormalities.

Rubella virus belongs to the family Togaviridae. It is a spherical virus 60 nm in diameter and consists of a nucleocapsid surrounded by a lipoprotein envelope. The RNA of the rubella virus is single-stranded. The virus also contains a hemagglutinin that interacts with erythrocytes from day-old chicks, geese, or pigeons. The virus can be cultivated on a large number of cell types, and isolation from clinical specimens is not difficult.

Pathogenesis

Postnatal Rubella Infection. Postnatal rubella infection is transmitted via the upper respiratory tract. The incubation period for the disease is 14 to 21 days. The virus multiplies in the mucosa of the respiratory tract and spreads to the bloodstream. During the viremic stage the virus is routinely found in the throat, blood, and feces. As the antibody level increases during infection, circulating virus decreases, a rash appears, and virus is found only in the nasopharynx. Maximal shedding of virus occurs 1 to 2 days before and 3 to 5 days after onset of rash. In addition to the rash, symptoms include fever, leukopenia, and suboccipital lymphadenopathy. The disease is self-limiting although complications such as arthritis and arthralgia are commonly encountered by young women.

Congenital Rubella Infection. Congenital rubella results from infection of the fetus during the viremic stage in the pregnant mother. Disease is more prevalent when infection occurs during the first trimester. More than 30 percent of fetuses infected during the first trimester will be stillborn, aborted, or deformed at birth. Congenital anomalies of the infant may include cataracts and glaucoma, heart defects, deafness, and encephalitis. The virus is not lethal to fetal tissue but does cause inhibition of mitosis, which culminates in underdeveloped organs or tissues. The mortality for babies symptomatic at birth is 20 percent.

Epidemiology

Rubella is worldwide in distribution and occurs more frequently during the winter and spring months. The virus is harbored in the upper respiratory tract of infected individuals and is transmitted by person-to-person contact. Both symptomatic and asymptomatic persons can shed virus and be a source of infection to others. In congenital rubella syndrome, for example, the virus is shed for several months after delivery.

This is a particularly important aspect of rubella infection because infant viral carriers are a constant source of infection to unimmunized nurses and other female personnel who come in contact with them.

The incidence of rubella and congenital rubella syndrome has steadily declined since 1969, the year rubella vaccine was first made available to the public (Fig. 31-16). Before 1969 approximately 50,000 cases per year were reported in the United States. In 1974 more than 62 percent of the children aged 1 to 12 years had received the rubella vaccine. In 1976, 12,000 cases were reported, but since then the number of cases has declined dramatically. In 1989 only 396 cases were reported. Congenital rubella syndrome has also delcined precipitously and in 1989 only 3 cases were recorded.

Laboratory Diagnosis

There are relatively few situations in which viral isolation is necessary for laboratory diagnosis. Serological diagnosis is the preferred method for accessing the state of acute and congenital disease. The standard test has been hemagglutination inhibition (HI) since HI antibodies are detected throughout the life of the patient following infection. The HI test, however, is time-consuming and highly technical, and requires removal of nonspecific inhibitors from the serum. Rapid commercially prepared test kits such as ELISA, enzyme immunoassay, latex agglutination, and passive hemagglutination have provided laboratories with accurate alternative methods to the HI test.

Immunity

Immunity to rubella infection is apparently lifelong, but not enough years have elapsed since licensure of the vaccine to determine the effect of vaccination. Recent studies have indicated that vaccine-induced antibody persists up to 16 years in the majority of those vaccinated. However, up to 10 percent of those vaccinated have low levels of antibody six years after vaccination. Subclinical infection can take place with wild rubella virus, but such infections are associated with those who have vaccine-induced immunity. The virus can be isolated from the upper respiratory tract in subclinical infections, but the period of virus shedding is short and the risk of viremia is not evident. Viremia may be possible in those with vaccine-induced immunity. Susceptible contacts are not believed to be at risk, and immune women reinfected are unlikely to infect their fetuses.

Prevention and Treatment

There is no treatment for either congenital or postnatal rubella infection. If infection occurs during the first trimester of pregnancy, therapeutic abortion is recommended by many doctors. Control of rubella rests primarily on vaccination procedures aimed at protecting women of childbearing age. Immunization in the United States is advised for children between the age of 1 year and puberty, and for adolescent girls and adult women who are seronegative and in whom pregnancy can be avoided for at least 3 months after vaccination. Although the risk of rubella may be minor, pregnant women can become infected and should avoid contact with rubella patients.

An attenuated rubella vaccine (RA 27/3) developed in 1979 has replaced older vaccines (Cendehill or HPV-77) for use in the United States. The vaccine may be given intranasally or by injection. It is used either in monovalent form or in combination with measles or measles-mumps vaccines. The trivalent vaccine is recommended in infant vaccination programs but should be given at 15 months of age to achieve maximum measles seroconversion.

The vaccine is not given to women during early pregnancy since fetal infection may occur. However, no teratogenic effects have been reported and termination of pregnancy is not considered under these conditions. Postpartum women who

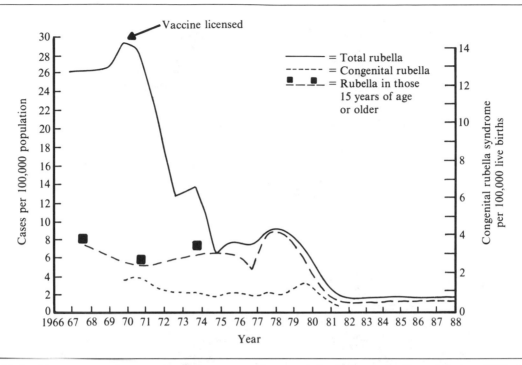

Fig. 31-16. Incidence rates of reported rubella cases and congenital rubella cases, United States, 1967–1988. (From Centers for Disease Control, *M.M.W.R.* 38:173, 1989.)

lack evidence of immunity should be vaccinated before discharge from the hospital. This procedure is believed to reduce the incidence of congenital rubella syndrome by 30 to 50 percent.

Vaccine side effects are more severe in adults, particularly women, than in children. Arthralgia and transient arthritis are the major complaints, but the symptoms seldom last more than 2 to 3 weeks. Recurrences of arthritis, especially in the knee joint, can prevail up to 24 months after vaccination.

It is estimated that 20 to 30 percent of women of childbearing age lack rubella antibody. Recommendations by hospital advisory committees on immunization of hospital personnel who have contact with female patients of childbearing age have not always been followed. Currently, only four states have laws requiring proof of immunity to rubella for hospital personnel.

INFLUENZA

The influenza viruses belong to the family of RNA viruses called the Orthomyxoviridae. They are usually spherical, although filamentous forms are known, and measure 80 to 100 nm in diameter (Fig. 31-17). Surrounding the internal ribonucleoprotein is a lipid envelope from which project *hemagglutinin* (*HA*) and *neuraminidase* (*NA*) peplomers. Hemagglutinin is responsible for attachment of the virus to host cell receptors and for penetration of virus into the cell. Proteolytic cleavage of HA glycoprotein into two subunits is necessary if the virus is to engage in these infectious activities. The source of the proteolytic enzyme is not known but it may be present in respiratory secretions. The exact function of neuraminidase is not known. Since the substrate of NA is neuraminic acid, a component of the mu-

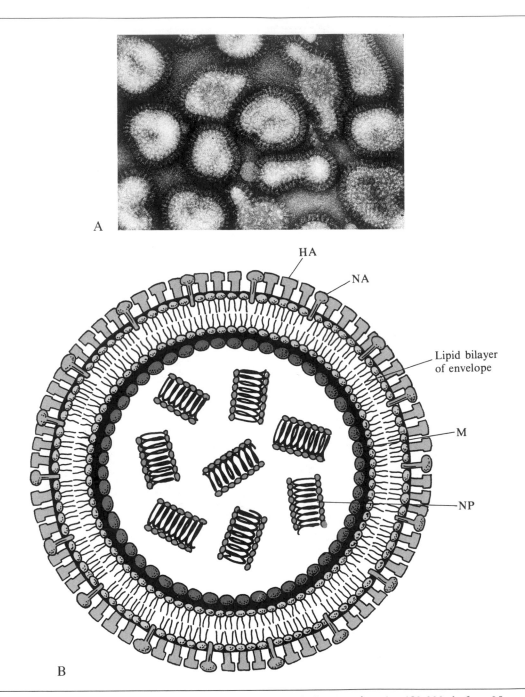

Fig. 31-17. Influenza virus. A. Electron micrograph of human influenza virus (× 180,000, before 25 percent reduction). (Courtesy R. C. Williams.) B. Diagrammatic illustration of influenza virus. HA = hemagglutinin peplomer; NA = neuraminidase peplomer; M = protein shell; NP = ribonucleoprotein. (From R. C. Compans and P. C. Choppin, *Compr. Virol.* 4:179, 1975.)

cosa, the NA peplomer may cause liquefaction of the mucosa. This leaves the underlying epithelial layer unprotected from infection by other microbial agents and promotes spread of virus.

The RNA genome of the influenza virus is unique among RNA viruses in that it consists of eight distinct RNA molecules that may be linked as a complete unit only in the mature virion. The presence of these distinct RNA units during replication in the animal host explains the high rate of genetic recombination observed when cells are infected with different strains of influenza virus. Recombination is the genetic mechanism responsible for the major antigenic differences in pandemics caused by the influenza virus.

The virus is stable to freezing and thawing but is inactivated by heat and ultraviolet light.

Classification

There are three types of influenza viruses: *A, B,* and *C*. Types B and C have been isolated only from humans, while type A has been found in horses, swine, and birds as well as humans. The separation of these viruses into types is based on differences in the antigenicity of their ribonucleoprotein and M protein, which is part of the inner surface of the lipid layer of the envelope (see Fig. 31-17). Strain specificity resides in the peplomers (that is, hemagglutinin and neuraminidase). Four types of hemagglutinin (H0, H1, H2, H3) and two types of neuraminidase (N1, N2) are recognized among influenza A strains causing illness in humans. These antigens are the basis for classifying new strains. The classification items used to describe, for example, the strain A/duck/Tokyo/5/69/(H2N2) of influenza A are as follows:

1. Antigenic type of nucleocapsid: A, B, or C; for example, influenza A
2. Source of the isolate if from a species other than humans: A/duck
3. Geographical location or origin of the isolate: A/duck/Tokyo
4. Strain number: A/duck/Tokyo/5
5. Year of isolation: A/duck/Tokyo/5/69

6. In parentheses, the antigenic identity of the hemagglutinin (H) subtype and neuraminidase (N) subtype: A/duck/Tokyo/5/69(H2N2) (The numbers after the hemagglutinin and neuraminidase subtypes [H2N2] are antigenic variants of earlier strains.) The designations indicating the species of origin of the HA and NA antigens are now omitted.

Pathogenesis

Influenza A and B cause the same spectrum of illness. Influenza is a disease of the upper respiratory tract. Infection is acquired primarily by inhalation of aerosols produced by infected individuals. Influenza is usually a benign disease characterized by no symptoms or very mild symptoms, but viral pneumonia resulting in death can be the outcome of infection. In uncomplicated infections the virus does not penetrate into the lower respiratory tract but remains in the upper or middle tract, resulting in necrosis and desquamation of the respiratory epithelium.

The incubation period for influenza is 24 to 48 hours; it is usually followed by fever, cough, headache, muscular aches, sore throat, and conjunctivitis. Acute symptoms last for approximately 3 to 5 days. Children infected by virus have symptoms similar to adults but the former are more likely to develop otitis media, croup, and pneumonia than healthy adults. Loss of the mucociliary blanket during infection makes the individual susceptible to infection by bacterial agents such as *Staphylococcus aureus, Streptococcus pneumoniae*, and *Hemophilus influenzae*. These agents plus the influenza virus may cause pneumonia. Other complications of influenza virus infection are encephalitis and meningitis. Elderly persons and those with underlying illnesses are at increased risk for complications of influenza infection.

A complication of influenza A and B infections as well as varicella is called *Reye's syndrome*. The syndrome occurs in children between the ages of 6 and 11 who are recovering from infection by these viruses. Manifestations of the disease include intractable vomiting, lethargy, and delirium. Untreated, the disease may progress to coma and death. Brain damage has been reported in some survivors, but most recover without affliction. Several studies have suggested that treatment of respiratory infections with salicylates to reduce fever may be a contributing factor to the syndrome. One of the features of Reye's syndrome is injury to mitochondria, especially hepatic mitochondria, which become disrupted. This characteristic is verified by the elevated levels of mitochondrial enzymes in the serum as well as elevated amounts of ammonia, lactate, pyruvate, alanine, and free fatty acids. These products are produced in part by reactions localized in the mitochondria. Metabolites such as ammonia and fatty acids are toxic to the central nervous system and thus could be responsible for encephalopathy. The risk of Reye's syndrome appears to be highest after influenza B infection, followed by varicella-zoster and influenza A infections.

Epidemiology

Influenza is an endemic disease in which epidemics take place every 2 to 5 years. The pandemics that occur approximately every 8 to 10 years are caused by influenza A virus. The first human influenza virus was isolated in 1934 and was the prototype, designated influenza A (A0). In the 1957 influenza pandemic, the infecting isolate was placed in a new serotype called Asian influenza (A2). Other than an antigenic relationship to the nucleocapsid, the A2 isolate exhibited no antigenic similarities to any of the influenza viruses isolated from 1933 to 1956. The Asian isolate has been shown to be related to swine, fowl, and horse influenza viruses in addition to human strains, but it is unrelated to influenza B or C viruses.

In the 1957 pandemic more than 80 million cases of influenza were recorded. In the United States alone, an estimated 88,000 deaths were pneumonia- and influenza-related. Most deaths were among the elderly and people seriously debilitated with chronic cardiovascular and lung diseases.

In 1968 an outbreak of influenza occurred in Hong Kong and spread throughout the world. In the United States nearly 20,000 deaths were attributed to the Hong Kong strain. A new antigenic subtype H3N2 of influenza A was responsible for this pandemic, and it remained the prevalent antigenic type until 1978. In 1976 a new type A influenza virus that was similar to swine influenza (Hsw1N1) appeared in Fort Dix, New Jersey. Many epidemiologists feared that a major epidemic would soon follow, and mass vaccination was initiated. The epidemic, however, never materialized.

In 1977 the Soviet Union reported large-scale outbreaks of influenza caused by viruses antigenically related to H1N1. H1N1 viruses had been a source of disease in the Soviet Union and China from 1947 to 1956. The prototype was designated A/USSR/90/77/(H1N1), and this strain has replaced H3N2 viruses in China and the Soviet Union as the major strain causing disease. In the United States H3N2 strains are still responsible for approximately 80 percent of the cases of influenza, while H1N1 strains account for 10 percent, and 10 percent are caused by type B isolates. H3N2 strains are nearly always associated with outbreaks in hospital settings or nursing homes, while H1N1 strains are more frequently associated with outbreaks in schools.

Epidemics caused by influenza B viruses are less frequent than those caused by influenza A. Influenza B viruses show more antigenic stability and are more easily handled in epidemics. Influenza B appears in the United States more frequently in local epidemics. Vaccines containing the B type antigens are available.

Type C influenza is prevalent throughout the world, and infection occurs early in life. Outbreaks caused by type C virus are rarely reported and are usually discovered retrospectively by serological studies associated with other types of influenza. Thus little is known of the pathogenesis or epidemiology of the type C influenza.

Between major epidemics, antigenic changes

take place in the virus. These changes may involve minor alterations (called *antigenic drift*) or major alterations (called *antigenic shift*) in the HA and NA peplomers. Antigenic drift is the result of two or more point mutations in which the amino acid composition of the peplomers is changed. The new viral strain is able to escape neutralization by antibodies of preceding viruses that caused infection in a population. Antigenic drift therefore leads to infections in which the population has antibodies with low affinity for the virus. Antigenic shift represents a more drastic change in the antigenic characteristics of the virus. The new virus strain may have been derived by genetic reassortment between human influenza virus and influenza virus of lower animals. A second possibility is that an animal or bird virus became infectious for humans through a series of mutations. For example, the swine flu virus isolated on a farm in Wisconsin in 1976 was identical to the virus isolated from humans. Antigenic shift ultimately leads to influenza infections (pandemics) in which there are few or no antibodies in the population that can neutralize the virus. As the population develops an immunity to the new strain there are likely to be periodic small epidemics among those who did not come in contact with the new strain and thus did not develop an immunity against it (Fig. 31-18).

Laboratory Diagnosis

Diagnosis of influenza is based on isolation and identification of the virus or by observation of

Fig. 31-18. Scheme for occurrence of influenza pandemics and epidemics in relation to level of immunity in the population. (— = incidence of clinically manifest influenza; – – – – = mean level of population antibody against A/HxNx/; – – – ··· = mean level of population antibody against A/HyNy/.) (From R. G. Douglas. In G. J. Galasso, T. C. Merigan, and R. C. Buchanan [eds.], *Antiviral Agents and Viral Diseases of Man.* New York, Raven, 1979.)

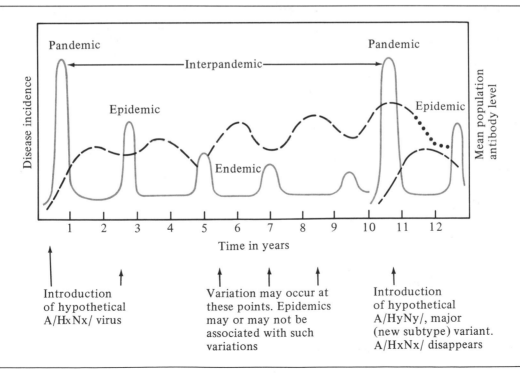

changes in the antibody titer of affected individuals. Throat and nasal specimens (swab or washings) are first treated with antibiotics and then clarified by centrifugation before inoculation into embryonated eggs or cell culture. After approximately 5 days of incubation the cultivated virus can be identified by hemagglutination using chick or guinea pig erythrocytes. Hemagglutination inhibition, neutralization, and complement fixation tests can also be employed for identification. In tissue culture, such as monkey kidney cells, presumptive identification of influenza B can be made because of the virus's characteristic cytopathic effect. Typing of the influenza virus into A, B, or C can be made by identification of the ribonucleoprotein (soluble antigen) in fluorescent-antibody staining or by immunoassays.

Serological diagnosis is based on a fourfold rise in antibody titer between the acute and convalescent sera as determined by the complement fixation test. During suspected epidemics, presumptive diagnosis is made by comparing the sera of recovered influenza patients and of those in the acute phase of the illness. Sera from both groups are tested for A and B ribonucleoproteins. If an epidemic has been caused by the influenza virus, the antibody titer to the A or B antigens should be higher in sera from convalescents than from the acutely ill. Direct fluorescent antibody detection is a rapid diagnostic technique for confirming infection by influenza viruses.

Immunity

Infection results in the production of antibodies to several viral proteins including HA and NA molecules. These antibodies are associated with resistance to infection. After infection, immunity lasts for only 1 or 2 years. Reinfection depends on the antigenic characteristics of the infecting virus strain and the patient's prior contact with related strains. Resistance to one strain does not always confer resistance to other strains. A person's serological response to influenza A is dominated throughout life by the type of antibody produced as a result of his or her first experience

with the virus. A person challenged with one antigen and then rechallenged with an influenza virus containing related and unrelated antigens will exhibit two immunological responses: First, an anamnestic response is initiated by the related antigen. Second, the unrelated antigen stimulates a primary response. Repeated challenges with related antigen will result in the production of antibodies against the first strain. This has been called the *doctrine of original antigenic sin*.

Prevention and Treatment

Amantadine hydrochloride can be used therapeutically and prophylactically for infection caused by all type A strains. It is most beneficial when administered within the first 2 days of the illness and should be continued as long as there is exposure to virus. This antiviral drug is recommended for persons at high risk during epidemics, that is, those with chronic pulmonary, heart, or kidney disease and those older than 65.

The influenza vaccine has been shown to afford protection during serious epidemics. The most widely used commercial preparation is the formaldehyde-inactivated vaccine. This is prepared from infected chick embryo and consists of three virus strains (two type A and one type B). The viruses represent those recently circulating worldwide and thought to circulate in the United States the following winter. The vaccine is administered intramuscularly.

A major problem with influenza virus vaccine preparation is that the hemagglutinin antigen that induces protective antibodies is constantly changing (antigenic drift). Close observation of the prevalent infecting influenza virus during epidemics and pandemics is therefore important so that effective viral antigens can be used in vaccine preparations.

It is generally recommended that only people who are most likely to be at risk be vaccinated: the aged, those debilitated by pulmonary and cardiac diseases, those with diabetes mellitus or other metabolic diseases, those with chronic renal disease, and those with conditions that compromise the immune mechanism. Split virus is used for children from 6 months to 12 years of age, while whole or split virus can be administered to those over 12 years of age. A single dose is administered, followed by a booster dose in 2 months. For those over 12 years of age who receive yearly vaccines, boosters are not advised unless the antigenic characteristics of the virus have changed enough to warrant them.

Most of the side effects from vaccine administration appear in children. They include fever, allergic response to vaccine components, and the *Guillain-Barré syndrome*. This syndrome is a self-limited paralysis that occurs within 8 weeks after vaccination in 10 of every million vaccinations. Roughly 5 to 10 percent of the persons with Guillain-Barré syndrome have residual weakness, and approximately 5 percent die.

POLIOMYELITIS

Epidemics of paralytic poliomyelitis were first described in the early 1800s. Not until 1949 was the poliovirus first cultivated in monkey kidney cells by Enders, Robbins, and Weller. Once sufficient virus could be cultivated, further research eventually led to the development of inactivated and attenuated vaccines in 1955 and 1956, respectively. Because of these vaccines, poliomyelitis in the developed countries of the world is almost a clinical oddity.

The poliovirus belongs to the family Picornaviridae, whose members also include the human hepatitis A virus, foot-and-mouth disease virus, and rhinoviruses. They are among the smallest of viruses, measuring approximately 25 to 30 nm in diameter (Fig. 31-19). They are nonenveloped and their genome is a single-stranded RNA molecule. The poliovirus belongs to the genus enterovirus. The other enteroviruses will be discussed later.

Pathogenesis

In more than 99 percent of persons infected with the poliovirus, clinical symptoms are very mild

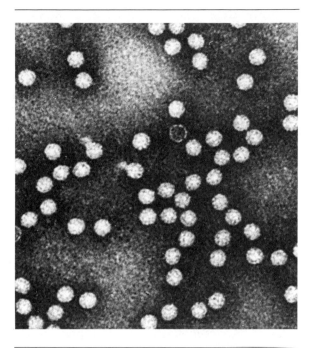

Fig. 31-19. Electron micrograph of poliovirus. (From J. L. Melnick, *Intervirology* 20:61, 1983.)

or inapparent. The virus is, under most circumstances, taken into the mouth through contaminated food, water, or milk. It multiplies in the tonsils, lymph nodes of the neck, and intestinal mucosa of the small intestine and from these sites of multiplication can be disseminated via the bloodstream. During the incubation period, which lasts 10 to 15 days, virus can be shed in the feces and will continue to be shed despite high titers of humoral antibodies. Virus is also present in the pharynx 1 to 2 weeks after infection. At the onset of illness the patient has fever, headache, and stiffness in the neck. In nonparalytic polio these symptoms subside in a few days and recovery is complete. In about one percent of the cases paralysis occurs. Paralysis is the result of invasion of the CNS by the virus from the bloodstream or along the axons of peripheral nerves to the anterior horn cells of the spinal cord. The virus may also affect the posterior horn and dorsal root ganglia. Multiplication of the virus in the neurons causes their destruction; as a result, nerve cells innervating the voluntary muscles are no longer functional and the muscles atrophy. Full or partial restoration of muscle function depends on the number of uninjured neurons that remain to innervate the muscle and the ability of unaffected muscles to hypertrophy and assume motor function.

Involvement of the CNS during infection by the virus may be enhanced under certain predisposing conditions such as tonsillectomy, pregnancy, steroids, fatigue, or conditions that may introduce virus into peripheral nerve fibers.

Epidemiology

Poliomyelitis is a human disease caused by three serotypes of poliovirus. Most infections in the United States have been caused by type 1. Permanent immunity is acquired only to the serotype causing the infection. Poliovirus is spread by the fecal-oral route and can infect any age group. Paralytic cases occur primarily in young adults and adolescents. Infection in the very young and infants often produces an asymptomatic disease that brings complete immunity. It is a paradox that before the discovery of polio vaccines improvement in sanitation practices had actually increased the risk of paralytic polio. Before improvements in sanitation the poliovirus was transmitted to infants through feces-contaminated food, milk, or water. Infection in the infant invariably resulted in asymptomatic disease that provided permanent immunity. In addition, most women of childbearing age had been exposed to the three poliovirus types, and passive immunity was transferred from mother to infant. As sanitation practices improved, many of the unvaccinated were not exposed to the virus until adolescence or adulthood, the period when infection most often causes paralysis or death.

Since the introduction of the inactivated vaccine in 1955 the number of cases of paralytic polio has decreased from 18,308 in 1954 to 5 in 1989 (Fig. 31-20). Polio is still very active in tropical and semitropical countries, occurring in 3-year cycles. In 1979 over 37,000 cases were reported to the World Health Organization, but it is estimated that only one-fifth to one-tenth of all cases are reported. Unfortunately, even with the availability of the polio vaccine, many countries do not have the budget or personnel to vaccinate all the people who require vaccination.

Laboratory Diagnosis

Isolation of the virus is the preferred method of diagnosis. In the laboratory, clinical specimens, usually fecal, are prepared in suspension and treated with penicillin and streptomycin to inhibit bacterial growth. The suspension is then clarified by centrifugation. Aliquots of the viral suspension are inoculated into tissue culture tubes containing monkey kidney or human cells. The culture tubes are observed daily for CPE (that is, rounding and shrinking of cells). Presumptive diagnosis of poliomyelitis is made from the clinical history of the patient and the CPE produced in tissue culture. Since other enteroviruses may have similar effects, identification of poliovirus rests on neutralization of the cultivated viral agent by antipoliomyelitis serum.

Serological diagnosis of infection can be made by using paired sera, one collected at the onset of illness and the other 2 to 4 weeks later. The microneutralization test is the preferred technique for determining the antibody titer against all three poliovirus types. Indirect immunofluorescence, however, appears to be as sensitive as microneutralization.

Prevention and Treatment

Since 1955 two vaccines have been employed in the prevention of poliomyelitis infection: an inactivated polio vaccine (IPV) and a trivalent oral polio vaccine (OPV). IPV was licensed in 1955, OPV in 1963. Both vaccines produce immunity in more than 90 percent of the recipients, but OPV has a higher benefit-to-risk ratio. IPV, which contains types 1, 2, and 3 poliovirus, is administered by injection and can be given si-

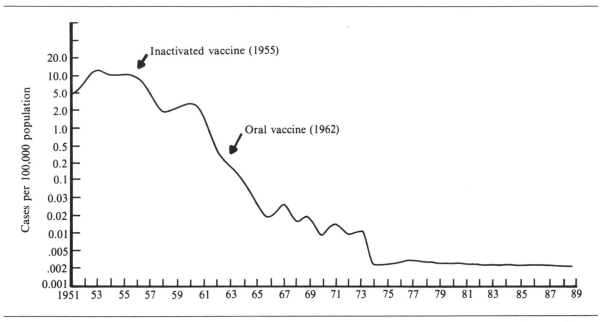

Fig. 31-20. Reported paralytic poliovirus attack rates by year, United States, 1951–1988. (From Centers for Disease Control.)

multaneously with diphtheria, tetanus, and pertussis antigen (DTP). Recipients can be infected with and become intestinal carriers of wild poliovirus or attenuated virus vaccine strains. For primary vaccination of children in the United States, OPV is the vaccine of choice because (1) it multiplies in the intestinal tract and establishes intestinal immunity to reinfection, thus breaking the chain of transmission; (2) it is simple to administer; (3) it does not require periodic boosters; (4) it is well accepted by patients; and (5) it has a record of having eliminated disease associated with wild poliovirus.

OPV is administered in three doses; the first two are given not less than 6 weeks apart, and the third dose should follow in 8 to 12 months. For infants the first dose is often given with the first dose of DTP. On entrance to kindergarten a single booster dose should be administered. Routine vaccination of adults in the United States is not necessary; the risk is small unless one is traveling to another country. Oral polio vaccine poses some risks. The vaccine contains live virus and

is able to cause disease in those exposed either by active immunization or by contact with a vaccinated person. Most vaccinated persons who acquire poliomyelitis are less than 4 years of age, whereas those who acquire disease after contact with a vaccinated person are over 20 years of age. The risk of vaccine-associated paralysis from attenuated vaccine is one case per 15 to 20 million vaccinations. If there is a risk for the vaccinated person, for example, those with immunodeficiency (e.g., AIDS), the killed vaccine can be substituted for the attenuated vaccine. Another disadvantage with the attenuated vaccine is the necessity of maintaining cool temperatures. The oral vaccine is very susceptible to heat. At 20 to 25°C inactivation occurs in less than 2 weeks; at temperatures greater than 37°C, in 1 to 3 days. Vaccine can be stored safely for 6 months under refrigeration.

OPV, although a success story in developed countries, has been a disappointment in tropical countries. Several factors may be involved: (1) children in developing countries harbor a substantial microflora in their upper small intestine, compared to the almost sterile upper small intestine in children in developed countries, which may prevent colonization by vaccine virus; (2) other enteroviruses may interfere with the poliovirus; (3) antibodies in breast milk interfere with poliovirus colonization; and (4) there is a breakdown in temperature storage of the vaccine. IPV so far has been shown to be more beneficial to children in the tropics.

A more potent IPV with greater antigenic content (N-IPV) was developed in 1978 and licensed in the United States in 1988. This enhanced-potency vaccine, when administered at a reduced number of doses, has been shown to be as effective as IPV. Enhanced-potency IPV is recommended for unvaccinated adults at increased risk of exposure to poliovirus—for example, those traveling to areas endemic for poliomyelitis. N-IPV is being used in clinical trials in children throughout the world, but in general OPV is recommended for those less than 18 years of age in the United States.

Although the risk of poliomyelitis is small, recent studies show over 30 percent of children 1 to 4 years old have not had primary vaccination. Because inapparent infections caused by wild strains of poliovirus have diminished, the risk of poliomyelitis in children is greatly increased. It is very important that parents have their children immunized as recommended.

OTHER ENTEROVIRAL DISEASES

The enteroviruses, which include the poliovirus discussed previously, inhabit the alimentary tract. Other important members of the genus enterovirus include hepatitis A virus, to be discussed later, as well as group A coxsackieviruses, group B coxsackieviruses, echoviruses, and human enteroviruses types 68 to 71.

Pathogenesis

The pathogenesis of the enteroviruses is similar to that of the poliovirus except that different tar-

get organs are involved. Most infections are mild and symptoms include respiratory tract involvement, fever, and sometimes rash. However, more serious illnesses may occur and include:

Aseptic meningitis is caused primarily by echoviruses but coxsackieviruses A and B may also be involved. The symptoms of aseptic meningitis include headache, fever, and vomiting, followed by stiffness of the neck and muscular weakness. The disease is self-limiting.

Herpangina is an infection of the throat caused primarily by group A coxsackieviruses. The disease is characterized by fever and sore throat with ulcerated lesions appearing on the mucous membranes of the oral cavity. Herpangina occurs primarily in children between the ages of 3 and 10 and is self-limiting.

Myocarditis is caused primarily by group A and B coxsackieviruses. Infection occurs in the newborn as well as in children and adults. Infection in neonates, which is often fatal, results from dissemination of the virus to a variety of organs. Rapidly developing cyanosis and circulatory collapse precede death. Most older children and adults recover from myocarditis, but permanent heart injury may occur.

Pleurodynia is a muscular disease caused primarily by group B coxsackieviruses. The illness occurs in children between the ages of 5 and 15 and their parents. Pain over the lower rib cage or upper abdomen is the most characteristic symptom. The illness is self-limiting, and most patients do not require bed confinement. The average length of illness is 4 to 7 days.

Hand-foot-and-mouth disease has been associated primarily with group A coxsackievirus type 16. Initially an eruption is seen on the buccal mucosa and this is followed by a vesicular rash on the hands and feet.

Respiratory illness includes several coxsackieviruses and echovirus types that are associated with pharyngitis. Illness has been observed among military recruits and, unlike other viral respiratory illness, appears during summer months.

Conjunctivitis can be caused by both echoviruses and coxsackieviruses. Very explosive epidemics of disease called *acute hemorrhagic conjunctivitis* occur frequently in tropical coastal cities. Symptoms may last for 3 to 5 days. Outbreaks may affect 50 percent or more of persons in a community with a low socioeconomic status within a one- to two-month period. Major outbreaks are associated with enterovirus 70 and group A coxsackievirus type 24.

Neonatal disease may be acquired transplacentally but is usually acquired in the hospital. The infection may result in an asymptomatic response or may cause cardiac or respiratory distress and death. Aseptic meningitis is one of the most frequent clinical syndromes. Coxsackievirus B serotypes and echoviruses are the principal etiological agents of disease.

Epidemiology

Humans are the only reservoir of the human enteroviruses, which can be found in the oropharynx and intestine. Virus can be shed in the stools; thus fecal contamination of food, water, and utensils is the most frequent source of infection. Some viral isolates, however, can be spread by contamination of fomites from nasal or conjunctival secretions. Nearly 60 percent of the cases of enteroviral disease are found in those under 10 years of age, while 25 percent of the cases are found in those under 1 year of age.

Virus is more easily spread in warm weather and isolates are more frequently recovered during the summer months. Enteric viruses are found in wastewater, and in underdeveloped countries this is a frequent source of infection. In the period 1970 to 1983 in the United States 52 percent of the nonpolio enterovirus isolates were echoviruses, 20 percent were group B coxsackieviruses, and 5 percent were group A coxsackieviruses. Data from several viral watch studies suggest that 10 to 15 million illnesses due to nonpolio enteroviruses occur each year in the United States.

Laboratory Diagnosis

Presumptive diagnosis of enteroviral disease can be established on the basis of the symptoms of the illness, the time of year the viral isolate was recovered, the type of cell culture system that supports viral growth, and the characteristic cytopathic effect in culture. Specific identification of the isolate can be accomplished by viral neutralization tests with antiserum containing antibodies to several specific viral serotypes.

Treatment

There are no satisfactory antiviral agents for treatment of enteroviral disease (excluding poliomyelitis) other than providing supportive care, which includes bed rest. Hospital-associated outbreaks of disease, especially in neonates, necessitate isolation techniques to prevent transmission.

RHINOVIRUSES AND THE COMMON COLD

A number of viruses, both respiratory and nonrespiratory, produce symptoms that resemble the common cold. The rhinoviruses account for approximately 50 percent of these upper respiratory tract infections. About 20 percent of colds are caused by coronaviruses. Very little is known about coronavirus pathogenesis; therefore a discussion of them will not be provided.

The rhinoviruses are a subgroup of the picornaviruses. There are about 89 serotypes of the rhinovirus subgroup, with biophysical and biochemical properties similar to those of the other picornaviruses. The rhinoviruses can be separated from the enteroviruses by determining their acid stability. Rhinoviruses lose their infectivity when they are subjected to pH's between 3 and 5, while enteroviruses are unaffected. The structure of rhinovirus has been recently determined, and this has provided scientists with very useful information (see Boxed Essay, p. 702).

Rhinovirus infections are spread from person to person by viral-contaminated respiratory secretions. The highest incidence of rhinovirus-associated illness occurs in September and October. The incubation period for rhinovirus infec-

RHINOVIRUS STRUCTURE AND DRUG DESIGN

In 1986 the x-ray crystallographic structure of the rhinovirus was solved by Rossman and colleagues. The capsid of the virus was shown to be made up of four barrel-shaped proteins that assemble into an icosahedron. So what is the big deal? Shortly after the structure of the virus had been determined, some scientists developed drugs that prevent viruses like the rhinovirus (other picorna viruses) from infecting cells. However, they could not determine how the drugs affected the virus. They asked Rossman and colleagues to find out how the drugs interacted with the virus. What they learned was that the drugs diffused into the barrel cavity of one of the capsid proteins. The drugs stabilized the capsid to such an extent that it could not release the RNA of the virus once the latter had entered the cell. The pH inside the host cell is different from outside the cell, and this difference is enough to cause the capsid to fall apart once the virus has entered the cell. The drug, however, stabilized the capsid to such a degree that it was unaffected by the change in pH. The data was then sent to scientists working with supercomputers to determine how the drugs were bound within the barrel-shaped capsid protein. The intramolecular interactions were calculated. This data also gave hints as to what portions of the drug are required for most efficient binding and what portions of the molecule might be modified without affecting antiviral activity.

Having the 3-dimensional crystal structure of a virus provides the scientist with a shape into which a drug could be designed to fill that space. Computer programs are being designed to match drugs with target shape. A library of drug structures could then be screened quickly by computer to determine what drugs might be the best candidates for clinical trials. This approach will hopefully speed up the search and discovery of clinically useful antiviral agents, which, to date, are few in number.

tions is 1 to 3 days. The most frequent symptoms of infection are coryza, sore throat, and cough. Fever is usually not present. In children rhinovirus infection may cause more severe respiratory disease such as bronchitis. Infection from one serotype provides protection from challenge with the same serotype for up to 2 years. Persons with low levels of type-specific antibody are asymptomatic but shed virus upon reinfection. Those with high antibody titers are immune to infection.

Diagnosis of the cold is made from observations of clinical symptoms. There are no procedures for direct examination of clinical specimens or for serological diagnosis. Rhinovirus can be isolated from clinical specimens. The latter are made into suspensions, then inoculated into tubes containing human fetal diploid cells. Cultures are observed daily for CPE, a rounding up of the cells.

Because of the mildness of colds and the great number of serotypes that may be involved, vaccine prophylaxis is not practical. Preliminary experiments with human volunteers, however, indicate that vaccines prepared from some serotypes are protective for up to 6 months while others elicit no immunological response.

RESPIRATORY SYNCYTIAL VIRUS (RSV)

Respiratory syncytial virus is the major cause of lower respiratory tract disease in infants and children. RSV is an enveloped, pleomorphic virus that ranges in size from 150 to 300 nm in diameter. The RNA genome is nonsegmented and single-stranded. RSV is a member of the genus called Pneumoviruses.

Our knowledge of the mechanism(s) of pathogenesis of RSV infection is incomplete. One pathogenic factor is probably the site of infection, the terminal respiratory airways (bronchioles). In infants inflammation from RSV infection causes the airways, whose diameter is very small in infants, to become obstructed, thereby preventing entry of oxygen to the lungs. It is also believed that some segment of the immune system also plays a role in the development of illness. One of the prevailing theories is that the relative concentration of IgE at the time of infection influences the outcome. Production of a small amount of IgE at the time of infection is normal and plays a role in recovery. Production of large amounts of IgE at infection appears to have a negative effect on the outcome of illness, probably because of the release of mediators such as prostaglandins, and leukotrienes by immune cells.

In normal infants RSV infection usually causes only upper respiratory symptoms that resolve without incident. In lower respiratory tract involvement there may be a cough, sneezing, wheezing, and fever that resolves within one to two weeks. In more severe cases the child has trouble breathing and becomes cyanotic. These latter cases require hospitalization. The pathology of severe RSV infection is similar to that of the bronchiolitis or pneumonia caused by other viruses.

In temperate zones, epidemics of RSV occur in late fall, winter, or spring. In the northern hemisphere the virus is rarely isolated during August or September. Antibody passively transferred from mother to fetus is of protective value during the first 6 weeks after birth, but the antibody titer decreases by a factor of two each month thereafter. Thus, children after 2 months are especially susceptible to infection by RSV. Infection does not confer a permanent immunity, and reinfections are common but also milder. In hospitalized infants the risk of infection is directly related to the length of hospitalization. The hospital staff play an important role in transmission of virus. Through the handling of infants, staff members acquire infection, probably by self-inoculation with contaminated secretions carried on their hands or on fomites.

One study has shown that more than 50 percent of children between the ages of 6 months and 4 years have no demonstrable antibody to RSV. Approximately 12,000 infants each year will require hospitalization for bronchiolitis and pneumonia associated with RSV infection.

Diagnosis of RSV infection on clinical grounds is difficult because so many other agents may produce similar symptoms (adenovirus, parainfluenza virus, rhinovirus, enterovirus, and *Chlamydia trachomatis*). Definitive diagnosis can be obtained by laboratory tests. Rapid diagnosis of RSV infection can be obtained by utilizing ELISA or indirect fluorescent antibody tests on nasopharyngeal aspirates. Virus culture can be used as a backup technique if the rapid tests are negative. Cell cultures, however, may be difficult because RSV is considered to be one of the most labile of human viruses.

Bronchiolitis can be managed by providing supplemental oxygen to the patient and by replacing fluids. Mortality from infection is very low. Ribavirin supplied in the form of an aerosol is used only in severe forms of disease. The drug prevents respiratory failure and shortens the course of hospitalization.

PARAINFLUENZA VIRUSES

Parainfluenza viruses, like RSV, are important respiratory pathogens in infants and children. Parainfluenza viruses are enveloped, pleomorphic viruses whose diameter ranges from 150 to 200 nm. They belong to the genus Paramyxovirus, family Paramyxoviridae, and share antigens with the mumps virus.

There are four parainfluenza antigenic types, but only types 1, 2, and 3 cause medically important infections. These three types account for nearly 40 percent of all viral isolates from lower respiratory tract disease. Types 1 and 2 cause epidemic outbreaks with peak occurrences in January and February, but type 3 is isolated throughout the year. Type 1 infections occur in the fall of years ending in an even number, while type 2 are observed in odd-numbered years. The reason for this is that infection by one virus interferes with the replication of the other virus type. At birth maternally acquired antibody is sufficient to prevent disease in infants by types 1 and 2, but this is not true for type 3.

Primary infection with types 1, 2, and 3 usually causes coryza,* pharyngitis, bronchitis, or a combination of them. The temperature of the patient is usually elevated to 100°F for 2 to 3 days. Types 1 and 2 viral infections may extend to the larynx and trachea, producing croup. *Croup* is the most severe manifestation of infection and is characterized by a coarse cough and hoarseness. Croup can lead to fatal pneumonia. Type 3 virus produces disease that primarily affects the bronchi, producing bronchiopneumonia or bronchitis. Reinfections with parainfluenza viruses are common and may occur within 3 months to a year after primary infection. The symptoms of disease are less severe with reinfection.

Direct examination of respiratory secretions is the preferred method for identification of parainfluenza viruses. Rapid viral diagnostic tests are now used extensively to detect the antigens of parainfluenza viruses 1 and 3. These tests include immunofluorescence and ELISA. If these rapid methods are not successful, culture of virus may be required.

Therapy for severe infections caused by parainfluenza viruses consists primarily of supportive care. No vaccine has yet proved to be effective in clinical trials.

RABIES

Rabies is an infectious viral disease that affects the central nervous system. Even before the discovery of viruses, Pasteur recognized in the 1880s that the causal agent of rabies was not a bacterium but a submicroscopic microorganism. He prepared the first rabies vaccine by intracerebral passage of the infectious agent in rabbits. The vaccine was first administered to a French peasant boy who was later to become the gatekeeper at the Pasteur Institute in Paris. In 1904 Negri made the first histological diagnosis of rabies when he observed inclusion bodies in the

---

* *Coryza* is defined as the appearance of common cold symptoms such as sneezing and watery eyes.

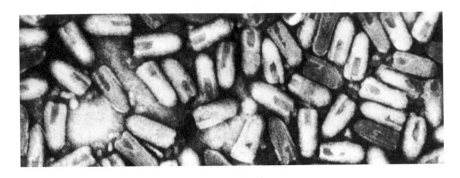

Fig. 31-21. Electron micrograph of a purified preparation of rhabdovirus particles. Note the bullet shape of the particles. (From R. W. Horne, *Virus Structure*. New York: Academic Press, 1974.)

cytoplasm of nervous tissue. These inclusion bodies bear his name: *Negri bodies* (see Plate 18 and Chap. 30).

The rabies virus is an RNA virus belonging to the family Rhabdoviridae. It is bullet-shaped and measures 180 × 75 nm (Fig. 31-21). A lipoprotein envelope encompasses the nucleocapsid and contains glycoprotein peplomers that constitute the hemagglutinins of the virus.

The rabies virus can infect most warm-blooded animals, including humans. Wild virus isolated from nature is termed *street virus*. When wild virus is attenuated in the laboratory it is referred to as *fixed virus*. Fixed virus has a higher infectivity titer and shorter incubation period than street virus.

Pathogenesis

Rabies is usually transmitted to people through the bite of infected animals, although exposure of virus to open wounds or membranes occasionally occurs. There are cases of infection by aerosols created by infected bats, and five cases of rabies-infected corneal grafts had been reported as of 1988. The incubation period for the disease is long and variable, depending on the site of infection, the infectious dose of virus, and the length of time required for the virus to migrate to the spinal cord or brain. The incubation period in humans varies from 2 to 16 weeks, but in a few

cases has lasted 2 to 3 years. The virus leaves the site of invasion and travels to the spinal cord. Virus replicates in the spinal ganglia and then migrates up the spinal cord to reach the medulla and brain. In the brain virus causes severe nerve cell damage. Demyelination occurs in the white matter.

Pain at the site of the bite is one of the first prodromal symptoms in 60 percent of the cases. In about 40 percent of the cases itching occurs at the site of the bite or involves the whole bitten limb. Nonspecific symptoms of infection include fever, changes in temperament, and coryza. Patients may demonstrate the furious (agitated) type or paralytic (dumb) type of rabies when symptoms become evident. *Hydrophobia* (fear of water) is the best-known symptom of furious rabies and is pathognomonic of this condition. Hydrophobia is a violent, jerky contraction of the diaphragm and accessory muscles of inspiration that is triggered by the patient's attempt to swallow liquid. Other features of the infection are terror and excitement and generalized convulsions. During the last stages of disease before death the patient becomes comatose and hydrophobia is replaced by an irregular pattern of respiration.

Epidemiology

Rabies is now rare in industrialized nations of the temperate zone. In many tropical areas, how-

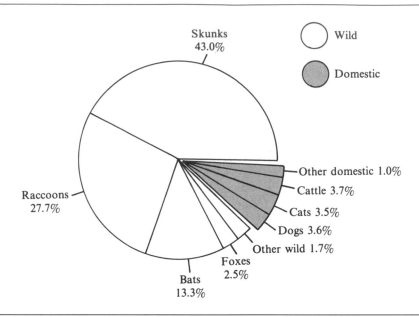

Fig. 31-22. Animal rabies, United States, 1987. (From Centers for Disease Control.)

ever, rabies is still a familiar and no less frightening disease than it was nearly 2000 years ago. From 1980 to 1989 only 10 cases of human rabies were reported in the United States. In Latin America the incidence of human rabies varies from 0.3 to 2.8 per 100,000 population, and in Brazil as many as 1000 deaths from human rabies are recorded each year.

In nature the virus's permanent host is the skunk, weasel, or mongoose. The virus is maintained in wildlife because of its ability to invade and replicate in various tissues and organs such as kidneys, lungs, and salivary glands without invading neural tissue and causing encephalitis. Various wild animals are a source of infection for domestic animals such as dogs and cats and even occasionally cattle and horses. Domestic dogs are still the most important source of human disease in areas where domestic animal rabies has not been controlled by animal vaccination. In those areas where domestic animals have been vaccinated most cases of human rabies result from wild animal bites or from imported cases of

rabies. In the United States human rabies has been associated with rabies among animals such as skunks, raccoons, foxes, and bats (Fig. 31-22). The most susceptible domestic animals are cattle. Transmission of the virus from cattle to humans is not uncommon.

Laboratory Diagnosis

Microscopic examination of brain tissue for rabies virus is the most common laboratory diagnostic technique. The fluorescent antibody test provides a rapid diagnostic procedure and has replaced other tests such as Negri body determination and isolation of virus by mouse inoculation.

When a person is bitten by a dog or other animal the latter is placed in quarantine for 7 to 14 days. If the animal is without symptoms it is released, but if it develops symptoms of rabies, its brain tissue is examined for rabies virus by fluorescent antibody. If this test is not conclusive, a suspension of brain or submaxillary gland tissue is inoculated intracranially into test animals such as suckling hamsters, rabbits, or mice. The experimental animals are later examined for the appearance of rabies antigen by the fluorescent antibody test, as well as for any clinical symptoms suggestive of rabies.

In humans diagnosis of rabies is dependent on clinical illness and epidemiological evidence of potential rabies exposure. Serological techniques are of little value since antibody does not appear until the eighth day of the illness. Sometimes viral antigen can be detected in smears prepared from corneal or nasal swabs by the direct fluorescent antibody technique. High levels of antibody in the cerebrospinal fluid (CSF) can be accepted as diagnostic of rabies even after administration of vaccine. Clinical rabies, but not vaccine, can stimulate production of antibodies in the CSF.

Immunity

The fact that antibody is not present in the infected individual until the eighth day of illness indicates that rabies does not stimulate the host immune response until the virus reaches the brain. A person receiving no therapy within this period will die before his or her own immune system can respond. Only three persons with clinical rabies have ever been known to survive.

Prevention and Treatment

Although rabies is rare in the United States, the management and treatment of persons infected is extremely important. The Public Health Service recommends that each exposure to possible rabies infection be evaluated individually. Thus the attending physician must take into account the animal initiating the attack, the epidemiology of rabies in the community, the circumstances under which the attack occurred, and the vaccination status of the attacking animal.

After attack by a rabid animal or one suspected of being rabid, the bite wound should be cleansed by flushing with soap and water followed by application of 40 to 70 percent alcohol, tincture of iodine, or 0.1 percent quaternary ammonium compounds. Vaccine and immune serum are administered according to the schedule indicated in the next paragraph. During the hospitalization of the patient, many complications involving vital functions may occur. Pulmonary and cardiovascular problems are common, and these vital systems must be monitored continually. Sedation of the patient is imperative if seizures are to be controlled. Such procedures protect not only the patient but attending hospital personnel from bodily injury and possible infection.

Vaccine and immune serum are available for prevention and control of rabies in humans. The vaccine currently available for administration is prepared from human fibroblasts and is called human diploid cell virus (HDCV). This is an inactivated vaccine that produces high levels of antibody. Immune serum globulin prepared from immunized human volunteers is also available in prevention. Both vaccine and immune serum are used in preexposure and postexposure prophylaxis. Preexposure prophylaxis consists of vaccination before exposure to the virus. Two intramuscular doses of HDCV are given after exposure, one each on days 0 (day of exposure) and 3. (Intradermal administration has been used to reduce the cost; however, antibody titers should be monitored because of less satisfactory antibody response in some cases.) For those individuals who do not receive preexposure prophylaxis, five doses of HDCV, one each on days 1, 3, 7, 14, and 28, and human rabies immune globulin (HRIG) on day 1 should be administered. The postexposure administration of HRIG is particularly important since vaccine alone cannot prevent rabies. Persons continually exposed to the risk of rabies should receive booster doses of vaccine at two-year intervals. Postexposure vaccine is administered to over 35,000 individuals per year in the United States.

Immune serum may occasionally suppress the immune response of a vaccinated person. It is therefore important to monitor the antibody response in case additional boosters of vaccine are required.

Success in the prevention of human rabies has been directly related to the prevention of rabies in domestic animals. All dogs and cats should be vaccinated. Stray dogs and cats should be removed from the community, especially in areas where rabies is epizootic. Stray animals should be impounded for at least 3 days to give owners sufficient time to reclaim the animals and to determine if human exposure has occurred. Prevention of wild animal rabies in foxes has been attempted in Europe with a great deal of success. Baits laced with an oral vaccine have been distributed by hand or by air in large-scale field trials. Whether this method will work in large areas of North America, where there is a complex system of rabies vectors, remains to be resolved.

HEMORRHAGIC FEVER (HF) VIRUSES

Viral hemorrhagic fevers are a group of illnesses characterized by the common feature of hemorrhage. There are 12 known viral hemorrhagic fevers (see Table 31-3) and all are capable of causing life-threatening illnesses. Most hemorrhagic fevers are zoonoses, with the major exception of dengue viruses. The majority of these diseases are seldom seen in the United States. Transmis-

Table 31-3. Characteristics of the Hemorrhagic Fever (HF) Viruses

Family and virus	Disease	Distribution	Means of transmission
Arenaviridae			
Lassa	Lassa fever	West Africa	Rodent; human-to-human transmission important in hospital-associated outbreaks
Junín	Argentine HF	Argentina	Rodent; exposure primarily in rural areas
Machupo	Bolivian HF	Bolivia	Rodent; human-to-human transmission occasionally occurs
Bunyaviridae			
Rift Valley fever	Rift Valley fever	Sub-Saharan Africa	Mosquito; human disease most often during epizootics
Crimean-Congo HF	Crimean-Congo HF	Africa, Asia, southern U.S.S.R.	Tick or contact with infected animal
Hantaan and related viruses	HF with renal syndrome	Asia, Balkans, U.S.S.R., Europe	Rodent; highly seasonal—disease found primarily in farmers during grain harvesting
Filoviridae			
Marburg	Marburg HF	Sub-Saharan Africa	Unknown
Ebola	Ebola HF	Sub-Saharan Africa	Unknown
Flaviviridae			
Yellow fever	Yellow fever	Tropical Americas, sub-Saharan Africa	Mosquito (see page 713)
Dengue	Dengue fever, dengue HF	Asia, Africa, Pacific, Americas	Mosquito (see page 714)
Kyasanur Forest disease	Kyasanur Forest disease	India	Tick
Omsk	Omsk HF	U.S.S.R.	Tick; disease primarily among muskrat trappers and skinners

Yellow fever and dengue are discussed in more detail on pages 711 and 713, respectively.

sion to humans is frequently by the bite of an infected tick or mosquito or via the aerosolized excreta of infected rodents. Human-to-human transmission is possible and is important in the epidemiology of some illnesses.

Two important hemorrhagic fevers associated with the Americas are yellow fever and dengue, both of which are transmitted by mosquitoes. These two viral diseases will be discussed separately under the Arboviruses. We will not discuss in detail all the remaining hemorrhagic fevers, but only four of them: (1) Lassa fever, (2) Ebola hemorrhagic fever, (3) Marburg hemorrhagic fever, and (4) Crimean-Congo hemorrhagic fever.

Lassa Fever

Lassa fever was first described in 1969 in northern Nigeria. The virus is morphologically and antigenically related to the lymphocytic choriomeningitis virus and to the viruses causing hemorrhagic fever in Bolivia (*Machupo virus*) and Argentina (*Junín virus*). Only the last two are implicated in human viral hemorrhagic fevers. The Lassa virus is an enveloped singled-stranded RNA virus, classified in the family Arenaviridae (*arena* means "sand" in Latin and electron micrographs of the virus give this appearance; see Fig. 31-23).

The natural host of Lassa fever virus is a ubiquitous African rat (*Mastomys natalensis*), which lives in close proximity with humans in rural areas. Human infection is acquired by contact with rats or its aerosolized excreta. Human-to-human transmission can occur by close personal contact or contact with contaminated blood or excreta. Recent studies in West Africa indicate that 100,000–300,000 cases of Lassa fever occur annually.

Fig. 31-23. Electron micrograph ($\times 90,000$) of arenavirus (arrow) cultivated in Vero cells. Note the sand-like electron-dense particles in the virus. (Courtesy R. Graham and P. Jahrling.)

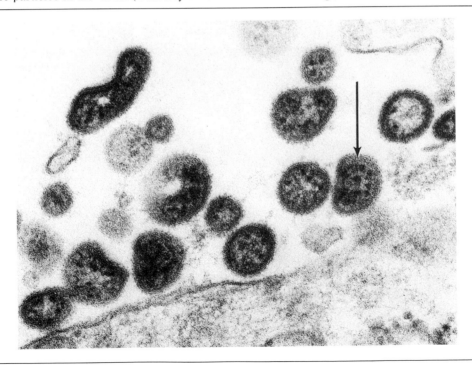

The incubation period is 1 to 3 weeks and symptoms appear initially as fever, sore throat, and weakness. Later there are pains in the joints and lower back together with a nonproductive cough, vomiting, and diarrhea. In milder cases the patient may suffer symptoms for one week and then recover, but in severe cases there are edema of the face and neck, conjunctival hemorrhage, cyanosis, encephalopathy, and shock. One of the most notable findings in severe cases is platelet dysfunction, which is characterized by reduced ability to aggregate in the presence of adenosine diphosphate. The mortality rate for patients hospitalized with Lassa fever is 15 to 20 percent. The prognosis is poor for pregnant women and fetal damage is frequent if the infection occurs in the third trimester.

Specific diagnosis is made by (1) isolating the virus from blood, urine, or throat washings, (2) demonstrating the presence of IgM antibody to Lassa virus, and (3) measuring antibody in acute and convalescent serum using the indirect fluorescent antibody technique.

Human-to-human transmission can be prevented by avoiding contact with infected tissue, blood secretions, and excretions. Ribavirin is the drug of choice for treatment of the disease.

Ebola Hemorrhagic Fever (EHF)

The Ebola virus, named after a small river in Zaire, Africa, is a single-stranded, enveloped RNA virus that has been placed in a new family, called Filoviridae. The reservoir of the virus in nature is not known.

EHF was first recognized in 1976. The method of acquiring natural infection is not known but transmission from human to human can occur through close personal contact. In the first recognized epidemic of the disease 284 patients acquired infection from the index case and 53 percent of them died.

The incubation period ranges from 2 to 21 days. Initial symptoms resemble those of influenza— that is, fever, myalgia, joint pain, and sore throat. These symptoms are followed by diarrhea and abdominal pain in most cases. A transient skin rash appears at the end of the first week and is frequently accompanied by an exudative pharyngitis. Hemorrhagic manifestations occur about the third day of illness and include petechiae as well as bleeding from the gastrointestinal tract and from multiple other sites.

Specific diagnosis requires isolation of virus from blood or demonstrating rising antibodies by indirect fluorescent antibody.

Treatment is supportive and no specific antiviral drug has been shown to be effective. No vaccine is available.

Marburg Hemorrhagic Fever

Marburg virus, named after a town in Germany, is a single-stranded, enveloped virus that is morphologically similar to the Ebola virus but antigenically distinct from it. Marburg virus is now classified in the family Filoviridae. The reservoir of the virus is not known.

How infection is acquired naturally is not known. The first outbreak occurred after 25 people had handled infected material of African green monkeys. Secondary spread occurs by close personal contact or contact with blood secretions or excretions. Sexual transmission is also possible. Marburg disease appears to be endemic in Central and East Africa.

The incubation period is 3 to 10 days and the clinical and laboratory features are virtually the same as for Ebola virus infection. The treatment for the disease is also the same as that for Ebola virus disease.

Crimean-Congo Hemorrhagic Fever (CCHF)

CCHF virus is a single-stranded RNA virus that belongs to the family Bunyaviridae. The disease has been recognized in Asia since the 1940s. Several domestic animals such as cattle, sheep, goats, and hares are reservoirs for the virus. Ixodid (hard) ticks act as reservoirs and vectors for the virus.

CCHF is endemic in eastern Europe, especially the Soviet Union, but it has also appeared in Africa, India, and China and around the Mediterranean. Humans acquire infection by being bitten by ticks or by crushing ticks on abraded skin. Transmission to humans may occur by contact with blood, secretions, or excretions of infected animals or humans.

The incubation period for the disease is 2 to 9 days. Symptoms include fever, headache, myalgia, arthralgia, abdominal pain, and vomiting. A petechial rash is common and frequently precedes abnormal bleeding and hemorrhage from multiple other sites. The case–fatality rate ranges from 15 to 70 percent but mild infections do occur.

Diagnosis requires viral isolation from the blood during the first week of illness or detecting rising antibody titer by indirect fluorescent antibody or other methods, such as ELISA.

Treatment is supportive and no antiviral drug has yet proved effective in vivo.

THE ARBOVIRUSES

The term *arbovirus* refers to *ar*thropod-*bo*rne viruses, which are a heterogeneous group belonging to several viral genera. The most important of the arboviruses belong to three major groups: (1) Alphavirus, (2) Flavivirus, and (3) Bunyavirus. The specific viruses in these groups cause several important types of infection, only three of which will be discussed: *viral encephalitis, yellow fever*, and *dengue fever*.

Viral Encephalitis
Encephalitis caused by measles, mumps, and herpes simplex virus is not considered epidemic in nature. Some flaviviruses, however, are responsible for *epidemic encephalitis*. Epidemic encephalitis in humans is not common but some viruses cause a highly fatal disease. The principal causes of epidemic viral encephalitis are *western equine encephalitis (WEE) virus, eastern equine encephalitis (EEE) virus, St. Louis encephalitis (SLE) virus*, and *Japanese B encephalitis virus*. *LaCrosse virus* also causes a mild form of the disease that is endemic in the eastern United States. Characteristics of some of the major viral agents causing encephalitis are outlined in Table 31-4.

Pathogenesis. Human viral encephalitis results from the bite of mosquitoes. The virus multiplies in local tissues and regional lymph nodes following the bite of the mosquito. Virus is carried via the thoracic duct into the bloodstream, from whence virus is seeded into other tissues and further viral replication takes place. How virus reaches neural tissue is still a matter of controversy, but in humans the thalamus and cerebellum are most vulnerable. Infections by the LaCrosse virus are rarely fatal but infections by the EEE virus often result in 30 percent of the cases being fatal. In JBE, the mortality rate in older age groups may be as high as 80 percent.

Recovery from some viral encephalitides may be prolonged in 30 to 50 percent of the cases. Some of the symptoms incurred during convalescence include sleeplessness, depression, memory loss, and headaches lasting up to three years. As many as 20 percent of these patients have symptoms that persist even longer and include speech and gait disturbance.

Diagnosis and Treatment. Isolation of the virus is extremely difficult and most laboratory diagnosis is based on serology and examination of acute and convalescent serum. Fluorescent antibody, hemagglutination inhibition, and complement fixation methods can be used to measure serum antibodies.

There is no antiviral treatment for viral encephalitis and only supportive care can be utilized.

Yellow Fever
Yellow fever, a disease transmitted to humans via the bite of a mosquito, is caused by a flavivirus.

Table 31-4. Some of the Major Viral Agents Causing Encephalitis in the United States*

Viral group	Virus	Mosquito vector	Reservoir in nature	Vertebrate host	Distribution	Other characteristics
Alphavirus	Venezuelan encephalitis (VEE) virus	*Aedes* species	Rodent	Horses, humans	Northern South America, Caribbean, Florida	Most infections are inapparent; encephalitis not common
	Eastern equine encephalitis (EEE) virus	*Aedes* species	Bird	Horses, pheasants, humans	Eastern U.S.A., Caribbean, South America	Rare disease in U.S.A.; incidence greater in children; case–fatality ratios between 50 and 80 percent
	Western equine encephalitis (WEE) virus	*Culex tarsalis*	Bird	Horses, sparrow, finches, pheasants, humans	Western U.S.A., Canada, Caribbean, South America	One-third of patients are infants, in whom 50 percent will have brain damage
Flavivirus	St. Louis encephalitis (SEE) virus	*Culex* species	Birds	Birds (e.g., sparrows, finches), humans	Central U.S.A.	Principal cause of endemic encephalitis in U.S.A.; case–fatality rate highest in elderly
Bunyavirus	LaCrosse encephalitis (LEE) virus	*Aedes triseriatus*	Small mammals	Small mammals, humans	U.S.A., endemic in eastern states	Cases primarily in young boys; rarely fatal

* The Japanese B encephalitis virus (JBE) is the principal cause of most cases of epidemic encephalitis. JBE causes annual epidemics among children in Asia. *Culex* species are the mosquito vector for JBE, while birds are the principal reservoir in nature.

Flaviviruses are single-stranded RNA viruses that are spherical and enveloped and have a diameter of 30 nm. Yellow fever is found primarily in the Americas and sub-Saharan Africa.

Pathogenesis. Yellow fever produces a hemorrhagic fever that is similar to other viral hemorrhagic fevers such as dengue hemorrhagic fever, Crimean-Congo hemorrhagic fever, and Lassa fever. There are three clinical periods in yellow fever: (1) *infection*, (2) *remission*, and (3) *intoxication*.

The infection period follows a 3- to 6-day incubation period and is characterized by fever, headache, lumbosacral pain, nausea, and vomiting. The infection period lasts about three days and virus is present in the bloodstream, which may be a source of virus for mosquitoes. Symptoms of the infection stage may remit for as long as 24 hours. During the intoxication phase virus is cleared from the blood and infects various organs, especially the liver, spleen, kidneys, and heart. Symptoms during this period include jaundice, albuminuria, hemorrhagic manifestations (for example, of liver, heart, and kidney), and central nervous system symptoms such as stupor, delirium, convulsive seizures, and coma. Death usually occurs between 7 and 10 days after infection. The case–fatality rate is 20 percent. Patients who survive show renal failure and a slow convalescence.

Epidemiology. There are two yellow fever cycles in nature. One cycle involves humans and the *Aedes aegypti* mosquito and is associated with epidemics in urban areas (*urban yellow fever*). Urban yellow fever has not been observed in the Americas in over 30 years because of vector control measures. The second cycle involves virus infection of monkeys with the latter acting as a source of virus for the mosquitoes of the genus *Haemagogus* (*jungle or sylvatic yellow fever*). This genus of mosquito can transmit the virus to other monkeys or to humans.

Vector control measures that led to the eradication of *A. aegypti* and urban yellow fever are almost impossible to implement in forested areas where yellow fever is endemic. There is great concern that urban yellow fever may reappear because of the reinvasion of countries by *Aedes aegypti*.

The actual number of cases of yellow fever that occur each year is difficult to evaluate because most epidemics occur in areas where surveillance is not adequate.

Laboratory Diagnosis. Diagnosis on clinical grounds is almost impossible in the infection phase of the disease. Severe forms of yellow fever resemble other hemorrhagic fevers. It is possible to detect yellow fever viral antigen in serum, blood, and liver tissue by enzyme immunoassays in which monoclonal or polyclonal IgM antibodies are used. IgM antibodies can be detected in the patient's serum by using enzyme immunoassays.

Treatment and Prevention. There is no specific treatment for yellow fever other than supportive care. Liver failure and shock can be treated by introducing 10 to 20 percent glucose intravenously to maintain adequate nutrition and prevent hypoglycemia. Renal changes must be monitored and treated since many patients die of renal tubular necrosis.

Prevention of yellow fever depends on control of the mosquito vector. A live attenuated virus vaccine, 17D, induces an effective antibody level that persists for at least 10 years and is recommended for anyone traveling to areas where yellow fever is endemic. Since the vaccine is produced in chick embryo cell culture, it should not be administered to persons who are hypersensitive to eggs.

Dengue Fever and Dengue Hemorrhagic Fever

Dengue is a disease caused by a flavivirus transmitted to humans primarily by the *Aedes aegypti* mosquito but other mosquito vectors can be involved. There are four serologic types of virus that are involved in two types of syndromes: *classical dengue fever* and *dengue hemorrhagic fever* (*DHF*).

Pathogenesis. Classical dengue fever produces a self-limiting infection in humans. There is an incubation period of 2 to 7 days following the mosquito bite. The initial symptoms include high fever, headache, and lumbosacral pain. Later there is soreness in the joints, myalgia, nausea, and vomiting. A macular rash may appear on the first or second day and this is followed by a maculopapular rash a few days later. Classical dengue is rarely fatal unless complications occur.

Dengue hemorrhagic fever is a serious and frequently fatal disease. Hemorrhages with leakage of plasma and erythrocytes lead to severe necrosis. DHF is considered an immune complex disease. It is believed that DHF follows a previous infection with a heterologous viral serotype. The nonneutralizing antibodies produced in the previous infection enhance the replication of newly acquired virus in mononuclear phagocytes and lymphatic tissue. The increased replication of virus sets off an immune response in which vasoactive mediators are released that cause vascular permeability, decreased blood volume, and shock. Activation of the clotting system may result in intravascular coagulation. Without physiologic treatment up to 50 percent of patients with severe disease die.

Epidemiology. Dengue fever and DHF occur wherever the mosquito vector is present. Most cases of the disease are associated with tropical areas: the Americas and tropical Asia. Infection by one serologic type of virus produces classical dengue fever. This results in lifelong protection against infection by the same virus type but not other virus types. Reinfection by another virus type often produces DHF.

Aedes aegypti is the most important vector in transmission of the dengue fever virus throughout all tropical areas. *Ae. albopictus*, which is an important vector in Asia and the Pacific, is now appearing in the Americas. *Ae. albopictus* commonly breeds in water found in tires stored outside. Infestations of this mosquito in the United States and other areas were the result of shipments of used tires from Asia. The tires contained eggs and larvae of the mosquito vector.

A total of 88,750 cases of dengue were reported in the Americas in 1986. Nearly half of these cases were from Brazil and the remainder primarily from Mexico, Puerto Rico, and Colombia. Most of these cases were of the classic type but there are increasing numbers of cases of DHF. One of the reasons for the appearance of severe disease is the simultaneous circulation of multiple virus serotypes in specific geographic areas. A second reason is the importation of *Ae. albopictus* from Asia in used tires and other water-holding containers. This mosquito vector is believed to increase the efficiency of virus maintenance in infested areas and hence increase the incidence of dengue.

In Asia classical dengue was the primary manifestation of infection until the 1960s, when dengue hemorrhagic fever began to appear. Today DHF is the leading cause of hospitalization and death among many children in Asian countries.

Laboratory Diagnosis. Specific diagnosis of dengue depends on virus isolation and serologic tests. Mosquito cell culture inoculated with clinical specimens and examined by immunofluorescence provides an early diagnosis. Serologic diagnosis relies on use of hemagglutination inhibition, complement fixation, or neutralization tests on acute and convalescent serum.

Treatment and Prevention. Treatment for classical dengue is only supportive and includes bed rest and electrolyte replacement in cases of dehydration. For DHF, fluid replacement is necessary to replace plasma volume. Oxygen should be administered and if intravascular coagulation occurs heparin therapy may be necessary. Blood transfusions may be necessary if hemorrhaging is severe.

Prevention of dengue relies on eradication of *Ae. aegypti* and other species via larvicides and spraying of insecticides. Eradication was begun in the 1920s and 1930s in the Americas but reinfestation seems to be occurring in certain regions. Reinfestation may be due to importation of new mosquito vectors, as well as to increased insecticide resistance of some mosquito vectors.

ROTAVIRUSES AND OTHER AGENTS OF GASTROINTESTINAL DISEASE

In developing countries viral gastroenteritis is the second most important clinical entity, second only to viral upper respiratory tract disease. Acute gastroenteritis affects over 500 million children yearly and is a leading cause of death of children in developing countries.

The principal viral agents causing gastroenteritis are RNA viruses; however, DNA viruses such as adenovirus types 40 and 41 plus Norwalk virus may also be associated with this syndrome. Rotaviruses are the most important viral agents as causes of morbidity and mortality, and most of our discussion will center on this group.

Rotaviruses

Rotaviruses belong to the family Reoviridae and they infect a wide variety of mammals, including humans, and birds. The virus (*rota* means "wheel" in Latin) possesses a double-shelled capsid that encloses a double-stranded RNA composed of 11 segments. The outer capsid gives the appearance of the rim of a wheel (Fig. 31-24).

Pathogenesis. The rotavirus is transmitted by the fecal-oral route. The virus is acid labile but can survive the pH of the stomach if the latter is buffered or can survive in the stomach after a meal. The incubation period is 48 hours. Fever, vomiting, and diarrhea are present at the onset of symptoms. The virus infects the small intestine and confines its activities to the epithelial cells on the tips of villi. During infection there are abnormally low levels of maltase, sucrase, and lactase in children with the disease. Most infected

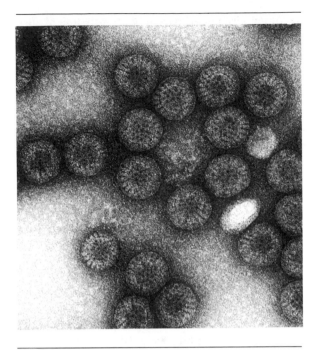

Fig. 31-24. Electron micrograph of rotavirus. (Courtesy H. Gelderblom.)

children also have lactose malabsorption and intolerance. If they are fed lactose, diarrhea actually increases; thus, a non-lactose–containing formula is given during rotavirus gastroenteritis. Normal lactose tolerance returns from 10 to 14 days after onset of symptoms.

Loss of fluids during gastroenteritis leads to severe dehydration and even death. In developing countries recurrent bouts of gastroenteritis cause protracted diarrhea, food intolerance, and malnutrition. In countries where many infants and children are already malnourished, rotavirus infection can be devastating.

Epidemiology. Rotaviruses infect nearly every child within the first four years of life and are considered the most important cause of morbidity and mortality in small children and infants. The virus can also cause gastroenteritis in adults, particularly the elderly.

The source of infection for the infant is often

an older sibling or parent with subclinical disease. In developed countries rotavirus infection and disease occur primarily in the colder months. Results from some studies have suggested that the low relative humidity in homes is a factor facilitating survival of the virus on surfaces. This seasonal pattern does not hold true in other settings; for example, in South Africa infection is observed throughout the year. Rotavirus infection is prevalent in many settings such as day-care centers and the virus can be spread to family contacts. Rotavirus infection in the elderly, such as those in nursing homes, can be severe. In nursing homes infection can become extensive and reports from these institutions indicate that outbreaks of the disease usually involve 50 percent or more of the patients.

Laboratory Diagnosis. Rotavirus cultivation is usually not carried out in clinical laboratories. Stool samples contain from 10^7 to 10^9 rotavirus particles per gram and can be detected by electron microscopy or immunoelectron microscopy (IEM). These techniques are time-consuming when a large number of samples have to be analyzed. The two most important tests for detecting viral antigen are the enzyme immunoassay and latex agglutination tests. Commercial kits are available.*

Treatment and Prevention. Replacement of fluids and electrolytes lost through dehydration is the most effective means of treatment. Fluid replacement can be accomplished by either oral or intravenous administration of water and electrolytes. Oral glucose-electrolyte solutions are preferred for routine use while intravenous solutions may be required for more severe forms of the disease.

A vaccine is needed, particularly for developing countries, where rotavirus infection is a leading cause of morbidity and mortality among

---

* In Europe, electrophenotyping is the principal diagnostic technique. RNA extracted from virus in the stool is run on a gel. An electric field will cause the separate rotavirus genes to migrate in a characteristic pattern.

children. As yet no vaccine has been licensed but several vaccines are under investigation.

Other Agents of Gastrointestinal Disease

Caliciviruses. Caliciviruses are single-stranded RNA viruses that have a distinctive morphology when examined by electron microscopy. They derive their name from the 32 cup-shaped depressions on the surface of the virions.

Caliciviruses cause gastroenteritis in infants and young children but are not an important cause of sporadic or epidemic gastroenteritis. Most individuals are infected by these viruses at an early age and infections may occur throughout the year. The symptoms of disease are as severe as those caused by rotaviruses with diarrhea the most prominent feature of the disease. Vomiting is also a common feature of infection in some outbreaks. Caliciviruses can also cause disease in the elderly.

Caliciviruses have not been isolated in routine cell cultures. Virus detection in stools is accomplished by electron microscopy and by radioimmunoassay (RIA).

Treatment of calicivirus infection is the same as for rotavirus infection. No vaccine is available.

Astroviruses. Astroviruses are responsible for about 5 percent of the cases of infantile gastroenteritis. The virus is a single-stranded RNA virus that has a star-shaped configuration. Children from infancy to 5 to 7 years of age are most likely to develop symptomatic disease with astroviruses.

The incubation period is 24 to 36 hours and the symptoms are similar to those of gastroenteritis caused by other viruses: vomiting, diarrhea, and fever. Most acute infections, unlike rotavirus infection, do not require hospitalization. There is no treatment for infection other than maintaining fluid and electrolyte balance.

Astroviruses can be detected in stool suspensions by electron microscopy. The virus can be propagated in tissue culture and infected cells can be observed by immunofluorescence.

ACQUIRED IMMUNE DEFICIENCY SYNDROME (AIDS)

Acquired immune deficiency syndrome (AIDS) has recently become the single most important challenge to public health since it was first reported in 1979 (to date AIDS is an incurable disease and a vaccine is not yet available). The causative agent of AIDS is a retrovirus called the *human immunodeficiency virus* (*HIV*). HIV belongs to a class of retroviruses called human T-lymphotropic viruses (HTLVs). HTLV-I and II are associated with human T cell leukemia and lymphoma while HTLV-III (now called HIV) is the cause of AIDS. HIV consists of a central core in which are enclosed two identical strands of RNA and enzymes such as reverse transcriptase, protease, and integrase (Fig. 31-25). Surrounding the core is a bilayered envelope, the inner side of which is adjacent to a protein shell. Embedded in the envelope are glycoprotein spikes that protrude from the surface of the virus. The glycoprotein of the spike that is found on the surface is called *gp 120*. As we shall see later, the gp 120 protein plays an important role in the disease process.

Fig. 31-25. Basic structure of the human immunodeficiency virus (HIV).

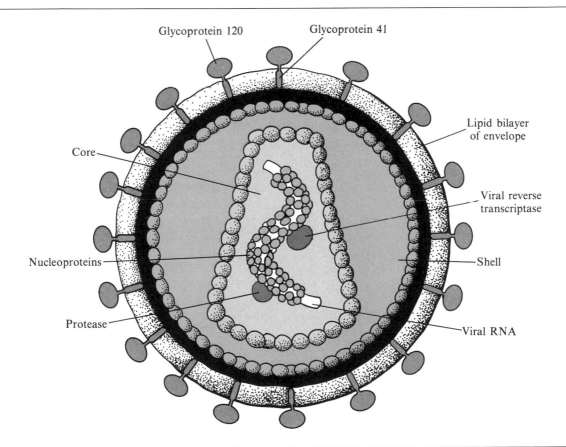

Pathogenesis

The first step in the pathogenesis of HIV infection is the binding of the virus to a target receptor molecule, called the *CD 4 antigen* of T cells. The CD 4 antigen is found primarily on cells of the immune system, especially helper T4 cells. The viral component that interacts with CD4 antigen is the gp 120 glycoprotein. The initial binding of the virus results in the uncovering of the viral glycoprotein, called gp 41, which is the protein to which gp 120 is anchored (Fig. 31-25). Gp 41 protein embeds itself in the cell membrane of the host cell and thus a fusion of viral and cell membranes takes place. During the fusion process the virus core is believed to be injected into the cell (the molecular biology of virus assembly was discussed previously on page 623).

HIV-infected cells produce gp 120 molecules and carry some of them on their cell membrane. If the infected cell meets an uninfected cell with a CD4 antigen it can fuse with it. When this process is repeated a syncytium of up to 50 healthy cells can be formed. The cells fuse to produce a single giant multinucleated cell.

After HIV enters the cell its genetic material (RNA) is converted to DNA by the enzyme reverse transcriptase. The viral DNA is then integrated into the genome of the cell. The integrated virus may manifest itself in one of three ways:

1. Virus may persist in the cell—a condition in which perhaps a few virus particles are produced and only a few cells are killed.
2. Infection may lead to formation of syncytia, which die soon after they are formed.
3. Infection may cause rapid death of cells without formation of syncytia. What viral component, or possibly host immune response, causes death of cells is not known. The CD antigen is present on a number of cells other than T4 cells and this may explain some of the clinical features of AIDS. Cells known to possess CD 4 antigen are macrophages, antigen-presenting cells in lymph nodes, skin, and other organs, some B cells, and probably somatic cells in the brain and gut.

The clinical picture of HIV infection is a long progression of symptomatic manifestations, the last of which is AIDS. The interval between infection with HIV and onset of AIDS is 5–10 years. During the course of HIV infection the patient's immune system is disrupted because of depletion of T4 lymphocytes. Among their important functions, T4 cells activate B lymphocytes that are responsible for antibody production and also effect cell-mediated immunity by their influence on cytotoxic cells and natural killer cells. In addition, T4 cells influence the activity of macrophages whose products modulate the activity of many cell types, including T and B cells. Once T4 cells become depleted, the patient's ability to ward off infectious agents becomes thwarted. HIV-infected patients are especially prone to infectious agents that require a strong cell-mediated immune response to destroy them—that is, intracellular infectious agents such as viruses, parasites, fungi, and bacteria such as the mycobacteria. Indicators of how far the disease has progressed can be determined from measuring T4 cell count and functions such as lymph node involvement, skin tests, and presence of opportunistic infections.

HIV infection can be broken down into six stages. Following contact with the virus and infection in the host, a period of 6 weeks to 1 year may be required before the virus or virus antibodies can be detected by laboratory procedures (*stage 1*). The T4 cell count during this period is usually normal (i.e., approximately 800 per cubic millimeter of blood). When HIV is first diagnosed there may be no symptoms or the patient may appear to have mononucleosis (fever, headache, fatigue, and swollen lymph glands). Many of the symptoms disappear but the lymph glands become chronically enlarged (*stage 2*). Lymph node enlargement is due to overstimulation of B cells, which are abundant in lymph nodes. Overstimulation of B cells causes a decrease in the

Table 31-5. Opportunistic Diseases That are Guidelines in Providing Presumptive Diagnosis of AIDS and Do Not Require Laboratory Evidence of HIV Infection*

1. Candidiasis of esophagus, trachea, bronchi, or lung (see page 778)
2. Cryptococcosis, extrapulmonary (see page 768)
3. Cryptosporidiosis, chronic intestinal (see page 825)
4. Cytomegalovirus disease (other than liver, spleen, or nodes. See page 668)
5. *Mycobacterium avium* complex or *M. kansasii*, disseminated or extrapulmonary (see page 543)
6. *Pneumocystis carinii* pneumonia (see page 787)
7. Toxoplasmosis of the brain (see page 822)
8. Herpes simplex: chronic ulcers (less than one month duration) or bronchitis, pneumonia, or esophagitis (see page 673)
9. Kaposi's sarcoma (see plate 21)
10. Progressive multifocal leukencephalopathy

* According to CDC AIDS case definition

number of resting cells that are needed to produce antibodies. Stage 2 may last from 3 to 5 years, a period during which the patient feels well, but then progresses into *stage 3*, accompanied by a persistent drop in T4 cell count (<400 cells/mm³).* The T4 cell count (less than 400 per cubic millimeter) near the end of stage 3 is low enough that cell-mediated functions show signs of severe impairment, as evidenced by skin tests for delayed hypersensitivity. Stage 3 lasts about 12 to 14 months. During *stage 4* the patient shows some hypersensitivity but by *stage 5* there is total lack of hypersensitivity and T4 cell count is usually less than 200 per cubic millimeter of blood. Stages 4 and 5 last from 12 to 24 months. During stage 5 opportunistic infections of the mucous membranes are characteristic of the disease. One of the first opportunistic infections to appear is called *thrush*—a fungal infection. Thrush, which is caused by *Candida albicans*, is manifested as whitish patches of the mucous membranes of the tongue and oral cavity (see Fig. 32-28). In addition to thrush, there are other infections involving the mucous membranes including chronic herpes virus infection of the skin surrounding the anus, genital area, or mouth. As the patient's T4 cell count is further diminished (200/mm³ or less) op-

portunistic infectious agents are capable of disseminating in the patient. Disseminated opportunistic infections appear in *stage 6* and can occur from 1 to 2 years after stage 5. Disseminated infection, which indicates almost total loss of T4 cell function, is considered the stage called *opportunistic-infection–defined AIDS*. Several opportunistic infections and conditions can be found at this stage (Table 31-5). Some of the more frequently observed infections are *Pneumocystis carinii* pneumonia**, Kaposi's sarcoma (Plate 21), cryptosporidiosis, and toxoplasmosis. In the terminal stages of HIV infection many patients suffer *AIDS dementia complex*, a syndrome characterized by gradual loss of mental control over thought and motion. The affected individuals are usually unable to effectively communicate or walk. A prominent manifestation of HIV infection is called *HIV wasting syndrome*: Involuntary weight loss greater than 10 percent of baseline body weight plus either chronic diarrhea or chronic weakness and fever not caused by other conditions (for example tuberculosis, cancer, or various enteric diseases). In addition to Kaposi's sarcoma, which produces tumors in the skin and linings of internal organs, there also appear lym-

* A normal T4 cell count is 800/mm³ of blood.

** About 70 percent of AIDS patients die of pneumonia caused by *P. carinii*.

phomas (cancer of lymph tissue) and cancers of the rectum and tongue.

Epidemiology

HIV is similar in morphology to the human T cell leukemia virus (HTLV-I), the first virus shown to cause cancer in humans. HIV is related to a virus, called *simian immunodeficiency virus* (*SIV*), which is found in African green monkeys. Based on genetic sequence analysis, SIV is only 50 percent related to the HIV strain that causes infection in people of Central Africa, Europe, and the United States. SIV, however, is more closely related to an HIV strain that is causing infection in West Africa. The HIV strain causing disease in all populations, except those from West Africa, is called *HIV-1*, while the virus causing infection in West Africa is called *HIV-2*. The relationship between SIV and the strain from West Africa is so similar that it is impossible to distinguish between them on the basis of serological criteria. In addition, the genetic material of the two viruses is also very similar. HIV-2 appears to be less virulent than HIV-1 since West Africans infected with HIV-2 are at a lower risk for development of AIDs than individuals infected with HIV-1. We still do not know if HIV-2 infections result in resistance of HIV-1 infections and vice versa.

As of December 1989 over 110,000 AIDS cases in the United States were reported to the CDC. More than half of the 100,000 patients reported in the United States have died. Epidemiologists predict that by 1992 from 400,000 to 500,000 cases of AIDS will be reported in the United States. HIV is transmitted primarily through sexual contact or exposure to blood and blood products, and from mother to child during the perinatal period. The population groups accounting for the adult cases of AIDS in the United States are:

1. Homosexual or bisexual men: 63 percent
2. Heterosexual IV drug abusers: 19 percent
3. Homosexual or bisexual IV drug abusers: 7 percent
4. Heterosexual men or women: 4 percent
5. Recipients of blood or blood product transfusions: 3 percent
6. People with hemophilia or other coagulation disorders: 1 percent
7. Undetermined: 3 percent

HIV infections have been increasing rapidly in children and 75 percent of these cases can be traced to IV drug use by the mother or her sexual partner. Most of the remaining pediatric cases result from blood transfusions or treatment of hemophilia.

There has been considerable concern that transmission of HIV may occur by casual contact or by insect vectors. Although HIV may appear in the saliva, the concentration of virus is much lower than in the blood. Studies have shown that skin or mucous membrane exposure of health care personnel to saliva of HIV-infected people has not yet resulted in infection. Studies of families in whom one member was infected with HIV have demonstrated that daily household contact with the infected member has as yet not resulted in any reported cases of disease (except for the sexual partners of infected persons and children born to infected mothers). Transmission of HIV is not caused by insect vectors.

HIV transmission by sexual contact is still a very inefficient process. When monogamous sex partners of HIV-infected persons were examined in the United States only 15 percent were infected with HIV (on the basis of 100 or more unprotected sexual contacts). This percentage figure is one-half that for transmission of gonorrhoea or syphilis from an infected female prostitute in a single sexual encounter. Some persons, however, become HIV infected after a single or few sexual encounters. Thus, HIV infection is affected by intrinsic properties of the HIV-infected partner, the virus itself, or the noninfected partner.

Fifty-six percent of all AIDS patients and 85 percent of those diagnosed before 1986 are reported to have died. In 1989, HIV infection/AIDS ranked fifteenth among the leading causes of death.

The epidemiology of AIDS in areas such as central, eastern, and southern Africa and in the Caribbean differs from that in the United States. Most AIDS cases in the former countries occur among heterosexuals and the ratio of infected males to females is 1:1. Transmission through homosexual activity or IV drug use is absent or very low; and because many women are infected, perinatal transmission is common. The AIDS problem is especially severe in urban areas of the Congo, Tanzania, Zaire, and Zambia. In some of those areas as many as 20 percent of the sexually active age group are infected by HIV. In some urban areas as many as 88 percent of the prostitutes are HIV infected.

Laboratory Diagnosis

Isolation and identification of whole virus from infected patients is difficult to perform, expensive, and a potentially hazardous procedure for laboratory personnel. Serological assays are the mainstay for determining prior exposure to HIV or HIV antigens. Serological testing is performed primarily in blood banks for the screening of potentially infected blood donors and for individuals at risk of acquiring AIDS.* The principal serological assays for detecting anti-HIV antibodies are the enzyme-linked immunosorbent assays (EIAs). The EIA tests use protein fragments or peptides from cultured AIDS viruses, which bind to and label AIDS antibodies in sampled blood. EIAs require lengthy incubations and produce erroneous results that necessitate use of a confirmatory test. The principal confirmatory test, approved by the FDA in 1987, is called the *immunoblot or western blot assay* (other confirmatory tests include indirect immunofluorescence or radioimmunoprecipitation assay). In the immunoblot assay HIV antigens are dotted onto

* People who test negative for AIDS antibodies may, in fact, be infected. Recent studies indicate that infected individuals may test negative for antibodies to HIV for up to 36 months after infection. These individuals may have a mechanism for suppressing viral activity or they may be infected with mutant viruses incapable of replicating.

a strip of nitrocellulose. The strip is then inoculated with the serum from the individual suspected of HIV infection. The strip is then placed in anti-human immunoglobulin G alkaline phosphatase conjugate. The strip is washed to remove excess reagents and then developed with a substrate of the enzyme that will react and produce a colored reaction—a dark blue dot with a double rim is a positive reaction. HIV antigen detection employing enzyme immunoassays has now been developed that may provide a more sensitive marker than routine antibody screening during the early stages of infection. These assays also appear useful for confirming neonatal infection in the presence of passively transferred maternal HIV IgG. HIV antigen assays, however, are not of value after seroconversion because most HIV-infected individuals become HIV antigen negative.

A promising generation of AIDS antibody tests now seems imminent with the aid of genetic engineering. These tests use either synthetic proteins or proteins made by genetically engineered microorganisms instead of protein from real AIDS viruses. The advantage of these new tests is that pure proteins are used, the proteins can be mass produced, no cell cultures are used, and infection among laboratory personnel is prevented. In addition, it may be possible with the new tests to differentiate closely related viruses such as HIV-1 and 2.

Treatment and Prevention

Like all retroviruses the HIV is capable of hiding in the cells it infects. HIV is also able to infect a wide range of cells; thus treatment of AIDS is a monumental task. In addition, the complications of HIV infection are in themselves difficult to treat. The only licensed drug currently used in the treatment of AIDS patients is called *AZT* (*azidothymidine* or *zidovudine*). AZT is not a cure but it can prolong the lives of certain AIDS patients. AZT, like other dideoxynucleosides, prevents the transcription of viral RNA and viral

DNA (see Chapter 8). AZT is a very toxic drug, producing a variety of side effects, some of which are potentially serious. In addition to causing insomnia, headache, and fatigue, AZT also adversely affects bone marrow cells, causing anemia and making transfusions necessary. The positive effects of AZT have not been well documented, but the drug appears to reduce opportunistic infections and can lessen HIV-induced dementia. A variety of drugs are recommended to treat the opportunistic infections associated with AIDS patients. Treatment for some of the more important opportunistic infections is outlined in Table 31-6.

A number of drugs with activity similar to AZT—for example, dideoxycytidine and dideoxyinosine—are now under study. Researchers are also examining the use of AZT in combination with other drugs, since prolonged use of AZT results in strains of HIV resistant to the drug. The drugs used in combination with AZT include alpha-interferon, acyclovir, and a genetically engineered form of CD4 (rs CD4). The last drug is a soluble preparation of the receptor molecule on the T4 lymphocyte. The CD4 preparation binds to healthy T4 cells and prevents binding of HIV to the lymphocyte receptor.

A vaccine is not yet available to prevent AIDS. Several types of vaccines are currently being evaluated but their potential is not assured. Reasons for this lack of assurance include:

1. The virus is able to hide in cells where antibodies cannot penetrate.
2. The virus is able to change the composition of its surface antigens, such as gp 120. Apparently these mutations can occur several times during the course of infection in the host.
3. There are people who have produced high levels of neutralizing antibodies to HIV but who still develop AIDS.
4. No one yet knows what are the protective antibodies that would provide permanent immunity.
5. The vaccine must not only kill free virus but

somehow stimulate cell-mediated immunity so that infected cells could also be killed.
6. Some virus particles can be trapped inside cells and not have viral proteins expressed on their surfaces, thus making infected-cell recognition impossible.
7. It has been difficult to find a good animal model for the disease. However, new mouse models may be useful for vaccine evaluation.

The vaccines undergoing trial include killed virus, HIV subunit with adjuvant, HIV subunit in a virus vector, and anti-idiotype. So far, subunit vaccines appear to be the most popular. HIV envelope, pieces of envelope proteins such as gp 120, or other structural antigens made by genetically engineered microorganisms or synthesized in the laboratory are being developed by several companies throughout the world. Some viral subunits are being inserted into viruses such as vaccinia virus and the recombinant used as an immunogen.

At present, worldwide prevention of AIDS is best accomplished through education. Various guidelines to minimize the risk of HIV transmission, particularly among the sexually active, include the following:

1. Avoidance of sexual contact with persons suspected of having AIDS or a positive HIV-antibody test
2. Avoidance of anal intercourse
3. Avoidance of sexual contact with multiple partners
4. Avoidance of sexual contact with people who use intravenous drugs
5. The use of condoms during sexual intercourse
6. Avoidance of oral-genital contact and open-mouthed, intimate kissing

In addition, any man having sex with any other man in the past 10 years should not donate blood, plasma, organs, or other tissues. Further, seropositive women should not breast-feed their babies.

Prevention of HIV transmission among labo-

Table 31-6. Current Regimens in the Treatment and Management of Some Important Opportunistic Infections in HIV-infected Patients

Opportunistic infection	Therapy	Prevention of primary disease	Prevention of relapse
Pneumonia by *Pneumocystis carinii*	Trimethoprim-dapsone; corticosteroids	Zidovudine (AZT); aerosolized pentamidine/trimethoprim-sulfamethoxazole/dapsone	Aerosolized pentamidine/trimethoprim-sulfamethoxazole/dapsone
Candidiasis	Fluconazole; ketoconazole	None	Fluconazole; ketoconazole
Cryptococcosis	Fluconazole	None	Fluconazole
Cytomegalovirus disease	Ganciclovir; foscarnet	None	Ganciclovir; foscarnet
Herpes simplex/herpes zoster (acyclovir resistant)	Vidarabine or foscarnet	None	None
Cryptosporidiosis	None	None	None
Toxoplasmosis	Clindamycin-pyrimethamine	None	None
Isosporiasis*	Trimethoprim-sulfamethoxazole; pyrimethamine	None	Trimethoprim-sulfamethoxazole; pyrimethamine

* Isosporiasis is caused by the animal parasite, *Isospora belli. I. belli* infection causes chronic diarrhea in immunocompromised patients, but it can cause a mild diarrhea in normal hosts (usually in tropical and subtropical areas). This parasite is related to the organism causing toxoplasmosis and is *not* discussed in Chapter 33.

ratory personnel can be obtained by utilizing biosafety procedures that would be used to prevent hepatitis B infection. These procedures including using latex or vinyl gloves, handwashing with soap and water after handling infectious material, and using protective clothing, including face masks and protective eyewear.

THE HEPATITIS VIRUSES

Viral hepatitis is a disease involving the liver. Sporadic hepatitis can result from infection by several viruses including the cytomegalovirus and yellow fever virus. Acute hepatitis, however, is caused by four viral agents designated *hepatitis A virus* (*HAV*), *hepatitis B virus* (*HBV*), and *hepatitis C* (*HCV*) and *E* (*HEV*). Another distinct type of hepatitis, *delta hepatitis*, is an infection dependent on the hepatitis B virus. The infection caused by HAV is also called infectious epidemic or short-term hepatitis, while infection caused by HBV is termed serum, transfusion, or long-incubation hepatitis. The worldwide impact of these viruses is tremendous. Several hundred thousand people each year die from the late manifestations of hepatitis.

Although the hepatitis viruses include both DNA and RNA types they are discussed together in this chapter because of their similar pathogenicity.

General Characteristics

Hepatitis A Virus. Direct visualization of a virus-like particle associated with hepatitis A infection was not reported until 1973. The particles were prepared from stool specimens and observed by immunoelectron microscopy (IEM) (Fig. 31-26). In IEM the virus particles are coated with specific antibody from convalescent serum. This treatment produces large antigen-antibody aggregates that can be visualized.

HAV is a nonenveloped icosahedral virus that is approximately 28 nm in diameter. The viral

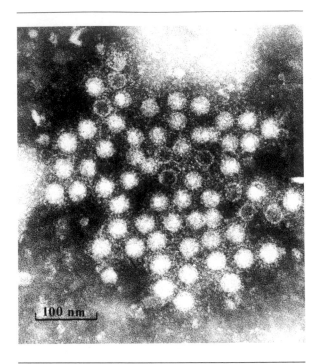

Fig. 31-26. Immunoelectron microscopy of hepatitis A virus. (From A. MacGregor et al., *J. Clin Microbiol.* 18:1237, 1983.)

genome consists of a single-stranded RNA molecule. The virus had not been appreciably characterized until 1982. At that time it was recommended that the agent be classified as enterovirus 72 but retain its original name, hepatitis A virus.

HAV is stable to treatment with acid and heat (60°C for at least one hour). Only one serotype of the virus has been defined and it does not cross-react with hepatitis B virus.

Hepatitis B Virus. The hepatitis B virus belongs to the genus Hepadna virus. HBV is a double-shelled virion 40 to 50 nm in diameter (originally called *Dane particles* because of their discovery in 1970 by Dane) with a core 27 nm in diameter. The core contains a double-stranded DNA molecule together with DNA polymerase. Tubular or filamentous forms up to 200 nm in length are also observed; they have a diameter of 22 nm. A third particle form, which is characteristically observed in the blood during persistent infection, is 22 nm in diameter (Fig. 31-27). These particles are composed of the same material as the surface antigen of HBV, which is called hepatitis B surface antigen (HBsAg). HBV is resistant to acid

Fig. 31-27. Electron micrograph ($\times 210,000$) of hepatitis B virus, (HBV). Three morphological forms are observed: spheres 22 ± 2 nm in diameter, filamentous forms approximately 22 nm in diameter and varying in length, and 42-nm particles. (Courtesy G. A. Cabral and M. Patterson.)

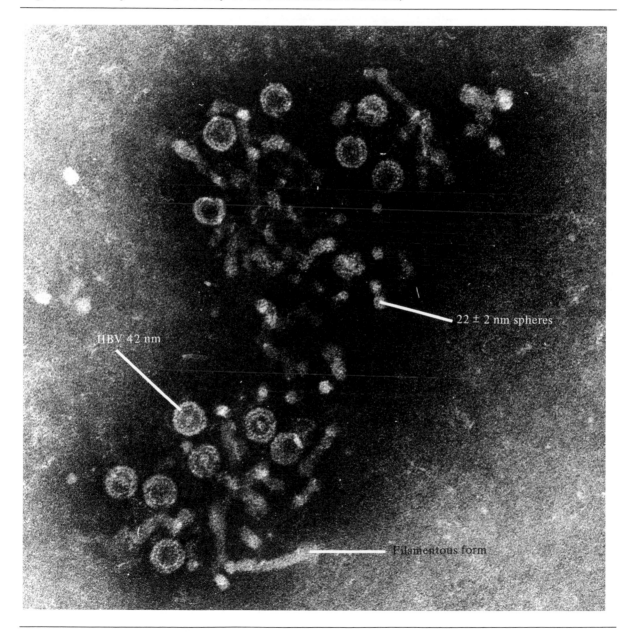

(pH 2.4 for 6 hours); heat (60°C for 10 hours) and up to 40 cycles of freezing and thawing.

A recently discovered antigen called the *delta antigen* is found only in those with HBsAg. The delta agent, which is now called *hepatitis D virus (HDV)* is a defective RNA virus that requires a helper function of HBV in order to replicate. HDV is, therefore, delta antigen wrapped in a HBsAg coat.

The surface antigen (HBsAg) manifests a group-specific determinant, *a*, and subtype-specific determinants *d* or *y* and *w* or *r*. With few exceptions, subtypes *d* and *y* have not been found simultaneously in the same patient, and subtypes *w* and *r* are also mutually exclusive. Of the four possible antigenic combinations—*adw, ayw, adr,* and *ayr*—the first three are epidemiologically predominant.

During the course of hepatitis B infection, several antigens and antibodies will appear. The following is a suggested system of nomenclature:

Hepatitis B virus—HBV, a 40- to 50-nm particle with a 27-nm core

Hepatitis B surface antigen—HBsAg, found on the surface of the HBV, tubular forms, and the unattached 22-nm particles

Hepatitis B core antigen—HBcAg, found within the core of HBV

Hepatitis Be antigen—HBeAg, closely associated with nucleocapsid of HBV

Hepatitis D virus—HDV, a 35- to 37-nm particle consisting of a delta antigen core wrapped by HBsAg

Antibody to HBsAg—anti-HBs

Antibody to HBcAg—anti-HBc

Antibody to HBeAg—anti-HBe

Hepatitis C and E (Formerly Non-A, Non-B [NANB] Hepatitis Virus). Serologically negative tests for HAV and HBV led to the discovery of a hepatitis caused by a serologically and morphologically unknown virus. The virus, which can be transmitted to chimpanzees, was originally referred to as non-A, non-B (NANB) hepatitis. Studies have now shown, however, that at least two distinct viral agents are involved, each with a different mode of spread. One virus type is transmitted parenterally and is associated with both post-transfusion and sporadic cases of acute hepatitis. The agent of parenterally transmitted NANB is now called the *hepatitis C virus* (*HCV*). In 1988 virus-like particles were found in the stools of patients with acute enterically transmitted NANB and this agent is now called the *hepatitis E virus* (*HEV*).

Pathogenesis

It is impossible to differentiate the clinical features of HAV, HBV, HCV, and HEV infection. Hepatitis viruses have an affinity for hepatocytes (liver cells). In the case of HBV infection, core components are apparently synthesized in liver nuclei, whereas the surface antigens are produced in the cytoplasm. The coat antigen is produced in excess and is sometimes passed into the bloodstream as an unassembled 22-nm particle. It is responsible for the antigenemia associated with hepatitis B infection.

The incubation period of HAV infection is 15 to 40 days; of HBV infection, 30 to 150 days (Table 31-7). The first clinical symptoms of hepatitis virus infection are usually fever, headache, and vomiting. The illness may be associated with jaundice (icteric) or there may be no jaundice (anicteric). HAV infection in children is usually not associated with jaundice but jaundice is associated with illness in adults. Jaundice is frequent in other hepatitis virus infections.

Hepatitic lesions caused by the hepatitis viruses are the same: parenchymal cell degeneration, necrosis, proliferation of reticuloendothelial cells, and inflammation. During the period of necrosis there is elevated serum amino transferase activity and bilirubin. Massive hepatic necrosis can lead to encephalopathy and death, but fortunately most patients recover from hepatitis B infections. HAV infection is much less severe than HBV infection and is associated with a self-limiting illness. HBV infections can lead to persistent infections and a severe outcome (a mor-

Table 31-7. Epidemiological and Clinical Features of Hepatitis Virus Infection

Characteristic	Hepatitis A	Hepatitis B	Hepatitis C[a]	Hepatitis D	Hepatitis E[b]
Transmission	Fecal-oral route (close personal contact; water and food as vehicles)	Parenteral (I.V. drug users); sexual contact (homosexual men primarily)	Parenteral (90% of posttransfusion-associated cases); I.V. drug use	Same as for hepatitis B (virus requires presence of hepatitis B virus)	Fecal-oral route
Incubation Period	15–50 days	30–150 days	50–70 days	Same as for hepatitis B	10–40 days
Immunity to reinfection	Solid immunity to homologous agent but not heterologous agents	Reinfection with homologous agent possible but seldom occurs; no immunity to heterologous agents	Reinfection believed to occur	Reinfection shown to be possible in animals	Reinfection possible
Complications	Usually none	10% or more become chronic and can lead to liver cancer	Chronic disease may develop	Chronic disease is possible	Chronic disease may develop
Mortality	Less than 1%	1%	Similar to hepatitis B virus	Similar to hepatitis B virus	1–2% in epidemics; 10–20% in pregnant women

[a] Hepatitis C formerly called *parenterally transmitted non-A, non-B hepatitis*
[b] Hepatitis E formerly called *enterically transmitted non-A, non-B hepatitis*

tality as high as 10 percent). Persistence is not associated with HAV infections. The immunological and biological events associated with infections by HAV and HBV are outlined in Figures 31-28 and 31-29, respectively.

A direct association between hepatitis B viral infection and hepatocellular carcinoma has been surmised for many years and has been recently detailed (see Epidemiology HBV).

Epidemiology

Hepatitis A. Hepatitis A is usually transmitted by the fecal-oral route. Fecally contaminated food, water, and milk are potential sources of infection. Improperly cooked shellfish obtained from waters contaminated with raw sewage have also been implicated in transmission. Many outbreaks of infection have been traced to food handlers who, being actively ill, have contaminated products such as potato salad, doughnuts, and frozen custard. Hepatitis A may also be spread by contaminated blood and blood products, just as hepatitis B is; however, this is not the usual means of transmission (see Boxed Essay, p. 730). The highest incidence of infection occurs in children and adolescents. In developing countries, where hygiene and sanitation may be poor, HAV infection occurs at an early age and 90 percent of the population have antibody to the virus. In developed countries only 20 percent of the population have antibodies to the virus. Sporadic outbreaks in the United States are frequently associated

Fig. 31-28. Immunological and biological events associated with viral hepatitis type A. (From F. B. Hollinger and J. L. Dienstag, *Hepatitis Viruses.* In E. H. Lennette [ed.], *Manual of Clinical Microbiology* [4th ed.]. Washington, DC: American Society for Microbiology, 1985.)

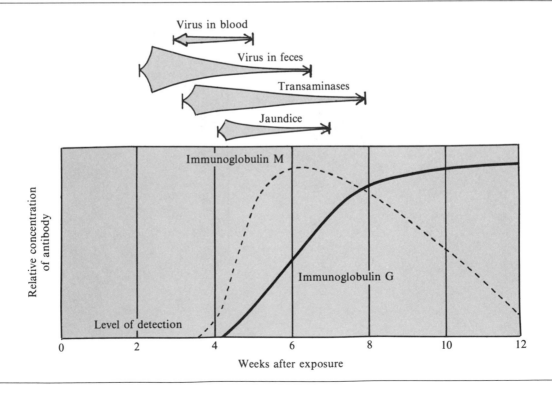

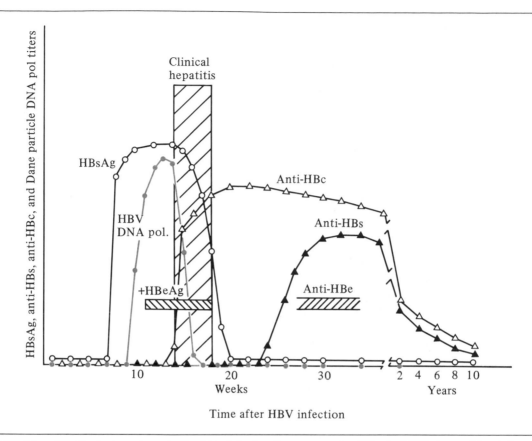

Fig. 31-29. Hepatitis B viral markers in the blood during the course of self-limited HBsAg-positive infection. (HBsAg = hepatitis B surface antigen; anti-HBs = antibody to HBsAg; anti-HBc = antibody to hepatitis B core antigen; DNA pol = DNA polymerase.) (From W. S. Robinson. In G. L. Mandell, R. G. Douglas, Jr., and J. E. Bennett [eds.], *Principles and Practices of Infectious Diseases*. New York: Wiley, 1979.)

with day-care centers. The risk for hepatitis A in day-care centers is highest when (1) the center accepts children less than 2 years old who are not toilet-trained and (2) the day-care center is large and accepts many children. Infected children readily transfer the virus to adults and other children.

Shedding of HAV occurs before the onset of jaundice and declines rapidly (see Fig. 31-28). No cases of shedding have been detected after the clinical stages of hepatitis A infection. In the United States, 35,821 cases of hepatitis A were reported to the CDC in 1989.

Hepatitis B. The major risk factors associated with reported cases of hepatitis B are, in order of importance: intravenous drug abuse, heterosexual activity, and homosexual activity (on the basis of 1988 and 1989 studies). In addition, health care professionals such as hemodialysis personnel, laboratory workers, oral surgeons, and dentists are high risks for hepatitis B infection. In 1989 the number of hepatitis B cases reported to the CDC was 23,419. Each year an estimated 300,000 people in the United States are infected with HBV. About 4000 persons die each year from hepatitis-related cirrhosis and more

HEPATITIS A AMONG DRUG ABUSERS

In the United States transmission of hepatitis A has usually been associated with crowding, poor personal hygiene, improper sanitation, and, less commonly, contamination of food or water. Recognized risk factors include intimate or close contact with children in day-care centers. The association of drug use and hepatitis A has been recognized only recently, especially in Scandinavian countries.

Two possible explanations for the association between hepatitis A and drug use have been proposed: HAV may be transmitted by (1) injection or ingestion* of contaminated drugs (common-source spread) or (2) direct person-to-person contact. Drugs could be contaminated with fecal material containing HAV at the cultivation site (for example, through use of human feces as fertilizer) or during transport, preparation, or distribution (for example, through smuggling in condoms concealed in the rectum or in baby diapers).

Person-to-person transmission of HAV between drug abusers could result from sharing needles, from sexual contact, or from generally poor sanitary and personal hygiene conditions, which have often been observed among drug abusers.

Drug abusers may be candidates for the vaccines against HAV that are currently being developed.

From *M.M.W.R.* 37:297,1988

* By tasting the drug to assess quality, for example.

than 800 die from hepatitis B–related liver cancer.

Mosquitoes carry HBsAg after contact with hepatitis B carriers. Transmission by mosquitoes probably takes place more often in tropical areas than in the United States.

Mother-to-infant transmission resulting in congenital hepatitis can occur in the following ways: transplacentally, by the oral route at delivery, from maternal blood or stool, or by mother–infant contact immediately after birth. Infants born to mothers positive for HBsAg and HBeAg have a 70 to 90 percent chance of acquiring perinatal HBV infection. About 90 percent of the infected infants will become chronic carriers and 25 percent of the carriers will die from cirrhosis of the liver or liver cancer. In the United States about 3500 infants become chronic carriers each year.

Infectious virus has been recovered from semen and saliva; thus, it is clear that venereal contact can lead to infection. The prevalence of HBV infection among homosexual men ranges from 51 to 76 percent. This is to be compared with 4.4 percent for blood donors, 40 percent of spouses and household members of HBsAg carriers, and 55 to 67 percent of parenteral drug abusers. The risk of infection among homosexuals is related to the frequency of sexual contact. Passive anal-genital intercourse is most strongly associated with HBV infection, followed by oral-anal intercourse and rectal douching in preparation for intercourse. Traumatized rectal tissue may serve as the portal of entry of HBV from infected semen. Oral-oral contact or oral-genital contact is not related to HBV infection.

As mentioned previously, HBV infection has been associated with liver cancer. In western Europe and the United States about 6000 cases of liver cancer are reported each year. In Africa and Asia, where HBV infection is endemic, liver cancer is one of the most widely recognized carcinomas. In those endemic areas the risk for primary liver cancer in the carrier group is 245 cases per 100,000 population. It is estimated that 500,000 deaths occur annually as the result of liver cancer. When all hepatitis B markers are included, 90 percent of liver cancer patients have evidence of present or past infection with HBV. The latent period from the time of HBV infection to the appearance of the cancer is approximately 30 years. Males are more likely to become and remain carriers. As liver disease progresses, males are more likely to develop liver cancer.

Patients who carry HBsAg for 20 weeks will usually become persistent or chronic carriers of HBV. There are believed to be from 750,000 to one million chronic carriers in the United States and 175 million chronic carriers worldwide. The most troubling aspect of these figures is that the mortality related to infection is highest in chronic carriers. Persistent carriers have high levels of HBsAg as well as anti-HBc in the serum. Chronic hepatitis can be divided into two types: *chronic persistent* and *chronic active*. Chronic persistent hepatitis is characterized by little liver damage, and there is no progression to severe liver damage. Chronic active hepatitis is characterized by chronic inflammation and necrosis of liver cells. The most important consequence of chronic active hepatitis is the progression to cirrhosis, which occurs in 50 percent of the affected individuals. Neonatal infection is associated with the highest rate of persistence (up to 90 percent). The rate decreases during childhood, but is still considerably higher than in adults (6–10 percent). Studies of those receiving hemodialysis indicate that altered immune response predisposes the patient to persistent infection. The more severe the primary infection, the less likelihood there is for the development of persistence. The more concentrated the viral inoculum, the less likely the person will become a carrier. Finally, males are more likely to become persistent carriers than females: the male-to-female ratio is greater than 2 to 1.

HDV, which requires helper functions from HBV, is frequently associated with progressive chronic liver disease or fulminant hepatitis. HDV, although first discovered in Italy in 1977, appears to have been in the United States as early as the 1940s, as determined by the detection of anti-HDV antibodies in a lot of immune globulin collected from United States Army soldiers during that period. Parenteral drug abusers appear to be responsible for the spread of HDV to non-endemic areas and constitute the major group in such areas to be exposed to HDV. The incidence of HDV infection varies in different parts of the world but is highest in Italy, where 90 percent of the patients with acute HBsAg-positive hepatitis are also infected with HDV. In this area transmission is thought to be by close personal contact.

Hepatitis C and E. As discussed previously, NANB is caused by at least two distinct forms of the virus. Parenterally transmitted NANB, or hepatitis C, is commonly seen in the United States and Europe. This type of infection may be the result of IV drug use (25–45 percent), blood transfusion (8–11 percent), and health-care occupational exposure (4–8 percent). A portion of the genome of hepatitis C has been cloned and an assay for its detection has been developed. The enterically transmitted form of the disease (hepatitis E) is transmitted by the fecal-oral route and causes large outbreaks in the Indian subcontinent, Burma, and parts of Africa, especially in refugee camps. These large outbreaks are frequently linked to fecally contaminated water supplies. Most patients recover but in pregnant women there is a high fatality rate (20 percent). Hepatitis E is much more common in adults than in children.

Laboratory Diagnosis

The clinical diagnosis of acute hepatitis is based on results from biochemical tests that assess liver damage. Several tests are used to determine: (1) presence and concentration of bilirubin in the urine and serum, (2) concentration of serum alanine and aspartate amino transferase as indicators of liver cell damage, and (3) alkaline phosphatase levels to measure intrahepatic and extrahepatic obstruction.

Hepatitis A is diagnosed by specific immunoassays for total and IgM antibodies to HAV. IgM antibody appears at the onset of illness and remains detectable for 6 weeks to 6 months (Fig. 31-28). The presence of IgM antibodies to HAV in serum is diagnostic of current or recent hepatitis. IgG antibody to HAV appears several weeks after onset of disease and lasts indefinitely; its presence is diagnostic of past hepatitis. Radioimmunoassay and ELISA are two of the most sensitive tests for diagnosis of HAV infection.

Diagnosis of HBV infection relies on detection of specific hepatitis B seromarkers: that is, HBsAg, HBeAg, and antibodies to hepatitis B core antigen (anti-HBc), e antigen (anti-HBe), and surface antigen (anti-HBs). Enzyme immunoassay kits are commercially available for detecting these seromarkers whose presence indicates the following:

1. Anti-HBs. Indicates past infection with and immunity to HBV. The antibodies may have also been derived from immune globulin (HBIG) prophylaxis or from vaccination. In carriers HBsAg persists and anti-HBs does not develop. Antibodies to HBs are a measure of recovery from HBV infection.
2. Anti-HBc. Indicates prior infection with HBV at some undefined time. In acutely infected individuals antibodies to HBcAg appear in serum after appearance of HBsAg and before onset of symptoms. IgM anti-HBc can persist at high levels for 6 months or longer and is a reliable marker of recent infection. Absence of IgM anti-HBc in HBsAg-positive individuals indicates the carrier state.
3. Anti-HBe. Antibody to HBeAg is infrequently observed in chronic infections. Patients with anti-HBe are usually not infectious because they have a low titer of HBV. In addition, they usually have normal liver histology, and have a good prognosis.
4. HBeAg. HBeAg at one time was considered a marker for infectivity and replication of HBV. HBV DNA is not considered the major predictor of infectivity (see below).
5. HBsAg and HBcAg. Any person positive for

HBsAg is potentially infectious. HBcAg is found in liver and intact virions but is not found free in the blood. The quantitative amount of HBcAg and HBsAg components in liver tissue, together with histological descriptions of liver cells, may be useful in determining the prognosis of infection. Low HBcAg or none in patients seropositive for HBsAg indicates persistent infection with little liver damage. A high level of HBcAg is associated with marked liver damage and doubtful prognosis. Determination of HBsAg only is recommended for universal screening of pregnant women.

6. HBV DNA. HBV DNA in the serum is now considered the major predictor of infectivity. The presence of HBV DNA in anti-HBe–positive patients with chronic HBV infection is associated with severe and progressive liver disease. Occasionally (fewer than 3 percent), patients with chronic hepatitis B have HBeAg but not HBV DNA.

Diagnosis of hepatitis C or E is based on the epidemiological characteristics of the outbreak, exclusion of hepatitis A and B viruses as causes of the outbreak, identification of 28- to 34-nm viruslike particles in stools of acutely ill patients (for HEV), and the aggregation of these particles by sera collected during the acute phase of illness from patients identified in previous outbreaks. There is as yet no available serological test for hepatitis C or E. However, a serologic assay for antibody to HCV has been developed and is undergoing evaluation. The assay appears to detect many persons with chronic infection and is being evaluated for screening potential blood donors. No serologic tests have been developed for HEV.

Immunity

Hepatitis A. Antibodies to HAV can be detected in the serum many years after infection. The appearance of various antibodies during the course of HAV infection has been discussed previously (see Fig. 31-28). HAV infection produces a solid immunity and reinfections do not occur; however, infection by HBV or NANB virus is possible.

Hepatitis B. From 4 to 8 weeks after infection HBsAg appears in the blood, yet antibodies to the surface antigen do not make their appearance until many months after the illness has terminated (see Fig. 31-29). Antibodies to the core antigen (anti-HBc) are produced and can be detected during the clinical manifestations of the disease. They decline with a decline in anti-HBs but can be detected 5 to 6 years after infection. Acute hepatitis B infection is usually of the *a* type specificity, which appears to confer resistance to reinfection by the same or different subtypes. Anti-HBs confers immunity to reinfections, but it has been observed that even when anti-HBs titers are undetectable, resistance to reinfections may still occur. This implies that cell-mediated immune responses are probably involved in resistance.

Hepatitis C and E. Infection with hepatitis C and E does not appear to confer a solid immunity. Studies with various animals have produced inconclusive results.

Prevention* and Treatment

No therapeutic measures have proved to be of any benefit during the course of acute hepatitis. Some drugs are under clinical investigation for treatment of HBV infection. These include alpha interferon, interleukin-2, and ara-AMP coupled to a serum albumin to reduce toxicity. Alpha interferon appears to be most promising for treatment of chronic HCV infection. The drug has been shown to greatly reduce liver damage.

Hepatitis A Prevention. Hepatitis A infections can be prevented by improvement of sanitation con-

---

* A more detailed discussion of hepatitis prevention can be found in *M.M.W.R.*, vol. 39, no. RR-2, February 9, 1990.

ditions and through the rapid detection of carriers. Careful handwashing after contact with a person with HAV or contact with contaminated objects is important in preventing infections. Food handlers should be screened for hepatitis infection before they are hired. Human gamma globulin affords some protection, if given during the incubation period of the disease, by reducing the severity of infection. Gamma globulin is recommended in preventing the spread of infection in crowded institutions or among people in high-risk occupations (military personnel, missionaries) and those traveling to areas where hepatitis A infection is endemic. HAV has been successfully cultivated in human diploid fibroblasts for use in vaccine studies. Safety and immunogenicity studies of formalin-inactivated hepatitis A vaccine with an adjuvant have been completed and a killed vaccine is expected to be licensed sometime in 1991.

Hepatitits B Prevention. Blood and blood products must be carefully screened for hepatitis B antigen (HBAg) to eliminate the risk of infection. To prevent posttransfusion hepatitis, blood donors must also be screened before their blood is collected. A great reduction in posttransfusion hepatitis has resulted from the use of volunteer blood donors. The use of dialysis units at home rather than in the hospital for known HBsAg carriers has also substantially reduced cross infections.

HBAg deposited on various surfaces is unusually resistant to chemical and physical agents and thus serves as a potential source of environmental contamination. Cross infection using dialysis equipment is very common since the monitoring devices contain connector elements that fit inside disposable blood tubing side arms. Connectors should be disposable, or they should be disinfected with sodium hypochlorite (0.5%). Dentists, oral surgeons, hospital personnel who work with dialysis equipment, drug addicts, and people who are likely to come in contact with blood or blood products should wear gloves and masks whenever possible (see Boxed Essay, p. 735). The equipment and instruments (e.g., syringes, needles) used in practice should be either disposable or sterilized to prevent infection.

Treatment of blood and blood products is difficult because of the unusual resistance of the virus. Sodium hypochlorite is virucidal when used on equipment containing minimal amounts of proteinaceous material. For whole serum an equal volume of full-strength sodium hypochlorite is sufficient to inactivate HBsAg.

The hepatitis virus heated for 1 minute at 90°C will lose its infectivity but not its antigenicity. Thus serum containing inactivated virus used as a prophylaxis before infection with HBV can reduce the severity of hepatitis B infection.

Studies of the effect of passive immunization are encouraging. Hepatitis immune globulin (HBIG) made from plasma pools containing high titers of anti-HBs is recommended for postexposure prophylaxis of individuals sustaining needle punctures or mucosal exposure to blood known to contain HBsAg, family members of acute or chronic carriers, and infants of chronically infected mothers.* HBIG is also given in conjunction with hepatitis B vaccine to health workers following exposure to blood containing HBsAg and to homosexual men following exposure to an HBsAg-positive man. Pre-exposure prophylaxis is advised for patients and staff in dialysis units, oral surgeons, physicians, dentists, drug addicts, family members of acute and chronic carriers, and infants of chronically infected mothers. Great care should be taken in determining who should be immunized because HBIG is expensive. Screening of individuals for antibodies to HBsAg and HBcAg should be performed. Those negative for anti-HBc should be vaccinated but those negative for HBsAg would have to be tested to determine if a carrier state exists.

Routine screening for HBsAg should be done early in pregnancy (to date, this policy has not

---

* HBIG and hepatitis B vaccine should be given as soon as possible after birth, followed by completion of hepatitis B vaccine series at 1 and 6 months of age. Infants should be tested at 12 to 15 months of age to monitor the effectiveness of therapy.

HEPATITIS B: A DISEASE NOT TAKEN SERIOUSLY EVEN AMONG HEALTH CARE WORKERS

A hepatitis B vaccine has been available since 1982. It is one of the safest vaccines ever made, and yet the number of cases of HBV infection in the United States continues to rise each year. Apathy, ignorance, and hard-to-reach populations are the principal reasons for the continued rise in hepatitis B. Health care workers are one of the high-risk groups for becoming infected with HBV. Yet many health care workers are unaware that, in addition to contact with blood or blood products, the virus can be transmitted by sexual contact. The majority of HBV infections (70 percent) occur in ''hard-to-reach'' populations—that is, IV drug abusers, homosexually active men, and heterosexual persons.

Risk of infection by the human immunodeficiency virus has received the most attention among health care workers. In the scientific literature, however, only 26 cases of occupationally acquired HIV infection have been reported. In the United States the CDC estimates that 12,000 health care workers become infected with hepatitis B virus each year. Of those infected individuals, 250 will die from cirrhosis of the liver or liver cancer. In addition, over 1200 infected individuals will become carriers of the virus.

New strategies have been suggested to control hepatitis B infection. For example, hepatitis B vaccine could be given at the same time as diphtheria, pertussis, and tetanus vaccines. In this way individuals who later in life may enter high-risk occupations or activities would be protected.

Health care workers should be more aware of the risks associated with HBV infection and utilize all the safety precautions available, which may include vaccination.

been fully implemented in the United States). Such testing would identify seropositive women and allow the immediate treatment of infants at birth. These infants should receive HBIG and hepatitis B vaccine treatment within 2 to 12 hours after birth. Such a procedure would prevent about 3500 infants from becoming HBV carriers. Immunization for posttransfusion hepatitis is of little value since most cases are caused by hepatitis C.

A hepatitis B vaccine licensed in 1981 was made available to the general public in 1982. The vaccine is a suspension of inactivated 22-nm surface antigen particles purified from human plasma. In 1986 a genetically engineered (recombinant) hepatitis B vaccine was licensed by the FDA. The vaccine was produced by first remov-

ing the gene that codes for the surface antigen of the HBV. The gene was inserted into a plasmid, which was then placed in a yeast cell. The transformed yeast cells were grown in synthetic medium and the antigen was then purified. These two vaccines produce comparable immunogenicity. Primary adult vaccination using either vaccine consists of giving 3 intramuscular doses over a 6-month period. The second dose is administered 1 month after the first and the third dose, 5 months after the second. The groups for whom hepatitis B vaccine is recommended are outlined in Table 31-8. Vaccine-induced antibody levels decline significantly after 5 years, yet protection against clinical HBV infection persists for more than 5 years. Booster doses after 5 years are generally not recommended. In hemodialysis patients, in whom vaccine-induced protection is less complete, booster doses may be necessary if antibody levels become too low.

Table 31-8. Persons for Whom Hepatitis B Vaccine is Recommended or Should be Considered

PRE-EXPOSURE
    Persons for whom vaccine is recommended:
        1. Health care workers having blood or needle-stick exposures
        2. Clients and staff of institutions for the developmentally disabled
        3. Hemodialysis patients*
        4. Homosexually active men
        5. Users of illicit injectable drugs
        6. Recipients of certain blood products
        7. Household members and sexual contacts of HBV carriers
        8. Special high-risk populations—e.g., dentists
    Persons for whom vaccine should be considered:
        1. Inmates of long-term correctional facilities
        2. Heterosexually active persons with multiple sexual partners
        3. International travelers to HBV-endemic areas

POSTEXPOSURE
        1. Infants born to HBV-positive mothers
        2. Health care workers having needle-stick exposures to human blood

* Recombinant vaccine is *not* recommended for hemodialysis patients.
Source: *M.M.W.R.* 36:353, 1987

Hepatitis C and E Prevention. There is no vaccine for hepatitis C or E. Blood donors with elevated levels of serum alanine aminotransferase are more likely to transmit hepatitis C virus to blood recipients than are donors with normal levels of enzyme.

SLOW VIRUS INFECTIONS

The history of slow virus diseases had its beginnings nearly 50 years ago in Iceland, where farmers observed pulmonary and neurological conditions in their sheep. These disorders, called *maedi* (an interstitial pneumonia) and *visna* (a paralytic disease) became epidemic and claimed the lives of over 100,000 animals. Scientists discovered that a filterable agent caused these diseases, whose overt symptoms did not appear until months to years after infection. The term ''slow infection'' was used to describe the long incubation period of these diseases. Later studies in the 1950s revealed that a slow infection in sheep called *scrapie* resembled in many ways an exotic neurological condition of the Foré tribe in

New Guinea, called *kuru*. A number of relatively uncommon neurological conditions such as *Creutzfeldt-Jakob disease, progressive multifocal leukoencephalopathy*, and *subacute sclerosing panencephalitis* are now considered slow infections.

We now recognize that slow infections in humans may be caused by conventional viral agents: for example, measles virus (subacute sclerosing panencephalitis, SSPE) and polyomavirus (progressive multifocal leukoencephalopathy) or unconventional agents, which cause the diseases kuru and Creutzfeldt-Jakob disease. The unconventional agents differ so radically from viruses that they have now been called *prions* (see Boxed Essay, p. 738). Let us briefly discuss some of the important slow infections.

Kuru and Creutzfeldt-Jakob Disease

Kuru is a chronic degenerative disease discovered in the Foré people of New Guinea. The disease was originally discovered to be transmitted during the ritualistic cannibalistic consumption of their dead relatives as a sign of respect. Women and children and not men handled liquefied brain tissue, which was the source of infection. Thus, the infectious agent gained entrance to the body through skin cuts, the nasal mucosa, or conjunctiva. Men rarely ate the flesh of dead kuru victims; thus, women and children were more likely to become infected. The latent period for kuru may be as long as 2 years, but once symptoms appear death occurs within 3 to 9 months. The first symptoms of disease are an unsteadiness in walking and a shivering tremor involving head, trunk, and legs. Later the patient begins to stammer and there is uncoordinated eye movement. These features worsen until the patient cannot walk and is unable to swallow.

Creutzfeldt-Jakob disease is a degenerative disease of the central nervous system affecting persons between 35 and 65 years of age. Most human cases are sporadic. The disease can be transmitted to nonhuman primates. The infected patient becomes uncoordinated and demented, and death occurs within 9 to 18 months of onset of symptoms. Accidental transmission of this disease has occurred, although infrequently, during transplantation procedures, which suggests that the infectious agent is not limited to the brain.

There is no treatment for kuru or Creutzfeldt-Jakob disease.

Subacute Sclerosing Panencephalitis

Persistent infection of the central nervous system with measles virus is recognized as the cause of SSPE. The disease occurs most often in children and appears with a frequency of one case per million but in the Southeast this ratio is 4 to 5 cases per million. The majority of patients with SSPE had measles at an early age, most before 2 years of age.

SSPE follows natural measles infection after a latent period of about 7 years. The virus apparently remains in the nervous tissue in a suppressed form and then spreads through the brain without the formation of mature viral particles. SSPE-infected cells can be observed to have nucleocapsids in the nucleus and cytoplasm, but none are aligned at the cytoplasmic membrane for budding. SSPE patients have high titers of measles antibody in the cerebrospinal fluid (CSF), a characteristic not associated with natural measles infection. Apparently some nerve cells in the CSF die and release viral antigens that stimulate antibody production. The suppression of virus formation in nerve cells is believed to be due to the absence of a virus-specific protein or presence of a suppressive factor. The immune system of the host is unable to neutralize the virus because most virus is hidden intracellularly. The precipitation of disease 7 years after measles infection is believed to be due to some hormonal factor associated with puberty, but this is only a hypothesis.

The clinical findings of SSPE can be divided

PRIONS AND SLOW INFECTIONS

We have become accustomed to the basic tenet of biology that all organisms carry nucleic acids that define their own identity. This tenet is being challenged by the discovery of *prions*—a term that means "proteinaceous infectious particle." Prions are not viruses or bacteria but proteins that are virtually impossible to identify by using any kind of classical technique. Prions were found to be the cause of an animal disease called *scrapie*. Scrapie is a common neurological disorder in sheep. In addition, prions are also the cause of a rare human dementia called Creutzfeldt-Jakob disease. This disease received public attention because it caused the death of the choreographer George Balanchine.

Scientists can transmit scrapie experimentally by taking brain tissue from sick animals and injecting it into healthy animals. Prions in the brains of infected animals form clumps called plaques. The plaques look like those common in the brains of people with Alzheimer's disease, the leading cause of senility. Scientists are now looking for prions in the brains of victims of multiple sclerosis, Lou Gehrig's disease, and Parkinson's disease.

The predominant questions about the prion is how it replicates and how it causes disease. One intriguing theory concerning the latter question is that prions are abnormal versions of some normal brain protein. According to this theory, everyone has the genetic potential to manufacture prions. When a prion invades the body it becomes attached to a cell and somehow turns on a gene that makes a normal protein. In the process, however, the prion alters cell metabolism in such a way that a modified form of the protein—more prions—are produced. The prions accumulate over several years and slowly interfere with neurological function.

In 1989 researchers at the Washington University of Medicine in St. Louis stumbled on a clue to the possible action of prions. They isolated a protein that stimulates the production of a receptor on chicken muscle fibers. These receptors subsequently become sensitive to chemical signals transmitted by nerves. When the researchers entered into their computer the amino acid sequence of the protein, the computer informed them that about one-third of their protein had amino acid sequences identical to prions. A high degree of sequence similarity indicates a similarity of function, even though the proteins are from different sources. One hypothesis is that prions, which are also found in normal cells, regulate production of neurochemical receptors in the nervous system. Mutant prions could possibly trigger neurodegenerative diseases.

into four stages: Stage I, cerebral changes; Stage II, convulsive motor signs; Stage III, coma and spasms of the head, back, and lower limbs; Stage IV, loss of cerebral-cortical function and inability to speak. Most patients live an average of 18 months after diagnosis of SSPE.

Some reports indicate that administration of transfer factor (see Chapter 12) can prevent the progression of symptoms. The drug isoprinosine has been reported to produce long-term remissions. The administration of measles vaccine in the United States has reduced SSPE greatly, but this is not true for developing countries, where measles is still a major cause of morbidity and mortality.

Progressive Multifocal Leukoencephalopathy (PML)

PML is a rare demyelinating disease associated with the polyoma viruses, JC virus, and BK virus, discussed earlier.

SUMMARY

Because of the length of this chapter the summary consists of Tables 31-9 and 31-10, which describe the characteristics of the viral diseases.

Table 31-9. Characteristics of Diseases Caused by DNA Viruses

Viral disease	Viral agent	Epidemiology	Clinical manifestations	Vaccine
Smallpox	Poxvirus	Person to person via direct contact; begins as respiratory infection	Lesions in internal organs and eruptions on skin	No longer available to general public: disease eradicated
Herpesvirus diseases				
Cytomegalovirus disease	Cytomegalovirus	Direct contact	Congenital disease can result in fetal abnormalities; opportunistic for transplant patients (jaundice, hepatosplenomegaly); mononucleosis-like disease from transfusions	Experimental vaccine for renal transplant patients
Chickenpox	Varicella-zoster virus	Direct contact with respiratory secretions	Viremia followed by rash; usually self-limiting	Yes*; immune globulins also available
Shingles	Varicella-zoster virus	Activation of latent varicella virus	Skin lesions similar to those of chickenpox but more painful	No
Cutaneous herpes	Herpes simplex virus 1	Direct contact; activation of endogenous virus	Lesions on face; encephalitis in neonate	No

Disease	Virus	Transmission	Symptoms	Vaccine*
	Herpes simplex virus 2	Activation of endogenous virus but can be transferred sexually	Lesions on genitalia; neonatal herpes may be cutaneous or disseminated	No
Infectious mononucleosis	Epstein-Barr virus	Direct contact with respiratory secretions	Fatigue, chills, fever, spleen and liver enlargement	No
Respiratory and ocular disease	Adenoviruses	Direct contact	Bronchitis, croup, pneumonia, conjunctivitis	Yes for military recruits
Epidemic acute gastroenteritis	Norwalk viruses; some adenovirus types	Fecal-oral	Diarrhea	No
Long-term hepatitis	Hepatitis B virus	Contact with contaminated blood or blood products; sexual transmission also possible	Jaundice, usually self-limiting, but chronic disease very serious	Yes; immunoglobulins also available
Warts	Papillomaviruses	Person to person, including sexual contact	Warts on areas of the body including genitalia	No

* Vaccine has not yet been licensed in the United States.

Table 31-10. Characteristics of Diseases Causes by RNA Viruses

Viral disease	Viral agent	Epidemiology	Clinical manifestations	Vaccine
Measles	Measles virus	Direct contact with respiratory secretions	Fever and rash associated with viremia; usually self-limiting; subacute sclerosing panencephalitis a rare sequela of measles	Yes; immune globulin also available
Mumps	Mumps virus	Direct contact with respiratory secretions	Salivary glands enlarged after viremia; usually self-limiting	Yes
Rubella	Rubella virus	Congenital rubella during viremia in mother; postnatal infection via respiratory secretions	Congenital disease can result in death of fetus or deformities at birth; rash in postnatal disease and usually self-limiting	Yes; immune globulin also available
Influenza	Influenza viruses A, B, and C	Contact with respiratory secretions	Cold-like syndrome but in compromised patients can be complicated by pneumonia	Yes
Poliomyelitis	Poliovirus	Fecal-oral	Fever and stiffness of neck; usually self-limiting: 1% develop paralytic disease	Yes; oral and parenteral types
Rabies	Rabies virus	Bite of infected arimal or inhalation of contaminated aerosols	Fever, difficulty in swallowing, convulsive seizures, coma, and almost invariably death	Yes for animals and humans; immune globulin also available
Yellow fever	Arbovirus	Bite of infected mosquito (*Aedes aegypti*)	Jaundice, extensive liver damage	Yes; immune globulin also available
Encephalitis	Arboviruses (western equine, eastern equine, LaCrosse, and St. Louis encephalitis viruses).	Bite of mosquito	Fever, headache, stiffness of neck; fatalities high in eastern equine encephalitis	No
Colds	Rhinoviruses	Contact with respiratory secretions or	Coryza, sore throat, and cough	No

Disease	Virus	Mode of transmission	Symptoms	Vaccine
Viral hemorrhagic fever	Lassa fever virus, Ebola virus, Marburg virus, Crimean-Congo hemorrhagic fever virus (CCHF)	contaminated fomites Contact with rats (Lassa fever); close personal contact (Ebola); tick bite (CCHF)	Fever, hemorrhaging from multiple sites	No
Dengue fever and Dengue hemorrhagic fever	Arbovirus	Bite of mosquito (*Aedes aegypti*)	Fever, arthralgia, myalgia (Dengue fever); hemorrhaging and intravascular coagulation (Dengue hemorrhagic fever)	No
Enterovirus disease	Polioviruses, coxsackieviruses A and B, echoviruses, and enterovirus types 68-71	Direct contact with respiratory secretions	Polio; aseptic meningitis, herpangina, myocarditis, and pleurodynia	Yes (polio virus); no (other viruses)
Lower respiratory tract disease	Parainfluenza viruses 1, 2, and 3; respiratory syncytial virus	Direct contact with respiratory secretions	Croup, bronchiolitis, pneumonia	No
Hemorrhagic fevers	Marburg virus, Ebola virus	Contact with blood (?)	Fever, headache, intravascular coagulation, and shock precede death	No
	Arenaviruses (lymphocytic choriomeningitis, Tacaribe group, and Lassa fever viruses)	Contact with rat secretions	High fever, headache, diarrhea, capillary leakage, and shock	No
Short-term hepatitis	Hepatitis A virus	Fecal-oral	Jaundice; recovery permanent and no persistence	In development; immune globulins available
Epidemic gastroenteritis	Rotavirus	Fecal-oral	Diarrhea accompanied by vomiting and fever	No
	Caliciviruses	Fecal-oral	Diarrhea and vomiting	No
	Astroviruses	Fecal-oral	Diarrhea and vomiting	No
Acquired immune deficiency syndrome (AIDS)	Retrovirus (human immunodeficiency virus)	Sexual contact; exposure to blood; mother to neonate	Long progression of symptoms terminating in death, usually from opportunistic infections	No

QUESTIONS FOR STUDY

Select the best response or responses for each of the following:

1. Which of the following viruses is considered of particular importance because of infection in the newborn?
   A. Herpes simplex virus
   B. Cytomegalovirus
   C. Rubella virus
   D. Papilloma virus

2. Which of the following viral agents is associated with gastroenteritis?
   A. Norwalk viruses
   B. Rotavirus
   C. Herpes simplex virus
   D. Adenovirus types 16 to 20

3. A child has a fever and small red macules with a bluish-white center on the inside of the cheek. Two days later the child is covered with a rash. The most likely of the following candidate viruses as the cause of the infection is
   A. Rubella virus
   B. Measles virus
   C. Mumps virus
   D. Varicella virus

4. All of the following cause persistent infections *except*
   A. Mumps virus
   B. Kuru agent
   C. Herpes simplex virus
   D. Measles virus

5. The most prevalent form of herpes simplex type I infection involves the
   A. Central nervous system
   B. Cervix of females and penis of males
   C. Lips
   D. Respiratory tract

6. Patients receiving blood transfusions are at risk for virus infections. Which of the following viruses causes the most posttransfusion viral infections?

   A. Human immunodeficiency virus
   B. Non-A, Non-B hepatitis virus
   C. Cytomegalovirus
   D. Hepatitis B virus

7. Which of the following viruses can be reactivated in the mother to cause perinatal or postnatal infection?
   A. Cytomegalovirus
   B. Rubella virus
   C. Varicella virus
   D. Hepatitis B virus

8. Which of the following is least likely to be the cause of influenza epidemics?
   A. Point mutations
   B. Genetic recombination
   C. Changes in population immunity
   D. Changes in core proteins

9. The principal reason that oral polio vaccine is used in the United States is
   A. It is an inactivated vaccine.
   B. It can be administered at the same time with other vaccines.
   C. Children find it more acceptable.
   D. It multiplies in the intestine and establishes intestinal immunity.

10. The major cause of lower respiratory infection in infants and children is
    A. Adenovirus
    B. Respiratory syncytial virus
    C. Parainfluenza viruses
    D. Rhinoviruses

11. The most important hemorrhagic fever in the Americas is
    A. Ebola hemorrhagic fever
    B. Lassa fever
    C. Marburg hemorrhagic fever
    D. Dengue hemorrhagic fever

12. The mosquito is a vector for all of the following diseases *except*

A. Yellow fever
B. Parvovirus-B19
C. Dengue hemorrhagic fever
D. Eastern equine encephalitis

13. The presence of IgG but not IgM antibodies to rubella virus in the newborn suggests
   A. Congenital infection
   B. Autoimmune disease
   C. Persistent infection
   D. Presence of maternal antibodies

14. All of the following concerning HIV infection are true *except*
   A. The T4 cell count declines over a period of years until the patient is unable to resist opportunistic infections.
   B. Most HIV infections are transmitted by sexual contact.
   C. The principal serological test is an enzyme-linked immunosorbent assay that detects HIV proteins in the serum.
   D. Azidothymidine is the primary drug used in treatment.

15. All of the following signs or symptoms may appear during the first stage of HIV infection *except*

A. Lymph node enlargement
B. Large numbers of B cells in lymph glands
C. T4 cell count that is still high
D. Disseminated opportunistic infections

16. Which of the following diagnostic markers persists in the bloodstream of HBV chronically infected individuals and is utilized as a measure of increased infectivity and persistent infection?
   A. HBcAg
   B. HBeAg
   C. anti-HBc
   D. anti-HBs

17. Which of the following best describes hepatitis A disease?
   A. Transmitted primarily by blood transfusion; incubation period, 50 to 70 days
   B. Transmitted by fecal-oral route; incubation period, 50 to 70 days
   C. Transmitted by sexual contact; incubation period, 50 to 70 days
   D. Transmitted by fecal-oral route; incubation period, 15 to 50 days

Match the specific viral disease or virus on the left with the principal method of transmission indicated on the right.

18. Hepatitis B
19. Kuru
20. Rotavirus
21. Yellow fever
22. Western equine encephalitis
23. Herpes cold sores
24. Poliomyelitis
25. Coxsackievirus
26. Influenza
27. Lassa fever
28. Rabies
29. Postnatal rubella
30. Zoster

A. Sexual contact
B. Bite of mosquito
C. Contact with rats or rat excrement
D. Bite of infected dog or other animal
E. Inhalation of, or contact with, contaminated aerosols
F. Handling of contaminated brain tissue
G. Fecal-oral route
H. Reactivation of latent virus

ADDITIONAL READINGS

DNA VIRUSES

Albert, M. J. Enteric adenoviruses: Brief review. *Arch. Virol.* 88:1,1986.

Behbehani, A. M. The smallpox story: Life and death of an old disease. *Microbiol. Revs.* 47(4):455,1983.

Brunell, P. A., et al. Risk of herpes zoster in children with leukemia: Varicella vaccine compared with history of chickenpox. *Pediatr.* 77:53,1986.

Cytomegalovirus infection and treatment with ganciclovir. *Rev. Infect. Dis.* 10 (Suppl. 3), 1988.

Dolin, R., Treanor, J. J., and Madore, H. P. Novel agents of viral enteritis. *J. Infect. Dis.* 155:356,1987.

Preblud, S. R., Orenstein, W., A., and Bart, K. J. Varicella: Clinical manifestations, epidemiology, and health impact in children. *Pediatr. Infect. Dis.* 3:505,1984.

Risks associated with human parvovirus B19 infection. *M.M.W.R.* 38(6):81,1989.

Whitely, R. J., and Alford, C. A., Jr. Neonatal herpes simplex infections. *Pediatr. Rev.* 7:119,1985.

RNA VIRUSES

CDC. ACIP: Poliomyelitis prevention: Enhanced-potency inactivated poliomyelitis vaccine—supplemental statement. *M.M.W.R.* 36(48):795,1987.

CDC. ACIP. Prevention and control of influenza. *M.M.W.R.* 37:361,1988.

CDC.ACIP. Prevention of perinatal transmission of hepatitis B virus: Prenatal screening of all pregnant women for hepatitis B surface antigen. *M.M.W.R.* 37:341,1988.

CDC. ACIP. Update on hepatitis B prevention. *M.M.W.R.* 36:353, 1987.

CDC. Management of patients with suspected viral hemorrhagic fever. *M.M.W.R.* 137 (No. S-3):February 26, 1988.

CDC. Measles—United States, 1987. *M.M.W.R.* 37:527,1988.

CDC. Mumps—United States, 1985–1986. *M.M.W.R.* 36:151,1987.

Christensen, M. L. Human viral gastroenteritis. *Clin. Microbiol. Revs.* 2(1):51,1989.

Hadler, S. C., and McFarland, L. Hepatitis in day care centers: Epidemiology and prevention. *Rev. Infect. Dis.* 8(4):548,1986.

McCormick, J. B., et al. A case control study of the clinical diagnosis and course of Lassa fever. *J. Infect. Dis.* 155(3):445,1987.

Monath, T. P. Yellow fever: A medically neglected disease. *Rev. Infect. Dis.* 9(1):165,1987.

Research towards rabies prevention. *Rev. Infect. Dis.* 10(Suppl. 4),1988.

Rubella. *Rev. Infect. Dis.* 6(Suppl. 1),1985.

Welliver, R. C. Detection, pathogenesis, and therapy of respiratory syncytial virus infections. *Clin. Microbiol. Revs.* 1(1):27,1988.

What science knows about AIDS. *Sci. Amer.* 259(4):1988.

Zuckerman, A. J. Current developments and issues in immunization against hepatitis A and B. *Curr. Opin. Infect. Dis.* 2(6):760,1989.

VII. MEDICAL MYCOLOGY

32. THE PATHOGENIC FUNGI

OBJECTIVES

To outline the major differences between fungi and bacteria in terms of structure and morphology, reproduction, and laboratory identification

To describe the relationship between dimorphism and fungal pathogenesis

To briefly list the major antifungal drugs and the types of diseases for which they are most frequently used

To make a list of the systemic, cutaneous, subcutaneous, and superficial mycoses and briefly describe the mechanisms of transmission for each

group, the body tissues affected, and how the diseases are treated

To describe the various types of candidiasis and aspergillosis as to the tissue affected, the groups of individuals most likely to be affected, and treatment

To briefly describe the importance of *Pneumocystis carinii* as an opportunistic pathogen

To describe the important mycotoxins and how humans become intoxicated

Fungi represent the first of the infectious eukaryotic microorganisms to be discussed. As you recall from Chapter 3, eukaryotes differ in many ways from prokaryotes such as bacterial (see Table 3-1, page 37). These differences influence the way in which eukaryotes cause disease and the way in which eukaryotic diseases are diagnosed and treated. The purposes of this chapter are (1) to briefly describe how fungal morphology, physiology, growth, etc. influence or affect the disease process, and (2) to outline some of the most important fungal diseases associated with humans.

CHARACTERISTICS OF THE FUNGI

Fungi are eukaryotes that encompass both macro- and microforms. Macroforms include the mushrooms while microforms include the single-celled yeasts. Most fungi are found in the soil, where they engage primarily in the degradation of organic matter. Many species of fungi are parasitic for plants but relatively few species are parasitic for humans. Fungal diseases in healthy humans are usually the result of occupational contact with the microorganism—for example, farmers, veterinarians, miners, nursery personnel, etc. Most human infections are caused by opportunistic fungi that are part of the microbial flora. It is in the setting of the hospital or situations in which the host is compromised that one sees most human fungal infections in the United States.

MORPHOLOGY AND STRUCTURE

The fungi are divided into two morphological forms: *yeast* and *molds*. Yeasts are typically round or oval single cells that measure approximately 4 to 5 μm in diameter (Plate 22), but some

may be as large as 25 μm in diameter. Molds are multicellular fungi composed of filamentous or tubular structures called *hyphae* (sing. *hypha*). A single hypha may be from 5 to 50 μm in length and 2 to 4 μm in diameter. Some hyphae are partitioned by cross walls called *septa* (Fig. 32-1) that divide them into individual compartments. Each compartment contains cytoplasm and one or more nuclei. Not all hyphae are septate. In hyphae without septa the cytoplasm and nuclei circulate freely. Thus each hypha may contain several nuclei. These hyphae are referred to as *aseptate* and represent a mass of nucleated protoplasm. As hyphae branch and grow they form

Fig. 32-1. Characteristic morphology of yeasts and molds. The filamentous molds illustrated are depicted with cross walls called *septa* (sing., *septum*), but not all molds possess septa.

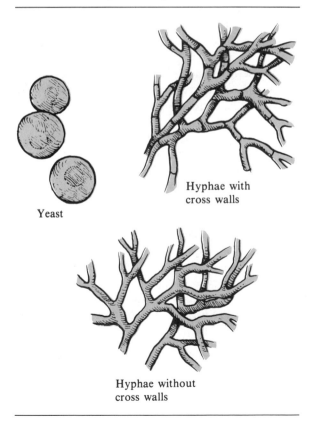

Yeast

Hyphae with cross walls

Hyphae without cross walls

a mat of intertwined hyphae called a *mycelium*. The mycelium may be divided into a *vegetative portion,* which remains attached to the substrate or penetrates it to obtain nutrients, and a *reproductive portion,* which is usually represented by aerial structures. The aerial structures give the mold a cottony appearance (Plate 23).

Not all fungi grow exclusively as yeasts or molds. Some fungi, which are called *dimorphic,* can exist in either state, depending on chemical and physical factors. Dimorphism plays an important role in the pathogenicity of certain fungi, as will be discussed later in the chapter.

Fungi possess cell walls that differ from those of bacteria. The fungal cell wall is relatively rigid and thick, and possesses no peptidoglycan layer. The major constituents of the fungal cell wall are polysaccharides (75 percent) and protein (25 percent). The polysaccharides are primarily chitin or cellulose. The absence of a peptidoglycan enables fungi to resist the actions of bacterial cell wall inhibitors such as the penicillins and cephalosporins.

The cytoplasmic membrane of eukaryotes is similar in structure and composition to that of prokaryotes. The principal difference between them is that eukaryotic cell membranes contain sterols and prokaryotes (except for *Mycoplasma*) do not contain them. Sterols are important stabilizing components; therefore, antimicrobials that interact with sterols cause permeability changes in the cytoplasmic membrane of the fungal cell. Eukaryotes possess an internal membrane system called the *endoplasmic reticulum* and important organelles, such as mitochondria, that are surrounded by a membrane system. These membrane systems also possess sterols, which are affected by antimicrobial agents that have no effect on prokaryotes such as bacteria.

Fungi differ from bacteria in that (except for some aquatic sex cells) they have no structures associated with locomotion and they do not produce capsules (except for *Cryptococcus neoformans*). Fungi, therefore, have fewer mechanisms than bacteria for attachment to host cells.

REPRODUCTION

Reproduction in fungi may be sexual or asexual, but asexual reproduction is the more important in propagating the organism. Sexual reproduction involves the union of two nuclei, sex cells, or sex organs. Asexual reproduction involves several mechanisms of propagation, which include:

1. *Fragmentation* of a hyphal filament with each fragment growing into a new individual
2. *Fission* of a cell into two daughter cells (similar to binary fission in bacteria)
3. *Budding* of the cells, each bud producing a new individual
4. Production of *spores,* each spore germinating into hyphae that grow into a mycelium.

Yeasts may reproduce asexually by *sporulation, fission,* or *budding,* but budding is the most common process. During the process of budding a protuberance, called a *bud,* is formed on the surface of the parent or mother cell (Fig. 32-2). As the bud enlarges it reaches a critical size and separates from the mother cell. Release of the bud

Fig. 32-2. Photomicrograph ($\times 1666$) of budding yeast cells. The large yeast cell at lower right shows multiple budding. (From M. Salazar, A. Restrepo, and D. A. Stevens, *Inf. Imm.* 56[3]:711, 1988.)

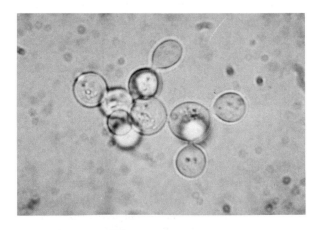

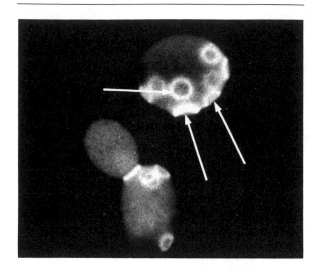

Fig. 32-3. Bud scars (*arrows*) on yeast *Saccharomyces cerevisiae*. (From K. Beran and E. Streiblova, *Adv. Microb. Physiol.* 2:143, 1968. Copyright Academic Press, Inc. [London], Ltd.)

leaves a permanent scar, called a *bud scar*, on the surface of the mother cell (Fig. 32-3). If the developing bud does not separate from the mother cell, it (developing bud) may also bud. As the budding process continues a chain of buds called *pseudohyphae* is formed (Plate 24).

Sporulation, which occurs in both yeasts and molds, may be brought about by sexual or asexual means. Asexual sporulation is the most important mechanism of reproduction and also the most important mechanism for propagating the species. Asexual sporulation produces numerous individuals and occurs repeatedly, as opposed to sexual spore formation, which occurs infrequently.

Sexual Sporulation

Sexual reproduction in fungi rarely occurs in the laboratory or in infected humans. The sexual phase (called the *perfect state*) of several species has not been detected and this is the basis of classification for one group of fungi called Deutero-

mycetes (Fungi Imperfecti) because they lack a sexual stage of reproduction. Sexual spores may be of various types:

1. *Oospores*. Oospores result from the fertilization of a specialized female structure called an *oogonium* by a male fungal structure called an *antheridium*.
2. *Zygospore*. Zygospores result from the fusion of two hyphae and their nuclear contents to form a single thick-walled spore.
3. *Ascospores*. Ascospores are formed within a sac called an *ascus*. The ascus is usually enclosed in a fruiting body called an *ascocarp*. Ascocarps vary in size and shape.
4. *Basidiospores*. Basidiospores are formed from the end of a club-shaped structure called a *basidium*. The fungi associated with such structures are mushrooms, puffballs, and other large fungi found in nature (Fig. 32-4).

Fig. 32-4. Edible mushrooms. (Courtesy Carolina Biological Supply Co.)

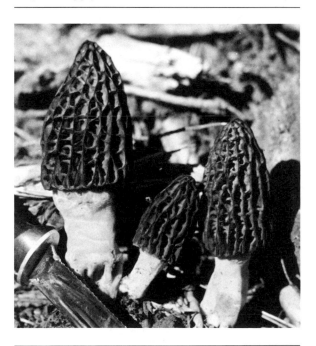

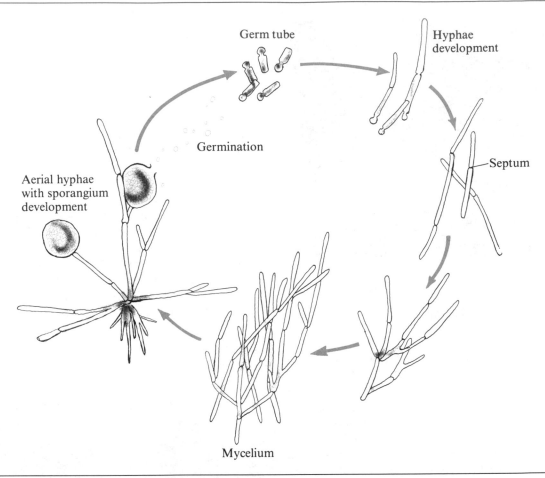

Fig. 32-5. Stages in the asexual production of a mold. Mycelium develops aerial sporangium in which spores are produced and later are released into the environment. Spores germinate and develop germ tubes, which later multiply and form hyphae.

Asexual Sporulation (Fig. 32-5).

Those fungi that form spores only asexually or not at all are referred to as being in the *imperfect state*. Until recently most human fungal pathogens were characterized as being in the imperfect state, but several species have been induced to produce spores by sexual means. Asexual spores may be produced in specialized structures that arise from hyphae, or they may be formed by modification of hyphae. *Conidia* are asexual spores produced on specialized stalks called *conidiophores* (Fig. 32-6) from which the spores are pinched off and released into the environment. Conidia vary in size, shape, and color (Fig. 32-6) a characteristic that lends itself to classification. Some asexual spores are produced within a specialized sac called a *sporangium* and are called *sporangiospores* (Fig. 32-7). Asexual

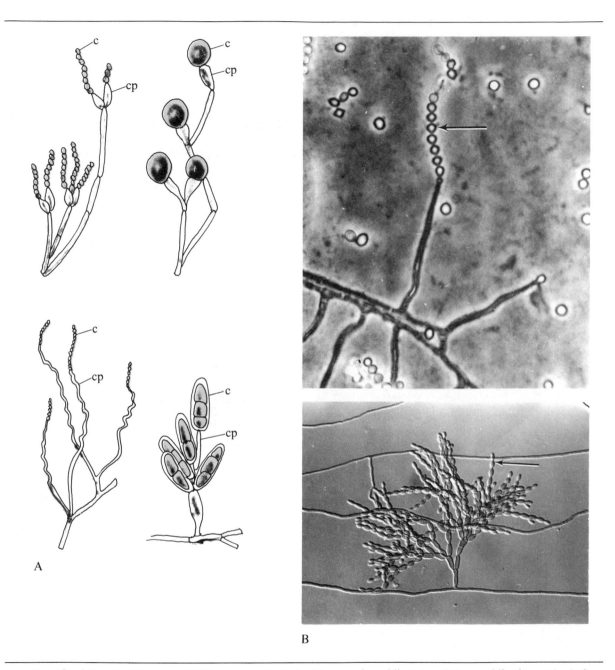

Fig. 32-6. Conidia. A. Diagram of different morphological forms of conidia (*c*) and the conidiophores (*cp*) that bear them. B. Photomicrographs of two types of conidia (*arrows*). Top, phase-contrast photomicrograph of *Gliomastix mucorum*. (From T. M. Hammill, *Mycologia* 73:229, 1981.) Bottom, differential interference phase-contrast micrograph of *Cladosporium* species. (From M. R. McGinnis, *Laboratory Handbook of Medical Mycology*. New York: Academic, 1980.)

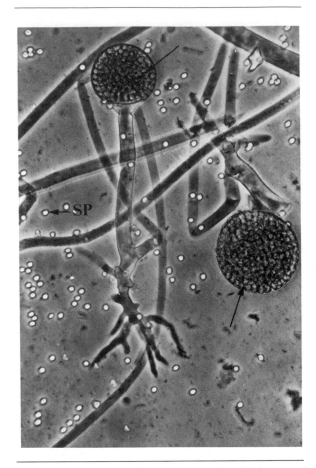

Fig. 32-7. Photomicrograph of a species of *Rhizopus* demonstrating the sporangium (*arrow*) and its encased sporangiospores (*SP*). (From E. J. Bottone, *J. Clin. Microbiol.* 9:530, 1979.)

spores arising directly from hyphae are collectively called *thallospores* and are divided into the following types:

1. *Arthrospores.* Arthrospores are barrelshaped, thick-walled spores produced by the fragmentation of hyphae (Fig. 32-8).
2. *Chlamydospores.* Chlamydospores are sometimes referred to as *resting spores* because they are produced in older, dried-out cultures. They are produced by a swelling of the hyphal fragment and development of a thick wall (Fig. 32-8).

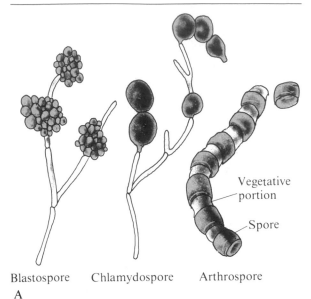

Blastospore   Chlamydospore   Arthrospore

A

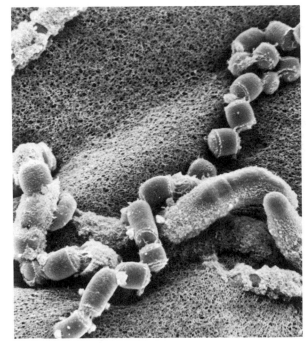

B

Fig. 32-8. Types of thallospores. A. Diagram. B. Scanning electron micrograph of arthrospores. (Courtesy D. J. Bibel.)

3. *Blastospores*. Blastospores represent a simple budding from the parent cell. They may appear as single daughter cells or as clustered cells, called *pseudophyphae*, that have not been detached (Fig. 32-8).

CULTURAL CHARACTERISTICS

All molds are aerobic, while yeasts are facultative anaerobes. Because of their biosynthetic potential fungi can grow on a variety of substrates that ordinarily would not support the growth of many bacteria. Fungi can tolerate pH's between 2.0 and 9.0, but abundant growth occurs between pH 5.0 and 6.0. In the laboratory fungi are cultivated on special media since they are recovered from specimens that are contaminated with bacteria. One of the most widely used isolation media for fungi is called *Sabouraud* agar, which contains maltose and peptone as its principal ingredients. It is selective against most bacteria because of its low pH. Antibiotics can be introduced into fungal media to inhibit bacteria since they are not active against fungi. Fungi can be differentiated into yeasts and molds by their appearance on growth media. Yeasts produce creamy opaque colonies, while mold colonies are fluffy and cottony (see Plate 23). Dimorphic fungi when cultivated at 37°C appear as yeasts, but at 30°C they exist in a mold-like state. Differentiation of some fungal species can be made by demonstrating thermal dimorphism.

PATHOGENESIS

Fungi, as we have already mentioned, are found primarily in the soil, where they degrade organic material. Hundreds of thousands of spores are released by fungi into the environment to be disseminated by air or water. Spores possess surface components that make them resistant to environmental factors (Fig. 32-9). The surface is usually a glycoprotein or glycoprotein-lipoprotein

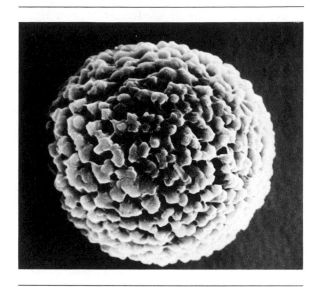

Fig. 32-9. Scanning electron micrograph ($\times 2500$ before 25 percent reduction) illustrating the surface characteristics of one type of fungal spore. (From J. S. Gardner et al., *Mycologia* 75:333, 1983.)

complex that is hydrophobic, thus permitting dissemination in the air. Spores are often inhaled or ingested by humans, yet fungal diseases are very rare in humans. Some spores are able to infect humans because of physical factors that force them into the host—for example, the lodging of spores in hair follicles. Some spores are present on sharp objects (wood, thorns) that can penetrate subcutaneous tissue. Inhaled spores are sorted out by the respiratory system on the basis of size and density. Only under unusual circumstances do ingested spores cause disease. When the infectious fungal unit, which may be an arthrospore, conidium, blastospore, or other type, makes contact with host tissue, it must germinate and, depending on host response, may or may not initiate infection. The diseases caused by fungi are called *mycoses*. Most fungal infections in humans result from occupational hazards. Infection is more likely to occur in those who are constantly in contact with the soil or those compromised by underlying disease or some condition that depresses the immune system. Laboratory workers who handle fungal cultures are at an increased risk of infection. Fungal spores are easily disseminated from a mold, but this is not a problem with yeast colonies. Mold cultures must therefore be handled with extreme care. Petri dishes containing mold colonies are handled in special hoods. Fungal infections can occur in the healthy adult only if the fungal infectious units are in excessive numbers and they make contact with a tissue that supports their growth.

Very little is known concerning the pathogenic mechanisms of fungi. None appear to produce toxins or toxic metabolites, which are characteristic of bacterial pathogens and which influence the outcome of infection. Most fungi that reach a mucosal surface are readily attacked by the host's immune system and are walled off. This response by the host prevents fungal reproduction and tissue invasion. Some fungi, when they make contact with the mucosal surface, induce an allergic response, but tissue invasion does not occur. Most of the research on the pathogenesis of fungi has been directed at the yeast *Candida albicans*. This organism apparently possesses external components that enable it to attach to mucosal surfaces. The attachment process occurs while the organism is in a yeast state, but invasion of tissue appears to require the formation of pseudohyphae. The appearance of pseudohyphae is believed to enable the fungus to escape phagocytosis, so the host must rely on other less efficient mechanisms of defense. This pleomorphic response is also characteristic of most fungi that cause systemic disease. Dimorphic fungi other than *Candida* are usually found in the yeast state in tissue, but outside the host they exist as filamentous forms. It appears that phagocytes are less efficient in killing yeast than the spore, which is the morphological form that is deposited on the mucosal surface. In addition, some yeast-like cells are approximately 20 to 25 μm in diameter, a size that prohibits efficient digestion by immune cells of the host. Not all fungal pathogens that invade the host tissue exist in the yeast state; for example, *Aspergillus* species exist as hyphae in tissue (this organism's pathogenesis will be dis-

cussed more extensively later). Another mechanism for resisting immune defenses is found in the yeast *Cryptococcus neoformans*. This organism is inhaled as a spore and germinates in the host to form a yeast, which quickly produces a capsule. Encapsulation apparently permits the organism to resist phagocytosis. Other examples of apparent pathogenic mechanisms will be discussed later with the individual organisms.

Fungal diseases can be broken down into four types on the basis of the tissue infected: *systemic, subcutaneous, cutaneous,* and *superficial*. In addition, a separate group, diseases caused by opportunistic fungal agents, will be discussed.

LABORATORY DIAGNOSIS

The manifestations of many fungal diseases are very similar to those of diseases caused by bacterial agents such as *Actinomyces*. Accurate diagnosis is made by direct microscopic observation, culture techniques, and serological tests.

Fungi can be observed directly in clinical specimens such as tissues, sputum, bronchial washings, hair, or skin scrapings. The specimens are usually treated with 10% potassium hydroxide and heated to destroy host cellular elements, leaving the KOH-resistant cell wall of the fungal agent unaltered. The structures (conidia, conidiophores) of many fungi are distinctive enough in the vegetative phase to permit presumptive diagnosis. Dried and fixed films may be stained with Gram's stain, periodic acid-Schiff stain, or Wright stain. The microscopic examination of filamentous molds can be performed by teasing apart a portion of the colony on a microscopic slide and adding a drop of lactophenol aniline blue stain.

Specimens are also cultured on laboratory media, even when direct examination provides almost positive results. Sabouraud agar and richer media are used with and without antibiotics to inhibit contaminating bacterial species. Growth at room temperature and at 37°C can be used to distinguish the yeast and mycelial phases of dimorphic fungi. Slide cultures can be made to observe fungal structures in their natural state, but this is not recommended for those agents of systemic mycoses that can cause fatal disease.

Serological tests have value in the diagnosis of mycotic disease, especially if culture or histologic results are negative. The results of intradermal injection of skin test antigens of *Aspergillus* species, for example, are important criteria in the diagnosis of disease, while other skin test antigens are sometimes used to assess the prognosis of disease. Serologic tests involving antibody determination can also be useful in determining the cause or prognosis of disease. Immunodiffusion, counterimmuno-electrophoresis, and complement fixation are the standard serologic tests in the laboratory.

IMMUNITY

Antibody is regarded as being less important than cell-mediated immunity as a protective device in response to fungal infections. This is best illustrated by the variety of fungal infections found in patients with defective T lymphocytes. In contrast, defects in B cells do not usually predispose the patient to fungal infections. Studies to date indicate that antibodies are protective only within a very narrow range of conditions in experimental animals and with only a few pathogens such as *Candida* and *Cryptococcus*. Antibodies act primarily to enhance the efficiency of the cell-mediated response. Those fungi that are allergenic when inhaled, such as *Alternaria* and *Cladosporium*, elicit an IgE-mediated hypersensitivity. The immune response triggered by these allergenic fungi is evidenced by enhanced activities by macrophages and lymphocytes. Again the morphology of the fungal agent in tissue influences the host response. Conidia of *Aspergillus fumigatus*, for example, are eliminated by macrophages, but neutrophils are more destructive to hyphae.

TREATMENT AND PREVENTION

Fungi are eukaryotic cells whose organelles and membranes are similar in composition to those of the host cells they infect. Most antifungal drugs are therefore very toxic to the host. The most devastating fungal infections are those that are systemic and require chemotherapeutic agents that not only are toxic, but have poor solubility in water and are poorly absorbed. Even though some of the major antifungal agents were discussed in Chapter 8, we will use Table 32-1 to provide a more detailed description of their clinical usefulness. Table 32-1 should be referred to during the discussion of the specific fungal diseases later in the chapter.

No vaccines are available to prevent fungal disease. One of the reasons for this is that fungal surfaces are poorly antigenic and, second, mycoses are rare in the general public. Antimicrobial prophylaxis, however, is being seriously considered because life-threatening fungal infections remain a major complication among immunosuppressed patients. Several antifungal agents in various formulations are now being evaluated in leukemic patients and others with depressed immune systems.

IMPORTANCE TO HUMANS

The fungi play a role in disease but, even more important, they are also of value in nature and industry. Fungi, because of highly developed enzymatic systems, can degrade organic material, a property that may be of immeasurable value or detriment to humans. Fungi are important in the recycling of carbon and other elements. In addition, they can degrade recalcitrant molecules and have an important role in the disposal of chemical wastes. Their metabolic activities are also responsible for the destruction of many grains, fabrics, and foods. Fungal contamination of grains, peanut crops, and fruits (apples) can lead to the production of *mycotoxins* that cause serious illness in humans and various domestic

Table 32-1. Antifungal Agents Currently Available for Clinical Use

Drug	Formulations	Indications for use
Amphotericin B	Oral, solutions for intravenous use, creams	Systemic infections caused by *Candida, Cryptococcus; Histoplasma, Blastomyces, Aspergillus, Sporothrix*
Nystatin	Oral, cream	*Candida* infections
Flucytosine	Solutions for I.V. use, oral	Systemic infections caused by *Cryptococcus* and *Candida.* Used in combination with amphotericin B
Griseofulvin	Oral	Infections caused by dermatophytes
Clotrimazole	Cream, vaginal tablets, solutions for I.V. use	Superficial fungal infections, including dermatomycoses, tinea versicolor, and cutaneous and vaginal candidiasis
Miconazole	Cream, vaginal suppositories, solutions for I.V. use	Systemic infections, including coccidioidomycosis, candidiasis, cryptococcosis, paracoccidioidomycosis, and chronic mucocutaneous candidiasis
Econazole	Topical and vaginal creams, sprays and powders	Superficial infections, including dermatomycoses, tinea versicolor, and cutaneous and vaginal candidiasis
Ketoconazole	Oral, creams, and solutions	Systemic infections including blastomycosis, some forms of coccidioidomycosis and histoplasmosis, chronic mucocutaneous candidiasis, chromoblastomycosis, paracoccidioidomycosis Superficial infections including dermatomycoses, tinea versicolor
Bifonazole	Creams and solutions	Superficial infections including dermatomycoses, tinea versicolor, and cutaneous candidiasis
Croconazole	Creams and gels	Superficial infections including dermatomycoses, tinea versicolor, and cutaneous candidiasis
Fenticonazole	Topical and vaginal creams	Superficial infections including dermatomycoses, tinea versicolor, and cutaneous and vaginal candidiasis
Isoconazole	Topical and vaginal creams	Superficial infections including dermatomycoses, tinea versicolor, and cutaneous and vaginal candidiasis
Sulconazole	Cream	Superficial infections including dermatomycoses, tinea versicolor, and cutaneous candidiasis
Terconazole	Vaginal cream	Vaginal candidiasis
Fluconazole	Oral, I.V.	Cryptococcal meningitis, thrush

animals (mycotoxins are discussed later in the chapter). Fungi play an important role in industry because they are used in the preparation of a variety of products beneficial to humans (Table 32-2), such as antibiotics, the most famous of which is penicillin, produced by the green mold *Penicillium.* Fungi such as mushrooms, truffles, and morels are also prized food delicacies.

CLASSIFICATION

Modern taxonomists place the fungi in the kingdom Fungi, making it distinct from the animal and plant kingdoms. The kingdom Fungi is separated into two divisions, Myxomycota and Eumycota. The Myxomycota, or slime molds, are nonpathogenic, while the Eumycota are the principal

Table 32-2. Industrial Products Obtained Through the Activities of Fungi

Organism	Product
VITAMINS	
Eremothecium ashbyi	Riboflavin
FOOD AND BEVERAGES	
Saccharomyces cerevisiae	Wine, ale, sake, baker's yeast
Penicillium species	Varieties of cheese
Saccharomyces rouxii	Soy sauce
Saccharomyces carlsbergensis	Lager beer
ORGANIC ACIDS AND SOLVENTS	
Aspergillus niger	Citric acid and gluconic acid
Saccharomyces cerevisiae	Ethanol from glucose
SINGLE-CELL PROTEINS	
Saccharomyces lipolytica	Microbial protein from petroleum alkanes
Candida utilis	Microbial protein from paper pulp waste
PHARMACEUTICALS	
Penicillium chrysogenum	Penicillins
Cephalosporium acremonium	Cephalosporins
Rhizopus nigricans	Steroid transformation

pathogens for humans. The Eumycota can be separated into five subdivisions, four of which are pathogenic to humans:

1. *Zygomycotina.* The Zygomycotina are the most primitive members of the fungi. They are filamentous and lack septa, a characteristic that separates them from other subdivisions. They reproduce sexually and asexually. The asexual spores or sporangiospores are produced in a sac called a *sporangium.* The members of this group are not primary pathogens but are opportunistic in certain predisposed patients.
2. *Ascomycotina.* The Ascomycotina produce asexual and sexual spores. The asexual spores

are called *conidia*, and the sexual spores produced by those species of medical interest are called *ascospores*. Some members of this group (dermatophytes) cause skin infections, while others are pathogenic yeasts.
3. *Basidiomycotina.* The Basidiomycotina produce septate hyphae and sexual spores called *basidiospores*. Mushrooms and puffballs belong to this subdivision.
4. *Deuteromycotina* (Fungi Imperfecti). The Deuteromycotina reproduce asexually. Sexual reproductive structures are unknown. Many species pathogenic to humans belong to this group.

FUNGAL DISEASES

SYSTEMIC MYCOSES

The agents of systemic mycoses are dimorphic fungi found in the soil and are acquired by humans by inhalation of spores. Initially there is a pulmonary infection, which may or may not be symptomatic, but eventually the organism is disseminated to other organs. The systemic mycoses to be discussed are histoplasmosis, coccidioidomycosis, blastomycosis, paracoccidioidomycosis, and cryptococcosis.

Histoplasmosis

Histoplasma capsulatum is the causal agent of histoplasmosis. Since the discovery of a sexual stage (asci and ascospores when properly noted) the perfect stage is classified as *Emmonsiella capsulatum*, but we will retain its original name. Histoplasmosis occurs worldwide. In the United States the incidence of infection is highest in the Mississippi Valley. Several million people in the United States are infected by *H. capsulatum*, but fewer than 5 percent are symptomatic.

Epidemiology. *H. capsulatum* is found in soil that is nitrogen-enriched, especially soils containing high levels of avian fecal material. The organism can easily be isolated from excrement in chicken houses and starling roosts and from guano in bat caves. The roosting of several hundred thousand starlings in a small midwestern town in the United States was responsible for a large outbreak of histoplasmosis in young children. Conidia are transmitted through the air when the avian excreta are disturbed and aerosolized, but there is no human-to-human transmission.

Pathogenesis. *H. capsulatum* is an intracellular parasite that preferentially attacks cells of the reticuloendothelial system. The host-parasite relationship in histoplasmosis is poorly understood. Tissue damage by *H. capsulatum* results in the formation of granulomatous lesions but no fungal toxin has been detected. The virulence of this organism is related to its ability to survive and proliferate within macrophages. One of the microorganism's defense mechanisms is its ability to prevent the macrophage from releasing the toxic oxygen metabolites (superoxide, hydrogen peroxide, etc.) that destroy parasites.

Histoplasmosis is primarily a pulmonary infection that is acquired by inhalation of conidia. The majority of cases are asymptomatic, as is readily evident since 60 to 90 percent of the adults in certain geographical areas show a delayed hypersensitivity reaction to the skin test antigen *histoplasmin*, which indicates prior exposure to the fungus. In acute asymptomatic cases the lung lesion may heal with calcification, a condition that resembles tuberculosis lesions. Pulmonary histoplasmosis sometimes becomes chronic and is almost indistinguishable from tuberculosis. Reactivation of the lesions is more frequent where the disease is endemic. Untreated chronic disease may lead to dissemination of the organism and invasion of the entire reticuloendothelial system. In areas where histoplasmosis is endemic, disseminated histoplasmosis occurs 400 times more often among leukemic patients than the rest of the population. The symptoms include

fever with liver, spleen, and lymph node enlargement. The phagocytic cells found in these tissues are gorged with small oval yeast cells, and the organs display small granulomas similar to those produced in miliary tuberculosis. In approximately 50 percent of individuals infected, mucocutaneous lesions of the oral cavity appear. The ulcerative oral lesions are often painful and are accompanied by regional lymph node enlargement.

In certain areas of the United States histoplasmosis is recognized as an important AIDS-associated opportunistic infection (see Chapter 31).

Laboratory Diagnosis. Sputum and gastric washings can be stained and examined for *H. capsulatum* in the benign stage of the disease. Direct fluorescent antibody technique can also be applied to clinical specimens for rapid identification. Because of the relatively few fungal cells in host specimens, however, microscopical identification of *H. capsulatum* in the benign stage is difficult if not impossible. During the disseminated stage of the mycosis, sputum, urine, bone marrow, and blood can be examined for the presence of the fungus. Staining these specimens with Giemsa's or Wright's stain reveals the fungus as small, oval, yeast-like cells crowded within the macrophages. Clinical specimens should also be inoculated onto Sabouraud agar with and without antibiotics at room temperature and observed for 1 to 2 weeks for the appearance of mycelial growth and the characteristic tuberculate conidia that develop from the hyphae (Fig. 32-10). Since the organism is dimorphic the yeast phase can be demonstrated by cultivation on enriched media such as brain-heart infusion or yeast extract containing antibiotics (penicillin and streptomycin) at 37°C.

Definitive diagnosis of histoplasmosis is established by serological methods. Complement fixation tests have been used but are both difficult to evaluate and expensive. High antibody titers to histoplasmin, the skin test antigen, may also be present in cases of cryptococcosis and blas-

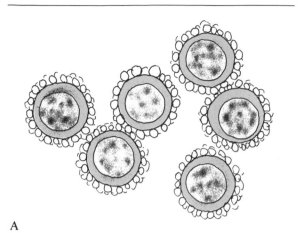

A

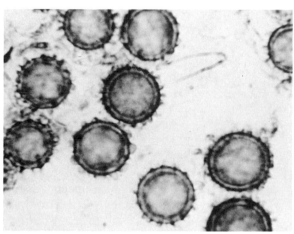

B

Fig. 32-10. *Histoplasma capsulatum.* A. Diagram of tuberculate macroconidia, which appear as round, thick-walled spores. Each spore has finger-like projections (tubercules) attached to it. B. Photomicrograph of cultured *H. capsulatum.* (Courtesy G. Roberts.)

tomycosis. Moreover, histoplasmin, which is injected intradermally to test for sensitivity to the fungus before serodiagnosis, increases the titer of complement fixation antibodies and makes the test unreliable. In disseminated histoplasmosis the immunological tests may be negative. The immunodiffusion test can be used on sera of patients who have or have not been skin-tested. In the test the patient's serum interacts with concentrated histoplasmin antigen, and a number of precipitin bands are formed, one of which is not influenced by previous skin testing.

Latex agglutination tests are useful for the detection of acute histoplasmosis. False-positives may occur and results should be confirmed by other serological tests such as immunodiffusion.

Treatment. Histoplasmosis is now considered a common benign infection rather than a rare fatal disease. Successful treatment of disseminated histoplasmosis is still dependent on early diagnosis. Amphotericin B and ketoconazole have been the standard therapeutic agents. Amphotericin B, administered intravenously (IV) slowly over a period of 6 to 8 hours, has been the best means of treatment. Such treatment must be repeated for several weeks. There has been considerable success using amphotericin B for several days, followed by ketoconazole treatment. Clinical trials with the drug itraconazole appear promising, particularly for those who are immunocompromised (e.g., AIDS patients).

Coccidioidomycosis

Coccidioidomycosis is caused by the agent *Coccidioides immitis.* Disease is initiated as an upper respiratory infection that usually resolves on its own, provided a cell-mediated immune response to the fungus is mounted by the patient. Dissemination of the agent, heralded by high antibody titers and absence of a cell-mediated immune response, often leads to a fatal outcome.

Epidemiology. Coccidioidomycosis is a highly endemic disease associated with hot, semiarid areas. In the United States the disease is endemic in areas of southern California, Arizona, New Mexico, and Texas. The fungus lives in the soil in a mycelium-arthroconidia (arthrospores) cycle. Autolysis of mycelia releases arthroconidia (Fig. 32-11), which are dispersed in the air as dust aerosols and inhaled by humans frequently during dust storms or during building construc-

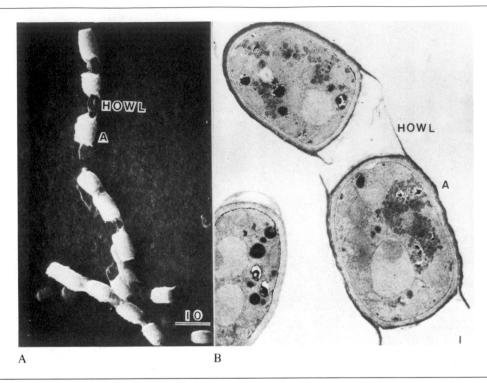

A   B

Fig. 32-11. *Coccidioides immitis.* A. Scanning electron micrograph of arthroconidia alternating with lysed vegetative component of the hypha. (HOWL = hyphal outer wall; A = arthroconidium; bar = 10 μm). B. Thin-section electron micrograph of a portion of A. (From M. Hupert et al., in D. Schlesinger [ed.], *Microbiology—1983.* Washington, DC: American Society for Microbiology, 1983.)

tion or excavation in dusty areas. Disseminated disease occurs more frequently among persons with pigmented skin: blacks, Filipinos, and American Indians. The fatality rate among American Indians is three to five times that of Caucasians, for reasons that are not immediately apparent.

Pathogenesis. After their deposition on pulmonary surfaces, the arthroconidia are first attacked by neutrophils and later by macrophages. Most infections are asymptomatic or produce mild pulmonary symptoms that resolve within a few weeks. These infected individuals are sensitive to coccidioidin, the fungal antigen, when the lat-

ter is injected intradermally, as evidenced by a delayed hypersensitivity reaction, heralding, as in primary histoplasmosis, the emergence of a cell-mediated immune response and a good prognosis. The principal symptoms of infection are fever, chest pain, cough, and other flu-like symptoms. Circumscribed nodules are observed by x-ray in symptomatic disease. Allergic responses are also observed in symptomatic disease. The pulmonary lesion may be a source of dissemination of the fungus with serious consequences. Disseminated disease is usually associated with an overwhelming exposure to fungal spores. The lungs, meninges, liver, kidneys, spleen, and deep lymph nodes are the major organs affected. Me-

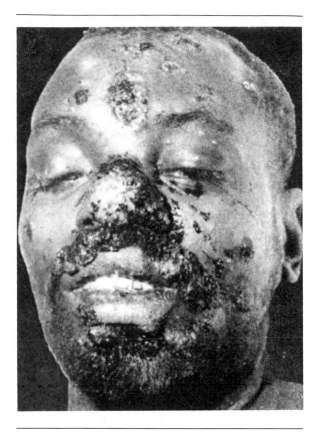

Fig. 32-12. Coccidioidomycosis. Disseminated disease with granulomatous crusted lesions of the face and nose. (Photograph by A. Gregerson, F.B.P.A. Reproduced with permission from G. M. Lewis, M. E. Hopper, J. W. Wilson, and O. A. Plunkett, *An Introduction to Medical Mycology* [4th ed.]. Copyright © 1958 by Year Book Medical Publishers, Inc., Chicago.)

ninges involvement usually results in a rapidly fatal course, particularly for dark-skinned individuals. Disseminated lesions may also appear on the skin, subcutaneous tissue, and bones (Fig. 32-12).

The virulence mechanisms for *C. immitis* are poorly understood. One possibility is that arthrospores, once they bind to the mucosal surface, transform into spherules that are more resistant to the inhibitory effects of PMNLs.

Laboratory Diagnosis. Depending on the immunological response of the host, the lesions found in the disseminated disease may be suppurative or granulomatous. Coccidioidomycosis resembles many other granulomatous diseases, and accurate diagnosis is based on laboratory identification of the fungus in pathological tissue in culture or by serological tests. *C. immitis* is a dimorphic fungus. The inhaled arthrospore is transformed into a large spherule in its tissue phase of development. Invagination of the inner layers of the spherule segments the protoplasm into smaller units or *endospores* (Plate 25). Clinical specimens of sputum, pus, or tissue can be examined for the presence of spherules. Clinical specimens should also be cultivated on Sabouraud and blood agar to demonstrate the mycelial phase of the organism. Arthrospores are easily disseminated; therefore laboratory techniques should be performed under a safety hood.

Skin test data using coccidioidin is not considered diagnostic, but if the test is negative it will help to exclude coccidioidomycosis.

Serological testing is an invaluable tool in diagnosis and prognosis. IgM antibodies are produced early in disease and can be detected by tube precipitin tests, latex agglutination, and immunodiffusion. IgG antibodies persist longer than do IgM antibodies and can be detected by complement fixation, counterimmunoelectrophoresis, and immunodiffusion. The titers detected in these tests reflect whether there is active infection or the disease is in the convalescent stage.

Treatment. To date, amphotericin B administered IV is the most effective antifungal agent in the treatment of systemic coccidioidomycosis. Itraconazole is effective in treating cutaneous lesions. Meningitis, which is an uncommon result of *C. immitis* infection, can be controlled. High doses of ketoconazole and intrathecal amphotericin B are the mainstays in management. Fluconazole may be the drug of the future because of its high cerebrospinal fluid penetration. Fluconazole is still in clinical trials.

Blastomycosis

Blastomycosis is caused by *Blastomyces dermatitidis*, a dimorphic fungus that initiates disease by infecting the lung. The disease is chronic and is characterized by granulomatous lesions that may give rise to a disseminated form.

Epidemiology. Blastomycosis appears to be endemic in southern Canada and in central midwest, southeast, and Atlantic coastal states of the United States. The organism has not, except for two or three instances, been isolated from the soil. The fungus is believed to remain dormant in the soil for most of the year and is then stimulated by climatic conditions to reproduce. The incidence of infection has been difficult to evaluate because antigen available for skin testing often gives false-positives. The incidence of disease is highest in blacks and in men, particularly those over 50 years of age, again for reasons unknown.

Most infections are believed to occur by inhalation of disseminated spores, but there are a few recorded cases of blastomycosis having been acquired by contact with fomites.

Pathogenesis. Blastomycosis generally takes two forms: pulmonary with dissemination, and chronic cutaneous disease. Pulmonary infection in many patients causes mild respiratory disease but is seldom acute. Pulmonary lesions may heal, but the organisms are usually disseminated and involve the skin (Plate 26). Chronic cutaneous disease is characterized by subcutaneous lesions that ulcerate. The lesions are found predominantly on the face, hands, and lower legs, or mucocutaneous areas such as the larynx. Untreated, the disease progresses and involves many unexposed areas of the body. The lesions are raised, crusty, and discolored. When the lesions heal they leave deforming scars that cover the face, neck, or other areas. Systemic blastomycosis occurs from unresolved infection but is rare. Disseminated disease involves most organs and may also be manifested as cutaneous or osseous (bone) lesions.

Laboratory Diagnosis. B. dermatitidis in the yeast phase exists as a spherical cell 8 to 15 μm in diameter. When observed in stained sections or preparations the cytoplasmic membrane of the fungus is seen to shrink and the cell appears double-walled. In addition, the buds of the dividing yeast remain attached to the parent cell, giving the appearance of a figure eight (Fig. 32-13).

Skin scrapings, sputum, and pus should be examined for typical thick-walled yeast forms. The features of the yeast are pathognomonic for blastomycosis. Specimens should also be cultured on Sabouraud and enriched media such as brain-heart infusion to detect the mycelial as well as

Fig. 32-13. Stained wet preparation of *Blastomyces dermatitidis*. The membrane shrinks during the staining, giving the appearance of a double wall. The smaller bud remains attached to the mother cell, which gives the appearance of a figure eight. (From H. W. Larsh and N. L. Goodman. Fungi of Systemic Mycoses, In E. H. Lennette, A. Balows, W. J. Hausler, Jr., and J. P. Truant [eds.], *Manual of Clinical Microbiology* [3rd ed.]. Washington, DC: American Society for Microbiology, 1980.)

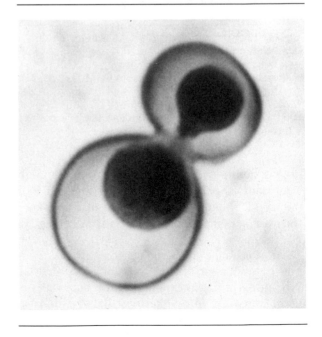

the yeast phase of the organism. The most useful serological test is an immunodiffusion test, which utilizes a specific *B. dermatitidis* antigen called the A antigen. The development of specific precipitin lines is indicative of disease. A decline or disappearance of these precipitin lines is evidence of a favorable prognosis. More recently, enzyme immunoassay (EIA) has been shown to have greater specificity than immunodiffusion.

Treatment. Many cases of acute pulmonary blastomycosis are self-limiting. Chronic symptoms or invasive disease requires therapy. Amphotericin B is effective in severely ill and immunocompromised patients. Ketoconazole is effective for chronic invasive disease. Cutaneous blastomycosis is never fatal, but untreated lesions may last for years. Systemic blastomycosis, if left untreated, is almost invariably fatal. Administration of hydroxystilbamidine isethionate over a 30-day period has proved successful. Although amphotericin B is apparently more effective, the nephrotoxic effect of the drug must be considered if it is used for prolonged periods.

Paracoccidioidomycosis

Paracoccidioidomycosis, also called *South American blastomycosis*, is a chronic, sometimes fatal disease characterized by lesions of the mucous membranes of the mouth. It is seldom seen in the United States. The causal agent of the disease is *Paracoccidioides brasiliensis*.

Epidemiology. *P. brasiliensis* is believed to be an inhabitant of the soil but has been only occasionally isolated from the soil. Most cases of disease have been reported from Brazil, Venezuela, Argentina, and other South American countries. The highest incidence of disease occurs among agricultural workers.

Pathogenesis. Paracoccidioidomycosis is an endemic disease whose mode of infection is not known. Many investigators believe that the res-

piratory tract and lungs are the first sites of infection; however, oral lesions and enlargement of regional lymph nodes are the first symptoms to be recognized. The oral lesions are granular but seldom ulcerative. The infection may become progressive, with development of lesions elsewhere on the body, including the skin, lymph nodes, and lungs. In the infected tissue a granuloma, similar to the granulomas encountered in tuberculosis, is the predominant pathological characteristic. In clinical specimens fungi may be found outside or inside phagocytic cells as oval, multiple budding cells averaging between 25 and 30 µm in diameter. Prognosis for the disseminated form of the disease is very poor, the fatality rate reaching 50 percent.

Laboratory Diagnosis. Clinical diagnosis can be made from the appearance of oral lesions, but confirmation depends on the finding of fungal parasites in clinical specimens. Procedures for laboratory diagnosis are the same as those employed in North American blastomycosis. The yeast phase cells show multiple buds, much resembling a ship's wheel, which distinguishes them from *B. dermatitidis*. The mycelial phase and characteristic conidia cannot be distinguished from those of *B. dermatitidis*. Serological tests are not totally reliable; however, the immunodiffusion, counterelectrophoresis, and complement fixation tests are reasonably specific.

Treatment. The sulfonamides, such as sulfadiazine and sulfisoxazole, have proved effective in treatment. Treatment must be continued for approximately 2 years to prevent relapses. If the fungal species encountered in the infection is resistant to sulfonamides, amphotericin B may be substituted. The advent of ketoconazole greatly facilitated and improved the treatment and prognosis of paracoccidioidomycosis. This drug is effective not only in suppressing symptoms but also in reducing the frequency of relapses.

Cryptococcosis

Cryptococcosis is a subacute chronic infection that involves mainly the lungs, brain, and meninges. The causative agent, *Cryptococcus neoformans*, has as its primary reservoir the soil where pigeon droppings containing organic nitrogen (urea) favor the growth of yeasts. It is capable of rapid growth and development in the feces. The fungus is not dimorphic, and only the yeast phase exists in the saprophytic and parasitic states.

Four serotypes of *C. neoformans* are present and two varieties are now recognized: *C. neoformans var. neoformans* (serotypes A and D) and *C. neoformans var. gatti* (serotypes B and C). *C. neoformans var. gatti* is found primarily in tropical and subtropical areas (Southern California, Australia, Brazil, Thailand, etc.), where it causes disease in healthy individuals. *C. neoformans var. neoformans* is found on the East Coast of the United States and in Europe, where it causes disease primarily in immunosuppressed patients.

Pathogenesis. Cryptococcus infection occurs more frequently in patients seriously debilitated by such conditions as Hodgkin's disease, tuberculosis, and various lymphomas than in healthy persons. The disease is believed to begin as a pulmonary infection that seldom goes beyond the subclinical stage. In many patients the pulmonary lesion heals without calcification and goes unrecognized. Systemic manifestations, in which the central nervous system or any organ of the body may become involved, occasionally follow pulmonary infection. Central nervous system involvement is characterized by the development of granulomatous lesions of the meninges; left untreated, they are usually fatal. Cutaneous lesions manifested as papules or abscesses may also be the result of systemic infection and can appear anywhere on the body (Fig. 32-14).

The pathogenesis of *C. neoformans* is related to a cell wall antigen and the capsule that surrounds the organism. It is well documented that the severity of cryptococcal disease is directly

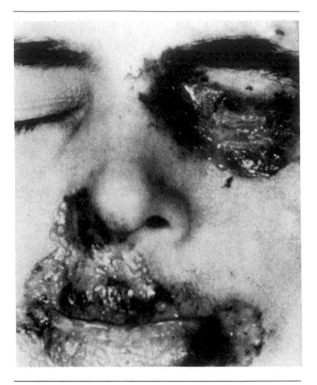

Fig. 32-14. Cryptococcosis. Extensive cutaneous involvement. The gelatinous material represents fungus in nearly pure culture. (Courtesy A. C. Curtis, Ann Arbor, MI. Reproduced with permission from G. M. Lewis, M. E. Hopper, J. W. Wilson, and O. A. Plunkett, *An Introduction to Medical Mycology* [4th ed.]. Copyright © 1958 by Year Book Medical Publishers, Inc., Chicago.)

related to the concentration of cryptococcal antigen in body fluids. The host's most important device in resisting infection is cell-mediated immunity but this mechanism is affected by cryptococcal antigen. Experimental studies have demonstrated that cryptococcal antigen suppresses the delayed-type hypersensitivity response and protective immunity to cryptococci. The most important property of the capsule is inhibition of phagocytosis.

Laboratory Diagnosis. India ink or nigrosin preparations of sputum, pus, urine, or infected tissue reveal *C. neoformans* as an oval, thick-walled yeast cell surrounded by a wide clear capsule

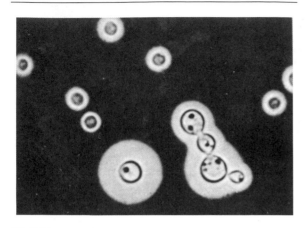

Fig. 32-15. *Cryptococcus neoformans.* A nigrosin-stained wet preparation of spinal fluid showing oval fungal cells surrounded by a clear capsule. (From M. Silva-Hunter and B. H. Cooper. Medically Important Yeasts. In E. Lennette, A. Balows, W. J. Hausler, Jr., and J. P. Truant [eds.], *Manual of Clinical Microbiology* [3rd ed.]. Washington, DC: American Society for Microbiology, 1980.)

(Fig. 32-15). After several days of incubation on Sabouraud agar, a slimy, mucoid, creamy colony containing budding cells with large capsules but no hyphae develops. *C. neoformans* can be differentiated from other *Cryptococcus* species by the former's (1) ability to grow at 37°C, (2) production of brown colonies on birdseed agar, (3) ability to assimilate specific sugars, (4) pathogenicity for animals, and (5) urease activity.

Treatment. Cryptococcal meningitis is treated with amphotericin B plus flucytosine, but there is a failure rate of over 40 percent if one employs only flucytosine. Both drugs are toxic, especially flucytosine, in patients with renal disease. Ketoconazole administered with subtherapeutic doses of amphotericin B has been demonstrated to increase the killing of *Cryptococcus*. Relapses have been known to occur, particularly among AIDS patients, in whom *C. neoformans* is a major fungal pathogen. In 1990, fluconazole was approved by the FDA for use in treatment of cryptococcal miningitis.

SUBCUTANEOUS MYCOSES

Subcutaneous mycotic infections are those that remain localized in subcutaneous tissue. Most infections are the result of puncture wounds by objects contaminated by fungal species found in decaying vegetation and in the soil. Several agents are associated with subcutaneous mycoses. We will elaborate on only one, *Sporothrix schenckii*, the most frequently associated with infection. Subcutaneous diseases caused by other fungal agents are outlined in Table 32-3.

Sporotrichosis and Other Subcutaneous Mycoses

Sporotrichosis is a subcutaneous infection that is seen most often in greenhouse workers, farmers,

Fig. 32-16. Chromomycosis involving arm. (From P. Lavalle et al., *Rev. Infect. Dis.* 9 [Suppl. I]:64, 1987.)

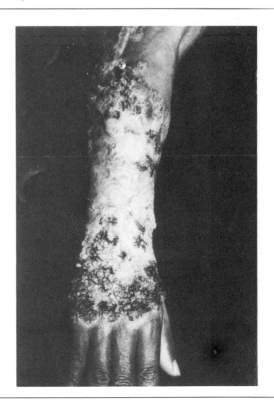

Table 32-3. Characteristics of the Subcutaneous Mycoses and Their Causal Agents

Disease	Agent	Clinical manifestations	Epidemiology	Treatment
Sporotrichosis	*Sporothrix schenckii*	Nodules along lymphatic channels that may ulcerate or superficial lesions not involving lymphatics; extracutaneous infections rare	Infection highest among agricultural workers	Potassium iodide for ulceroglandular and lymphatic forms of disease (itraconazole is also effective). Surgery plus amphotericin B may be required for joint and pulmonary disease.
Chromomycosis (Fig. 32-16)	*Phialophora verrucosa, Cladosporium carrioni, Fonsecaea* species, *Wangiella dermatitidis*	Infections usually on lower extremities with discolored lesions that become raised and cauliflower-like if untreated; systemic invasion rare	Predominant in tropical and subtropical regions among barefoot agriculturalists	Surgery in early disease, flucytosine for advanced cases
Mycetoma	*Petriellidium boydii, Madurella mycetomatis, Madurella grisea, Acremonium kiliense,* and others	Granulomatous lesions with multiple sinus tracts; feet, hands, and other exposed areas usually infected; scar tissue leads to disfigurement of affected area	Found worldwide but most frequently in Africa, Asia, and tropical and subtropical areas	Surgery to remove tissue that prevents drug penetration; nystatin, amphotericin B, and flucytosine
Rhinosporidiosis	*Rhinosporidium seeberi*	Lesions of mucous membranes of nose or soft palate; lesions become enlarged masses that can interfere with breathing	Found primarily in India and Sri Lanka and mostly in males	Surgery
Lobomycosis (Fig. 32-17)	*Loboa loboi*	Lesions localized primarily on feet, legs, or face; lesions spread as enlarged masses	Found primarily in Amazon basin	Surgery and sulfa drugs
Subcutaneous phycomycosis	*Basidiobolus haptosporus*	Nodule formation in subcutaneous tissue; infection usually in abdomen or a limb	Found primarily in Africa among children 5–9 years of age	Potassium iodide

ized and seldom becomes disseminated. Ulcerated lesions may heal, but new ones appear nearby. Infection in areas where sporotrichosis is endemic often results in a single lesion at the original site of inoculation (fixed sporotrichosis). These lesions may appear to heal spontaneously but usually reappear at the same location. Pulmonary disease is being increasingly recognized in hospitalized patients who inhale these spores. Like the systemic mycoses, pulmonary infections by *S. schenckii* mimic tuberculosis. Disseminated sporotrichosis is seldom observed but when it occurs usually involves the skeletal system and seldom organ systems (Fig. 32-18).

Laboratory Diagnosis. Aspirated pus from lesions should be cultured on Sabouraud agar or brain-

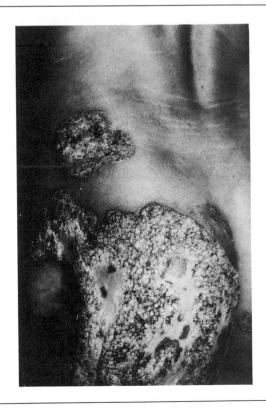

Fig. 32-18. Disseminated sporotrichosis on buttock. (From P. Lavalle et al., *Rev. Infect. Dis* 9 [Suppl. I]:64, 1987.)

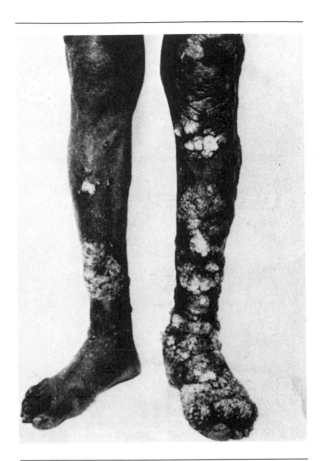

Fig. 32-17. Lobomycosis. Keloidal lesions of 30 years' duration. (From C. W. Emmons et al., *Medical Mycology* 3rd ed.]. Philadelphia: Lea & Febiger, 1977.)

and others who are constantly exposed to the soil (see boxed essay). The causative agent, *Sporothrix schenckii*, is found in the soil and vegetation and has a worldwide distribution. Sporotrichosis is endemic in parts of Brazil, South Africa, and Zimbabwe.

Pathogenesis. Cutaneous infection resulting from traumatization of tissue and contact with spores begins as a small, purplish, ulcerated lesion. The lesion becomes necrotic and soon spreads subcutaneously to local lymph nodes, causing them to become swollen and sometimes necrotic (Plate 27). The subcutaneous infection remains local-

Multistate Outbreak of Sporotrichosis in Seedling Handlers, 1988

Between April 23 and June 30, 1988, 84 cases of cutaneous sporotrichosis occurred in persons who handled conifer seedlings packed in Pennsylvania with sphagnum moss that had been harvested in Wisconsin. Confirmed cases occurred in 14 states, with the majority occurring in New York (29), Illinois (23), and Pennsylvania (12). Each of the victims handled seedlings from April 4 to May 16; symptoms developed between April 23 and June 30.

Thirty-one cases (37 percent) occurred in state forestry workers and garden club members who participated in annual tree distributions in which seedlings were separated from one another, repacked in moss, and distributed to area residents. In addition, 12 patients had received seedlings through these distributions, 38 had purchased seedlings directly from nurseries, and three were nursery workers. All the patients had contact with seedlings distributed by two Pennsylvania nurseries. *Sporothrix schenckii* was cultured from skin lesions of 38 persons and from five samples of unopened bales of moss obtained from one nursery.

Sphagnum moss harvested in Wisconsin is shipped to nurseries in more than 15 states, and the involved Pennsylvania nurseries ship seedlings and moss to 47 states. Previous outbreaks associated with Wisconsin sphagnum moss have occurred. The largest previously reported United States outbreak involved 17 forestry workers in 1976.

From *M.M.W.R.* 37:652,1988

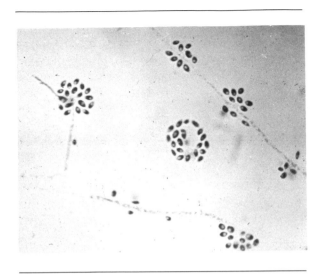

Fig. 32-19. Floweret arrangement of conidia on conidiophores of *Sporothrix schenckii*. (Courtesy G. Roberts.)

heart infusion agar at 37°C to demonstrate the yeast phase and on Sabouraud agar at room temperature to demonstrate the mycelial phase. The yeast phase cells are oval and sometimes cigar shaped. The mycelial phase is characterized by brown to black colonies in which conidia appear as flower-like clusters on conidiophores (Fig. 32-19).

The slide latex agglutination test is the preferred technique for serological diagnosis. An increasing or sustained titer is helpful in diagnosing pulmonary disease. The test is useful for monitoring disease but is of little prognostic value.

Treatment. Saturated solutions of potassium iodide in milk administered orally are the best treatment of the ulceroglandular type of sporotrichosis. Such treatments are often not well tolerated because they cause considerable skin irritation. Topical heat treatments have been used for treating skin lesions. This approach works presumably because the fungus prefers growth at relatively low temperatures. Ampho-

tericin B and itraconazole are used in the treatment of localized pulmonary and disseminated sporotrichosis.

DERMATOPHYTOSES (CUTANEOUS MYCOSES)

General Characteristics

The fungi that invade the keratinized and cutaneous areas of the body (nails, hair, and skin) are called the *dermatophytes*. The dermatophytes are represented by three major genera of pathogenic molds: *Microsporum, Trichophyton,* and *Epidermophyton*. In the United States, *Trichophyton rubrum* is the most frequently encountered causal agent of cutaneous mycoses. The diseases produced by these three genera are referred to as *tineas* (*ringworm*) of various parts of the body. Tinea capitis is ringworm of the scalp, tinea barbae, ringworm of the beard area; tinea pedis, ringworm of the feet; tinea cruris, ringworm of the groin; tinea corporis, ringworm of the body; tinea favosa, ringworm of the scalp; tinea unguium, ringworm of the nails; and tinea imbricata, ringworm of the torso.

Dermatophytes produce enzymes that enable them to degrade keratinized tissue. These enzymes include keratinase, elastase, and collagenase, which break down keratin, elastin, and collagen, respectively, all of which are components of epithelial and connective tissue. The reason for the inability of dermatophytes to invade deep tissue is not known but may be related to temperature, tissue conditions, oxidation-reduction potential, and other factors.

Dermatophytes abound worldwide as saprophytes in the soil, but many of them have evolved to a parasitic existence. Some dermatophytes are strict parasites of humans and are no longer found in the soil. Others no longer found in the soil are parasites of lower animals that can also infect humans. Finally some are found free in nature and accidentally cause infections in humans. The cutaneous mycoses are the only contagious fungous diseases in humans.

Laboratory Diagnosis

Dermatophytic infections of the hair, nails, and skin are sometimes diagnosed from the clinical symptoms—loss of hair, thickened and discolored nails, or generalized scaling. In ringworm of the scalp the patient can be examined directly for skin lesions or areas where there is loss of hair. In some scalp infections, particularly those caused by *Microsporum*, the infected hair fluoresces a bright yellow-green when exposed to Wood's lamp (ultraviolet). Hair, skin scrapings, or nail clippings can be examined directly if the infected material is placed on slides and 10% potassium hydroxide (KOH) is added. The preparation is gently heated to free the hyphae from keratinous material. The infected material is examined for the presence of septate hyphae or arthrospores. Identification of the specific dermatophyte can be accomplished by culturing the infected material on Sabouraud agar and examining the macroscopical colonial characteristics as well as the microscopical morphology of individual species. The Sabouraud agar should contain cycloheximide (Actidione), which suppresses growth of most saprophytic fungi but not dermatophytes, and an antibacterial agent such as chlortetracycline hydrochloride (Aureomycin) or chloramphenicol to give the slower-growing dermatophytes a chance to outgrow bacteria.

Fig. 32-20. Tinea capitis. (Courtesy G. Roberts.)

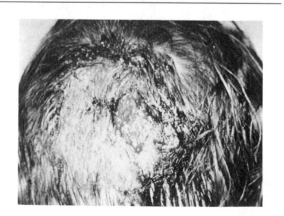

Treatment

Griseofulvin given orally has proved useful for eliminating scalp infections. For body infections, several antifungal ointments containing the following agents can be applied: 3% salicylic acid, 5% undecylenic acid, 5% benzoic acid, or 5% sodium thiosulfate. For foot infections, potassium permanganate (1:4000), 20% zinc undecylenate, 3% salicylic acid, or 5% benzoic acid is helpful in treatment. Drugs such as tolnaftate, miconazole nitrate, and clotrimazole are also available.

Tinea Capitis (Ringworm of the Scalp)

Most species of *Microsporum* and *Trichophyton* may be involved in ringworm of the scalp (Fig. 32-20). *M. canis,* transmitted by infected dogs and cats, is a major causal agent of this disease. The infection is usually acquired during childhood and begins with inflammation and itching of the scalp. The fungi spread on the keratinized areas of the scalp and may even involve the hair shaft, so that hair is broken off at the scalp level. If the hyphae are found growing only within the hair shaft, the infection is called *endothrix* infection. If the hyphae are found both within and on the external surface of the hair, the infection is called *ectothrix* infection.

Tinea Corporis (Ringworm of the Body)

Tinea corporis is a dermatophytosis involving the nonhairy areas of the body (Fig. 32-21). Fungal infections of the face are often misdiagnosed as connective tissue diseases such as lupus erythematosus or disorders caused by overexposure to sunlight. The lesions appear as reddened, scaly, papular eruptions. Pustules are often seen on the periphery of the lesion. Species of *Trichophyton* and *Microsporum* are commonly involved in tinea corporis infections.

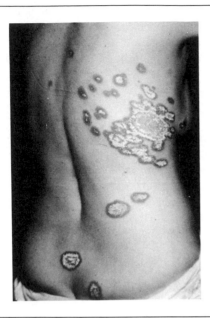

Fig. 32-21. Tinea corporis. (Courtesy G. Roberts.)

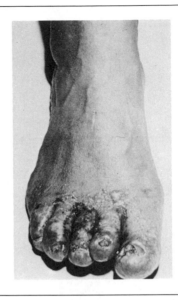

Fig. 32-22. Tinea pedis. (Courtesy G. Roberts.)

Tinea Pedis (Ringworm of the Feet)

Tinea pedis, usually called *athlete's foot*, is believed by many investigators to be spread primarily through the use of public showers, swimming pools, or other such facilities and is favored by failure to dry one's feet between the toes after bathing. The disease is characterized by itching and burning between the toes. Lesions releasing a watery fluid may later appear. Chronic infections show peeling and cracking of the skin, often resembling eczema (Fig. 32-22). The causative agents of athlete's foot may be any number of species of *Microsporum, Trichophyton,* or *Epidermophyton.*

Tinea Barbae (Ringworm of the Beard Area)

Tinea barbae is a dermatophytic infection of the bearded areas of the face. Infection may remain superficial or may become severe and involve deeper tissue. Superficial infection appears as a scaly lesion; the deeper infection is characterized

by deep pustules and nodular lesions (Fig. 32-23). Permanent loss of hair is common with the more severe infection. *T. rubrum* is the principal agent involved in superficial infections, while *T. verrucosum* is associated with the more severe form of the disease.

Tinea Favosa (Ringworm of the Scalp)

Tinea favosa is characterized by the formation of yellow, cup-shaped crusts of matted debris and mycelia on the scalp or torso. The crusts are called *scutula* (Fig. 32-24). The hair follicle is involved, and in more severe cases there is loss of hair. Most cases of disease are caused by *T. schoenleini.*

Tinea Unguium (Ringworm of the Nails)

Invasion of the nail plate is characteristic of tinea unguium. Infection may be of two types: (1) superficial involvement, in which the fungus invades only the pits of the nail and (2) involvement of the nail surface followed by invasion of the fungus beneath the nail plate (Fig. 32-25). Invasion of hyphae below the nail results in discoloration, keratinization, and distortion of the nail.

Tinea Imbricata (Ringworm of the Torso)

Tinea imbricata is restricted to certain areas of the world such as the Pacific Islands, Southeast Asia, and Central and South America. The infection is characterized by the formation of scaly, elevated concentric rings that may be scattered over most of the body (Fig. 32-26). The causal agent of disease is *T. concentricum*. The organ-

Fig. 32-25. Tinea unguium. A. Initial infection at distal edge of nail plate. B. Advanced disease showing grooved nails and dark brown coloration. (From W. Rippon, *Medical Mycology* [2nd ed.]. Philadelphia: Saunders, 1982.)

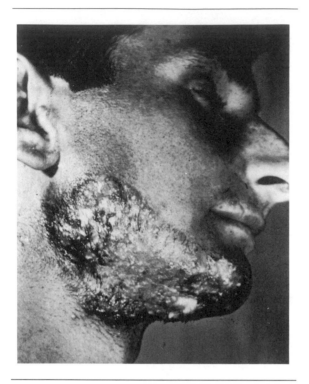

Fig. 32-23. Tinea barbae. Deep pustular folliculitis in patient with *Trichophyton verrucosum* infection. (From W. Rippon, *Medical Mycology* [2nd ed.]. Philadelphia: Saunders, 1982.)

Fig. 32-24. Tinea favosa. Seborrheic stage of disease showing matted hair and lesion with erythematous base. The infected hair is gray, whereas the normal hair is pigmented. (From W. Rippon, *Medical Mycology* [2nd ed.]. Philadelphia: Saunders, 1982.)

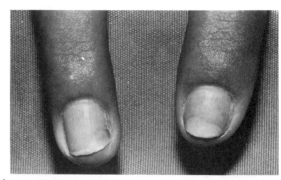

A

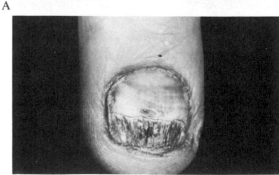

B

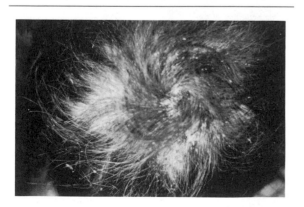

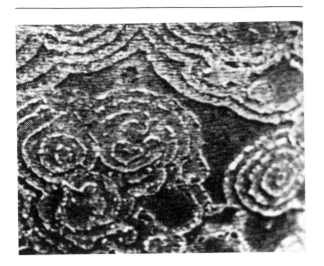

Fig. 32-26. Tinea imbricata produced by *Trichophyton concentricum* and manifested by concentric rings of scales. (From W. Rippon, *Medical Mycology* [2nd ed.]. Philadelphia: Saunders, 1982.)

ism is believed to be transmitted by direct contact from mother to infant.

Tinea Cruris (Ringworm of the Groin, Jock Itch)

Tinea cruris is a common dermatophytic infection that may appear in epidemic form, for example, in locker rooms. Careless exchange of clothing or towels may result in transmission of the fungus. The lesions may appear on the groin or perianal areas and are characterized as red, scaly, itchy, and often dry.

Dermatophytes and Allergy

Many fungi act as allergens, causing allergic skin reactions. Allergic manifestations that appear in response to dermatophytosis and candidiasis are often referred to as *ids*. They appear as vesicular lesions at sites distant from the primary site of fungal infection and give rise to severe itching, especially after antifungal treatment.

SUPERFICIAL MYCOSES

Infections of the most superficial layers of skin and hair are termed *superficial mycoses*. These infections are generally innocuous and frequently reappear with or without treatment.

Tinea Versicolor

The causal agent of tinea versicolor is *Malassezia furfur*. The lesions, generally on the chest, back, and shoulders, are tan and scaly (Fig. 32-27). There is little or no inflammation associated with them. Irradiation of the infected areas with Wood's light in the dark demonstrates orange-red

Fig. 32-27. Tinea versicolor. The pigmented areas represent the infected sites of the skin. (From W. Rippon, *Medical Mycology* [2nd ed.]. Philadelphia: Saunders, 1982.)

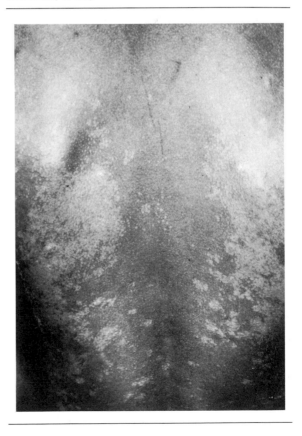

fluorescing hyphae. Scales can also be removed from the infected areas and examined microscopically for the hyphal elements. A saturated solution of sodium thiosulfate applied two to three times daily is effective in treatment of superficial mycotic infections. Tolnaftate 1% in various creams and in polyethylene glycol also provides good results. Other drugs that have proved effective are selenium sulfide (1%) and salicylic acid (10–15%). Miconazole nitrate and other imidazoles are also effective (see Table 32-1).

Tinea Nigra Palmaris

Tinea nigra palmaris is an asymptomatic infection that appears on the palms of the hands and fingers as dark brown or black macular areas. The condition is chronic and may last several years if left untreated. It is seldom seen in the United States. The causal agent is *Exophiala* (*Cladosporium*) *wernecki*. Scales removed from the skin should be examined microscopically on a wet mount containing 10% KOH. The wet mount is gently heated to break up keratinous cells, and this procedure allows one to see detached hyphae. The fungus appears in the form of highly branched hyphae. Treatment is the same as for tinea versicolor.

Black and White Piedra

Piedra is a fungus infection of the hair in the form of small nodules. *Black piedra* (caused by *Piedraia hortae*) affects the hair of the scalp, and the nodules produced are very dark. *White piedra* (caused by *Trichosporon beigelii*) affects the hairs of the beard, and the nodules produced are very light. These diseases are rarely seen in the United States. Over the past 10 years, however, sporadic disseminated infections have appeared in immunocompromised patients, especially those with leukemia. Infected hairs with attached nodules can be prepared in wet mounts containing 10% KOH. The nodules contain mycelia and can be examined microscopically. Treatment of black and white piedra is the same as for tinea

versicolor, except that amphotericin B is used for disseminated disease.

DISEASES CAUSED BY OPPORTUNISTIC FUNGAL PATHOGENS

In seriously debilitated and traumatized people, or those under treatment with broad-spectrum antibiotics and immunosuppressive drugs, nonpathogenic fungi may cause grave illness. These opportunistic fungi are found in the environment and belong to the following groups: *Candida, Aspergillus, Mucor, Rhizopus,* and *Pneumocystis.* (*Cryptococcus neoformans* is also an important opportunistic pathogen and was discussed previously.) These groups are the major opportunists, but remember that any of the fungi can also cause disease in the compromised host.

Candidiasis

General Characteristics. *Candida* species are yeasts capable of producing pseudohyphae (see Plate 24). They can be found as commensals in animals and humans, where they inhabit the respiratory tract, intestinal tract, skin, and female genital tract. Most infections are of the endogenous type (disease caused by one's own microbial flora), but transmission from mother to fetus and venereal transmission are also possible. The most important *Candida* species causing infection in humans is *C. albicans*, but other species such as *C. tropicalis, C. parapsilosis,* and *C. krusei* are occasionally involved.

Pathogenesis. The frequency of *Candida* infections has risen dramatically since the advent of antibiotics and the increase in the number of surgical procedures, including transplants, in which antibiotics and immunosuppressive drugs are used. Infections are either cutaneous or disseminated and reflect the type of compromising condition that affects the host. Cutaneous diseases are usually naturally occurring and arise because of some condition such as diabetes or other endocrine imbalances, natural immunological deficiencies, or exposure of the skin to moist environments over long periods of time (e.g., in dishwashers and laundry workers). Disseminated infections are most often iatrogenic (produced by physicians; resulting from diagnostic procedures or treatment). The administration of some antibiotics and immunosuppressive drugs encourages the growth of fungal species such as *C. albicans* at the expense of bacterial species. The proliferation of *Candida* in the intestinal tract, for example, can lead to the hematogenous spread of the microorganism. The use of catheters, the implantation of prosthetic devices, and various types of surgery also provide an avenue for dissemination of *Candida*.

The initial events in cutaneous infection involve the adherence of blastoconidia to epithelial surfaces, fungal proliferation, and invasion of epithelial tissue. Prior to invasion of the epidermis there is transformation by the organism from the conidial to the hyphal state. An inflammatory response on the part of the host helps to confine the infection to the superficial epidermis. During serious disseminated candida infections a polysaccharide, mannan, produced by the organism is introduced into the circulation. Mannan apparently has an immunosuppressive effect and interferes with the presentation of candidal antigens to monocytes.

Candida infections may be divided into three types: cutaneous, systemic or deep organ, and mucocutaneous.

CUTANEOUS CANDIDIASIS. Oral *thrush* is one of the most common cutaneous candidal infections. In thrush the surface of the tongue is covered by white patches or pseudomembranes, which, if removed, reveal a raw, bleeding undersurface (Fig. 32-28). The pseudomembranes are composed of fungal cells, both yeast and hyphal forms, and epithelial debris. Thrush is most often observed in infants but can occur in any age group. Many infants appear to acquire the disease from moth-

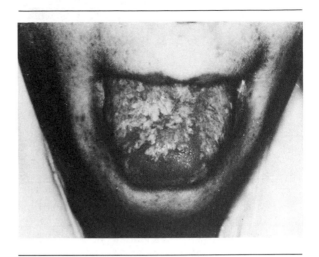

Fig. 32-28. Thrush. (From E. Drouhet, *Rev. Infect. Dis.* 2[4]:609, 1980.)

ers who have vaginal candidiasis. Endogenous thrush is a result of the administration of antibiotics, particularly broad-spectrum drugs, or various immunosuppressive agents that reduce the bacterial flora and permit *Candida* to divide unrestrictedly.

Vaginal candidiasis is frequently associated with diabetes, pregnancy, oral contraceptives, and antibacterial drugs. Lactobacilli in the vaginal tract are known to inhibit the growth of *Candida*. Women undergoing antibiotic therapy with drugs such as penicillin show reduced numbers of lactobacilli in the vagina. The reduction of these bacterial competitors permits the proliferation of *Candida*. The infection is characterized by inflammation of the vagina and the formation of a thick yellow-white discharge. Infection may spread to perianal areas and appear as a diaper rash in infants. Vaginal candidiasis may lead to candidiasis in a sexual partner after sexual intercourse. The condition in the male, called *candidal balanitis*, is characterized by superifical erosions and thin pustules on areas of the penis.

Individuals who have their appendages immersed in water for long periods of time or whose unexposed body sites are subject to a moist en-

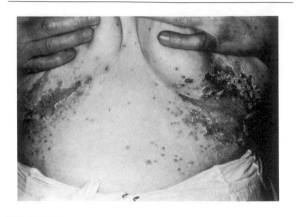

Fig. 32-29. Intertriginous candidiasis in a diabetic patient. Note "scalded skin" areas and satellite eruptions. (From W. Rippon, *Medical Mycology* [2nd ed.]. Philadelphia: Saunders, 1982.)

vironment are also subject to infection by *Candida* (*intertriginous candidiasis*). The feet, hands, groin, axillae, and intergluteal folds are the most commonly affected areas (Fig. 32-29). The lesions resemble eczema and may be scaly, creeping, and erythematous. Intertrigo may also be observed in diabetics, obese individuals, chronic alcoholics, or others with metabolic disorders.

Some of the most common cutaneous infections are those involving the nails (*onychia*) or around the nails (*paronychia*). These infections also result from immersion of appendages in water.

SYSTEMIC CANDIDIASIS. Systemic candidiasis results from hematogenous spread of the microorganisms and may involve any organ or tissue of the body. The most critical sites of infection are the heart (pericarditis, myocarditis, endocarditis), spinal cord (meningitis), and urethra (urethritis, cystitis). More recently recognized conditions resulting from dissemination are arthritis and osteomyelitis. Heart infections may be the result of the use of contaminated needles by heroin addicts (see Boxed Essay, p. 781), surgery involving the implantation of prosthetic valves, and prolonged catheterization with polyethylene

catheters. Neonates receiving hyperalimentation and broad-spectrum antibiotics are at an increased risk of candidemia, which often leads to meningitis, arthritis, or osteomyelitis.

CHRONIC MUCOCUTANEOUS CANDIDIASIS. Chronic mucocutaneous candidiasis (CMC) is associated with immunological deficiency. T cell immunodeficiency syndromes with failure in the cell-mediated immune response appear to be the initiating factor in disease. CMC is also frequently observed in patients with other underlying conditions that in some way affect the cell-mediated immune response. Patients are likely to lack delayed hypersensitivity to *Candida* and other skin test antigens. In addition, the lymphocytes of affected patients cannot be transformed in vitro by *Candida* antigen.

CMC infections involve the skin (Plate 28), mucous membranes, or any other epithelial surface including the respiratory tract, gastrointestinal tract, and genital epithelium. Most cases begin in infancy, but the disease may also involve those up to 30 years of age. The onset of disease seldom occurs after the age of 30. The disease is often refractory to treatment. Fatalities are rare, but when they occur they are usually due to bacterial sepsis.

Laboratory Diagnosis. Presumptive identification of *Candida* species can be made by direct microscopical examination of clinical material for the presence of yeast cells or pseudohyphae (see Plate 24). A valuable presumptive test is the germ tube test, in which a suspension of yeast cells from a colony is mixed with serum and incubated at 37°C for 2 to 4 hours. The mixture is then examined microscopically for the presence of *germ tubes.* Chlamydospore production in nutritionally deficient media such as rice extract agar and trypan blue agar is also used for identification of the fungus. If chlamydospores are not formed, it may be necessary to determine the sugar fermentation and sugar assimilation pattern to distinguish between *C. albicans* and other *Candida* species. *Candida* is the only fungus to produce both yeast cells and pseudohyphae in tissue.

HEROIN, LEMON JUICE, AND CANDIDA INFECTIONS

Heroin addicts are at risk for a variety of infectious diseases. Use of contaminated needles or injection of skin microflora are the most frequent methods of transmission. Candidiasis is not the usual microbial complication of drug abuse, but a very unusual circumstance in 1980 contributed to its appearance in this specialized group. Heroin is usually sold as a dry white powder that is relatively soluble in water. In 1980 a brand of heroin was available that was brown in color and poorly soluble in water. This type of heroin required acidification to make it soluble and the preferred method was to use lemon juice. A few drops of lemon juice was added to the heroin and the mixture was heated in a spoon over the flame of a lighter. The heat was removed as soon as the first bubbles appeared and the fluid was drawn into a syringe.

The marked increase of candidiasis in heroin abusers appeared only when the brown heroin appeared on the drug market. The lemon juice was apparently contaminated by the heroin abuser and served as a source of *Candida*. Lemon juice with its low pH is an excellent selective medium that supports the growth of *Candida* but inhibits bacteria such as *Staphylococcus aureus* and *Pseudomonas aeruginosa*.

Disseminated candidiasis in the heroin abuser can be manifested in several ways: cutaneous lesions, particularly on hairy parts of the body such as the scalp, ocular involvement such as chorioretinitis, and bone involvement such as osteoarthritis.

Blastospores and pseudohyphae can be demonstrated in biopsy tissue by staining techniques. For systemic *Candida* infections, the latex agglutination test has proved to be an invaluable diagnostic as well as prognostic tool. Latex agglutination tests detect *Candida* antigens in the serum.

Treatment. Most cutaneous infections are treated with creams or powders containing nystatin, gentian violet, or a variety of imidazoles (see Table 32-1); for example, miconazole or clotrimazole is recommended in the treatment of vaginal candidiasis. Amphotericin B has been used in severe systemic mycoses, but its therapeutic dose level is close to the toxic dose level and it must therefore be administered with caution. Amphotericin B is toxic to the kidneys and should not be given to persons suffering from systemic candidiasis after kidney transplantation. The drug flucytosine has been employed as a replacement for amphotericin B; however, some cases of fatal aplastic anemia have been reported when flucytosine was used. Its administration should be correlated with periodic patient hemograms during the course of therapy. Over 50 percent of clinical isolates of *C. albicans* develop resistance to flucytosine. Mucocutaneous candidiasis responds to treatment with ketoconazole, while esophageal candidiasis responds to amphotericin B. A recent development in the delivery system for amphotericin B may be a solution to the problems (see Boxed Essay, p. 783) in the treatment of *Candida* and other disseminated fungal infections.

Thrush is a common complication associated with AIDS. In 1990, fluconazole was approved for treatment of thrush.

Aspergillosis

Aspergillosis represents a spectrum of diseases caused by species of *Aspergillus*. These organisms are ubiquitous and are common to the soil, water, decaying vegetation, and any area that contains organic debris. The respiratory tract is the principal portal of entry, and inhaled spores can cause disease in healthy as well as compromised patients. The species most frequently associated with disease is *A. fumigatus*, but other species such as *A. flavus*, *A. niger*, and *A. terreus* are occasionally involved.

Pathogenesis. The clinical manifestations of aspergillosis can be divided into three types: allergic, colonizing (aspergilloma), and invasive.

Allergic aspergillosis is an asthma-like response to an allergen, which in this instance is the fungal spore. The spores usually fail to germinate unless the host is severely compromised. This asthma-like illness is characterized by fever, cough, and wheezing induced by the presence of reaginic IgE antibodies. The syndrome may become severe and chronic with bronchial plugging. Occasionally in the chronic form the spores will germinate and be released from fruiting heads (see Laboratory Diagnosis).

Colonizing aspergillosis, which may develop after allergic aspergillosis, is characterized by the formation of a fungus ball (*aspergilloma*), a dense collection of hyphae. The fungus grows out of and colonizes the pulmonary surfaces. Symptoms are similar to those of allergic aspergillosis, but spitting of blood (hemoptysis) is frequently encountered.

Invasive aspergillosis can develop from the allergic or colonizing forms of the disease, or it can arise independently. *Invasive* implies that *Aspergillus* hyphae have penetrated tissue as either a localized or a disseminated form of the disease. Several factors may predispose the patient to invasive disease: (1) cytotoxic chemotherapy, (2) therapy with broad-spectrum antimicrobial agents, (3) leukopenia, and (4) acute leukemia. Mortality is very high, especially among renal transplant patients and leukemia or lymphoma patients. Invasive disease affects primarily the respiratory tract. Usually the fungus colonizes the tracheobronchial tree, and this leads to bronchopneumonia. Hyphae invade the lumina and walls of blood vessels causing pulmonary hemorrhage. Lung tissue may also be invaded as a direct result of hematogenous spread, for ex-

AMPHOTERICIN B AND LIPOSOMES

The treatment of disseminated fungal infections in immunocompromised patients is difficult because the most efficacious drug, amphotericin B, has a narrow therapeutic index. Toxicity from the short-term effects of amphotericin B therapy includes fever, chills, vomiting, and cardiotoxicity, while long-term therapy is associated with hypomagnesemia,* renal toxicity, and anemia.

A promising new drug delivery system that results in more effective antifungal activity is now under investigation. The new technique involves the encapsulation of drugs such as amphotericin B in liposomes (L-AmB). Liposomes are synthetic vesicles; that is, they are bubbles composed of a phospholipid bilayer. Liposome preparations of amphotericin B are easily reproduced by dissolving the drug in methanol and adding this preparation to a phospholipid-chloroform solution.

Liposomes have an affinity for organs rich in endothelial cells such as liver, lung, spleen, kidney, and bone marrow. This attraction is particularly advantageous because disseminated fungal infections localize in these areas. Liposomes have an affinity for ergosterol, the steroid present in the fungal cell membrane.

Current studies in animal systems and in humans indicate that amphotericin encapsulated in liposomes is less toxic than free amphotericin B during the course of therapy. Thus, patients were shown to be capable of tolerating higher concentrations of the drug and to respond more favorably to therapy.

* Hypomagnesemia is a condition in which there is a deficiency of magnesium in the body that results in twitching and convulsions.

ample, after parenteral therapy. Untreated invasive disease results in death within 2 weeks of onset of symptoms. Invasive disease may also affect the nose and paranasal sinuses. This type of infection is endemic in the Sudan. Infections have also involved the ear canal, the eye, and the heart. Endocarditis caused by aspergilli is associated with prosthetic valve implantation.

Disseminated aspergillosis following invasive disease is the most severe form and invariably results in death. Either antimicrobial agents or glucosteroids have been implicated as predisposing factors, but occasionally even healthy individuals may develop disseminated disease. There is widespread organ involvement, with the lung as the principal target. Death usually results from bilateral pneumonia or intracerebral hemorrhage with fungal invasion and thrombosis.

Considerable research with murine and human cells in vitro has led to some important discoveries concerning the pathogenesis of aspergillosis. It appears that two lines of host defense must be breached before aspergilli can invade tissue. When spores of aspergillus are deposited in lung tissue they are metabolically inactive and are coated by a thick wall. Resting spores ingested by neutrophils are not killed because the respiratory burst is not sufficient to release oxidative metabolites. In contrast, if the resting spore begins to swell and germinate it can be killed by neutrophils. Neutrophils are therefore active against hyphal forms. Macrophages on the other hand can ingest resting spores and kill them. This dual defense by the host normally prevents *Aspergillus* (and other fungi) species from causing invasive pulmonary disease. In immunocompromised patients receiving corticosteroids the host's defenses are breached and invasive pulmonary disease is the rule rather than the exception. Corticosteroids impair the ability of macrophages to destroy resting spores. Spore germination leads to mycelial invasion of blood vessels, hemorrhage, and necrosis. When the dosage of corticosteroids in compromised patients (for example, renal transplant patients) is reduced, the frequency of fungal invasive disease also decreases precipitously.

Laboratory Diagnosis. Diagnosis of aspergillosis is dependent on demonstrating fungal elements in pathologic material and repeated isolation of *Aspergillus* from clinical specimens. Identification in tissue is dependent on (1) finding uniform-sized hyphae 3 to 4 μm in width (Fig. 32-30), (2) finding characteristic dichotomous branching of hyphae at 45-degree angles, (3) the staining of hyphae by special stains, (4) a positive fluorescent antibody response, (5) the presence of characteristic conidiophores (Fig. 32-31), and (6) the presence of septate hyphae. Tissue identification techniques should also be backed up by cultural tests since it may not be possible to evaluate all the criteria in tissue. In addition, some of these morphological characteristics are also found with other fungi. Because of the widespread occurrence of aspergilli in the environment, a positive culture of *Aspergillus* from human tissue must be carefully evaluated. Invasive disease is difficult to diagnose without biopsy, a procedure that many patients cannot withstand. Serological techniques therefore play an important role in diagnosis; however, in immunocompromised patients these tests are of limited value because antibody elaboration is minimal. An early, accurate diagnosis of invasive aspergillosis is important because early treatment is necessary to prevent a fatal outcome. Methods are being currently developed to detect *Aspergillus* antigen in serum. Assays of circulating antigen may also be useful for monitoring therapeutic responses.

Intradermal injection of *Aspergillus* antigens can produce skin reactions that are important criteria in the diagnosis of allergic pulmonary aspergillosis.

Treatment. Invasive aspergillosis is a highly fatal disease, and prompt therapy is required. The mortality rate for those with leukemia is approximately 70 percent but only 25 percent for those with pulmonary disease following transplanta-

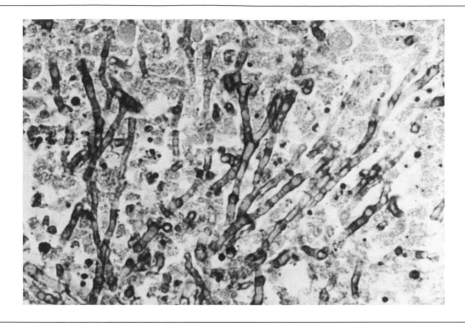

Fig. 32-30. *Aspergillus* hyphae in lung tissue. (Courtesy K. J. Kwon-Chung.)

tion. Amphotericin B alone or in combination with flucytosine has been used with some success in invasive disease. Studies with itraconazole indicate that this drug may, one day, be an alternative to amphotericin B. Allergic forms of the disease can be treated with corticosteroids (but not in immunosuppressed patients). Surgical resection may be necessary for aspergilloma.

Mucormycosis

Mucormycosis (also called *phycomycosis* or *zygomycosis*) refers to diseases caused by members of the order Mucorales. The causal agents of the disease include species of *Rhizopus*, *Absidia*, *Mucor*, *Saksenaea*, *Cunninghamella*, and others. The members of these genera are inhabitants of the soil and are commonly found on fruits and bread. Infections occur in compromised patients such as those with keotacidosis resulting from diabetes but also in leukemic patients, burn pa-

tients, and those undergoing immunosuppressive therapy (for example, during organ transplantation).

Pathogenesis. The most severe forms of mucormycosis involve the nasal region (rhinocerebral mucormycosis) and lung (thoracic mucormycosis). Sporangiospores of the causal agent are inhaled and germinate either in the nasal surfaces or in the lung. Nasal invasion takes place with the formation of hyphae that can spread and involve the orbit, face, meninges, and frontal lobes of the brain. Edema and necrotic tissue are found around the eye and in the nose (Fig. 32-32). Death can occur within a few days of onset. The overall mortality from rhinocerebral mucormycosis is 50 percent. Diabetics have the best survival rate.

Hyphae that invade the lung cause mass lesions and bronchopneumonia. Hyphae invade the walls of blood vessels and cause thrombosis. Dissemination of disease to the central nervous system is a frequent complication of pulmonary infec-

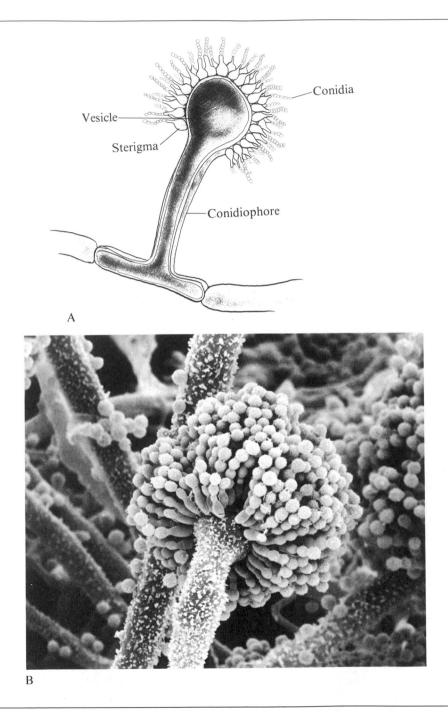

Fig. 32-31. *Aspergillus* conidiophore. A. Diagram. B. Scanning electron micrograph of the conidiophore, terminal vesicle, sterigma, and conidia of *Aspergillus flavus*. (From E. U. King and M. F. Brown, *Can. J. Microbiol.* 29:653, 1983.)

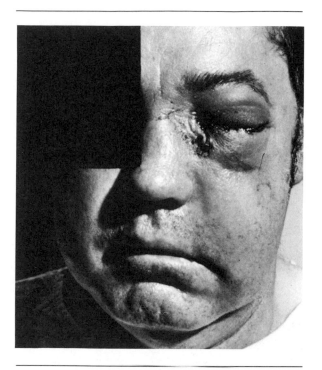

Fig. 32-32. Mucormycosis. (Courtesy G. Roberts.)

tion. Pulmonary infection occurs in patients with uncontrolled leukemia.

Laboratory Diagnosis. Diagnosis is usually made by the observation of broad (10- to 15-μm) aseptate hyphae in normally sterile body fluids or tissue scrapings or biopsy specimens (Fig. 32-33). Since *Rhizopus* is a common contaminant in the laboratory, recovery of this organism from culture is not diagnostic unless accompanied by clinical signs in the patient. Genera can be separated on the basis of morphologic characteristics such as sporangia, and presence or absence of rhizoids (root-like filaments used by the fungus to attach to a substrate).

Treatment. Viral and bacterial infections are frequently observed concomitantly with fungal disease and may be the cause of many fatalities. If recognized in time mucormycosis can be treated with amphotericin B administered IV.

Pneumocystis Pneumonia

Pneumocystis pneumonia is caused by *Pneumocystis carinii*, an organism that was originally thought to be a protozoan but is now considered a fungus on the basis of ribosomal RNA analysis. *P. carinii* has become a pathogen of increasing importance because of the appearance of AIDS.

The organism exists widely in nature as a saprophyte in the lungs of humans and a variety of animals. *P. carinii* causes pneumonia in premature, malnourished infants; patients receiving corticosteroids or other immunosuppressive drugs; and persons with AIDS. *Pneumocystis* pneumonia has been used as an index diagnosis of AIDS since in over 80 percent of AIDS patients this organism is a cause of pneumonia.

The most frequent symptoms of *Pneumocystis* pneumonia are fever, cough, and shortness of breath. The cough is usually nonproductive. Diagnosis of infection is difficult and may require different sampling options. These options include sputum examination, bronchioalveolar lavage, and transbronchial lung biopsy. Lavage specimens, for example, can be stained with methenamine silver, Gram-Weigert, and Giemsa stains. All these stains are nonspecific and *P. carinii* must be distinguished from other yeasts on the basis of morphology. These stains can detect pneumocystis organisms in cysts that measure 4 to 7 μm. Stained free cells, however, are difficult to differentiate from cell fragments. Recently an indirect fluorescent monoclonal antibody test has been described for the rapid detection of *P. carinii* in biopsies or bronchioalveolar lavage.

Three conventional treatment regimens for *pneumocystis* pneumonia are trimethoprim-sulfamethoxazole, parenteral pentamidine, and pyrimethamine-sulfadiazine. Trimethoprimsulfamethoxazole has also been shown to be an effective prophylactic agent. Recently (in 1989) the FDA approved the use of an aerosol version of pentamidine to treat and prevent *Pneumocystis* pneumonia. Aerosolized pentamidine is now being used in AIDS patients who either have had one bout of this pneumonia or whose helper T4 cell numbers go below a level of 200 per cubic

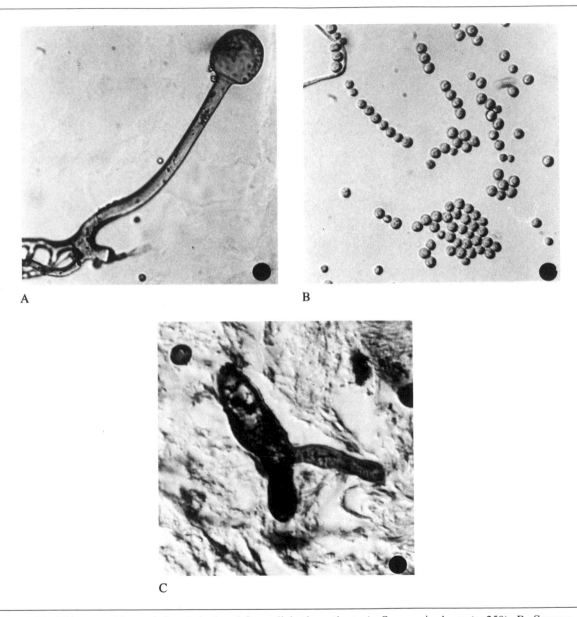

Fig. 32-33. *Rhizopus rhizopodoformis* isolated from diabetic patient. A. Sporangiophore (×250). B. Sporangiospores (×500). C. Stain of hyphae in abscess (×1000). (From B. C. West et al., *J. Clin. Microbiol.* 18:1384, 1983.)

millimeter in the blood. All of these drugs produce adverse reactions and other drugs are under investigation. Current epidemiologic studies indicate that by the year 1991 there may be more than 150,000 cases of *Pneumocystis* pneumonia in the United States.

MYCOTOXINS (MYCETISMUS AND MYCOTOXICOSIS)

MYCETISMUS

Mycetismus, or mushroom poisoning, is caused by the ingestion of certain poisonous fleshy field fungi. Mushroom poisoning is not so common in the United States as it is in areas of eastern Europe where mushroom gathering is a common family practice. The most common symptoms of mushroom poisoning involve the gastrointestinal tract and nervous system. Symptoms, which appear 1 to 2 hours after ingestion, include profuse sweating, violent gastrointestinal involvement, and convulsions. If the dose of toxin is sufficiently high, death may occur within 10 to 12 hours of onset. The most toxic mushrooms are those belonging to the genus *Amanita*.

MYCOTOXICOSIS

Unlike mycetismus, in which the toxic substance is part of the fungal tissue, mycotoxicosis is due to a toxin that is produced as a secondary metabolite. The mycotoxins of interest are produced by species of the genera *Penicillium, Fusarium, Streptomyces,* and *Aspergillus*. These organisms are a common contaminant of grains and foods. Mycotoxins are intimately associated with every food or feed and can be produced at every stage of harvesting, production, and storage of food. When certain environmental conditions prevail (moisture content, temperature, and others) the fungal contaminants grow and release toxic secondary metabolites. Some of the more widely recognized mycotoxins are *aflatoxins*, which are produced by *Aspergillus flavus* and *A. parasiticus*. Aflatoxin was first discovered in 1960 when 100,000 turkeys and several thousand other domestic birds died after ingesting contaminated Brazilian peanut meal. Investigations into the cause of death revealed that the bird feed was contaminated by *A. flavus*.

The animal population displays a wide range of susceptibility to aflatoxin. Young pigs and calves are more vulnerable to the action of the toxin than are other barnyard animals. Low levels of aflatoxin stunt their growth and increase their susceptibility to infectious disease. Aflatoxin B_1 is the most potent naturally occurring carcinogen. Studies show that liver cancers occur with greater frequency in countries or areas where aflatoxin is known to grossly contaminate stored grains. In parts of the Far East and India, maize, corn, rice, and other grains that have high concentrations of aflatoxin are consumed in large amounts. Autopsies on individuals there reveal that many organs contain high levels of aflatoxin.

The effects of aflatoxin on human metabolism have not been fully elucidated. Animal studies reveal, however, that lipid and vitamin metabolism are severely affected. During aflatoxicosis in chickens, fatty liver and steatorrhea (increased lipid in the excreta) appear to be associated with a decrease in bile salts and the main fat-digesting enzyme, pancreatic lipase. Aflatoxin also interacts with certain vitamins. Experiments in chickens and cattle indicate that aflatoxin reduces the vitamin A, vitamin D, and riboflavin content of vital organs and tissue. A natural or induced deficiency of these vitamins makes the animals more susceptible to the effects of aflatoxin.

Mycotoxins of current concern are produced by species of *Fusarium*. Two of these toxins are called *T-2* and *vomitoxin*. Like aflatoxin these toxins are also produced by growth of the fungal species on various grains and have been implicated in animal disease. *Fusarium*-infected feed has caused disease in humans in countries outside the United States. There have been reports from Southeast Asia that *Fusarium* toxins have been used in chemical warfare. The term *yellow rain* has been used because of the color of these toxic materials allegedly released from aircraft. Contact with the toxin causes vomiting, skin irritations, bleeding, and death. Some scientific agencies, however, identify the cause of the problem as a natural occurrence of the toxins resulting from prior defoliation or the use of napalm.

SUMMARY

1. Fungi are eukaryotic microorganisms that can be divided into two morphological forms: spherical yeasts and filamentous molds. The filaments of molds are composed of units called *hyphae* that may or may not be compartmentalized. Some fungi can exist in both morphological forms and are called dimorphic.

2. The fungal cell wall is primarily polysaccharide and possesses no peptidoglycan and is not affected by bacterial cell wall inhibitors such as penicillin. Cell membranes of fungi possess sterols that distinguish them from bacterial cell membranes.

3. Fungi can reproduce by sexual or asexual means, but asexual processes are the more important. Sporulation is the most important reproductive technique used by fungi to propagate the species and can occur by sexual or asexual means. Asexual sporulation results in the release of more individuals than sexual sporulation.

4. Sexual spores include oospores, zygospores, ascospores, and basidiospores. Conidia and sporangiospores are asexual spores produced on specialized hyphal structures while arthrospores, chlamydospores, and blastospores are asexual spores arising directly from hyphae.

5. Fungi grow best at pH's between 5 and 6 but they can tolerate and grow at pH's between 2 and 9. Sabouraud agar is the most widely used isolation medium for fungi. Yeasts produce creamy opaque colonies while mold colonies are cottony on agar media.

6. Most fungal diseases are primarily due to occupational exposure to large numbers of fungal spores. The highest mortality from fungal diseases is found in those compromised by some underlying disease or condition. Most fungi can be observed directly in tissue via staining or by cultivation of specimens in the laboratory. If culture and histologic results are negative, serological tests have value in diagnosis.

7. Immunity to fungal diseases is primarily by cell-mediated immunity. Antibodies appear to play a minor role in protecting the host; thus, diagnostic serological techniques are difficult to evaluate. Some fungi produce an allergic response mediated by IgE antibodies. Drugs used to treat fungal disease are outlined in Table 32-1.

8. Fungal diseases can be divided into five types: systemic, subcutaneous, cutaneous, superficial, and opportunistic. The systemic diseases are outlined in Table 32-4. The subcutaneous mycoses were outlined previously in Table 32-3.

9. Cutaneous fungal infections, or dermatophytoses, are caused primarily by three genera: *Microsporum, Trichophyton,* and *Epidermophyton.* They invade keratinized areas of the body and are transmitted by contact with clothing or articles contaminated by human dermatophytes or by contact with infected animals. These infections are referred to as tineas or ringworms. Several topical solutions such as potassium permanganate, benzoic acid, and salicylic acid are available for treatment as well as orally administered drugs such as griseofulvin. The allergic manifestations caused by some dermatophytes are called ids.

10. Superficial mycoses involve superficial areas of the skin and usually do not require treatment. Lesions are usually scaly eruptions on the chest, back, and shoulders. Some pathogens can attack the scalp or beard hair. Three important infections are called tinea versicolor, tinea nigra palmaris, and black-and-white piedra.

Table 32-4. Characteristics of the Systemic Mycoses

Disease	Etiological agent	Transmission	Primary site of infection	Treatment
Histoplasmosis	*Histoplasma capsulatum*	Inhalation of conidia found associated with bird dung	Lung primary site but can be disseminated to organs via reticuloendothelial system	Amphotericin B and ketoconazole
Coccidioidomycosis	*Coccidioides immitis*	Inhalation of arthrospores from semi-arid and dusty areas	Lung primary site but if disseminated to meninges is invariably fatal	Amphotericin B for systemic disease; itraconazole for cutaneous disease and fluconazole for meningitis
Blastomycosis	*Blastomyces dermatitidis*	Inhalation of spores from contaminated soil	Lung primary site with dissemination to skin and organs; chronic cutaneous occasionally encountered	Hydroxystilbamidine isoethionate or amphotericin B
Paracoccidio-idomycosis	*Paracoccidioides brasiliensis*	Inhalation of spores (?)	Lungs primary site but can be disseminated to skin and lymph nodes	Ketoconazole and sulfonamides
Cryptococcosis	*Cryptococcus neoformans*	Inhalation of spores found in pigeon droppings	Lungs; but in compromised patients systemic involvement possible, including central nervous system	Amphotericin B plus flucytosine or ketoconazole; fluconazole

Table 32-5. Characteristics of Opportunistic Fungal Pathogens

Disease	Etiological agent(s)	Pathogenesis	Primary compromising situation or condition	Treatment
Candidiasis	Candida species (C. albicans, C. krusei, C. tropicalis, etc.)	CUTANEOUS A. Thrush	Antibiotic administration; acquired immune deficiency syndrome	Discontinue drug treatment; nystatin orally; fluconazole
		B. Vaginal	Antibiotic administration, pregnancy, diabetes, oral contraceptives	Discontinue drug treatment; creams and other topical ointments (see Table 32-1)
		C. Intertriginous	Body site exposure to moist environments	Topical creams and ointments (see Table 32-1)
		SYSTEMIC	Implantation of prosthetic devices, contaminated needles, prolonged catheterization	Amphotericin B
		CHRONIC MUCOCUTANEOUS	T-cell immunodeficiency	Usually refractory to treatment
Aspergillosis	Aspergillus species (A. fumigatus, A. flavus, A. niger)	ALLERGIC	Inhalation of spore	Corticosteroids, but not in immunocompromised patients
		COLONIZING	Formation of fungus ball in lung	Surgical resection
		INVASIVE	Can develop from allergic or colonizing and usually found in patients compromised by drugs	Amphotericin B alone or in combination with flucytosine
Mucormycosis	Species of Mucor, Rhizopus, Absidia, etc.	Rhinocerebral mucormycosis	Diabetes, burn wounds, immunosuppressive drugs	Amphotericin B
Pneumocystis pneumonia	Pneumocystis carinii	Pneumonia	AIDS patients, premature malnourished infants, patients on immunosuppressive drugs	Trimethoprim-sulfamethoxazole, pentamidine, pyrimethamine sulfadiazine
Cryptococcosis	Cryptococcus neoformans	Discussed under Systemic Mycoses; see page 768		

11. Opportunistic fungal pathogens cause disease primarily in compromised patients (those with metabolic disorders or those receiving immunosuppressive drugs or antimicrobial therapy). The opportunistic fungal diseases are outlined in Table 32-5.

12. Fungi can be toxic because of the nature of their own tissue (mycetismus) or because they produce secondary metabolites when growing on various foods or grains (mycotoxicosis). One of the most toxic secondary metabolites is aflatoxin B_1, which is believed to be a cause of liver cancer when contaminated grains are ingested over long periods of time.

QUESTIONS FOR STUDY

Select the best response or responses for each of the following:

1. The following are characteristics of fungi *except*
   A. They are eukaryotic.
   B. They can exist in a single-cell or filamentous state.
   C. They are inhibited by penicillins or cephalosporins.
   D. They demonstrate sexual and asexual reproduction in the laboratory.

2. All of the following are asexual spores *except*
   A. Conidia
   B. Ascospores
   C. Arthrospores
   D. Sporangiospores

3. Which of the following situations would not lead to dermatophyte infection?
   A. Inhalation of arthrospores
   B. Working as a horse groomer
   C. Walking barefoot in a shower area
   D. Playing with your cat

4. Which of the following fungi is part of the host's normal flora?
   A. *Blastomyces dermatitidis*
   B. *Sporothrix schenkii*
   C. *Candida albicans*
   D. *Microsporum* species

5. Most systemic fungal diseases resemble which of the following in terms of symptomatology?
   A. Measles
   B. Tuberculosis
   C. Leprosy
   D. Hepatitis

6. Amphotericin B could be used to treat all the diseases caused by the following infectious agents *except*
   A. *Histoplasma capsulatum*
   B. *Coccidioides immitis*
   C. *Cryptococcus neoformans*
   D. *Trichophyton rubrum*

7. Several weeks after pruning her rosebushes and mulching them with peat moss a housewife developed a necrotic lesion on her hand. The physician suspected the lesion was caused by a fungus. Which of the following treatments would the physician be likely to recommend?
   A. Ointments containing griseofulvin
   B. Potassium iodide
   C. Cream containing ketoconazole
   D. Tablets containing nystatin

8. *Candida* infections can be the result of
   A. Exposure of the skin to moist environments over a period of time
   B. Sexual transmission of the infectious agent
   C. Antibiotic administration over a prolonged period
   D. Catheterization

9. The presence of hyphae in the patient's sputum might lead one to suspect which of the following diseases?
   A. Sporotrichosis
   B. Aspergillosis
   C. Cryptococcosis
   D. Histoplasmosis

10. The fungus that is the most important cause of pneumonia in AIDS patients is
    A. *Candida albicans*
    B. *Trichophyton rubrum*
    C. *Pneumocystis carinii*
    D. *Histoplasma capsulatum*

Fill in the blank:

11. *Penicillium, Fusarium,* and *Aspergillus* species produce contaminants in grains called _____.

12. Studies with *Aspergillus* have demonstrated that drugs called_____impair the ability of macrophages to destroy resting spores.

13. The lipid preparations being evaluated as transporters of drugs such as amphotericin B are called_____.

14. Germ tube formation is an important presumptive test in the laboratory diagnosis of _____species.

15. The agar medium used to cultivate fungi is called_____agar.

16. Diseases produced by dermatophytes are collectively called_____.

17. The antifungal drug that is being used as a substitute for amphotericin B because of its high therapeutic index is called_____.

18. The fungus found as arthrospores in hot, semiarid areas of Southern California, Arizona, and New Mexico is called_____.

19. The ability of a fungal species to exist in either a yeast or mycelial form is referred to as_____.

20. Most of the fungal species pathogenic to humans belong to the subdivision called_____.

ADDITIONAL READINGS

Emmons, C. W., Binford, C. H., Utz, J. P., and Kwong-Chung, K. J. *Medical Mycology* (3rd ed.). Philadelphia: Lea & Febiger, 1989.

Epstein, J. B., Truelove, E. L., and Izutzu, K. T. Oral candidiasis: Pathogenesis and host defense. *Rev. Infect. Dis.* 6(1):96,1984.

Fromtling, R. A. Overview of medically important antifungal azole derivatives. *Clin. Microbiol. Revs.* 1(2):187,1989.

Gold, J. W. M. Opportunistic fungal infections in patients with neoplastic disease. *Am. J. Med.* 76:458,1984.

Goodwin, R. A., Lloyd, J. E., and des Prez, R. M. Histoplasmosis in normal hosts. *Medicine* 60:231,1981.

Kovacs, J. A., and Masur, H. *Pneumocystis carinii* pneumonia: Therapy and prophylaxis. *J. Infect. Dis.* 158(1):254,1988.

Lehrer, R. I. Mucormycosis (Review). *Ann. Intern. Med.* 93:93,1980.

McGinnis, M. R. *Laboratory Handbook of Medical Mycology.* New York: Academic, 1980.

Rinaldi, M. G. Invasive aspergillosis. *Rev. Infect. Dis.* 5:1061,1983.

Rippon, J. W. *Medical Mycology* (3rd ed.). Philadelphia: Saunders, 1986.

Shepherd, M. G., Poulter, R. T. M., and Sullivan, P. A. *Candida albicans:* Biology, genetics and pathogenicity. *Annu. Rev. Microbiol.* 39:579,1985.

Uraguchi, K., and Yamazaki, M. (eds.). *Toxicology, Biochemistry, and Pathology of Mycotoxins.* New York: Wiley, 1980.

VIII. MEDICAL PARASITOLOGY

33. THE PROTOZOA, HELMINTHS, AND ARTHROPODS

OBJECTIVES

To discuss parasitism and parasitic disease in terms of types of life cycles and hosts, adaptations, modes of transmission, factors that affect the geographic distribution and incidence, laboratory identification procedures, and control and treatment measures

To give the name of the parasite, the principal clinical manifestations, identification procedures, mode of transmission, and treatment and control measures of the various parasitic diseases

To associate with specific parasites: primary amebic meningoencephalitis, opportunistic pathogens in the immunodepressed, visceral and larval migrans, pinworm or seatworm, muscle worm, swimmer's itch; improperly cooked pork, cats, beavers, female anopheles mosquito

To comment on the importance of the changing of surface antigens by trypanosomes

To summarize the disease-related involvements of invertebrate arthropods

GENERAL CHARACTERISTICS OF PARASITES AND PARASITIC INFECTIONS

Medical parasitology deals with those members of the animal kingdom that sometime in their life cycle take up temporary or permanent abode in or on a human host. It includes consideration of arthropods that cause discomfort and sometimes death by the injection of venoms. Disease may occur during the period when the parasite is dependent on the human host for shelter and sustenance; this is the ecological niche where a part of the life cycle for many is spent. Other medically important infectious agents cause disease largely under the circumstances of a parasitic relationship, but, traditionally, the term *parasites* refers to organisms from the animal kingdom that cause disease.

Parasites are found in four divisions of the animal kingdom: the *Protozoa, the single-celled animals*; the *Nemathelminthes, the roundworms*; the *Platyhelminthes, the flatworms*; and the *Arthropoda, invertebrate animals with jointed appendages*. Most of the adult forms of the last

three phyla are macroscopic in size. It may seem incongruous that microbiology, which by definition is the study of microscopic forms, includes the study of organisms that are readily observable by the unaided eye. Ascaris worms are the size of earthworms. The large tapeworms attain a length of 25 to 30 feet. Medical microbiology encompasses the study not only of disease-causing microscopic forms but of all infectious agents, the macroscopic parasites included. However, the microscope does figure prominently in the identification of the eggs and larvae of these macroscopic organisms.

INCIDENCE OF PARASITIC INFECTION

Industrialized nations are not highly cognizant of the incidence of parasitic infections and how they affect the quality of the lives of a large segment of the human population. Millions of people, particularly in the tropics and subtropics, are debilitated, disfigured, blinded, and inconvenienced by such infections and die of parasitic infections (Table 33-1). Many of these infections are diseases of the poor, the lower socioeconomic

Table 33-1. Deaths Due to Parasitic Diseases in the Developing World (1990 WHO Figures)

Diseases	Deaths
Malaria	1–2 million
Schistosomiasis	200,000
Amebiasis	40,000–110,000
African trypanosomiasis (sleeping sickness)	20,000
Hookworm	50,000–60,000
Ascariasis	20,000

groups, those in primitive surroundings, and those in substandard living conditions. The disquieting statistics include the following facts: One in four people in the world suffers malaria or is exposed to it. One in five people suffers from hookworm infection, with energies depleted by bloodsucking worms attached to the intestinal wall. Fifty million Africans harbor trypanosomes, which cause an infection that occasionally develops into fatal sleeping sickness. One of every four inhabitants of the earth carries roundworms in the intestinal tract. Similar figures of the incidence of infection can be quoted for many of the parasites.

Parasitic infections in the United States are common enough, but their morbidity and mortality are very low. The better-known parasitic diseases are due to the protozoal infections of amebiasis, giardiasis, vaginal trichomoniasis, and toxoplasmosis and the helminthic infections of enterobiasis and trichinelliasis. Congenital toxoplasmosis seems to be the most serious of the indigenous infections on account of the occurrence of mental retardation and visual impairment or loss. The popularity of travel and the influx of immigrants account for the appearance of sporadic cases of exotic parasitic infections in this country.

SURVIVAL OF PARASITIC SPECIES

Certain requirements need to be fulfilled for parasitic infection to occur and on a broader scale for the parasitic species to survive. The parasite must *gain entrance to the host, survive and reproduce* there, eventually *leave the host, and chance upon suitable environmental conditions* (e.g., moisture, temperature) *or contact other appropriate hosts and vectors.* For many parasites other appropriate hosts are *intermediate hosts,* where a developmental stage in the life of the parasite (e.g., the larval form of worms) occurs. It is in the requirement for specific intermediate hosts that a number of parasites especially differ from the other infectious agents.

The ability of the parasite to multiply and survive in the host is related to *adaptations* undergone by the species in its evolution. *The gain or loss of structures and markedly increased reproductive capacities* are examples of differences between parasites and their free-living counterparts. Tapeworms do not have digestive tracts. They need only absorb nutrients from the host's digestive tract. Various species of parasites have holdfast structures such as hooks, adhesive disks, and suctorial grooves by which they become embedded in or attached to host tissues. The movement of food and the contractile waves of the host's intestine do not dislodge the anchored parasite.

INFECTIVE FORMS AND LIFE CYCLES OF PARASITES

Most parasites undergo a series of developmental stages during which they grow, mature, and reproduce. Many exist in more than one form. Many of the protozoa exist not only in the active, feeding, proliferative form, the *trophozoite*, but also in a resistant, quiescent form, the *cyst*, or as *sporozoites*. The trophozoite causes the disease; the cyst or sporozoite serves as the infective, transmitted form. Most of the worms produce eggs (are oviparous) from which *embryos or larval forms* develop. Others directly produce *live larvae* (are viviparous). The fertilized eggs or the larvae are the infective forms from which the adults develop. The adult worms are usually responsible for the symptoms and pathological conditions of the disease. The eggs, as in schistosomiasis, and the larvae, as in trichinelliasis, however, may cause the pathology and the symptoms.

Some parasites spend their lives in the same host, generation after generation. Some leave the host and remain quiescent in nature until they enter another host. Others undergo active growth and metamorphosis outside the final host. In some parasites there are sexual and asexual forms. In some the parasite is able to develop in more than one host or requires more than one host to complete its life cycle (Fig. 33-1).

Examples of parasitic life cycles reflect their diversity and their complexity. The protozoon *Entamoeba histolytica* is transmitted via its cyst directly from one host to another or through fecally contaminated soil, water, and plants. Most of the intestinal roundworms are transmitted in a similar manner, except that the infective forms are fertilized eggs or larvae. No intermediate hosts and no alternative hosts are involved.

In another type of life cycle the parasite completes its stages in a single host. There is no survival apart from a host. In trichinelliasis ingested larvae develop into adult worms. The adult female within the same host produces live larvae that embed in muscle. The worm reaches a dead end here unless the flesh is consumed by another host.

The more complex life cycles involve intermediate and definitive (final) hosts. *Intermediate*

Fig. 33-1. Overview of the life cycles of parasites of importance to humans. (From E. W. Koneman et al., *Color Atlas and Textbook of Diagnostic Microbiology*. Philadelphia: Lippincott, 1979.)

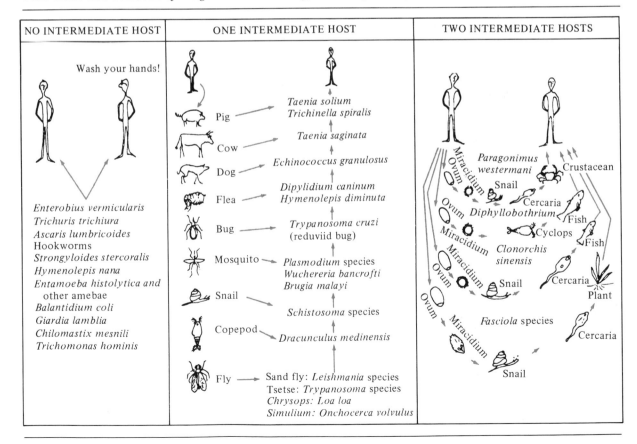

hosts are those in which the asexual or larval stages occur. *Definitive hosts* are those that contain the sexual forms or the mature adult forms or sometimes, arbitrarily, the most important host. Arthropods serve as intermediate hosts for some parasites and occasionally as definitive hosts for others. The very same arthropods, especially the biting and bloodsucking arthropods, also serve as the vectors of certain parasitic diseases. Humans and other vertebrates are definitive hosts to most parasites.

Some parasites have a succession of developmental forms and of intermediate hosts. The fish tapeworm, which has a complex life cycle, leaves the definitive host—a human, say—in the form of a fertilized egg. In cool fresh water a ciliated embryo (coracidium) hatches out after 2 weeks. The coracidium, when ingested by a copepod (crustacean), the first intermediate host, transforms in 2 to 3 weeks into the first larval stage, the procercoid larva. The cycle is continued when the infected copepod is ingested by a fish. In the tissues of the fish, the second intermediate host, a second larval stage forms, the plerocercoid larva. Consumption of raw or improperly cooked plerocercoid-containing fish by a human or some other animal completes the cycle. The adult tapeworm develops, and the eggs shed in feces into fresh water initiate another cycle. It is evident that continuation of the species is at an even greater risk for parasites that have so complex a life cycle. They are subjected to an increased number of host and environmental changes while completing the full circle of developmental and maturational changes. Little wonder that some parasites produce prodigious numbers of eggs and that some cycles include a stage in which larval forms also multiply.

FACTORS THAT INFLUENCE THE INCIDENCE OF PARASITIC INFECTION

The incidence of infection is related to such factors as climate, the availability of suitable intermediate and definitive host and vectors, the eating and sanitary habits of the human population, and their mode of dress, occupation, and nutritional status. The occurrence of hookworm infection, for example, is dependent on the sanitary habits of the population, climate, soil texture, and mode of dress. Hookworm eggs that are shed in the feces on the ground develop into the infective larval form only when the temperature is in the range of 70 to 85°F and in areas where the average rainfall is more than 40 inches per year. Lack of vegetation and a hard, clay-like soil adversely affect the development of the parasite. The filariform (thread-like) hookworm larvae lurk on vegetation or moist soil awaiting contact with a warm-blooded animal. A barefoot child is a likely candidate to provide opportunity for the larva to contact bare skin, the portal of entry for the parasite.

The eating habits of various population groups have a bearing on the incidence and persistence of certain parasitic diseases. The consumption of uncooked vegetables, particularly leafy vegetables, where human excrement ("night soil") has been used as fertilizer is a mode of transmission of the protozoal infections of amebiasis and giardiasis and of the helminthic infections of ascariasis and trichuriasis. The ingestion of raw fish may lead to anemia caused by infection with the fish tapeworm or to liver and gastrointestinal tract pathology caused by flukes. Raw beef may transmit the beef tapeworm and *Toxoplasma* organisms and, indirectly, the pork tapeworm and the muscle worm.

THE NATURE OF PARASITIC DISEASE

The occurrence of disease is often correlated with the number of parasites present and the complicating effects of multiparasitic infection, bacterial infections, malnutrition, age, and immune status. Many people in the tropics and subtropics, where parasites abound, suffer a multiplicity of parasitic infections. The triad of roundworm (ascariasis), whipworm (trichuriasis), and hookworm infection within the same person is not uncommon. Other parasitic combinations also occur. Singly, the infections might be comparatively benign.

Asymptomatic infections sometimes escalate into serious chronic disease. In chronic Chagas' disease, the patient may have heart disease or enlargement of the esophagus or colon years after the inception of an asymptomatic infection. Severe parasitic disease in life may lead to retardation of growth and mental retardation, especially when compounded with malnutrition.

The pathogenesis of parasitic disease is varied. In addition to tissue invasion and destruction and toxic products, parasites create symptoms and pathology by obstruction, exertion of pressure, competition for host nutrients, and induction of hypersensitivities. The toxins are not devastating, as are the bacterial exotoxins.

The symptoms and pathogenesis of some parasitic infections are associated with the migrations within the body that are the normal mode of spread of some parasites. In trichinelliasis, for example, the early manifestations appear in the GI tract during the time adult females are producing live larvae. In heavier adult-stage infections, it appears that the patient has acute food poisoning. There may be fever, malaise, diarrhea, vomiting, and other GI complaints. In the next stage, larval migration, the chief complaint stems from myositis (inflammation of the muscles). There may be difficulty in breathing, speaking, use of extremities, chewing, eye movement, and so forth. There may be central nervous system (CNS) disturbances, congestive heart failure, and general wasting owing to loss of appetite.

LABORATORY DIAGNOSIS

Early diagnosis is important for those diseases that develop into chronic, disabling forms: filariasis, leishmaniasis, schistosomiasis, trypanosomiasis, and others. Once chronic inflammatory responses have produced scar tissue, little can be accomplished by drug treatment to undo the dam-

age. Palliative drugs (analgesics, corticosteroids) or surgical intervention may be the only form of treatment applicable once unalterable tissue damage has occurred.

Definitive diagnosis of parasitic infections depends largely on laboratory findings. Diagnosis based solely on clinical signs and symptoms is rarely possible or justified without laboratory confirmation, especially in nonendemic areas.

Parasitic infection, especially exotic parasitic infection, may not be suspected in areas where parasitic diseases are not prevalent. Inquiry into the geographical and dietary history of the patient may reveal the opportunity for parasitization. Has the patient resided in or visited areas where parasitic infections are endemic within the incubation period? Does the patient recall an insect bite? Did the patient eat raw fish or uncooked vegetables?

Direct Examination

The *major mode* of laboratory identification is *morphological identification*, that is, recognition of the various forms of the parasite as they appear in clinical specimens. The diagnostic procedures of culturing, biochemical and serological tests, and animal inoculations that are commonly used in bacteriology and virology are much less frequently used in routine diagnosis of parasitic infections. The microscope is extensively used in the laboratory identification of parasitic infections because the forms most often sought are the microscopic cysts, trophozoites, and tissue forms of the protozoa and the typical, distinctive eggs and larvae of the helminths.

Identification of Intestinal Parasites

The GI tract is the site of infection for many parasites, or it is the site where the infection is initiated, with subsequent migration from the tract. The laboratory usually examines at least three fecal specimens serially collected at 24- to 48-hour intervals. Fecal specimens, collected in dry, clean containers, are first grossly inspected for blood, mucus, adult forms of worms, and consistency. Stools that are liquid or that contain blood or mucus should be kept warm and examined as soon as possible after evacuation. A technique for sampling duodenal contents introduced in 1970 avoids the previously used patient-discomforting method of duodenal intubation. A number of parasites establish themselves in the duodenum. In the *Entero-Test method*, the patient swallows a gelatin capsule that is packed with a nylon thread 140 cm long. The free end of the thread is fastened to the patient's face. After the capsule dissolves, the thread is carried by peristaltic action to the duodenum. The thread is gently retrieved after 4 hours. The droplets of duodenal contents on the distal end of the thread (composed of porous material) are then examined for parasites. Most of the laboratory procedures are directed toward making suitable preparations for microscopical examination.

Blood Smears

Blood films are prepared to detect parasites such as trypanosomes, leishmanias, microfilarias, and plasmodia (malaria parasites). In the diagnosis of malaria, for example, films are prepared as thin smears and thick smears and are stained. In thin smears the red blood cells are spread out into a monocellular film. The red blood cells remain intact to better reveal the typical morphology of the infecting parasites and their effects on the red blood cells. In thick smears the drop of blood that is deposited at one end of the thin smear slide is not spread out. The cells are lysed so that the parasites are concentrated, making it easier for the trained observer to spot a light infection.

Examination of blood smears may disclose *eosinophilia*. Eosinophilia is a common finding in helminthic (worm) infections.

Tissue Examination

Wet mounts, stained tissue sections, and smears are also prepared from other body fluids and tissues. The material for such preparations is obtained by scrapings of skin and mucosal lesions, by biopsy, and by aspiration of the fluids of ulcers, abscesses, and bone marrow.

Serology of Parasitic Infection

The use of serological tests in parasitic disease is increasing as the sensitivity and specificity of the tests are being constantly improved. Not all parasitic diseases elicit an appreciable antibody response. Generally speaking, the immune response is greater with parasites that invade the tissues than with those that remain in the lumen of the intestine or those that are ectoparasitic (live on the outside of the host). Serological tests are especially useful in extraintestinal amebiasis, toxoplasmosis, Chagas' disease, visceral leishmaniasis, trichinelliasis, schistosomiasis, visceral larva migrans, and cysticercosis.

TREATMENT AND CONTROL

The control of parasitic infection requires an understanding of how infections are acquired and the pathogenesis and clinical manifestations of the parasitic diseases; the role of hosts, especially intermediate hosts, including the environmental circumstances that determine the intermediate host's ecological niche; and the availability of control measures and the realistic chances of applying those measures. Eradication of many of the parasitic diseases would entail the expensive and formidable task of totally regulating intermediate host (insects, molluscs) and strictly managing environmental conditions (breeding places of insects, soil contamination with excreta). A reasonable goal with helminth infections it to reduce infectious doses by a combination of measures. Helminths do not multiply in the form of adults in the definitive human host, and so with a reduced infectious dose the worm burden often would not reach the level to cause disease. Ways to reduce the infectious dose include applying insecticides, molluscicides (snail killers), and other agents that destroy intermediate hosts and vectors; managing environmental conditions, such as insect breeding places; making foods and water supplies safe for consumption; and using therapeutic and prophylactic drugs in those populations or segments of populations that experience the highest rate of infection.

Travelers to places where parasitic infections are endemic, especially when the itinerary or temporary residence is away from urban areas, should be knowledgeable about the types of foods, beverages, insects, and other factors that are involved in the transmission of endemic infectious diseases. In addition to the required immunizations, recommended prophylactic drugs and immunizations should be given thoughtful consideration. The Centers for Disease Control (CDC), Atlanta, Georgia, annually publishes Health Information for International Travel.

Development of vaccines for some parasitic diseases (e.g., against malaria) is under way, but problems that stem from the characteristics of parasites make the attainment of an effective vaccine generally more difficult than with bacterial and virus vaccines. The parasites are antigenically very complex, they appear in different forms (trophozoites and cysts or adult worms, larvae, and eggs), and assessment of the host's immunological response is difficult. Significant active immunity has not been attained in humans or experimental animals except in limited studies in which irradiated organisms or irradiated crude extracts were used. Such preparations are unsatisfactory as vaccines. The multiple antigens present in parasites and the changes (shifts) in the composition of a given antigen make it difficult to define the antigens that evoke protective responses. Currently, a major approach to defining the relevant antigens is the development of monoclonal antibodies against antigens that appear at various stages of the parasite life cycle. In some instances the antibodies provide partial passive immunity and indicate candidate antigens for vaccine development.

Chemotherapy ordinarily should not be undertaken when the diagnosis of parasitic disease is provisionally based on clinical signs and symp-

toms. The clinical signs and symptoms often are too diverse, too nonspecific, for a conclusive diagnosis to be made. Some of the antiparasitic drugs, especially those used for tissue infections, are toxic, and so the need for therapy must be weighed against the toxicity of the drug.

The effects of the antiparasitic drugs, as might be expected, are varied. Some are curative; they terminate the parasitosis. Some destroy the adult form of the parasite but are not able to eliminate the cysts or larvae. Some halt the multiplication of the parasite, an action which can be tantamount to curing the disease but not ridding the patient of the infection. Some are palliative; that is, they only lessen the patient's discomfort.

Popular drugs that are used on a somewhat broad spectrum basis include the azole drugs *mebendazole, metronidazole, thiobendazole,* and *niclosamide and praziquantel.* The azole drugs and niclosamide are particularly effective against lumen-dwelling parasites.

The appearance of drug-resistant strains sometimes impedes progress in the treatment and control of a parasitic disease. A notable example is that of the plasmodial protozoon that causes falciparum malaria. Strains that do not respond to first-choice antimalaria drugs are constantly evolving and relentlessly spreading globally.

THE PROTOZOA

The parasitic protozoa are customarily divided into four groups, variously termed subphyla, classes, or subdivisions: *Sarcodina, Mastigophora, Ciliata or Ciliophora, and Sporozoa.* A summary (Table 33-2) of the protozoal diseases described in this chapter is presented on page 806.

SARCODINA—THE AMEBAE

Amebae that regularly parasitize humans (Fig. 33-2), *Endolimax nana, Iodamoeba bütschlii,*

Table 33-2. Characteristics of Protozoal Diseases

Disease name and agent	Clinical condition	Infective form; mode of transmission	Specimen examined; diagnostic form	Comments	Treatment
Amebiasis *Entamoeba histolytica*	Intestinal: diarrhea, dysentery Extraintestinal: related to abscess formation in liver, brain, lung	*Cyst* Food (night soil), water; anal intercourse	*Stool, serum* Cysts or trophozoites; antibodies		Iodoquinol (intestinal); metronidazole followed by iodoquinol (extraintestinal)
Primary amebic meningoencephalitis (PAM) *Naegleria fowleri*	Fever, severe headache, nausea, disorientation, coma	*Cysts and trophozoites* Warm stagnant water entering nares	*CNS fluid* Trophozoites	Soil-water ameboflagellate; swimmers in warm stagnant water	Amphotericin B (questionable effectiveness)
Acanthamebiasis *Acanthamoeba* species	Keratitis (eye) may lead to blindness Chronic granulomatous amebic encephalitis	*Trophozoites* Eye: improper cleaning of contact lens Other: soil, water, sewage	*Specimen from infected tissue* Cysts or trophozoites	Free-living ameba	Topical miconazole for eye infections
Giardiasis, lambliasis *Giardia lamblia*	Protracted diarrhea, malabsorption syndrome	*Cyst* Person to person (day-care centers, gays) contact; food, water	*Stool, duodenal contents* Cyst or trophozoite	Animal reservoirs: beavers, muskrats Entero-Test	Quinacrine HCl; metronidazole
Trichomoniasis (vaginal) *Trichomonas vaginalis*	Vaginitis with itching, burning, inflammation, discharge	*Trophozoite* Venereal	*Vaginal discharge/ scrapings* Trophozoite	Sometimes found in Pap smear; Males usually asymptomatic No cyst form	Metronidazole
African trypanosomiasis (sleeping sickness) *Trypanosoma b. gambiense* *Trypanosoma b. rhodesiense*	Skin lesion at site of bite; fever, lymph node enlargement CNS involvement: progressive mental deterioration, coma; death due to pneumonia, starvation, sepsis	*Metatrypanosomes:* bite of tsetse fly	*Blood, cerebrospinal fluid, aspirates of lymph nodes* Trypanosomes	Winterbottom's sign; variation of surface antigens	Suramin for early stages; melarsoprol for CNS stage

Disease / Organism	Disease	Infective stage / Transmission	Diagnostic specimen / Form	Comments	Treatment
American trypanosomiasis *Trypanosoma cruzi*	Chagas' disease; acute disease (especially in children) in visceral organs and heart; chronic disease in adults, megacolon, megaesophagus, enlarged heart	*Trypomastigotes* Feces of reduviid bugs	*Blood* Trypomastigotes	Romana's sign; xenodiagnosis; domestic and wild animals as hosts and reservoirs	Nifurtimox; benznidazole
Leishmaniasis *Leishmania donovani*	Visceral (Kala azar) leishmaniasis; destruction of macrophages; liver, spleen, lns enlargement; protracted fever	*Promastigotes* Bite of sandfly	*Bone marrow aspirate* Leishmania in macrophages	Dogs and foxes, important reservoirs; thatched roofs as breeding places for sandflies	Antimony gluconate
Leishmania tropica *Leishmania mexicana*	Cutaneous leishmaniasis; ulcerating lesions at site of insect bite	*Promastigotes* Bite of sandfly	*Biopsy or scrapings of ulcer* Leishmania	Dogs, forest rodents, anteaters important reservoirs; thatched roofs as breeding places for sandflies	Antimony gluconate
Leishmania brasiliensis	Mucocutaneous leishmaniasis; cutaneous lesions followed by multiple lesions, usually at border of mouth, nose; may be disfiguring	*Promastigotes* Bite of sandfly	*Culture of ulcer or biopsy* Leishmania	Dogs, forest rodents, sloths important reservoirs	Antimony gluconate
Balantidiasis *Balantidium coli*	Diarrhea, dysentery	*Cysts* Food, water contaminated by pigs	*Stool* Cyst	Largest protozoal parasite	Tetracycline
Plasmodiasis (Malaria) *Plasmodium vivax, malariae, falciparum, ovale*	Periodic fever, chills, sweats; enlargement of spleen, liver; anemia	*Sporozoites* Bite of female Anopheles mosquito	*Blood* Cyclical plasmodial forms in red blood cells	Drug resistance is a major problem in falciparum malaria	Chloroquine phosphate; primaquine phosphate

Table 33-2. (continued)

Disease name and agent	Clinical condition	Infective form; mode of transmission	Specimen examined; diagnostic form	Comments	Treatment
Toxoplasmosis *Toxoplasma gondii*	Primary infection usually asymptomatic or mild; in immuno-compromised, a disseminated infection often involving CNS; congenital infections—anomalies of CNS, eye	*Oocysts or tissue cysts* Ingestion of oocysts or meat containing tissue cysts	*Serum and tissues* Organism not readily observed or cultured from humans	Members of cat family only definitive hosts	Pyramethamine plus trisulfapyrimidines
Babesiosis *Babesia microti*	Nantucket fever; resembles malaria	Bite by nymph of hard ticks	*Blood* Organism in red blood cells	Long recognized as an important infection of domestic and wild animals; deer, mice, and field mice important reservoirs	Clindamycin plus quinine
Cryptosporidiosis *Cryptosporidium* species	Profuse, watery diarrhea	*Oocysts* Feces of animals; respiratory secretions of humans	*Stool, gut tissue* Oocysts observed via phase contrast microscopy or in acid-fast stained material	Fatal intractable diarrhea in immunocom-promised; dehydration and parenteral nutrition as supportive therapy	Vancomycin (questionable effectiveness)

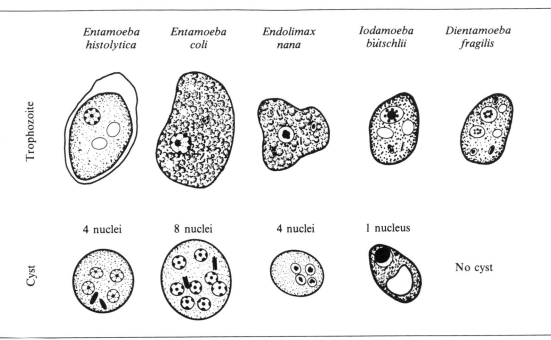

Fig. 33-2. Amoebae found in human stool specimens.

Entamoeba coli, Entamoeba hartmanni (considered by some to be a nonvirulent strain of *E. histolytica*), and *Dientamoeba fragilis*, are commensal, nonpathogenic amebae that colonize the intestinal tract. They have a direct life cycle (no invertebrate or intermediate host) and are cosmopolitan (worldwide) in their distribution. They are important because they must be differentiated from the one intestinal amebic pathogen, *E. histolytica. Entamoeba gingivalis* appears in the oral cavity in trophozoite form only. It is of uncertain pathogenicity but is generally regarded as a nonpathogen whose numbers increase the more unhygienic the condition of the oral cavity.

There are two genera of free-living amebae, *Naegleria* and *Acanthamoeba*, that do not require an animal host but occasionally cause serious infections of humans, especially of the CNS.

Amebiasis and Amebic Dysentery

The term *amebiasis* generally indicates a condition caused by *E. histolytica*, the only frank pathogen of the amebae. *E. histolytica* is best known as the causal agent of *amebic dysentery*. The clinical response to *E. histolytica* infection, however, is variable.

Pathogenesis. Overt infections are in the forms of a *diarrhea* that tends to be protracted, *dysentery* of varying severity, *amebic abscesses* that form in various organs, and an *amebic granuloma* (*ameboma*).

INTESTINAL AMEBIASIS. The ameba exists largely as a commensal in the colon. There is some question as to whether the parasite initiates disease on its own or invades and causes disease once tissue is damaged by other means. *E. histolytica* has gelatinase, hyaluronidase, amylase, and trypsin activities, but how these enzymes relate to the invasive behavior has not been clearly demonstrated. The species name implies tissue-dissolving activity. Whatever the pathogenic mechanism, once *E. histolytica* has breached the intestinal mucosa, it spreads and undermines the subjoined areas. Tissue sections of such affected areas reveal a flask-shaped configuration, giving rise to the term *flask-shaped ulcers*. The formation of multiple and coalescing ulcers causes a violent dysentery with stools that typically contain blood-stained mucus. Clinically, intestinal amebiasis can easily be mistaken for ulcerative colitis. Sometimes a space-occupying lesion in the form of a granuloma (more specifically called an ameboma) occurs in the cecum or colon. Clinically and radiologically it may resemble cancer.

EXTRAINTESTINAL AMEBIASIS. The amebae may penetrate all the way through the intestinal wall and be carried via mesenteric venules and lymphatic vessels to other organs to cause extraintestinal amebiasis. The organ most likely to be so affected, usually by *amebic abscesses*, is the liver. Amebic liver abscess is a serious public health problem in developing nations. Other sites of amebic invasion are the lungs, skin, brain, and pericardium.

Laboratory Diagnosis. Bloody mucous stools that are examined within a half hour after evacuation may contain the living, motile trophozoites. Trophozoites may also be found in ulcer scrapings, rectal biopsy specimens, and aspirated material. Cysts may be found in formed stools. The diagnosis of extraintestinal amebiasis rests on the clinical evaluation along with laboratory findings. Cultivation of aspirated material and especially serological tests such as the ELISA test are used in the diagnosis of extraintestinal amebiasis.

Epidemiology. According to the World Health Organization, an estimated 10 percent of the world population is infected with *E. histolytica*. The greater incidences and the more serious infections are usually found in warmer climates and in communities and institutions where personal hygiene is neglected or is difficult to supervise. It is estimated that there is a 3 to 5 percent prevalence rate in the United States. The majority of infected individuals have no clinical manifestations. These persons are important to the continued transmission, however, in their role as cyst passers. Transmission is usually attributable to poor sanitary conditions, but in the United States person-to-person contact is probably a common mode, especially among male homosexuals. Most epidemics in the United States are traceable to fecal contamination of a faulty water supply system. The level of chlorination used in most municipal water supplies does not destroy the cysts. Poor sanitation, including the use of "night soil" (human excreta) as fertilizer, is mainly responsible for the high incidence of amebiasis in the tropics.

Treatment and Control. A variety of chemotherapeutic agents are used to treat amebiasis: emetine, iodine-containing compounds such as iodoquinol (diiodohydroxyquin) and chiniofon, tetracyclines, and chloroquine. The choice of drug is determined by the clinical type of the infection. Metronidazole or iodoquinol is applicable to the various types of infections: asymptomatic, mild to severe intestinal disease, and hepatic abscesses. Diloxanide furoate (furamide) is used for asymptomatic cyst passers.

Control of *E. histolytica* infections depends on improved hygiene, sanitation, and water treatment; isolation of patients; and education about the risks of anal-oral contact.

Primary Amebic Meningoencephalitis

The causative agent of primary amebic meningoencephalitis (PAM) is *Naegleria fowleri*. It is a free-living, soil-water ameboflagellate (an ameba that can transform into a flagellate). The infection typically is seen in young, healthy persons and *usually is associated with a history of swimming in warm bodies of fresh water* that are either natural or man-made. The parasite gains entrance to the brain via the nasal passages and from there travels along olfactory nerve fibers through the cribriform plate to the olfactory bulbs. Spread within the gray matter and multiplication of the parasite are rapid, and unless early diagnosis is made and treatment initiated, the patient dies within a week to 10 days from the time of exposure. Inflammation and tissue damage can lead to severe frontal headache; disturbances of smell, taste, and vision; anorexia; nausea, fever; and stiff neck. The patient may experience or exhibit convulsions, irrational behavior, seizures, and coma. All in all, the patient's condition resembles fulminant septic meningitis. Diagnosis is made by identifying the living or stained amebae in cerebrospinal fluid or in postmortem brain tissue. No satisfactory treatment for PAM exists. One patient, an 8-year-old girl from California who swam in a hot springs pool that had a water temperature of 105°F, was diagnosed early and was successfully treated with amphotericin B, miconazole, and rifampin.

Acanthamoebiasis

Members of the genus *Acanthamoeba* and of other genera of free-living soil amebae are facultatively parasitic, especially in individuals whose health is compromised. The cysts of the amebae probably enter and infect a human host via the lungs, conjunctivae, or skin. The infection may spread from those sites to other tissues. Infections usually are in the form of chronic granulomatous abscesses. Occasionally spread is to the CNS, where the condition is called *granulomatous amoebic encephalitis (GAE)*. Foci of necrotizing encephalitis develop in days to months with manifestations such as headaches, mental status alterations, and seizures.

Acanthamoeba keratitis is a rare, serious infection of the cornea (see Boxed Essay, p. 812.)

MASTIGOPHORA—THE FLAGELLATED PROTOZOA

The Mastigophora at some time in their life cycle have whip-like flagella as locomotory organelles. Some possess undulating membranes. Parasitic flagellates appear in the oral cavity (*Trichomonas tenax*), in the intestine (*Giardia lamblia, Trichomonas hominis, Chilomastix mesnili, Enteromonas hominis, Retortamonas intestinalis*), in the genitourinary tract (*Trichomonas vaginalis*), and in the circulation and tissues (the hemoflagellates and tissue flagellates of the genera *Trypanosoma* and *Leishmania*).

Giardiasis (Lambliasis)

Giardia lamblia is a flagellated intestinal protozoon that was regarded as a borderline pathogen for many years. It is now known to cause significant morbidity. It is the *causal agent of the most common waterborne diarrheal disease* in the United States. The trophozoite, when viewed from the ventral side, is a pear-shaped organism 9 to 16 μm in length, 9 to 12 μm in width, and 2 to 5 μm in thickness (Fig. 33-3). It contains four pairs of flagella; two prominent nuclei; a stiff, rod-like structure, the axostyle; and an anterior, oval, concave, adhesive (sucking) disk that occupies most of the flat ventral surface. It has a falling-leaf type of movement. The tough-walled cyst, which is the infective stage, is an ovoid form 9 μm by 12 μm containing two to four nuclei and

Fig. 33-3. *Giardia lamblia.*

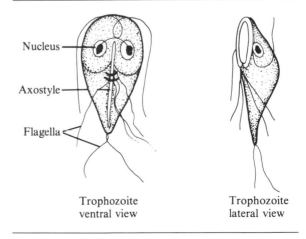

Nucleus

Axostyle

Flagella

Trophozoite
ventral view

Trophozoite
lateral view

ACANTHAMOEBA *KERATITIS IN SOFT CONTACT LENS WEARERS*

Within a 9-month period, from mid-1985 to February 1986, the CDC received reports of 24 cases of *Acanthamoeba* keratitis, a much higher number than previously reported during similar time periods.

Acanthamoeba keratitis is a serious infection of the cornea caused by amoebae of the genus *Acanthamoeba*. The mechanism by which *Acanthamoeba* infects the human cornea is unknown. Historically, the infection has been associated with penetrating corneal trauma. More recently, an association with contact lens wear has become apparent.

The risk factors identified in this study suggest deviations from contact lens wear and care procedures recommended by lens manufacturers and health-care professionals. Current United States Food and Drug Administration licensure of commercial salt tablets (used to make homemade saline solution) applies only to using the saline solutions before and during thermal disinfection of lenses, not as a postdisinfection rinse or wetting agent. Thermal disinfection of soft contact lenses is effective in killing *Acanthamoeba* trophozoites and cysts, suggesting that use of homemade saline solutions before and during the thermal disinfection phase is safe.

Persons wearing contact lenses should be reminded to adhere closely to recommended contact lens wear and care procedures. These include using sterile solutions after disinfecting lenses, using solutions and disinfection methods appropriate for the specific lens type, cleaning and disinfecting lenses each time they are removed, and hand washing before handling lenses. Contact lens wearers who do not comply with these recommendations may be increasing their risk for infection with *Acanthamoeba* and other organisms. As a result, they could develop partial or total loss of vision.

From *M.M.W.R.* 36:397, 1987.

many of the structures that are seen in the tro-phozoite.

Pathogenesis. The spectrum of infection ranges from asymptomatic colonization to a severe per-sistent malabsorption syndrome (Table 33-2). The parasite is found in the upper part of the du-odenum and jejunum. It does not ordinarily in-vade the tissues but is a lumen dweller. Watery diarrhea, flatulence, and abdominal cramps are common complaints in acute infections. In sub-acute and chronic infections there may be epi-sodic diarrhea; malodorous, bulky, greasy stools; abdominal distention; flatus (gassiness); loss of appetite; and weight loss. The *malabsorption syndrome*, in which there is interference with the absorption of fats, carbohydrates, and vitamins, includes wasting, reduction in serum albumin (hypoalbuminemia), diarrhea, and steatorrhea (high fat content of feces). Possible mechanisms through which *Giardia* damages intestinal epi-thelial cells include formation of a tightly joined network of parasites on the mucosal surface that interferes with the passage of nutrients, inflam-mation that leads to cell injury, damage to mi-crovilli by the overlying trophozoites (electron microscopical studies show deformation of mi-crovilli—Fig. 33-4), alteration of bacterial flora that are coinfectors, production of as yet un-identified toxins, and competition for nutrients.

Laboratory Diagnosis. Diagnosis is made by find-ing trophozoites or cysts in feces, intestinal as-pirates, or material retrieved via the Entero-Test method (see Identification of Intestinal Parasites earlier in this chapter). The trophozoite is found in feces only in cases of profuse diarrhea because this more delicate form is usually destroyed in the sojourn from the upper intestine. The phy-sician should consider the possibility of giardiasis in patients who have diarrhea that persists longer than 1 week, especially if the diarrhea is accom-panied by any two of the following: foul-smelling stools, bloating, abdominal cramps, loss of ap-petite, or loss of weight. A history of the patient's travels, a history of drinking untreated water from surface bodies of water, and community outbreaks of diarrhea should alert the physician to rule out giardiasis.

Epidemiology. Infection occurs via the ingestion of cysts from fecally contaminated sources. Known routes of transmission to humans are con-taminated water and food and person-to-person spread. Waterborne outbreaks have occurred via community water supplies in over two dozen mu-nicipalities that use surface water sources. Fail-ures in the filtration aspect of the water purifi-cation systems appear to be the determining fac-tor in failure to eliminate the parasite. Chlorine levels routinely used to disinfect municipal water supplies (0.4 mg/L free chlorine) do not kill *Giar-dia* cysts in the usual exposure times. Among wild animals *Giardia* has been found in beavers, muskrats, and water moles. These animal sources probably explain how it is that back-packers and mountain climbers who drink from mountain streams acquire *Giardia* infections. A human source in such areas is remote. Trans-mission through person-to-person contact is sug-gested by the observations of high frequency of giardiasis among children in day-care centers, by the 15 to 30 percent incidence in children below the age of 2 in developing countries, and by the incidence in promiscuous male homosexuals. It is estimated that 2 to 20 percent of the population in the United States harbor this protozoan, de-pending on the age group and community sur-veyed.

Treatment and Control. *Quinacrine hydrochloride* is the drug of choice. Alternative reliable drugs are metronidazole and furazolidone for children. Adequate treatment with these drugs usually re-sults in prompt resolution of symptoms. In sit-uations where giardiasis is transmitted by con-taminated water, prevention of outbreaks re-quires proper maintenance of community water supplies. In situations of person-to-person con-tact, control includes screening of food handlers, routine stool examinations, followed by treat-ment, where outbreaks occur among the insti-

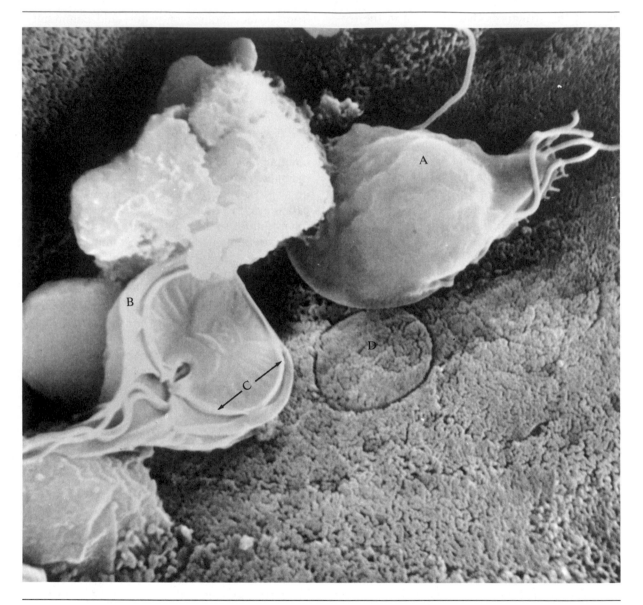

Fig. 33-4. Scanning electron micrograph of *Giardia muris* trophozoites in a mouse intestine. A. Dorsal view. B. Ventral view. C. Adhesive disk on the ventral surface. D. Circular mark left by the adhesive disk on the columnar cell microvilli of intestine (×8026). (From R. L. Owen, P. C. Nemanic, and D. P. Stevens. Ultrastructural observations of giardiasis in a murine model. *Gastroenterology* 76:757, 1979.)

tutionalized, and instructions about and insistence on good hygienic practices among the institutionalized and their caregivers.

Trichomoniasis
Trichomonads are globular protozoa possessing three to five anterior flagella (see Fig. 33-5).

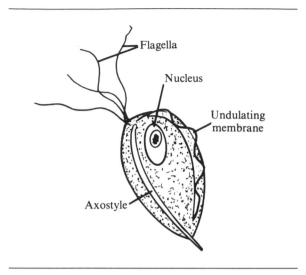

Flagella

Nucleus

Undulating membrane

Axostyle

Fig. 33-5. Trichomonad.

There is a single prominent oval nucleus. An internal, stiff, rod-like structure called an axostyle runs the length of the protozoon and emerges posteriorly as a caudal spine. An undulating membrane, a thin filmy structure, extends along the longitudinal axis. Trichomonads appear only in the trophozoite form, the transmissible form. Three morphologically similar *Trichomonas* species are found in humans: *T. tenax, T. hominis*, and *T. vaginalis*. Differentiation among the three is possible on morphological and cultural grounds. Each has a specific habitat in humans.

Trichomonas tenax *and* Trichomonas hominis. *T. tenax* and *Entamoeba gingivalis* are the only animal parasites that have the oral cavity as their regular habitat. They apparently occur in only a low percentage of healthy mouths. Most investigators regard them as scavengers or commensals that flourish best when there is disease of the periodontium, the supporting soft tissue of the teeth. Neither forms demonstrable cysts, and neither appears to have tissue-invasive tendencies. Transmission probably occurs through saliva-soiled fomites (e.g., tableware) and through kissing.

T. hominis, found in the human intestinal tract, is clinically unimportant.

Trichomonas vaginalis. *T. vaginalis* is regarded as a pathogen and causes an estimated 2 to 3 million cases of sexually transmitted disease annually. Hygienic practices and promiscuity have a bearing on the incidence of infection.

PATHOGENESIS. *T. vaginalis* is one of the three main causes of vaginitis, the other two being the bacterium *Gardnerella vaginalis*, which causes a frothy discharge and a fishy odor, and the endogenous yeast, *Candida albicans*, which causes vulvovaginal irritation with itching and a curd-like discharge. *T. vaginalis* infections are normally limited to the vagina, cervix, urethra, and vulva. Only about 15 percent of those infected experience symptoms. Vaginal discharge is the most common complaint and is often associated with burning, itching, or chafing. A thick, yellow, blood-tinged discharge may accompany a heavy infection. Cervical involvement may cause dyspareunia (painful coitus). There may be pruritus and chafing of the vulva.

Men, usually symptomless, may have urethritis, epididymitis, or prostatovesiculitis. They may note a slight discharge, especially with the first urination in the morning. There may be dysuria (painful urination) and increased urination.

LABORATORY DIAGNOSIS. *Saline wet mounts* are prepared from genitourinary tract specimens and examined microscopically for the typical jerky, swift movements of the living trichomonad. The edges of the undulating membrane look like a cogwheel as they come into and move out of focus. Stained trichomonads are not uncommonly discovered in routine *Papanicolaou (Pap) smears* prepared for cancer detection.

EPIDEMIOLOGY. Transmission is generally by sexual intercourse, although it can occur via fomites such as unclean toilet facilities and contaminated garments.

TREATMENT AND CONTROL. The approval of metronidazole in 1963 revolutionized treatment. Metronidazole is taken orally, and sometimes a metronidazole-containing vaginal suppository is prescribed simultaneously. Regular sex partners of women with vaginal trichomoniasis should also be treated with metronidazole.

Trypanosomiasis

There are seven species of blood and tissue flagellate protozoa (collectively referred to as *hemoflagellates*) that infect humans. They appear in two genera: *Trypanosoma* and *Leishmania*. These parasites live alternately in vertebrate hosts and in bloodsucking insects where they undergo a cyclic development. There are four distinct cyclic morphological types: the *amastigote* (leishmanial form), the *promastigote* (leptomonad form), the *epimastigote* (crithidial form), and the *trypomastigote* (trypanosomal form) (Fig. 33-6).

African Trypanosomiasis (African Sleeping Sickness). The Trypanosoma species that is medically and economically important is *T. brucei*. It contains three subspecies: *T. brucei gambiense* (chronic sleeping sickness in humans), *T. brucei rhodesiense* (acute sleeping sickness in humans), and *T. brucei brucei* (nagana in cattle).

Fig. 33-6. The body forms of members of the genera *Trypanosoma* and *Leishmania*.

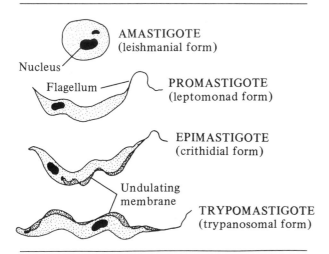

AMASTIGOTE (leishmanial form)

Nucleus

Flagellum

PROMASTIGOTE (leptomonad form)

EPIMASTIGOTE (crithidial form)

Undulating membrane

TRYPOMASTIGOTE (trypanosomal form)

PATHOGENESIS. The parasites first lodge in the local tissues where they were introduced by the bite of the tsetse fly. After 2 to 3 days there is local inflammation and itching, followed about 4 days later by the development of a chancre. Approximately a week or two after infection the parasite is detectable in the blood. Episodes of parasitemia that last for 2 to 3 days follow at intervals of 2 to 10 days. Headaches, joint pain, malaise, and enlarged lymph nodes and spleen accompany the recurring episodes of parasitemia. The second stage of the disease—the sleeping sickness phase—involves the CNS. Insomnia, irritability, personality changes, and decreasing mental acuity precede a gradual loss of CNS function. In the advanced stages the victim suffers convulsions and becomes somnolent and comatose before eventually expiring from malnutrition and secondary infection. Untreated rhodesiense infections run a course from weeks to months; gambiense, from months to years.

The relapsing parasitemia and the longevity of infections despite an elevated IgM response by the patient were for many years unexplained. Observations on *T. b. brucei* infections in experimental animals provided the answer. *Trypanosoma* parasites evade existing antibodies by a continual variation of surface coat glycoprotein antigens. Many antigenic types sequentially derived from the same organisms have been detected. The variation is believed to be due to gene rearrangement, just as occurs for antibody diversity, rather than to random mutation.

LABORATORY DIAGNOSIS. A presumptive diagnosis is made on the basis of geographical history and clinical signs and symptoms. A clinical sign, named *Winterbottom's sign*, is enlarged lymph nodes of the posterior cervical triangle. In the laboratory, stained preparations of blood, spinal fluid, and lymph node and bone marrow aspirates are examined for the typical spindle-shaped parasites. If the smears are negative, 1 ml of the patient's blood is injected intraperitoneally into rats and their blood is examined in 2 weeks for the parasites. A variety of serological tests can be used to test for IgM levels. Indirect fluorescent antibody testing is the most commonly used technique.

EPIDEMIOLOGY. *Tsetse flies* transmit rhodesiense and gambiense to humans. A wide range of wild game animals and domestic animals serve as reservoir hosts for *T. b. rhodesiense*. *T. b. gambiense* supposedly is not maintained in nature by animal reservoir hosts, so its cycle involves only humans and tsetse flies.

TREATMENT AND CONTROL. Suramin sodium administered intravenously is used for the bloodstream and lymphatic stage and melarsoprol for late disease with CNS involvement. Control consists of medical surveillance, chemoprophylaxis, and vector control through the use of insecticides and modification of the tsetse fly principal habitat, namely, the dense vegetation along rivers and in forests.

American Trypanosomiasis (Chagas' Disease)

PATHOGENESIS. The parasites multiply in the tissues rather than in the blood. In the tissues (reticuloendothelial system [RES], heart, and CNS) they multiply in the leishmanial form, whereas in the blood they appear in the trypanosomal form. Infections are usually subclinical. In a small percentage of cases, usually in children, infection takes an acute form. The early lesion, usually on the face, is called a *primary chagoma*. It is often accompanied by unilateral palpebral edema (swelling of one eyelid). The *palpebral edema* of Chagas' disease is called *Romana's sign*. About 5 percent of acute infections are fatal, usually because of infections of the heart or CNS. It is not unusual for the infection to remain asymptomatic for years and then to become gradually manifest as chronic Chagas' disease. The parasites localize in various tissues and organs. Infections of the heart, a typical site of localization, are a leading cause of cardiac disease and sudden death in endemic areas. Grossly enlarged hearts and congestive heart failure are characteristics of Chagas' disease. Another manifestation of chronic disease is dilation and enlargement of the esophagus and colon (megaesophagus and megacolon, respectively).

LABORATORY DIAGNOSIS. A positive geographical history, residence under conditions in which transmission is known to occur, and typical clinical signs and symptoms suggest American trypanosomiasis. The trypanosomal morphological form may be observed in stained blood films obtained during the febrile stages of infection. The leishmanial trypanosomal morphological form may be observed in stained blood films obtained during the febrile stages of infection. The leishmanial morphological form may be found within macrophages that are aspirated from RES tissue. Cultivation on modified blood agar or infection of mice and serological tests are also employed. A definitive diagnosis is not easily accomplished. The parasite is scarce in circulating blood, the most accessible specimen. An indirect technique, called *xenodiagnosis*, is used in areas where trypanosomiasis is endemic. Laboratory-reared reduviid bugs (see under Epidemiology below) that are free of *T. cruzi* parasites ("clean bugs") are allowed to feed on the patient. Ten days later the rectal contents of the bugs are examined for active stages of the parasite. The sensitivity of xenodiagnosis is only 50 percent in those with chronic infections.

EPIDEMIOLOGY. *Trypanosoma cruzi* is transmitted by various species of *reduviid bugs*, which are known as assassin bugs or kissing bugs in the United Sates, as barbieros in Brazil, and as vinchucas in Spanish-speaking South America. They are called kissing bugs presumably because of their predilection for alighting on the face and lips. Human beings, domesticated animals, and wild animals are the most important vertebrate hosts. Cats and dogs serve as the main reservoirs for humans. The insect vectors and infected raccoons and opossums have been found in the southwestern and southeastern United States. It is estimated that 10 to 12 million people in South America and Central America are infected. The lower economic groups who dwell in thatched adobe huts are the population group most likely to be affected, because the adobe huts provide breeding places for the insect vectors.

TREATMENT AND CONTROL. Nifurtimox and benznidazole appear to eradicate the parasites in the blood and prevent spread from tissue to tissue. Treatment is not completely satisfactory. Education, construction of reduviid-proof housing, and spraying for insect control are among the preventive measures being pursued.

Leishmaniasis

In definitive hosts, such as humans, *Leishmania* species appear as oval parasites 3 to 5 μm in length. They are intracellular parasites of macrophages. In culture they are motile flagellates. Transmission is predominantly by *sandflies* (*Phlebotomus* and *Lutzomyia* flies), the intermediate host. Reservoir hosts include dogs, cats, wild rodents, horses, sheep, and cattle. Four morphologically indistinguishable species—*L. donovani, L. tropica, L. mexicana*, and *L. braziliensis*—infect humans, producing visceral leishmaniasis, cutaneous leishmaniasis, and mucocutaneous leishmaniasis. There is considerable overlap or intergradation of clinical manifestations caused by the four species. Diagnosis of leishmaniasis is made by demonstrating the organisms in stained smears from lesions or in biopsy specimens. Aspirated specimens from bone or lymph nodes are cultured on diphasic blood agar or injected intraperitoneally into hamsters. Antimony gluconate is the drug of choice for all four types of leishmanial infection.

Visceral Leishmaniasis (Kala-Azar). Visceral leishmaniasis, or kala-azar, is found in foci in most tropical and subtropical countries. It is a diffuse parasitization of the entire reticulo-endothelial system, usually caused by *L. donovani*. Phagocytic cells are stuffed with the amastigote parasites, bringing about enlargement of the spleen (Fig. 33-7, panel 5), liver, lymph nodes, and other parasitized tissues and organs. There is an accompanying reduction of neutrophils (granulocytopenia), rendering the patient subject to intercurrent infections of the lungs and digestive tract that may be fatal.

Cutaneous Leishmaniasis. In cutaneous leishmaniasis (also called Oriental sore), an ulcerating lesion develops at the site of each inoculating insect bite (Fig. 33-7, panel 1). The ulcer may become secondarily infected. A permanent depigmented scar develops 9 to 12 months later in untreated cases. *L. tropica* is associated with the Old World infection; *L. mexicana*, with the New World version.

Mucocutaneous Leishmaniasis. The primary lesion of mucocutaneous leishmaniasis (also called espundia and chichlero ulcer) resembles the lesion of cutaneous leishmaniasis. The parasite may metastasize to secondary foci, particularly to mucocutaneous junctions—for example, in the vicinity of the nares. Lesions of the oronasal mucosa also occur (Fig. 33-7, panel 4). The lesions that develop at the secondary foci are often extensive, erosive, destructive, and disfiguring. *L. braziliensis* is the species responsible.

CILIATA—THE CILIATED PROTOZOA

The organelles for locomotion of the Ciliata are short, bristle-like cilia.

Balantidiasis (Ciliary Dysentery)

Balantidium coli is the only ciliated protozoon that is a bona fide pathogen of humans. It is the largest protozoon to infect humans.

B. coli is a common parasite of swine and of several lower primates. From 60 to 90 percent of hogs harbor *B. coli* or *B. suis*. The latter, which does not infect humans, is the more common in hogs. Infection of humans is rare. The chief symptom is *diarrhea* in varying severity. Occasionally a dysentery, termed balantidial dysentery or ciliary dysentery, develops. Diagnosis is based on the identification of the characteristic trophozoites and cysts in diarrheic or formed stools. Iodoquinol and oxytetracyclines are used for treatment.

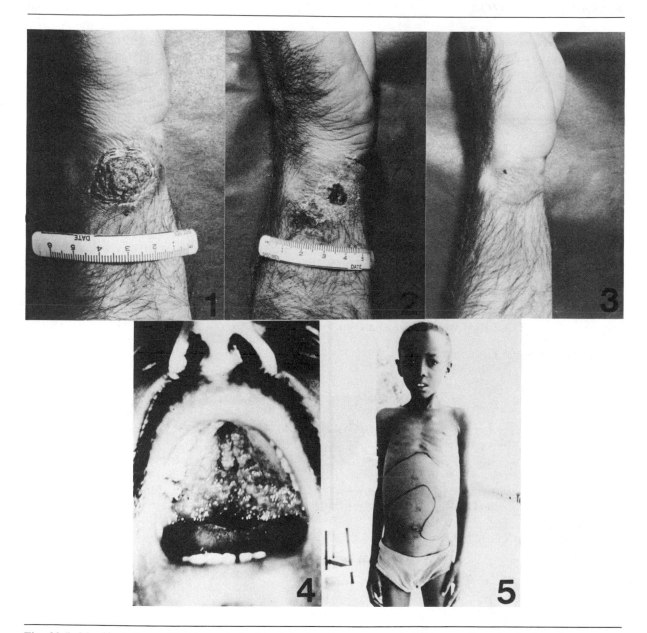

Fig. 33-7. Manifestations of leishmaniasis. Panel 1: American cutaneous lesion on the wrist before therapy. Panel 2: Same lesion after 20 days of Pentostam therapy. Panel 3: Same lesion six weeks after the end of therapy. Panel 4: Mucosal lesion of the pharynx. Panel 5: Visceral lesion before therapy. Hepatosplenomegaly is outlined. (From J. Berman, *Rev. Infect. Dis.* 10[3]:560, 1988.)

SPOROZOA—THE SPOROZOITE-FORMING PROTOZOA

Sporozoa have no special organelles of locomotion. They have a complex life cycle that includes sexual and asexual generations. The most important sporozoite (animal spore)-forming genera are *Plasmodium*, which contains species that cause malaria, and *Toxoplasma*.

Plasmodiasis—Malaria

At least four species of *Plasmodium* infect humans: *P. vivax, P. malariae, P. falciparum,* and *P. ovale*. Essentially, most of the information and incidence relate to the first three species. Falciparum malaria is regarded as the most serious form of malaria.

Life Cycle. A knowledge of the malaria life cycle (Fig. 33-8) aids in understanding the clinical events, treatment, and control measures. The two phases in the life cycle of the malarial parasite are sporogony and schizogony. The sexual phase, *sporogony*, occurs in the *female Anopheles mosquito*. It is initiated when the mosquito, while consuming a "blood meal" from an infected individual, takes in red blood cells that contain the male and female gametocytes of the malaria parasite (Fig. 33-8, lower right). The gametocytes mature in the midgut of the mosquito and form *zygotes*. Growth results in the formation of *oocysts*, which come to locate on the outside of the mosquito stomach. Hundreds of *sporozoites* develop in each oocyst, whence they are released into the body cavity. Eventually they reach the salivary glands.

Fig. 33-8. Malaria life cycle.

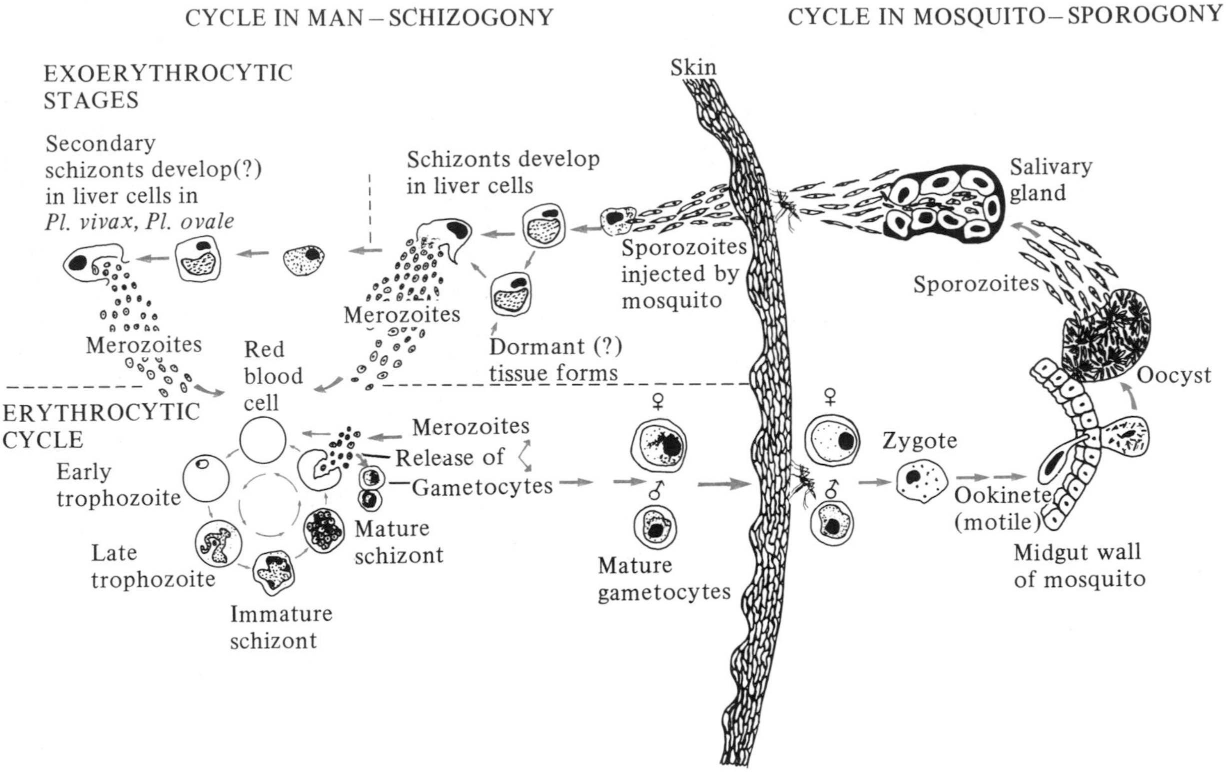

CYCLE IN MAN—SCHIZOGONY

CYCLE IN MOSQUITO—SPOROGONY

EXOERYTHROCYTIC STAGES

Secondary schizonts develop(?) in liver cells in *Pl. vivax, Pl. ovale*

Schizonts develop in liver cells

Skin

Salivary gland

Sporozoites injected by mosquito

Sporozoites

Merozoites

Dormant (?) tissue forms

Oocyst

Merozoites

Red blood cell

ERYTHROCYTIC CYCLE

Early trophozoite

Merozoites Release of Gametocytes

Zygote

Ookinete (motile)

Late trophozoite

Mature schizont

Mature gametocytes

Midgut wall of mosquito

Immature schizont

The asexual phase, known as *schizogony*, takes place in the vertebrate host. It is initiated when the sporozoite-laden saliva of the mosquito is introduced at the time of the mosquito bite. There are two stages in the development of malaria once the sporozoites enter the body. Plasmodial infection is primarily an infection of the red blood cells. Before the infection of the red blood cells there is a liver stage; it is termed the preerythrocyte stage, and it may include exoerythrocytic cycles (see Fig. 33-8, upper left). The parasites are called *cryptozoites* (hidden forms) in the liver stage. The entrance of the sporozoites into the liver cells begins the incubation period, which lasts 10 to 28 days, depending on the plasmodial species. *Schizonts* are formed. The liver cells rupture, yielding cytoplasm-enveloped schizonts (now called *merozoites*) that infect either other liver cells (to produce the exoerythrocytic cycle) or red blood cells. In *falciparum* malaria there is only one preerythrocytic liver cell infection. In *malariae* and *vivax* malaria the liver cell infection can be repeated in the exoerythrocytic cycle. Knowledge of the exoerythrocytic cycle is important in chemotherapy for malaria.

The release of merozoites from the liver cells and their entry into red blood cells initiates the erythrocytic stage (see Fig. 33-8, lower left). The merozoites develop into trophozoites, which eventually segment to give rise to a new crop of merozoites, The merozoites infect other red blood cells. In falciparum malaria as many as 40 percent of the red blood cells become infected. The release of the merozoites usually becomes synchronized; that is, infected red blood cells rupture at approximately the same time. The paroxysms of chills and fever experienced by the patient are closely related to that release. During the erythrocyte sequences some of the trophozoites develop into gametocytes. The ingestion of the gametocytes by the mosquito initiates the sporogenous phase.

Pathogenesis. The infected individual experiences the paroxysms of malaria in conjunction with the synchronous release of the merozoites. In vivax malaria synchronous showers of merozoites are released every 48 hours. Vivax malaria is therefore called *tertian malaria* because the interval spans three calendar days. *Falciparum* malaria is also a tertian malaria, although the interval may be less than 48 hours, giving rise to the sometimes-applied term *subtertian malaria*. Malaria caused by *P. malariae* is called *quartan malaria* because the episodes occur every 72 hours. *Vivax malaria* is furthermore called benign tertian malaria and falciparum malaria malignant tertian, reflecting the difference in the severity of the disease caused by the two.

In a malaria attack the patient initially experiences chills for 15 to 60 minutes coincident with the release of a brood of merozoites. This is usually accompanied by headache, nausea, and vomiting. Succeeding the chills is a febrile stage of several hours' duration. Temperatures sometimes spike to 105°F or higher. Profuse sweating concludes the paroxysm. The exhausting episode induces sleep, from which the patient awakens with a feeling of comparative well-being. The infections may be asymptomatic, severely enfeebling, or fatal. When the red blood cells rupture, malarial pigments, hemoglobin, and metabolites of the parasite are also released. These products are taken up, especially by the RES, and account for the marked pigmentation and enlargement seen in the spleen, liver, lymph nodes, and bone marrow. The parasitized red blood cells become sticky and plug up the smaller vessels, especially in falciparum malaria. The obstructing action of the "sludge blood" has a variety of effects: tissue anoxia (lack of oxygen) and necrosis, bursting of vessels, electrolyte imbalance, and other vessel-associated pathology. Many organs may be affected. Some of the more dramatic pathological changes associated with malaria occur in the brain and the kidneys.

Laboratory Diagnosis. The definitive diagnosis of malaria rests on discovery of the typical parasite forms in stained blood smears. The experienced malariologist is able to differentiate the plasmodial species because of differences in trophozoite forms, malarial pigment, numbers of merozoites, character of the infected red blood cells, and other differences.

Epidemiology. Malaria is one of the truly major infectious diseases of humankind. Although it is limited largely to the tropics and the subtropics, 50 percent of the world's population reside in malarious regions. It is estimated that more than 200 million persons have malaria. According to the WHO, malaria is responsible annually for the death of 1 million children below the age of 5 in Africa. The incidence of malaria in the United States and Puerto Rico among civilians showed an upward trend from 139 cases in 1969 to 1,023 cases in 1988. Most civilian cases are imported through travelers and immigrants. Malaria transmitted by drug addict practices falls into the category of *transfusion malaria.* Such an infection, incidentally, occurs only in the erythrocytic cycle; that is, there is no liver stage to the infection.

Treatment and Control. Chemotherapy for malaria is complex. It may be applied for prophylaxis, for the suppression or prevention of an attack in an infected individual, or for cure. Two mainstays of malaria chemotherapy are chloroquine, a 4-aminoquinoline (used for the erythrocytic stage) and primaquine phosphate, an 8-aminoquinoline (used for the exoerythrocytic stage). It is necessary to eliminate the tissue phase in malaria in types in which the parasite persists in the liver because the plasmodia that survive in the liver can reestablish clinical malaria. Chloroquine-resistant strains, notably strains of *P. falciparum,* pose continuing challenges. The treatment of resistant strains consists of quinine sulfate, pyrimethamine, and sulfadiazine. Mefloquine is recommended as a prophylactic measure for travelers at risk of infection with chloroquine-resistant *P. falciparum.*

Considerable efforts are being made in a network of more than 30 malaria research centers to develop an antimalaria vaccine. A successful vaccine would do much to reduce the immensity of malaria control problems, which include the parasites' resistance to chemotherapeutic agents, the resistance of mosquito vectors to insecticides, and the cost of current control measures. As of early 1990, experimental malaria vaccines, many of which were developed using molecular biology techniques, have not been effective. Among the difficulties in developing an effective vaccine is the surprising degree of immunological variability of the parasite's antigens.

Mosquito control measures include the destruction of mosquito larval forms, the elimination of mosquito breeding places, and the use of netting and repellents.

Toxoplasmosis

Toxoplasma gondii occurs in all hosts as *tachyzoites* (rapidly dividing forms) that accumulate in host cells and as *bradyzoites* (slowly dividing forms) that accumulate within a parasitic membrane called a cyst. Tachyzoites are often crescent- or bow-shaped (*toxon:* bow or arc) organisms, 4 to 8 μm in length and 2 to 3 μm in width, with the anterior end pointed and the other end round or blunted. The bradyzoite-containing cysts are from 5 μm to 1000 μm in size and may house hundreds of parasites. The cysts are found mainly in the brain, eye, and muscles, where usually they persist harmlessly after the host has acquired immunity.

Life Cycle. Members of the cat family (Felidae) serve as the *definitive host* in the life cycle of *Toxoplasma* organisms (Fig. 33-9). Cats are the only animals in which oocysts are formed. Cats become infected by eating warm-blooded animals such as mice and birds or by ingestion of oocysts from cat feces. After ingestion sporogony and gametogony occur, leading to the formation of oocysts in the epithelium of the cat ileum. The zygote-containing oocysts are shed in the feces. In 3 to 4 days (under suitable climatic conditions) the zygote divides into two sporoblasts, each of which gives rise to four sporozoites. Each mature oocyst thus contains eight infective sporozoites. The mature oocyst can survive for up to 18 months in nature. Cats probably shed oocysts

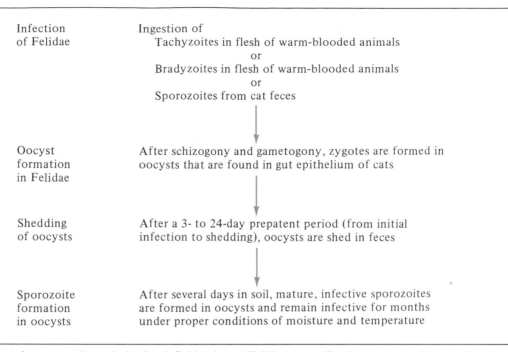

Infection of Felidae	Ingestion of Tachyzoites in flesh of warm-blooded animals or Bradyzoites in flesh of warm-blooded animals or Sporozoites from cat feces
Oocyst formation in Felidae	After schizogony and gametogony, zygotes are formed in oocysts that are found in gut epithelium of cats
Shedding of oocysts	After a 3- to 24-day prepatent period (from initial infection to shedding), oocysts are shed in feces
Sporozoite formation in oocysts	After several days in soil, mature, infective sporozoites are formed in oocysts and remain infective for months under proper conditions of moisture and temperature

Fig. 33-9. *Toxoplasma gondii* cycle in the definitive host. (Felidae = cat family.)

only once in their lives for a period of about 2 weeks. They appear to be resistant to reinfection. One authority estimated that 30 to 60 percent of adult cats harbor tissue cysts and that as few as 1 percent of domestic cats are shedding oocysts at any one time. A single cat may excrete millions of oocysts. Cats that hunt for all or some of their food are much more likely to be infected than cats that are highly domesticated (eat prepared diets, are declawed). Overt disease in cats includes pneumonia, hepatitis, pancreatitis, myocarditis, myositis, and other clinical conditions that result from the inflammation or necrotization of affected tissues. Congenitally acquired infection probably does not occur.

Pathogenesis. The most common outcome of primary infection in humans is asymptomatic infection (Fig. 33-10). A very small percentage of primarily infected individuals develop clinical disease, which is usually mild and rarely fatal. Most often an overt primary infection resembles mononucleosis: enlarged cervical lymph nodes, hepatosplenomegaly, myalgia, and atypical lymphocytes. Tissue cysts develop in various organs after primary infection and are accompanied by immunity. The tissue cysts are dormant (latent) and are probably of no further consequence except when reactivation occurs in immunocompromised transplant recipients, in those who are immunosuppressed because of cancer therapy, in victims of acquired immune deficiency syndrome (AIDS), and in those in whom cancer affects the lymphatic system. Reactivation can lead to *disseminated toxoplasmosis*, which can be fatal. Disseminated infection in transplant recipients may not necessarily be due to reactivation but could originate from parasites that are present in the transplant. These opportunistic infections often involve the CNS, which is the dominant site of *Toxoplasma* infection. The lungs and myocardium are other common targets of disseminated toxoplasmosis.

Transplacentally acquired (congenital) infec-

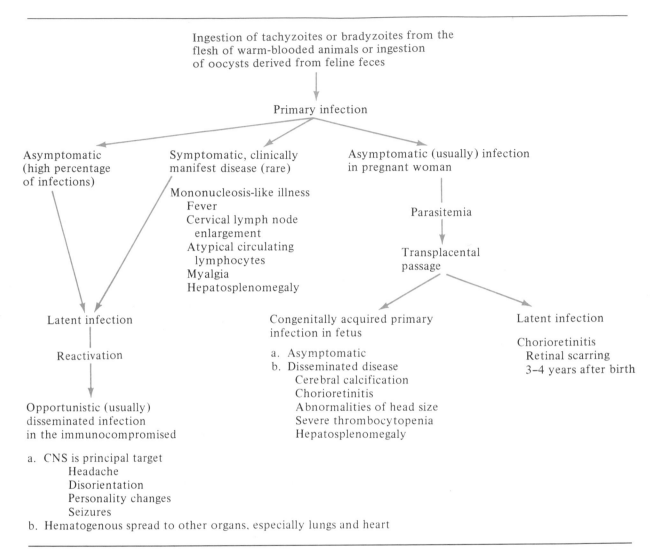

Fig. 33-10. *Toxoplasma gondii* infections in humans (an intermediate host). (CNS = central nervous system.)

tions can occur when a woman has a primary infection during pregnancy. The mother rarely is symptomatic but in the period when she has parasitemia, *Toxoplasma*-containing cysts may form in the placenta, where the parasite causes a generalized infection of the fetus. Infection of the fetus, according to one study, occurs in about 50 percent of cases in which the mother has a primary infection during pregnancy. A high per-

centage of children who were congenitally infected have no disease sequelae and remain well. It is estimated that less than 1 percent are born with clinical disease. A wide range of illnesses results from congenitally acquired toxoplasmosis. The seriously diseased have chorioretinitis, cerebral calcifications, hydrocephalus, severe thrombocytopenia, and convulsions. Mental retardation and grave visual handicaps are among the outcomes of these conditions. Some congenitally infected children who are normal at birth are latently infected and progressively develop retinal scarring around the age of 3 to 4 years.

Laboratory Diagnosis. Diagnosis may be made by identifying the organisms in body fluids and biopsy tissues or by infecting mice with material from appropriate specimens. Diagnosis is usually based on serological tests, however. The serological test specifically used in *Toxoplasma* infection is the Sabin-Feldman dye test, in which anti-*Toxoplasma* antibodies in the patient's serum prevent the uptake of methylene blue dye by living *Toxoplasma* test organisms. The living organisms are stained by the dye in the absence of specific antibodies. Other serological tests include direct and indirect fluorescent antibody, complement fixation, and enzyme-linked immunosorbent assay (ELISA).

Epidemiology. *T. gondii* infects a wide range of mammals and birds. Infection of humans is common, ranging from 5 to 80 percent in various populations through the world. Human infection is believed to stem primarily from the ingestion of raw or undercooked meat. Ingestion of oocysts is another route.

Treatment and Control. The drugs of choice are trisulfapyrimidines (combinations of sulfadiazine, sulfamerazine, and sulfamethazine) plus *pyrimethamine*. Spiramycin is an alternative drug that is especially prescribed during pregnancy to avoid the teratogenic effect of sulfadiazine and pyrimethamine.

Practical recommendations that can reduce the incidence of acquisition by as much as 90 percent are especially pertinent for pregnant women. The recommendations include careful handling of raw meat and the heating of meat to 150°F throughout, daily cleaning of cat litter boxes, disinfection of litter pans with boiling water, covering of sandboxes when they are not in use, wearing of gloves for gardening, and thorough washing of homegrown vegetables if they are to be eaten raw.

Babesiosis (Nantucket Fever)

There are 71 species of *Babesia* that infect wild and domesticated animals. Hard ticks are intermediate hosts and vectors. Texas cattle fever, an economically important disease, was first shown to be a babesiosis in 1893 by T. Smith and F. L. Kilbourne.

B. microti has been known for a long time as a parasite of a variety of animals. An endemic focus in 1975 on Nantucket Island and vicinity called attention to it as a human pathogen. Deer mice and field mice appear to be consistent reservoirs for *B. microti*. Human babesiosis resembles malaria clinically in its pathogenesis. The parasite propagates in red blood cells. The infection ranges from asymptomatic to severe and sometimes fatal disease. Signs and symptoms include chills, fever, drenching sweats, fatigue, nausea, myalgia, and emotional changes.

Cryptosporidiosis

Until recently cryptosporidiosis was considered a rare animal disease that was even more rarely transmitted to humans. *Cryptosporidium* species are now well known to veterinarians because they are important causes of gastroenteritis and diarrhea in animals (Fig. 33-11).

Pathogenesis. Cryptosporidiosis causes fatal, intractable watery diarrhea in compromised individuals, but a self-limited enteritis in normal hosts. The most common symptoms in normal hosts are profuse, watery diarrhea that lasts 3 to 12 days, nausea, vomiting, abdominal cramping, low-grade fever, and headache. The disease assumes particular severity in patients with AIDS. The average fluid loss in immunodeficient patients is about 3 to 6 liters per day, but as much as 17 liters per day has been reported.

Laboratory Diagnosis. *Cryptosporidium* can be found in the pharynx, esophagus, and stomach as well as the upper and lower intestine of immunodeficient patients. A modified acid-fast staining technique is used to detect and differ-

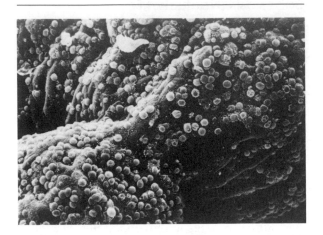

Fig. 33-11. SEM of tips of two fused atrophied villi from ileum of *Cryptosporidium*-infected calf. (From J. Heine, J. Pohlenz, H. Moon, and G. Woode. *J. Infect. Dis.* 150:768, 1984.)

entiate this protozoan from yeast. Fluorescent antibody techniques can also be applied to stool preparations to detect oocysts.

Epidemiology. Cryptosporidiosis is transmitted to humans by *oocysts* that are present in the feces of farm animals, mice, birds, and other animals. Several waterborne outbreaks have been documented. Human-to-human transmission is by direct or indirect contact with contaminated feces or by contact with respiratory secretions. Cryptosporidiosis is a frequent cause of diarrhea in children from developing countries.

Treatment. The prognosis for immunocompromised patients with cryptosporidiosis is poor. Spiromycin treatment is somewhat effective, but fewer than half the patients show an improvement. Supportive therapy, such as rehydration therapy and parenteral nutrition, is the only intervention available. Treatment usually is not necessary for immunocompetent individuals infected with the parasite.

THE NEMATHELMINTHES

Members of the animal phylum Nemathelminthes are referred to as roundworms because they are round or oval in cross section. Their body form is elongated and cylindrical, tapering at both ends. Unlike the earthworm, they are nonsegmented. They have a well-developed digestive tract. The sexes are separate. A summary of the helminth diseases described in this chapter is presented on page 827 (Table 33-3).

ASCARIASIS (ROUNDWORM INFECTION)

Ascaris lumbricoides is the largest intestinal nematode to infect humans. The adult worms are 8 to 12 inches long. They resemble the earthworm in size and overall configuration. The males, which are smaller than the females, have an incurved tail.

Pathogenesis
The larvae in ingested eggs hatch out in the duodenum, penetrate the mucosa, enter the blood and lymph vessels, and are transported to the lungs. At this juncture the larvae, if present in large enough numbers, elicit hemorrhage and inflammation to a degree sufficient to cause pneumonitis or an asthma-like response. Since *Ascaris* eggs are not found in the feces at this time, the pneumonitis is difficult to diagnose. From the lungs the larvae move up the respiratory tree, enter the esophagus, and are swallowed. Adult worms develop in the intestine, where they may cause vague abdominal symptoms. Because of their proclivity to probe and meander, they may obstruct the excretory ducts of the pancreas or the biliary tract, or they may appear in many other parts of the body. The majority of people rarely are symptomatic. Heavy infections, more

Table 33-3. Characteristics of Helminth Diseases

Disease name and agent	Clinical condition	Infective form; mode of transmission	Specimen examined; diagnostic form	Comments	Treatment
Ascariasis *Ascaris lumbricoides*	Most common in children; abdominal pain; occasionally symptomatology due to obstruction or worm migration	*Eggs* Feces-contaminated food or soil	*Stool* Eggs		Mebendazole or pyrantel pamoate
Hookworm *Necator americanus* *Ancylostoma duodenale*	Epigastric pain, anemia	*Larvae* Larvae in soil or on vegetation penetrate skin	*Stool* Eggs	Sanitary disposal of human feces is most effective control measure	Mebendazole or pyrantel pamoate
Strongyloidiasis *Strongyloides stercoralis*	Watery, mucous diarrhea	*Larvae* Larvae in soil or on vegetation penetrate skin	*Stool* Eggs	Only nematode worm that can reproduce in host; free-living phase and parasitic phase	Thiobendazole
Enterobiasis *Enterobius vermicularis*	Anal pruritus	*Eggs* Ingestion of eggs	*Anal contact specimen* Eggs	Called *pinworm* or *seatworm infection*	Mebendazole or pyrantel pamoate
Trichinelliasis *Trichinella spiralis*	Fever, myalgia, periorbital edema	*Larvae* Ingestion of meat from pigs, bear, walrus	*Muscle biopsy, serum* Curled-up larvae in muscle; antibodies	Called *muscle worm infection*	Steroids for severe symptoms; thiabendazole for adult stage
Schistosomiasis *Schistosoma mansoni,* *haematobium*	Fever, lymph node and liver enlargement; obstruction of venous vessels of urinary bladder, liver, intestines	*Larvae (cercariae)* Larvae in snail-infested waters penetrate skin	*Stool, rectal biopsy* Eggs		Praziquantel
Taeniasis *Taenia saginata* (beef) *Taenia solium* (pork)	Tapeworm infection; adult worm infection usually asymptomatic; symptoms (beef): epigastric fullness, nausea	*Larvae (cysticercus)* Ingestion of raw or undercooked beef or pork	*Stool* Eggs or worm segments	Cysticercus larva of *T. solium* (bladderworm) may cause serious CNS infection (cysticercosis)	Niclosamide; praziquantel for cysticercosis
Diphyllobothriasis *Diphyllobothrium latum*	Fish tapeworm; usually asymptomatic; abdominal discomfort, diarrhea, anemia	*Larvae (plerocercoid)* Ingestion of raw or undercooked fish	*Stool* Eggs or worm segments		Niclosamide

likely to be found in children, may produce toxic symptoms or intestinal obstruction. Combinations of *Ascaris, Trichuris*, and hookworm infections in the same individual are not uncommon in areas of hyperendemism. These vitality-sapping parasitic infections, compounded by the malnutrition that is ever present in economically depressed areas, may produce physical and mental retardation.

Laboratory Diagnosis
The identification of the typical fertilized or unfertilized eggs in the feces is diagnostic (Fig. 33-12).

Epidemiology
A. lumbricoides is found worldwide. It is thought to infect some one billion people. Virtually all members of the population in some areas of the world harbor the parasite. Fecal contamination and the use of human excreta as fertilizer are mainly responsible for the maintenance of the parasite in regions where ascariasis is endemic. Each female worm produces 200,000 eggs per day. Infective larvae develop in about 2 to 4 weeks in fertilized eggs that have been deposited in the soil. The eggs remain viable for months, possibly as long as 10 years. Immigrants from areas where ascariasis is highly endemic do not pose a threat because adequate sewage disposal prevents exposure of the public to the infective eggs.

Treatment and Control
Mebendazole or pyrantel pamoate is the drug of choice. If there is a heavy *Ascaris* worm burden, the compacted worms may cause intestinal obstruction requiring surgical intervention. There is no specific anthelmintic (anti-worm) drug for the larvae during the period of migration. The control of ascariasis, as of other helminthic infections, depends on education and chemotherapy.

Visceral Larva Migrans
Larvae of nematodes that infect other mammalian species sometimes infect humans, but they are unable to develop into adult worms. They survive for a period of time to migrate through organs of the body (visceral larva migrans) or to tunnel through the skin (cutaneous larva migrans; see under Hookworm Infection). In visceral larva migrans (VLM) there may be fever, infiltration of the lungs, hepatomegaly (enlargement of the liver), hyperglobulinemia (increased globulin in the blood), and granuloma formation in the brain, eye, lungs, and other organs. VLM is most likely to occur in children between the ages of 1 and 5 years who are in contact with pets or who have

Fig. 33-12. Nematode eggs.

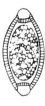

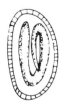

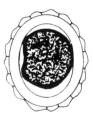

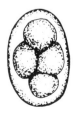

Trichuris trichiura　　*Enterobius vermicularis*　　*Ascaris lumbricoides*　　Hookworm

pica (an unnatural craving for bizarre foods such as dirt). Most often implicated in VLM are dog and cat ascarids (close relatives of *A. lumbricoides*) in the genus *Toxocara*. *Toxocara canis* is found in at least 20 percent of the 30 million dogs in the United States.

HOOKWORM INFECTION

Human hookworm infection is usually caused by one of two nematodes, *Necator americanus* (New World hookworm) or *Ancylostoma duodenale* (Old World hookworm). Infection is acquired when filariform larvae (larval forms of certain nematodes) that have developed from eggs deposited in the soil penetrate the skin. The larvae find their way to tops of grass blades, rocks, and so on, increasing their chances to contact skin. They enter the venous circulation, sojourn through the lung, migrate up the respiratory tract over the epiglottis, and are swallowed, thereby reaching the jejunum, where they develop into adults.

Pathogenesis
Classically, individuals who carry a heavy hookworm burden are markedly anemic and have low serum iron. Loss of proteins of the blood in already malnourished people adds to the debility. Severe, protracted, or repetitive infections, of children especially, may lead to physical stunting and mental retardation.

Laboratory Diagnosis
Routine diagnosis is based on identification of the eggs in feces (see Fig. 33-12).

Epidemiology
Hookworm is prevalent in tropical and temperate climates. In the United States it is found primarily along the Atlantic seaboard. Hookworm infection in the United States has declined so that it is no longer a public health problem.

Treatment and Control
Mebendazole is the drug of choice, as it is for most non-tissue–invasive, lumen-dwelling parasites. Pyrantel pamoate likewise is effective. It is necessary to remedy the malnutrition and the loss of iron in the severely diseased. Control is difficult where hookworm is hyperendemic because the soil in areas of human habitation is constantly being contaminated with human excreta and the wearing of footwear is not customary. Chemotherapy is, therefore, only temporarily effective and will probably remain so until the population is educated to dispose of human excreta properly.

Cutaneous Larva Migrans
Filariform larvae of dog and cat hookworm species (*Ancylostoma braziliense* and *Ancylostoma caninum*) and larvae of nonhuman species of *Strongyloides* penetrate the skin of children, farmers, craftsmen, and others who have contacted warm, moist, sandy soil, especially where dogs and cats have defecated. The larvae burrow into the subcutaneous tissues and produce linear, pruritic, papulovesicular lesions (Fig. 33-13). The condition is referred to as *serpiginous dermatitis, creeping eruption, or ground itch.* Secondary bacterial infection may occur as a consequence of the scratching that is done in response to the intense itching. *Thiabendazole* applied topically is the drug of choice.

STRONGYLOIDIASIS

Strongyloides stercoralis is an intestinal parasite of humans.

Life Cycle
The life cycle and distribution resemble those of the hookworm. There are two larval forms, the *rhabditiform* (so-called because of a bulb-like prominence in the esophagus) larva and the *filariform* larva. The filariform larva is the infec-

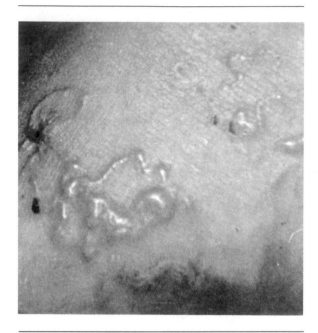

Fig. 33-13. Creeping eruption in a human being. This dermatosis is caused by larval hookworms of the species *Ancyclostoma braziliense, Uncinaria stenocephala,* and perhaps *A. caninum*, all of which are natural parasites of dogs and cats. The infective larvae apparently penetrate the skin but are unable to pierce through the dermis. Instead, they migrate between dermis and epidermis. (From W. Orris, In A. A. Fisher [ed.], *Atlas of Aquatic Dermatology*. New York: Grune & Stratton, 1978. Copyright 1978 American Cyanamid Company, Lederle Laboratories Division.)

tive (transmission) form. In the usual mode of infection filariform larvae penetrate the skin and pass via the venous circulation to the lungs, whence they are coughed up to the level of the epiglottis and subsequently swallowed, thereby gaining entrance to the upper intestinal tract. The female larva burrows into the mucosa, matures, and ovideposits (lays eggs). The eggs hatch, liberating rhabditiform larvae, which transform into filariform larvae in the intestine, on the perianal skin, or in the shed feces. The three sites of transformation are reflected in the three modes of infection: internal autoinfection through the intes-

tinal mucosa, reinfection through the skin of the perianal area, and (most commonly) contact with feces or fecally contaminated soil. *S. stercoralis* is the only nematode that can reproduce within the host (internal autoinfection), leading to chronic infection. Rhabditiform larvae shed in the feces either transform into filariform larvae directly or mature and form a free-living generation including adults that copulate and produce infective larvae. *S. stercoralis* is unusual among nematodes because it has both a free-living generation and a parasitic generation.

Pathogenesis

Most infections are asymptomatic, but heavy infections can cause anorexia, diarrhea, ulceration of the mucosa, and anemia. In internal autoinfection, filariform larvae may disseminate throughout the body of a compromised host, leading to a life-threatening situation. Bacterial infections that accompany strongyloidiasis frequently cause death in the immunocompromised.

Laboratory Diagnosis

Diagnosis is made by microscopic examinations of the stool, duodenal fluid (obtained by the Entero-Test technique), and mucosal biopsies. Immunological tests are based on the ELISA technique.

Epidemiology

S. stercoralis is found especially in warm, moist, tropical climates. It is estimated that the number of infected people in the world is 100,000 to 200,000 million. In the United States it is most common in the rural Southeast.

Treatment

Uncomplicated strongyloidiasis is effectively treated with thiabendazole. Use of antibiotics and intravenous fluid and other supportive measures are also required in the disseminated syndrome.

ENTEROBIASIS (PINWORM OR SEATWORM INFECTION)

Infections by *Enterobius vermicularis* are called *enterobiasis or oxyuriasis* and in the vernacular *pinworm or seatworm infections*. The worms are yellowish-white in color. Males are 2 to 5 mm long; females, 8 to 13 mm, with pointed tails.

Pathogenesis

Infections caused by *Enterobius* are comparatively innocuous. The adult worms inhabit the cecum, ileum, and appendix, where they may cause a mild inflammatory reaction. The chief complaint of seatworm infection is anal pruritus. Restless sleep is another common symptom. Discomfort in the perianal area occurs when the gravid female migrates out of the anus, usually during the night, to deposit eggs in the perianal, perineal region. The intense itching encourages scratching, which in turn may abrade the area sufficiently to introduce secondary bacterial infection. Scratching, furthermore, collects eggs under the fingernails and on the fingers, thence to produce autoinfections or to contaminate articles that will spread the infection to others. The eggs are found on clothing, bedding, windowsills, floors, and elsewhere in the environment of an infected individual.

Laboratory Diagnosis

The *transparent tape swab method* or digital rectal examination is used to obtain specimens. In the swab method parents frequently are asked to obtain the specimen when the child first awakens in the morning. The sticky side of the tape is applied several times to the anal area. The tape is then fastened, adhesive side down, to a glass slide. The contact areas are examined under the microscope for the presence of the typical conspicuously flat-sided eggs (see Fig. 33-12). The same technique is sometimes used in tapeworm infections.

Epidemiology

Distribution is worldwide. Humans are the only natural hosts. Enterobiasis is the most common worm infection in temperate climates. The greatest incidence is in children between the ages of 5 and 9.

Treatment and Control

Several highly effective and relatively nontoxic drugs can produce a 90 to 100 percent cure rate. Mebendazole and pyrantel pamoate are the drugs of choice. The life span of the worm is about 1 month. Reinfection is not uncommon, so retreatment may be necessary. Scrupulous hygienic practices such as boiling bed linens and disinfecting toilet seats at one time were recommended to rid a family of the pinworms. It is questionable how effective and how necessary these practices are, especially in view of the psychological trauma such admonitions may initiate in embarrassed parents. Rather, parents should be told of the commonness of pinworm infection, its relative innocuousness, and the effectiveness of drug treatment.

TRICHINOSIS (MUSCLE WORM INFECTION)

Life Cycle

A number of animals serve as hosts for *Trichinella spiralis*, the adult and larval forms appearing in the same animal. When flesh that contains live encysted larvae is ingested, the larvae emerge in the duodenum and mature into adults. Impregnated females penetrate the wall of the intestine and start to produce live larvae after about 1 week. Each female produces about 500 larvae over a 2-week period. The shower of larvae enters the capillaries and lymphatics and they migrate through the lungs into the heart and the systemic circulation. No tissues are immune to invasion. The heaviest infections are in the striated muscles, but the heart, the CNS, and the serous cavities are also favored sites of localization. The larvae coil up in muscle fibers, and the body surrounds the area with a calcified wall in 6 months to 2 years (Plate 29—Trichinella larva encysted in muscle). The encysted larvae may remain viable for as long as 10 years. They are at a dead end here unless the flesh is ingested by another host.

Pathogenesis

The symptoms of trichinosis are related to the clinical phase of the infection. During establishment of the adult worms in the intestine, the symptoms—diarrhea, abdominal discomfort, and vomiting—suggest food intoxication or infectious diarrhea. Beginning about the tenth day and reaching a peak in the second to third week, when the larvae are migrating and being filtered out in the muscles, periorbital swelling occurs in about 80 percent of symptomatic cases, fever in 90 percent, myalgia in 80 percent, and rash in about 10 percent. It is estimated that at least 100 larvae are required to initiate symptoms. In the third clinical phase, when the larvae are encysted and the body responds with repair measures, the patient experiences muscle pain, weakness, and cachexia (wasting). The symptoms just described are related primarily to muscle invasion, but no tissue or organ is immune.

Laboratory Diagnosis

Trichinelliasis should be suspected in patients who have periorbital edema, fever, and myalgia. The likelihood of trichinelliasis is increased if others who shared the same diet have the typical signs and symptoms. A definitive diagnosis can be made only by detection of the larvae in a muscle biopsy. The biopsy material is taken from a tender swollen muscle. Biopsy is not always necessary if the clinical signs and symptoms are fortified with a positive dietary history, high eosinophilia, and positive serology. There is a skin test, but it does not differentiate between past and recent infections.

Epidemiology

Trichinosis (trichinelliasis) formerly was one of the more prevalent worm infections in the United States. Autopsies conducted in the 1930s and early 1940s revealed an incidence of about 16 percent. From 1980 to 1985 the reported morbidity averaged 89 cases each year. There was an average of fewer than two deaths per year in that time. Rodents are largely responsible for maintaining the infection in nature. A wide variety of carnivores is infected. Humans contract the infection by eating meat that contains viable encysted larvae. During the period 1975 to 1985 pork was implicated in 78.7 percent of reported cases, ground beef in 6 to 7 percent, and wild animals (wild boar, bear, walrus) in 13.8 percent (see Boxed Essay, p. 833).

Treatment and Control

There is no satisfactory treatment for trichinelliasis. Thiabendazole is useful in the very early intestinal phase of the infection, but the infection is rarely diagnosed at this juncture. Treatment is largely for symptomatic relief: salicylates as a mainstay for pain and corticosteroids, with questionable effectiveness, for the inflammation. Human muscle worm infection has declined in the United States because of education of the public, use of deep freezers, and a decrease in the prevalence of infection in swine. The public is repeatedly urged to cook pork thoroughly, to the point at which none of the meat is pink. An internal temperature of at least 137°F kills trichinae. Deep-freezing of pork at a temperature of the average home freezer (5°F or −15°C) for 20 days destroys the trichina larvae in cuts of meat that are less than 6 inches thick. The enactment in 1952 of a law that required garbage fed to hogs to be cooked reduced the incidence of Trichinella infections in swine from between 5 and 10 percent to 0.3 percent in garbage-fed hogs. The incidence in grain-fed swine has decreased from the former 1 percent to 0.1 percent.

About 70 percent of the pork products are processed through federally inspected meat-pro-

TRICHINOSIS—HAWAII

In January 1986, three cases of trichinosis were reported to the Hawaii Department of Health. The cases occurred among persons who had eaten wild boar meat given to them by a local Hawaiian who had killed the animal. Because the meat had been distributed among several family members and friends of the hunter, an investigation was conducted to determine the extent of the outbreak.

Among all of those who had received some of the wild boar, health officials identified 28 persons who had eaten the meat. Seven of these had illnesses that met the standard case definition for trichinosis. All seven patients had at least four of the following symptoms: myalgia, malaise, fever, headache, diarrhea, nausea, periorbital edema, vomiting, trunk and limb edema, and cutaneous rash. One patient was hospitalized; three were treated with mebendazole, and two were treated with thiabendazole. All patients recovered.

Samples of the implicated boar meat were sent to the Centers for Disease Control for study. An artificial digestion procedure performed on the meat revealed from 2 to 9 *Trichinella* larvae per gram of the frozen meat.

Four of the 21 persons interviewed ate the meat after it had been microwaved at high for two minutes, the remaining 17 persons ate the meat fried. All four of those eating microwaved meat became ill, and three of those who had eaten fried meat became ill. The two people with the most severe illness had eaten the largest amounts of wild boar meat.

Trichinella spiralis continues to be a persistent public health problem in the United States. During the period between 1975–1985, pork was implicated in 78 percent of the reported cases in which the implicated meat was identified. Improper cooking was implicated in all seven cases of illness. The USDA recommends cooking pork in a microwave until it attains a temperature of 76.7°C (170°F) throughout.

From *M.M.W.R.* 36:14, 1987

cessing firms. The meat, however, is inspected only macroscopically, since microscopical examination is impractical in the automated American abattoirs. Some infections are traceable to homemade sausages, to small, local meat firms, and to the culinary preferences for raw pork by some ethnic groups. Infected pork may adulterate other types of meats if it is mixed with them, as in hamburger or through the use of a common meat grinder. Smoking, heavy spicing, salting, pickling, and drying of meats do not reliably destroy trichinae.

FILARIASIS

Seven species of roundworms are categorized as filariform worms. They constitute a major health problem in many areas of the world. None, however, is endemic to the United States. Filariform worms are transmitted by bloodsucking arthropods such as mosquitoes, midges, blackflies, and deerflies. The adult worms preferentially inhabit certain tissues in humans, who are their principal definitive hosts. *Wuchereria bancrofti* and *Brugia malayi* parasitize the lymphatics. *Onchocerca volvulus* and *Acanthocheilonema streptocerca* are found in tumor-like subcutaneous nodules, usually at bony protuberances or in the deeper connective tissue, whence the larvae frequently emigrate to congregate in the eye, thus leading to blindness or disturbances of vision. Loa loa, the "eye worm," migrates throughout the connective tissue, often passing across the cornea. *Mansonella ozzardi* and *Acanthocheilonema perstans* are found in the body cavities, such as the pericardial, pleural, and peritoneal cavities.

Female filariform worms produce live larvae called microfilariae. These are ingested by the bloodsucking insects and are transformed into infective larvae that are transmitted to the definitive host.

Pathogenesis

In general usage, filariasis, unless otherwise qualified, refers to Bancroft's filariasis (*W. Bancrofti*) and filariasis malayi (*B. malayi*). It is an insidious disease that takes years to develop. Repeated bites of mosquitoes over many years are necessary to build up a population of adult worms to produce the pathology. The adult parasites localize in the lymph nodes and lymph vessels, producing host cell infiltration and the proliferation of the endothelial cells of the lymphatics. Eventually the worms die and the affected area is patched over by fibroblasts, as in scar formation. Obstruction of lymph channels leads to lymphedema (accumulation of lymph fluid in the tissue). When this is extensive, grotesque enlargement of limbs or of the external genitalia occurs. The descriptive term *elephantiasis* is applied to the condition. (Short-term visitors to areas where filariasis is endemic do not experience such consequences, as World War II military personnel sometimes feared.)

Laboratory Diagnosis

Microfilariae are sought for conclusive evidence *in the blood* of individuals who have a geographical history of residence in endemic areas. The microfilariae are not regularly present in the blood. Blood specimens are customarily drawn around midnight because of the *nocturnal periodicity* of the microfilariae. They exit from the deep tissues into the peripheral blood during the hours that the arthropod vector habitually takes a blood meal.

Treatment

The administration of diethylcarbamazine citrate reduces the number of microfilariae in the blood and appears to have some effect on the adults in the tissues. Chronic obstruction in the less advanced stages is sometimes improved by surgery.

THE PLATYHELMINTHES

Members of the animal phylum Platyhelminthes collectively are termed the *flatworms*. They are characteristically flat when viewed in dorsoventral section. They are bilaterally symmetrical. Nearly all are hermaphroditic. The medically important flatworms appear in two classes, the *Trematoda*, or *flukes*, and the *Cestoidea*, or *tapeworms*.

TREMATODA (FLUKES)

Discussion of the medically important flukes is generally organized on the basis of the habitat of the adult worm in the host. Thus, *Fasciola hepatica, Clonorchis sinensis, Opisthorchis felineus* and *Opisthorchis viverrini* are the *liver flukes*; *Fasciolopsis buski* is the *intestinal fluke*; *Paragonimus westermani* is the *lung fluke*; and species of the genus *Schistosoma* are the *blood flukes*.

The liver, intestinal, and lung flukes are leaf-shaped, hermaphroditic worms that attach to the host by means of ventral suckers. Their life cycles are among the most complex found in animal species. Specific species of snails (always) and crustacea (sometimes) serve as intermediate hosts for the flukes' several larval forms (such as miracidia, cercariae, and metacercariae). *F. hepatica*, which infects ruminants primarily, is cosmopolitan. It is the only one of the flukes that is enzootic in the United States. Human infection is rarely reported in the United States. The other hermaphroditic flukes are found mainly in the Orient, where millions of persons are infected. Infections are transmitted to humans largely through the ingestion of raw or poorly cooked fish, crabs, crayfish, and aquatic plants. The symptoms are related to the site of infection. Clinical diagnosis is guided by the anatomical location of the symptoms and by the dietary and geographical history of the patient. Definitive laboratory diagnosis is made through the identification of the typical operculated (having a lid) eggs.

The blood flukes are an exception in that they are not hermaphroditic and the body configuration of the adults is not leaf-like. They produce a major parasitic disease of humans, schistosomiasis, or bilharziasis.

Schistosomiasis (Bilharziasis)

Life Cycle. Schistosome eggs, discharged in the feces or urine of humans, hatch into ciliated miracidia. The miracidium must enter a specific snail species to continue its development. Hundreds of thousands of the next larval form, the free-swimming cercariae, develop and emerge from the snail. Upon contacting human skin, they penetrate within seconds to minutes, to migrate through the lungs to the hepatoportal system. After maturing and mating in the blood vessels of the hepatoportal system, the adults settle in the mesenteric or vesical venules. The adults themselves do not multiply, so the number of adults is determined by the number of cercariae that entered the host. Blood fluke infections may persist as long as 25 years. One explanation for the persistence, as discovered in *Schistosoma mansoni* infections, is that adult blood flukes evade the host's immune system by camouflaging their surfaces with host proteins (serum proteins, blood group antigens, immunoglobulins), thereby preventing recognition by the host's immune system.

Pathogenesis. Pathology is due to a large extent to the masses of eggs (300 to 3000 per day per female, depending on the *Schistosoma* species) produced. Hypersensitivity reactions also account for some of the pathology. Less than 50 percent of the eggs are shed in the feces or urine. The remaining eggs are found in the tissues or move along the blood vessels until they become lodged in veins of a smaller caliber. The eggs have protruding spines and knobs that abet such lodgment. The blood vessels and tissues react to the entrapped or embedded eggs with a marked granulomatous reaction and tissue destruction. The liver and spleen enlarge, with esophageal varices (enlarged and tortuous vessels) as an occasional complication. *S. haematobium* may cause urinary tract disease in the form of fibrosis, strictures, or stones. Chronic disease has been implicated as a factor in the development of urinary bladder malignancies. In addition to the classic infections just described, schistosomes cause dermatitis and acute schistosome infections (Katayama fever).

Laboratory Diagnosis. In most cases diagnosis is made by the detection of the characteristic eggs in the feces or urine. Fecal and bladder biopsies, skin testing, and serological tests may also be valuable.

Epidemiology. The definitive geographical distribution of the schistosomes is related to the geographical presence of particular species of snails. There has to be a more than casual contact with fresh water for a sufficient number of cercariae to penetrate the skin. Cases of schistosomiasis are seen in the United States in persons who have traveled to areas where the disease is endemic, and especially in immigrants from Puerto Rico and the Philippines. The absence of the specific species of snails in the continental United States prevents the completion of the parasite's life cycle.

Treatment and Control. *Praziquantel* is effective against the schistosome species that infect humans. Control is difficult. Education is the only practical avenue at this time. People in the endemic areas, however, can hardly avoid repeated exposure in snail-infested waters. Such waters often are the only kind available for bathing, washing clothes, and planting crops. The use of human excrement as fertilizer also is a practical economic matter in some parts of the world.

Schistosome Dermatitis. In a schistosomal disease entity that occurs commonly in the United States, humans serve as the accidental hosts to the cercariae of blood flukes of birds and mammals. The condition is called *schistosome dermatitis, swimmers' itch, clam diggers' itch,* or *sea bathers' itch*. When infected birds (especially migratory fowl) and mammals pollute lakes, ponds, and streams, the miracidia that emerge from the schistosome eggs infect snails. The free-swimming furcocercous (fork-tailed) cercariae that emerge from the snails penetrate the skin of humans, lose their tails, and become schistosomulae (juvenile worms). The parasite is at a dead end because maturation of animal schistosomes does not occur in humans. The larval infestation of skin rarely leads to a serious condition. The erythematous pustular lesions (accompanied by intense itching) appear within hours of exposure and subside gradually after the second or third day (Fig. 33-14). Antihistamines and antipruritics may alleviate discomfort.

Fig. 33-14. Cercarial (schistosome) dermatitis. The eruption appeared on the arms of a patient exposed to avian schistosome cercariae while he was sitting on a dock jutting out over a lake. (From H. D. Blankespoor. In A. A. Fisher [ed.], *Atlas of Aquatic Dermatology*. New York: Grune & Stratton, 1978. Copyright 1978 American Cyanamid Company, Lederle Laboratories Division.)

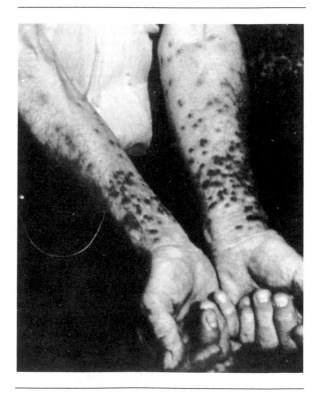

CESTOIDEA (TAPEWORMS)

Members of the other class of flatworms that contains worms of medical importance, the *Cestoidea*, are dorsoventrally flat, ribbon-like worms collectively referred to as *tapeworms*. Tapeworm infections occur less commonly and their pathogenic potential is considerably less than roundworm or trematode (fluke) infections.

The ribbon-like tapeworms can be divided into regions. The *head or scolex* is a pinhead-size structure that anchors in the mucosa by means of a holdfast organ. The holdfast structures are cup-shaped suckers or suctorial grooves (bothria) or hooks. The latter emanate from a raised, crown-like structure, the *rostellum*. The head tapers into the narrow neck region, which is the proliferative zone. Segments called *proglottids* proliferate from the neck zone and are known collectively as the strobila. Some tapeworms consist of only several segments; others, such as the fish tapeworm, may reach extraordinary lengths of 3000 to 4000 segments. As long as the head region with the proliferative neck region remains attached, new segments will continue to be formed. The series of proglottids progresses from immature proglottids immediately behind the neck region through sexually mature proglottids to the gravid (egg-laden) proglottids at the distal end of the worm. The proglottids contain both male and female reproductive organs. There are no digestive, skeletal, circulatory, or respiratory organs. Niclosamide is the drug of choice for all tapeworms that are in the adult stage.

Six tapeworms cause disease in humans: (1) *Taenia saginata*, the beef tapeworm; (2) *Taenia solium*, the pork tapeworm; (3) *Diphyllobothrium latum*, the fish tapeworm (Fig. 33-15); (4) *Hymenolepis nana*, the dwarf tapeworm; (5) *Hymenolepis diminuta*, the rat tapeworm; and (6) *Dipylidium caninum*, the dog tapeworm.

Taeniasis (Beef and Pork Tapeworms)

Infections with adult beef and pork tapeworms (taeniasis) are seldom of themselves serious.

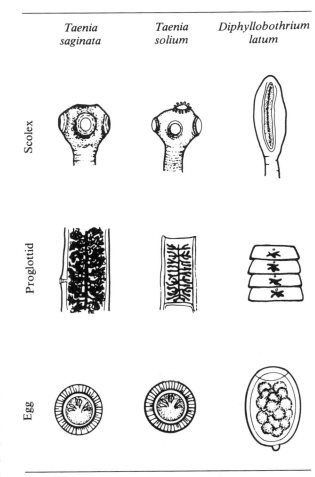

Fig. 33-15. Important stages and diagnostic characteristics of the major tapeworms that parasitize humans.

Symptoms, if present, usually take the form of epigastric pain or vague abdominal discomfort.

Cysticercosis or Larval Tapeworm. The principal danger to humans occurs when they become the intermediate hosts to the larval form, the *cysticercus larva*, commonly called the *bladder worm*. Most known cases of cysticercosis in humans are due to the pork tapeworm larva (*Cysticercus cellulosae*). The tissues of infected swine contain the larvae. Ingestion of the larvae in raw or inadequately cooked pork leads to the development of the adult tapeworm in humans. Sometimes, mature eggs get into the small intestine of humans and hatch. The eggs may come from an external source such as food, or autoinfection may occur in individuals who have an adult tapeworm infection. The hatched larvae that enter the blood stream settle in one of many tissues, where they encyst. No matter where they settle, the effect is that of a space-occupying lesion. Eventually the cysticerci die and become calcified in about two years. Cerebral cysticercosis can mimic a tumor. The patient may present with symptoms such as seizures, hydrocephalus, and focal neurological abnormalities. Cysticercosis is the most common parasitic disease to affect the CNS. Cysticercosis is a serious health problem in eastern Europe, Thailand, and, especially, Mexico (3 percent of autopsies in Mexico show the presence of larvae). Specific diagnosis of cysticercosis is difficult to establish. Biopsies, radiograms, CAT scans, magnetic resonance imaging, and ELISA-based serological tests comprise the diagnostic approaches. Cysticercosis responds well to treatment with praziquantel.

Diphyllobothriasis (Fish Tapeworm)

The fish tapeworm (*Diphyllobothrium latum*) is found in temperate climates where the eating of freshwater fish is common—in the Great Lakes regions of the United States and Canada, in Alaska, and in Europe, especially Finland. Infection, which is acquired by ingestion of plerocercoid larvae (see Representative Life Cycles earlier in this chapter), usually is clinically asymptomatic, but abdominal discomfort, diarrhea, constipation, and, most important, *anemia* do occur. About 1 percent of infected individuals suffer a macrocytic, hyperchromic anemia. Most carnivores can serve as reservoir hosts for *D. latum*.

Cooking fish at a temperature of 56°C (135°F) for 5 minutes or freezing to −18°C (0°F) for 24 hours or to −10°C (14°F) for 72 hours prevents infection. Fish properly brined before smoking should not constitute a source of infection.

THE ARTHROPODA

Arthropods are the most highly organized of the invertebrate animals. Sometime during their life cycle they have paired, jointed appendages, a chitinized (horny polysaccharide) exoskeleton, and a hemocele (body cavity through which a blood-like fluid circulates). The majority of the medically important arthropods are found in the classes *Insecta* and *Arachnida*. Flies, fleas, lice, bees, and wasps are members of the class Insecta, arthropods with three pairs of walking legs. Spiders, ticks, and mites are arachnids, arthropods with four pairs of walking legs.

Arthropods periodically shed (molt) the entire exoskeleton. The stages between moltings are called *instars*. Immature instar forms that resemble the adults are called *nymphs*; those that are morphologically quite distinct from the adult form are called *larvae*. Larvae are worm-like in character. In some arthropods there is a non-feeding form, the *pupa*, that appears between the larval form and the adult form.

The medical importance of arthropods will only be noted here. The larvae and adults may affect humans in a number of ways; as *ectoparasites*, as *intermediate or definitive hosts* of other animal parasites, as *venom-producing agents*, or as *vectors* of infectious disease.

As ectoparasites they cause disease while feeding or taking up abode on the skin and underlying tissues. That association is an *infestation*. Examples of arthropods that cause infestations of humans are the itch mite (which causes *scabies*—see Boxed Essay) and the larval mites known as chiggers; fleas (which have backward-projecting bristles and spines that enable them to proceed through hair and fur without becoming entangled), often from infested pets; ticks (Fig. 33-16), bedbugs, and kissing bugs; the body louse, the head louse, and the pubic or crab louse (Fig. 33-17); and larval forms of flies (maggots) that infest the body (myiasis).

The role of arthropods as intermediate and definitive hosts should have been apparent in the

SCABIES IN HEALTH CARE FACILITIES—IOWA

Scabies continues to occur among residents and staff of Iowa nursing homes and hospitals. For the eight-year period between July 1979 and June 1987, the Iowa Department of Public Health confirmed scabies in 25 nursing homes, one hospital, one state institution, and one county residential care facility.

Scabies becomes pandemic at approximately 30-year intervals. Evidence suggests that community scabies peaked in the mid-1970s but has persisted at high levels for the past ten years. Scabies is a major problem in nursing homes, particularly among patients who are debilitated and require extensive hands-on care. Because treatment failure is common with approved scabicides (10 percent crotamiton cream/lotion, 1 percent lindane, and 10 percent sulfur in petrolatum), lengthy, intensive retreatment may be necessary.

The scabies mite is probably introduced when infested patients are transferred between institutions. The quantity of mites carried by these patients expedites transmission, which can occur directly (through contact between residents) or indirectly (through contact with staff).

Skin scraping is the only consistent means of detecting mites, assessing the degree of transmissibility, and evaluating treatment when skin lesions persist or reappear. Any red, raised, pruritic skin lesions (especially on the upper back) that are not obviously due to other causes are suspect and should be scraped to detect mites. Treatment of residents, especially those with atypical, crusted rashes, should be aggressive (for example, lindane lotion for one day, followed by 10 percent crotamiton lotion for five days, followed by a second lindane treatment). Treatment should include the entire body from the neck down, with special attention to the underside of well-trimmed fingernails.

Nursing personnel frequently acquire scabies, especially on the upper arms and abdomen, but rarely on the hands and wrists. Standard treatment will usually eliminate the problem and should be given to the staff's family members.

From *M.M.W.R.* 37:178, 1988.

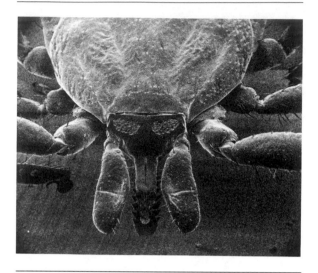

Fig. 33-16. Forepart of the tick. When biting, the tick thrusts the serrated biting organ (center) through the skin into deeper-lying tissues. It is the serrations that make dislodgment so difficult. (From P. B. Armstrong, D. W. Deamer, and J. J. Mais. What's biting you? *J. Natl. Hist.* June/July 1972.)

Fig. 33-17. A human crab louse from underneath. The thick legs and large claws are used to grasp hair shafts on the host. (From P. B. Armstrong, D. W. Deamer, and J. J. Mais. What's biting you? *J. Natl. Hist.* June/July 1972.)

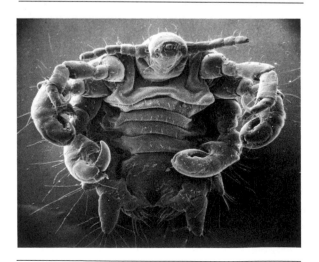

preceding descriptions of the parasitic diseases. As venom producers, arthropods such as bees, wasps, spiders, and tarantulas produce substances that are toxic or that induce allergic reactions (see Chapter 14 under Agents of Human Anaphylaxis). The importance of arthropods as mechanical and biological vectors of bacterial, viral, rickettsial, and mycotic disease agents is evident in the descriptions of those diseases. In summary, arthropods directly cause medical problems as ectoparasites and as venenators, or they do so by fulfilling a role in the development or transmission of other disease agents.

SUMMARY

1. Traditionally the term *parasites* is applied to the infectious disease agents that are found in four divisions of the animal kingdom: the Protozoa, the Nemathelminthes (roundworms), the Platyhelminthes (flatworms), and the Arthropoda.

2. The distribution and incidence of parasitic disease is governed by such factors as availability of suitable definitive and intermediate hosts and appropriate vectors, climate, socioeconomic conditions, sanitary practices, and ethnic eating habits.

3. The infective forms that are involved in the transmission of parasites are the trophozoites, cysts, and sporozoites of protozoa and the eggs and larvae of worms.

4. The major mode of laboratory diagnosis is identification by microscope of the various morphological forms of trophozoites, cysts, eggs, and larvae.

5. Control of parasitic disease includes the destruction of vectors and intermediate hosts and

management of their breeding places, education of the populace, proper sanitation, and the use of appropriate drugs.

6. For summaries of the parasitic diseases described in this chapter, see Tables 33-2 and 33-3.

QUESTIONS FOR STUDY

Select the best response or responses for each of the following:

1. The hardy form in the life cycle of some protozoa that is responsible for the spread of diseases such as amoebiasis and giardiasis is the
   A. Trophozoite   D. Larva
   B. Ovum   E. Zygote
   C. Cyst

2. Which *Plasmodium* species produces the most severe form of malaria and is ever developing more drug-resistant strains?
   A. *malariae*   C. *falciparum*
   B. *vivax*   D. *ovale*

3. Primary amebic meningoencephalitis (PAM) is usually seen in young, healthy persons and it is usually associated with a history of swimming in warm bodies of water. The free-living, soil-water ameba that causes this usually fatal infection is
   A. *Dientamoeba fragilis*   D. *Entamoeba gingivalis*
   B. *Naegleria fowleri*   E. *Iodamoeba bütschlii*
   C. *Entamoeba histolytica*

4. A camper who drank untreated water from a mountain stream developed diarrhea that persisted for more than one week. Questioning of the patient by the physician revealed that the patient had noted flatulence and foul-smelling, bulky stools. The patient's geographical history and symptomatology are strongly suggestive of
   A. Enterobiasis
   B. Fish tapeworm infection (diphyllobothriasis)
   C. Giardiasis or lambliasis
   D. Trichinelliasis
   E. Toxoplasmosis

5. "Of the 31 people who ate the smoked sausage, 19 became ill. The incubation period ranged from 5 to 31 days. The illness was characterized by periorbital edema, fever, and myalgia. Twelve of the 19 patients had elevated eosinophilia counts." The preceding findings are typical of the disease:
   A. Trichinosis (trichinelliasis)   D. Staphylococcal enteritis
   B. Brucellosis   E. Amebiasis
   C. Toxoplasmosis

6. Which protozoon or the disease it causes has these characteristics? The acquired form of the disease may resemble infectious mononucleosis; congenital infections may be seriously teratogenic; domestic cats are the definitive or final host; infections of humans (and warm-blooded animals) is of cosmopolitan distribution.
   A. *Toxoplasma gondii*   D. *Plasmodium falciparum*
   B. *Trichomonas vaginalis*   E. *Entamoeba histolytica*
   C. *Giardia lamblia*

7. Which group of antimicrobial agents is used therapeutically primarily against animal parasites?
   A. Amoxacillin, chloramphenicol, rifampin
   B. Amphotericin B, Nystatin, ketoconazole
   C. Mebendazole, metronidazole, praziquantel
   D. Hexachlorophene, sodium hypochlorite, 70 percent alcohol
   E. Acyclovir, amantadine, ARA-AMP

Match the test on the left with the disease for which it is used on the right.

8. Transparent tape swab method

9. Enterotest (gelatin capsule containing nylon thread)

10. Papanicolau (PAP) smear

11. Stained thick and thin blood smears

12. Exposure of patient to the bite of a "clean" reduviid (kissing) bug (xenodiagnosis)

A. Plasmodiasis
B. Retrieval of specimen from upper intestinal tract (e.g., for giardiasis)
C. Vaginal trichomoniasis
D. Chagas disease
E. Enterobiasis and taeniasis

Match the term on the left with its definition on the right.

13. Female Anopheles mosquito

14. Cysticerciasis

15. Infestation

16. Antihelminthic

17. Trophozoite

A. An agent (usually a drug) that inhibits or destroys worms
B. Infection (frequently of the CNS) caused by tapeworm larvae
C. Actively feeding/metabolizing form of protozoa
D. Skin-associated infection caused by ectoparasites
E. Transmission of malaria

ADDITIONAL READINGS

Amin, N. M. Giardiasis. *Hosp. Med.* 20:39,1984.
Ash, L. R., and Orihel, T. C. *Parasites: A Guide to Laboratory Procedures and Identification.* Chicago: American Society of Clinical Pathologists Press, 1987.

Current, W. L. The biology of *Cryptosporidium*. *A.S.M. News.* 54:605,1988.
Feldman, H. A. Epidemiology of Toxoplasma infections. *Epidemiol. Rev.* 4:204,1982.
Jones, J. E. Pinworms. *Amer. Family Physician.* 38:159,1988.

Katz, M., Despommier, D. D., and Gwadz, R. W. *Parasitic Diseases*. New York: Springer-Verlag, 1989.

Markell, E. K., Voge, M., and John, D. T. *Medical Parasitology* (6th ed.). Philadelphia, Saunders, 1986.

Warren, K. S. Algorithms in the diagnosis and management of exotic diseases (serial feature). *J. Infect. Dis.* 131:613,1975, through 136:465,1977.

Yamaguchi, T. (ed.). *A Color Atlas of Clinical Parasitology*. Philadelphia: Lea & Febiger, 1981.

IX. SELECTED TOPIC

34. HOSPITAL-ACQUIRED DISEASES

OBJECTIVES

To outline the various ways in which hospital-associated diseases can be acquired

To list the sites of infection in the host and the microbial agents most frequently isolated from them

To list those predisposing factors that contribute to hospital-associated infections

To understand the relationship of antibiotic use and hospital-associated infections

To list those hospital procedures that contribute to hospital-associated infections

To outline the techniques and practices that help to prevent hospital-associated infections

Infections acquired in the hospital are referred to as *nosocomial* (Greek: *nosa*, disease; *komeion*, to take care of). One of the reasons that we have a separate chapter on hospital-associated diseases is that their epidemiology differs dramatically from community-associated diseases, discussed in Chapter 10. Ironically, hospital-associated diseases have become a major health problem because of our advances in medicine. The services now provided by hospitals are complex and involve such practices as organ transplantation, implantation of foreign devices, and replacement and repair of defective tissues. In addition, a variety of invasive devices for therapeutic or diagnostic purposes provide vehicles for transmission of infectious agents.

The purpose of this chapter is to briefly outline those factors that contribute to hospital-associated diseases and how they may be prevented and/or controlled. A knowledge of these factors is an important aspect of the health professional's education.

EPIDEMIOLOGY

TRANSMISSION

The percentage of nosocomial infections acquired from community sources is not easily es-

tablished in the hospital setting. Infectious microorganisms may reach the patient by direct contact with other patients and with hospital personnel, contact with contaminated fomites, or contact with contaminated air.

Direct Contact

Upon entry into the hospital, individuals who are considered infectious require some type of isolation. Handwashing is the single most important isolation precaution because it removes organisms acquired from infected patients. If the patient can transmit microorganisms by air it may be necessary to place him/her in a private room to prevent cross infection between patients. Direct contact between hospital personnel and the patient, however, remains a major avenue of infection, with transmission by hands the most important route for transfer of the infectious agent. For example, a physician removing a dressing from a bacterially contaminated wound could accidentally contaminate his or her hands with infectious microorganisms and transfer them to other patients.

Infections may also be caused by microorganisms of low virulence that are members of one's own microbial flora (*endogenous*). In endogenous infections the virulence of the pathogen is not so important as the number of microorganisms present in the host and the physiological state of the host. For example, *Escherichia coli* is considered a nonpathogen or an opportunistic pathogen. It exists in equilibrium with other residents in the gut as well as the host tissue. There is no dramatic increase in the numbers of *E. coli* and no pathological response of the host to its presence. *E. coli* displaced into the genitourinary tract, however, finds itself in a new environment, where ecological and physiological pressures may not be exerted on it. Depending on the site of infection and the immunological response of the host, *E. coli* can become highly pathogenic. Endogenous infections are often the result of surgical manipulation, chemotherapeutic treatment, and diagnostic or therapeutic procedures (iatrogenic infections). Frequently in these procedures microorganisms are accidentally displaced from their normal habitat into other areas of the host.

Contaminated Fomites and Fluids

The contact of any instrument with open wounds, mucous membranes, or internal organs of the body represents a mechanism for transmission of infectious agents to the patient. Various solutions or fluids such as intravenous fluids, drugs, blood, or blood products may also be contaminated either by the distributor or by the hospital pharmacy. In other words, a common vehicle may be the source of disease and can result in hospital epidemics. Most infections caused by contact with inanimate objects are incurred during various hospital procedures such as surgery, catheterization, hypodermic injection, and diagnostic procedures.

Many inanimate objects within the hospital environment can act as sources of infection to hospitalized patients. These include potted flowers, bed linen, fruits and vegetables, carpeting, and walls and floors and other smooth surfaces. These objects, however, are not the most frequent sources of infection.

Airborne Spread

Air is a major vehicle for the dissemination of microorganisms. Usually the airborne microbes are derived from nasal carriers or from the desquamated epithelium of patients and personnel. Individuals with upper respiratory tract infections, or asymptomatic carriers, can infect others by means of discharged air droplets that carry potentially pathogenic microorganisms. These contaminated mucous discharges can make direct contact with the patient, or they may settle on various surfaces to remain infectious for anyone coming in contact with them. Aerosolized bacteria can also be generated by inanimate disseminators. Many cases of pneumonia, for example, have been traced to the use of inhalation equipment. Such instruments are used to generate aerosols of medication for patients with respiratory problems. If equipment or medication becomes contaminated, the nebulizer in the unit will generate bacterial aerosols that are inhaled by the patient. *Pseudomonas* species such as *P. cepacia* and *P. aeruginosa* can proliferate in relatively pure water. *P. cepacia*, for example, has been shown to multiply to levels of 10^7 per milliliter and remain at those levels for weeks in distilled water. Outbreaks of Legionnaire's disease have been traced to the aerosolization of potable water, for example, in shower heads.

Microorganisms on the skin have been found on desquamated epithelium, which is readily shed onto bedclothes and thus dispersed into the air on bed making. Individuals with skin diseases such as eczema are prolific disseminators of skin microorganisms because they have more skin scales and because the smaller size of the scales facilitates their transmission. In addition, humans normally liberate 3×10^8 scales per day and most *Staphylococcus aureus* organisms are carried on these skin flakes. Outbreaks of *S. aureus* surgical wound infections have been linked to airborne spread from human dispensers in the operating room.

Microorganisms dispersed into the air from any source can be acquired by the patient through inhalation, by deposition on the skin, or indirectly by contaminated fomites. In the hospital airborne infections are therefore related to the kind of disseminator in operation, the type of filtration system, and the velocity of air and airflow patterns in the hospital.

Laboratory techniques used to trace hospital-associated infections are discussed in Chapter 10.

NOSOCOMIAL INFECTION RATES AND AGENTS INVOLVED

Data have been collected from hospitals in the United States to determine the rates of infection for hospital services as well as the agents implicated in the infection. The microbial groups, in order of importance, involved in nosocomial disease are bacteria, fungi, viruses, and animal parasites. Over 80 percent of nosocomial infections are caused by bacteria while very few are ever caused by animal parasites such as protozoa. The

isolation rates of the 15 most frequently encountered pathogens are outlined in Table 34-1. Table 34-2 illustrates the incidence of selected pathogens by site of infection. These tables clearly demonstrate the importance of gram-negative species in nosocomial disease. *Escherichia coli*, for example, is the most frequently isolated pathogen, followed by *Pseudomonas aeruginosa*, *enterococci*, and *Staphylococcus aureus*. The dominance of gram-negative species is due to the abundant number of currently available antibiotics that affect gram-negative species. Increased use of these antimicrobials has selected for antibiotic-resistant strains of the offending species.

Even though Table 34-1 indicates the importance of bacteria in nosocomial disease, fungi and viruses also play an important role, particularly

Table 34-1. The 15 Most Frequently Isolated Pathogens and Their Percentage Distribution on Each Service, 1984

Pathogen	Percentage distribution for Service						
	MED	SURG	OB	GYN	PED	NEW	Percentage, all services
E. coli	19.6	16.2	21.2	29.8	11.4	9.3	17.9
P. aeruginosa	11.4	13.0	1.3	4.3	9.7	6.7	7.7
Enterococci[a]	9.6	10.5	16.6	18.1	5.3	5.7	10.9
S. aureus	9.2	10.4	8.0	5.8	16.6	24.8	12.4
Klebsiella species	9.0	6.9	2.1	4.8	6.6	6.7	6.0
Coagulase-negative staphylococci	5.6	6.1	5.7	5.2	13.2	15.3	8.5
Enterobacter species	4.7	7.5	2.1	3.7	4.2	3.7	4.3
Candida species	7.0	4.9	1.1	2.2	7.6	3.8	4.4
Proteus species	5.6	5.4	3.4	5.3	0.3	1.0	3.5
Serratia species	2.1	2.9	0.2	0.3	1.4	1.3	1.4
Other fungi	2.3	1.5	0.1	0.1	1.2	1.0	1.0
Citrobacter species	1.5	1.5	1.1	0.8	1.0	0.8	1.2
Bacteroides species	0.6	1.4	4.6	2.8	0.3	0.2	1.6
Group B *Streptococcus*	0.8	0.5	7.9	3.8	1.2	6.2	3.4
Other anaerobes	0.9	0.9	4.8	2.0	0.3	0.2	1.05
All others[b]	10.1	10.4	19.8	11.0	19.7	13.3	14.0

MED = medicine; SURG = surgery; OB = obstetrics; GYN = gynecology; PED = pediatrics; NEW = newborn.
[a] Enterococci includes group D streptococci.
[b] No other pathogen accounted for more than 3 percent of the isolates on any service.
Source: CDC Surveillance Summaries, 1986. Nosocomial Infection Surveillance, 1984. *M.M.W.R.* 35 (No. 1SS). (Data come from 51 hospitals located throughout the United States that regularly report their surveillance studies to the National Nosocomial Infections Surveillance System (NNISS)).

Table 34-2. The 15 Most Frequently Isolated Pathogens and Their Percentage Distribution for Each Site of Infection, 1984

Pathogen	Percentage distribution						Percentage, all sites
	UTI	SWI	LRI	BACT	CUT	Other	
E. coli	30.7	11.5	6.4	10.1	7.0	7.4	12.2
P. aeruginosa	12.7	8.9	16.9	7.6	9.2	6.7	10.3
Enterococci[a]	14.7	12.1	1.5	7.1	8.8	7.0	8.5
S. aureus	1.6	18.6	12.9	12.3	28.9	14.6	14.8
Klebsiella species	8.0	5.2	11.6	7.8	3.8	4.6	6.8
Coagulase-negative staphylococci	3.4	8.3	1.5	14.9	11.5	11.6	8.5
Enterobacter species	4.8	7.0	9.4	6.3	4.5	3.9	6.0
Candida species	5.4	1.7	4.0	5.6	5.8	14.1	6.1
Proteus species	7.4	5.2	4.2	0.8	3.3	2.1	3.8
Serratia species	1.2	2.1	5.8	3.0	2.2	1.5	2.6
Other fungi	2.2	0.4	1.4	1.3	0.9	2.8	1.5
Citrobacter species	1.8	1.4	1.4	0.7	0.7	0.9	1.2
Bacteroides species	0.0	3.7	0.2	3.4	1.2	1.4	1.7
Group B *Streptococcus*	0.9	1.3	0.7	2.3	1.1	1.9	1.4
Other anaerobes	0.0	1.7	0.1	1.8	0.8	4.4	1.5
All others[b]	5.2	10.9	22.0	15.0	10.3	15.1	13.0

UTI = urinary tract infection; SWI = surgical wound infection; LRI = lower respiratory infection; BACT = primary bacteremia; CUT = cutaneous.
[a] Enterococci belong to group D streptococci.
[b] No other pathogen accounted for more than 3 percent of the isolates at any site. (From CDC Surveillance Summaries, 1986. Nosocomial Infection Surveillance, 1984. *M.M.W.R.* 35 [No. 1SS].)

in the past few years. The emergence of acquired immune deficiency syndrome (AIDS) and the increased used of corticosteroids for specialized groups of patients are the principal reasons for these increases. Each one affects cell-mediated immunity, the major host defense mechanism against fungi and viruses.

Candida and *Aspergillus* species are the most frequently encountered fungal pathogens in the hospital but others may also be involved (Table 34-3). *Candida albicans* is the *Candida* species most frequently isolated from the hospital. *Candida* is indigenous to the skin and gastrointestinal tract. Patients exposed to antimicrobials that suppress the bacterial flora of the gastrointestinal tract are subject to overcolonization by *C. albicans*. The yeast may become invasive if the pa-

tient is undergoing surgery or is receiving cytotoxic chemotherapy. Intravenous catheterization may permit cutaneous colonization and subcutaneous invasion by *Candida*. *Aspergillus* species are ubiquitous in the environment. In the hospital air is the principal route of transmission of *Aspergillus* and the respiratory tract the most common portal of entry. The conidia of *Aspergillus* are so small that they easily reach the lungs. Contamination of air ventilation systems is usually involved in nosocomial aspergillosis. Hospital construction is occasionally another source of airborne transmission of *Aspergillus*. In 1974 and 1975 the National Cancer Institute in Baltimore, Maryland, experienced 8 cases of aspergillosis in the process of relocating to a new facility. All those cases were due to *A. flavus*, which had col-

Table 34-3. Most Frequently Isolated Fungal Pathogens in the Hospital

Mycoses or fungal groups	Clinical manifestation; type of individuals affected	Treatment
Candidiasis (*Candida albicans, C. tropicalis, C. torulopsis, glabrata, C. parapsilosis*)	Onychomycosis; HIV-infected patients	Ketoconazole
	Chronic mucocutaneous; acquired T-lymphocyte deficiency	Ketoconazole
	Thrush; HIV-infected and other T-lymphocyte deficiency states	Oral nystatin, oral ketoconazole
	Gastrointestinal—acute leukemia	Amphotericin B
	Genitourinary tract—indwelling catheter	Amphotericin B with or without flucytosine
	Disseminated—leukemia patients, intravascular catheterization	Amphotericin B with or without flucytosine
Aspergillosis (*Aspergillus fumigatus, A. flavus, A. niger, A. terreus*)	Pulmonary—patients with acute leukemia, those undergoing bone marrow transplantation	Surgical debridement, amphotericin B
Zygomycosis (species of *Mucor, Rhizopus, Absidia, Cunninghamella, Saksenaea*)	Pulmonary—uncontrolled leukemia, organ transplantation	Amphotericin B
	Rhinocerebral—uncontrolled diabetes, organ transplantation	Debridement and amphotericin B
Cryptococcosis (*Cryptococcus neoformans*)	Meningitis—those receiving high doses of corticosteroids	Amphotericin B
Trichosporonosis (*Trichosporon* species)	Disseminated (lesions in skin, kidney, liver, eyes, lung) hematologic malignancies	Amphotericin B, ketoconazole, miconazole
Pseudallescheriasis (*Pseudallescheria boydii*)	Pulmonary; disseminated involving kidney, thyroid, brain and heart; local lesions in paranasal sinuses	Surgical debridement, amphotericin B
Fusarium infection (*Fusarium solani, F. moniliforme, F. proliferatum*)	Disseminated skin lesions—patients with leukemia	Amphotericin B

onized the fireproofing material used to coat the steel and cement superstructure.

Viruses are not included in nosocomial statistical studies but their importance in nosocomial diseases cannot be overlooked. Most viruses can cause nosocomial disease, but the ones that either are highly transmissible or have devastating effects in the host are:

1. Rubella virus
2. Respiratory syncytial virus
3. Varicella-zoster virus
4. Herpes simplex virus
5. Hepatitis A virus

Endogenous viruses such as the cytomegalovirus, Epstein-Barr virus, and herpes simplex virus are activated in the host by physical and chemical factors that may include trauma, immunosuppression, and hormonal imbalances. Latent viruses, when activated, replicate and are shed by the host.

FACTORS IMPORTANT IN NOSOCOMIAL INFECTIONS

MICROBIAL FACTORS

Recent findings indicate that most nosocomial infections are associated with microorganisms previously described as opportunistic—for example, *E. coli, Staphylococcus epidermidis,* and *Serratia marcescens.* In the compromised host all microorganisms must be considered potentially pathogenic, partly because changes in medical procedures have brought about changes in the microorganism, its environment, and its disease manifestations. New or unusual microorganisms now appear as permanent residents of the hospital atmosphere, and each must be treated as a potential pathogen. Most microbial changes have been the result of the increased use of antibiotics, both medical and nonmedical.

Microorganisms that inhabit human bodies are in various ecological niches (respiratory tract, intestinal tract, and other sites), where they are in equilibrium with other microorganisms as well as the host. Under normal healthy conditions this relationship does not allow for the indiscriminate increase in numbers of one species over another. For example, there is an independent mutual antagonism between gram-positive cocci and gram-negative bacilli in the human respiratory tract, and together they are antagonistic to the fungi. A microbial imbalance is evident in the host when broad-spectrum antibiotics are administered over a long period of time. In this situation the numbers of gram-negative and gram-positive bacteria are greatly reduced, and secondary fungal infections tend to occur because of the uninhibited multiplication of the fungal species. Since the advent of antibiotics and other drugs the intermicrobial environment of the microorganism in the host has been constantly challenged. Drugs are now a part of people's food, drink, and cosmetics, and because of their antimicrobial activities

they have selected for the infrequent low-grade pathogens.

The increasing use of new procedures and instruments has also changed the pattern of microorganisms in the hospital. Some microorganisms are equipped to survive in and around these new instruments. Together these factors can lead to the replacement of normal microbial inhabitants in the host with infrequently encountered microorganisms. Such altered relationships are likely to lead to serious infection.

Organisms causing nosocomial infections are frequently resistant to antimicrobials. This resistance involves not only microorganisms of low virulence but also the more frequently isolated pathogens such as *Staphylococcus aureus.* As many as 75 percent of hospital personnel can be described as carriers of antimicrobial-resistant *S. aureus.* The resistance of this organism was for many years confined to the antibiotic penicillin G, but the organism is now resistant to several aminoglycosides as well as methicillin. Gram-negative organisms such as *Serratia, Klebsiella,* and *Pseudomonas* are resistant to a variety of antimicrobials including many of the important aminoglycosides. Still there are some microbial species that have remained uniformly susceptible to specific antimicrobials—for example, group A streptococci, meningococcus, and *Treponema pallidum,* all of which are susceptible to penicillin. In addition, the resistant organisms that inhabit the host do not usually persist when the antimicrobial is removed. Despite these positive signs antimicrobial resistance does affect the outcome of infection in the patient.

Two factors leading to increasing prevalence of antimicrobial resistance as a cause of nosocomial infections are the frequent use of antimicrobials and the mechanisms of resistance transfer in microorganisms. Chromosome-mediated resistance is a problem, but most of our concern today is with resistance mediated by plasmid transfer factors and transposons. Resistance transfer occurs not only between members of the same genus and species but between species and within genera. Microorganisms regarded as nonpathogenic can be the source of resistance factors. The most common sites of resistance transfer are the gastrointestinal tract and the skin. Resistance transfer in the bowel does not depend on the affected individual's receiving antimicrobial agents at the time of transfer. Transfer on the skin, however, appears to occur more frequently in the presence of topically applied antimicrobial agents. Because plasmids can carry multiple resistance markers, selection of resistance to one drug used in treatment may be accompanied by resistance to unrelated drugs. Within the hospital environment the selective pressures for survival of the multiply resistant strain are related to frequency of use of each of the drugs. Even when antimicrobial usage is decreased, resistant microorganisms are capable of persisting. The fact that hospital-associated strains are also transferred to those in the community (and vice versa) is of great concern to the medical community. Many examples now exist in which some microorganisms have developed resistance to antimicrobials outside the hospital: *Hemophilus influenzae* to ampicillin, *Salmonella typhimurium* to ampicillin, *Staphylococcus aureus* to methicillin, pneumococcus to penicillin and tetracyclines, and *Shigella* species to sulfonamides and tetracyclines. The hospitalized patient undergoing drug therapy, therefore, represents a source of multiply resistant microorganisms not only to other hospitalized patients and hospital staff but to the community as well.

IMMUNOLOGICAL STATE OF THE HOST

The single most important factor determining susceptibility to infection is the relative immunological state of the host at the time of infection. The immunological state can be depressed under certain conditions.

Age

In the few months after birth, the child is very susceptible to bacterial infection—especially the premature child. It is well known that the serum of the newborn does not exert the bactericidal activity that the maternal serum does. The infant serum shows little opsonic activity against such gram-negative bacteria as *E. coli* and *S. marcescens*. Diarrhea caused by enteropathogenic *E. coli* is a major affliction of infants in the hospital nursery. Neonatal sepsis occurs more frequently in premature infants, and fatalities are as high as 50 percent. *E. coli* is the most frequent cause of neonatal sepsis. Up to 6 years of age pediatric patients remain highly susceptible to infection with *Hemophilus influenzae*. Their serum is particularly deficient in antibody for this species of bacteria. Recent extensive use of ampicillin in pediatric diseases has triggered the appearance of unresponding, antibiotic-resistant varieties of *H. influenzae*. In consequence, the number of cases of fatal meningitis among infants has risen.

Older patients with cardiovascular disease, urinary tract abnormalities, or respiratory conditions are especially prone to infections while in the hospital. So are older patients kept alive with immunosuppressive drugs and immunosuppressive procedures. When catheterization, positive pressure apparatus, or anesthesiology equipment is applied to these compromised patients, they are often unable to withstand the challenge of the microbe.

Metabolic Disorders

Patients with leukemia or any hematological disorder that involves the immune system must be considered likely candidates for hospital-acquired infections. In leukemic patients the problem is often compounded because of the need for radiation or drug therapy to reduce the number of leukocytes. This kind of therapy leads to immunological deficiencies.

Diabetics are also highly susceptible to nosocomial infections. Their susceptibility is related to secondary effects of the disease such as renal insufficiency, acidosis, and vascular insufficiency, particularly of the lower extremities. Insulin-dependent patients with diabetes mellitus suffer more frequent and severe staphylococcal infections than nondiabetics.

Immunosuppressive Drugs

Immunosuppressive drugs are used therapeutically for immunological disease in which there is a need to reduce the level of leukocytes in the host system. They are also used prophylactically to prevent the rejection of transplant tissue in the immunologically sensitive recipient. The three classes of immunosuppressive agents are (1) the lymphocytolytic agents such as the corticosteroids; (2) the metabolic analogues, such as azathioprine, which interfere with DNA synthesis of lymphoid tissue; and (3) the alkylating agents, such as nitrogen mustard, which depurinate nucleic acids. The function of these agents is to suppress the cellular or humoral immune systems of the host. Corticosteroids, for example, generally depress the formation of antibodies and suppress the delayed hypersensitivity reaction that is believed to be responsible for transplantation immunity. A recent addition to immunosuppressive drug regimens is *cyclosporine*. This is a partially selective drug, which has reduced the incidence of infection as well as decreased the incidence of graft loss.

In the immunosuppressed state the patient is literally at the mercy of any opportunistic pathogen. In renal transplantation, for instance, pneumonia is the most common cause of death, with bacteria causing about 60 percent of the infections, followed by viruses (25 percent) and fungi (15 percent). Most fatalities of fungal origin in immunocompromised patients are associated with species of *Candida* and *Aspergillus*. Fatal septicemias of bacterial origin are attributed to the gram-negative bacilli, particularly species of *Pseudomonas*. Hepatitis is often the most serious viral complication. Cytomegalovirus (CMV) in-fection is also a frequent complication in renal transplantation but is seldom fatal.

Trauma

Individuals in accidents that cause trauma are susceptible to infection. Traumatic wounds, by crushing and tearing, produce large amounts of dead fat with poor vascularity. In addition, burn wounds appear to depress numerous immune resistance factors such as neutrophil function. This type of condition lends itself to microbial contamination and sepsis by microorganisms usually considered to be noninvasive. Microorganisms associated with burn wound infections are *Pseudomonas aeruginosa, S. aureus,* and enterococci. *P. aeruginosa* and other *Pseudomonas* species thrive in moist environments, and in the hospital they are frequent contaminants of humidifiers and nebulizers. *Pseudomonas* species are also resistant to many antimicrobials and disinfectants. The mortality from *Pseudomonas* septicemia in burn wound patients can be greatly reduced with the administration of a polyvalent vaccine in conjunction with an immunoglobulin prepared from the serum of vaccinated healthy volunteers.

HOSPITAL PROCEDURES

Surgery

Unsterilized instruments, sutures, sponges, and irrigating solutions as well as the surgical team itself are the main sources of infection related to surgery. Only sterile equipment and solutions are used during surgical activities. In addition, the surgical team wear sterile gowns, masks, and gloves. The patient has many nonspecific mechanisms for resisting infection. Surgery and related procedures can interfere with these natural resistance factors and may be responsible for severe and sometimes fatal infections. Since tissue is being cut, the normal host defense mechanisms are breached, and the reduction in host resistance is worsened by anesthesia. The number of microorganisms that gain entrance to the traumatized tissue and the site of the surgical operation greatly influence the rate of infection. Wounds can be divided into four types: clean, clean-contaminated, contaminated, and dirty (Table 34-4):

1. *Clean wounds* are those in which no hollow muscular organ (gastrointestinal or respiratory tract) was opened and no break in aseptic technique occurred.
2. *Clean-contaminated wounds* refers to the opening of a hollow muscular organ with minimal spillage of contents.
3. *Contaminated wounds* refers to the opening of hollow organs with gross spillage of contents and acute inflammation without pus formation.
4. *Dirty wounds* refers to the presence of pus or perforated viscera.

The probability of infection goes up further if the patient has been compromised by immunosuppressive drugs, malnutrition, or an underlying illness. Studies with animals show that within the first 3 hours of bacterial contamination of tissue the host's antimicrobial defenses are at their peak. This 3-hour peak activity can be strengthened through the use of antibiotics. If the peak antimicrobial activity of the antibiotic can be coordinated with the host's, there is a better chance of resisting infection.

Table 34-4. Rates of Infection of Various Types of Wounds

Type of wound	Total number of wounds	Number of wounds infected (%)
Clean	47,054	732 (1.5)
Clean-contaminated	9,370	720 (7.7)
Contaminated	4,442	676 (15.2)
Dirty	2,093	832 (35.0)
Total	62,959	2,960 (4.7)

Source: P. Cruse, *Surg. Clin. North Am.* 60:27, 1980.

Most postoperative infections occur when surgery has been performed on the alimentary, respiratory, or genitourinary tract. In recent years the number of postoperative infections caused by gram-negative species, especially species of *Pseudomonas, Klebsiella, Proteus,* and *Serratia,* has increased (Table 34-1). Much of this increase is directly correlated with the prophylactic use of antibiotics. The major problems result from the extended use of antibiotics after surgery. When antibiotics are continued longer than one week after surgery, the incidence of infection rises dramatically.

A number of procedures, in addition to the ones already mentioned, can help to reduce the incidence of infection following surgery, and these are outlined in Table 34-5.

Catheterization

Catheterization is a process in which a tabular device (catheter) is inserted into a blood vessel

Table 34-5. Procedures That Help Reduce the Incidence of Infection in Patients Undergoing Surgery

1. Sterilized gloves, instruments, and solutions used by the surgical team
2. Hand scrubbing by surgical team with an antiseptic solution containing chlorhexidine (Hibitane)
3. Preparation of the patient's skin by using a solution such as 0.5 percent chlorhexidine in 70 percent alcohol (Hibiscrub)
4. Surgeries carried out in operating rooms in which there is ultraclean air; restriction of traffic in the operating room and restriction of passage to anyone with a skin infection
5. Mechanical bowel preparation through use of laxatives, low-residue diet, and enemas for patients who will be subjected to large-bowel surgeries
6. Oral antibiotics, such as erythromycin plus neomycin, administered to patients prior to bowel surgeries
7. Prophylactic antibiotics for any operation in which contamination is expected or infection could be catastrophic (for example, implantation of orthopedic prostheses)

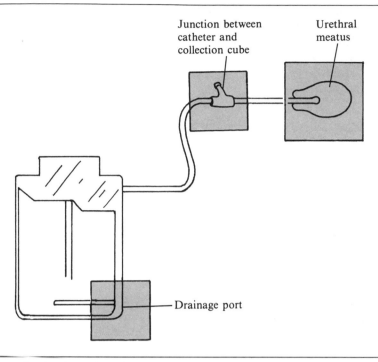

Junction between
catheter and
collection cube

Urethral
meatus

Drainage port

Fig. 34-1. Sites of contamination in catheterization.

or the urinary tract. Catheters may be used diagnostically or therapeutically. Improper sterilization of the catheter or contamination of sterilized catheters by attending hospital staff represents a potential risk to the patient. The catheter is the single most important predisposing factor in nosocomial infections. Nearly 10 percent of all hospitalized patients receive a urinary catheter. Most catheter-associated infections occur at the time of insertion of the catheter when microorganisms on the body surface are inserted into the urethra (extraluminal—Fig. 34-1). In addition, infections occur when the juncture between catheter and collecting tube is broken, permitting microbial contamination. Indwelling catheters are used for the drainage of urine in patients whose urine flow is obstructed. Bacteria can pass into the bladder urine along the catheter tubing by a backward flow of voided urine from a contaminated drainage bottle (intraluminal). The development of the closed sterile drainage system equipped with a nonreturn valve that prevents the reflux of urine from the drainage bag into the drainage tube has markedly reduced the number of urinary tract infections. Despite this development, infections do occur because of breaches in aseptic technique on the part of hospital personnel. Most infections are caused by the gram-negative bacilli (see Tables 34-1, 34-2). These infections are increased when the patient is being treated with antibiotics. Most catheter-associated urinary tract infections are benign if the catheterization lasts less than 10 days.

Intravenous catheters not inserted aseptically and left in place for more than 48 hours are a source of infection. Skin microorganisms can enter the tip of the catheter at the time of insertion. However, contamination can occur at insertion by microorganisms on the hands of hospital personnel. The mechanisms of microbial colonization of I.V. catheters is influenced by many factors, including type of device used. Intravenous catheters made of polyvinylchloride are more susceptible to adherence by coagulase-negative staphylococci than catheters made of te-flon. Coagulase-negative staphylococci are the most common cause of I.V. device–related infection. Bacteremia caused by these organisms is associated with prolonged hospital stay and results in excess mortality. Many hospital-associated coagulase-negative staphylococci are resistant to semisynthetic penicillins and vancomycin may be the drug of choice.

Catheter-related *Candida* infections can also occur when broad-spectrum antibiotics are applied at the site of catheterization. Topical antibiotic treatment reduces the number of bacteria without affecting the fungal population.

Though rare, septic infections due to contamination of infusion fluids are more likely to be caused by microorganisms introduced during infusate preparation and administration to the patient than during the manufacturing process. Sources of contamination of infusion fluids are illustrated in Figure 34-2. Other sources of contamination of infusion fluids are illustrated in Fig. 34-2.

Antibiotic Chemotherapy

The areas within the hospital having the highest usage of antimicrobials are the intensive care units, burn units, and special surgery care areas. These areas also have the highest prevalence of antimicrobial-resistant bacteria. Colonization with these antimicrobial-resistant bacteria will occur even in those who are not being treated with antimicrobials. This is related to the individual's time of exposure to patients who are being treated with antimicrobials.

There has been considerable debate concerning the prophylactic use of antimicrobials for surgical techniques. Antimicrobial-resistant microorganisms can arise endogenously if the antimicrobials are improperly used. In surgical operations in which there is no contamination, the administration of antimicrobials is not recommended. The following procedures are currently considered acceptable for antimicrobial prophylaxis:

1. Cardiovascular—valve and open heart, coronary artery bypass
2. Orthopedic—prosthetic joint
3. Intestinal—colonic
4. Biliary tract—patient over 70 years of age, acute cholecystitis, obstructive jaundice, or stones in common bile duct
5. Gynecological—vaginal hysterectomy, caesarian section
6. Urological—patients bacteriuric before urological procedures

The antimicrobial agent should be administered 1 to 2 hours before surgery, and the last dose (doses should not exceed six) should be administered less than 24 hours after surgery.

Some techniques that have supplanted surgery may also require antibiotic prophylaxis (see Boxed Essay, p. 860).

Hypodermic Injections

Hypodermic injections can be a source of infection in three ways: (1) use of contaminated needles or syringes, (2) displacement of an infectious agent from the surface of the skin into the bloodstream or underlying tissue in the injection process, and (3) use of contaminated solutions for injection. Of the three, injection of contaminated solutions is the principal source of infection. Any kind of injectable fluid such as blood, vitamins, and vaccines may be contaminated before injection and thereby transmit infectious microorganisms to the patient. Blood transfusions remain a constant means of infecting the compromised patient. In the United States from 20,000 to 30,000 cases of viral hepatitis are reported each year arising from transfused blood acquired from donors infected with the hepatitis virus. Blood donors are now being screened for hepatitis B surface antigen, and whenever possible washed packed red blood cells should be used for transfusions. These procedures alone can reduce the incidence of transfusion hepatitis.

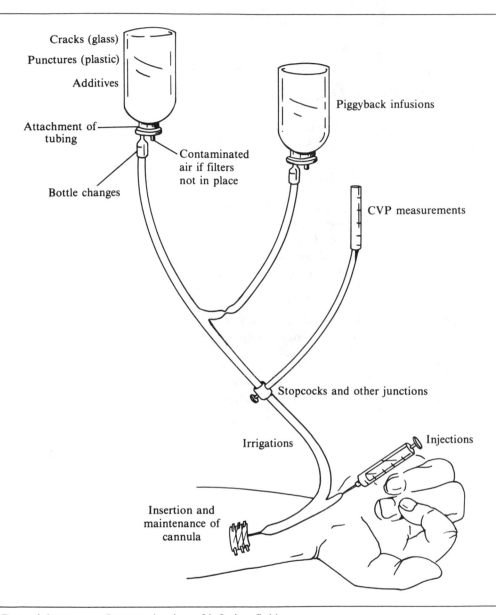

Fig. 34-2. Potential sources of contamination of infusion fluid.

Diagnostic Procedures

Diagnostic procedures or equipment used on patients by physicians or other medical personnel have been implicated as sources of nosocomial infection. The reason is that the devices or instruments are often not decontaminated before use on the next patient. In addition, endogenous microorganisms may be displaced into abraded tissue, thereby giving rise to infection. Among the instruments implicated are cystoscopes, urometers, cannulas of urinary catheters, gastrointestinal fiberoptic endoscopes, and pressure-

A NEW HOSPITAL TECHNIQUE—LITHOTRIPSY

Lithotripsy is a new technique that has become the preferred method for the treatment of urinary stones or calculi. The treatment, which involves the use of shock waves, has almost completely supplanted open surgery and, to a lesser extent, endourological approaches. When the stones are broken up, thousands of minute fragments are released, which can remain in the collecting system of the patient for weeks to months. Many of these stones are infected with urea-splitting microorganisms that may cause urinary tract infections, obstructive pyelonephritis, and septicemia.

Recent studies have demonstrated that there may be a need for antibiotic prophylaxis in a select group of patients: those with staghorn or struvite calculi, a large stone burden, infected urine, or a documented history of recurrent urinary tract infections. In the absence of complicating factors there is no indication of antibiotic prophylaxis. Characterization of organisms and their antibiotic sensitivities, before lithotripsy is initiated, is necessary should infection occur in those with complications.

These studies once again demonstrate that with each new hospital procedure the risk of hospital-associated infection increases.

monitoring devices such as venous and arterial pressure transducers.

PREVENTION AND CONTROL OF NOSOCOMIAL INFECTIONS

ENVIRONMENTAL SURVEILLANCE

One of the keys to the management and control of hospital-acquired infections is surveillance. In the past few years it has become evident that antibiotics have not reduced the risk of hospital-associated infections. The only important change brought about by the use of these drugs is a shift in the type of infectious agent involved in infections. Today the gram-negative bacilli have replaced the gram-positive cocci in the number of hospital-acquired infections. Many hospitals now have resident epidemiologists or infection-control nurses whose duty it is to determine the frequency and kind of nosocomial infections. Attempts to reduce infection by surveillance and control of environmental factors, however, have shown only moderate success. Culturing of the entire hospital environment is not practical and in many instances is of little value. There are procedures that are believed to be of maximum benefit, and these should be performed in all hospitals:

1. Environmental culturing only as part of an investigation of a disease outbreak or other problem of patient infection.
2. Testing the effectiveness of steam and ethylene oxide sterilizers.
3. Testing the sterility of products prepared in the hospital that have been shown to present risk of contamination. These products include infant formula, hyperalimentation fluids prepared in the hospital, and breast milk collected for group use.
4. Testing the effectiveness of decontamination

and disinfection of instruments such as endoscopes, inhalation therapy equipment, and physical therapy equipment.

Environmental surveillance is but one of the roles of the infection-control nurse, who must also become involved in control, teaching, and implementation of policy.

The effect that infection control programs has had on the prevention of nosocomial disease is described in Table 34-6.

HYGIENIC PRACTICES

It is important that housekeeping practices as well as patient-related medical procedures be evaluated. The maintenance of a satisfactory standard of hygienic practices is the duty of all hospital personnel from physician to kitchen cook. Disinfectants and antiseptics are used in the hospital to maintain a standard of hygiene. The use of a particular disinfectant or antiseptic depends on a number of factors (Table 34-7):

1. The nature of the object to be treated and the presence or absence of residual material on the object that might neutralize the effect of the agent, such as soap or other organic material.
2. The type of pathogen to be treated—spores, vegetative bacteria, viruses.
3. The antimicrobial spectrum of the disinfectant or antiseptic.
4. The strength of the agent and the time required for it to exert a bacteriostatic or bactericidal effect.

Hygienic practices are extremely important in controlling and preventing nosocomial infections. It is necessary to maintain aseptic technique in handling instruments, catheters, intravenous therapy equipment, and any other type of device that may come in contact with the hospitalized patient. The one practice that probably reduces the incidence of nosocomial infection more than any other, and yet is often overlooked,

Table 34-6. Percentage of Nosocomial Infections Prevented by the Most Effective Infection Surveillance and Control Programs

Type of infection	Components of most effective programs	Percent prevented
Surgical wound infection	An organized hospitalwide program with intensive surveillance and control Reporting surgical wound infection rates to surgeons *Plus*	20
	An effectual physician with special interest and knowledge in infection control	35
Urinary tract infection	An organized hospitalwide program with: Intensive surveillance in operation for at least one year An Infection Control Nurse per 250 beds	38
Nosocomial bacteremia	An organized hospitalwide program with intensive control alone *Plus*	15
	Moderately intensive surveillance in operation for at least one year An Infection Control Nurse per 250 beds An infection control physician or microbiologist	35
Postoperative pneumonia in surgical patients	An organized hospitalwide program with intensive surveillance An Infection Control Nurse per 250 beds	27
Pneumonia in medical patients	An organized hospitalwide program with intensive surveillance and control	13
All types of nosocomial infections	An organized hospitalwide program with all of the components listed above	32

The data in this table were obtained by reviewing the records of approximately 339,000 patients in 338 hospitals in the United States from 1970, before any of the hospitals had infection control programs, to 1975–1976, a period after infection control programs had been instituted.
Source: R. W. Haley and J. S. Garner, in J. V. Bennet and P. S. Brachman (eds.), *Hospital Infections* (2nd ed.). Boston: Little, Brown, 1986.

is *handwashing*. It is estimated that at least 50 percent of hospital infections could be prevented by handwashing. Although cross contamination by hand transmission occurs frequently in the hospitalized patient, handwashing is not consistently performed. The microflora of the skin harbors an indigenous population of microorganisms such as *S. epidermidis* and *Propionibacterium* species, both of which are considered relatively nonvirulent. Because of constant contact with patients and the perpetuation of certain species in the hospital, large numbers of more virulent microorganisms are also carried on the skin—for example, *S. aureus* and gram-negative species.

It is very important, therefore, during the handling of patients, particularly when medical personnel are going from one patient to another, that contaminating microorganisms be removed from the skin. Washing one's hands with soap and water is sufficient to reduce the microbial population of the skin, but, because of the drying effect of soap and the failure of soap to remain bacteriostatic for any length of time, other antiseptic agents are more suitable. Iodophors and 3 percent hexachlorophene are two agents that are extensively used today. In 1976 the FDA approved the use of chlorhexidine gluconate (CG) with 4% isopropyl alcohol in a sudsing base (Hib-

Table 34-7. Useful Disinfectants and Antiseptics Employed in the Hospital

| Compound* | Activity against | | | | Uses (and limitations) |
	Vegetative bacteria and fungi	TB bacillus	Hepatitis virus	Spores	
Alcohols					
Ethyl	+	+	−	−	Skin antiseptic
Isopropyl	+	+	−	−	Skin antiseptic
Iodine					
Tincture of iodine	+	?	−	−	Skin antiseptic
Iodophors	+	+	−	−	Unstable, skin antiseptic
Phenols and cresols					
1–2% Phenols	+	+	−	−	Disinfectant, stable in solution
Chlorophenol	+	+	−	−	More active than phenol but more toxic
Hexachlorophene	+	−	−	−	Antiseptic, good surgical scrub
Chlorhexidine	+	−	−	−	Skin antiseptic
Chlorine					
Chloramine	+	−	−	−	1–2% solution for wounds
Sodium hypochlorite	+	+	+	?	Disinfectant, unstable in solution
Formaldehyde	+	+	+	+	Disinfectant, noxious fumes
Glutaraldehyde	+	+	+	+	Disinfectant, unstable, toxic
Ethylene oxide	+	+	+	+	Disinfectant, toxic, absorbed by porous material
Quaternary ammonium compounds	+	−	−	−	Antiseptic, ineffective against gram-negatives

* 0.2% Sodium nitrite added to alcohols, formalin, quaternary ammonium compounds, and iodophors prevents corrosive actions of these agents; 0.5% sodium bicarbonate added to phenolic compounds reduces the corrosive action of those compounds.

iclens). It has been approved for use as a surgical scrub, patient-care handwashing agent, and superficial wound cleanser. This preparation appears to achieve a more immediate reduction in the skin flora than the other agents and has a more sustained antimicrobial effect.

HOSPITAL PERSONNEL SURVEILLANCE

The immunization records of all hospital personnel should be checked and vaccinations given or recommended if they have not been done. Certain personnel should be vaccinated for tuberculosis and offered immunization against polio-

myelitis, tetanus, diphtheria, and rubella. The rubella vaccination is especially important for members of hospital staff who come in contact with nurses, doctors, patients, and pregnant women (see Chapter 34). Every one of these procedures is important, not only to hospital personnel but also to the patient, who in the compromised condition is most susceptible to infection.

PATIENT SURVEILLANCE

When patients are admitted to the hospital, their medical files should include an infection "report card." During their stay, data regarding disease treatment should be recorded. This information should include

1. The type of infection, if any, the patient had on admission to the hospital
2. The kind and site of any hospital-acquired infection
3. The organism isolated from the infection
4. Any surgical procedure or chemotherapy that preceded the development of the infection
5. The antibiotic regimen employed to combat the infection
6. The length of time required to control the infection

The information gathered from the report card could be compiled each week and a monthly report distributed to the infection control committee. The data would thus include statistics on infections as to site (urinary tract, respiratory tract), causative agents isolated, and antibiotic regimen employed. An increase in the rate of infection could then be investigated and the source of infection uncovered.

If an infectious disease is detected in the patient on admission to the hospital, he or she may require isolation. Isolation is necessary for persons who have such diseases as meningococcal meningitis, staphylococcal pneumonia, tuberculosis, diphtheria, whooping cough, measles (rubella and rubeola), smallpox, chickenpox, mumps, influenza, or pneumonic plague. Patients who have been compromised by hospital procedures should also be isolated from other patients. This group would include patients recovering from open-heart surgery, transplantation, and burns, and those requiring renal dialysis. It is very important to protect these individuals from airborne microbes that are easily transferred in an open ward. Isolation can be accomplished by means of plastic tents and laminar airflow, in which a positive current of filtered air is directed at the patient. The positive pressure of this airflow prevents access of contaminated air from other sources.

SUMMARY

1. The term *nosocomial* is a synonym for hospital-associated disease. Nosocomial diseases differ from community-associated diseases primarily in their epidemiology.

2. The microbial agents responsible for nosocomial diseases can be transmitted from patient to patient indirectly via hospital personnel, directly by contact with hospital staff, by contact with contaminated fomites or solutions, and by airborne spread. However, most nosocomial infections are caused by species that are part of the victim's own microbial flora.

3. The most prevalent microbial groups causing infection are the gram-negative bacilli, which inlude *Escherichia coli, Pseudomonas aeruginosa*, and species of *Klebsiella, Serratia*, and others. *Staphylococcus aureus* is still the most frequently isolated species, primarily because most hospital personnel are carriers of the microbial species. Coagulase-negative staphylococci are the most frequent cause of morbidity and mortality in primary bacteremias.

4. *Candida* and *Aspergillus* are the two most frequently isolated genera of fungi causing disease, while viruses such as rubella, respiratory syncytial virus, varicella-zoster virus, herpes simplex virus, and hepatitis A virus are the most frequent causes of viral nosocomial disease. Some viruses such as herpes simplex virus and cytomegalovirus are endogenous viruses that may be activated by hospital procedures or conditions of the host.

5. Microbial factors contributing to nosocomial disease have been brought about by the frequent use of antimicrobials, which select for resistant strains of a microbial species. Many of these resistant strains can readily transfer their resistance factors, via plasmids, to other species.

6. The immunological state of the host is the single most important factor determining an individual's susceptibility to infection. Age, met-

abolic disorders, use of immunosuppressive drugs, and burn wounds reduce one's resistance to infection, particularly to infection by the opportunistic microorganisms.

7. Hospital procedures including surgery, antibiotic chemotherapy, hypodermic injection, and diagnostic and therapeutic techniques lead to the introduction of microorganisms into host tissue. Most of the time the organisms are part of the host's flora that are displaced by surgery or diagnostic procedures.

8. Catheterization, which is performed on many patients, is the single most important procedure causing predisposition to infection. Most urinary tract infections resulting from catheterization are benign if the catheter is not left in over 10 days.

9. Antibiotic prophylaxis is necessary in surgeries in which microbial contamination is certain and infection could be catastrophic.

10. Hypodermic injections can be a source of infection in three ways: by (1) use of contaminated needles, (2) displacement of infectious agents from the skin, and (3) use of contaminated solutions. Blood transfusions, for example, can cause hepatitis.

11. Diagnostic procedures that utilize devices such as cystoscopes, fiberoptic endoscopes, etc. can be causes of nosocomial disease. The infections may arise because of contamination of the instrument or displacement of endogenous microorganisms.

12. Studies have demonstrated that hospital infection control programs headed by an infection-control nurse and/or physician can bring about significant reductions in nosocomial diseases. These programs include techniques for environmental surveillance, maintenance of hygienic practices, and surveillance of patient and hospital personnel.

QUESTIONS FOR STUDY

Select the best response or responses for each of the following:

1. A patient develops a severe bacteremia following parenteral nutrition. Which of the following microbial agents would you suspect is most likely responsible?
   A. Enterococci
   B. *Bacteroides* species
   C. *Proteus* species
   D. *Staphylococcus epidermidis*

2. The two most frequently isolated causes of urinary tract infections in the hospital are
   A. *Klebsiella* and *Proteus* species
   B. *Klebsiella* and *E. coli*
   C. *E. coli* and enterococci
   D. *Candida* and *Proteus* species

3. Most hospital staff are carriers of antibiotic-resistant

   A. *E. coli*
   B. Enterococci
   C. *Staphylococcus aureus*
   D. *Candida albicans*

4. The groups of bacteria most commonly associated with burn wound infections are
   A. *Pseudomonas aeruginosa*, *S. aureus*, and enterococci
   B. *S. aureus*, *K. pneumoniae*, and *Bacteroides* species
   C. *P. aeruginosa*, *K. pneumoniae*, and *Bacteroides* species
   D. *S. epidermidis*, *S. aureus*, and enterococci

5. The microbial agent(s) responsible for most hospital-associated infections is (are)

A. *S. aureus*
B. Enterococci
C. *P. aeruginosa*
D. *E. coli*

6. Under which of the following conditions would antibiotics *not* be used as a prophylactic measure?
   A. Surgery involving the bowel
   B. Coronary bypass surgery
   C. Implantation of an orthopedic device
   D. Cosmetic surgery involving the face

7. Which of the following procedures contributes to the majority of hospital-associated diseases?
   A. Surgery
   B. Intravenous catheterization
   C. Urinary catheterization
   D. Hypodermic injection

8. The single most important factor determining one's susceptibility to nosocomial infection is

A. Patient age
B. Type of hospital procedure performed on the patient
C. Type of microorganism involved
D. The immunological state of the host

9. The hospital practice that can reduce over 50 percent of hospital-associated infections is
   A. Disinfection of hospital surfaces
   B. Air filtration
   C. Handwashing
   D. Administration of antibiotics to all patients undergoing surgery

10. Which of the following compounds is believed to have a more sustained antimicrobial effect when present in antiseptic preparations?
    A. Chlorhexidine
    B. Formaldehyde
    C. Alcohol
    D. Iodine

ADDITIONAL READINGS

CDC. *CDC Surveillance Summaries. Nosocomial Infection Surveillance, 1984. MMWR* 35 (No. 1SS), 1986.

Mayer, K. H., and Zinner, S. H. Bacterial pathogens of increasing significance in hospital-acquired infections. *Rev. Infect. Dis* 7(Suppl.3):771,1985.

Musial, C. E., Cockerill, F. R. III, and Roberts, G. A. Fungal infections of the immunocompromised host: Clinical and laboratory aspects. *Clin. Microbiol. Revs.* 1(4):349,1988.

Nosocomial Viral Infection: Incidence and Control. *Microbiology—1985* (page 121). Washington, DC.: American Society for Microbiology, 1985.

Sacks, T., and McGowan, J. E., Jr. International Symposium on control of nosocomial infection. *Rev. Infect. Dis.* 3:4, 1981.

Walsh, T. J., and Pizzo, P. Z. Nosocomial fungal infections: A classification for hospital-acquired fungal infections and mycoses arising from endogenous flora or reactivation. *Annu. Rev. Microbiol.* 4:517,1988.

Wenzel, P. P. The evolving art and science of hospital epidemiology. *J. Infect. Dis.* 153:462,1986.

Wenzel, R. P. (ed.). *Prevention and Control of Nosocomial Infections*. Baltimore: Williams & Wilkins, 1986.

APPENDICES

APPENDIX A. TABLES OF INFECTIOUS DISEASE BASED ON BODY SITE

The following tables bring together all the different infectious agents that can affect one body site. It is important to note that many diseases that are acquired through various body sites can cause major pathologic responses at other body sites. For example, several helminths penetrate the skin but affect internal organs. In some diseases more than one body site may be involved, and for this reason you may see a microbial agent listed more than once. For example, the organism causing plague affects the lymph and cardiovascular systems but pneumonic plague may also be a result of infection. Thus plague can be considered to affect the respiratory tract as well as the lymph and cardiovascular systems. For your convenience the text page where the specific disease is discussed in detail is also included in the tables.

Table A-1. Diseases Affecting the Skin and Eyes

	Microbial agent	Mode of transmission	Treatment and or prevention	Discussion page
BACTERIAL				
Skin				
Impetigo	*Staphylococcus aureus, Streptococcus pyogenes*	Contact with infected person	None usually required	396, 406
Folliculitis, boils	*Staphylococcus aureus*	Infection of hair follicles by commensals	Methicillin, oxacillin, cephalosporins	396
Scalded skin syndrome	*Staphylococcus aureus*	Infection of infant skin by certain commensal strains	None	396
Erysipelas	Group A beta-hemolytic streptococci	Infection of skin by toxin-producing species	Penicillin	406
Leprosy	*Mycobacterium leprae*	Repeated exposure to infected person	Dapsone, clofazimine	544
Eye				
Pink eye (conjunctivitis)	*Hemophilus aegyptius*	Person-to-person contact with infected secretions	None usually required	522
Trachoma	*Chlamydia trachomatis*	Person to person via contaminated fingers or objects	Erythromycin, tetracycline	590
Ophthalmia neonatorum	*Neisseria gonorrhoeae*	From mother to fetus	Tetracycline, erythromycin, silver nitrate	426
VIRAL				
Skin				
Smallpox	Smallpox (variola) virus	Contact with pustules or contaminated objects	Disease eradicated in 1977	662
Chickenpox-shingles	Varicella-zoster virus	Contact with skin lesions or respiratory secretions	Vidarabine in complicated cases	670
Measles	Measles (rubeola) virus	Contact with oral secretions	None; vaccine available	684
German measles (rubella)	Rubella virus	Contact with respiratory secretions	Vaccine available	689
Warts	Papilloma viruses	Contact with infected person	Podophyllum, surgery	681
Cold sores	Herpes simplex virus type 1	Contact with eye secretions?	Acyclovir	673

	Organism	Transmission	Treatment	Page
Eye				
Herpetic keratoconjunctivitis	Herpes simplex virus type 1	Contact with eye secretions	Vidarabine	673
Epidemic keratoconjunctivitis	Adenoviruses	Contact with eye secretions	None required	679
Acute hemorrhagic conjunctivitis	Echoviruses and coxsackieviruses	Contact with eye secretions	None required	701
FUNGAL				
Skin				
Superficial mycoses	*Malassezia furfur, Exophiala (Cladosporium) wernecki, Trichosporon beigelii, Piedraia hortae*	Person to person via direct or indirect means	Tolnaftate	777
Subcutaneous mycoses	(See Table 32-3, page 770)	Puncturing of skin by soil-contaminated objects		
Cutaneous mycoses (tineas)	*Trichophyton, Microsporum, Epidermophyton* species	Contact with infected animals; human-to-human transmission via direct or indirect means	Miconazole, clotrimazole	773
Candidiasis	*Candida albicans*	Allergic response to organism (dermatophytid); appendages in water or moist environment; debilitated patients subject to infection	Nystatin, miconazole, clotrimazole	778
PROTOZOAL				
Skin				
Leishmaniasis	*Leishmania tropica, L. braziliensis*	Bite of sandfly	Antimony sodium gluconate	818
HELMINTH				
Eye				
Loiasis (eye worm)	*Loa loa*	Bite of tabanid fly	Diethylcarbamazine	834
Onchocerciasis (river blindness)	*Onchocerca volvulus*	Bite of black fly	Suramin, mectizan	

Table A-2. Diseases Affecting the Respiratory Tract

	Microbial agent	Mode of transmission	Treatment and or prevention	Discussion page
BACTERIAL				
Tuberculosis	*Mycobacterium tuberculosis*	Contact with respiratory secretions, ingestion of contaminated milk	Isoniazid, streptomycin, ethambutol, and rifampin in various combinations; vaccine available	535
Pneumonia	*Streptococcus pneumoniae*	Primarily a complication following respiratory distress	Penicillin; polyvalent vaccine available	412
	Klebsiella pneumoniae	Primarily in those with upper respiratory complications (alcoholics)	Cephalosporins	495
	Mycoplasma pneumoniae	Contact with respiratory secretions	Erythromycin, tetracycline; vaccine available	574
	Legionella pneumophila	Inhalation of contaminated aerosols	Erythromycin	609
	Francisella tularensis	Inhalation of contaminated aerosols generated by animals	Streptomycin; vaccine for lab personnel	529
	Staphylococcus aureus	Primarily a secondary infection following viral infection	Methicillin, cloxacillin, and cephalosporins	397
	Hemophilus influenzae	Primarily a secondary infection following viral infection	Ampicillin, chloramphenicol	520
	Yersinia pestis	A complication of bubonic plague caused by bite of infected rat flea	Streptomycin, chloramphenicol, tetracycline; vaccine available in areas endemic for disease	490
	Coxiella burnetii	Ingestion of contaminated milk, inhalation of contaminated aerosols from barnyard animals	None usually required	585
	Chlamydia psittaci (see also *C. pneumoniae*, p. 592)	Inhalation of aerosols from infected birds	None usually required	592
Whooping cough	*Bordetella pertussis*	Contact with respiratory secretions	Erythromycin; vaccine available in DPT	523
Diphtheria	*Corynebacterium diphtheriae*	Contact with respiratory secretions	Penicillin; vaccine available in DPT	459

Disease	Organism	Transmission/Source	Treatment	Page
Pharyngitis	*Streptococcus pyogenes*	Contact with respiratory secretions	Penicillin, erythromycin	406
Scarlet fever	Toxin-producing strain of *S. pyogenes*	Contact with respiratory secretions	Penicillin, erythromycin	405
VIRAL				
Common cold	Rhinovirus	Contact with respiratory secretions	None specific	701
	Parainfluenza virus	Contact with respiratory secretions	None specific	704
	Coronavirus	Contact with respiratory secretions	None specific	701
Pneumonia	Influenza viruses	Contact with respiratory secretions	Amantadine; vaccine available	693
	Respiratory syncytial virus	Contact with respiratory secretions	None specific	703
FUNGAL				
Histoplasmosis	*Histoplasma capsulatum*	Inhalation of aerosols from contaminated bird feces	Amphotericin B, ketoconazole	761
Cryptococcosis	*Cryptococcus neoformans*	Inhalation of aerosols from contaminated pigeon droppings	Amphotericin B plus flucytosine	768
Coccidioidomycosis	*Coccidioides immitis*	Inhalation of spores from soil	Amphotericin B, ketoconazole	763
Paracoccidioidomycosis	*Paracoccidioides brasiliensis*	Inhalation of spores from soil	Ketoconazole	767
Blastomycosis	*Blastomyces dermatitidis*	Inhalation of spores from soil	Amphotericin B, ketoconazole	766
Aspergillosis	*Aspergillus* species	Inhalation of spores from soil	Amphotericin B	782
Mucormycosis (zygomycosis)	*Rhizopus, Mucor,* and *Absidia* species	Inhalation of spores from soil	Amphotericin B, flucytosine	785
Pneumocystis pneumonia	*Pneumocystis carinii*	Opportunistic (in AIDS patients, for example)	Trimethoprim-sulfamethoxazole, pentamidine, and pyrimethamine-sulfadiazine	787
PROTOZOAL				
African sleeping sickness	*Trypanosoma* species	A complication following initial nervous system involvement	Suramin, pentamidine isethionate	816
HELMINTH				
Paragonimiasis	*Paragonimus westermani*	Ingestion of raw contaminated crustaceans	Dichlorophenol	835

Table A-3. Diseases Affecting Internal Organs and Digestive System

	Microbial agent	Mode of transmission	Treatment and/or prevention	Discussion page
BACTERIAL				
Caries (tooth decay)	*Streptococcus mutans*	Indigenous species initiates plaque formation on sucrose diet	Flossing, brushing, fluoridation to prevent plaque, reduction of dietary intake of sucrose	52, 410, 602
Periodontal disease	Many species, including those of *Bacteroides* and *Actinomyces*	Presence of plaque inflames gingiva, which become infected	Flossing, brushing, fluoridation to prevent plaque; antimicrobials in mouthwashes	602
Actinomycosis (lumpy jaw)	*Actinomyces* species	Opportunistic infection resulting from compromising condition such as jaw fracture, pulled tooth	Penicillin	600
Gastroenteritis	*Escherichia coli* strains	Ingestion of contaminated food or water	Fluid and electrolyte replacement	478
	Salmonella species	Ingestion of contaminated food or water	Fluid and electrolyte replacement	481
	Staphylococcus aureus	Ingestion of toxin-contaminated food	Fluid and electrolyte replacement	397
	Vibrio parahaemolyticus	Ingestion of contaminated shellfish	Fluid and electrolyte replacement	513
	Shigella species	Ingestion of contaminated food or water	Fluid and electrolyte replacement	487
	Clostridium perfringens	Ingestion of contaminated food	Fluid and electrolyte replacement	449
	Campylobacter jejuni	Ingestion of contaminated food	Fluid and electrolyte replacement	565
	Yersinia enterocolitica	Ingestion of contaminated food	Fluid and electrolyte replacement	494
	Bacillus cereus	Ingestion of contaminated food	Fluid and electrolyte replacement	442
	Vibrio cholera (see Cholera)			
	Aeromonas hydrophila	Ingestion of contaminated water	Fluid and electrolyte replacement	514
	Plesiomonas shigellosis	Ingestion of contaminated food or water	Many cases require antibiotic therapy (chloramphenicol, tetracycline)	514

Disease	Organism	Transmission	Treatment	Page
Pseudomembranous colitis	*Clostridium difficile*	Associated with antimicrobial therapy	Vancomycin	452
Gastritis and duodenal ulcer	*Helicobacter pylori*	Not known	None yet available	566
Typhoid fever	*Salmonella typhi*	Ingestion of contaminated food or water	Chloramphenicol, ampicillin, amoxicillin; vaccine available	481
Cholera	*Vibrio cholerae*	Ingestion of contaminated food or water	Fluid and electrolyte replacement	510
Brucellosis (liver, spleen, bone)	*Brucella* species	Ingestion of contaminated food or water	Ampicillin, streptomycin, tetracycline	527
Rheumatic fever (heart)	*Streptococcus pyogenes*	Complication following pharyngitis	Penicillin	406
VIRAL				
Infectious hepatitis	Hepatitis A virus (HAV)	Ingestion of contaminated food or water	None	726
Serum hepatitis	Hepatitis B virus (HBV)	Hypodermic injection (drug addicts), sexual contact	None; vaccine available	726
Mumps (parotid glands)	Mumps virus	Contact with oral secretions	None; vaccine available	686
Cytomegalovirus inclusion disease (kidney, spleen, liver)	Cytomegalovirus (CMV)	Congenital transfer, transplantation	None	665
Gastroenteritis	Astroviruses	Fecal-oral or ingestion of contaminated food or water	Fluid and electrolyte replacement	716
	Adenovirus types 40 and 41	Fecal-oral or ingestion of contaminated food or water	Fluid and electrolyte replacement	679
	Caliciviruses	Fecal-oral or ingestion of contaminated food or water	Fluid and electrolyte replacement	716
	Rotavirus	Fecal-oral or ingestion of contaminated food or water	Fluid and electrolyte replacement	715
	Norwalk virus	Ingestion of contaminated food or water	Fluid and electrolyte replacement	682
Yellow fever (liver, spleen, kidney)	Yellow fever virus	Bite of infected *Aedes aegypti* mosquito	None; vaccine available	713
Infectious mononucleosis	Epstein-Barr virus (EBV)	Contact with oral secretions (kissing)	None	677

Table A-3. (continued)

	Microbial agent	Mode of transmission	Treatment and/or prevention	Discussion page
FUNGAL				
Mycotoxicosis	Species of *Penicillium*, *Fusarium*, *Streptomyces*, and *Aspergillus*	Ingestion of toxin-contaminated foods	None	789
PROTOZOAL				
Giardiasis	*Giardia lamblia*	Ingestion of contaminated food or water	Metronidazole, quinacrine	811
Amoebic dysentery	*Entamoeba histolytica*	Ingestion of contaminated food or water	Metronidazole, iodoquinol	809
Cryptosporidiosis	*Cryptosporidium* species	Animals to humans	None suitable	825
Balantidial dysentery	*Balantidium coli*	Ingestion of contaminated food or water	Oxytetracyclines iodoquinol	818
Chagas' disease	*Trypanosoma cruzi*	Abraded skin contaminated with feces of reduviid bug	None totally suitable	817
Malaria (kidney, spleen, liver)	*Plasmodium* species	Bite of infected female *Anopheles* mosquito	Chloroquine, primaquine phosphate	820
Visceral leishmaniasis	*Leishmania donovani*	Bite of sandfly	Antimony sodium stibo-gluconate	818

HELMINTH

Tapeworm	*Taenia saginata* (beef) *Taenia solium* (pork) *Diphyllobothrium latum* (fish)	Ingestion of larvae-contaminated fish	Niclosamide or praziquantel	837
Trichinosis	*Trichinella spiralis*	Ingestion of larvae-contaminated meat	Thiabendazole	832
Pinworm	*Enterobius vermicularis*	Person to person via fecal-oral route	Mebendazole and pyrantel pamoate	831
Fascioliasis	*Fasciolopsis buski*	Ingestion of aquatic plants contaminated with larvae	Hexylresorcinol	835
Clonorchiasis	*Clonorchis sinensis*	Ingestion of larvae-infected fish	Chloroquine-phosphate	835
Schistosomiasis (liver)	*Schistosoma mansoni, S. haematobium, S. japonicum*	Larvae penetrate skin	Praziquantel	835
Whipworm	*Trichuris trichiura*	Ingestion of eggs from contaminated soil	Mebendazole	—
Ascariasis	*Ascaris lumbricoides*	Ingestion of eggs from contaminated soil or water	Mebendazole	826
Strongyloidiasis	*Strongyloides stercoralis*	Larvae in soil penetrate skin	Thiabendazole	829

877

Table A-4. Diseases Affecting Lymph and Cardiovascular Systems

	Microbial Agent	Mode of Transmission	Treatment and/or prevention	Discussion page
BACTERIAL				
Subacute bacterial endocarditis	Alpha-hemolytic streptococci	Follows bacteremia resulting from displacement of microbes from oral cavity	Penicillin, erythromycin	410
Acute bacterial endocarditis	*Streptococcus pneumoniae*, *Staphylococcus aureus*	Bacteremia following primary infection	Penicillin (*S. pneumoniae*), methicillin, oxacillin (*S. aureus*)	397, 412
Rheumatic fever	*Streptococcus pyogenes*	Complication of heart following primary infection (pharyngitis)	Penicillin for primary infection	406
Anthrax	*Bacillis anthracis*	Inhalation of spores, contact of abraded skin with spores	Penicillin, streptomycin, tetracycline	439
Gas gangrene	*Clostridium perfringens* and other clostridia	Spore contamination of open wounds	Wound debridement, antiserum, penicillin therapy	447
Plague	*Yersinia pestis*	Bite of infected rat flea	Streptomycin, chloramphenicol, tetracycline; vaccine for endemic areas of plague	490
Brucellosis	*Brucella* species	Contact of abraded skin with infected animal carcasses, ingestion of contaminated milk	Ampicillin, streptomycin, tetracyclines	527
Tularemia	*Francisella tularensis*	Contact of abraded skin with contaminated animal carcasses, bite of infected ticks or deerflies	Streptomycin; vaccine for lab personnel	529
Rat bite fever	*Spirillum minor*	Bite of infected rat	Penicillin, tetracycline	564, 607
Lyme disease	*Borrelia* species	Bite of infected tick	Penicillin	561
Relapsing fever	*Borrelia* species	Bite of infected body louse	Tetracycline, chloramphenicol	561

Disease	Causative organism	Mode of transmission	Treatment	Page
Rickettsial disease				
Epidemic typhus	*Rickettsia prowazekii*	Contamination of wound with louse feces	Tetracycline, chloramphenicol	582
Endemic typhus	*R. typhi*	Bite of infected flea	Tetracycline, chloramphenicol	584
Rocky Mountain spotted fever*	*R. rickettsii*	Bite of infected tick	Tetracycline, chloramphenicol	584
Scrub typhus	*R. tsutsugamushi*	Bite of infected mite	Tetracycline, chloramphenicol	585
VIRAL				
Myocarditis	Coxsackieviruses	Ingestion of contaminated food or water	None	700
Yellow fever	Yellow fever virus	Bite of *Aedes aegypti* mosquito	None; vaccine available	713
Dengue fever	Dengue fever virus	Bite of *Aedes aegypti* mosquito	None	714
Marburg and Ebola virus disease	Marburg and Ebola viruses	Contact with infected humans (but may be transmitted from African green monkey)	None	710
Infectious mononucleosis	Epstein-Barr virus	Contact with oral secretions	None	677
PROTOZOAL				
Malaria	*Plasmodium* species	Bite of female *Anopheles* mosquito	Chloroquine, primaquine, or quinine sulfate for resistant strains	821
Chagas' disease	*Trypanosoma cruzi*	Contamination of wound with feces of reduviid bug	Nifurtimox, benznidazole	817
Nantucket fever	*Babesia microti*	Bite of infected tick	Chloroquine phosphate	825
HELMINTH				
Filariasis	*Brugia malayi, Wuchereria bancrofti*	Bite of infected mosquito	Diethylcarbamazine	834
Schistosomiasis	*Schistosoma* species	Contact of skin with contaminated water	Praziquantel	835

* Other spotted fevers of minor interest are outlined in Table 27-1, page 583.

Table A-5. Diseases Affecting Nervous System

	Microbial agent	Mode of transmission	Treatment and/or prevention	Discussion page
BACTERIAL				
Meningitis	*Neisseria meningitidis*	Contact with respiratory secretions	Penicillin, chloramphenicol; vaccine available	422
	Hemophilus influenzae	Contact with respiratory secretions	Ampicillin, chloramphenicol; vaccine available	520
	Listeria monocytogenes	To fetus from infected mother	Chloramphenicol, ampicillin	465
	Streptococcus agalactiae	To fetus from infected mother	Penicillin	408
Botulism	*Clostridium botulinum*	Ingestion of toxin-contaminated food	Antitoxins; prevention of respiratory failure	444
Tetanus	*Clostridium tetani*	Contamination of deep wound with spores	Antitoxin followed by penicillin; vaccine (DPT) available	450
Leprosy	*Mycobacterium leprae*	Contact with nasal secretions	Dapsone, clofazimine	544
VIRAL				
Encephalitis	Western equine encephalitis (WEE) virus	Bite of infected mosquito	None	711
	Eastern equine encephalitis (EEE) virus	Bite of infected mosquito	None	711
	St. Louis encephalitis virus	Bite of infected mosquito	None	711
	Venezuela encephalitis virus	Bite of infected mosquito	None	711
	California encephalitis virus	Bite of infected mosquito	None	711
Rabies	Rabies virus	Bite of infected animal or contact with contaminated saliva	Antirabies serum and vaccination	705
Aseptic meningitis	Echoviruses and coxsackieviruses	Ingestion of contaminated food or water	None	700
Poliomyelitis	Poliovirus	Ingestion of contaminated water	None; vaccine available	697

Disease	Causative agent	Mode of transmission	Treatment	Page
Creutzfeldt-Jakob disease	Prion	Ingestion of contaminated meat; transplantation procedures	None	737
Kuru	Prion?	Contact with infected tissues	None	737
Nervous system complications of acute viral disease				
Subacute sclerosing panencephalitis (SSPE)	Measles virus	Reactivation of latent measles virus		737
Progressive multifocal encephalopathy	Papovaviruses	Reactivation of virus in immunocompromised adults		739
Zoster	Varicella virus	Reactivation of latent virus	Vidarabine in compromised patients	670
Guillain-Barré syndrome	Influenza and varicella viruses	Disease follows influenza vaccination or varicella infection		697
Reye's syndrome	Influenza viruses (A and B) and varicella	Disease occurs in children recovering from varicella or influenza infection		693
FUNGAL				
Cryptococcosis	*Cryptococcus neoformans*	Inhalation of spore-contaminated pigeon droppings	Amphotericin B, flucytosine	768
PROTOZOAL				
Primary amebic meningoencephalitis	*Naegleria fowleri*	Inhalation of contaminated water	Amphotericin B	810
African sleeping sickness	*Trypanosoma* species	Bite of tsetse fly	Suramin and pentamidine isethionate	816
Toxoplasmosis	*Toxoplasma gondii*	Congenital infection	Sulfadiazine, sulfamerazine, and sulfamethazine in combinations	822

Table A-6. Diseases Affecting Genitourinary Tract

	Microbial agent	Mode of transmission	Treatment and/or prevention	Discussion page
BACTERIAL				
Gonorrhea	*Neisseria gonorrhoeae*	Sexual contact	Penicillin; spectinomycin for resistant strains	425
Syphilis	*Treponema pallidum*	Sexual contact	Ceftriaxone plus doxycycline, or spectinomycin and doxycycline	—
Lymphogranuloma venereum	*Chlamydia trachomatis*	Sexual contact	Tetracycline	591
Soft chancre	*Hemophilus ducreyi*	Sexual contact	Erythromycin	—
Granuloma inguinale	*Calymmatobacterium granulomatis*	Sexual contact	Streptomycin, tetracycline	607
Gardnerella vaginitis	*Gardnerella vaginalis*	Opportunistic commensal	Metronidazole	607, 608
Acute glomerulonephritis	*Streptococcus pyogenes* (immune reaction to microbial antigen)	Complication following infection at another body site (cutaneous, respiratory)	Penicillin or erythromycin for eradicating microbe	407
Nongonococcal urethritis	*Chlamydia trachomatis*	Sexual contact	Tetracyclines or erythromycin	591
Pelvic inflammatory disease (PID)	*Neisseria gonorrhoeae* and *Chlamydia trachomatis* most important	Sexual contact—complication of primary infection by microbe	Carbenicillin or two to three drug combinations including an aminoglycoside	426
Leptospirosis	*Leptospira interrogans*	Ingestion of contaminated water or direct contact with infected animals	Penicillin	563
VIRAL				
Genital warts	Human papilloma virus	Sexual contact	Podophyllotoxin, trichloroacetic acid, or surgery	681
Genital herpes	Herpes simplex virus type 2	Sexual contact	Acyclovir	675
FUNGAL				
Vaginal candidiasis	*Candida albicans*	Opportunistic commensal but can be sexually transmitted	Miconazole, clotrimazole	779
PROTOZOAL				
Trichomoniasis	*Trichomonas vaginalis*	Sexual contact	Metronidazole	815

882

APPENDIX B. TABLES OF HUMAN MICROFLORA

Table B-1. Microorganisms Found on the Skin, Ear, and Eye

Organism	Diseases with which microorganism may be implicated
BACTERIA	
Acinetobacter calcoaceticus	Skin; postoperative wound infections
Bacillus spp.	Skin; panophthalmitis, meningitis
Corynebacterium spp.	Skin, eye, ear; bacterial endocarditis, skin lesions
Hemophilus aegyptius	Eye infections
Micrococcus spp.	Skin; pneumonia, meningitis
Moraxella spp.	Eye infections
Mycobacterium spp.	Skin; mycobacteriosis (see page 543)
Neisseria spp.	Eye; none
Propionibacterium acnes	Skin; pimples, acne, bacterial endocarditis
Staphylococcus aureus	Skin, ear; boils, furuncles, impetigo, mastitis, toxic shock syndrome (see page 396)
Staphylococcus epidermidis	Skin, ear, eye; pimples, acne, endocarditis (see page 401)
FUNGI	
Candida albicans and other yeasts	Skin; candidiasis (see page 779)
Trichophyton spp.	Skin; dermatophytoses (see page 774)
Pityrosporium spp.	Skin; tinea versicolor and other cutaneous lesions, including folliculitis (see page 777)
Epidermophyton floccosum	Skin; skin infections such as athlete's foot (see page 775)

Table B-2. Microorganisms Found in the Respiratory Tract

Organism	Diseases with which microorganism may be implicated
BACTERIA	
Acinetobacter spp.	Meningitis, pneumonia
Actinomyces spp.	Actinomycosis (see page 598)
Arachnia propionica	Actinomycosis (see page 598)
Bacteroides spp.	Lung abscess
Bifidobacterium spp.	Actinomycosis (see page 598)
Corynebacterium spp.	Subacute bacterial endocarditis
Enterococcus spp.	Meningitis, pneumonia, bacterial endocarditis
Fusobacterium spp.	Lung abscess
Hemophilus spp.	Laryngotracheobronchitis, meningitis
Lactobacillus spp.	Bacterial endocarditis
Leptotrichia buccalis	No definitive implications
Micrococcus spp.	No definitive implications
Moraxella spp.	Conjunctivitis
Mycoplasma spp.	Primary atypical pneumonia (see page 574)
Neisseria spp.	Meningitis (see page 422)
Peptococcus spp.	Lung abscess
Peptostreptococcus spp.	Lung abscess
Propionibacterium acnes	Pimples, acne
Rothia dentocariosa	Abscess
Selenomonas sputigena	No definitive implications
Staphylococcus aureus	Pneumonia, otitis (see page 397)
Staphylococcus epidermidis	Subacute bacterial endocarditis (see page 402)
Streptococcus pneumoniae	Pneumonia, meningitis, otitis media (see page 412)
Treponema denticola	No definitive implications
Veillonella spp.	Bacterial endocarditis
Vibrio sputorum	No definitive implications
Viridans streptococci	Subacute bacterial endocarditis
FUNGI	
Candida albicans and other yeasts	Thrush (see page 779)
Torulopsis glabrata	No definitive implications
ANIMAL PARASITES	
Entamoeba gingivalis	No definitive implications
Trichomonas tenax	No definitive implications

Table B-3. Microrganisms Found in the Genitourinary Tract

Organism	Disease with which microorganism may be implicated
BACTERIA	
Acinetobacter spp.	Urethritis
Bacteroides spp.	Complication of surgery
Bifidobacterium spp.	None
Chlamydia spp.	Urethritis, cervicitis, neonatal disease (see page 591)
Clostridium spp.	Complications of surgery
Corynebacterium spp.	No definitive implication
Enterobacteriaceae	Pyelonephritis, cystitis
Enterococcus spp.	Pyelonephritis, cystitis
Fusobacterium spp.	No definitive implications
Gardnerella vaginalis	Vaginitis (see page 607)
Lactobacillus spp.	None
Moraxella spp.	Postoperative complications
Mycobacterium spp.	None
Mycoplasma spp.	Nonspecific urethritis (see page 575)
Neisseria spp.	None
Peptococcus spp.	Postoperative complications
Peptostreptococcus spp.	Puerperal fever
Sarcina spp.	Postoperative complications
Staphylococcus aureus	Urethritis, furunculosis (see page 396)
Staphylococcus saprophyticus	Urinary tract infection in women
Streptococcus agalactiae	Neonatal disease, meningitis, endocarditis, osteomyelitis, myocarditis (see page 408)
Viridans streptococci	None
FUNGI	
Candida albicans and other yeasts	Candidiasis (see page 779)
ANIMAL PARASITES	
Trichomonas vaginalis	Vaginitis

Table B-4. Microorganisms Found in the Gastrointestinal Tract

Organism	Diseases with which microorganism may be implicated
BACTERIA	
Achromobacter spp.	Postoperative wound infections
Acidaminococcus fermentans	No definitive implications
Acinetobacter calcoaceticus	Postoperative complications
Aeromonas spp.	Osteomyelitis, postoperative complications
Alcaligenes faecalis	No definitive implications
Bacillus spp.	Wound infections
Bacteroides spp.	Peritonitis, abscess, cholecystitis
Bifidobacterium spp.	Peritonitis
Campylobacter spp.	Diarrhea
Clostridium spp.	Pseudomembranous colitis, cholecystitis
Corynebacterium spp.	No definitive implications
Enterobacteriaceae	Peritonitis, diarrhea, postoperative complications, typhoid fever, meningitis, endocarditis
Enterococcus spp.	Peritonitis, postoperative complications
Eubacterium spp.	Peritonitis
Flavobacterium spp.	Meningitis
Fusobacterium spp.	Abscess
Lactobacillus spp.	No definitive implications
Mycobacterium spp.	None
Mycoplasma spp.	No definitive complications
Peptococcus spp.	Peritonitis, abscess
Peptostreptococcus spp.	Cholecystitis, abscess
Propionibacterium spp.	Endocarditis
Pseudomonas aeruginosa	Meningitis, postoperative complications
Ruminococcus bromii	No definitive implications
Sarcina spp.	No definitive implications
Staphylococcus aureus	Pancreatic abscess, enteritis
Veillonella spp.	No definitive implications
Viridans streptococci	No definitive implications
Vibrio spp.	None
FUNGI	
Candida albicans and other yeasts	Postoperative complications

GLOSSARY

GLOSSARY

ABATTOIR   slaughterhouse

ABSCESS   a localized collection of pus

ACCESSORY CELLS   macrophages and other antigen-presenting cells that express, along with Class II MHC glycoproteins, antigen on their surfaces in a form recognizable by lymphocytes

ACQUIRED PELLICLE   the thin, structureless film of salivary glycoproteins that forms on the tooth surface

ACTIVE IMMUNITY   the acquired immune status that develops as a consequence of an infection or of immunization with vaccines

ACUTE   having a short and relatively severe course

ADAPTIVE IMMUNITY   antigen-specific protection resulting from the formation of antibodies and effector T cells

ADCC   antibody-determined cell-mediated cytotoxicity; the destruction of IgG-coated cells by K cells

ADHESINS   components on the microbial surface that are used for attachment to host cells or tissue

ADJUVANT   a substance administered with an antigen (especially with a vaccine) to enhance the immune response to the antigen

AEROBIC   requiring oxygen for growth

AEROSOL   a solution delivered as a fine mist

AEROTOLERANT   referring to the ability of obligate anaerobes to tolerate the presence of oxygen

AFLATOXIN   a fungal toxin produced by certain species of *Aspergillus*

AGGLUTINATION   a reaction in which cells are clumped, as occurs in the interaction of a particulate antigen with antibody

AGGLUTININ   antibody that can cause agglutination

AIDS   acquired immune deficiency syndrome, an often fatal disease that especially strikes multicontact male homosexuals; probably a defect in cell-mediated immunity in which there is a preponderance of T suppressor cells over T helper cells; nonpathogens or Kaposi's sarcoma or both often cause the fatality

ALLERGEN   an antigen that elicits allergic reactions

ALLERGY   commonly refers to harmful/unpleasant reactions of immunological or seemingly immunological origin; in the strict sense, a Type I reactivity (atopy, anaphylaxis)

ALLOGRAFT (HOMOGRAFT)   a tissue or organ graft between members of the same species who are not identical

ALLOSTERIC ENZYME   an enzyme whose reactivity with another molecule such as its substrate is altered because of interaction of the enzyme with other molecules

ALOPECIA   loss of hair due to disease

ALPHA HEMOLYSIS   a type of blood agar plate hemolysis in which there is partial destruction of RBCs and some leakage of hemoglobin resulting in a greenish discoloration of the medium surrounding the microbial colony

ALTERNATIVE (ALTERNATE) COMPLEMENT PATHWAY   the complement pathway that is activated at the C3 level; does not require immune products for activation and is therefore important for nonspecific host resistance

ALVEOLAR   pertaining to the small sac-like structures in the lung

ALVEOLAR BONE   the type of bone supporting the teeth

AMPHITRICHOUS   having one flagellum at each pole of the cell

AMYLOPECTIN   intracellular storage polysaccharide synthesized by bacteria in dental plaque

ANABOLISM   metabolic process involved in the synthesis of cell material

ANAEROBIC   growing only in the absence of molecular oxygen

ANAEROBIOSIS   life in the absence of oxygen

ANALOGUES   closely similar compounds that can sometimes replace an essential metabolite

ANAMNESTIC RESPONSE   a rapid increase of antibodies or effector T cells due to immune memory cells following subsequent exposures (e.g., booster doses) to the same antigen

ANAPHYLATOXIN   complement fragments C3a or C5a that mediate intense inflammatory reactions by causing the degranulation of mast cells

ANAPHYLAXIS   a type I reactivity in which a hypersensitive individual is sensitized against a specific antigen; reaction primarily involves vasodilation and smooth muscle contraction

ANEURYSM   a sac formed from the dilation of the walls of an artery or vein and filled with blood

ANHEMOLYTIC   having no hemolytic activity on blood agar media

ANOREXIA   a condition in which the person has no appetite

ANTIBIOGRAM   pattern of results obtained from tests used to determine a microorganism's susceptibility to antimicrobials

ANTIBIOTIC   a chemical compound produced by microorganisms that can inhibit or kill other microorganisms

ANTIBODY   a glycoprotein produced by mammalian hosts in response to a foreign body called the antigen; the antibody reacts specifically with the antigen that induced it

ANTICODON   the triplet of nucleotides in a transfer DNA molecule that complements a specific codon on the messenger RNA

ANTIGEN   a substance that induces an immune response and that reacts with the products of the immune response

ANTIGEN-BINDING SITE   the variable region of the Fab portion of the immunoglobulin molecule that binds a specific or closely related antigenic determinant

ANTIGENIC DETERMINANTS   small, discrete chemical groups on the antigen surface that combine with the antigen-binding site on an immunoglobulin molecule or on a lymphocyte receptor

ANTIGEN-PRESENTING CELL (APC) (See accessory cells.)

ANTI-IDIOTYPE   an immune product that reacts with the antigenic determinants of the antigen-binding site

ANTIMETABOLITE   a molecule that bears a strong resemblance to one required in a normal physiological reaction

ANTISEPTIC   a chemical compound that can be

used on the surface of living tissue and that inhibits bacterial growth

ANTISERUM a serum containing specific antibodies

ANTITOXIN a specific antibody capable of neutralizing the exotoxin that stimulated its production

ANUG acute necrotizing ulcerative gingivitis

ARTHRALGIA painful swollen joints

ARTHROPOD invertebrate with jointed limbs

ARTHROSPORE an asexually produced fungal spore that is thick-walled and barrel-shaped

ARTHUS REACTION a type III hypersensitivity that is produced when antigen-antibody complexes activate complement; it leads to hemorrhage and inflammation resulting in necrosis

ASCOSPORE a sexual spore of the Ascomycetes

ASEPTIC free of living microorganisms

ASPERGILLOMA a ball of hyphae of the genus *Aspergillus* that accumulates at the site of infection

ASPHYXIA suffocation

ASPIRATION a process in which fluids are removed from body cavities

ASSIMILATION transformation of nutrients into biologically useful compounds or structures

ASTHMA a respiratory condition causing difficulty in breathing

ATOPIC ALLERGIES common clinical allergies involving IgE

ATROPHY the wasting away of a tissue, organ, or limb

ATTENUATION lessening; reduction of the virulence of microorganisms as in a vaccine

AUSTRALIA ANTIGEN hepatitis B surface antigen associated with serum hepatitis (hepatitis B); originally discovered in an Australian aborigine (hence the name)

AUTOCATALYSIS a process in which the product of a reaction acts as a catalyst to accelerate the reaction

AUTOCLAVE sealed chamber used for sterilizing

AUTOGRAFT tissue graft from one site to another in the same person

AUTOIMMUNE DISEASE disease in which the host's immune system destroys its own tissue

AUTOLYSIS digestion of a cell by enzymes produced by that cell at time of death

AUTOTROPH an organism that obtains energy by the oxidation of inorganic compounds

AUXOTROPH a mutant microorganism that will grow only on minimal media supplemented with growth factors not required by the normal parent

AXENIC a culture of organisms containing but one strain; also called pure culture

BACILLUS an organism of the genus *Bacillus*; also used to designate rod-shaped bacteria

BACTEREMIA presence of bacteria in the bloodstream

BACTERICIDE an agent that kills bacteria

BACTERIOCIN antimicrobial substance produced by bacteria that kills sensitive members of related strains

BACTERIOPHAGE a bacterial virus, sometimes referred to as phage

BACTERIOSTATIC AGENT an agent that inhibits the growth of bacteria

BACTERIURIA presence of bacteria in the urine

BACTOGEN see CHEMOSTAT

BASIDIOSPORE a sexually produced fungal spore of the subdivision Basidiomycotina

BCDF B cell differentiation factor, a lymphokine secreted by antigen-activated T_H cells that stimulates the conversion of activated B cells into plasma cells; also called IL-6

BCGF B cell growth factor, a lymphokine secreted by antigen-activated T_H cells that stimulates B cell proliferation

B CELLS the lymphocyte population involved in the production of antibodies (humoral immunity)

BENIGN not malignant; subject to recovery

BETA HEMOLYSIS complete hemolysis of red blood cells resulting in a clear zone around the microbial colony

BETA OXIDATION a degradation process of lipids resulting in the release of two carbon fragments

BIOLOGICAL MONITORS preparations of bacterial spores of a known resistance (to heat and ethylene oxide) that are used as sterilization indicators

BIOSYNTHESIS   the building up of chemical compounds

BIOTRANSFORMATION   a process of detoxification of drugs, primarily by the liver

BIOTYPE   a strain of a species differing from other strains in a biochemical property

BIOVAR   a strain within a species having one or more biochemical characteristics that differ from other strains within the species

BLASTOSPORE   a spore formed by budding, as occurs in yeast cells

BLOCKING ANTIBODY   an antibody that interferes with the binding of other antibodies or immune cells to antigen

BOIL   a localized abscess resulting from infection of a hair follicle; also called a furuncle

BOOSTER DOSE   an amount of immunogen given some time after primary immunization to sustain the immune response at a high level

BRONCHIECTASIS   chronic dilatation of the bronchi marked by repeated coughing spells

BROWNIAN MOVEMENT   dancing motion of particles in a liquid caused by thermal agitation

BUBOES   swollen, inflamed lymph nodes

BUCCAL   pertaining to the cheek

BUDDING   in virology, release of virus through cellular membranes and acquisition of cell envelope components; asexual division in prokaryotes

BULLA   a blister or vesicle filled with fluid

BURSA OF FABRICIUS   lymphoid organ in avian cloaca from which B cells are derived

CACHEXIA   physical wasting due to ill health and/or malnutrition

CALCULUS   a mineralized form of plaque on the surface of teeth in which organic components have been replaced by inorganic ones

CAPNEIC   requiring elevated concentrations of CO_2 for growth

CAPSID   the protein coat of a virus

CAPSOMERE   an aggregate of polypeptides forming a unit of the viral capsid

CAPSULE   a slimy envelope that surrounds the cell wall of certain microorganisms

CARBUNCLE   a circumscribed infection of the skin or subcutaneous tissue containing multiple draining sinuses

CARIES   a disease of the calcified tissue of teeth; tooth decay

CARRIER   a host that harbors infectious microorganisms and can transmit them to others but shows no disease symptoms

CASEATION   a type of necrosis in which the tissue resembles an amorphous mass of cheese

CATABOLISM   a metabolic process in which foodstuffs are broken down to release energy

CATALYST   a substance that increases the rate of a chemical reaction without being consumed in the reaction

CATARRHAL   a stage during infection in which there is a discharge from inflamed mucous membranes

CATHETER   a tubular device used to withdraw fluids from or introduce them into the body cavities

CELL-MEDIATED IMMUNITY (CMI)   an acquired immunity in which the T lymphocytes play a major role; responsible for resistance to infectious disease, some autoimmune diseases, and certain allergies

CELLULITIS   diffuse inflammation of connective tissue

CHANCRE   the primary lesion of syphilis

CHEMIOSMOSIS   a process in which energy is harnessed to produce an electrochemical gradient across cell membranes

CHEMOPROPHYLAXIS   preexposure administration of drugs to prevent disease

CHEMOSTAT   an apparatus used to maintain bacterial cultures in a state of continuous division

CHEMOTAXIN   a leukoattractant such as an antibody or C3a and C5a

CHEMOTAXIS   the attraction of microorganisms or phagocytes to chemicals released in the environment or in tissues

CHEMOTHERAPY   treatment of disease through the administration of drugs

CHORIORETINITIS   inflammation of the choroid and retina of the eye

CHROMATIN BODY   a network of DNA fibers giving the appearance of a distinct body in the cell

CHROMOSOME   a rod-shaped mass of DNA that carries hereditary characteristics

CHRONIC   lasting a long period of time

CIRRHOSIS   a disease of the liver

CLASS I MAJOR HISTOCOMPATIBILITY [MHC] ANTIGENS   genetically determined cell membrane proteins that (1) provoke the immune response in graft rejection; (2) are self markers that must be complexed with foreign antigens on target cell surfaces before effector T cells can destroy the target cells

CLASS II MAJOR HISTOCOMPATIBILITY [MHC] ANTIGENS   genetically determined cell membrane proteins that (1) provoke the immune response in graft rejection; (2) are self markers that must be complexed with antigens on antigen-presenting cells before immunocompetent B and T cells can recognize and respond to antigen

CLASSIC COMPLEMENT PATHWAY   the complement pathway that is activated at the C1 level, usually by the reaction of an IgG or IgM antibody with antigen

CLONAL SELECTION   the theory that for each antigenic determinant there is a specific, genetically predetermined receptor on the surface of an immunocompetent lymphocyte; the combination of the determinant with the receptor activates the formation of a clone of cells, each of which forms immune products of the same antigen-binding specificity

CLONE   a group of identical organisms or cells derived from a single cell or organism

COCCOBACILLUS   an oval bacterial cell resembling both coccus and rod shapes

COCCUS   spherical bacterium

CODON   a nucleotide triplet in messenger RNA that specifies a particular amino acid

COENZYME   an organic molecule that is loosely bound to the enzyme and necessary for the activity of the enzyme

COFACTOR   in enzymology, an organic or inor-
ganic molecule that is required by an enzyme to become totally active

COLICIN   a protein secreted by certain strains of *Escherichia coli* and lethal to other strains of the same species

COLITIS   inflammation of the colon

COLONY   a uniform mass of cells derived from a single cell growing on a solid surface

COMMENSALISM   a symbiotic relationship between different species of organisms in which neither is harmed

COMPLEMENT   a series of complex thermolabile plasma proteins; also, the lyophilized preparation of fresh serum that is used in the complement fixation test

COMPLEMENT SYSTEM   a system of plasma proteins that upon activation proceeds in a serial (cascade) fashion to generate biologically active fragments including opsonins, chemotaxins, anaphylatoxin, and membrane attack units

CONDYLOMATA ACUMINATA   warts on the genitalia

CONDYLOMATA LATA   moist syphilitic papules

CONIDIA   asexual fungal spores produced on specialized mycelial branches called conidiophores

CONIDIOPHORE   a hyphal filament on which spores, called conidia, are borne

CONJUGATION   the act of joining together; in bacteria a process in which genetic information is transferred from one cell to another

CONJUNCTIVITIS   inflammation of the membrane that lines the eyelids and the exposed surfaces of the sclera of the eye

CONSTANT REGION   the relatively unchanging portion of H or L chains that is identical for each immunoglobulin class or the α, β, γ, and δ chains of the T cell receptor

CONSTITUTIVE ENZYME   an enzyme produced by a cell under any environmental conditions

CONVALESCENCE   period of recovery

COPROANTIBODIES   antibodies occurring in the intestinal tract, consisting primarily of the IgA class

CORYZA   inflammation of the nasal mucosa characterized by nasal discharge and watery eyes

COUNTERIMMUNOELECTROPHORESIS (CIE)   serological procedure in which antigen and antibody are made to migrate toward each other, under the influence of charged buffer ions, to facilitate precipitation

C-REACTIVE PROTEIN   a plasma protein that appears in response to inflammation in the body

CRISTAE   the inner folded membrane found in the mitochondrion

CROSS-REACTIVE ANTIGENS   antigens that share antigenic determinants or have similarly structured determinants

CROUP   a condition of children in which there is coughing and hoarseness

CRYOSURGERY   use of extreme cold to destroy tissue

CULTURE   a population of microorganisms growing in a nutrient medium

CUTANEOUS   pertaining to the skin

CYANOSIS   bluish tinge to the skin due to excessive amounts of reduced hemoglobin (lack of oxygenated hemoglobin)

CYSTITIS   inflammation of the urinary bladder

CYCLOSPORIN   drug used to suppress graft rejection

CYST (OF PARASITES)   the resistant quiescent form of some parasites that serves as the transmission, infective stage

CYTOCHROME   a respiratory pigment involved in oxidation-reduction reactions

CYTOKINES   soluble molecules such as lymphokines and monokines that mediate interactions between cells

CYTOPATHIC   characterized by pathological change in a cell

CYTOPATHIC EFFECT (CPE)   morphological alteration of host cells that usually results in cell death

CYTOPHILIC ANTIBODY   antibody that binds to receptors on cells (macrophages, neutrophils, mast cells) via the Fc portion of the antibody molecule

CYTOTOXIC T LYMPHOCYTES (T_{CTL})   effector (sensitized) T cells that specifically destroy target cells that bear antigens complexed with Class I MHC markers

DEAMINATION   removal of amino groups

DEBILITATED   characterized by loss of strength or health

DEBILITATION   loss of normal function

DEBRIDE   remove devitalized tissue

DECARBOXYLATION   removal of carboxyl groups

DECUBITUS ULCERS   bedsores

DEFINITIVE (FINAL) HOST   the host in which the sexually mature or adult stage of parasites occurs; or the most important host

DEGENERATE   in genetics, a code in which more than one code word specifies an amino acid

DEGRANULATION   the extracellular release of granules that contain physiologically active or antimicrobial substances

DEHYDROGENATION   a process in which hydrogens are removed from a compound

DELAYED-TYPE HYPERSENSITIVITY (DTH)   inflammatory reaction mediated by T_{DTH} cells; skin test reaction develops fully 24 to 72 hours after challenge dose in a sensitized person

DELETION   in genetics, loss of genetic material

DEMENTIA   mental deterioration

DEMYELINATION   removal of the myelin sheath around nerve fibers

DENATURATION   a process in which a macromolecule loses its configuration and often its biological activity

DERMATOPHYTE   fungi that invade keratinized tissue

DESENSITIZATION   the process of reducing an individual's sensitivity

DESICCATE   to dry

DESQUAMATION   shedding of the superficial layers of skin

DETERGENT   a synthetic cleansing agent

DETERMINANT GROUP (EPITOPE)   the chemical grouping of the antigen molecule that binds specifically with the antibody combining site or to the receptor on T cells

DEXTRO-   to the right

DIARRHEA   abnormal fluidity of fecal discharge

DIMORPHIC   in mycology the ability of the fungus to exist in the yeast or mold state

DIPHTHEROID   resembling the diphtheria bacillus

DIPLOPIA double vision

DISEASE an abnormal condition of the body having characteristic symptoms

DISINFECTANT an antimicrobial agent applied to inanimate objects that destroys harmful microorganisms except spores

DTP a vaccine consisting of toxoids of diphtheria and tetanus plus a pertussis bacterial antigen

DYSURIA painful urination

ECTATIC distended

ECTOPIC not in the normal place

ECTOTHRIX fungal infection in which hyphae remain on external surface of the hair shaft

ECZEMA an inflammatory skin disease characterized by scales, crusts, and watery lesions

EDEMA a swelling due to accumulation of fluids in tissues

EFFECTOR CELL a lymphocyte that has a direct (e.g., killer T cell) or a mediated (e.g., via lymphokines) effect on an antigen (compare REGULATOR CELL)

ELECTROPHORESIS the separation of differently charged molecules in an electric field

ELISA enzyme-linked immunosorbent assay, a serological test in which enzyme-linked antibodies allow antigen-antibody reactions to become visible upon addition of a color-producing enzyme substrate

EMETIC an agent causing vomiting

EMPYEMA pus accumulation in a body cavity

ENDEMIC continually present in a community

ENDOCARDITIS inflammation of the endocardium of the heart

ENDOCYTOSIS the phase of phagocytosis when the extracellular material is entering the phagocyte

ENDOENZYME an enzyme produced by a cell whose activity is associated with intracellular processes or an enzyme that attacks the interior of macromolecules

ENDOGENOUS produced within the cell; coming from within

ENDOMETRITIS inflammation of the endometrium of the uterus

ENDONUCLEASE an enzyme that attacks the interior of nucleic acid molecules

ENDOPLASMIC RETICULUM a protoplasmic network in eukaryotic cells consisting of a continuous double membrane system that courses throughout the cytoplasm

ENDOSPORE a spore occurring within the cell

ENDOTHELIUM epithelial lining of heart, blood vessels, and lymph vessels

ENDOTHRIX fungal infection resulting from hyphal invasion of the hair shaft

ENDOTOXIN a toxin derived from the cell wall of gram-negative bacteria

ENTERIC occurring in the gastrointestinal tract

ENTEROCOLITIS inflammation of small intestine and colon

ENTEROTOXIN a toxin that gives rise to gastrointestinal symptoms when ingested or formed in the intestine

ENVELOPE a host cell-derived membrane, containing virus-specific antigens, which is acquired during virus maturation

EOSINOPHIL a granular leukocyte readily stained red by eosin; prominent in atopic allergies and parasitic infections

EPIDEMIC an outbreak of a disease affecting a large number of individuals in a community

EPIDEMIOLOGY the science that deals with the incidence, transmission, and prevention of disease

EPIDIDYMITIS inflammation of the epididymis, which is part of the seminal duct lying posterior to the testes

EPINEPHRINE (ADRENALIN) a drug that is a vasoconstrictor and smooth muscle relaxant

EPISOME a piece of DNA that may be an autonomous unit in the cell or may be integrated into the chromosome

EPITHELIOID CELLS macrophage cells in granulomas that resemble epithelial cells

EPITOPE antigenic determinant

EPIZOOTIC an outbreak of disease affecting a large number of animals

ERYSIPELAS   a contagious disease of the skin resulting from infection by *Streptococcus pyogenes*

ERYTHEMATOUS   having red eruptions on the skin

ERYTHROGENIC   able to produce redness

ESCHAR   a dry mass of necrotic (dead) tissue

ETIOLOGY   study of the causation of a disease

ETO   ethylene oxide, a gas used for sterilization

EUKARYOTIC   a cell type in which the nuclear material is bounded by a membrane

EXANTHEM   eruptive disease or fever characterized by nodular eruptions on mucous membrane

EXFOLIATIN   a staphylococcal toxin that causes necrosis of epidermis

EXFOLIATION   shedding of layers of the skin

EXOENZYME   an enzyme secreted by the cell and associated in activity with the extracellular process

EXON   in eukaryotic genetics, an mRNA sequence that codes for information

EXOTOXIN   toxin produced in the cell and released into the environment

EXUDATE   material (fluids, cells, etc.) that has escaped from blood vessels

FAB   the fraction of the immunoglobulin molecule that contains the antigen-binding site

FACULTATIVE ANAEROBES   organisms that grow best under aerobic conditions but can grow anaerobically

FAUCIAL   pertaining to the upper part of the throat

FC   the crystallizable fragment of the immunoglobulin molecule, composed of the constant regions of the H chains; roles include binding of complement, attachment of immunoglobulin to phagocytes and other cell types, and transplacental passage

FC RECEPTORS   receptors on the surface of various cells that bind the Fc portion of antibody molecules

FEBRILE   pertaining to or characterized by fever

FERMENTATION   an anaerobic metabolic process that uses an organic compound as the final electron acceptor

F FACTOR   a fertility factor that determines the sex of a bacterium

FIBRONECTIN   glycoprotein receptors on cells; believed to be important in binding microorganisms

FIBROSIS   formation of fibrous tissue

FILAMENTOUS   composed of long thread-like structures

FIMBRIA   fringe; in microbial genetics, a small protein projection on the surface of bacteria

FISSION   the act of splitting, a form of asexual reproduction

FISTULA   an abnormal passageway providing organisms with communication between tissues during infection

FIXED VIRUS   an attenuated variant of the virulent "street" rabies virus

FLAGELLA   hair-like projections on the cell that aid in locomotion

FLATULENCE   presence of air or gases in the stomach or intestine

FLATWORMS   worms that are flat when viewed in cross section

FLOCCULATION   a phenomenon in which suspended components form visible discrete particles

FLORA   the resident organisms in a particular area

FLUORESCENCE   the emission of light while being exposed to light of shorter wavelength than the emitted light

FLUORESCENT ANTIBODY   an antibody conjugated with a dye that fluoresces on ultraviolet irradiation; used in serological techniques to detect antigens

FOCUS   in virology, an accumulation of transformed cells

FOLLICULITIS   inflammation of follicles (for example, hair follicles)

FOMITE   an inanimate object that may be involved in disease transmission

FRAMEWORK REGIONS   the less variable regions

of the antigen-binding site of the antibody molecule that flank the hypervariable subregions where antigen contact actually occurs

FULMINATING   occurring very suddenly and with intensity

FUNGICIDE   an agent capable of destroying fungi

FURUNCLE   a boil

GAMETE   sex cell

GAMMA GLOBULIN   a blood protein fraction with which antibodies are associated

GENETIC ENGINEERING   type of recombinant DNA technology in which foreign genes can be inserted into the DNA of related and unrelated organisms

GENETIC RESTRICTION   (See MHC restriction.)

GENOME   the complete set of hereditary factors

GENOTYPE   the genetic constitution of an organism

GENUS   a taxonomic category

GERMICIDE   an agent that destroys pathogenic microorganisms

GERMINATION   the sprouting of a spore and the formation of a vegetative cell

GERM TUBE   in fungal reproduction a hyphal element arising from a germinating spore

GINGIVAE (GUMS)   soft tissue surrounding the teeth

GLOBULINS   a class of proteins found in the blood

GLOMERULONEPHRITIS   renal disease affecting primarily glomeruli

GLOSSITIS   inflammation of the tongue

GLUCAN   extracellular glucose polymers (dextran, mutan)

GLYCOLYSIS   the anaerobic process in which carbohydrates such as glucose are oxidized to pyruvic or lactic acid

GNOTOBIOTIC ANIMALS   animals originally germ free, harboring one or more known microorganisms

GOLGI   membranous complex found in eukaryotes that packages proteins and lipids for transfer to selected sites in the cell

GRAFT-VS.-HOST REACTION (GVHR)   a reaction in which the immunocompetent cells of a graft tissue attack the tissues of the graft recipient

GRANULOMA   a tumor-like mass of granulation tissue containing macrophages and fibroblasts and caused by chronic inflammation

GUARNIERI'S BODIES   acidophilic intracytoplasmic inclusion bodies in epidermal cells infected with smallpox virus

GUMMA   granuloma found in tertiary stage of syphilis

HALOPHILIC   (of bacteria) requiring high concentrations of salt to maintain the integrity of the cell

HAPTEN   a partial or incomplete antigen that alone does not induce antibody formation but can react with certain antibodies

H CHAIN   heavy chain, one of the pair of identical polypeptides that represent two of the four polypeptide chains of the basic immunoglobulin molecule; differences in H chain composition are the basis for classification of immunoglobulins into five classes.

HELPER T CELLS (T_H)   a regulator T cell that initiates most immune responses by specifically recognizing the antigen fragment-class II MHC complex on the surface of an antigen-presenting cell and then promotes the proliferation and differentiation of antigen-specific B and T cell clones

HELMINTH   worm

HEMAGGLUTINATION   clumping of red blood cells

HEMAGGLUTININ (VIRAL HEMAGGLUTININ)   a nonantibody protein on the outer surface of some viruses (e.g., orthomyxoviruses) that reacts with surface determinant(s) on red cells to cause agglutination of the red cells (hemagglutination)

HEMATOGENOUS   derived from the bloodstream

HEMATURIA   presence of blood in the urine

HEMOLYSIN   any agent that can cause the lysis of red blood cells

HEPATOMA   tumor involving the liver

HETEROPHILE ANTIGEN   an antigen common to more than one species such as lens protein antigen

HETEROTROPH   an organism requiring organic material for energy and biosynthesis

HEXON   a capsomere surrounded by six capsomeres

HINGE REGION   a flexible H chain region between the Fc and Fab portions of the immunoglobulin molecule that allows the two antigen-binding sites to attach to identical antigenic determinants located at different sites

HISTAMINE   a physiologically active substance released by certain cell types, especially mast cells, that affects capillary permeability and smooth muscle contraction

HISTOCOMPATIBLE   said of cells or tissues that share or have like transplantation antigens

HISTONE   a protein containing many basic amino acids and associated with the DNA of eukaryotic cells

HLA   human leukocyte antigens; human transplantation antigens—first discovered on leukocytes

HOMOGRAFT   see ALLOGRAFT

HUMORAL IMMUNITY   antibody-mediated immunity

HYBRIDOMA   a cell that results from the fusion of two cells; usually refers to a cell fused from a cancerous (myeloma) cell and an antibody-producing cell and that is a source of monoclonal antibodies

HYDROLASE   an enzyme that catalyzes the hydrolysis of compounds

HYDROLYZE   to split a compound by the addition of water

HYDROPHILIC   attracted to water

HYDROPHOBIC   repelled by water

HYPERCHROMIC   highly stained

HYPERPLASIA   increase in the number of cells in a tissue

HYPERTONIC   a solution in which the concentration of solutes is higher outside the cell than inside the cell

HYPERVARIABLE REGIONS   extremely variable regions of the variable H and L regions of immunoglobulins; the "hot spots" where antibodies bind antigenic determinants

HYPHA (PL. HYPHAE)   one of the filaments that make up a fungal mycelium

HYPOSENSITIZATION   a process in which an allergen is injected to reduce the allergic state

HYPOTONIC   a solution in which the concentration of solute is lower outside the cell than in the cell

ICOSAHEDRAL   20 sided

ICTERUS (JAUNDICE)   a condition characterized by excess of bile pigments in the blood and tissues that leads to a yellow color of the surface integuments

ID   an allergic skin reaction to fungi or fungal products

IDIOTOPE   a single determinant of the idiotype

IDIOTYPE   the set of antigenic determinants that are part of the antigen-binding site of the immunoglobulin molecule

IMMEDIATE HYPERSENSITIVITY   a hypersensitivity in which there is a response within seconds to minutes when a sensitized individual is again exposed to the corresponding antigen

IMMUNE COMPLEX   aggregate of soluble antigen and antibody

IMMUNE GLOBULIN   a preparation of purified antibody used to confer passive immunity

IMMUNE SURVEILLANCE   a postulated function of the immune system: that it constantly destroys newly formed cancer cells

IMMUNITY   state of being protected, especially to microorganisms or their products

IMMUNODIFFUSION   a serological technique in which antibodies and antigens form lines of precipitate as they diffuse toward each other in an agar gel support medium

IMMUNOFLUORESCENCE   fluorescence resulting from the conjugation of an immunoglobulin to a fluorescent dye

IMMUNOGEN   an antigen or a substance that induces an immunity

IMMUNOGENICITY   that property of an antigen that makes it capable of stimulating an immune response

IMMUNOGLOBULINS   a class of blood proteins with which antibodies are associated

IMMUNOSUPPRESSIVE   inhibiting the normal immunological response of an organism

IMMUNOTOXIN   in cancer immunotherapy, a toxin (e.g., ricin A) attached to a monoclonal antibody that poisons the cell against which the antibody is specific

IMPETIGO   a streptococcal or staphylococcal infection of the skin

INCLUSION BODIES   in virus infection, the highly stainable components, usually virus, found in the cytoplasm or nucleus of the infected cell

INDIGENOUS   native to a particular place

INDUCER   a molecule capable of stimulating the formation of compounds such as enzymes involved in cellular metabolism

INDUCIBLE ENZYME   an enzyme synthesized only in response to an inducer

INDURATION   a hardened area or lesion

INFANT   a child usually up to 2 years

INFECTIOUS   able to cause disease

INFECTIOUS DOSE (ID_{50}; $TCID_{50}$)   that amount of virus required to cause a demonstrable infection in 50 percent of the inoculated animals or tissue culture cells, respectively

INFLAMMATION   nonspecific response to irritants (chemical, physical, microbial, antigenic) characterized by pain, heat, redness, and swelling

INFUSION   a preparation in which important components of a substance have been extracted with water

INNATE IMMUNITY   state of protection or resistance to infection due to factors other than immune system products

INOCULUM   a substance (microorganisms, serum, etc.) introduced into the tissues or culture media

INSERTION   in genetics, the addition of nucleotides or genes to the chromosome

INSERTION SEQUENCE   small nucleotide sequences that are capable of movement on the DNA

INSPISSATE   to dry by evaporation

INTERFERON   a class of proteins produced by vertebrate cells in response to viruses, endo-toxins, and certain chemicals; associated primarily with antiviral activity

INTERLEUKIN-1 (IL-1)   protein secreted by macrophages that signals the activation of T_H cells in an immune response; also, the endogenous inducer of fever

INTERLEUKIN-2 (IL-2)   a protein derived from activated T_H cells that promotes the proliferation of other activated T cells and B cells

INTERLEUKIN-6 (IL-6)   same as BCDF

INTERMEDIATE HOST   a host that is required in the life cycle of some parasites in which the asexual or larval stage occurs

INTOXICATION   state of being poisoned by some chemical

INTRADERMAL   within the skin

INTRAPERITONEAL   within the peritoneum, which is the membrane lining the abdominal cavity

INTRON   in eukaryotic genetics, a mRNA sequence that does not code for information

INTUBATION   insertion of a tube

IN UTERO   within the uterus

INVASIVE   able to invade or penetrate the body

IN VITRO   outside the body or performed in artificial environments

IN VIVO   within the body or within a living organism

IODOPHORS   disinfectants consisting of iodine combined with a carrier molecule

ISCHEMIA   blood deficiency in a body part

ISOAGGLUTININS   antibodies specific for antigenic sites on red blood cells of the same species and causing their agglutination; also called alloagglutinins

ISOANTIBODY   an antibody that reacts with alternate forms of an intraspecies antigen (e.g., A and B blood group antigens)

ISOANTIGEN   an intraspecies antigen that appears in alternate forms

ISOMER   a molecule having the same atoms or groups of atoms as another molecule, but with different arrangement

JAUNDICE   see ICTERUS

J CHAIN   a polypeptide chain that joins basic monomer immunoglobulin units of the same immunoglobulin class to form polymers, as in secreted IgM and secretory IgA

K CELL   a lymphocyte with Fc receptors that binds to and kills antibody-coated target cells

KAPOSI'S SARCOMA   a relatively benign skin cancer that often takes a more aggressive fatal form in AIDS victims

KARYOTYPE   chromosomal makeup of a cell

KERATITIS   inflammation of the cornea

KERNICTERUS   a condition associated with high levels of bilirubin in the blood that affects the nervous system

KININS   inflammatory vasoactive peptides produced following tissue injury

KOPLIK'S SPOTS   small bluish spots surrounded by a reddened area in the mucous membrane of the mouth and characteristic of measles

KUPFFER'S CELLS   macrophages lining the hepatic sinusoids

KURU   a chronic, progressive, degenerative disorder of the central nervous system caused by a virus, found among certain natives of New Guinea

L CHAINS (LIGHT CHAINS)   the two smaller identical polypeptide chains of the four-chain immunoglobulin molecule

LABILE   unstable or susceptible to various chemical or physical agents

LABIUM   a lip; for example, labia in females are two folds of skin of the genitalia

LARVA   worm-like immature form of arthropods and helminths (worms)

LATENCY   a state of inactivity

LD$_{50}$ lethal dose 50; the dose lethal to 50 percent of the subjects

LECTIN   glycoprotein found on the surface of plant cells

LEUKEMIA   a blood disease characterized by high levels of leukocytes

LEUKOCIDIN   a substance produced by some pathogenic bacteria and toxic to white blood cells

LEUKOCYTE   white blood cell

LEUKOPENIA   a smaller than normal number of circulating leukocytes

LEUKOTRIENES   secondary or lipoid mediators that arise from changes in cell membrane phospholipids (arachidonic acid) especially when antigen combines with IgE on mast cell surfaces; leukotrienes increase vascular permeability, contract smooth muscles, and attract neutrophils

LEVO-   to the left

L-FORMS   bacteria with deficient cell walls

LIGASE   an enzyme that catalyzes the joining together of two molecules coupled with the breakdown of adenosine triphosphate to adenosine diphosphate

LIMULUS LYSATE   an extract from the amoebocytes of horseshoe crabs that gels with minute quantities of endotoxin

LIPOSOME   synthetic phospholipid sac having properties of biological membranes

LOCAL (TOPICAL) IMMUNITY   mucous surface immunity primarily owing to secretory IgA

LOCHIA   vaginal discharge that appears after childbirth

LOGARITHMIC GROWTH   the uniform doubling of a population of cells per unit time

LOPHOTRICHOUS   having a tuft of flagella at one end of the cell

LUMBAR REGION   lower region of the back, where cerebrospinal fluid usually is drawn ("spinal tap")

LYMPHADENOPATHY   infection of a lymph node

LYMPHOCYTE   a white blood cell devoid of cytoplasmic granules, associated with immune response and chronic inflammation

LYMPHOKINES   soluble products, especially of sensitized T cells, that are released upon antigen contact and that have among their varied actions the mobilization of uncommitted macrophages, neutrophils, lymphocytes, and other cells

LYMPHOMA   any neoplasia (abnormal growth) associated with the lymph system

LYOPHILIZATION   process of freeze-drying

LYSIN   an agent (bacterial, chemical, antibody) capable of causing the destruction of cells

LYSIS   dissolution (as in cell destruction)

LYSOGENIC CONVERSION   a change in characteristics of an organism due to carriage of a prophage

LYSOGENY   a state in which a bacteriophage genome is integrated or firmly associated with the host genome

LYSOSOME   a cell organelle derived from the Golgi apparatus containing hydrolytic enzymes collectively termed acid hydrolases

LYSOZYME   an enzyme that degrades peptidoglycan, a compound of the cell wall

MACROPHAGE   a versatile cell of the mononuclear phagocyte system (MPS) whose two major functions are (1) processing and presentation of antigens and (2) phagocytosis and destruction of antigens

MACROPHAGE ACTIVATION FACTOR (MAF)   a general term that signifies several lymphokines, including gamma interferon, that enhance the phagocytic and cytotoxic activities of macrophages

MACULA   a spot; often associated with a type of rash (macular) in which the lesion is not elevated

MAJOR HISTOCOMPATIBILITY COMPLEX   the genes of a specific chromosome region that code for the majority of cell membrane surface glycoproteins that serve as transplantation antigens and that guide antigen recognition and cell interactions, especially by T cells

MALADSORPTION   faulty absorption of nutrients through the intestine

MALAISE   a general feeling of "not being well"

MAST CELL   a connective tissue cell that is a major source of vasoactive and muscle-contracting compounds; for example, histamine; has Fc receptors for IgE and is the principal intermediate in anaphylactic reactions

MEDIUM   a substance that provides nutrients for the growth of microorganisms

MEMBRANE ATTACK COMPLEX (MAC)   the complex of C_5–C_9 factors of complement that inserts into and destroys cell membranes

MEMBRANE FILTERS   paper-thin filters composed of cellulose esters and other materials

MEMORY CELLS   a reserve of antigen-sensitive immune cells developed in the primary immune response that respond swiftly and to higher levels in the secondary immune response

MENINGES   membranes that cover the brain and spinal cord

MENINGITIS   inflammation of the membranes (meninges) of brain or spinal cord

MESOPHILE   a microorganism that grows best at temperatures between 20° and 45°C

MESOSOME   involuted membrane of the bacterial cell

METABOLISM   the sum total of physical and chemical changes that take place in a cell and maintain the cell's integrity

METABOLITE   a product of metabolic processes

METACHROMATIC GRANULES   cytoplasmic inclusions that are polymetaphosphates; also called Babès-Ernst bodies or volutin

METASTASIS   transfer of disease from primary site of infection

MHC ANTIGENS   genetically determined major histocompatibility antigens that are markers of self and provoke the immune response to foreign grafts

MHC (GENETIC) RESTRICTION   the requirement that antigens be complexed with MHC proteins in order to be recognized and responded to by cells of the immune system

MICROAEROPHILE   an organism requiring less than 1 atmosphere of oxygen

MICROTUBULE   cylindrical hollow protein tubes found in eukaryotic cells and associated with motility as well as spindle organization during cell division

MIGRATION INHIBITING FACTOR (MIF)   a lymphokine that prevents macrophages from leaving the site of cell-mediated immunological reaction

MILIARY   resembling millet seeds; said of lesions

MISSENSE   refers to a mutation that results in a codon's being translated into a different amino acid

MITOCHONDRION   rod-shaped organelle found in

eukaryotic cells and involved in energy production

MOLD another name for fungi that exhibit branching

MONOCLONAL ANTIBODY antibody obtained from an isolated clone of cells (e.g., hybridoma); preparations containing monoclonal antibodies have a highly precise specificity for a given antigenic determinant and are therefore valuable in diagnosis and therapy

MONOCYTE a macrophage of the circulating blood

MONOKINES soluble molecules produced by macrophages that mediate interactions between cells (see IL-1)

MONOMER a basic molecule that is repeated in polymers

MONOTRICHOUS having one flagellum

MORBIDITY sickness; the ratio of sick to well individuals of a community

MORDANT a chemical that binds dyes to cells or tissues

MORPHOLOGICAL related to shape or structure

MORTALITY fatality; the ratio of the number of deaths to a given population in a defined situation

MUCOUS secreting mucus; for example, mucous gland

MUCOLYTIC capable of dissolving mucus

MUCUS the viscous liquid secreted by mucous glands

MULTINUCLEATED GIANT CELL a large cell containing the nuclei of fused macrophages and found in chronic inflammatory lesions

MUTAGEN a substance that increases the mutation rate of an organism

MUTATION a process in which a gene undergoes structural changes

MYALGIA pain in the muscles

MYCELIUM a mat of intertwined hyphae of fungi

MYCETISMUS mushroom poisoning

MYCETOMA a chronic infection, usually involving the foot; but other parts of the body may be involved

MYCOTOXIN toxic secondary metabolite resulting from the growth of fungi on grains

MYELOMA PROTEINS homogenous immunoglobulin molecules or parts of immunoglobulin molecules produced by malignant plasma cells

MYOCARDITIS a condition involving the heart muscle (myocardium)

MYOMETRIUM the uterine muscular structure

MYOSITIS inflammation of muscle

NATURAL KILLER (NK) CELLS probably a subclass of lymphocytes that occur without antigen stimulation and that serve as effectors of nonspecific immunity (e.g., against malignant cells)

NECROSIS death of tissue or cells

NEGRI BODIES inclusion bodies found in brain cells infected with the rabies virus

NEMATODE roundworm

NEONATAL pertaining to the first 4 weeks after birth

NEOPLASIA formation of tumors

NEPHROTOXIC toxic to the kidney

NEONATORUM pertaining to the newborn

NEUROTOXIN toxin that affects the nervous system

NEUTROPHIL a leukocyte in which granules do not stain with basic or acid dyes

NITROGEN FIXATION the union of nitrogen gas with other elements to form chemical compounds

NK CELLS natural killer cells

NONSENSE a mutation that results in a codon's not being translated into an amino acid

NOSOCOMIAL pertaining to the hospital

NUCLEOCAPSID a unit of viral structure consisting of a protein coat (capsid) and the nucleic acid it encloses

NUCLEOID area of DNA concentration in the bacterial cell

NUCLEOLUS a small body within the nucleus rich in ribonucleic acid

NUCLEOSIDES a class of compounds consisting of a carbohydrate and a purine or pyrimidine base

NUCLEOTIDES a class of compounds consisting of a purine or pyrimidine base, phosphoric acid, and carbohydrate

NUTRIENT a substance removed from the environment by cells and used in various metabolic processes

OBLIGATE   necessary or required

OCCLUSAL SURFACE   area of the tooth associated with grinding

OKAZAKI FRAGMENT   short pieces of DNA synthesized during replication

OLIGURIA   secretion of a diminished amount of urine

ONCOGENIC   able to cause tumors

ONYCHIA   infection involving the nails

OPERATOR GENE   a chromosomal region that is capable of controlling adjacent structural genes

OPERON   a unit on the chromosome consisting of adjacent genes controlled by an operator

OPHTHALMIA   inflammation of the eye

OPPORTUNISTIC PATHOGEN   a nonpathogen capable of infection only under the most favorable conditions

OPSONIN   an antibody or complement fragment C3b that attaches antigens to phagocytes, thereby facilitating endocytosis

ORCHITIS   inflammation of the testes

ORNITHOSIS   a bird disease, transmissible to humans

OSMOSIS   passage of fluids through a semipermeable membrane

OSTEITIS   inflammation of a bone

OSTEOCLAST   a bone-resorbing cell

OSTEOMYELITIS   inflammation of the marrow of the bone

OTITIS MEDIA   inflammation of the middle ear

OXIDATION   loss of electrons by a compound

OXIDATIVE PHOSPHORYLATION   enzymatic addition of phosphate to adenosine diphosphate to form adenosine triphosphate, which is coupled to the electron transport system

OZENA   chronic inflammation of the nose

PALINDROMIC   in genetics, nucleotide sequences that are repeated but inverted on the opposite ends of a double-stranded nucleic acid molecule

PANDEMIC   a worldwide epidemic

PAPILLOMA   a benign tumor derived from the epithelium

PAPULE   a small, firm, circumscribed, raised lesion of the skin

PARASITE   an organism that survives on or at the expense of a living host

PARESIS   a slight paralysis

PARONYCHIA   infection involving areas around nails

PAROXYSM   a state of intensified symptoms

PARTURITION   the process of birth

PASSIVE IMMUNITY   the temporary acquired immune status that results from the transfer of antibodies from an outside source

PASTEURIZATION   a process in which fluids are heated at temperatures below boiling to kill pathogenic microorganisms in the vegetative state

PATHOGEN   an organism capable of habitually causing disease in a percentage of healthy persons

PATHOGENESIS   the progression of tissue, biochemical, and functional alterations that occur during the development of a disease

PATHOGNOMONIC   refers to a sign or symptom that is so characteristic of a disease that a diagnosis can be made from it

PENTON   a capsomere surrounded by five capsomeres

PEPLOMER   a projection (spike) extending from the outer surface of a virus envelope

PEPTIDE BOND   a bond that unites two amino acids

PEPTIDOGLYCAN   the relatively rigid structural component of most bacterial cell walls that consists of layers of polysaccharide made up of N-acetylglucosamine and N-acetylmuramic acid

PERCUTANEOUS   performed through the skin

PERINATAL   pertaining to a period of time shortly before and just after birth

PERIODONTITIS   inflammation of the periodontium or tissue surrounding and supporting the teeth

PERIOSTITIS   inflammation of the periosteum, the specialized connective tissue covering all bones

PERIPLASM   contents of a space (periplasmic) that lies between the cell wall outer membrane and cytoplasmic membrane of gram-negative bacteria

PERITRICHOUS   having flagella that cover the entire bacterial surface

PERMEASE   an enzyme found in cell membranes that transports compounds into the cell cytoplasm

PETECHIAL   pinpoint hemorrhages in skin and mucous membranes

PHAGOCYTOSIS   the process of ingestion of foreign particles

PHAGOLYSOSOME   intracytoplasmic vesicle in phagocytic cells formed by the fusion of lysosome and phagosome membranes

PHAGOSOME   a cell vacuole resulting from phagocytosis of particulate materials

PHENOTYPE   the genetic makeup of an organism; its observable properties

PHLEBITIS   inflammation of a vein

PHOSPHORYLATION   joining of phosphoric acid to a compound

PHOTOPHOBIA   literally, fear of light; painful sensitivity to light

PHOTOSYNTHETIC   able to convert light to chemical energy

PHOTOTROPH   an organism that uses light for energy

PHYLOGENETIC   pertaining to the evolutionary history of an organism

PILUS   small protein projection on the bacterial cell involved in conjugation or adherence

PINOCYTOSIS   the engulfment of liquid droplets by a cell

PLAQUE   a clear area produced by the lytic action of viruses on an opaque lawn of bacteria or on a monolayer of tissue culture cells

PLAQUE (DENTAL)   the structureless accumulation of bacteria, extracellular polysaccharides (e.g., glucans), and host proteins found on the surface of teeth

PLASMA   the fluid portion of the blood containing elements necessary for clot formation

PLASMA CELL   a fully differentiated B lymphocyte that produces antibodies

PLASMID   an extrachromosomal piece of DNA

PLASMOLYSIS   shrinkage of the cell caused by osmotic removal of water

PLASMOPTYSIS   swelling or bursting of a cell caused by osmotic inflow of water

PLATELETS (THROMBOCYTES)   small non-nucleated cytoplasmic elements in blood responsible for activating blood coagulation, and a source of vasoactive agents

PLEOMORPHISM   the state of having more than one form or shape

PMN   polymorphonuclear leukocyte (neutrophil)

POCK   a pit, spot, or pustule

POLYGENIC   a messenger RNA coding for more than one gene

POLYMERIZATION   formation of a polymer from monomeric molecules

POLYPEPTIDE   a polymer made up of amino acids linked by peptide bonds

POLYSACCHARIDE   a carbohydrate; for example, starch produced from the polymerization of many monosaccharides

POLYSOME (POLYRIBOSOME)   several ribosomes bound to a single mRNA strand

POLYURIA   frequent urination

PORINS   channels in the cell wall for solute transport

POSTPARTUM   referring to the period after birth

POTABLE   suitable to drink

PRECIPITIN   an antibody that causes precipitation

PREDISPOSING   conferring a tendency

PROCTITIS   inflammation of the rectum

PRODROMAL   pertaining to early manifestation of disease before specific symptoms appear

PROKARYOTIC   characterized by lack of nuclear membrane and organelles (e.g., bacteria)

PROMOTER   a site on DNA that initiates the transcription of an operon

PROPERDIN   a bactericidal protein component of the blood

PROPHAGE   state of a virus in which the viral genome is integrated into the host genome

PROPHYLAXIS   protection, for example, against disease

PROSTATITIS   inflammation of the prostate gland

PROTEOLYTIC   able to break down proteins

PROTO-ONCOGENE   a normal cellular gene capable of conversion to an oncogene

PROTOPLAST   a viable bacterial cell without its cell wall

PROTOTROPH   an organism capable of synthesizing cell material from inorganic compounds

PROVIRUS   virus integrated into host chromosome and transmitted from one generation to another

PRURITUS   itching

PSITTACOSIS   a bird disease, transmissible to humans

PSYCHROPHILE   a microorganism that grows best at temperatures between 0° and 20°C

PUERPERAL   related to the period after childbirth

PURINE   an organic base found in nucleic acids

PURPURA   dusky, blotchy hemorrhages in the skin or mucous membrane

PURULENT   associated with the formation of pus

PUS   creamy yellow fluid that is a product of inflammation and consists primarily of leukocytes and serum

PUSTULE   an elevated lesion filled with pus

PUTREFACTION   decomposition of proteins resulting in foul odors

PYOCIN   bacteriocin produced by *Pseudomonas aeruginosa*

PYODERMA   pus-containing lesion in the skin

PYOGENIC   pus forming

PYRIMIDINE   an organic base found in nucleic acids

PYROGEN   an agent that induces fever

QUARANTINE   to detain or isolate individuals because of suspicion of infection

QUELLUNG REACTION   a test in which the bacterial capsule swells as a result of combining with specific antibody

RADIO ALLERGOSORBENT TEST (RAST)   a radioimmunoassay test used for detecting IgE antibodies against a specific allergen

REAGIN   the nonprotective antibody found in the blood and produced in response to a number of different diseases; also, the antibody of immunoglobulin class IgE, involved in anaphylaxis and atopic allergies

RECALCITRANT   resistant to change

RECOMBINATION   in genetics, a process in which genetic information is exchanged

RECRUDESCENCE   recurrence of symptoms after their abatement

REDUCTION   gain of electrons or hydrogen

REGULATOR CELL   a T helper or T suppressor cell that regulates an immune response

REGULATOR GENE   a genetic unit on the chromosome that controls the synthesis of the repressor protein

REPLICATION   a duplication process requiring a template

REPLICON   any genetic unit capable of autonomous replication

REPRESSIBLE ENZYME   an enzyme whose synthesis can be decreased by certain metabolites

REPRESSOR PROTEIN   a protein whose function is to control the operator gene; the regulator gene controls the synthesis of the repressor protein

RESOLVING POWER   the ability of a lens (or the eye) to distinguish two closely associated objects as distinct structures

RESPIRATION   an oxidative process in which energy is released from foodstuffs

RESPIRATORY BURST   the generation of toxic oxygen products by activated phagocytes

RETICULOENDOTHELIAL SYSTEM (RES)   a network of phagocytic cells produced and residing in the bone marrow, spleen, lymph nodes, and liver of vertebrates

RHEUMATOID FACTOR   a distinctive gamma globulin found in the serum of patients with rheumatoid arthritis

RHINITIS   inflammation of the nose

RHIZOID   filamentous appendage used by organisms such as fungi to attach to the soil

RIBOSOME   a ribonucleoprotein particle found in the cell cytoplasm and involved in protein synthesis

RINGWORM   a common name for ring-shaped

patches appearing anywhere on the body surface and caused by a group of fungi called dermatophytes; tinea

ROUNDWORMS worms that are round or oval in cross section

RUBELLA German measles

RUBEOLA measles

SACCHAROLYTIC capable of breaking down sugars

SALPINGITIS inflammation of the uterine (fallopian) tube

SANITIZE to reduce the number of bacteria to a nonhazardous level

SAPROBE an organism that derives its nourishment from dead or decaying material

SARCOMA a solid tumor growing from derivatives of embryonal mesoderm such as connective tissue, bone, muscle, and fat

SCLEROSING undergoing a hardening

SCRAPIE an infectious, usually fatal, disease of sheep

SCROFULA tuberculosis of the lymph glands

SECRETORY IgA polymerized IgA with a secretory piece that appears on mucous membranes where it provides local immunity

SEPSIS a toxic condition resulting from the presence of microbes or microbial products in the body

SEPTICEMIA a systemic disease in which microorganisms multiply in the bloodstream

SEPTUM a dividing wall or partition

SEQUELA a morbid (abnormal) condition that develops as a consequence of a disease

SEROCONVERSION the induction of specific antibodies in the serum after their apparent absence from the serum

SEROLOGY the study of antigen-antibody reactions in vitro

SEROTYPE a taxonomic subdivision of microorganisms based on the kind of antigens present

SERUM the clear portion of the blood minus the factors necessary for clotting

SERUM SICKNESS a Type III hypersensitivity in which there are fever, rash, and painful joints due to immune complex formation and the activation of complement following the injection of large amounts of soluble antigen such as an antiserum

SIMIAN pertaining to apes or monkeys

SKIN-SENSITIZING ANTIBODY IgE antibody that attaches to mast cells in the skin

SLOW-REACTING SUBSTANCE OF ANAPHYLAXIS (SR—A) leukotrienes derived from mast cells during anaphylaxis that induce protracted contraction of smooth muscles

SLOW VIRUS a virus that causes subacute or chronic disease with an incubation period that lasts several weeks to years before the onset of clinical symptoms

SMEAR a film of material such as a bacterial suspension spread on a glass slide

SNUFFLES the nasal discharge from mucous patches associated with congenital syphilis

SPECIFICITY that property of a relationship that restricts an agent or a reactant to combine with or to affect a particular group, subject, substance, cell, or molecule

SPECTROPHOTOMETER an instrument used to measure the absorption of light in test liquids

SPHEROPLAST in bacteriology, a gram-negative cell in which the cell wall has been removed but some cell wall components remain

SPIKES surface projections of various lengths spaced at regular intervals on the virus envelope

SPIROCHETE a corkscrew-shaped bacterium

SPLENOMEGALY enlargement of the spleen

SPONDYLITIS inflammation of one or more vertebrae

SPORANGIOSPORES asexual fungal spores produced in a sac called a sporangium

SPORANGIUM a structure that holds asexual spores

SPORE the resistant form of a bacterium derived from the vegetative cell; the reproductive cell of certain organisms

SPORICIDE an agent that destroys spores

SPOROGENESIS production of spores

SSS scalded skin syndrome, caused by *Staphylococcus aureus*

STAPHYLOCOCCAL PROTEIN A   a protein linked to the cell wall of *Staphylococcus aureus* strains; basis for coagglutination test

STEATORRHEA   excessive loss of fats in the feces

STEM CELL   a pluripotential precursor cell that can develop into functionally and morphologically different cell types

STERILIZATION   the process that destroys or removes all living microorganisms

STOMATITIS   inflammation of the oral mucosa

STREET VIRUS   the virulent type of rabies virus isolated in nature from domestic or wild animals; see FIXED VIRUS

STREPTOLYSIN   a hemolysin produced by streptococci

SUBACUTE   between acute (short course) and chronic (persisting over a long period)

SUBCLINICAL   without clinical manifestations of the disease

SUBSTRATE   a specific compound acted on by an enzyme

SUBUNIT VACCINE   a vaccine containing purified antigenic components of a microorganism—for example, capsular polysaccharides

SUPERINFECTION   an infection superimposed on an already existing infection; for example, a bacterial infection on top of a viral infection

SUPPRESSOR T CELLS (T_S)   a regulatory T lymphocyte that suppresses the responses of immune cells

SUPPURATIVE   pus forming

SURFACTANT   agent that reduces surface tension; a wetting agent

SVEDBERG   the relative sedimentation constant of a component being centrifuged at high speed

SYNCYTIUM   a mass of cytoplasm with many nuclei and resulting from the fusion of many cells

SYNDROME   a group of symptoms that characterize a disease

SYNERGISM   a phenomenon in which the action of two components together is more than the sum of the two alone

SYNOVIAL FLUID   a thick transparent fluid found in the joints of bones

SYNTHESIZE   to build up a chemical compound from its individual parts

SYSTEMIC   relating to the entire organism and not any individual organ

TAUTOMERISM   existing in a state of equilibrium between two isomeric forms

TAXONOMY   the orderly classification into distinct categories based on some suitable relationship between groups or individual organisms

T CELLS   thymus-dependent lymphocytes involved in cell-mediated immunity

T (THYMUS)-DEPENDENT ANTIGEN   an antigen that requires recognition by T_H cells before B cells can produce antibody to the antigen

TEMPERATE PHAGE   a nonvirulent bacteriophage

TEMPLATE   a mold for the synthesis of new material

TERATOGENIC   capable of inducing abnormal development and congenital malformations

THERMOLABILE   sensitive to heat

THERMOPHILES   microorganisms growing best at temperatures between 45° and 70°C

THROMBOCYTOPENIA   a decreased number of blood platelets

THROMBOPHLEBITIS   inflammation of a vein associated with thrombosis

THROMBOSIS   formation of a clot within a blood vessel

THRUSH   fungal infection involving the oral mucous membrane

THYMUS   the central lymphoid organ, where T cells differentiate and mature

T (THYMUS)-INDEPENDENT ANTIGEN   an antigen that can directly elicit antibody formation by B cells without antigen recognition by T_H cells

TINCTURE   an alcoholic solution of a particular substance, for example, tincture of iodine

TINEA   a name applied to fungal infections of the skin; ringworm

TITER   the concentration of animate or inanimate agents in a medium

TOLERANCE (IMMUNOLOGICAL)   the lack of response to a specific antigen, thereby allowing the antigen to persist

TOXEMIA   a condition in which toxins are in the blood

TOXIN   an organic (usually) poisonous substance produced by living organisms

TOXOID   a modified exotoxin that has been treated to destroy its toxicity and retain immunogenicity

TRACHOMA   ocular disease caused by *Chlamydia trachomatis*

TRANSAMINATION   a chemical reaction in which an amino group is transformed to a keto-acid

TRANSCRIPTION   the formation of messenger RNA from a DNA template

TRANSDUCTION   the transfer of bacterial genetic information from one cell to another by a virus

TRANSFERASE   an enzyme that catalyzes the exchange of functional groups between compounds

TRANSFORMATION   in genetics, a process in which the genetic constitution of a cell is altered through the uptake of free DNA from the environment

TRANSITION   a mutation caused by substitution of one purine for another or one pyrimidine for another

TRANSPLANTATION ANTIGENS   major histocompatibility antigens

TRANSPOSITION   in genetics, the ability to be transferred to different sites on the nucleic acid molecule

TRANSPOSON   an element of DNA containing insertion sequences as well as genetic information

TRIPLET CODE   a code in which a set of three nucleotides specifies one amino acid

TRISMUS   spasm of the masticatory muscles resulting in difficulty in opening the mouth (lockjaw)

TROPHOZOITE   the active vegetative stage of a protozoon

TROPISM   the involuntary movement of an organism toward or away from a stimulus

TSS   toxic shock syndrome, caused by *Staphylococcus aureus*

TUBERCLE   a nodule

TUBERCULOPROTEIN (TUBERCULIN)   protein extract derived from *Mycobacterium tuberculosis*

TUMOR   a new growth of tissue in which the multiplication of cells is uncontrolled; a swelling

TYPE I REACTIONS   local and systemic anaphylactic reactions

TYPE II REACTIONS   cytotoxic reactions

TYPE III REACTIONS   immune complex reactions

TYPE IV REACTIONS   delayed hypersensitivity reactions

ULCER   a circumscribed area of inflammation characterized by necrosis and found in the epithelial lining

URTICARIA   hives—a vascular reaction of the skin characterized by elevated patches (wheals)

VACCINE   a suspension of organisms, usually killed or attenuated, used for immunization

VARICELLA   chickenpox

VARIOLA   smallpox

VASCULAR   containing blood vessels

VASOACTIVE   affecting vessels, especially blood vessels

VECTOR   a carrier of pathogenic microorganisms

VEGETATIVE   concerned with the growing stage of a microorganism as opposed to the spore state

VENEREAL   transmitted by sexual contact

VENOM   poisonous substance produced and injected, for example, by arachnids, insects, and snakes

VESICLE   a blister; also a membranous unit derived from Golgi and involved in transport

VIREMIA   presence of virus in the bloodstream

VIRION   a complete virus particle consisting of a core of nucleic acid and a protein capsid

VIROGENE   a viral gene incorporated in the host genome

VIROID   an infectious subviral particle consisting of nucleic acid without a protein capsid

VIRULENCE   the relative ability of an organism to cause disease

VISCERAL LARVA MIGRANS   a condition in which larvae that are unable to develop into adult worms invade and migrate through organs of the body

VOLUTIN   see METACHROMATIC GRANULES
VULVA   the external female genitalia

WHEAL   a flat elevated area of skin caused by edema of underlying tissue

WILD TYPE   in microorganisms the most frequently observed phenotype and often referred to as normal (as opposed to mutant) phenotype

XENOGRAFT   a graft between members of a different species

YAW   a lesion associated with the disease yaws

YAWS   an infectious nonvenereal disease occurring in the tropics

YEAST   a unicellular fungus

ZOONOSIS   a disease of animals that can be transmitted to humans

ZOSTER (SHINGLES)   an inflammatory response due to activation of the varicella-zoster virus

INDEX

INDEX